Pharmacology
Essentials
for Allied Health

Jennifer Danielson, PharmD, MBA, CDE
Jill Marquis, PharmD, MFA
Skye A. McKennon, PharmD, BCPS

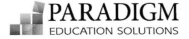

PARADIGM
EDUCATION SOLUTIONS

St. Paul

Director of Editorial: Christine Hurney
Managing Editor: Brenda M. Palo
Senior Developmental Editor: Nancy Papsin
Digital Developmental Editor and Production Editor: Eric Braem
Contributing Editor: Carley Fruzzetti
Assistant Developmental Editors: Bethany Gazelka and Katie Werdick
Director of Production: Tim Larson
Cover and Text Designer: Jaana Bykonich
Senior Design and Production Specialist: Jaana Bykonich
Copy Editor: Catherine A. Minick
Indexer (subject index): Terry Casey
Indexer (drug index): Schroeder Indexing Services
Director of Digital Projects: Chuck Bratton
Digital Projects Manager: Tom Modl
Digital Editorial Intern: Mamie Clark
Director of Marketing: Lara Weber McLellan
Product Marketing Specialist: Shealan Eldredge

ISBN 978-0-76385-859-9 (print)
ISBN 978-0-76387-110-9 (digital)

© 2017 by Paradigm Publishing, Inc.
875 Montreal Way
St. Paul, MN 55102
Email: educate@emcp.com
Website: http://ParadigmCollege.com

Brief Contents

Contents

Unit 2: Pharmacology in the Practice Setting 93

Unit 5: Pharmacotherapy for the Cardiovascular and Respiratory Systems   385

Unit 6: Pharmacotherapy for the Gastrointestinal and Endocrine Systems 479

Unit 7: Pharmacotherapy for the Genitourinary System   579

Preface

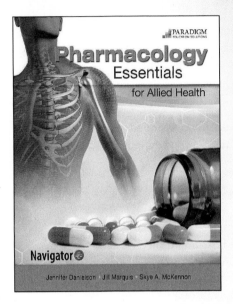

Pharmacology Essentials for Allied Health is an up-to-date textbook—written by three doctors of pharmacy—to introduce allied health students to the fundamentals of and correlations among three specialty areas: anatomy and physiology, pharmacology, and pharmacy practice. Using an accessible and meaningful approach, this textbook provides students entering the dynamic and growing allied health field a firm foundation in learning these concepts and their applications to real-world settings.

The textbook is designed to meet the pharmacology course requirement of allied health students who are enrolled in two-year associate's degree programs or six-month certification programs at community colleges, technical schools, or private career schools. To receive the greatest benefit from this textbook and its associated courseware, students should have completed and passed courses in basic algebra, medical terminology, and anatomy and physiology.

Student Textbook Features

Units

The 29 chapters of *Pharmacology Essentials for Allied Health* are grouped into 10 units that provide a logical, stepped approach to learning pharmacology:

- Units 1 and 2 provide an introduction to pharmacology and the implementation of pharmacology concepts in the practice setting. Some of the topics include the history and principles of pharmacology, sources of drugs, drug classification and nomenclature, pharmaceutical development, dosage forms and routes of administration, prescriptions and medication orders, pharmacy calculations, medication safety, and the important role of the allied health professional in the practice setting.

- Units 3 through 9 cover the major body systems to help students understand the connections between particular body systems, their disorders, and the drug therapies used to treat these disorders.

- Unit 10 addresses two patient populations—pediatrics and geriatrics—that have unique characteristics and challenges that affect drug selection and therapy.

Chapters

Each chapter contains several engaging in-text and in-margin features created to aid student learning. These features, as outlined below, challenge students to expand their knowledge, think critically, work collaboratively, test their mastery of chapter content, learn professional expectations, and explore allied health careers.

Chapter Openers

Each chapter begins with a Chapter Opener that includes the following elements:

- a **Pharm Facts** feature that provides unusual or surprising information related to the chapter content

- a **professional quotation** feature that offers wisdom and advice from an allied health veteran who works in an allied health specialty related to the chapter content

Learning Objectives

The **Learning Objectives** listed at the beginning of each chapter establish clear goals for allied health students as they begin their chapter study. These Learning Objectives are correlated with the assessment questions provided on the online Navigator+ learning management system.

Key Terms

The boldfaced **key terms** in each chapter are defined both in context and in the online Navigator+ learning management system.

Career Exploration

The **Career Exploration** feature provides students with a list of allied health positions related to the chapter topic. This feature serves as a catalyst for a related career research activity located on the Navigator+ learning management system.

Checkpoints

Throughout each chapter are **Checkpoints**, or stopping points, where students pause in their reading to test their comprehension of the content just presented. These best-practice features provide a stepped-learning approach to understanding chapter concepts.

Kolb's Learning Styles

The **Kolb's Learning Styles** feature boxes are sprinkled throughout each chapter. These activities provide students with tips for learning textbook content based on their learning styles, which students determine by taking the Kolb's Learning Style Inventory located in Appendix B.

Drug Alert

Drug Alert feature boxes focus on unusual or harmful drug effects; look-alike, sound-alike drugs; drug interactions and medication safety; and drugs in the news.

Patient Teaching

The **Patient Teaching** feature boxes offer students communication strategies for patient instruction, a key responsibility of allied health professionals. Patient teaching boxes address topics such as medications, treatments, and procedures.

Work Wise

Work Wise margin tips focus on professional soft skills in the workplace. Topics include communication skills, medical terminology and jargon, ethics, professional dress, and patient privacy.

Quick Study

The **Quick Study** margin tips provide fast strategies for learning—and remembering—chapter concepts.

In the Know

In the Know margin tips offer interesting insights on topics related to chapter concepts. Topics may include items in the news, historical figures, or pharmacology trivia.

Name Exchange

The margin tip **Name Exchange** allows students to learn the generic name and corresponding brand names of many of the most popular drugs on the market.

Chapter Summary

The **Chapter Summary** provides an overview of the key points from the chapter. This feature offers students an opportunity to review all chapter concepts at a glance.

Appendixes

In addition to the many helpful in-text and in-margin features, *Pharmacology Essentials for Allied Health* has two appendixes that enhance student comprehension and learning: Checkpoint Answer Keys and Kolb's Learning Styles Inventory.

Appendix A: Checkpoint Answer Keys

The **Checkpoint Answer Keys** allow students to check their answers to the Checkpoint questions posed throughout each chapter of the textbook.

Appendix B: Kolb's Learning Styles Inventory

The **Kolb's Learning Styles Inventory** offers a detailed explanation of Kolb's Learning Styles and their applications to the learning environment. Students have the opportunity to take a brief assessment to determine their predominant learning styles and use that information in their chapter study.

Indexes

Two indexes provide students with easy references for locating specific pharmacology-related topics: a Generic and Brand-Name Drugs Index and a Subject Index.

Generic and Brand-Name Drugs Index

The **Generic and Brand-Name Drugs Index** contains the nomenclature for both generic and brand-name drugs mentioned in the textbook. Having a separate drug index allows students to locate information about a specific drug quickly and efficiently.

Subject Index

The **Subject Index** offers students an easy-to-use reference for locating specific pharmacology topics within the textbook.

ebook

For students who prefer studying with an **ebook**, the *Pharmacology Essentials for Allied Health* textbook is available in an electronic format. The web-based, password-protected ebook features dynamic navigation tools, including bookmarking, a linked Table of Contents, and study tools such as highlighting and note-taking. The student ebook is available online at http://Paradigm.bookshelf.emcp.com and through the Navigator+ learning management system.

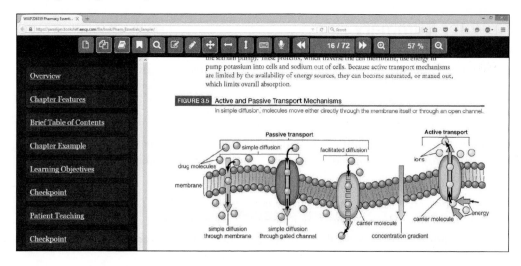

Navigator+ Learning Management System

Integrated with the *Pharmacology Essentials for Allied Health* textbook is the **Navigator+ Learning Management System.** This rich, web-based system offers students a variety of learning and practice opportunities related to course content. Students will observe the Navigator+ logo tucked into the margins of the book. This logo alerts students to go to Navigator+ for related learning activities.

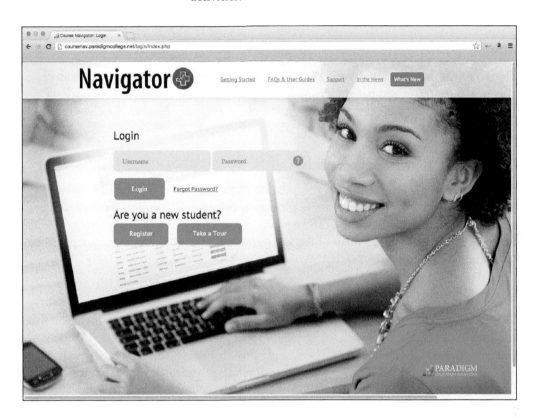

Student Practice Opportunities

Navigator+ provides students with a variety of engaging activities to support their learning of chapter concepts. These activities include end-of-chapter exercises, an interactive glossary and accompanying flash cards, web projects, interactive games, practice assessments, and case studies.

End-of-Chapter Exercises

The end-of-chapter exercises provide a scaffolding of difficulty and correlate with the revised Bloom's taxonomy. These exercises include Review the Basics, Know the Drugs or Know the Terms, Put It Together, and Think It Through.

Review the Basics

The **Review the Basics** exercise offers a set of 15 multiple-choice questions that test students' recall and comprehension of major chapter concepts.

Know the Drugs or Know the Terms

The **Know the Drugs** or **Know the Terms** activity provides five to eight matching exercises to test students' recall of generic and brand-name drugs or key terms and their definitions.

Put It Together

The **Put It Together** exercise offers 8 to 10 short-answer questions that gauge students' synthesis of chapter material.

Think It Through

The **Think It Through** activity focuses on critical-thinking and research skills. Students are given three real-world patient scenarios to consider and are asked to think critically before responding. Students are also assigned a research topic related to the chapter content and tasked with creating an appropriate response.

Glossary and Flash Cards

The digital, interactive **glossary** is a compilation of the boldfaced key terms from each chapter of the textbook. This interactive glossary provides audio of the pronunciation and a definition for each key term and can be viewed by chapter or by the entire book. The **flash cards** provide reinforcement of the key terms and their definitions and are student-scored and timed.

Web Projects

Two types of **web projects** are offered on Navigator+: a **Career Form** that provides students with a research opportunity to explore an allied health specialty listed in each chapter's Career Exploration feature box, and a **Pharm Fact Follow-up** activity that invites students to use one of the Pharm Facts listed in the Chapter Opener as a catalyst for further research.

Games

Navigator+ provides four games for each chapter of *Pharmacology Essentials for Allied Health*. These interactive games challenge students to apply their knowledge of pharmacology concepts in a fun learning environment. Basic games such as **Unscramble** and **Crossword** are offered as well as more challenging, timed games such as **Chart It Out**, **Drag Race**, and **Photo Synthesis**.

Student-Practice Assessments

Student-practice assessments are gradable and provide opportunities for students to gauge their learning of chapter content.

Case Studies

The **case studies** simulate real-world patient scenarios drawn from a variety of practice settings. These case studies require students to integrate communication and professional skills with clinical knowledge to determine the best approach for resolving the situations.

Instructor Resources

Navigator+ provides instructors access to students' work and allows them to track students' progress in the course. Most of the available student resources are automatically gradable and can be exported to instructors' grade books.

The **instructor resources** that accompany this textbook are located on Navigator+ and are visible only to instructors. These resources offer instructors a number of tools such as course-planning guidelines, chapter lessons, and handouts and their answer keys.

Course-Planning Guidelines

The **course-planning guidelines** provide instructors with assistance in shaping a pharmacology course. **Syllabus models** are tailored specifically to the achievement of course outcomes within a designated time frame.

Chapter Lessons

Chapter lessons feature instructional tips and activities to integrate into a pharmacology course. Written by healthcare instructors, these activities enhance students' comprehension of chapter topics.

Handouts and Answer Keys

Each textbook chapter offers related handouts and their answer keys to supplement student learning.

Instructor-Controlled Test Banks

Instructor-controlled test banks provide instructors with additional assessment questions with which they can create gradable exams. Students' test scores can be exported to the grade book.

Supplemental Resources

Lastly, Navigator+ provides a variety of resources to supplement a pharmacology course. Resources located there or offered separately include:

- BioDigital™ Human: Students are provided with a link within Navigator+ that allows them to view and interact with three-dimensional human anatomy images to enhance their study of anatomy and physiology.

- Top 200 drugs

- Greek and Latin root words used in healthcare settings

- List of medical abbreviations

- Additional pharmacy calculations practice

- Tips for working in multicultural environments

- Paradigm's *Pocket Drug Guide* print book and mobile applicaiton

About the Authors

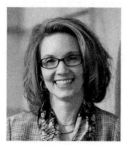

Jennifer Danielson, PharmD, MBA, CDE

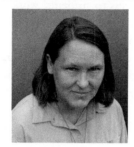

Jill Marquis, PharmD, MFA

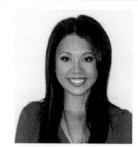

Skye A. McKennon, PharmD, BCPS

Jennifer Danielson has been a pharmacist since 1993 and a recognized leader in pharmacy education since 1996. She has spent most of her academic career serving as Director of Experiential Education at four pharmacy schools (University of Washington, University of Colorado, Campbell University, and Oregon State University). In 2004–2006, Dr. Danielson served as chair of the pharmacy technician program at Pikes Peak Community College in Colorado Springs where she taught pharmacology. It was her work in Colorado that formed the basis for her approach to teaching this topic to pharmacy technician students in both this textbook and her previous book, *Pharmacology Essentials for Technicians.*

Dr. Danielson has presented and published on various topics in pharmacy education on the national, regional, and local levels. Her current teaching and scholarship responsibilities are in interprofessional education and diabetes-related topics. Her practice background in diabetes care in the ambulatory clinic setting provides inspiration for her teaching and writing. Her most recent work at the University of Washington involves the provision of collaborative learning opportunities between pharmacy and allied health students.

Dr. Danielson lives with her family in Mill Creek, Washington.

Jill Marquis received her doctor of pharmacy (PharmD) degree from the University of Washington in 2012, and a master of fine arts (MFA) degree in writing from the University of Montana in 1996. Dr. Marquis is a pharmacist at Propac, a long-term care pharmacy based in Vancouver, Washington. She has also worked as a drug information pharmacist, writing about new drugs for clients in the pharmaceutical industry, and about drug interactions for an online database. Her retail pharmacy experience includes a stint at a pharmacy based in the public health clinic of Missoula, Montana. Her practice interests are geriatrics, drug interactions, and effective pharmacy communication.

Skye A. McKennon is a licensed pharmacist, board-certified pharmacotherapy specialist (BCPS), group exercise instructor, certified lifestyle coach, and preventionist. Dr. McKennon completed her bachelor's degree and doctor of pharmacy (PharmD) degree from Washington State University. She also completed postdoctoral residency training at Swedish Medical Center in Seattle, Washington.

After residency, Dr. McKennon practiced in the institutional and ambulatory pharmacy settings. Notably, she was instrumental in the development of a lipid management clinic at Evergreen Health. In 2009, her passion for teaching and education led her to a position as a clinical faculty member at the University of Washington School of Pharmacy. Courses designed and directed by Dr. McKennon include applied pharmacotherapeutics, institutional pharmacy practice, and diabetes prevention. She has been both an instructor and a guest lecturer of various courses for pharmacy and other health science students, including therapeutics, pharmacotherapy for older adults, global health brigades, and law and ethics.

Dr. McKennon has presented her work at international and national symposiums such as the Seventh International Conference on Interprofessional Practice and Education and the American Association of Colleges of Pharmacy annual meeting. She is also a contributor to her regional pharmacy community and regularly provides live and online continuing education.

In 2015, she relocated to Salt Lake City where she joined the University of Utah's College of Pharmacy as a clinical faculty member. Her role includes teaching pharmacotherapy to health professional students and practicing in an ambulatory clinic.

Authors' Acknowledgments

I would like to thank my coauthors, Jill and Skye, for their hard work on this book. They were the primary driving force behind so much of this book's content and the real heart of this work. I appreciate their attention to detail and constant momentum to keep going. Just keep swimming, just keep swimming. . . .

I would like to acknowledge the following pharmacists (who were all students at the time) for their contributions to textbook content: Katelin Brooks, PharmD; Anne Kim, PharmD, MPH; Chi Mac, PharmD; and Mitul Patel, PharmD. They helped me with revising and updating specific chapters or pieces of chapters. As they learned, so did I learn. I appreciate their hard work, and I wish them well in their careers.

Lastly, I would like to acknowledge my family for putting up with my late nights and weekends working. I love you and want you to be as proud of me as I am of you.

—Jennifer Danielson

I'd like to thank my family (Ed Skoog, and Oscar too)! Many marvelous pharmacists mentored me at the University of Washington, Partnership Health Center, Idyllwild Pharmacy, Group Health, and Propac Pharmacy. I'm especially thankful I got to work with Raina White, Brent Dehring, Barry Shapiro, Micki Kedzierski, and Jennifer Danielson! I'm grateful to Nancy Papsin and the expert editorial team at Paradigm Publishing for shepherding this project to completion. I'd also like to thank the many wonderful pharmacy technicians and med aides whom I work with every day.

—Jill Marquis

There are so many people in my professional and personal journey that made writing and production of this book possible. To all my mentors (including Nanci and Paul), a heartfelt thank-you for your energy and investment to make me the pharmacist and teacher I am today. I am appreciative of the Paradigm team, notably Nancy Papsin, Carley Fruzzetti, Brenda Palo, the copy editor, and my coauthors, Jennifer and Jill, for their hard work in making this book a reality.

I am eternally grateful to my family; my father (Kelly) and mother (Michi), who ceaselessly give and sacrifice for me and my well-being. To my grandfather, Satoru, whose gentle and unwavering love helped me face adversity with a smile. Thank you to Tom, my caring husband, who supports me with the freedom to pursue my dreams. To my friends, especially Lucia, the Arnolds, and Heidi, who give me encouragement and many reasons to laugh and enjoy life. I am truly blessed.

—Skye A. McKennon

Acknowledgments

The quality of this body of work is a testament to the many contributors and reviewers who participated in the creation of *Pharmacology Essentials for Allied Health*. We offer a heartfelt thank-you for your commitment to producing high-quality instructional materials for allied health students.

Contributing Writers, Textbook Content

Katelin Brooks, PharmD

Erik Hare, BS
Writer and Consultant
St. Paul, MN

Andrea Iannucci, PharmD
Assistant Chief Pharmacist
Oncology and Investigational Drugs
    Services
UC Davis Medical Center
Sacramento, CA

Anne Kim, PharmD, MPH

Len Lichtblau, PhD
University of Minnesota
Minneapolis, MN

Chi Mac, PharmD

Shawn McPartland, MD, JD
Azure College - School of Nursing
Boca Raton, FL

Tanja B. Monroe, CPhT
Hematology/Oncology Clinical Pharmacy
    Technician III
Student Pharmacy Technician Internship
    Coordinator
University of California Davis Health
    System (UCDHS)
Sacramento, CA

Kit Naylor, BA
Writer/Editor
Kittridge Communications
Minneapolis, MN

Mitul Patel, PharmD

Aaron Reed, MSN, CRNA
Great Lakes Anesthesia
South Bend, IN

Reviewers, Textbook Content

Natasha Freeman Cauley, MPH, RHIA

Karen Garcia, MS, RMA, RAHI, RPT
Front Range Community College
Westminster, CO

Patricia Gavin, MS, RN
Brunswick Community College
Boliva, NC

Shawn McPartland, MD, JD
Azure College - School of Nursing
Boca Raton, FL

Andrea R. Redman, PharmD, BCPS
Emory Healthcare
Atlanta, GA
and
Walden University
Minneapolis, MN

Contributing Writers, Navigator+ Learning Management System

ansrsource
5440 Harvest Hill Road
Suite 234
Dallas, TX

Natasha Freeman Cauley, MPH, RHIA

Michelle C. McCranie, AAS, CPhT, CMA
(AAMA)
Ogeechee Technical College
Statesboro, GA

Andrea R. Redman, PharmD, BCPS
Emory Healthcare
Atlanta, GA
and
Walden University
Minneapolis, MN

Interactive Image Programs, Navigator+ Learning Management System

Aaron Oliker
BioDigital Systems
594 Broadway
Suite 1101
New York, NY

Tim Spaid
  and Dan Johnson
Ebix, Inc./A.D.A.M.
10 10th Street, Suite 500
Atlanta, GA

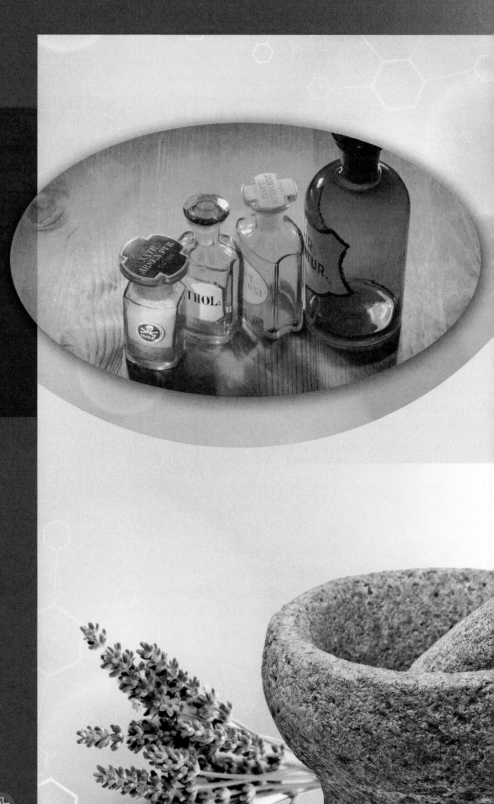

Pharmacology Overview

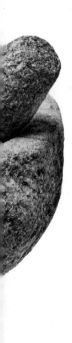

1

Introduction to Pharmacology

Pharm Facts

- Smallpox was common in the 1700s. Its name was derived from the small pockmarks that scarred the faces of its victims. To cover these scars, aristocrats used white lead—a powdered mixture that was corrosive to the skin and required even more powder to cover.

- As the number of Chinese immigrants in the United States rose during the 1800s, they brought with them a tradition for treating joint inflammation: omega-3–rich snake oil. Many traveling hucksters saw an opportunity and sold mineral-oil tonic disguised as rattlesnake oil. This fraudulent practice was outlawed in 1906, but these peddlers made their mark in folklore: An individual who is the purveyor of any fraudulent, deceptive, or unreliable product is still referred to as a *snake-oil salesperson*.

- Up until the middle of the twentieth century, the most common ingredient in many of the most popular "medicines" in the United States was alcohol. Therefore, it is no surprise that these medicines were touted as cure-alls, given the numbing effects of alcohol.

- Penicillin saved many lives during World War II. Prior to that time, more soldiers died from infection than from battlefield injuries. For example, in World War I, the death rate from bacterial pneumonia was 18%; by World War II, that rate fell to less than 1%.

"As a pharmacy technician, I understand the important role that I play in protecting the safety and well-being of patients. I rely on my knowledge of pharmacology in every decision that I make in the prescription-filling process. Having a strong pharmacology foundation allows me to foresee potential issues with certain medication combinations and alert the pharmacist. I recognize that my education and training are paramount to a positive patient outcome, and I remind myself with every task that I hold a person's life in my hands."

—**Elina V. Pierce**, MSP, CPhT
Program Director and Pharmacy Technician

Learning Objectives

1 Define the terms *pharmacology* and *drug*.

2 Discuss the major advancements in medicine throughout the history of pharmacology.

3 Understand ways in which drugs are classified.

4 Understand the importance of having a working knowledge of the drugs used in the workplace.

5 Obtain strategies for learning pharmacology.

6 Discuss the importance of being able to communicate effectively with the proper understanding or use of medical terminology.

7 Describe the Kolb's Learning Styles Inventory and its significance to an individual's learning and processing of information.

8 Learn where to obtain drug information from reliable resources and how to use this information in a health information toolkit.

Pharmacology is the study of the effects of drugs on the body. A **drug** is a substance that affects the normal functioning of humans or animals and may be used to diagnose, treat, mitigate, cure, or prevent disease. **Drug therapy** plays a large role in modern medicine. In fact, according to a report published in the journal *Mayo Clinic Proceedings* (2013), more than 50% of US citizens take two prescription medications and 20% take at least five prescription medications. In light of these statistics, healthcare personnel will certainly encounter and care for patients with complex drug therapy regimens. To provide these patients with optimum care, allied health professionals need to have a general understanding of how the history of pharmacology has affected current medication practices. In addition, healthcare personnel should be aware of some strategies for learning pharmacology as well as several valuable resources that provide reliable drug information.

History of Pharmacology in Europe and Asia

The study of ancient documents shows that people have been treating physical and psychological ailments with medicines for thousands of years. Clay tablets found in Babylonia date back to the eighteenth century BCE and list more than 500 medicinal remedies made from plant, animal, and mineral sources. In these ancient civilizations, sickness or disease was thought to be a form of punishment or curse placed on individuals by evil spirits or demons. Consequently, medical treatment was largely controlled by religious leaders—shamans, priests, and priestesses—who guarded their healing knowledge closely. By using trial-and-error methods, these ancient practitioners extracted the healing properties of natural substances to prepare medicinal treatments for the diseases that afflicted early inhabitants. These preparations were often accompanied by prayers, chants, incantations, rituals, and magic.

As mentioned earlier, for thousands of years, the only substances used to treat illnesses were extracted from plants, animals, and minerals. With time and experience, ancient practitioners learned to formulate recipes to treat various disorders. These recipes were the precursors to modern-day **formularies**, or drug lists. The most famous drug compendium is the **Ebers Papyrus**, a collection of medicinal recipes written around 1550 BCE. This Egyptian medical source lists more than 700 different herbal remedies used by healers. These remedies consisted of botanical drugs drawn from the natural environment, such as castor bean, garlic, and poppy seed. The most common mixtures were laxatives and enemas administered rectally; however, other naturally occurring substances were administered in some of the same ways used today: orally, topically, and through inhalation.

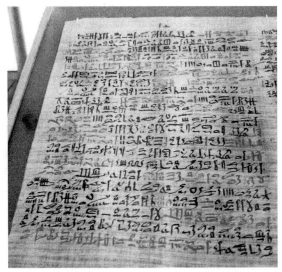

The 110-page Ebers Papyrus contains more than 700 remedies for ailments that affected early Egyptians.

Roots of Traditional Eastern Medicine

In East Asia, early cultures relied mainly on the healing properties of plants to treat common ailments and restore harmony to the body. The use of botanicals as a healing method became the basis of **traditional Eastern medicine**, a practice that continues today in India and China. Two well-known figures who laid the foundation for traditional Eastern medicine are Sushruta and Li Shizhen.

Sushruta

In the sixth century BCE, a Hindu surgeon named Sushruta wrote a medicinal work called the *Sushruta Samhita* that discussed 300 surgical procedures, 1,120 medical conditions, and the medicinal uses of more than 600 plants. Sushruta's collection of medicinal recipes is one of the three foundational texts of Indian traditional medicine called Ayurveda. (The other two texts are *Caraka Samhita* and *Astanga Hridaya*.) In **Ayurvedic medicine**, doctors prescribe treatments such as herbs, exercise (yoga), and diet and lifestyle changes to maintain a balance of the natural forces in a patient's body. In this system, the elements of nature combine in the body to form three components called *doshas* (Vata, Pitta, and Kapha). Good health depends on maintaining balance among the doshas. Ayurveda is a holistic approach to medicine that includes a patient's spiritual well-being.

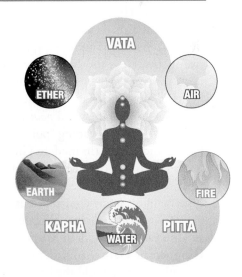

According to Ayurveda, an individual is dominated by three dosha types: Vata-Pitta (a volatile air-fire element), Pitta-Kapha (a stable fire-water-earth element), and Vata-Kapha (a passive, dependent ether-earth element).

Li Shizhen

The roots of Chinese traditional medicine rest on the extensive body of knowledge produced by Li Shizhen, a sixteenth-century Chinese physician who lived during the Ming Dynasty. Li Shizhen compiled a resource called *Ben Cao Gang Mu (Compendium of Materia Medica)* that lists more than 1,000 plants and 8,000 recipes used in the treatment of illnesses. This work, which also describes the causes of various illnesses, is considered the most comprehensive text in traditional Chinese medicine.

Roots of Traditional Western Medicine

The ancient Greeks shifted the practice of medicine from a spiritual-based approach to a more logical, scientific-based approach. This approach laid the foundation for **traditional Western medicine**, a practice in which an illness is identified and then treated with drugs. In fact, Greek physicians had such a profound influence on the field of medicine that knowledge of the Greek alphabet is vital to an understanding of many medical and pharmacologic terms. Three influential figures in traditional Western medicine are Hippocrates, Dioscorides, and Galen.

Hippocrates

The famous Greek physician Hippocrates of Kos, who lived in the fourth century BCE, was the first practitioner to propose that disease was caused by natural rather than supernatural causes. Although he practiced herbal medicine like his predecessors, he rejected unsupported theory and superstition in favor of observation and classification, or empirical learning. He believed that the four **humors** of the body (blood, phlegm, yellow bile, and black bile) must be in the correct balance to maintain optimal health. His hypothesis formed the basis of traditional Western medicine. During his lifetime, Hippocrates published more than 70 medical texts that scientifically categorized diseases, their signs and symptoms, and their treatments. He is also credited with establishing a **lexicon** for the medical terminology that healthcare professionals continue to use in their practices. In fact, the word *pharmacy* comes from *pharmakon*, meaning "poison" (in classic Greek) and "drug" (in modern Greek). Hippocrates was also the first to dissect the human body to study the functions of specific organs. Because of his many contributions to the practice of Western medicine, Hippocrates is known as "The Father of Modern Medicine," and the **Hippocratic Oath**—an oath taken by medical practitioners to uphold the highest standards of medical ethics—is named in his honor.

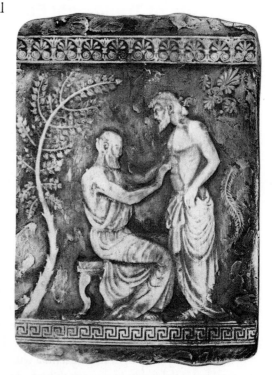

Hippocrates proposed that disease came from an individual's internal state (imbalance among the four humors) or from an individual's lifestyle (environment, hygiene, diet, and activity).

Dioscorides

Pedanius Dioscorides, another early Greek physician, is credited with writing one of the world's greatest pharmaceutical texts: ***De Materia Medica (On Medical Matters)***. Compiled by Dioscorides in the first century CE, this text scientifically described and classified more than 1,000 substances—mainly botanicals—that had medicinal value. Dioscorides included descriptions of the botanicals, their uses, quantities, dosages, side effects, and storage guidelines. For 15 centuries, *De Materia Medica* served as the standard reference text for drugs.

Galen

Another Greek physician, Aelius Galenus (better known as Galen of Pergamon), lived in Rome during the second century and built on Hippocrates's ideas of empirical learning. Galen also studied the effects of herbal medicine on the body, which led to the coining of the term **galenical pharmacy**, or the process of creating extracts of active medicinals from plants. For his extensive work in extracting, identifying, and classifying active ingredients from natural sources, Galen is considered "The Father of Pharmacy," and his research influenced medical knowledge for more than 1,000 years.

Galen's position as a surgeon for gladiators contributed to his knowledge of anatomy. For example, Galen described the aorta as "a trunk divided into many branches and twigs" and discovered that these branches (arteries) contained blood, not air as previously thought.

Emergence of Apothecaries

During the Middle Ages, the pharmacy profession was evolving in the Persian and European empires. Early Arabic civilizations introduced various dosage formulations for drugs, such as syrups, elixirs, and pills. They are also credited with identifying the pharmacist as a qualified healthcare professional and for establishing the **apothecary** or pharmacy concept.

Europeans during this period adopted this apothecary model. Apothecary shops sprang up in villages across the continent. Residents of these villages received both diagnosis and treatment from the practitioners who worked in these shops. Typically, the apothecary shop had several rooms: The outermost room contained shelves and display cases filled with prepared medicines and bottles of tinctures and elixirs; the two innermost rooms were devoted to patient diagnosis and compounding of medicines. The **mortar and pestle** were the apothecary's main tools for grinding and mixing ingredients by hand.

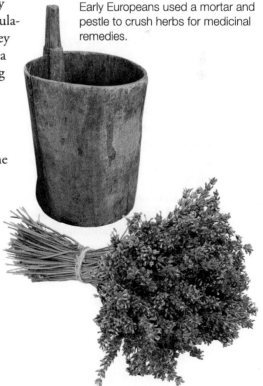

Early Europeans used a mortar and pestle to crush herbs for medicinal remedies.

To train chemists and pharmacists to work in apothecaries, guilds were established. These guilds were the forerunners of universities and professional organizations devoted to the pharmaceutical sciences.

Rise of Alchemy and Anatomy

By the Renaissance period, the Roman Catholic church had become a dominating cultural force in Europe, and the practice of medicine and pharmacy passed again from lay practitioners to religious leaders. Monasteries became centers of treatment. There, monks wrote medical texts and grew herb gardens of medicinal plants. In addition, many hospitals and pharmacies were run by religious orders. These facilities provided free health care and medicines to the poor, thus serving as the archetypes of community healthcare clinics, public health departments, and charity hospitals.

Alchemy

During the Middle Ages and the Renaissance, the practice of alchemy became popular. **Alchemy** combined elements of chemistry, metallurgy, physics, and medicine with astrology, mysticism, and spiritualism in order to turn something ordinary into something

extraordinary. For example, alchemists would attempt to change base metals such as iron, nickel, or lead into silver or gold. They would also apply the principles of alchemy to developing medicine. One famous alchemist, the Swiss surgeon Paracelsus, thought diseases that were rampant during the Renaissance—such as typhus, syphilis, and the plague—needed to be fought with stronger medicines than those derived from botanicals. He used metals such as mercury, arsenic, and lead to purge the body of these disorders. Today, ironically, these metals are considered toxic. Paracelsus was also the first individual to challenge the teachings of Galen. He denounced the philosophy of humors in medicine and advocated the use of individual drugs rather than mixtures or potions. He reasoned that treating diseases with individual drugs would make it easier to determine which agent helped, which made the patient worse, and how much of a drug was needed. These concepts are still used today.

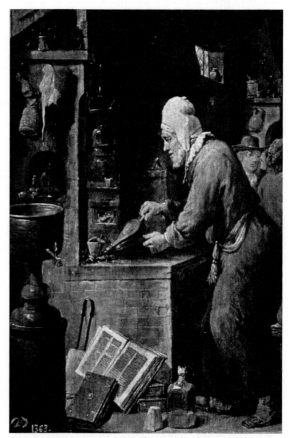

The experimentation of early alchemists laid the foundation for the fields of chemistry, pharmacology, and metallurgy.

Anatomy

Major strides were made as well in the understanding of human **anatomy** during the sixteenth and seventeenth centuries. Italian painter, inventor, and anatomist Leonardo da Vinci used human corpses to study anatomy and render drawings of what he observed. The intricate drawings of Flemish physician and anatomist Andreas Vesalius were published in his book *De Humani Corporis Fabrica (On the Fabric of the Human Body)*, laying the foundation for the continued study of human anatomy and its disorders. In addition, William Harvey, a sixteenth-century English physician and anatomist, created drawings from his research on the human circulatory system. His drawings led other scientists to view the circulatory system as a potential route for carrying medication to different parts of the body.

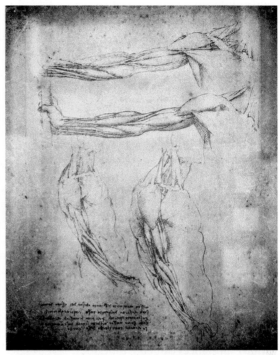

Leonardo da Vinci's study of human anatomy is captured in his detailed illustrations, such as this drawing of the human arm.

Advances in Pathology, Immunology, and Medical Treatments

Late in the seventeenth century, Italian scientist Marcello Malpighi pioneered the use of microscopes and discovered the role of capillaries in circulation in 1661. That discovery closed a key gap in what was known about the circulatory system. Over the next two decades, Malpighi made many important observations about pathology by using microscopes to examine the layers of the skin and various organs.

Italian physician and professor of anatomy Giovanni Battista Morgagni published his groundbreaking text on pathology *De Sedibus et Causis Morborum per Anatomen Indagatis (The Seats and Causes of Disease)* in 1761. The text detailed the dissections of hundreds of corpses and described the symptoms each patient had prior to death.

Several new medications and medical treatments were also developed in the eighteenth century. In 1754, English physician James Lind published *A Treatise on Scurvy*, which proposed that eating lemons and other citrus fruits would help sailors fend off scurvy, a treatment that eventually eradicated the problem. Joseph Priestly discovered nitrous oxide, oxygen, and several other gases. Nitrous oxide and oxygen are used to treat many patients today. Late in the century, another English physician, William Withering, used the foxglove plant to treat dropsy (edema). The drug derived from that discovery, digoxin, is still used today to treat patients with heart failure.

The spread of infectious diseases was also a major problem in the eighteenth century, when the Industrial Revolution prompted mass migrations of people from the country to large cities in Europe. One of those diseases, smallpox, was epidemic in Europe. In fact, more than three-fourths of infants in cities such as London and Berlin died of this disease.

An English physician and scientist named Edward Jenner discovered the first vaccine for smallpox in 1796. He had observed that milkmaids who were exposed to cowpox did not become infected with smallpox. By transferring matter from a cowpox lesion on a milkmaid to a healthy patient, he prevented the healthy patient from contracting smallpox. The smallpox vaccine was one of the wonder drugs of the nineteenth century.

Meanwhile, in Germany, Samuel Hahnemann began to promote his theory of **homeopathy**, publishing his first paper on the subject in 1796. Hahnemann had observed that quinine, which is used to treat

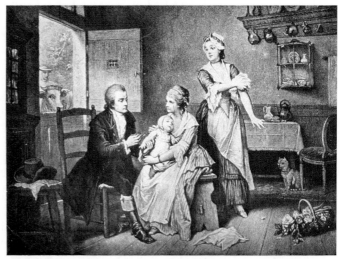

Until Jenner discovered the smallpox vaccine, many children succumbed to the "speckled monster," whose name was derived from the small pockmarks (pox) on the faces of its victims.

malaria, causes symptoms similar to malaria when given to healthy people. He concluded that "likes are cured by likes." Proponents of homeopathy believe that miniscule doses of various substances can cure illnesses.

An Understanding of Pharmacology, Pain Relief, and Infection Control

As practitioners gained a better understanding of human anatomy, they focused their research on how these body systems functioned and responded to medications. Their anatomic knowledge also led to the refinement of surgical techniques.

Connection between Physiology and Pharmacology

In the nineteenth century, the French scientist Claude Bernard laid the foundation for the study of **physiology**, or the science that explores the normal functions of living organisms and their parts. His research focused on the idea that the human body has an internal environment (what he called *milieu intérieur*) or **homeostasis** that must be maintained. Bernard advanced the knowledge of how drugs work in the body when he demonstrated that certain drugs (such as curare) have specific sites of action within the body. Curare, a plant-based poison once used by hunters in South America to paralyze their prey, blocks the transmission of nerve impulses, which causes skeletal muscle relaxation. Bernard's use of laboratory methods to study drugs

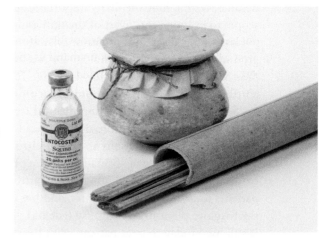

Intocostrin was the first commercial preparation of curare, a medication used for skeletal muscle relaxation during surgical procedures. Indigenous inhabitants of the Amazon rainforest would dip their darts into the pot of curare (shown here) and propel the darts toward their prey.

led him to be credited as one of the founders of the field of **experimental pharmacology**, which is the science of drugs and their interactions with the systems of living animals.

The field of experimental pharmacology continued to develop when several European universities recognized pharmacology as a field of study and established laboratories and a course of study for individuals interested in scientific research. One notable professor was Oswald Schmiedeberg, whose research at the University of Strasbourg in Germany formed the basis of his text *Outline of Pharmacology* published in 1878. Schmiedeberg's work contributed to Germany's dominance in the pharmaceutical industry prior to World War II and his subsequent recognition as "The Father of Modern Pharmacology."

Surgical Advances

Surgical advances were also made in the nineteenth century. Ether, chloroform, and nitrous oxide were administered by healthcare practitioners for sedation, and cocaine was administered as a local anesthetic. Narcotics such as opium and morphine were used as painkillers during and after hospital surgical procedures. With these advances, surgery was no longer considered by practitioners as a last-resort procedure when other treatment options failed but rather a first-line treatment to restore a patient's health.

Infection Control Measures

An understanding of the importance of sanitary conditions and **infection control** measures was also a hallmark of the nineteenth century. The work of Hungarian obstetrician Ignaz Semmelweis in 1847 influenced hospital awareness of infection control. At Vienna General Hospital in Austria, Semmelweis recognized the role that hand washing played in reducing infection and mortality among maternity patients. To encourage such results, Semmelweis insisted that all obstetric interns wash their hands with chlorinated lime before they examined patients.

Notable English nurse Florence Nightingale observed the importance of cleanliness and sanitary conditions firsthand as she provided treatment for wounded soldiers during the Crimean War. Upon her return to England, Nightingale compiled her observa-

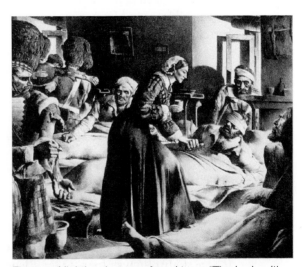

Florence Nightingale was referred to as "The Lady with the Lamp" because she carried a lamp as she worked through the night tending to soldiers' wounds.

tions and a plan for infection control and sanitation improvements into a 500-page document and submitted the report to the British government. Her research provided the catalyst for healthcare reform in England.

Finally, British surgeon Joseph Lister used the sterile practices set forth by Semmelweis and Nightingale for his research on the germ theory of disease. Lister's experiments with sterilization techniques proved that cleansing hands, donning gloves, and using germicides such as carbolic acid on surgical instruments and sutures greatly reduced infection.

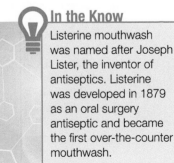

In the Know

Listerine mouthwash was named after Joseph Lister, the inventor of antiseptics. Listerine was developed in 1879 as an oral surgery antiseptic and became the first over-the-counter mouthwash.

Widespread Use of Aspirin and Cocaine

By the second half of the nineteenth century, pharmacology had become a scientific discipline. Several medications were marketed: Some are still in use today and others are deemed dangerous by today's standards. In 1897, German scientist Felix Hoffmann combined salicylic acid, a natural plant derivative, with an acetyl group that buffered some of the acidic properties to form **acetylsalicylic acid (ASA)**—a drug commonly known as *aspirin*. In 1915, aspirin was sold as an over-the-counter (OTC) remedy to treat pain and inflammation. Although this drug continues to be used worldwide for these indications, aspirin is now also recommended by healthcare practitioners as a **prophylactic** for heart attacks. Chloral hydrate (a sedative) and **cocaine** (a local anesthetic) were also marketed for their curative properties. In fact, cocaine was a key ingredient in several cough syrups and toothache remedies that were advertised for use in children until further studies proved its harmful effects.

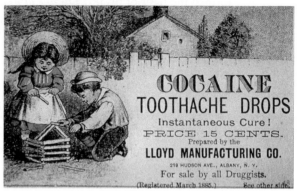

Cocaine became a component in several patent medicines, including these toothache drops manufactured in 1885.

Checkpoint 1.1

Take a moment to review what you have learned so far and answer these questions.

1. What contributions to medicine were made by the Greek physician Hippocrates?

2. Who is considered "The Father of Modern Pharmacology"?

3. What was the contribution of the Swiss surgeon Paracelsus to modern medicine?

History of Pharmacology in the United States

In the Know

Several famous individuals once worked as apothecaries. Physicist and mathematician Sir Isaac Newton (1643–1727), US statesman Benjamin Franklin (1706–1790), US general Benedict Arnold (1741–1801), and English poet John Keats (1795–1821) all worked as apothecaries.

In colonial United States, herbal medicine was commonly practiced by both Native Americans and settlers. Preparations made from natural vegetation such as echinacea (used to prevent infection), ginger (used to treat a stomachache), lavender (used for insomnia), and willow bark (used for pain and fever) were common remedies for restoring harmony to the body, mind, and spirit. These remedies were prepared in the homes, for early North American colonies had few medical personnel. As the colonies grew in the eighteenth century, they attracted a broader range of immigrants, including physicians and apothecaries.

Early Drug Compounding

Like their European counterparts, most colonial physicians owned a dispensary or pharmacy. They prescribed, prepared, and dispensed drugs imported from England. The American Revolution forced American physicians, druggists, and wholesale distributors of drugs to manufacture their own chemical-based drugs and to make common preparations of crude drugs. In 1820, the first official listing of drugs in the United States, the *Pharmacopoeia of the United States*—known today as the **US Pharmacopeia (USP)**—was published by the Massachusetts Medical Society, with approval from a national convention of physicians. A revision of this early formulary exists today and is written by the US Pharmacopeial Convention, an independent, nonprofit organization that sets quality standards for prescription medications and OTC drugs and dietary supplements. The publication also sets national drug standards for all pharmaceutical manufacturers of brand-name and generic drugs.

Unregulated Medicine

Despite the publication of an official drug list, drug distribution in the nineteenth century went largely unregulated in the United States. The rapid expansion of both large cities and isolated rural communities became a gold mine for small-time con men and big-time drug companies. Consumers became the victims of these fraudulent practices, buying the miracle drugs and bogus vaccines that were advertised. Factories could produce and distribute medicines in huge quantities without quality control or inspections and claim medicinal properties based on faulty research or outright lies. Small-time hucksters crisscrossed the country promoting fabulous cure-alls and would often be accompanied by circus-like entertainment. These traveling medicine shows promoted **quack medicine** products that were typically elixirs consisting of large amounts of alcohol or opium often laced with random herbs. Still, it would be well into the twentieth century before the US government would begin to implement controls on the production and distribution of medicine.

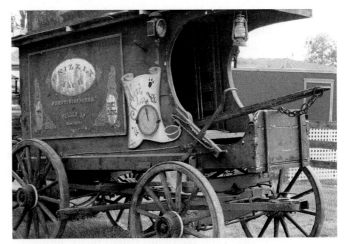

Traveling medicine shows crisscrossed the United States during the nineteenth century. Peddlers, often referred to as *professors*, rolled into small towns in their wagons and hawked their fabulous cure-alls. Circus-like entertainment, such as jugglers, fire-eaters, and musicians, were used to lure crowds to the event.

Pharmacy as a Profession

In the United States in the 1880s, as many errant drug peddlers continued to hawk their potions, healthcare practitioners who were newly trained by medical schools set up practices and prepared their own medications. Like their European counterparts, these practitioners slowly moved away from compounding drugs and focused solely on the diagnosis and treatment of their patients. In 1852, the American Pharmaceutical Association (now known as the **American Pharmacists Association** or APhA) was formed, releasing physicians from the task of compounding medicines and allowing pharmacists the opportunity to hone their skills and increase their professional stature. However, the boundaries between the professions of physician and pharmacist were not clearly established until after the US Civil War (1861–1865).

Community pharmacy practice in the United States in the late 1800s involved the compounding of many herbs and chemicals for medicinal use. Pharmacists often experimented by compounding refreshing drinks served at a soda fountain, a mainstay of pharmacies at that time. For example, in 1886, John Pemberton, a pharmacist by trade in Atlanta, Georgia, began to sell a compounded tonic called Coca-Cola. Its name was derived from the main active ingredient, cocaine, and the caffeine-containing kola nut. For more than two decades, the Coca-Cola formula contained this plant alkaloid, until growing concerns over the effects of cocaine forced its manufacturer to remove this ingredient. Another compounding medication that had spread from Europe to the United States was laudanum. This preparation was made by combining ground opium powder with alcohol and was used to alleviate pain from migraines, cure intestinal upset, and induce sleep.

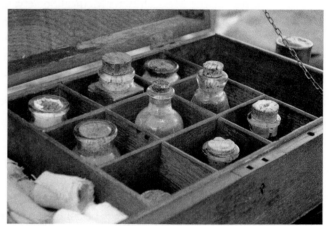

Community pharmacists concocted several herbal remedies, placed the preparations in small jars with cork stoppers, and packed a traveling case such as the one shown here.

Beginnings of Pharmaceutical Manufacturing

By the beginning of the twentieth century, pharmaceutical manufacturing began to take hold. Although many pharmacists continued to rely on plants as ingredients in their compounded preparations, they now incorporated mass-manufactured ingredients as well. Pharmacists formulated their own liquids and powders and rolled their own pills.

In 1906, in reaction to the lack of oversight of drug distribution, the US Congress passed the **Pure Food and Drug Act**, setting standards for both the food and drug industries. This act forbade the manufacture, sale, and transportation of adulterated food products and poisonous patent medicines. It also mandated accurate content and dosage labeling of certain drugs and established the Bureau of Chemistry—the predecessor of the US Food and Drug Administration (FDA).

Important Drug Discoveries

Several drugs were discovered during the first half of the twentieth century. These drugs were created on foreign ground and imported to the United States and other countries. German scientist Emil von Behring discovered the diphtheria antitoxin at the turn of the century and was awarded the Nobel Prize in Physiology or Medicine in 1901 for his research. In 1907, Paul Ehrlich, a German bacteriologist, introduced arsphenamine, or Salvarsan, to treat syphilis. This rudimentary antimicrobial was the first chemical agent used to treat an infectious disease. In 1923, Sir Frederick Banting, a Canadian physiologist, and his assistant Charles Best, successfully extracted the hormone insulin from the pancreas to create the first effective treatment for diabetes. Finally, in 1934, German scientist Hans Andersag discovered chloroquine to combat malaria; chloroquine is still part of the antimalarial drug arsenal today.

Age of Antibiotics

The introduction of **antibiotic medications** early in the twentieth century revolutionized health care in developed countries. In 1929, **penicillin** was discovered by Scottish bacteriologist Sir Alexander Fleming at St. Mary's Hospital in London. In 1935, the first sulfa drug, Prontosil, was introduced by German biochemist Gerhard Domagk who worked for Bayer Laboratories. Domagk was so confident in his research results that he used Prontosil to treat his own daughter's streptococcal infection. Thankfully, his daughter made a complete recovery. Finally, in 1949, Filipino scientist Abelardo Aguilar sent a soil sample to his employer, Eli Lilly and Company. Company scientists were able to use this sample to isolate the antibacterial substance **erythromycin** from a strain of *Streptomyces erythreus*. With the emergence of these antibiotics, the twentieth century is sometimes referred to as "The Golden Age of Antibiotics."

Revolutionary Medicine

Several drug discoveries during the twentieth century had a significant impact on health care. The development of vaccines for infectious diseases saved the lives of countless children—most notably, the **polio vaccine** discovered by Jonas Salk. Many new antibiotics were introduced, continuing to improve patients' ability to combat infectious diseases. Other revolutionary drugs in this era included the introduction of the first **oral contraceptive**, Enovid (first patented in 1960), which changed women's lives, and the emergence of the **antidepressant** fluoxetine (1987) and the **antipsychotic** chlorpromazine (1951), which changed the lives of individuals coping with mental illness. In 1949, mechlorethamine was developed for the treatment of cancer, followed by methotrexate in 1953. That same year, the discovery of **deoxyribonucleic acid (DNA)** by Francis Crick, James Watson, and Maurice Wilkins allowed scientists to understand the functions of genes and the role of defective genes in the development of cancer.

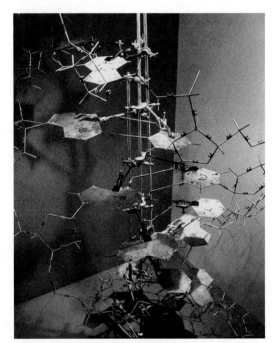

This replica of the DNA helix is housed in the Science Museum of London and contains the original plates that Crick, Watson, and Wilkins used in their model.

The latter half of the twentieth century brought a flood of significant drug discoveries in pharmacology. Drug development focused on treatments for chronic diseases such as cardiovascular and cerebrovascular diseases and diabetes—a trend that continues today. Drugs for hypertension were introduced, including beta blockers such as atenolol, angiotensin-converting enzyme inhibitors such as lisinopril, and diuretics such as hydrochlorothiazide. The first-line oral drug for Type 2 diabetes, metformin, was approved by the FDA in 1995, and other diabetes drugs including glipizide were also approved late in the century. Finally, research for a treatment for the **human immunodeficiency virus (HIV)** led to the discovery of zidovudine.

Most recently, biotechnology has improved the treatment of some serious disorders, including diabetes, hemophilia, rheumatoid arthritis, and some cancers. **Biotechnology** is the study and manipulation of living things or their component molecules, cells, tissues, or organs. This science has led to the creation of drugs designed to target specific biomarkers on cancerous tumors. Biotechnology has also advanced the field of genetics. Patients can now undergo tests to reveal genetic variations in the major drug metabolic pathways. The results of these tests allow prescribers to personalize drug therapy. For example, genetic testing is now recommended prior to prescribing abacavir, an HIV medication. Currently, more than 900 biotechnologically engineered drugs are under development to treat more than 100 diseases.

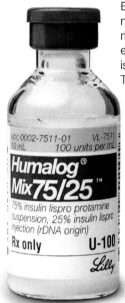

Biotechnologically engineered drugs can treat many serious illnesses. An example is Humalog, which is used primarily to treat Type 1 diabetes.

 ## Checkpoint 1.2

Take a moment to review what you have learned so far and answer these questions.

1. Can you name two drugs that were developed in the first half of the twentieth century?

2. What are some important drug classes that were developed in the second half of the twentieth century?

3. What is the *US Pharmacopeia*?

Pharmacology Study for the Allied Health Professional

Today's scientists, like their predecessors, continue to build on past knowledge to discover new, innovative drug treatments for the disorders and diseases that affect the human body. Consequently, pharmacology continues to change, which means that the allied health professional must stay current with these advancements.

Knowledge of pharmacology has many practical applications for allied health professionals. For example, in your work, you may find the following skills useful:

- being able to determine the correct dose of a drug

- learning strategies for avoiding common medication errors

- knowing the common side effects of different classes of drugs

- knowing which drugs are controlled substances, that is, which are more tightly regulated because they have a higher potential for abuse

- knowing the common routes of drug administration (oral, intravenous, topical)

- being aware of which drugs have special administration requirements (e.g., a drug that must be taken with food or a drug that must be given with a full glass of water)

- knowing which drugs have special storage requirements (e.g., a drug that requires refrigeration or a drug that must be protected from light)

- knowing the different classes of drugs and their indications

- recognizing the generic and brand names of the most commonly prescribed medications

- being able to easily find more information about specific drugs

Knowledge of drugs, their actions, their interactions, their side effects, and their adverse reactions is necessary for appropriate patient care. All allied health professionals must have a working knowledge of all medications used in their workplace, including new drugs that become available and new applications of established drugs. Accurate pharmacology knowledge, when shared with the patient, improves the patient's understanding and helps to establish patient trust and cooperation.

Learning Pharmacology

You may have heard that pharmacology is a challenging and demanding subject in allied health programs. In fact, many students would probably admit that the volume of information and new terminology to remember is daunting. You are being asked to learn hundreds of drug names and understand the uses of different drugs. There is an additional complication: Each drug you must learn has two names, a **generic name**, which is assigned by the United States Adopted Names Council and is similar to the names of other drugs in the same drug class, and a **brand name**, which is assigned by the manufacturer and is often easier to pronounce. To further complicate matters, once a drug's patent expires, it can be sold as a generic drug under a variety of different brand names. Each manufacturer of a generic form of a drug may choose a different brand name (although some simply use the generic name).

This textbook will help you adopt some systematic and logical strategies for learning pharmacology. **Best practices** indicate that the study of pharmacology must go hand-in-hand with the study of the body systems.

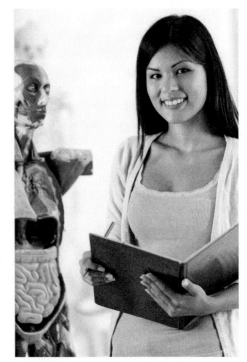

Learning the body systems and their associated drugs provides a logical approach to the study of pharmacology.

Having an understanding of the body systems and their associated drugs provides a context for learning the names of drugs as well as their drug classes, indications, mechanisms of action, side effects, contraindications, and cautions and considerations.

Using anatomy and physiology as a foundation for learning pharmacology can be challenging in other ways. As an allied health student, you may find that you have entered a scientific discipline that has its own language—and indeed it does. **Medical terminology** is based largely on Greek and Latin root words and is used extensively in the study of anatomy and physiology. This text does not attempt to teach medical terminology because there are many other quality texts and programs with that purpose. However, this text does define many key terms in the study of physiology because knowing these terms helps allied health students learn pharmacology essentials.

Strategies for Learning Pharmacology

To best learn pharmacology, first break up the material into categories. For instance, pharmacology tends to be discussed in terms of **drug classes**—categories of drugs having similar characteristics. All the drugs in a class work by a particular mechanism of action and cause many of the same side effects. Fortunately, drugs within a specific class are often given similar generic names, which can help your learning process. For example, all of the beta blocker medications have generic names that end in *–olol* (atenolol, metoprolol, and propranolol), and all of the HMG coenzyme A reductase inhibitors (cholesterol-lowering drugs) have generic names that end in *–statin* (atorvastatin, rosuvastatin, and simvastatin). Once you learn common similarities for a drug class, you can then focus on learning the drug names associated with that class. (Admittedly, you must also memorize the brand names that go with the generic drug names.)

In effect, you will learn a set of rules for each drug class and then connect the individual drugs to that set of rules. For example, all of the benzodiazepine medications (which are used for anxiety) have names that end in *–pam* or *–lam*, and all of them can be sedating. When studying this class of drugs, it would be useful to learn which ones are long-acting (clonazepam), which ones are short-acting (lorazepam), which ones are also indicated for the treatment of seizures (diazepam), which ones are available in injectable forms, and which ones have the safer drug-interaction profiles. When you approach the learning of drug classes in this way, you will instantly know what a particular drug does and how it works by simply seeing or hearing its name. Once you are aware of the drug-class rules, you only have to remember the few exceptions, which typically apply to side effects.

To learn pharmacology, you will benefit from both independent and group activities. For example, some students download smartphone applications (apps) to make their own flash cards and quiz themselves. Other students may find it useful to turn to YouTube to watch videos on pharmacology that reinforce what they learned in class. Still others like to create tables to organize and help them memorize drug information. In addition to these activities, students can access several online tools to help them study pharmacology. Learning management systems, such as Navigator+ that accompanies this textbook, enable delivery of multiple interactive practice tools for students to use. Finally, group activities can be very helpful for students learning pharmacology—whether working with a partner and using flash cards or creating pharmacology versions of the game *Jeopardy!*

Navigator⊕

Checkpoint 1.3

Take a moment to review what you have learned so far and answer these questions.

1. What are the two types of names associated with each drug?
2. What is one strategy for learning the generic names of drugs?

Understanding Learning Styles

Because pharmacology is a complex topic that involves learning a large vocabulary of unfamiliar terms, it is useful for students to take a few moments to think about how they learn and to use that understanding to develop strategies for studying.

Everyone learns in different ways. Some individuals prefer to learn independently by reading alone, whereas others prefer group interaction and discussion. Concrete learners like facts and details rather than abstract concepts, and auditory learners need to hear new material read aloud. Still other types of learners grasp new concepts best through the following means:

- kinesthetic methods (hands-on learning, pacing or dancing while reviewing)
- logical reasoning and math
- music (playing music or putting new material into a catchy tune)
- speaking and writing
- visual presentations (needing to see words on a page to process them)
- visual-spatial methods (drawing pictures or diagrams)

Kolb's Learning Styles Inventory

In 1984, the American educational theorist David Kolb, a professor of organizational behavior at Case Western Reserve University in Cleveland, Ohio, theorized that each individual has a preferred way of learning and processing new information. In his learning model, known as **Kolb's Learning Styles Inventory**, he described four learning styles: Accommodator, Diverger, Assimilator, and Converger (see Table 1.1).

TABLE 1.1 Kolb's Learning Styles Inventory

Learning Style	Preferences
Accommodator	Concrete experience and active experimentation: practical, adventurous, and intuitive
Diverger	Concrete experience and reflective observation: imaginative and aesthetic, interested in people and the ideas of others
Assimilator	Abstract conceptualization and reflective observation: theoretical, interested in abstract connections and ideas
Converger	Abstract conceptualization and active experimentation: practical, unemotional, and rational

The categories in Kolb's Learning Styles are based on the idea that students tend to be better at two of the four learning stages:

- learning by being involved in the world (concrete experience)

- thinking about those experiences (reflective observation)

- making generalizations and developing theories based on those experiences (abstract conceptualization)

- testing those theories while solving problems (active experimentation)

For example, in Kolb's theory, students who learn best by being involved in the world (concrete experience) and then thinking about those experiences (reflective observation) are considered Divergers.

Kolb also theorized that individuals learn a task by following a cycle of steps or stages (see Figure 1.1) and most likely require more than one rotation through the cycle. In addition, Kolb postulated that individuals start their learning at different stages of the cycle, excel at different steps, and spend more time at their preferred stages of learning in order to obtain new knowledge and skills.

FIGURE 1.1 Kolb's Learning Cycle

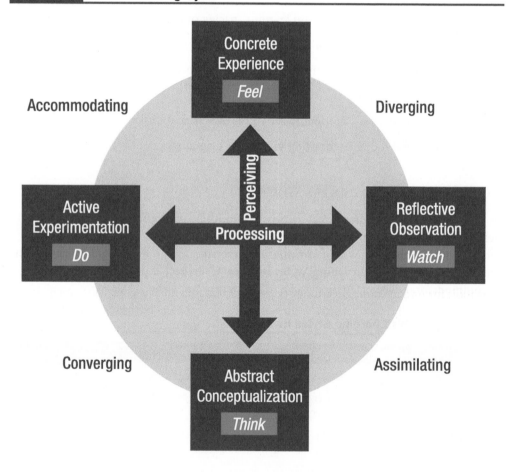

Preferred Learning Styles

Preferred learning styles can be determined, in part, by understanding and applying the Kolb's Learning Styles Inventory to a self-assessment and by identifying personal preferences based on experience. For example, some learners want to think about a task and observe someone else performing that task before trying it on their own. Others prefer to dive in and learn from trial and error. Take a few minutes to consider your learning preferences. When you buy a new electronic gadget, do you read the manual, or do you just try to figure out how to use it on your own? Do you find it difficult to master a task without watching someone else do it first? Do you find it easier to learn by doing, or do you prefer to start by thinking about the best way to approach a task?

You can apply the same self-assessment to learning pharmacology. For example, if you had to memorize the list of the 200 most frequently prescribed medications, how would you approach it? Would you write them all out alphabetically? Make flash cards? Form a study group and quiz one another? Develop mnemonic devices to help you learn all the terms? Make a chart? Sort all the drugs by disease state, and then memorize them in groups? In addition to learning the names of drugs, you will need to memorize a lot more information about the most commonly used drugs, such as common dosages, side effects, and dangerous drug interactions.

> **Quick Study**
>
> *MONA* is an example of a mnemonic device. Medical practitioners use the acronym MONA to remember the treatment steps for a myocardial infarction: **M**orphine, **O**xygen, **N**itrates, **A**spirin.

Depending on your intended career path, in the course of your healthcare education and training you may also need to memorize large amounts of information about anatomy and physiology, such as the names of the 206 bones in the body, the dozens of muscles of the legs, the names and purposes of the different cranial nerves, and the hormonal controls of different systems in the body. Knowing your learning preferences will help you learn and retain this knowledge.

Even after you complete your formal studies in the allied health curriculum, you will find that lifelong learning is essential in practice. Health care is always changing and expanding, with new drugs coming to market regularly. Appreciating how you learn will help you to find ways to retain large amounts of information as a student and to develop new skills for learning and adapting in the workplace.

You can perform a learning styles inventory to gain insight into how your brain works and how you prefer to receive, understand, and commit information to memory. Numerous tools for understanding learning styles are published and available. Most are easy to use, and each has its unique take on learning styles. For the purposes of this text, the Kolb's Learning Styles Inventory will be used to identify your preferences. To discover how your learning approaches correspond with the Kolb's Learning Styles Inventory, go to Appendix B and take the self-assessment. Once you determine which of the four learning styles is your dominant method, look for the Kolb's Learning Styles feature boxes interspersed throughout this textbook.

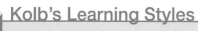

Kolb's Learning Styles

To apply Kolb's Learning Styles to your own learning, think about your approach to understanding new material and then consider which learning style (Assimilator, Converger, Diverger, or Accommodator) most closely matches your own. Finally, determine which of the following methods would help you in your study of pharmacology:

- Read pharmacologic content on your own. Then write notes or make a list to organize your thoughts about drugs: their drug class, generic and brand names, indications, side effects, contraindications, cautions and considerations, and common dosages.
- Make flash cards and use them with a classmate to remember specific information about drugs.
- Draw pictures or diagrams of how drugs work, and record pertinent information about the medications under the illustrations. Then present your drawings or discuss them with a study group.
- Work with others in a group to discuss common uses of drugs as well as other detailed information. Then, as a group, create an electronic document that lists and describes the drugs, their indications, and other important information.

Information Resources

Recognizing preferred learning styles provides individuals with an awareness of how they approach learning and what methods are conducive to their knowledge acquisition and retention. Learning new content in any field of study also requires relevant, accurate, and current information resources. In addition to this textbook, there are several print and online resources available to aid the study of pharmacology and the body systems.

Evaluation of Online Information

There is a wealth of healthcare information available online. A simple web search for a body system, disorder, or drug will yield results, but the accuracy and quality of the information available varies widely. Consequently, individuals must evaluate each source of information before using it. One good practice for determining content quality is to ask two questions:

1. Is the information credible?

2. Is the information understandable?

The first question is more important than the second question because information you understand is not useful if it is not true.

Assessing Credibility

Health information that is posted in a blog or on a message board is not likely to be as reliable or useful as information published on a more established website, such as a site associated with a medical school, major hospital, medical journal, healthcare organization, or medical society devoted to a particular health problem. For example, a blog or online forum entry may tell you that one individual who took acetaminophen experienced hemorrhoids. However, the blog may not address these important overriding concerns: Does acetaminophen commonly cause hemorrhoids? Does acetaminophen cause hemorrhoids in more than 10% of the individuals who use it? The answer to each question is *no*. Therefore, it is not likely that acetaminophen would cause hemorrhoids.

Determining Understandability

It can also be challenging to find solid medical information that is written in plain language. For example, articles in medical journals are typically written for their target audience—physicians. Thus, the articles tend to contain too many technical details to be useful to many allied health professionals. However, a website sponsored by a medical society concerned with a particular disease is often a good source of reliable medical information that is written in plain language. Information posted on a medical society's website is typically aimed at both healthcare practitioners and consumers seeking healthcare information. For example, the website of the American Diabetes Association is user-friendly and contains excellent information on diabetes. The website of the American Cancer Society features a glossary of terms to orient readers to this large and complex topic; it also contains information on the treatment options for different types of cancer.

Medical Society Websites

As mentioned earlier, medical society websites are sources of reliable healthcare information. For a list of common medical societies and their descriptions, see Table 1.2.

TABLE 1.2 **Medical Society Websites**

Organization	Go To	Description
American Cancer Society (ACS)	http://PharmEssAH .emcp.net/ACS	Contains information on the types of cancer and treatment options for each type as well as a glossary of terms used in cancer treatment
American Diabetes Association (ADA)	http://PharmEssAH .emcp.net/ADA	Features an overview of diabetes, a glossary of terms related to the disease, and news on recent research
American Heart Association (AHA)	http://PharmEssAH .emcp.net/AHA	Contains information on hypertension, high cholesterol, congenital heart defects, heart failure, heart attacks, and arrhythmias
American Lung Association (ALA)	http://PharmEssAH .emcp.net/ALA	Features information on asthma, chronic obstructive pulmonary disease, lung cancer, smoking cessation, and current research on respiratory disorders

US Government Healthcare Websites

US government websites devoted to health care, such as the websites of the Centers for Disease Control and Prevention (CDC) and the US Food and Drug Administration (FDA), also contain reliable information; much of it is written in layperson's terms. Table 1.3 provides a list of common US government websites related to health care and their descriptions.

TABLE 1.3 US Government Healthcare Websites

Organization	Go To	Description
Centers for Disease Control and Prevention (CDC)	http://PharmEssAH.emcp.net/CDC	A website that includes information on vaccinations, immunizations, and common disease states
National Institutes of Health (NIH) and the National Library of Medicine (NLM)	http://PharmEssAH.emcp.net /MedlinePlus	A website known as MedlinePlus that contains consumer information about different drugs and medical conditions
National Plan & Provider Enumeration System (NPPES)	http://PharmEssAH.emcp.net /NPIRegistry	A website known as the NPI Registry, which can be used to look up a prescriber's National Provider Identifier (NPI), which may be needed for filing an insurance claim or ordering a prescription
US Department of Health and Human Services (HHS)	http://PharmEssAH.emcp.net/HHS and http://PharmEssAH.emcp.net /HHSHealthTopics	Websites that offer prevention and wellness information on more than 100 disease states, as well as dietary guidelines, exercise guidelines, and information about government initiatives to improve patient health and safety
US Food and Drug Administration (FDA)	http://PharmEssAH.emcp.net /FDAdrugs	A website that provides drug product inserts or detailed information about drugs such as dosage, indications, and warnings about potential side effects

Health Information Toolkit

Knowing that credibility and understandability are important qualities of reliable pharmacology resources, allied health professionals should develop their own health information toolkit. A **health information toolkit** is a set of trusted sources to use when searching for medical information. The toolkit should include a medical dictionary, a pocket guide of

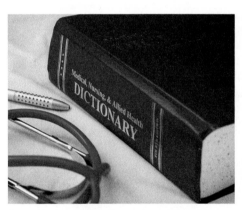

A medical dictionary is a great resource for learning medical terms, including their pronunciations, definitions, and word roots.

brand and generic drugs, a drug handbook or smartphone app, and other resources to help answer the questions that frequently arise in the workplace. Bound volumes such as the *Physicians' Desk Reference* and the *Handbook of Nonprescription Drugs* are excellent sources of drug information. In addition, your employer may have a subscription to one of the comprehensive, online drug information databases currently on the market, such as *Facts & Comparisons eAnswers*, *Clinical Pharmacology*, *Micromedex*, or *UpToDate*. Table 1.4 contains an example of a health information toolkit.

If your health information toolkit is complete, you will not have to rely on additional sources very often, which means you will not put yourself in the risky position of turning to unreliable sources of information.

Having good tools close at hand will protect you from inaccurate information. Keep in mind, too, that many knowledgeable sources of information work alongside you in the healthcare setting, including pharmacists, the drug information experts on the healthcare team. Rely on their pharmacologic expertise and guidance as needed.

Table 1.5 describes what resources might be used to field some questions about drugs that commonly arise in healthcare practice.

Work Wise

To access drug information easily, allied health professionals may want to bookmark useful drug information websites in their web browsers.

TABLE 1.4 | Suggested Health Information Toolkit Resources

Resource	Examples
Drug handbook	• *Nursing2016 Drug Handbook*
Major hospital websites	• Children's Hospital of Philadelphia website • Mayo Clinic website
Medical dictionary	• *Merriam-Webster's Medical Dictionary* • *Stedman's Medical Dictionary* • Various online medical dictionaries such as the *MedlinePlus* dictionary
Medical society websites	• American Cancer Society website • American Diabetes Association website • American Heart Association website • American Lung Association website
Pocket guide of brand-name and generic drugs	• Paradigm Education Solutions' *Pocket Drug Guide* (available in print, ebook, and smartphone-app formats)
Smartphone apps	• *Epocrates* • *Lexicomp* • *Micromedex Drug Reference Essentials* • *MobilePDR*
US government websites	• Centers for Disease Control and Prevention (CDC) website • Department of Health and Human Services (HHS) website • National Institutes of Health (NIH) website • US Food and Drug Administration (FDA) website

TABLE 1.5 | Toolkit Resources for Common Drug Questions

Common Questions	Toolkit Resources
What does that medical term mean? *Example: What is pruritus?*	• *Merriam-Webster's Medical Dictionary* • *Stedman's Medical Dictionary* • Various online medical dictionaries such as the *MedlinePlus* dictionary
What is that drug used to treat? *Example: Is lisinopril used to treat asthma?* What is a normal dose for that drug? *Example: Is 10 mg of lisinopril a reasonable dose?* What are the common side effects? *Example: Is coughing a side effect of lisinopril?*	• *Epocrates* smartphone app • *Micromedex Drug Reference Essentials* smartphone app • *MobilePDR* smartphone app • *Nursing2016 Drug Handbook* • Other online drug databases
What is the other name for that drug? *Example: Is Abilify the same drug as clonazepam?*	• *Epocrates* smartphone app • *Micromedex Drug Reference Essentials* smartphone app • *MobilePDR* smartphone app • Online drug databases • Paradigm Education Solutions' *Pocket Drug Guide*
How can I find more information about a specific health problem? *Example: What are the symptoms of diabetes?*	• Website for a major hospital, such as the Mayo Clinic or the Children's Hospital of Philadelphia • Website for a society devoted to a specific health problem—in this case, the American Diabetes Association

TABLE 1.5 Toolkit Resources for Common Drug Questions *(continued)*

Common Questions	Toolkit Resources
What is that pill? *Example: Is this little green pill warfarin or levothyroxine?*	• *Epocrates* smartphone app • *Lexicomp* smartphone app • *Physicians' Desk Reference (PDR)* • *MobilePDR* smartphone app • RxList Pill Identification Tool (online)
How much does this medication cost? *Example: What is the cost of a 30-day supply of lisinopril?*	• *Epocrates* smartphone app • *Red Book* • http://drugs.com/price-guide
What nonprescription drugs could be used to treat my patient's symptoms? *Example: What over-the-counter product is best for treating itching caused by bug bites?*	• *Handbook of Nonprescription Drugs* • *Facts & Comparisons eAnswers*
Do the drugs my patient is taking interact with each other? *Example: Will this new antibiotic my patient is starting change the efficacy of her ongoing warfarin treatment?*	• *Epocrates* smartphone app • *Facts & Comparisons eAnswers* • *Micromedex Drug Reference* smartphone app

 Checkpoint 1.4

Take a moment to review what you have learned so far and answer these questions.

1. What are the four learning styles described by Kolb? Based on these learning styles, what is Kolb's theory on how individuals learn?

2. What are two reliable medical society websites for allied health professionals to use?

Chapter Review

Chapter Summary

The study of ancient documents shows that individuals have been treating physical and mental ailments with medicines for thousands of years. Early texts, such as the *Ebers Papyrus* written in 1500 BCE, focused on the medicinal uses of plants, animals, and minerals. This well-known document, a predecessor of the drug formularies that are used today, contains more than 700 different herbal recipes. The discovery of this ancient papyrus marks the beginnings of pharmacology. To view a timeline of significant discoveries and events in the pharmacology field, refer to the "Pharmacology Historical Review" that follows.

A review of the history of pharmacology underscores the idea that pharmacology is an ever-changing field. Consequently, individuals who work in the healthcare field must keep apprised of a vast number of drugs that enter and exit the market. To best learn pharmacology, allied health professionals should break up the drug information into categories. Learning drug classes first is an effective approach to learning the names of medications because these drugs have similar generic names, mechanisms of action, and associated side effects. Once individuals learn the drug classes, they should focus their attention on learning the names of the generic drugs within those classes, including the brand names of those drugs.

Because pharmacology is a complex topic that involves learning a large vocabulary of unfamiliar terms, it is useful for allied health students to take a few moments to think about how they learn, and then to use that knowledge to develop strategies for studying. David Kolb first described four learning styles (Accommodator, Diverger, Assimilator, and Converger) in his well-known learning styles inventory in the 1980s and 1990s. Being aware of one's preferred learning styles can be useful for finding effective ways to study and learn new material.

There is a wealth of information about drugs and medical conditions available in books and online, but the quality of the information available varies widely. It is a good idea for allied health professionals to develop their own health information toolkit: a set of trusted sources to use when searching for medical information. The toolkit should include a medical dictionary, a pocket guide to brand-name and generic drugs, a drug handbook or smartphone app, and other resources to help answer the questions that will arise most frequently in the workplace.

Chapter Checkup

The Navigator+ learning management system that accompanies this textbook offers many opportunities to help you master chapter content, including end-of-chapter exercises, a glossary of key terms, flash cards, and additional interactive activities.

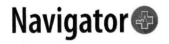

Career Exploration

If you enjoyed learning about pharmacology basics in this chapter, you may want to explore the following career options:

- emergency medical technician (EMT)/paramedic
- medical assistant
- pharmacy technician

Pharmacology Historical Review

c. 1550 BCE The Ebers Papyrus was compiled in Egypt and lists more than 700 herbal remedies used by healers. → 4th century BCE Sushruta, a Hindu surgeon, wrote the *Sushruta Samhita* in India. → 460–370 BCE The Greek physician Hippocrates proposed that disease was caused by natural rather than supernatural causes and that the four humors of the body (blood, phlegm, yellow bile, and black bile) must be in balance to maintain optimal health.

50–70 CE Dioscorides, a Greek physician, compiled *De Materia Medica*, a text that described and classified more than 1,000 substances—mainly botanicals—that had medicinal value. For 15 centuries, *De Materia Medica* served as the standard reference text for drugs. → c. 130–201 CE The Greek physician Galen studied the effects of herbal medicine on the body, which led to the coining of the term *galenical pharmacy*, or the process of creating extracts of active medicinals from plants. → c. 13th century CE Apothecary shops sprang up in villages across Europe. Residents of these villages received both diagnosis and treatment from the practitioners who worked in these shops.

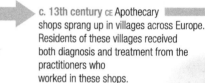

1493–1541 CE Paracelsus, a Swiss surgeon, denounced the theory of the four humors and advocated the use of individual drugs rather than mixtures to treat diseases. → 1507–1513 CE Leonardo da Vinci, an Italian painter, inventor, and anatomist, studied human corpses to create anatomic drawings. → 1543 CE Flemish physician and anatomist Andreas Vesalius compiled his intricate anatomic drawings for his book *De Humani Corporis Fabrica (On the Structure of the Human Body)*, laying the foundation for the continued study of human anatomy and its disorders.

1578 CE Chinese physician Li Shizhen compiled *Ben Cao Gang Mu (Compendium of Materia Medica)*, a text that lists more than 1,000 plants and 8,000 recipes used in the treatment of illnesses. → 1628 CE English physician and anatomist William Harvey's research on human blood circulation was presented in *De Motu Cordis*. → 1661 CE Italian scientist Marcello Malpighi pioneered the use of microscopes, discovering the role of capillaries in circulation and making many observations about pathology over the next two decades.

1754 CE English physician James Lind treated scurvy in sailors by adding citrus fruits to their diets. → 1761 CE Italian physician Giovanni Battista Morgagni published his groundbreaking text on pathology *De Sedibus et Causis Morborum per Anatomen Indagatis (The Seats and Causes of Disease)*. → 1772–1790 CE English clergyman and scientist Joseph Priestly discovered 10 gases including oxygen and nitrous oxide (laughing gas), which are used in medicine today.

1785 CE English physician and botanist William Withering first described the medicinal use of the foxglove plant (the source of digoxin) to treat edema. → 1796 CE German physician Samuel Hahnemann introduced the medical theory of homeopathy. → 1796 CE English physician Edward Jenner developed the first vaccine, preventing smallpox in a healthy patient by inoculating a young boy with cowpox.

1813–1878 CE Claude Bernard, French scientist, demonstrated that certain drugs have specific sites of action in the body. → 1820 CE The *Pharmacopoeia of the United States*, the first official listing of drugs in the United States, was published by the Massachusetts Medical Society. → 1838–1921 CE Oswald Schmiedeberg established a department of pharmacology at the University of Strasbourg, Germany, where he worked. His research, published in *Outline of Pharmacology*, coupled with his contributions to the advancement of the pharmacology field led to his recognition as "The Father of Modern Pharmacology."

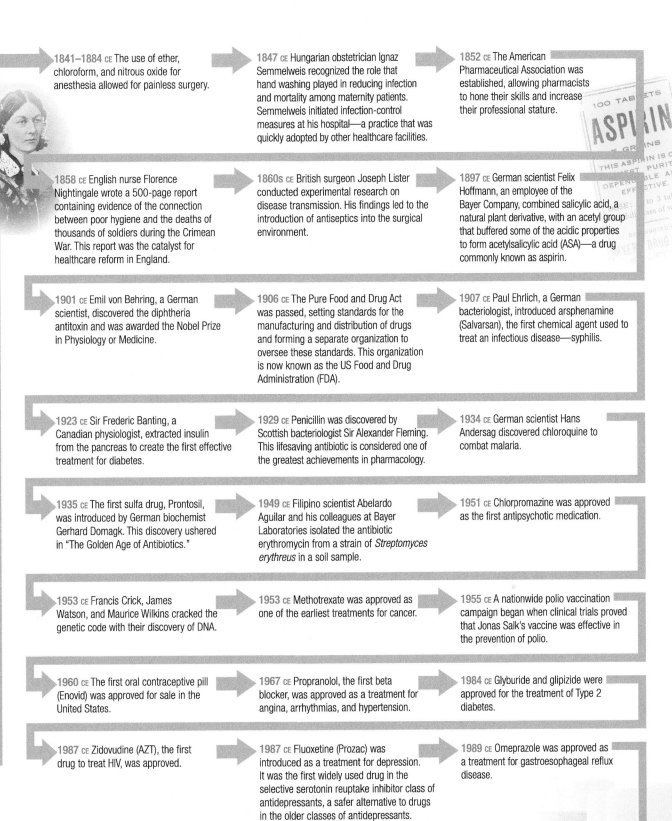

1841–1884 CE The use of ether, chloroform, and nitrous oxide for anesthesia allowed for painless surgery.

1847 CE Hungarian obstetrician Ignaz Semmelweis recognized the role that hand washing played in reducing infection and mortality among maternity patients. Semmelweis initiated infection-control measures at his hospital—a practice that was quickly adopted by other healthcare facilities.

1852 CE The American Pharmaceutical Association was established, allowing pharmacists to hone their skills and increase their professional stature.

1858 CE English nurse Florence Nightingale wrote a 500-page report containing evidence of the connection between poor hygiene and the deaths of thousands of soldiers during the Crimean War. This report was the catalyst for healthcare reform in England.

1860s CE British surgeon Joseph Lister conducted experimental research on disease transmission. His findings led to the introduction of antiseptics into the surgical environment.

1897 CE German scientist Felix Hoffmann, an employee of the Bayer Company, combined salicylic acid, a natural plant derivative, with an acetyl group that buffered some of the acidic properties to form acetylsalicylic acid (ASA)—a drug commonly known as aspirin.

1901 CE Emil von Behring, a German scientist, discovered the diphtheria antitoxin and was awarded the Nobel Prize in Physiology or Medicine.

1906 CE The Pure Food and Drug Act was passed, setting standards for the manufacturing and distribution of drugs and forming a separate organization to oversee these standards. This organization is now known as the US Food and Drug Administration (FDA).

1907 CE Paul Ehrlich, a German bacteriologist, introduced arsphenamine (Salvarsan), the first chemical agent used to treat an infectious disease—syphilis.

1923 CE Sir Frederic Banting, a Canadian physiologist, extracted insulin from the pancreas to create the first effective treatment for diabetes.

1929 CE Penicillin was discovered by Scottish bacteriologist Sir Alexander Fleming. This lifesaving antibiotic is considered one of the greatest achievements in pharmacology.

1934 CE German scientist Hans Andersag discovered chloroquine to combat malaria.

1935 CE The first sulfa drug, Prontosil, was introduced by German biochemist Gerhard Domagk. This discovery ushered in "The Golden Age of Antibiotics."

1949 CE Filipino scientist Abelardo Aguilar and his colleagues at Bayer Laboratories isolated the antibiotic erythromycin from a strain of *Streptomyces erythreus* in a soil sample.

1951 CE Chlorpromazine was approved as the first antipsychotic medication.

1953 CE Francis Crick, James Watson, and Maurice Wilkins cracked the genetic code with their discovery of DNA.

1953 CE Methotrexate was approved as one of the earliest treatments for cancer.

1955 CE A nationwide polio vaccination campaign began when clinical trials proved that Jonas Salk's vaccine was effective in the prevention of polio.

1960 CE The first oral contraceptive pill (Enovid) was approved for sale in the United States.

1967 CE Propranolol, the first beta blocker, was approved as a treatment for angina, arrhythmias, and hypertension.

1984 CE Glyburide and glipizide were approved for the treatment of Type 2 diabetes.

1987 CE Zidovudine (AZT), the first drug to treat HIV, was approved.

1987 CE Fluoxetine (Prozac) was introduced as a treatment for depression. It was the first widely used drug in the selective serotonin reuptake inhibitor class of antidepressants, a safer alternative to drugs in the older classes of antidepressants.

1989 CE Omeprazole was approved as a treatment for gastroesophageal reflux disease.

1992 CE Zolpidem (Ambien) was approved as a short-term treatment for insomnia, the first in the class of Z-drugs to be approved (the others are zaleplon and eszopiclone).

1995 CE Metformin was approved as a treatment for Type 2 diabetes.

1998 CE Sildenafil (Viagra) was introduced as the first oral medication for erectile dysfunction.

Pharmaceutical Development

Pharm Facts

- According to Sigurdur Olafsson of Teva Pharmaceutical Industries, the leader of the generic drug industry in sales, "Nearly every therapeutic class and disease state has at least one generic medicine available."

- Many pharmaceutical manufacturers, including Merck and Pfizer, spend twice as much money on advertising and marketing than they do on research and development.

- The average period between the launching of a brand-name drug and the arrival of its first generic counterpart is about 12 years.

- More than 90% of drugs tested in clinical trials fail to make it to market.

- In 2015, the FDA launched an electronic version of informed consent, known as *eIC*. This form allows interested individuals to access electronic media (animated videos, podcasts, interactive quizzes, etc.) to gain a clearer understanding of a particular drug study prior to granting consent for participation.

"As a pharmacy technology educator, I have noticed that students who truly learn the top 200 generic and brand-name drugs—including the common prefixes and suffixes of generic drugs—become successful pharmacy technicians in the workplace. Committing this knowledge to memory provides pharmacy technicians with a solid medication foundation and saves time in the prescription-filling process, thus improving overall customer service. Most importantly, learning the top 200 generic and brand-name drugs improves patient safety, the guiding principle of the pharmacy profession."

—**Shelina Hardwick-Moses**,
MBA, MSHCA, CPhT, PhTR
Pharmacy Technician

In the last six decades, technologic advances in the synthesis and production of pharmaceuticals have transformed lives, providing improved antibiotics, vaccines, and other medications to better control chronic diseases such as hypertension, hyperlipidemia, and diabetes. The development of these drugs was built on the scientific framework provided by earlier major research discoveries that have defined and shaped pharmacology. Along with the emergence of these lifesaving medications came improvements in the regulation of these drugs, including lengthy drug trials that test the efficacy and safety of medications before they are marketed.

This chapter provides insight into medications by exploring the process of pharmaceutical development, including the sources of drugs, their classifications, and their approval by various regulatory agencies. For allied health professionals, understanding how drugs are developed and named is useful not only for following regulations and drug handling requirements but also for learning the different classes of medications.

Sources of Drugs

Drugs are derived from various sources and can be classified as natural, synthetic (created artificially), semisynthetic (containing both natural and synthetic components), and synthesized (created artificially but in imitation of naturally occurring substances). The development of lifesaving and life-altering biogenetically engineered drugs is a major source of new drug development in the twenty-first century.

Natural Sources of Drugs

Some drugs are naturally occurring biologic products and can be made or taken from single-celled organisms, plants, animals, minerals, and humans. Many herbal products come from natural sources, and two lifesaving drugs, insulin and penicillin, are also derived from nature. Other examples of modern-day drugs from natural sources include the following:

- The antibiotic streptomycin is produced from cultures of the bacterium *Streptomyces griseus*.

- Digitalis, a drug used to strengthen the heart and regulate its rhythm, is formulated from the foxglove plant.

- The narcotic opium and its derivatives (morphine and codeine) come from the opium poppy plant.

- Quinine, used to treat malaria, and colchicine, used to treat gout, both come from the bark of the cinchona tree.

- Acetylsalicylic acid, more commonly known as aspirin, is derived from the bark of the white willow tree (which contains salicylic acid).

- Thyroid extract is derived from the desiccated (dried) thyroid glands of pigs.

- The salts of minerals such as iron and potassium, which are commonly found in nature, are used for the treatment of iron deficiency and electrolyte replacement therapy.

- Milk of magnesia, an aqueous suspension of magnesium hydroxide, is used as an antacid or a laxative. Magnesium hydroxide is produced from seawater or the mineral brucite.

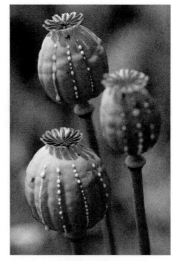

Scoring of the capsules of poppy heads releases a milky sap called *latex*. This exudate, known as raw opium, is used in the creation of morphine and codeine.

Laboratory Sources of Drugs

In the modern era, many naturally occurring substances have been combined with other ingredients in a laboratory setting to produce synthetic, semisynthetic, and synthesized drugs.

Synthetic Drugs

A **synthetic drug** is a drug that has been created from a series of chemical reactions to produce a specific pharmacologic effect. Phenobarbital—a barbiturate prescribed for seizure, nerve, or headache disorders—is an example of a synthetic drug. Another example would be a sulfa antibiotic. Both phenobarbital and sulfa are considered synthetic drugs because these substances do not exist in nature.

Semisynthetic Drugs

A **semisynthetic drug** is a natural drug that has been modified chemically in the laboratory to do one or more of the following actions: (1) improve the efficacy of the natural product; (2) reduce its side effects; (3) overcome developing bacterial resistance; or (4) broaden the spectrum of bacteria against which a product can be effective. Many current antibiotics such as amoxicillin/clavulanate, azithromycin, and ampicillin are modifications of existing natural drugs. These antibiotics are more effective against different strains of bacteria or bacteria that have developed resistance to the natural product.

Synthesized Drugs

A **synthesized drug** is a drug created artificially in the laboratory but in imitation of a natural drug. Epinephrine hydrochloride is an example of a synthesized drug. A single dose of this lifesaving drug is contained in an auto-injector device called an EpiPen and is used by hypersensitive patients to treat severe allergic reactions to insect stings or other triggers. Epinephrine hydrochloride mimics the pharmacologic action of the naturally occurring hormone adrenaline. Digoxin, aspirin, and quinine are all considered synthesized drugs that mimic the pharmacologic action of their naturally occurring sources—foxglove, white willow (weeping willow) tree, and the cinchona tree, respectively. In addition, many antibiotics are produced by or derived from certain fungi, bacteria, and other organisms in the laboratory.

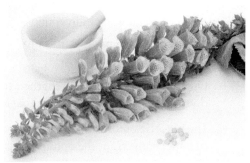

The foxglove plant is the source for digoxin (digitalis), a medication that increases the contractility of the heart in congestive heart failure. Foxglove is highly toxic, and ingestion of any part of the plant may be fatal. For that reason, foxglove is sometimes called "dead man's bells," "witch's gloves," and "bloody fingers."

Synthesized drugs have also found their way into the illegal drug market. Known as "designer drugs," these illegal drugs are produced in home chemistry laboratories by individuals who skirt drug control laws by modifying the chemical structure of existing drugs. The new drugs they create offer pharmacologic effects similar to those of their drug counterparts. For example, a synthesized version of marijuana exerts an effect that is similar to that of the natural product but also produces more hallucinations. Methamphetamine, also known as "meth" or "speed," is another example of a synthesized drug. Because methamphetamine is produced from the common decongestant pseudoephedrine hydrochloride, community pharmacies are required by law to place restrictions on the sale of products containing this key ingredient.

Biotechnology and Drugs

Biotechnology combines the sciences of biology, chemistry, and immunology to produce synthetic, unique drugs with specific therapeutic effects. These drugs can be created by means of the recombinant deoxyribonucleic acid (recombinant DNA) techniques of genetic engineering. **Deoxyribonucleic acid (DNA)** is the complex, helically shaped molecule that carries the genetic code (see Figure 2.1). DNA is made up of pairs of nucleotides. Each nucleotide contains one of four bases, which are abbreviated as A, T, C, and G. Combinations of these pairs are repeated millions or billions of times throughout a genome.

A **genome** is the complete set of DNA base pairs in an organism. DNA contains the instructions, or recipe, for creating messenger **ribonucleic acid (RNA)**, which in turn contains arranged sequences for making amino acids into proteins for living organisms. These proteins determine everything about how an organism works. A person's DNA determines the body's physical appearance, metabolic and immune functions, and predisposition for the development of certain diseases or disorders. By conducting research to unravel the DNA code, geneticists have allowed other scientists to design drug therapies that address

FIGURE 2.1 Modeling DNA

(a) A single nucleotide. (b) A short section of a DNA molecule consisting of two rows of nucleotides connected by weak bonds between the bases adenine (A) and thymine (T) and between the bases guanine (G) and cytosine (C). (c) Long strands of DNA twisted to form a double helix.

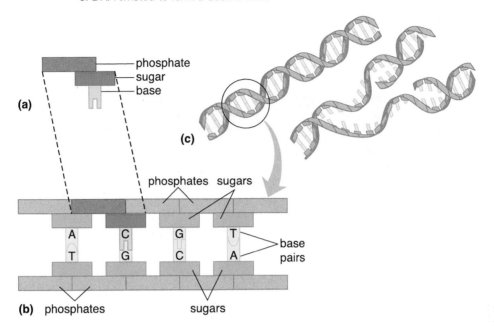

specific sections or abnormalities in this code. The process of utilizing DNA biotechnology to create a wide variety of drugs is called **genetic engineering**. Drug therapies that have resulted from these coordinated research efforts include insulin for diabetes; clotting factors for hemophilia; potent anti-inflammatory drugs for rheumatoid arthritis; and drugs for combating viral and bacterial infections, anemia, and some cancers.

The development of biotechnology drugs has led to a new field of study that blends two other scientific areas: pharmacology and genomics. Known as **pharmacogenomics**, this field of study examines the relationship between an individual's genes and his or her body's response to drugs. One goal of pharmacogenomics is to design and produce drugs that cater to an individual's genetic makeup. For example, blood thinners are metabolized by patients at different rates, thus altering the pharmacologic and toxic effects of the drugs. Pharmacogenomics could potentially specify a blood-thinner formula for a physician to prescribe that would produce the intended pharmacologic effect in a particular patient without the additional risk of adverse effects. The role of biotechnology in the development of drugs catered to patients' genetic profiles holds promise for the prevention and treatment of various disorders.

Biologic Products

A **biologic product** is created in a living organism such as a plant or animal cell. Many biologic products use **recombinant DNA (rDNA) technology**, or the process of combining DNA strands from two or more different organisms to produce a new genetic form. Examples of biologic products include vaccines, gene therapy, certain insulin products (see Figure 2.2), and recombinant therapeutic proteins such as the injectable rheumatoid arthritis drug etanercept (Enbrel). Unlike synthetic and semisynthetic drugs, which are well defined, biologic products are complex mixtures, not easily identified or characterized. They tend to have large chemical structures and are often heat sensitive (require refrigeration). A

biosimilar drug is something that is similar to, but not the same as, a biologic drug product. (A biosimilar drug is the generic form of a biologic drug product.) Filgrastim (Zarxio) is the first biosimilar approved by the US Food and Drug Administration (FDA).

FIGURE 2.2 Medication Label for the rDNA Drug Humalog

Humalog is an rDNA drug and is identified as such on the label. Used primarily to treat Type 1 diabetes, this form of insulin—called *insulin lispro*—is synthesized from a genetically altered, nonpathogenic strain of *Escherichia coli (E. coli)*.

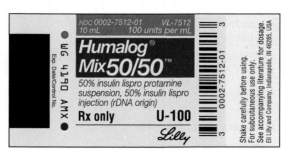

 Checkpoint **2.1**

Take a moment to review what you have learned so far and answer these questions.

1. What are some examples of naturally occurring drug therapies?

2. What is the difference between synthetic and semisynthetic drugs?

3. What is pharmacogenomics?

Drug Nomenclature

Prior to understanding the drug development process, allied health professionals must be familiar with **drug nomenclature**, or a naming system used to classify drugs. Drug names are assigned according to principles of consistency, logic, and safety in using the name for prescribing, ordering, dispensing, and administering a drug. Every drug has three names: a chemical name, a generic name, and a brand name or trade name.

 Drug Alert

Healthcare personnel must be vigilant in their selection and handling of all medications because there are a number of drugs with similar names. The Institute for Safe Medication Practices (ISMP) maintains a list of drugs whose names are commonly confused (http://PharmEssAH.emcp.net/ConfusedDrugs). It is recommended that healthcare personnel who handle medications keep a list of this type handy in their workplace setting.

Chemical Name

The **chemical name** describes the chemical makeup of a drug based on its molecular structure and traditional chemical nomenclature. The chemical name of a drug is typically long and difficult to pronounce, such as *N-acetyl-p-aminophenol*. This name is used early in a drug's development by a pharmaceutical chemist. Later in the development process, the chemical name will be assigned a generic name by a US healthcare agency.

Generic Name

The **generic name** is a shorter name that identifies the drug without regard to what company is manufacturing and marketing the drug. Also referred to as a **USAN (United States Adopted Name)** or the **nonproprietary name**, the generic name is often a shortened version of the chemical name and always begins with a lowercase letter. An example of a generic name is *acetaminophen* (derived from the chemical name *N-acetyl-p-aminophenol*).

In the United States, the **United States Adopted Names Council (USANC)** assigns the generic names of drugs. The USANC is sponsored by the **American Medical Association**, the **US Pharmacopeial Convention**, and the **American Pharmacists Association**. The USANC selects simple, unique names based on a chemical or pharmacologic relationship.

Brand Name

The **brand name** or **trade name** is the name under which a manufacturer markets a drug. This name is chosen by the manufacturer and is exclusive to the company. For that reason, a brand name has a registered mark (®) after the name, indicating that the name has been registered with a national trademark office and is the property of the drug manufacturer. An example of a brand name is Tylenol.

At first, a drug is sold only under its brand name. Once a drug's **patent** has expired, other manufacturers can make and sell the same drug under its generic name. The same generic drug can be manufactured by different drug companies, each of which can give the drug a different brand name. For example, Prinivil and Zestril are two brand names under which the generic drug lisinopril is marketed by pharmaceutical companies.

Consequently, knowing both the brand and generic names of a drug is necessary because **generic substitution** is a regular practice. Although the prescriptions of healthcare practitioners are often written in brand names, prescriptions are often filled with generic products. It is common for a patient to only know one of the two names of a drug they have been prescribed. However, it is important for allied health professionals to know both the brand and generic names of the most commonly prescribed drugs so that they can help patients use the proper medications appropriately.

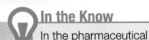

In the Know

In the pharmaceutical industry, a *patent* is an intellectual property right granted by the US government that gives the manufacturer exclusive authority to manufacture a drug and sell it in the United States for a limited period, usually 20 years. While under patent protection, a product is available only as a brand-name drug and is sold at a premium price. Once the patent expires, cheaper, generic forms of the drug are produced by several manufacturers, and sales of the brand-name drug plummet. Consequently, drug manufacturers work hard to secure and maintain patents for their products.

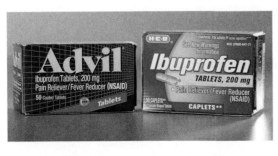

Ibuprofen, a medication that reduces pain and inflammation, is sold as a generic drug (ibuprofen) and as a brand-name drug (Advil).

Work Wise

Allied health professionals should be aware that prescribers often continue to use brand names in their orders even after the patents have expired.

Kolb's Learning Styles

If you enjoy group collaboration, as Convergers do, work with classmates to create a drug chart. Using a list of the top 100 prescribed drugs, record the generic name, brand name, and source of the drug (natural, synthetic, semisynthetic, or synthesized). When you are finished with the chart, you and your group will have a convenient drug resource to use.

Drug Review and Approval Process

The FDA requires that the manufacturer of any new drug provides evidence of its safety and effectiveness before the drug will be allowed to enter the US market. The drug must be shown to be safe through an intensive testing process that is undertaken by a **drug sponsor**, which is usually a pharmaceutical company. A drug sponsor must obtain permission from the FDA before testing any new drugs. Any hospital, physician, or researcher involved in experimental drug testing must also get FDA approval.

The FDA has regulations for manufacturers to follow while researching new chemical entities and developing those chemicals into brand-name drug products for the market. A manufacturer must first conduct extensive preclinical animal laboratory research using the new chemical formulation. Once this preclinical phase is completed, the manufacturer then submits an **investigational new drug (IND) application** to the **Center for Drug Evaluation and Research (CDER)**, a division of the FDA. CDER and the institutional review board review and grant permission for human studies to begin. The **institutional review board (IRB)**, also known as the Human Use Committee, comprises scientists and practitioners from various disciplines as well as consumers from an institutional setting such as a university or hospital. The committee is charged with the responsibility of reviewing, approving, and monitoring all medical research involving humans, including new drugs in development. The proposed research must meet both scientific and ethical standards.

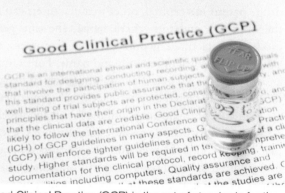

Good Clinical Practice (GCP) is the set of standards for the design, conduct, monitoring, and analysis of clinical drug trials. These standards, endorsed by the FDA, protect the rights, safety, and welfare of human participants and ensure the integrity of the collected data.

Preclinical Testing

Drug sponsors are responsible for testing the efficacy and safety of their drugs on animals and, later, on human subjects through controlled clinical trials. Before the clinical testing begins, researchers analyze the main physical and chemical properties of the drug in the laboratory and study its pharmacologic and toxic effects in laboratory animals. At this phase of drug development, the drug is known by its chemical name.

Clinical Trials

Once animal studies have been completed, scientists conduct three phases of clinical trials as part of the drug approval process: Phase I, Phase II, and Phase III. Protocols for testing are typically developed by researchers and are subject to approval by the FDA. These protocols describe what type of people may participate in the trial, the schedule of tests and procedures, medications and their dosages, and the length of the study. Allied health professionals may help researchers follow the protocols of a drug trial. For example, they may be responsible for taking a subject's vital signs during each study visit.

Once a drug has been approved for marketing, Phase IV studies continue to collect information about a drug's effects and side effects as long as the drug is still in clinical use. For more information on Phase IV studies, refer to the section titled "Postmarketing Surveillance" later in this chapter.

Phase I Drug Review Studies

Phase I drug review studies are conducted on a small group (usually 20 to 80) of healthy volunteers and are designed to evaluate a drug's safety, determine a safe dosage range, and identify side effects. Each volunteer must sign an **informed consent**, a document that states, in easily understandable terms, the purpose and risks of the research (see Figure 2.3).

During this phase, a drug is given its generic name, which is assigned by the USANC. If there are already drugs on the market that work in a way that is similar to the new drug, the new drug will be assigned a generic name that is similar to the names of those other drugs.

Phase II Drug Review Studies

In **Phase II drug review studies**, an experimental drug is tested on a group of patients (typically a few dozen to 300) who have the disease or condition the drug is intended to treat. This clinical phase determines whether the drug has a favorable effect on the disease state. Tests in Phase II trials are well controlled and closely monitored by the FDA.

Phase III Drug Review Studies

In **Phase III drug review studies**, a drug is also tested on individuals (several hundred to 3,000) who have the condition or disease. However, the experimental drug is now tested on a large number of patients to further assess efficacy and to study potential side effects a drug could have once it reaches the market and is used by many individuals.

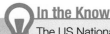
In the Know

The US National Library of Medicine at the National Institutes of Health (NIH) has a website that provides information to the public on clinical studies that are ongoing or completed on a variety of diseases and conditions. Data posted on the website is provided and updated by a drug sponsor of the clinical trial. Currently, the database offers information on more than 190,000 clinical trials conducted in the United States and around the world. To access the website, go to http://PharmEssAH.emcp.net/ClinicalTrials.

New Drug Application for Brand-Name Drugs

If an investigational drug shows promise after Phase III studies are completed, the pharmaceutical manufacturer can apply to the FDA for a **new drug application (NDA)**. The NDA contains details on the entire history of the development and testing of the drug. It documents results of clinical trials; describes components and composition of the drug; explains how the drug behaves in the body; proves the safety and effectiveness of the drug; and provides the details of manufacturing, processing, and packaging, with a special emphasis on quality control. The FDA also requires that the NDA include samples of the drug and its labels. The results of the scientific studies are evaluated by an advisory panel of experts, and recommendations are forwarded to the FDA. If the benefits of the drug outweigh the risks, generally the drug is approved (see Figure 2.4). The FDA may also request that additional studies be completed.

FIGURE 2.3 Informed Consent

This selection of pages comes from an informed consent document for a drug trial for the combination drug pemetrexed/cisplatin, a medication used to treat advanced nonsquamous non–small-cell lung cancer. In addition to addressing the purpose and the participant profile of the drug trial, the 14-page document also covers the procedures, possible benefits and harms to the participants, potential side effects from the drug, and treatment and compensation for any injury incurred.

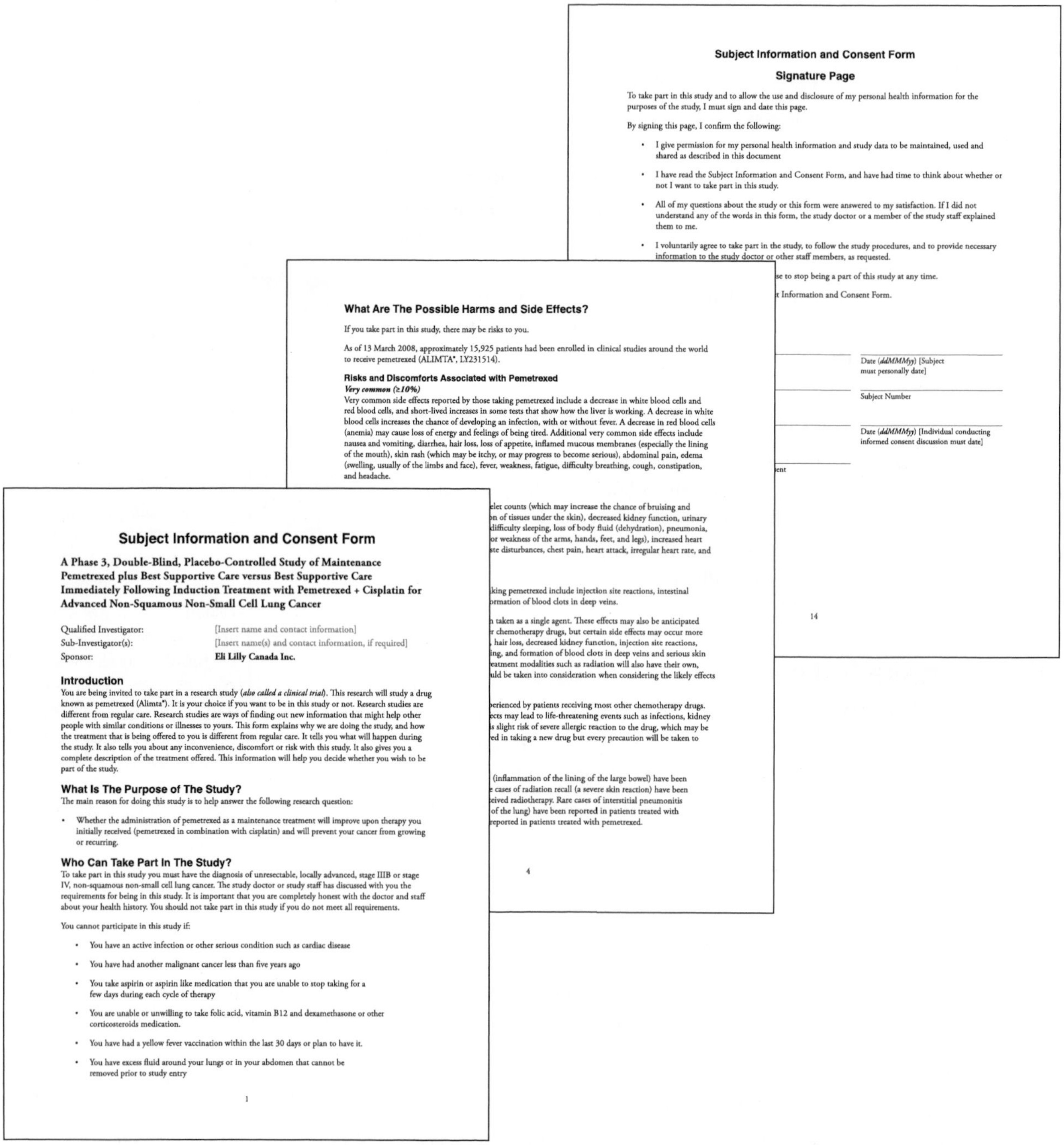

Subject Information and Consent Form

Signature Page

To take part in this study and to allow the use and disclosure of my personal health information for the purposes of the study, I must sign and date this page.

By signing this page, I confirm the following:

- I give permission for my personal health information and study data to be maintained, used and shared as described in this document

- I have read the Subject Information and Consent Form, and have had time to think about whether or not I want to take part in this study.

- All of my questions about the study or this form were answered to my satisfaction. If I did not understand any of the words in this form, the study doctor or a member of the study staff explained them to me.

- I voluntarily agree to take part in the study, to follow the study procedures, and to provide necessary information to the study doctor or other staff members, as requested.

...se to stop being a part of this study at any time.

...t Information and Consent Form.

Date (ddMMMyy) [Subject must personally date]

Subject Number

Date (ddMMMyy) [Individual conducting informed consent discussion must date]

14

What Are The Possible Harms and Side Effects?

If you take part in this study, there may be risks to you.

As of 13 March 2008, approximately 15,925 patients had been enrolled in clinical studies around the world to receive pemetrexed (ALIMTA®, LY231514).

Risks and Discomforts Associated with Pemetrexed

Very common (≥10%)
Very common side effects reported by those taking pemetrexed include a decrease in white blood cells and red blood cells, and short-lived increases in some tests that show how the liver is working. A decrease in white blood cells increases the chance of developing an infection, with or without fever. A decrease in red blood cells (anemia) may cause loss of energy and feelings of being tired. Additional very common side effects include nausea and vomiting, diarrhea, hair loss, loss of appetite, inflamed mucous membranes (especially the lining of the mouth), skin rash (which may be itchy, or may progress to become serious), abdominal pain, edema (swelling, usually of the limbs and face), fever, weakness, fatigue, difficulty breathing, cough, constipation, and headache.

...let counts (which may increase the chance of bruising and ...on of tissues under the skin), decreased kidney function, urinary ...difficulty sleeping, loss of body fluid (dehydration), pneumonia, ...or weakness of the arms, hands, feet, and legs), increased heart ...te disturbances, chest pain, heart attack, irregular heart rate, and

...king pemetrexed include injection site reactions, intestinal ...ormation of blood clots in deep veins.

...n taken as a single agent. These effects may also be anticipated ...r chemotherapy drugs, but certain side effects may occur more ..., hair loss, decreased kidney function, injection site reactions, ...ing, and formation of blood clots in deep veins and serious skin ...treatment modalities such as radiation will also have their own, ...ld be taken into consideration when considering the likely effects

...erienced by patients receiving most other chemotherapy drugs. ...cts may lead to life-threatening events such as infections, kidney ...s slight risk of severe allergic reaction to the drug, which may be ...ed in taking a new drug but every precaution will be taken to

...(inflammation of the lining of the large bowel) have been ...e cases of radiation recall (a severe skin reaction) have been ...eived radiotherapy. Rare cases of interstitial pneumonitis ...of the lung) have been reported in patients treated with ...reported in patients treated with pemetrexed.

4

Subject Information and Consent Form

A Phase 3, Double-Blind, Placebo-Controlled Study of Maintenance Pemetrexed plus Best Supportive Care versus Best Supportive Care Immediately Following Induction Treatment with Pemetrexed + Cisplatin for Advanced Non-Squamous Non-Small Cell Lung Cancer

Qualified Investigator: [Insert name and contact information]
Sub-Investigator(s): [Insert name(s) and contact information, if required]
Sponsor: **Eli Lilly Canada Inc.**

Introduction

You are being invited to take part in a research study (*also called a clinical trial*). This research will study a drug known as pemetrexed (Alimta®). It is your choice if you want to be in this study or not. Research studies are different from regular care. Research studies are ways of finding out new information that might help other people with similar conditions or illnesses to yours. This form explains why we are doing the study, and how the treatment that is being offered to you is different from regular care. It tells you what will happen during the study. It also tells you about any inconvenience, discomfort or risk with this study. It also gives you a complete description of the treatment offered. This information will help you decide whether you wish to be part of the study.

What Is The Purpose of The Study?

The main reason for doing this study is to help answer the following research question:

- Whether the administration of pemetrexed as a maintenance treatment will improve upon therapy you initially received (pemetrexed in combination with cisplatin) and will prevent your cancer from growing or recurring.

Who Can Take Part In The Study?

To take part in this study you must have the diagnosis of unresectable, locally advanced, stage IIIB or stage IV, non-squamous non-small cell lung cancer. The study doctor or study staff has discussed with you the requirements for being in this study. It is important that you are completely honest with the doctor and staff about your health history. You should not take part in this study if you do not meet all requirements.

You cannot participate in this study if:

- You have an active infection or other serious condition such as cardiac disease

- You have had another malignant cancer less than five years ago

- You take aspirin or aspirin like medication that you are unable to stop taking for a few days during each cycle of therapy

- You are unable or unwilling to take folic acid, vitamin B12 and dexamethasone or other corticosteroids medication.

- You have had a yellow fever vaccination within the last 30 days or plan to have it.

- You have excess fluid around your lungs or in your abdomen that cannot be removed prior to study entry

1

FIGURE 2.4 The Drug Review Process

After the government approves a manufacturer's IND application, a drug must pass through three phases of testing on human subjects before it is ready for final review by the FDA.

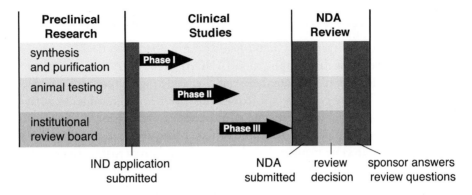

Timeline for Drug Approval

The drug approval process may take a year or longer in most cases. Occasionally, when a medication appears to be very promising early on in the testing, the FDA may opt to fast-track the drug and grant early approval within six months. A recent example of this accelerated process can be seen with the quick approval of sofosbuvir (Sovaldi), a drug used to treat hepatitis C. The FDA may also grant accelerated approval to drugs that fulfill an unmet need or treat rare but serious disease states for which little treatment is available. These drugs are called **orphan drugs**.

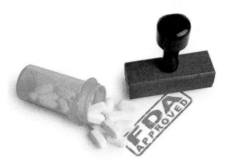

When determining the order of new drug applications, the FDA considers drugs for life-threatening diseases as top priority.

A classification system helps to determine the order in which new applications are reviewed. Priority is given to drugs with the greatest potential benefit. Drugs that offer a significant medical advantage over existing therapies for any given disease state are assigned *priority status*.

Once the NDA for a drug has been reviewed, the FDA then checks the medication's labeling and inspects the facilities where the drug will be manufactured. If all requirements have been met, the FDA grants approval for the manufacturing and marketing of the new medication.

Risk and Cost of Drug Development

Drug development is risky as well as costly. Of every 5,000 to 10,000 screened compounds, only 250 enter preclinical research testing, 5 enter human clinical trials, and 1 new compound is approved by the FDA. The cost of developing a drug is more than $1.2 billion, and it can take 10 to 15 years of research and development to bring a new medication from the laboratory to the pharmacy shelf.

Although the lengthy approval process and exorbitant costs can be daunting for pharmaceutical manufacturers, the financial incentive of patent protection on new drugs allows manufacturers to continue with their research and development of breakthrough drugs. As mentioned earlier, the patent for a brand-name drug is granted for an extended period, which allows the manufacturer sufficient time to recover the costs of clinical research. For this reason, brand-name prescription drugs are costly for consumers.

Abbreviated New Drug Application for Generic Drugs

Once the patent is due to expire on a brand-name drug, a pharmaceutical company may submit an **abbreviated new drug application (ANDA)** to the FDA for approval to manufacture a generic form of the patented drug. Generic drug applications are called *abbreviated* because they are generally not required to include preclinical (animal) and clinical (human) data to establish safety and effectiveness. Instead, generic applicants must scientifically demonstrate that their products are **bioequivalent**, meaning that these products perform in the same manner as their brand-name counterparts. The generic drug must meet the following requirements:

- contain the same active ingredients as the original brand-name drug

- be identical in strength, dosage form, and route of administration

- have the same indications for usage

- meet the same batch requirements for identity, strength, purity, and quality

- yield similar blood absorption and urinary excretion curves for the active ingredient

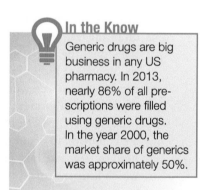

In the Know

Generic drugs are big business in any US pharmacy. In 2013, nearly 86% of all pre-scriptions were filled using generic drugs. In the year 2000, the market share of generics was approximately 50%.

One way that scientists demonstrate bioequivalence between a brand-name drug and a generic drug is to measure the generic drug's **bioavailability**. This study gives scientists the objective data necessary to compare the absorption and distribution of the generic drug with the brand-name drug. The generic version must deliver approximately the same amount of active ingredient into a patient's bloodstream as the brand-name drug.

FDA's Role in Drug Development

As mentioned earlier in this chapter, the FDA has the important responsibility of ensuring the American public that approved drugs are both safe and effective. As a watchdog agency for public safety, the FDA also enforces the packaging, labeling, marketing, and advertising guidelines for medications. Finally, once a drug has been marketed, the FDA conducts postmarketing surveillance on approved medications and, if necessary, oversees the recall of products that are deemed dangerous to the public.

Safety and Efficacy of Drugs

Stringent regulations regarding a drug's safety and efficacy were developed in response to a medication tragedy in the early 1960s. During that period, a sedative called *thalidomide* was a popular sleep aid marketed in 46 countries, particularly in Europe. When an Australian doctor discovered that the medication could also alleviate morning sickness in pregnant women, the drug was also marketed as a treatment for nausea and vomiting. In the United States, one FDA drug inspector was not convinced that thalidomide was adequately tested for this new therapeutic use and refused to approve this medication.

Thalidomide was later proven to cause severe birth defects in fetuses, a discovery that spurred the FDA to tighten their drug approval process by requiring that all medications pass trials for both safety and efficacy.

It is important to remember that no drug is absolutely safe. The FDA's approval is based on a judgment about whether the benefits of a new drug to users will outweigh its risks (risk-benefit analysis). The FDA will allow a product to present more of a risk when its potential benefit is great, especially if the product is used to treat a life-threatening condition.

FDA Pregnancy Labeling System

Although drugs are not tested on pregnant women, the FDA uses all available information (mainly from animal studies) to assess the risks each drug marketed in the United States poses to pregnant and lactating women. Prior to December 2014, the FDA categorized risks of taking a medication during pregnancy under a five-letter system (*A, B, C, D,* and *X*). Based on healthcare practitioner and consumer feedback, the five-letter system was replaced with a new labeling system. The new system provides more helpful information about a medication's risks to the expectant mother, the developing fetus, and the breast-fed infant. In addition, contact information for registries that collect and maintain information regarding the effects of medication on pregnant women are provided. Lastly, the new labeling system contains a subsection called "Females and Males of Reproductive Potential" and includes information on pregnancy testing, birth control, and a medication's effect on fertility.

Drugs approved after December 2014 utilize the new labeling requirements. Removal of the letter categories and revision of labeling is needed for drugs approved prior to December 2014, an undertaking that will require several years to complete.

Although no drug is completely without side effects or 100% safe during pregnancy, some drugs are considered safe during pregnancy because they do not significantly cross through the placenta and enter the bloodstream of a developing fetus. Typically, the patient and her prescriber must weigh the urgency of and need for treating a particular condition with the potential adverse effects the medication may cause for the fetus.

Work Wise

Allied health professionals may continue to be exposed to the old five-letter pregnancy-labeling system for any drugs that are awaiting the update or by healthcare practitioners who are more accustomed to the old system. For these reasons, allied health personnel should familiarize themselves with both the old and new labeling systems.

Packaging and Labeling of Drugs

In addition to providing oversight for the development of safe and effective generic and brand-name drugs, the FDA is also responsible for ensuring that drug manufacturers adhere to strict packaging and labeling guidelines for medications. These guidelines were put into place with the passage of the Federal Food, Drug, and Cosmetic (FD&C) Act of 1938. Up until that time, no manufacturing standards existed for the labeling of medications, and many manufacturers made false claims on their drug labels.

The FD&C Act identified two types of products whose false claims would result in legal action against the products' manufacturers if distributed: adulterated products and misbranded products. An **adulterated product** is a product that differs in drug strength, quality, and purity. For example, an adulterated product may be a drug contaminated with other drugs or chemicals that may or may not be harmful. A recent example of an adulterated product was a contaminated drug that was prepared in a sterile compounding facility in Massachusetts and then administered to patients, resulting in many deaths due to fungal meningitis. A **misbranded product**, on the other hand, is a product whose label includes false statements about the identity or ingredients of the container's contents.

Dietary supplements are commonly misbranded. The amount of active ingredient in the supplement may not always match the labeled amount because of inconsistencies in quality control or product contamination. The FDA does not approve dietary supplements; however, if the supplements are not safe and accurately labeled, the FDA can act to remove the supplements from the market. (For more information on dietary supplements, see the "Dietary Supplements" section later in this chapter.)

Labeling of Prescription Drugs

A prescription drug label (also known as a **drug-package insert**) must include the FDA-approved indications for the medication and must disclose the drug's side effects, adverse reactions, and contraindications. It also must contain information on drug interactions, pharmacology, drug administration, pregnancy risk, and the results of the clinical trials for the drug. The information in a drug-package insert contains a lot of medical jargon and is intended for use mainly by healthcare professionals.

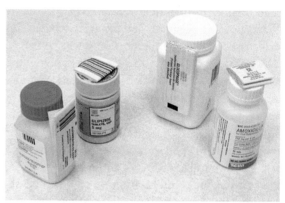

Drug-package inserts are attached to or placed inside stock bottles. These inserts provide detailed information about the medication for the pharmacist, pharmacy technician, and other healthcare professionals.

Black Box Warning

Quick Study

Black box warnings are the sternest warnings put on drug labels. As you are learning pharmacology, you should commit these warnings to your memory.

Some drug-package inserts feature a **black box warning**. Inside this clearly marked box, which is always located on the first page of the document, the manufacturer describes a serious or life-threatening adverse effect of the drug. The FDA mandates this labeling only on drugs that have the most serious adverse effects. The black box is designed to ensure that prescribers and consumers are informed of the most important risks posed by a drug. For example, the antidepressant Prozac contains a black box warning (see Figure 2.5).

FIGURE 2.5 Black Box Warning

The FDA requires a specific format for a black box warning: The text must be in boldfaced type and have bullets or subheads that highlight the serious adverse effects of the drug.

> **WARNING: SUICIDAL THOUGHTS AND BEHAVIORS**
> *See full prescribing information for complete boxed warning.*
> - **Increased risk of suicidal thinking and behavior in children, adolescents, and young adults taking antidepressants (5.1).**
> - **Monitor for worsening and emergence of suicidal thoughts and behaviors (5.1).**
> *When using PROZAC and olanzapine in combination, also refer to Boxed Warning section of the package insert for Symbyax.*

Medication Guide

The FDA requires that patients receive a paper handout called a **medication guide** whenever they receive a prescription for certain drugs that pose serious risks, such as the drugs that have black box warnings. Each medication guide must be written in plain language so that consumers can understand the content. Medication guides describe the risks posed by a drug and provide information that may be necessary to avoid adverse effects. Medication guides also contain information about how to take the drug (e.g., with or without food) and about potential drug interactions.

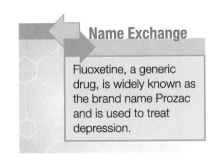

Name Exchange

Fluoxetine, a generic drug, is widely known as the brand name Prozac and is used to treat depression.

National Drug Code Number

Once a brand name or generic name receives FDA approval, each one is assigned a unique **National Drug Code (NDC) number** that appears on all drug stock labels as well as on copies of duplicate prescription labels filed in the pharmacy. The 10- to 11-digit NDC number contains the following components:

- a four- or five-digit *labeler code*, identifying the manufacturer or distributor of the drug

- a three- or four-digit *product code*, identifying the drug (active ingredient and its dosage form)

- a one- or two-digit *package code*, identifying the packaging size and type

The FDA is responsible for assigning the labeler code to the product. The product and package codes are assigned by the drug manufacturer or distributor. The NDC number plays a critical role in the checks and balances of preventing avoidable medication errors during the dispensing process. The pharmacist or pharmacy technician focuses on the product code, or the middle number of the NDC, when filling a prescription (see Figure 2.6).

FIGURE 2.6 NDC Number and Bar Code

For both of these labels for Strattera (an attention-deficit/hyperactivity disorder [ADHD] drug for adults), the first four digits of the NDC number (0002) indicate *Eli Lilly and Company*. The second four digits of the NDC number indicate the product code, and the last two digits define the packaging size and type.

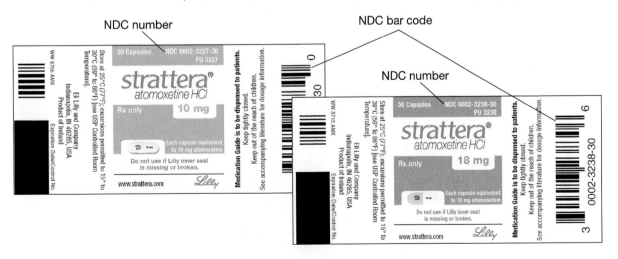

Marketing and Advertising of Drugs

Truthfulness in the packaging and labeling of medications extends into the marketing and advertising arenas. The FDA regulates the advertising of prescription drugs, and the Federal Trade Commission regulates the advertising of over-the-counter (OTC) drugs. The FDA has been known to ask a manufacturer to cancel advertising campaigns and even to instruct the manufacturer to present a new advertising campaign to clear up any misconceptions about a particular medication.

Pharmaceutical manufacturers have also been found guilty and paid hefty fines for promoting the "off-label" marketing of approved prescription drugs. An **off-label use** is the use of a drug to treat a disease or condition that is not described in the drug-package insert. For example, if a drug is FDA-approved for the treatment of high blood pressure but is not approved for the treatment of Alzheimer's disease, representatives of the manufacturer are not allowed to promote and market its use for Alzheimer's disease.

Postmarketing Surveillance

Postmarketing surveillance of a medication is considered Phase IV of the drug approval process. In this phase, the FDA continues to gather information about approved medications—in particular, about any serious adverse reactions that were not identified from research studies in the drug approval process. An **adverse drug reaction (ADR)** is defined as a negative consequence to a patient caused by taking a particular drug. Despite many years of research and clinical studies, some medications will enter the marketplace and place patients at risk for serious ADRs. These events may not always be preventable or predictable.

FDA Adverse Event Reporting System

Due to these potential risks, the FDA recognized the need to establish a nationwide postmarketing surveillance system to serve as a conduit for reporting serious adverse effects of medications. The **FDA Adverse Event Reporting System (FAERS)** is a centralized database that stores information from two separate programs: MedWatch and VAERS. This safety system allows any healthcare professional or consumer to report a serious adverse event associated with a drug, biologic device, or dietary supplement. Additional information on MedWatch and VAERS can be found in Chapter 7 and Chapter 24, respectively.

Drug Recall Process

Once a drug is approved, FDA oversight continues. A drug's manufacturer is required to report any serious side effects and adverse reactions to the FDA. Using this data, as well as the data from FAERS or from other independent sources, the FDA has the authority to obtain a court injunction and order a **drug recall**. The basis for the drug recall might be a poor quality or contaminated product or a drug that produces serious adverse effects. In some cases in which the risk is greater than the perceived benefit, the FDA may issue a drug recall and withdraw the drug from the market; in other cases, the manufacturer may voluntarily withdraw the drug due to future liability concerns. When a drug recall occurs, an allied health professional may be asked to remove all recalled medications from the medication carts in a long-term care facility. The FDA's role is to monitor the pharmaceutical company's recalls and assess the adequacy of the company's action. After a recall is completed, the FDA ensures that the product is destroyed or suitably reconditioned and investigates why the product was defective. To keep apprised of drug recalls, allied health professionals can access the following link: http://PharmEssAH.emcp.net/DrugRecalls.

Recall Classes

Three classes of recalls exist (see Table 2.1), and the FDA determines which class of recall is issued based on reports from the particular manufacturer and from healthcare practitioners. A Class I recall is serious and requires immediate action by pharmacy personnel. In case of a drug recall, consumers can return a recalled drug for refund or credit per pharmacy policy. In 2014, certain lots of mitoxantrone, an injectable cancer medication manufactured by Hospira, underwent a worldwide Class I recall because the drug failed stability tests, was subpotent, and contained impurities.

TABLE 2.1   Recall Classes for Drugs

Class	Risk
I	A reasonable probability exists that use of the product will cause or lead to serious adverse health events or death. An example of a product that could fall into this category is a label mix-up on a lifesaving drug.
II	The probability exists that use of the product will cause adverse health events that are temporary or medically reversible. One example is a drug that is understrength but that is not used to treat life-threatening situations.
III	The use of the product will probably not cause an adverse health event. Examples might be a container defect, odd flavor, or wrong color in a liquid.

Drug Classifications

Medications are grouped into major **drug classes** according to their **mechanism of action**. All drugs that work in the same way are put into a particular class and are usually given similar names with a common stem. For example, several cholesterol-lowering medications that use a similar mechanism of action all have generic drug names that end in the suffix *–statin*: atorvastatin, simvastatin, rosuvastatin. This stem in the generic drug name helps to classify the drug with other drugs that have the same mechanism of action. Learning these common drug name stems can help when learning pharmacology and how various drugs work within the body. Table 2.2 shows the generic nomenclature of several major drug classes.

Individual drug classes are then grouped into **therapeutic classes** according to their use on a particular body system. Drug classes in this textbook are discussed in relation to their therapeutic class. For example, antihypertensive medications (therapeutic class) are discussed together in Chapter 15. The major drug classes that are used to treat cardiovascular conditions include beta blockers, angiotensin-converting enzyme (ACE) inhibitors, calcium-channel blockers, and HMG-CoA reductase inhibitors (statins).

Drugs are also classified by the FDA as *prescription* or *over the counter*. Vitamins, minerals, and herbs (discussed in Chapter 19 and the "Herbal and Alternative Therapies" sections throughout this textbook) are technically considered dietary supplements (not drugs) and, as mentioned earlier in this chapter, are not directly regulated by the FDA.

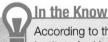

In the Know

According to the IMS Institute for Healthcare Informatics, the top 10 therapeutic classes for dispensed prescriptions in the US market in 2013 are as follows:

1. Antihypertensives
2. Mental health
3. Pain
4. Antibacterials
5. Lipid regulators
6. Antidiabetics
7. Nervous system disorders
8. Antiulcerants
9. Respiratory
10. Antithyroid

TABLE 2.2 Common Drug Name Stems

Drug Class	Stem	Examples
ACE inhibitors	–pril	Enalapril, lisinopril
Angiotensin receptor inhibitors	–sartan	Losartan, valsartan
Antifungals	–azole	Fluconazole, miconazole
Antivirals	–vir	Acyclovir, ganciclovir
Benzodiazepines	–pam or –lam	Alprazolam, lorazepam
Beta blockers	–olol	Atenolol, propranolol
Cephalosporins	cef– or ceph–	Cefuroxime, cephalexin
Corticosteroids	–sone or –lone	Prednisone, triamcinolone
HMG-CoA reductase inhibitors	–statin	Lovastatin, simvastatin
Macrolides	–thromycin	Azithromycin, erythromycin
Penicillins	–cillin	Amoxicillin, ampicillin
Proton-pump inhibitors	–prazole	Lansoprazole, omeprazole
Quinolones	–floxacin	Ciprofloxacin, levofloxacin
Selective serotonin receptor agonists	–triptan	Sumatriptan, zolmitriptan
Tetracyclines	–cycline	Doxycycline, minocycline
Thiazolidinediones	–glitazones	Pioglitazone, rosiglitazone
Tricyclic antidepressants	–triptyline	Amitriptyline, nortriptyline

Healthcare professionals must have a solid understanding of the federal and state laws and regulations regarding the ordering, preparing, and administration of the drugs that fall into these classifications. They should also have a working knowledge of the top 200 generic and brand-name drugs and their indications. To help allied health professionals learn the names of these top 200 drugs, the Navigator+ learning management system that accompanies this textbook provides a complete list to use as a study aid.

Prescription Medications

A **prescription drug**, formerly known as a *legend drug*, can be dispensed only upon receipt of a prescription from a healthcare professional licensed to practice in that state. Consequently, all prescription drugs are labeled with the legend "Rx only." A prescription drug may be available as a generic product (for example, clopidogrel), or it may be available as a brand-name product (for example, Plavix).

Controlled Substances

Some prescription drugs are classified as **controlled substances** by the Controlled Substances Act of 1970. This law promoted drug education and research into the prevention and treatment of drug dependence; strengthened enforcement authority; and designated five **schedules**, or categories, for drugs based on their degree of potential for abuse and addiction. Schedule I substances are illegal or available only for research or experimental purposes. Schedule II–V drugs can be legally dispensed but have restrictions on numbers of refills and quantities. The US Drug Enforcement Administration (DEA) is the primary agency responsible for enforcing the laws regarding controlled substances.

Dispensing procedures and inventory control measures for controlled substances are strictly regulated at both the federal and state levels. Schedule II has the most stringent restrictions for patient dispensing. See Table 2.3 for a description of these controlled substances schedules.

Allied health professionals should have a good understanding of the scheduled drugs and should learn the restrictions placed on these drugs. They should also be aware that the labels of controlled substances use a symbol to designate them as such (see Figure 2.7).

TABLE 2.3 Schedules of Controlled Substances

Schedule	Description	Examples	Restrictions
I	Drugs with no accepted medical use having the highest potential for abuse/dependence. Illegal to possess, except for a few substances that can be used for research purposes (special registration and restrictions apply).	Lysergic acid diethylamide (LSD), marijuana (cannabis),* opium derivatives such as heroin, peyote, phencyclidine (PCP)	**Greatest**
II	Drugs with accepted medical use having high potential for abuse. May lead to high risk of physiologic and psychological dependence.	Codeine, depressants (pentobarbital, secobarbital), fentanyl, hydromorphone, meperidine, methadone, morphine, oxycodone, stimulants (amphetamines such as methylphenidate [Ritalin])	
III	Drugs with accepted medical use having some potential for abuse. May lead to moderate physiologic but high psychological dependence.	Anabolic steroids, barbiturates, codeine combination products (e.g., codeine/acetaminophen), dronabinol	
IV	Drugs with accepted medical use having lower potential for abuse. May lead to low physiologic but moderate psychological dependence.	Appetite suppressants (phentermine), benzodiazepines, phenobarbital, sleep aids (eszopiclone, zaleplon, zolpidem)	
V	Drugs with accepted medical use with low potential for abuse. May lead to limited physiologic or psychological dependence.	Codeine combination products in oral liquid forms (mostly cough syrups)	**Least**

* Although the use of marijuana is illegal according to federal law, many states now have laws that allow its use for medical purposes. A few states have also legalized marijuana's recreational use.

FIGURE 2.7 Prescription Drug Label

Schedule II controlled substances, such as narcotics and amphetamines, have the highest potential for abuse, drug tolerance, and psychological or physical dependence among drugs with accepted medical use.

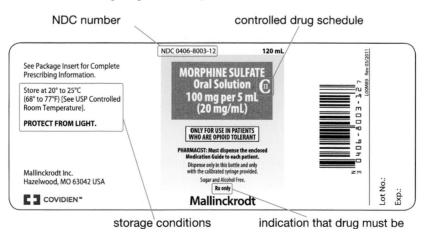

NDC number

controlled drug schedule

storage conditions

indication that drug must be dispensed by prescription only

Controlled-Substance Responses

Patients who are taking controlled substances are at a higher risk for drug tolerance, psychological and/or physical dependence, or addiction. Allied health personnel should be familiar with the distinctions among these adverse effects.

Drug tolerance is a condition in which the body adapts to a drug so that higher doses are needed to produce the same therapeutic effect achieved earlier with smaller doses. For example, a patient who is taking a Schedule II or Schedule III narcotic on a continuous basis for pain relief may build up a drug tolerance, resulting in less pain relief at the prescribed dosage. Consequently, that patient may take higher doses or more frequent doses to achieve the pain relief he or she once had. Drug tolerance can lead to psychological or physical dependence, or even to drug addiction.

Drug Alert

All healthcare practitioners must ensure that controlled substances are used for legitimate medical purposes. With that in mind, personnel should be on the alert for patients who exhibit drug-seeking behaviors in order to obtain narcotics or other controlled substances for illicit use. These drug seekers may be tolerant, psychologically or physically dependent, addicted to these medications, or may be illegally selling these drugs. To aid healthcare personnel in identifying a drug seeker, the Office of Diversion Control of the US Drug Enforcement Administration (https://PharmEssAH.emcp.net/DrugSeekers) has compiled a list of these behaviors:

- must be seen right away
- wants an appointment toward the end of office hours
- calls or comes in after regular hours
- states he/she is traveling through town, visiting friends or relatives (not a permanent resident)
- feigns physical problems, such as abdominal or back pain, kidney stone, or migraine headache, in an effort to obtain narcotic drugs
- feigns psychological problems, such as anxiety, insomnia, fatigue, or depression, in an effort to obtain stimulants or depressants
- states that specific nonnarcotic analgesics do not work or that he/she is allergic to them
- contends to be a patient of a practitioner who is currently unavailable or will not give the name of a primary or reference physician
- states that a prescription has been lost or stolen and needs replacing
- deceives the practitioner, such as by requesting refills more often than originally prescribed
- pressures the practitioner by eliciting sympathy or guilt or by direct threats
- utilizes a child or an elderly person when seeking methylphenidate or pain medication

Psychological dependence is defined as a condition in which a patient takes a drug on a regular basis because it produces a sense of well-being. If the patient stops taking the drug, he or she may experience anxiety or **withdrawal symptoms** due to a psychological dependence on the medication. For example, a patient who takes a sleeping pill every night may experience disruptive sleep patterns, yet the patient feels that he or she must take the medication to get a good night's sleep.

Physical dependence is defined as taking a drug continuously so that when the medication is stopped, physical withdrawal symptoms such as restlessness, anxiety, insomnia, diarrhea, vomiting, and goose bumps occur. Withdrawal symptoms commonly occur with high doses of Schedule II and Schedule III drugs and, for some patients, may occur after four weeks of continuous use.

Addiction is defined as compulsive and uncontrollable use of controlled substances, especially narcotics. Addicted patients will do anything to support their drug habit.

OTC Medications

An **over-the-counter (OTC) drug** is a drug that can be purchased without a prescription. Before an OTC drug is approved for sale, the FDA must first recognize it as safe and effective when the labeled directions on the container—with regard to dose, frequency, precautions and contraindications, and duration of therapy—are followed. Most OTC drugs are indicated for self-limiting conditions requiring accurate self-diagnosis and short-term therapy (usually less than seven days). Other OTC drugs such as baby aspirin or allergy medication may be used on a long-term basis with direction from a healthcare practitioner.

The FDA has approved many OTC drugs after the expiration of the manufacturer's patent on the prescription drug. Such examples include Advil (ibuprofen), Aleve (naproxen), Claritin (loratadine), Benadryl (diphenhydramine), Zyrtec (cetirizine), and hydrocortisone. These drugs have been proven relatively safe over the years when appropriately used and sold as OTC medications. If used inappropriately, these drugs can cause side effects, adverse reactions, and interactions with prescription drugs.

Behind-the-Counter Products

Some OTC drugs and supplies are only sold behind the counter of a pharmacy. These **behind-the-counter products** are confined to that area because they have certain dispensing restrictions. These restrictions may include the following:

- federal or state laws and regulations (to control the dispensing of pseudoephedrine or codeine cough syrups)

- possible product abuse/diversion (to monitor the use of insulin syringes)

- medications that require pharmacist counseling (to discuss the use of certain asthma medications)

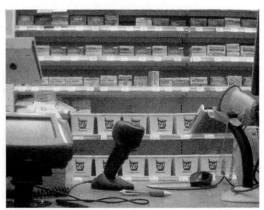

Behind-the-counter products, such as those containing pseudoephedrine, have strict dispensing regulations. Sale of these products requires a photo ID as well as completion of a sales logbook (name and address of customer, quantity of drug sold, date and time of the sale, and signature of the customer).

Product Labeling

OTC drugs must have adequate product labeling, written in easily understood terms, to assist the consumer in properly using the product, as there may be no contact with a pharmacist or any typed instructions from a physician or other healthcare practitioner. The FDA requires that OTC labels contain a prominent "Drug Facts" box that lists the active ingredients, purposes, and use of the product, with any warnings and directions including age-appropriate dosing. This "Drug Facts" box allows the consumer to compare active ingredients and assess the benefits and risks of various OTC products. For example, if a customer is considering the purchase of multiple cold medications, a comparison of active ingredients can identify any overlap or duplication of drugs that may cause adverse effects. This information may be critically important if the medication is being purchased for a child or an elderly adult. In fact, many OTC medications have age restrictions on their package label such as, "Do not use < age 4 years," or, "Use under physician's care if under age 2 years." In addition to this information, drug labels are also required to have an expiration date as well as a list of inactive ingredients for those patients with allergies.

Kolb's Learning Styles

When studying pharmacology, Assimilators and Divergers may find it helpful to look through their own medicine cabinets to reinforce their learning. They should examine each bottle or package and determine whether the product is a prescription or an OTC drug. They should also recall the generic name for each brand-name drug and its drug class.

Homeopathic Medications

Another group of products under FDA control is called **homeopathic medications**. The term *homeopathy* is derived from the Greek root words *homos*, meaning "similar," and *pathos*, meaning "suffering or disease." Homeopathic practice uses subclinical doses of natural extracts or alcohol tinctures in which the active ingredient is diluted from one part

Drug Facts

Active Ingredients .... Purpose

Conium maculatum 6X ....redness
Graphites 12X...dryness
Sulphur 12X .... tearing, burning

Uses:

According to homeopathic principles, the active ingredients in this medication temporarily relieve minor symptoms associated with styes, such as:
• redness   • burning   • dryness   • tearing

Homeopathic medications contain one or more ingredients in a diluted form to stimulate the immune system. As with OTC medications, "Drug Facts" labeling is required.

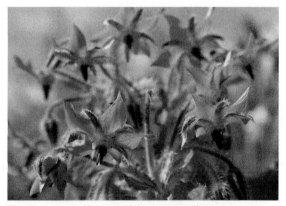

The flowers and leaves of the borage plant are used as a homeopathic remedy to treat fever, cough, and depression. The seed oil of the plant is used to treat skin conditions such as eczema and seborrheic dermatitis.

per ten (1:10) to more than one part per thousand (1:1,000), or even higher. The concept is that these small doses are sufficient to stimulate the body's own immune system to overcome the specifically targeted symptom.

Homeopathic medications are available over the counter. An OTC homeopathic medication is labeled for a self-limiting condition, or a condition that does not require medical diagnosis or monitoring, and is nontoxic. The use of homeopathic medications was popular in the United States in the early nineteenth century and remains popular in many areas of Europe today. These medications are sometimes considered "natural treatments," and the risk of side effects is minimal.

Dietary Supplements

A **dietary supplement**, especially an herb, exerts a weak pharmacologic effect on the body similar to that of drugs. Consequently, dietary supplements may cause side effects, adverse reactions, and drug interactions. Glucosamine is an example of a dietary supplement that provides nutrients for bone cartilage to treat mild arthritis symptoms. As with OTC drugs, consumers can purchase dietary supplements without a prescription and should read the labels carefully. Because dietary supplements are considered "food supplements" that maintain health, consumers should not exceed the recommended daily dose or serving size. (For more information on dietary supplements, see Chapter 19.)

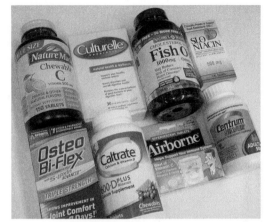

Manufacturers of dietary supplements are not permitted to make claims of curing or treating ailments. They may only state that the products are supplements to support health.

Allied health professionals should be aware that dietary supplements do not have the same stringent controls as prescription medications and are loosely regulated by the Dietary Supplement Health and Education Act (DSHEA) of 1994. The FDA can only regulate dietary supplements when patient safety concerns exist, as in the case of weight-loss drugs. Consumers should know that the quality of many of these products is suspect when tested by independent consumer laboratories.

The use of herbs by patients poses a particular challenge to healthcare practitioners. Quite often, patients take herbal supplements and fail to disclose that information when asked about their medication history. As a result, some patients, particularly the elderly, may have an adverse reaction between their herbal supplements and their prescription medications. Therefore, allied health personnel can assist prescribers and pharmacists by gathering and recording information about the patient's use of herbs or other dietary supplements.

 Checkpoint 2.2

Take a moment to review what you have learned so far and answer these questions.

1. What is the difference between prescription and OTC drugs?

2. What are *controlled substances*? Provide two examples of drugs in each of the schedules.

3. What are two examples of behind-the-counter products?

Chapter Review

Chapter Summary

Drugs are derived from various sources and can be classified as natural, synthetic (created artificially), synthesized (created artificially but in imitation of naturally occurring substances), and semisynthetic (containing both natural and synthetic components). Biologic products comprise large complex molecules that are often made using recombinant DNA technology.

To understand the drug development process, allied health professionals must know drug nomenclature, or a naming system used to classify drugs. Drugs are assigned three names: a chemical name, a generic name, and a brand name. A drug's chemical name is used during the preclinical testing. During Phase I of clinical trials, a drug is assigned a generic name by USANC. Generally, the designated generic name will resemble the names of other drugs that work in a similar way. The brand name of a drug is chosen by the manufacturer during clinical trials.

In the United States, drug development is regulated by the FDA, which requires that each prescription drug undergo three phases of testing on human subjects before it can be approved for sale. Phase I tests are conducted on a small group of healthy volunteers and are designed to evaluate a drug's safety, determine a safe dosage range, and identify side effects. In Phase II of the clinical trials, an experimental drug is tested on a group of patients (typically a few dozen to 300) who have the disease or condition the drug is intended to treat. This clinical phase determines whether the drug has a favorable effect on the disease state. Phase III tests are also conducted on individuals (several hundred to 3,000) who have the condition or disease. However, the experimental drug is now tested on a large number of patients to further assess efficacy and to study potential side effects a drug could have once it reaches the market and is used by many individuals. Once the three phases of clinical tests are complete, the manufacturer completes an NDA. This document provides the results of clinical trials; describes components and composition of the drug; explains how the drug behaves in the body; proves the safety and effectiveness of the drug; and provides the details of manufacturing, processing, and packaging. An ANDA allows a pharmaceutical company to manufacture a generic drug that is bioequivalent to a brand-name drug.

In addition to regulating the safety and efficacy of drugs during their development, the FDA requires that drug labels include information on the pregnancy risks of each drug. The FDA also ensures that manufacturers adhere to other labeling and packaging standards, oversees the advertising of prescription drugs, and conducts postmarketing surveillance initiatives.

Drugs are sorted into groups based on how they work (drug classes) and based on how they are used (therapeutic classes). Drugs are also classified by the FDA as *prescription* or *over the counter*.

Medications available only by prescription are referred to as *prescription drugs*. Controlled substances are considered *prescription drugs* as well. These medications have the potential for abuse and dependence and are categorized by the DEA into five schedules based on their degree of potential for abuse. Among the other controlled substances, Schedule II drugs have the most stringent restrictions for patient dispensing.

Medications that can be bought without a prescription are called OTC medications. Behind-the-counter products are considered OTC products but are confined to that area because they have certain dispensing restrictions. Other OTC products include homeopathic medications and dietary supplements. Homeopathic medications provide subclinical doses of natural extracts or alcohol tinctures to treat self-limiting conditions. Dietary supplements are considered "food supplements," and consumers should not exceed the recommended daily dose.

Chapter Checkup

The Navigator+ learning management system that accompanies this textbook offers many opportunities to help you master chapter content, including end-of-chapter exercises, a glossary of key terms, flash cards, and additional interactive activities.

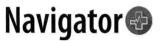

 ## Career Exploration

If you enjoyed learning about pharmaceutical development in this chapter, you may want to explore the following career options:

- medical assistant
- pharmacy technician
- quality control coordinator
- research laboratory technician

3 Medications and the Body

Pharm Facts

- The blood-brain barrier (BBB) helps protect the brain from dangerous toxins and viruses. Sometimes, though, this barrier impedes the treatment of brain disorders. For example, patients with Parkinson's disease require dopamine, a drug that does not cross the BBB. Fortunately, scientists discovered that the amino acid levodopa *does* cross the BBB and is then converted to dopamine. Levodopa is now a mainstay in the treatment of Parkinson's disease.

- Despite what is depicted on medical television shows, a patient does not lose consciousness immediately after the administration of an intravenous injection. It takes several seconds for a drug to arrive at its targeted site of action.

- No matter what route of administration is used (oral, inhalation, injection, etc.), all drugs eventually enter the bloodstream and pass through the liver, where enzymes break apart or link the molecules.

- Black licorice can cause a serious drug-food interaction in individuals over age 40 who eat two ounces of licorice a day for two weeks. Black licorice contains glycyrrhizin, a compound that causes a dramatic drop in the body's potassium levels. This effect may produce a heart arrhythmia.

"I chose the healthcare field several years ago because of my fascination with how drugs get to where they need to go in the body. Learning about the lock-and-key system of drugs and receptors gave me my answer to this question and helped me understand why so many medications have an extensive list of side effects. Having a pharmacist explain this concept to patients gives them a clearer understanding of how their medications work."

—**Sandi Tschritter**, MEd, CPhT
Pharmacy Technician

Learning Objectives

1 Distinguish the classifications for uses of drugs, including therapeutic agents, pharmacodynamic agents, diagnostic agents, prophylactic agents, and destructive agents.

2 Understand the control and feedback mechanisms of homeostasis.

3 Describe factors that influence absorption, distribution, metabolism, and excretion of drugs from the body.

4 Distinguish routes of administration and common dosage formulations.

5 Understand the relationship between drug dosage and a patient's unique drug response factors, including age, weight, gender, nutritional status, and liver and kidney functions.

Today's medications are used not only to treat and cure illnesses but also to aid in their diagnosis and even prevent their onset. Because drugs serve a variety of purposes in a patient's healthcare regimen, allied health professionals must be knowledgeable about the uses of commonly prescribed drugs and their mechanisms of action. In addition, allied health personnel need to have an understanding of the dispensing and administration of drugs, such as the routes of administration, dosage formulations, and drug response factors that are critical for medication safety. This chapter provides the necessary foundational knowledge of the dynamics between medications and the body.

Uses of Drugs

Several classifications for uses of drugs exist, and most of these categories are not mutually exclusive. These classifications include therapeutic agents, pharmacodynamic agents, diagnostic agents, prophylactic agents, and destructive agents.

Therapeutic Agents

A **therapeutic agent** is a drug that targets a specific need in the body. Therapeutic agents are categorized according to the following functions:

- *Maintaining health*—Drugs with this purpose include vitamins and minerals to regulate metabolism and otherwise contribute to the maintenance of normal growth and functioning of the body. A specific example is the use of baby aspirin for patients identified as being at risk for a heart attack.

- *Relieving symptoms*—Drugs with this purpose include anti-inflammatory drugs such as ibuprofen used to treat fever, pain, or inflammation; narcotics to treat and prevent severe pain in terminally ill patients with cancer; and diuretics or "water pills" to control excess fluid or high blood pressure.

- *Combating illness*—Drugs with this purpose include antibiotics to treat pneumonia, strep throat, or a bladder infection. Although antiviral medications do not cure human immunodeficiency virus (HIV) or acquired immunodeficiency syndrome (AIDS), they may allow the immune system to remain sufficiently intact so as to delay disease progression. Drugs for Alzheimer's disease will not cure the patient but may delay both disease progression and loss of independence of the patient.

- *Reversing disease processes*—Drugs with this purpose include medications that control depression, blood pressure, or cholesterol levels.

Pharmacodynamic Agents

A **pharmacodynamic agent** is a medication that alters body functioning in a desired way. Pharmacodynamic agents can be used, for example, to stimulate or relax muscles, to dilate or constrict pupils, or to increase or decrease blood glucose levels. Caffeine found in coffee, tea, or a soft drink is considered a pharmacodynamic agent because it stimulates the nervous system, allowing the consumer to remain alert. Other examples of these medications include decongestants for nasal stuffiness, oral contraceptives that depress hormones to prevent pregnancy, expectorants to thin fluid or loosen mucus in the respiratory tract, anesthetics to cause numbness or loss of consciousness, glucagon to increase blood glucose levels in diabetics, and digoxin to increase heart muscle contraction or slow heart conduction in patients with heart disease.

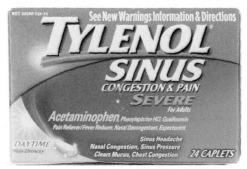

Tylenol Sinus contains a nasal decongestant that reduces the swelling in the nasal passages, thereby relieving pressure and improving airflow. Because of these physiologic changes, this medication is considered a pharmacodynamic agent.

Diagnostic Agents

A **diagnostic agent** is a chemical containing radioactive isotopes that is used to diagnose or treat disease. Isotopes are forms of an element that contain the same number of protons but different numbers of neutrons. Unstable, radioactive isotopes give off energy in the form of radiation. These isotopes act as radioactive tracers, helping healthcare practitioners to pinpoint, diagnose, and treat certain disorders. Nuclear medicine uses radioactive isotopes such as technetium (99mTc) and iodine (^{131}I) for imaging regional function and biochemistry in the body. Technetium is also commonly used for imaging and functional studies of the brain, thyroid, lungs, liver, gallbladder, kidneys, and blood. The radiation exposure from the use of these isotopes is minimal and, therefore, has no harmful effects on patients.

Prophylactic Agents

A **prophylactic agent** prevents illness or disease from occurring. Examples of prophylactic agents include the antiseptic and germicidal liquid chemicals used for preoperative

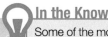
hand-washing procedures to prevent the spread of infection. Vaccines are also considered prophylactic agents; they prevent the onset of diseases such as influenza, pneumonia, shingles, tetanus, measles, mumps, rubella, chicken pox, smallpox, poliomyelitis, and hepatitis.

In certain situations, antibiotics are prophylactic agents as well. For example, a patient who has a history of rheumatic fever may be given a large, single dose of an antibiotic prior to a dental procedure. This preventive action decreases the patient's risk of acquiring a serious bacterial infection from the dental work.

Destructive Agents

A **destructive agent** has a *–cidal* action; that is, it kills bacteria, fungi, and viruses—even normal cells or abnormal cancer cells. Many antibiotics, especially those given in high doses and/or as intravenous (IV) infusions, are **bactericidal**, meaning that these agents kill rather than inhibit bacteria that are sensitive to these drugs. Penicillin is an example of a bactericidal drug, although resistance by some bacterial organisms has developed over the years. Another example of a destructive agent is radioactive iodine, which is used to destroy some of the excess hormone secreted by the thyroid.

An **antineoplastic drug**, or a drug used in cancer chemotherapy to destroy malignant tumors, is also an example of a destructive agent. Cancer is often caused by an unregulated growth of abnormal dysfunctional cells. Different antineoplastic drugs are used in combination to slow the growth of cancer cells at different phases of their cell growth cycles. Unfortunately, most of these drugs cannot effectively distinguish cancer cells from normal cells, so side effects such as hair loss, immunosuppression, and ulcerations of the mouth or gastrointestinal (GI) tract commonly occur.

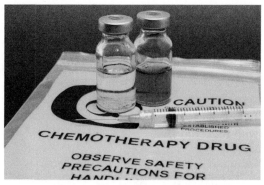

Chemotherapy drugs are powerful destructive agents that are used to treat malignant tumors. These agents target tissue cells that are rapidly growing and duplicating, such as those within tumors. GI cells and hair follicles also rapidly turn over, so the side effects of chemotherapy agents often include nausea, vomiting, and hair loss.

Homeostasis

To understand how drugs work in the body, allied health professionals need to grasp the concept of homeostasis. **Homeostasis** is a relatively stable state of equilibrium in the body. This state is achieved by a system of control and feedback mechanisms that enables the body to keep its living processes in balance. When the body's own processes cannot maintain a healthy state, drugs can be used to help the body restore and maintain homeostasis.

Messengers and Receptors

For the body to maintain a healthy control over its processes, it is essential that the cells that perform the various tasks needed for life have the ability to communicate with each other. The principal way in which cells communicate is through the action of **chemical messengers**, or chemical substances that cells produce and send out into the extracellular fluid. Histamine, prostaglandin, and bradykinin are some important **endogenous** chemical messengers (ones that originate within the body). Once the messenger has been released, it eventually reaches its target cell. The messenger recognizes and communicates with the target cell through a specific protein molecule, or **receptor**, on the surface of or within the cell. When the messenger molecule binds with the receptor, it triggers a series of reactions within the target cell. These reactions are the next step in the body's response to the condition (such as an illness or allergy) that caused the messenger to be produced. A good way to think about this process is to compare messengers and receptors to locks and keys: The cells of the body have many different receptors (or "locks") on their cell surfaces, and various messengers (or "keys") fit exactly into them.

Mechanisms of Drug Action

Many drugs exert their powerful and specific actions in the body by working in the same way as the chemical components the body itself uses for control and feedback. Generally, drug molecules mimic the molecular shape of the body's endogenous chemical messengers and then either stimulate or block the activity of substances that are already present in the body (see Figure 3.1). This action explains why drugs with similar molecular structures are categorized together in a drug class: The drug molecules interact with the same receptors and thus have similar activity.

FIGURE 3.1 **Drugs and Receptors**

Drug molecules are similar to but not the same as endogenous molecules. Their slight differences can be the reason that side effects occur.

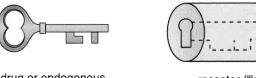

drug or endogenous substance ("key")

receptor ("lock")

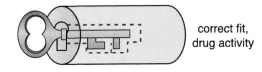

correct fit, drug activity

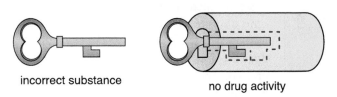

incorrect substance

no drug activity

Agonists and Antagonists

Sometimes drugs embed themselves in the cell membrane or combine with an enzyme or a protein. In most cases, however, drug molecules interact with receptors on the surface or inside of specific cells. Drugs that trigger the same cellular response as the body's own chemical messengers are called **agonists**. Drugs that block the action of the endogenous messengers when binding to receptors are called **antagonists**.

Antagonists block a response in one of two ways. They can either directly inactivate the receptor, blocking its ability to trigger a response, or bind to the receptor in a competitive fashion, keeping other agonist molecules from binding and triggering a response. When a drug binds with high affinity to a receptor, it sticks to the receptor longer—perhaps even permanently. Drugs with low affinity for a receptor may bind quickly and then fall off easily, which can lead to a short duration of action.

Dose-Response Relationship

For a drug to be effective, it must reach its site of action within the body in a sufficient concentration to produce a measurable effect. In other words, enough of the drug molecules must reach the site of action to produce a significant response. The time that the drug takes to reach its therapeutic concentration is called its **onset of action**.

Time-Response Curve

This relationship between dose and effect is depicted graphically as a **time-response curve** (see Figure 3.2). This graph displays the concentration of drug in the bloodstream over time once a dose is given. Proper drug dosing aims for blood concentrations in the middle of this curve, an area known as the **therapeutic range**. The lower threshold of this range is the **minimum therapeutic concentration**. Drug dosing must achieve at least this concentration to gain any measurable effect. The upper edge of this range is the **toxic concentration**; above this concentration, the incidence of toxic effects may outweigh any benefit of the drug and thus pose a risk to the patient.

Drug Concentrations and Steady State

For drugs with which a constant concentration in the therapeutic range is desired, timing of doses is important. Figure 3.3 shows how repeated doses are timed to produce an average drug concentration that remains in the therapeutic range. When this constant concentration is maintained, **steady state** is achieved, meaning that the drug concentration remains stable. Up to five doses, if timed appropriately, may be required before blood concentrations reach steady state. When it is important for a patient to receive treatment quickly, a loading dose is given. A **loading dose** is a dose that is large enough to bring blood concentrations up to the therapeutic range quickly. Subsequent doses then keep levels at steady state.

FIGURE 3.2 Time-Response Curve

Some drugs have a narrow therapeutic range: The minimum therapeutic and toxic levels are close to each other. In these cases, drug dosing must be monitored closely to ensure the appropriate amount of a drug is given to produce the desired effects without overshooting and causing toxic effects.

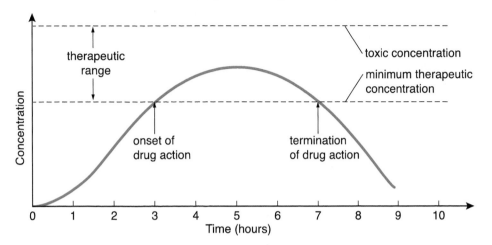

FIGURE 3.3 Steady State

Repeated IV doses must be given in order to maintain a steady concentration in the therapeutic range.

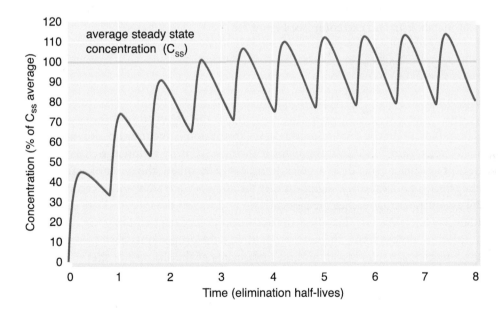

The point at which a drug is at its highest concentration between doses is called the **peak**. The **trough** is when the drug concentration is at its lowest. For some drugs, peaks and troughs are measured to be sure they are high enough and low enough. Measuring drug levels helps healthcare prescribers ensure that patients get maximum benefit but avoid toxicity. Once steady state has been reached and the prescriber is sure that peaks and troughs are appropriate, monitoring of drug concentration levels may become less frequent.

As an allied health professional, you may be involved in ordering, collecting, or reading drug concentration levels from the laboratory, or you may be involved in drawing blood for such tests.

Checkpoint 3.1

Take a moment to review what you have learned so far and answer these questions.

1. What is the difference between a drug used for relief of symptoms versus one used to combat illness? Give examples.

2. How do drug molecules interact with receptors? What is the difference between an agonist and an antagonist?

3. What is the therapeutic range of drug therapy, and how would you depict it graphically?

Pharmacokinetics

The study of pharmacokinetics uses mathematical modeling—in the form of time-response curves—to observe and predict how a drug enters, moves around, and leaves the body. In other words, **pharmacokinetics** studies how drugs are absorbed, distributed, and eliminated from the bloodstream. This entire process can be described in terms of four distinct phases: absorption, distribution, and elimination, which includes the two processes of metabolism and excretion (see Figure 3.4).

Absorption

Absorption is the process by which drugs enter the bloodstream. It is measured as the rate at which and extent to which a drug moves from the site of administration to the circulating blood. On the time-response curve, absorption is the upward-sloping part of the curve (see Figure 3.2). Absorption affects the onset of drug action as well as the extent of action. For instance, if a drug is quickly and easily absorbed, the onset of action is fast and the effect is noticeable and significant. If the absorption is slow and incomplete, only a small amount of drug reaches the bloodstream and targets the intended site of action.

There are several factors that affect the absorption of a drug including the route of administration, dosage form, chemical properties of the drug and its absorption site, drug transport mechanism, and bloodflow and surface area of the absorption site.

Route of Administration

The route of administration affects absorption by enhancing or limiting the medication's systemic effect. Using the oral route of administration, which is the most common route, typically results in good systemic absorption through the small intestine. IV administration skips the absorption step entirely by delivering drugs directly into the bloodstream. Topical routes do not always produce a measurable systemic effect because absorption is usually limited. Inhaled medications are absorbed in the lungs.

FIGURE 3.4 | Pharmacokinetic Process

Most oral drugs enter the bloodstream through the lining of the intestines, where all blood goes through the liver before entering the rest of the body.

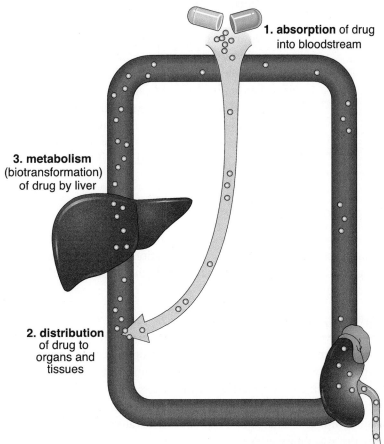

1. absorption of drug into bloodstream

3. metabolism (biotransformation) of drug by liver

2. distribution of drug to organs and tissues

4. excretion of drug in liquid waste by kidney, and solid waste by intestine

Dosage Form

Dosage form also affects absorption. Before a drug can enter circulation, it must dissolve. Therefore, solid dosage forms usually result in slower absorption rates than do liquids. Transdermal patches release drugs slowly, so that absorption through the skin is steady and incremental. Some tablets and capsules are specially manufactured or coated for specific solubility properties. Oral disintegrating tablets, also referred to as *rapidly dissolving tablets*, are quickly absorbed when placed on the tongue because they instantly dissolve in saliva. Coated tablets take longer to dissolve and absorb. Sublingual tablets are placed under the tongue for absorption, and buccal tablets are placed between the cheek and gums. Both sublingual and buccal tablets are absorbed in the oral mucosa.

Chemical Properties of Drugs and Their Absorption Sites

Acidic and basic properties (pH levels) of drugs and their environment affect drug solubility and ultimately drug absorption. When a drug with basic properties is in an acidic

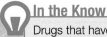
environment such as the stomach, it dissociates into ionic (charged) particles, which cannot cross membranes easily. Therefore, basic drugs do not get absorbed well when in the acidic environment of the stomach. Acidic drugs placed in an acidic environment do not easily dissociate; thus, more drug will be absorbed. For example, taking an antacid, which has basic properties, raises the pH of the stomach and, consequently, reduces the stomach's acidity. This change in pH can reduce the absorption of an acidic drug and can enhance the absorption of a basic drug. Therefore, certain drugs, such as cholesterol medications, should not be taken at the same time as antacids because the action of the antacids reduces the absorption of the medication. If less of the drug is absorbed into the bloodstream, it will not be as effective.

Drug Transport Mechanisms

The transport mechanisms that drugs use to cross membranes also affect absorption. Crossing membranes between the site of administration and the circulatory system is necessary for drug activity. Drug molecules cross membranes by active and passive transport mechanisms (see Figure 3.5).

Active Transport Mechanisms

Active transport mechanisms use energy to bring drug molecules across a membrane. An example of an active transport mechanism is the sodium/potassium exchange pump, which requires adenosine triphosphate (ATP) for energy (Na^+/K^+–ATPase, also known as the sodium pump). These proteins, which traverse the cell membrane, use energy to pump potassium into cells and sodium out of cells. Because active transport mechanisms are limited by the availability of energy sources, they can become saturated, or maxed out, which limits overall absorption.

FIGURE 3.5 Active and Passive Transport Mechanisms

In simple diffusion, molecules move either directly through the membrane itself or through an open channel.

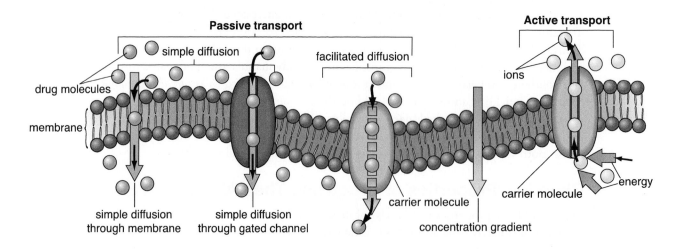

Passive transport mechanisms move drug molecules across a membrane on their own. Passive mechanisms are usually driven by **concentration gradients**. Drugs absorbed via passive transport move down a gradient from an area of high concentration (the site of administration) to an area of low concentration (the bloodstream). Thus, higher doses typically produce greater absorption. Diffusion is a passive transport mechanism by which many drugs are absorbed because molecules simply move down a concentration gradient.

Bloodflow and Surface Area of Absorption Site

Finally, the bloodflow and surface area of an absorption site affect drug absorption. For instance, the GI tract may not have a pH that is conducive to absorption of a particular drug. But the large surface area and good bloodflow of the small intestine overcome this limitation to absorption (see Figure 3.6). Surface areas that are large, thin, and have good blood supply, such as those of the small intestine and lungs, provide a good environment for drug absorption into the bloodstream. A drug can easily move across the membranes of the intestines or lung tissue into the circulation. Once in the bloodstream, the drug can travel to the site of action and produce the desired response.

FIGURE 3.6 | **Villi of the Small Intestine**

The inner surface of the small intestine is a mucous membrane with circular folds. Finger-like projections from these folds, called *villi*, are rich in capillary beds and allow more surface area for the absorption of a drug into the bloodstream.

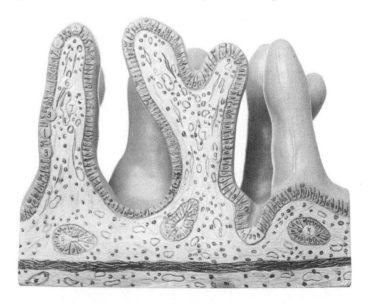

Distribution

Distribution is the process by which drugs move around in the bloodstream and reach other tissues of the body. Consequently, distribution is highly affected by bloodflow. If bloodflow is poor in a particular tissue or area of the body, few drug molecules are able to reach it. On the other hand, organs with high bloodflow (for example, the heart, kidneys, liver, and lungs) are exposed to drugs easily. Three factors affect a drug's distribution: its solubility, affinity for protein molecules, and ability to cross the blood-brain barrier.

Drug Solubility

The distribution of a drug in the body depends on the drug's **solubility**. A drug can be highly water-soluble or highly fat-soluble or lipid-soluble. If a drug is highly water-soluble, it will tend to stay in the bloodstream. If a drug is highly fat-soluble or lipid-soluble, it can accumulate in fatty tissue and then slowly be released back into the bloodstream over time.

Drug's Affinity for Protein Molecules

A drug's affinity for protein molecules also affects the distribution process. Some drug molecules have a high affinity for protein that circulates in the blood, such as albumin, and bind to these molecules. When drug molecules are bound to proteins in the blood, they are not free to reach the intended site of action. If a drug binds to a large extent (90% or more), distribution is affected. If two highly protein-bound drugs are administered together, they compete with each other for binding sites, leaving more of both drugs to roam freely in the blood. Therefore, they are more easily distributed. If dosing is not adjusted accordingly, both drugs can cause toxic effects.

Disease states can also affect protein binding. Renal failure and liver disease, for example, may result in a loss of plasma proteins to transport drugs. These conditions can increase both the therapeutic and toxic effects of a drug.

Drugs and the Blood-Brain Barrier

The **blood-brain barrier (BBB)** is a physical layer of cells that affects the distribution of drugs to the central nervous system. Although oxygen and carbon dioxide molecules easily pass across the BBB to reach brain cells, most larger drug molecules do not. This barrier is structured to allow only select molecules through. The BBB serves as a good defense mechanism for preventing harmful substances from reaching delicate brain tissue; however, it may also limit access to desired drug therapy (see Figure 3.7).

FIGURE 3.7 Blood-Brain Barrier

The blood vessels of the brain have a lining of endothelial cells that block many molecules from entering the brain. Scientists are working on new drug delivery systems that attach drugs to molecules that are capable of crossing this blood-brain barrier.

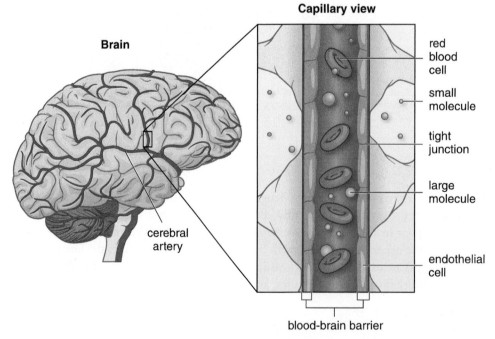

Elimination is the process by which drugs leave the body. Elimination can be measured as the rate and the extent to which a drug leaves the bloodstream. The elimination process occurs primarily in the kidneys and liver, but other routes of elimination exist, including exhalation and perspiration.

On the time-response curve, elimination is the downward-sloping part of the curve (see Figure 3.2). **Half-life** ($t_{1/2}$) refers to the time it takes for half (50%) of a drug to be cleared from the blood. This rate is referred to as the drug's **clearance**. It takes approximately eight half-lives for a drug to be completely eliminated from the blood, and thus from the body. Two processes, metabolism and excretion, affect elimination half-life. Drugs can either be deactivated via metabolism and then excreted from the body, or excreted from the body unchanged.

Metabolism

Metabolism is the process by which drugs are converted to other biochemical compounds and then excreted through metabolic pathways. The liver is considered the primary site of drug metabolism. This organ contains enzymes that metabolize drugs and other substances in the body, thus detoxifying the blood.

Metabolism converts drugs to more water-soluble (less lipid-soluble) forms. Once in a more water-soluble state, drugs may be more easily excreted by the kidneys. Drug metabolism is, therefore, highly dependent on bloodflow to the liver as well as the efficiency and function of enzymes located there. Other factors that affect the metabolism process include disease states, age, and genetic predisposition.

First-Pass Effect

Because blood coming from most of the GI tract goes through the liver before entering the rest of the body's circulation, many drugs undergo the first-pass effect. The **first-pass effect** refers to the process whereby the liver metabolizes (breaks down) some percentage of a drug during the "first pass" through the liver, before the drug reaches its intended site of action. As a result, the full drug dose does not reach the body, and its systemic effect is lessened. For those drugs that are quickly and easily metabolized by liver enzymes, this first-pass effect is especially problematic, and alternative routes of administration that bypass the liver must be used.

Drug Interactions

Many liver enzymes are involved in metabolism; the **cytochrome P450 (CYP450) enzyme system** most frequently deactivates drugs. CYP450 enzymes that metabolize drugs are numbered. Common ones include CYP1A2, CYP2A6, CYP2C9, CYP2D6, and CYP3A4. Drugs that interfere with these enzymes can affect other drugs that need these enzymes for proper elimination. Two drugs that use the same enzyme system, when given together, can compete for elimination, which increases the potential for drug toxicity. It is easy to see how the CYP enzyme system is a common source of drug interactions.

Excretion

Excretion is the process by which drug molecules are removed from the bloodstream. The process occurs primarily in the kidneys, the organs responsible for filtering substances from the blood and making urine. Excretion can also occur via bile, feces, sweat, and exhalations. Usually, excretion is highly dependent on bloodflow through the kidney as well as kidney function itself. Like transport mechanisms that control entry into the bloodstream, excretion can occur by active or passive mechanisms. The pH (acidity) of urine can also affect elimination rates.

Patient Teaching

When caring for patients with liver or kidney disease, allied health professionals should encourage them to establish honest communication with their prescribers and pharmacists. Tell patients to report any unwanted side effects they experience with their medication regimens to their prescribers so that doses and dosing schedules can be adjusted as needed. In addition, advise these patients to report all drug therapy (prescription drugs, over-the-counter [OTC] medications, and alternative therapies and supplements) to their prescribers and pharmacists so that potential drug interactions can be determined.

Drug Effects

The pharmacokinetic models described earlier provide critical insight for predicting the effects of each specific drug. Some effects are beneficial, whereas others can be detrimental or dangerous. Just as each individual is different, each person's reaction to a drug may be different. Thus, each patient must be monitored closely to ensure that his or her response to the drug is appropriate.

Indications and Contraindications

A disease, symptom, or condition for which a drug is known to be of benefit is termed an **indication** for the drug; that is, if the patient has the condition, it may be a good idea to prescribe the drug. This desired action is referred to as a **therapeutic effect**. In selecting a drug for an individual patient, the healthcare practitioner considers its medically accepted uses and situations in which it should or should not be given. A disease, symptom, or condition for which the drug will not be beneficial and may do harm is termed a **contraindication** for the drug; that is, if the patient has such a condition, the drug should not be prescribed, even when indications for the drug are present.

Side Effects

A **side effect** is a secondary response to a drug other than the primary therapeutic effect for which the drug was intended. On occasion, drugs can be prescribed for their side effects. For example, many antihistamines cause drowsiness and, consequently, they are found in many OTC insomnia preparations. Sometimes, two drugs are prescribed together because the combination has fewer or more easily tolerated side effects than a high dose of the individual drug. Nausea, skin rash, and constipation are the most common side effects and are usually fairly benign. Other side effects can be bothersome and even serious.

Allergic Responses

An **allergic response** is a local or general reaction of the immune system to an otherwise harmless substance. A substance that produces an allergic response is known as an **allergen**. In general, a molecule that causes an immune response, whether allergic or not, is known as an **antigen**. The first exposure to an allergen generally gives little or no observable response. Rather, what is critical about the initial exposure is the resulting "memory storage" that characterizes active immunity. Upon subsequent exposure, the body recognizes the antigen and responds with a more potent antibody response. This response can elicit reactions that range from uncomfortable to life-threatening. Some responses start within minutes of exposure; others may be delayed. Exposure to the allergen may cause mild, moderate, or, in some cases, severe inflammation. Some common allergic reactions to drugs include nasal secretions, swelling, wheezing, an excessively rapid heart rate, **urticaria** (hives), **pruritus** (itching), **angioedema** (abnormal accumulation of fluid in tissue), **wheals** (red, elevated areas on body), and, in rare cases, even death. An **anaphylactic reaction** is a severe allergic response resulting in life-threatening, immediate respiratory distress, usually followed by vascular collapse and shock and accompanied by hives. An **idiosyncratic reaction** is an unusual or unexpected response to a drug that is unrelated to the dose given.

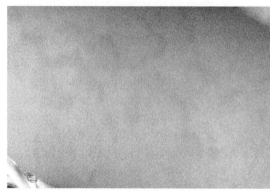

Urticaria (hives) is a common allergic reaction to a drug.

Work Wise

Allied health professionals who are administering injections to patients in clinical settings must detain them for 20 minutes after the injection procedure to observe for signs of anaphylaxis.

Drug Interactions

There are several types of **drug interactions**, but two common types are drug-drug interaction and drug-food interaction.

Drug-Drug Interaction

A **drug-drug interaction** occurs when one drug interferes with the action of another drug when administered together. Several factors determine the likelihood of a patient having a drug-drug interaction:

- age
- lifestyle
- physiology
- genetic makeup
- underlying disorders

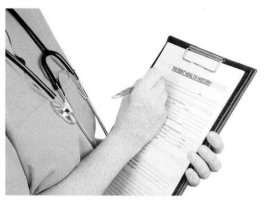

When obtaining a patient's health history, an allied health professional must encourage the patient to divulge all prescription drugs and OTC remedies that he or she takes. Providing a complete list of drugs and supplements helps prevent potential drug-drug interactions.

For example, hydrochlorothiazide (a medication used to treat hypertension) can interact with lithium (a medication used to treat bipolar disorder).

For this reason, allied health professionals should encourage their patients to provide a complete list of their prescription drugs, OTC medications, vitamins, and herbal remedies to their healthcare practitioners and pharmacists.

Drug-Food Interaction

A **drug-food interaction** occurs when either a drug interferes with a nutritional element or when the pharmacokinetic or pharmacodynamic properties of a drug are altered due to the consumption of a nutritional element. A common example of a drug-food interaction is the concurrent use of warfarin (Coumadin) with the intake of foods rich in vitamin K, such as green, leafy vegetables.

Grapefruit is also the source of a potential drug-food interaction. Grapefruit juice contains certain chemicals that inhibit a form of CYP that is found primarily in the intestines. Because of this inhibition, less of the drug undergoes first-pass metabolism, so more active drug is absorbed into the bloodstream, thereby increasing the risk of overdose. The effect of grapefruit juice on intestinal enzymes is partially irreversible; thus, enzyme levels do not return to normal immediately after the juice is cleared from the intestines. Absorption of drugs from the intestines may be affected for up to a day following ingestion of grapefruit juice.

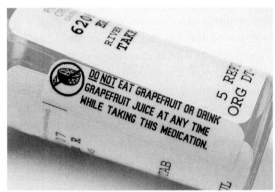

To avoid a possible drug-food interaction, an auxiliary warning label is affixed to certain medications. For example, this label warns patients to avoid the ingestion of grapefruit or grapefruit juice while taking this medication.

Other Responses to Drugs

Other dangerous effects of drugs involve drug dependence, addiction, and abuse. **Drug dependence** is a state in which a person's body has adapted physiologically to a drug and cannot function without it. Dependence should not be confused with **addiction**, which is a dependence characterized by a perceived need to take a drug to attain the psychological and physical effects of mood-altering substances. One sign of addiction is a decrease in psychological well-being and social or vocational functioning. Patients who are being treated for various disease states may become dependent on medications without exhibiting the signs of addiction.

Drug abuse is the use of a drug for purposes other than those prescribed and/or in amounts that were not directed. Abusive use of drugs can be, but is not always, linked to addiction. After a patient has been taking a drug over a significant period, he or she may begin to develop a decreased response to the drug. This decrease in response to the effects of a drug with continued administration is referred to as **tolerance**. As tolerance develops, the dosage of the drug may need to be increased to maintain a constant response.

Checkpoint **3.2**

Take a moment to review what you have learned so far and answer these questions.

1. What are the four phases of pharmacokinetics? Provide a summary of the actions that occur in each phase.

2. What is the first-pass effect?

3. How do enzymes in the liver (such as the cytochrome P450 enzyme system) cause drug interactions?

4. What are some common allergic reactions to drugs? List at least three examples.

Kolb's Learning Styles

Grasping concepts related to pharmacokinetics can be difficult. Assimilators and Convergers may find it useful to redraw the time-response curve to represent the influence of various factors on absorption and elimination. Accommodators and Divergers may find group discussion valuable for considering the effects that changes in absorption, distribution, and elimination have on the time-response curve and drug behavior.

Routes of Drug Administration

A **route of administration** is a way to get a drug into or onto the body. The route, as well as the dosage form, is determined by many factors, including the disease being treated, the area of the body that the drug needs to reach, and the chemical properties of the drug itself.

For a medication to be effective, it must be administered in a way that allows it to reach the appropriate site of action in a sufficient amount to produce the desired effect. Drugs can produce two different types of effects: a systemic effect and a localized effect. A **systemic effect** is a generalized effect on the entire body (e.g., using lisinopril to lower blood pressure). To achieve a systemic effect, a drug must be administered or absorbed directly into the bloodstream via a systemic route of administration. Whenever a drug is absorbed into the bloodstream, it travels throughout the body and can exert an effect everywhere. A **local effect** is an effect on a specific part of the body (e.g., using lidocaine to numb an area for sutures). To achieve a localized effect, a drug must be administered directly at the site of action via a local route of administration.

Systemic Routes of Administration

Systemic routes of administration are used when a drug needs to enter the bloodstream and travel to its site of action. Oral, sublingual, buccal, transdermal, rectal, parenteral, and implant routes are all considered systemic routes (see Table 3.1). A variety of dosage forms is available for each systemic route to enhance drug delivery and to provide patients with options if they are having difficulty using a particular route of administration.

TABLE 3.1 Systemic Routes and Corresponding Dosage Forms

Route of Administration	Common Dosage Forms
Buccal (between the cheek and gum) or sublingual (under the tongue)	Lozenge, spray, tablet, troche
Implant (under the skin)	Drug encasement carrier
Oral (into the mouth)	Capsule, liquid, suspension, tablet
Parenteral (into the body as an injection)	Injectable, solution, some suspensions
Rectal (into the rectum)	Solution, suppository
Transdermal (through the skin)	Cream, ointment, paste, patch

Oral Route

The **oral route of administration** (also known as **per oral** or **PO**, meaning "giving a drug by mouth") is the most convenient and cost-effective method of systemically delivering a drug. The majority of medications given through the oral route are pills (tablets and capsules). Liquid medications, such as solutions and syrups, are commonly given to children and other patients who have difficulty ingesting oral drugs. The oral dosage form of a drug is typically swallowed and absorbed into the bloodstream through the GI tract. However, the oral route also includes two routes in which a medication enters the oral cavity but is *not* swallowed. These routes are called the *sublingual route* and the *buccal route* and are discussed in detail below.

Medications that are ingested via the oral route may enter the blood circulation at a variety of sites along the GI tract, depending on the drug formulation. Certain medications may be absorbed into the bloodstream as soon as they reach the stomach. Other drugs are absorbed in the small intestine, with a few drugs undergoing absorption in the large intestine. Some drugs need to be digested by GI enzymes before absorption. All drugs that are absorbed into the blood through the GI system will undergo a first-pass effect through the liver. **Prodrugs** rely on this first-pass effect to work. When swallowed, prodrugs are not in an active form. They must first be metabolized into an active form in the liver before entering the bloodstream to produce the desired effect. Codeine is an example of a prodrug.

The absorption process of the oral route of administration takes time and is affected by several factors, including the presence of food (which slows the process) or digestive disorders. Therefore, allied health professionals who are involved in dispensing medication must be aware of whether a medication should be given with or without food and whether any specific patient assessments should be done before dispensing it.

Sublingual Route

Quick Study

The word *sublingual* comes from two Greek roots: *sub*, meaning "under," and *lingua*, meaning "tongue."

The **sublingual route of administration** involves placing a drug under the tongue to allow it to dissolve and be absorbed in the bloodstream through the underlying tissues. Medications given sublingually avoid the first-pass effect and go directly into the bloodstream, which allows for quick drug action. One common medication administered through the sublingual route is the lifesaving drug nitroglycerin. A patient who is experiencing angina (chest pain) places one nitroglycerin tablet under the tongue every five minutes until the pain is relieved or until three tablets have been administered.

Buccal Route

In the **buccal route of administration**, a drug is absorbed by the blood vessels in the lining of the mouth. A patient places a buccal tablet right next to the gum lining, between the teeth and cheek. A medication given via the buccal route acts quickly because it enters the bloodstream through the tissues of the mouth. A common example of a drug administered through the buccal route is nicotine gum. This gum is slowly and carefully chewed and then "parked" in the buccal area for absorption.

Transdermal Route

The **transdermal route of administration** involves application of a drug delivery system to the skin, such as a patch with adhesive backing, so that the drug is slowly absorbed through the skin over time (see Figure 3.8). Transdermal patches can be applied and left in place for hours to days to allow a gradual and even absorption of a drug. Examples include nicotine patches used for smoking cessation and birth control available as a patch. Occasionally, a cream or paste is used for transdermal delivery.

FIGURE 3.8 | Transdermal Drug Delivery

Transdermal drug delivery has become popular among patients who find it difficult to remember to take a pill every day. The convenience enhances their ability to adhere to therapy.

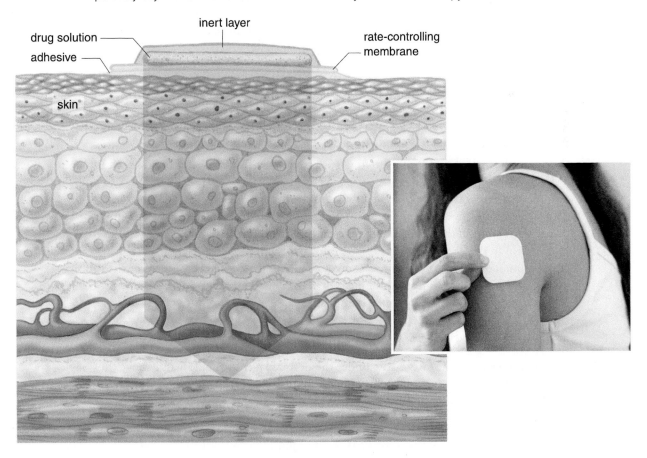

Rectal Route

Drugs delivered via the **rectal route of administration** are inserted into the rectum and allowed to melt or dissolve in place. Systemic absorption usually occurs through the mucosal lining; consequently, many dosage forms given this way are intended for systemic effect. There are, however, a few medications intended solely for local activity, such as drugs that treat hemorrhoids or colon cancer. Some products that are used rectally to cleanse the bowel also have local effects. Dosage forms include suppositories, enemas, solutions, foams, and ointments.

Parenteral Route

Drugs delivered via the **parenteral route of administration** are administered by injection. Usually, the intention is to deliver the drug systemically by injecting the medication into veins, skin, muscles, or the spinal column. These routes are useful when rapid drug delivery is needed or when a patient's condition warrants (for example, lack of consciousness or inability to swallow). This route is also useful for administering drugs that have a large first-pass effect because absorption through the GI tract is bypassed.

Use of the parenteral route for drug administration provides immediate access to the circulatory system, which results in a quick onset of drug effects. Many injections are given in emergencies and in hospital settings where patients are closely monitored. Some drugs that have a large **volume of distribution** (V_d) require a loading dose and continuous infusion before any drug effects are seen. When administering a drug via the parenteral route, healthcare personnel must exercise caution not to exceed toxic threshold levels because it is difficult to "take back" a dose that is already in the blood. Three parenteral routes that allow for slower absorption rates than the IV route are the subcutaneous (sub-Q), intradermal (ID), and intramuscular (IM) routes of administration.

Intravenous Route

The **intravenous route of administration** allows for injections to be given directly into a vein (see Figure 3.9). When repeated or continuous infusion of a drug into a vein is needed, a small catheter (plastic tube) is inserted into a vein and left in place while IV fluid containing the drug runs through the catheter and into the blood. IV solutions are the dosage form of choice for this route. A **peripheral IV line** is most often inserted into a vein in the arm, wrist, or hand. A peripheral IV line is used when small amounts of fluid need to be given or the time over which the fluid will infuse is only a few days or less. Most IV medications are given via a peripheral line. A **central IV line** is inserted into one of the larger veins in the upper chest area near the clavicle (collarbone) or into the internal jugular vein in the neck.. This type of line must be inserted surgically and is used when large volumes of fluid must be given, many repeated infusions will be needed, or the time over which the infusion is needed is longer than a few days. Cancer chemotherapy is one example of a medication that is often administered via a central IV line.

Subcutaneous Route

Injections given into the fatty tissue under the dermal layer of the skin and above the muscular tissue are given through the **subcutaneous (sub-Q) route of administration** (see Figure 3.10). Common sub-Q injection sites are the abdomen, upper thigh, and back of the upper arm. A drug administered via the sub-Q route is absorbed into the blood supply at the area of the injection over the next few minutes to hours, depending on the drug. Dosage forms used in the sub-Q route are solutions and some suspensions. Common medications that are administered subcutaneously include epinephrine (or adrenaline) for emergency asthmatic attacks or allergic reactions, heparin to prevent blood clots, sumatriptan (Imitrex) for migraines, and the shingles vaccine. In addition to these medications, almost all insulins and insulin-like products for diabetes are administered by the sub-Q route.

FIGURE 3.9 | Intravenous Injection

The size and angle of the needle used for IV injections depend on the area of the body and the vein into which the drug is delivered.

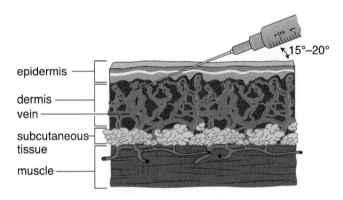

FIGURE 3.10 | Subcutaneous Injection

Some subcutaneous injections, such as those for insulin, use a very fine, short needle and are injected at a 90-degree angle. For others, a 1-inch needle injected at a 45-degree angle ensures that the drug is delivered into subcutaneous tissue, not the underlying muscle.

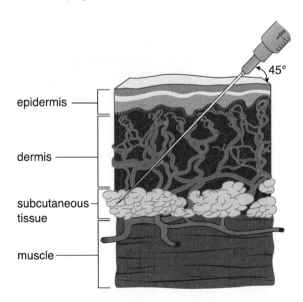

Intramuscular Route

The **intramuscular (IM) route of administration** involves giving an injection directly into a muscle, which can absorb a greater volume of medication than the subcutaneous tissue can (see Figure 3.11). The most common muscles used for IM injection are the deltoid (upper arm) and gluteus medius (buttocks) in adults and the vastus lateralis (thigh) in infants and toddlers. The drug is absorbed into the blood supply within the muscle and distributed throughout the body. The most common dosage form injected via the IM route is a solution. The IM route is used to administer antibiotics, narcotics, medications for migraine headaches, vitamins, iron, male and female hormones, anti-psychotic medications, and several vaccines including the influenza or flu vaccine. This route is also used to deliver lifesaving medication, such as epinephrine, in an emergency. An EpiPen, an autoinjector device used for administering epinephrine, is available in both pediatric and adult dosages and can be administered intramuscularly (including through clothing) or subcutaneously.

FIGURE 3.11   Intramuscular Injection

Typically, a 1-inch needle is used and is injected at a 90-degree angle to ensure that the drug is administered within the muscle tissue.

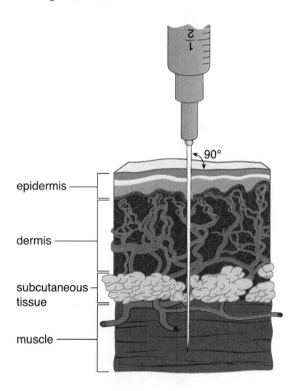

Intradermal Route

Injections that are given just underneath the top layer of skin (epidermis) use the **intradermal (ID) route of administration**. (see Figure 3.12). This type of injection is used for tuberculosis (TB) skin tests (known as purified protein derivative [PPD] tests) that are given on the forearm, local anesthesia at the site of pain or injection, and allergy skin testing on the back. ID injections should produce a wheal—a transient, raised area of skin at the injection site.

| FIGURE 3.12 | Intradermal Injection |

After an intradermal TB injection, the patient must return within two to three days to have an appropriate healthcare professional examine the injection area. Induration (firmness) at the site indicates possible previous exposure to TB.

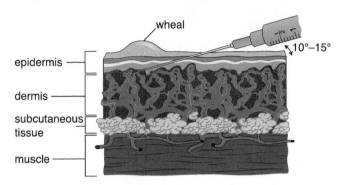

Intrathecal and Epidural Routes

Injections that are given into the spinal column between the vertebrae in the back use the **intrathecal (IT) route of administration**. Injections administered via the **epidural route of administration** require a small catheter to deliver the drug directly between the vertebrae of the spinal column over a certain period. These types of injections are used most often for regional anesthesia, such as in childbirth and delivery. IT and epidural injections must be mixed and administered using strict aseptic technique so as not to introduce pathogens into the central nervous system. Only anesthesiologists and anesthetists are permitted to perform these types of injections.

Implantation Route

The **implantation route of administration** involves the insertion of a drug delivery device, known as an *implant*, just below the skin to release a drug slowly over time (months to years). This route is effective for long-term treatments (such as birth control or a stent placed inside a coronary artery) because a sustained, consistent effect is produced. Improved adherence to a medication regimen is one of the benefits of implants. Various forms of implants are available for systemic drug delivery. The only implant product that does not produce a systemic effect is an intravitreal implant. This implant is inserted inside the eyeball to treat cytomegalovirus (CMV) infection in patients with AIDS.

Local Routes of Administration

Local routes of administration are typically used with the intention that the drug will not be systemically absorbed. In many cases, the potential for systemic absorption exists with these routes but typically occurs to such a small extent that—for all intents and purposes—the effect is local. Some local routes of administration include dermal, inhalation, intranasal, ophthalmic, otic, and vaginal. A variety of dosage forms is available for each local route to enhance drug delivery and to provide patients with options if they are having difficulty using a particular route of administration (see Table 3.2).

TABLE 3.2 Local Routes and Corresponding Dosage Forms

Route of Administration	Common Dosage Forms
Dermal	Cream, lotion, ointment, powder, solution
Inhalation	Dry powder inhaler, metered-dose inhaler, nebulizer solution
Intranasal	Solution, spray
Ophthalmic	Ointment, solution
Otic	Solution, suspension
Vaginal	Cream, gel, ointment, solution, suppository, tablet

Drug Alert

Some medications are used for their local effects but have the potential for unwanted systemic effects as well. For instance, inhaled bronchodilators are used primarily for their effect within the lungs in patients with asthma. However, these medications have some systemic absorption, which results in the presentation of side effects. Patients using inhaled bronchodilators often report nervousness, dizziness, and tremors after using their inhalers.

Dermal Route

The **dermal route of administration** is the topical application of drugs to the skin. Various creams, lotions, gels, ointments, powders, solutions, and pastes are spread or sprayed on the skin to treat local infections, wounds, sunburns, and rashes. Examples of dermal products include antibiotic cream applied to a cut or scrape, hydrocortisone cream applied to a rash or bug bite, and aloe vera lotion applied to a sunburn. If the drug is applied over a wide area in a large enough quantity, systemic absorption may occur. Therefore, patients must follow the labeling instructions of their medications closely.

Inhalation Route

The **inhalation route of administration** delivers medication into the lungs through patient inhalation. These medications can be inhaled through the mouth or through the nose, where they are then absorbed through the mucous membrane linings of the lungs and/or nostrils. The mucous membrane linings are filled with capillary blood vessels, which enable medications to enter the circulatory system rather

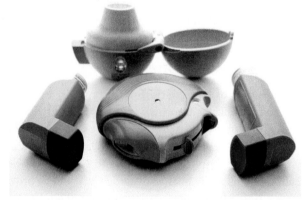

Several types of inhalers are used in delivering aerosolized and powdered medication through the inhalation route.

quickly. Note that a common issue with drugs administered via inhalation is that they can irritate mucous membrane linings.

The inhalation route is used primarily to deliver anti-inflammatory agents and bronchodilators to individuals with chronic lung disease or asthma. These patients inhale from a device—such as a metered-dose inhaler, dry powder inhaler, or nebulizer—that contains an aerosolized or powdered form of a drug. Although systemic absorption is possible, inhalation allows for direct treatment to lung tissue without significant systemic side effects in most cases. To ensure effective drug delivery, patients must learn the proper inhalation technique for their particular device.

Intranasal Route

Drug products that are sprayed into the nose use the **intranasal route of administration**. These products are typically used to offer relief from nasal congestion or prevention of allergy symptoms. In most cases, a liquid dosage form, such as a solution, delivers the drug to the nasal mucosa. Most intranasal products are intended for local activity, but a few are formulated to achieve systemic absorption. Patients should be cautioned to not sniff forcefully when using these products. Doing so pulls the drug too far back into the sinus cavities, which results in the medication draining down the back of the throat and, therefore, missing the intended site of administration. Patients should also be instructed to not blow their nose immediately after intranasal product administration. This action negates the intended effect.

Ophthalmic Route

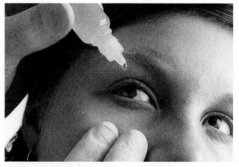

The **ophthalmic route of administration** delivers medication in the form of solutions and suspensions to the eye. Whereas solutions have a more rapid onset of action, suspensions have a longer duration of action. Eyedrops and eye ointments are examples of ophthalmic dosage forms that are used to treat eye disorders such as glaucoma and conjunctivitis, as well as to soothe the pain and discomfort from eye surgery. Systemic absorption of medication is possible but usually limited with ophthalmic dosage forms.

Lubricant eyedrops—administered via the ophthalmic route—relieve dry, irritated eyes.

Otic Route

Preparations delivered into the external ear canal use the **otic route of administration**. Otic preparations, usually eardrops, are instilled into the ear canal, but the eardrum prevents systemic absorption. Dosage forms include both solutions and suspensions that are used to treat ear infections and manage pain.

Vaginal Route

The **vaginal route of administration** involves the insertion or application of medication into the vagina. Typically, systemic absorption is not intended but is certainly possible. Only a few products delivered vaginally are intended for systemic absorption. Dosage forms given via the vaginal route include creams, gels, solutions, suppositories, ointments, and tablets. In most cases, patients use a vaginal applicator to aid delivery. Drugs delivered through this route are used for contraception, hormone replacement therapy, and treatment of common bacterial and yeast infections.

Checkpoint 3.3

Take a moment to review what you have learned so far and answer these questions.

1. What is the difference between a systemic drug effect and a local drug effect? Which routes of administration are used to achieve these two different effects?

2. What are the various parenteral routes of administration? Provide a brief description of each route.

3. What drug is used sublingually to provide relief from angina?

Dosage Formulations

In addition to route of administration, drug delivery is dependent on the **dosage formulation**, often referred to as *dosage form*. The choice of dosage form is based on many factors, including the disease being treated, the targeted area the drug needs to reach, the chemical composition of the drug, and—for some patients—the ease of administration. Dosage formulations can be classified into three categories: solid formulations, semisolid formulations, and liquid formulations.

Solid Formulations

Solid formulations include tablets, capsules, caplets, gelcaps, powders, troches/lozenges, and implants. These formulations are mainly for systemic use.

Tablet

A **tablet** is a solid dosage form produced by compression. Most tablets are swallowed whole, but some are intended to be chewed before swallowing. Onset of effect occurs approximately 30 minutes after swallowing.

Tablets are available in a wide variety of shapes, sizes, and surface markings. They are typically imprinted with a distinctive letter and/or numeric code as well as coloring from their manufacturers for drug identification purposes. Tablets are also available with coatings. A **tablet coating** is a special outside layer that is used to improve the appearance, flavor, or ease of swallowing. This coating is often designed to dissolve or rupture in a specific place, either the stomach or small intestine.

Types of Tablets

Tablets are designed by manufacturers to have properties that allow for patient adherence as well as effective drug delivery. Many tablets are available on the market, including compression tablets, multiple-compression tablets, chewable tablets, and oral disintegrating tablets.

Compression Tablet

A **compression tablet** is the most inexpensive and common dosage form used today. These tablets are made by compressing powder or granular ingredients together. Typically, these tablets are uncoated. Acetaminophen (Tylenol) is an example of a common compression tablet.

Multiple-Compression Tablet

A **multiple-compression tablet** is designed to have a tablet on top of a tablet or a tablet inside a tablet (see Figure 3.13). Each layer of the tablet contains a separate medication and is colored differently. This type of tablet is sometimes manufactured to combine two incompatible substances into a single medication. Ambien CR is a common example of a multiple-compression tablet; it combines an extended-release form and an immediate-release form of the drug in one tablet.

FIGURE 3.13 Multiple-Compression Tablets

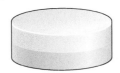
two layers or compressions

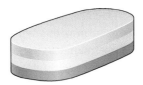
three layers or compressions

Chewable Tablet

A **chewable tablet** contains a base that is flavored and/or colored. The dosage form is designed to be chewed and absorbed quickly for a slightly faster onset of action. Chewing is preferred for antacids, antiflatulents, certain vitamins, and children's tablets. Other drugs that are available in a chewable tablet include montelukast (Singulair), used to control asthma symptoms, and amoxicillin, used to treat infection.

Oral Disintegrating Tablet

A tablet that is designed to dissolve quickly on the tongue and be absorbed directly in the mouth is known as an **oral disintegrating tablet**. This type of tablet starts acting within minutes and is useful for pediatric and geriatric patients who have difficulty swallowing, or for patients with nausea. Examples of oral disintegrating tablets include ondansetron (Zofran), for the treatment of nausea and vomiting, and donepezil (Aricept), for the treatment of Alzheimer's disease.

Capsule

A **capsule** is a granular powder or liquid gel that is enclosed in a gelatinous shell. The gelatin shell can be hard or soft and may be transparent, semi-transparent, or opaque. Like tablets, capsules contain both active and inert ingredients. Drugs that have a bitter taste or unpleasant odor are usually formed into capsules. For those who have trouble swallowing medications, capsules can be broken apart so that the medication contents can be sprinkled into food or dissolved into drinks. There are certain capsules, however, that must be swallowed so that their medication contents are released over a certain period. Extended-release formulations (which include both sustained-release [SR] medications and controlled-release [CR] medications) must be taken whole. The generic drug esomeprazole (Nexium), a proton pump inhibitor used to treat chronic gastroesophageal reflux disease, is marketed as the "purple pill" but is actually a capsule.

Caplet

A **caplet** is simply a tablet shaped like a capsule and sometimes coated to look like a capsule. The inside of the caplet is solid rather than filled with powder or granular material like the inside of a capsule. Caplets have many beneficial properties: They are easier to swallow than large tablets, have a longer shelf life than capsules, and—unlike capsules—are tamper proof. Caplet formulations on the market include the OTC drug naproxen (Aleve) and the prescription drug oxaprozin (Daypro).

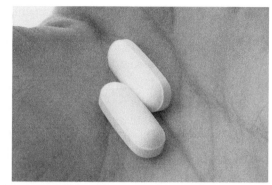
Caplets are easier to swallow than large tablets and can be easily scored (cut) with a tablet splitter if necessary.

Gelcap

A **gelcap** is a dosage form with a typically oil-based content that is surrounded by a soft gelatinous coat. Some prenatal vitamins come as gelcaps. One of the OTC versions of ibuprofen also comes in a gelcap formulation.

Powder

A medication that is ground into fine particles is a **powder**. Powders are helpful in keeping an area dry while simultaneously delivering drug to the site. Other powders, such as Goody's Headache Powder and Metamucil, are mixed with liquid and taken orally.

Lozenge or Troche

A medication that is intended to slowly dissolve in the mouth is called a **lozenge**, or **troche**. A lozenge is to be left in the mouth until the medication has completely dissolved; it should not be swallowed. It is important to note that there are some lozenges that are gummy-like and can be chewed. Lozenges generally have local therapeutic effects. OTC lozenges for relief of sore throats are common, although many other drugs, including such prescription drugs as nystatin, are also available in a lozenge form.

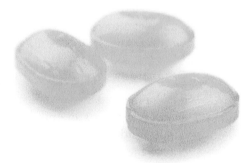
Cough drops are lozenges designed to release medication while slowly dissolving in the mouth.

Implant

An **implant** is a medication that is surgically inserted just below the skin surface. The medication may be encased in a nonirritating device (e.g., plastic polymers and degradable microspheres) that allows the drug to be released into the bloodstream over a specific period. The device must be removed once the medication therapy is complete or must be replaced if a "refill" is due. Examples of implants include Implanon and Nexplanon, two brand-name products that contain the birth control hormone etonogestrel.

Semisolid Formulations

Semisolid formulations include suppositories, ointments, creams, gels, lotions, pastes, and transdermal patches. These formulations are mainly for topical or local use.

Suppository

A medication that is shaped into the form of a bullet and that melts on insertion is called a **suppository**. Suppositories are formulated to be solid prior to insertion and then to melt at body temperature and release an active drug. They are designed for insertion into body orifices such as the rectum, vagina, or, less commonly, the urethra. These medications are meant for localized action, as in the treatment of hemorrhoids, or systemic action, as in the treatment of ulcerative colitis. Rectal suppositories are sometimes used in children or adults who are unable to take oral medications for nausea, vomiting, or constipation. For example, promethazine (Phenergan) suppositories are administered to treat nausea, and OTC glycerin suppositories are used to treat constipation.

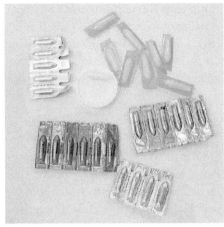

Suppositories use wax or another semisoft medium that liquefies when warmed to body temperature.

Ointment

An **ointment** is a medication that contains a small amount of water dispersed in oil. Consequently, ointments feel greasy. These medications are applied directly to external surfaces—most commonly to the skin. Although not as cosmetically acceptable as creams, ointments may be more therapeutically effective due to their skin adherence and moisturizing qualities. Many cortisone-like medications and topical antibiotics such as Neosporin are available in an ointment formulation.

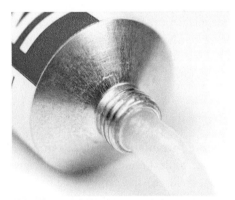

An ointment typically has an oily or greasy feel and a strong adherence to the skin.

Cream

Unlike an ointment, which is a small amount of water dispersed in oil, a **cream** is a medication that contains a small amount of oil dispersed in water. Therefore, a cream feels less greasy than an ointment. Creams are typically applied directly to the skin and are invisible once applied. Examples of creams include acne products containing benzoyl peroxide or salicylic acid, such as Clearasil or Salacyn, and hydrocortisone cream products used for skin rashes, such as Cortizone-10 or Instacort.

Gel

A **gel** is a semisolid formulation that consists of water, oil, and, sometimes, alcohol. It is applied directly to external surfaces or used to administer medications into body cavities. Gels usually thicken upon standing and liquefy when shaken. If a gel is alcohol based, it should be applied to unbroken skin. Application of a gel to broken skin can cause a stinging sensation. Unlike ointments, gels have a drying effect when applied to the skin. Examples of gels include prescription acne products such as azelaic acid (Finacea) and clindamycin (Cleocin T and ClindaMax).

Lotion

A **lotion** is a medication mixed with a combination of water, oil, and alcohol. The moisturizing property of lotions is difficult to generalize due to the wide variability of ingredients. Lotions are also most commonly applied to the external skin surface of the body and are easily absorbed. Examples of lotions include calamine lotion, used to soothe sunburn and relieve the itchiness associated with poison ivy, and benzoyl peroxide lotion, used to control acne.

Paste

Similar to an ointment, a **paste** is a medication in which powder has been suspended. Pastes are most commonly applied externally to the skin. Common examples of pastes include zinc oxide paste, which is used as a sunscreen, and triamcinolone acetonide dental paste, which is an anti-inflammatory preparation.

Transdermal Patch

A **transdermal patch** is designed to deliver a drug contained within a patch or disk to the bloodstream via absorption through the skin. The patch consists of a backing, a drug reservoir, a rate-controlling membrane, an adhesive layer, and a protective strip. Once the strip is removed, the adhesive layer is attached to the skin. Transdermal patches provide a slow release of a drug, and therapeutic effects last from 24 hours to 1 week. Drugs offered in a transdermal patch include nicotine, nitroglycerin, narcotic analgesics, and estrogen/progestin.

Liquid Formulations

Liquid formulations include syrups, solutions, elixirs, tinctures, emulsions, suspensions, and aerosols. Liquids can be advantageous for individuals who have difficulty swallowing (e.g., children) and can be used for either systemic or local effects. IV drug therapy also comes in liquid form, usually an **aqueous** (soluble in water) solution.

Syrup

An aqueous solution thickened with a high content of concentrated sugar water is called a **syrup**. This sweet, thick liquid medication is classified as medicated and nonmedicated. Medicated syrups include ranitidine hydrochloride, used for the treatment of heartburn, and cetirizine hydrochloride, used for the treatment of allergies. Nonmedicated syrups include cherry syrup and cocoa syrup. Most pediatric formulations are syrups that mask the taste and ease the swallowing of medication. Syrups are often the preferred vehicle of pediatric cough medicine because they do not contain alcohol.

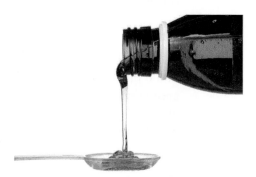

The flavor and consistency of children's cough syrups make patient adherence easier.

Solution

A **solution** is a liquid in which the active ingredients are completely dissolved in a liquid vehicle. Solutions may be classified by their vehicle as aqueous (water-based), alcoholic (alcohol-based), or hydroalcoholic (water-based and alcohol-based). The vehicle that makes up the greater part of a solution is known as the **solvent**. An ingredient dissolved in a solution is known as the **solute**. Examples of solutions include OTC saline solution, which is used to flush the eyes and moisten contact lenses, and the prescription drug promethazine hydrochloride, which is used to treat nausea.

Elixir

An **elixir** is a clear, sweetened, flavored solution containing water and ethanol (less than or equal to 20%). Elixirs are known for having a pleasant taste. An example of a drug in this dosage form is phenobarbital elixir, which is used to treat anxiety and seizures. Because this formulation contains sugar and alcohol, healthcare practitioners must exercise caution when prescribing elixirs for patients who have a history of diabetes and/or alcohol abuse.

Tincture

A liquid medication that has a high concentration of alcohol is called a **tincture**. These medications most often contain active ingredients originating from plant sources. Examples of tinctures include iodine, belladonna, and some herbal dietary supplements.

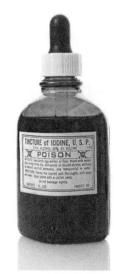

Tincture of iodine is 2% iodine and 2.4% sodium iodide diluted in 50% ethanol. This medication has corrosive effects on the GI tract if swallowed.

Emulsion

An **emulsion** is a liquid mixture of two unblendable substances. For that reason, an emulsion must be shaken well to mix it evenly before use. Emulsions can be oil preparations dispersed in water (more common) or water preparations dispersed in oil. Examples of emulsions include some OTC oral dosage formulations, such as Creomulsion cough-and-cold products.

Suspension

A **suspension** is a liquid medication that contains an ingredient that is not soluble in water but rather is suspended in the water-based solution as fine particles. Suspensions are often refrigerated, and they must be shaken well prior to use. Some suspensions are commercially available, such as Maalox, Mylanta, and Nystatin. Others are dry powders or granules that are mixed by the pharmacist or pharmacy technician with purified distilled water prior to dispensing to the patient.

Aerosol

A medication that is turned into a gaseous mist of fine particles is called an **aerosol**. Aerosols are usually based on liquid ingredients but, if a solid powder is fine enough, aerosols can be powder based. A propellant in the aerosol device allows for the release of the medication as a spray of fine particles. Aerosols such as Ventolin, Proventil, and ProAir HFA are metered-dose inhalers that are commonly prescribed to relieve the symptom of shortness of breath in acute asthma.

Kolb's Learning Styles

To learn routes of administration and corresponding dosage forms, try one of these methods. If you are an Accommodator, pull everything out of your medicine cabinet and categorize each product into its route of administration and dosage form. If you are an Assimilator, make a chart of all of the routes of administration on one axis and dosage forms on the other axis, and then place a check mark in each column and row where the dosage form makes sense to give by the corresponding route. If you are a Converger, take a trip to your local pharmacy and make a note of all routes and dosage forms available for OTC items familiar to you. Finally, if you are a Diverger, watch the national news and make note of all drug product advertisements; then look up the routes and dosage forms available for each product.

Checkpoint 3.4

Take a moment to review what you have learned so far and answer these questions.

1. What are the solid dosage forms of drug therapy?

2. What are the semisolid dosage forms of drug therapy?

3. What are the liquid dosage forms of drug therapy?

Drug Response Factors

The individual characteristics of patients can influence the effectiveness of drug therapy. Awareness of these differences is important when healthcare practitioners are choosing the appropriate drug and route of administration for each patient. Some **drug response factors** that must be considered include the patient's age, weight, gender, nutritional status, and liver and kidney functions. GI dysfunction can also affect drug response.

Age

Very young and very old patients pose the greatest risks to safe drug therapy because the pharmacokinetic behavior of drugs varies widely in these populations. Prescribers can use a variety of formulas when ordering medications for pediatric and geriatric patients.

Pediatrics

In **pediatric practice** (infants and children), infants are of greatest concern when prescribing medications because their body makeup and liver function are different from those of adults. Babies have higher body water content and strong blood circulation, so drugs that are highly water-soluble will distribute well, making toxicity an issue.

Liver function of pediatric patients also affects drug therapy. Remember that the liver is the site where many drugs are metabolized. Because liver function is not fully mature at birth, drugs are not quickly eliminated in pediatric patients. It takes months or years for all liver enzyme systems to become fully functional. Therefore, absorption, distribution, and metabolism of drugs in infants and children differ from those processes in the adult patient population, and drug dosages must be adjusted accordingly. For more information on pediatrics and drug therapy, refer to Chapter 28.

Geriatrics

In **geriatric practice** (elderly patients), healthcare practitioners must consider several effects that aging has on pharmacokinetic parameters. First, acidity in the stomach is usually decreased in older adults, which translates to a higher pH. Drugs that need a highly acidic (low pH) environment for absorption are affected. In addition, older patients tend to have higher body fat content, so drugs that are highly fat-soluble may distribute well and accumulate, leading to a higher risk of toxicity. Finally, as people age, both kidney and liver functions decrease, so drug elimination decreases dramatically. Bloodflow to these vital organs also decreases with age. Because of decreased ability to eliminate the drugs, doses may be decreased and dosing intervals increased to accommodate altered absorption, distribution, and elimination in older patients. For more information on geriatrics and drug therapy, refer to Chapter 29.

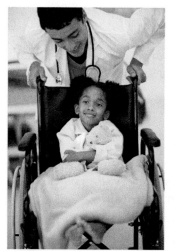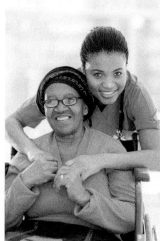

Pediatric patients and geriatric patients have anatomic and physiologic differences that must be considered when prescribing drug therapy. These two patient populations are most vulnerable to adverse drug reactions and drug toxicity.

Weight

Many medication dosages are based on the "average" adult weight. Thus, if a patient's weight is higher or lower than the average weight, the medication dose may need to be either increased or decreased to provide the intended effect. Dosing of medications for children is often weight based because weight changes quickly in that patient population and may vary substantially among children of the same age.

Gender

Some drugs work differently in male patients and female patients. The hormonal differences between men and women lead to more muscle mass in men and more fat content in women. The distribution of drugs will differ because of the varying amounts of muscle tissue and fatty tissue. Remember that fat-soluble drugs distribute well into fatty tissue, which means women will retain these drugs in their bodies longer than men will. Similarly, drugs that distribute well into muscle tissues will have quicker and more lasting effects in men than in women. Another point to consider is weight difference between men and women. In general, women tend to be smaller than men, which can affect dosing requirements.

Nutritional Status

A patient's nutritional status not only affects his or her weight (which can, in turn, affect drug response) but also affects the blood's protein levels. In malnutrition, patients may not have as much of the blood protein albumin circulating throughout the body. As mentioned earlier, blood protein such as albumin aids in drug distribution and response because some drug molecules bind to this substance. With a reduced level of albumin, more of the drug is left unbound and freely circulating in the blood. Consequently, higher levels enter tissues, which results in drug toxicity. Examples of highly protein-bound drugs include phenytoin, used to treat seizures, and digoxin, used to treat cardiac arrhythmia.

Liver Function

Because metabolism occurs primarily in the liver, problems in liver function can greatly affect drugs eliminated via metabolism. Cirrhosis, hepatitis, and other liver diseases can severely affect liver function. In these cases, doses must usually be adjusted downward.

Kidney Function

Because excretion happens most often through the kidneys, problems with kidney function greatly affect drug elimination. Both acute and chronic kidney failure make a difference in a drug's ability to leave the body. If doses are not adjusted accordingly, drug levels accumulate and can cause toxicity.

GI System Function

Because oral dosage forms depend on absorption into the bloodstream through the GI tract, severe dysfunction of this system can affect drug response. For instance, severe diarrhea or short-bowel syndrome (where part of the intestine has been removed) can reduce drug absorption. In these conditions, intestinal contents move so quickly or come into contact with less surface area available for absorption that adequate blood levels of a drug may be difficult to achieve. In some of these cases, alternative routes of administration may be needed.

Chapter Review

Chapter Summary

Drugs are used to maintain health, relieve symptoms, combat illness, and reverse disease. To learn how drugs work, an understanding of drug receptor theory is useful. Drug receptor theory helps explain drug activity. Drugs that are receptor agonists stimulate a response, whereas drugs that are antagonists block a response. Pharmacokinetics is the study of how drugs move around in the body. The four phases of pharmacokinetics are absorption, distribution, metabolism, and excretion. Mathematical models describe these phases, and graphical representation shows how drugs enter and exit the bloodstream. Drug dosing and response depend on these concepts. These pharmacokinetic models also predict the effects of drugs. The desired action of a drug is referred to as a *therapeutic effect*. Undesirable drug effects are referred to as *side effects*, *allergic responses*, or *drug interactions*.

This chapter reviews routes of administration and common dosage forms used for each route. Systemic routes of administration are used when a drug needs to enter the bloodstream and travel to its site of action. Local routes of administration are typically used with the intention that the drug will not be systemically absorbed. A variety of dosage forms is available for each route to enhance drug delivery and to provide patients with options. As you learn how various drugs work, you should also learn how they are delivered to the body to exert their activity. Various factors affect individual patient parameters for drug activity. Factors such as the patient's age, weight, gender, nutritional status, liver and kidney functions, and GI dysfunction affect how drugs are absorbed, distributed, and eliminated. Such characteristics are taken into account when choosing appropriate drug therapy and dosing.

Chapter Checkup

The Navigator+ learning management system that accompanies this textbook offers many opportunities to help you master chapter content, including end-of-chapter exercises, a glossary of key terms, flash cards, and additional interactive activities.

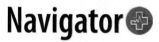

Navigator ✚

 ## Career Exploration

If you enjoyed learning about medications and the body in this chapter, you may want to explore the following career options:

- emergency medical technician (EMT)/paramedic
- medical assistant
- pharmacy technician

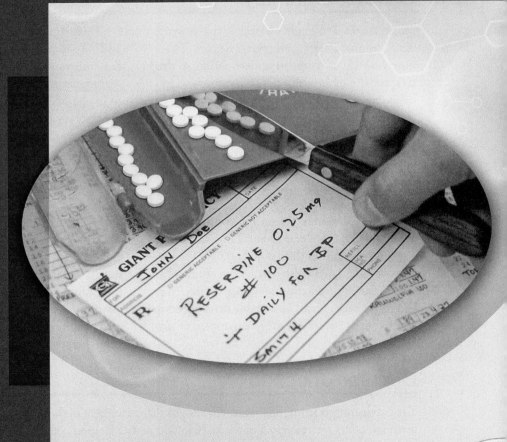

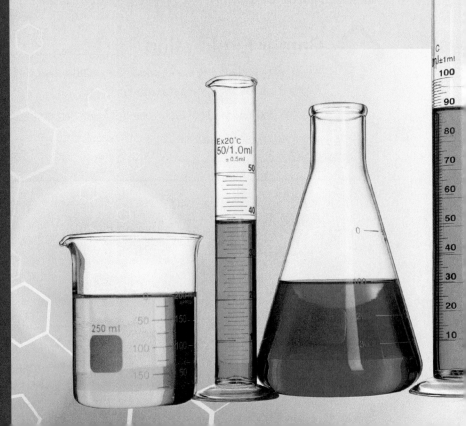

Pharmacology in the Practice Setting

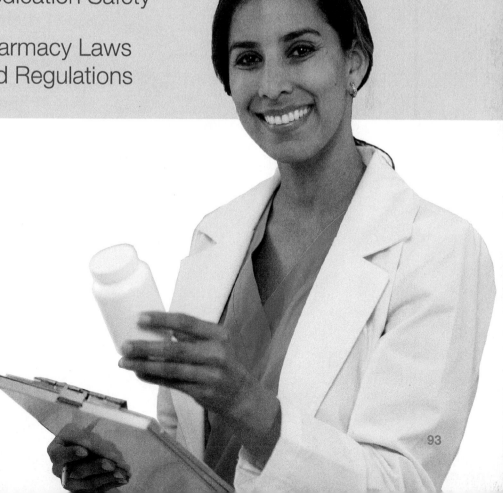

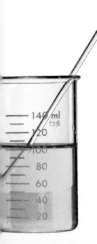

The Allied Health Professional

Pharm Facts

- The number of allied health professionals in the United States is twice the number of physicians and nurses combined.

- According to the US Bureau of Labor Statistics, the following allied health positions are projected to have the highest growth by 2022:
  - physical therapist (36%)
  - audiologist (34%)
  - dental hygienist (33%)
  - surgical technologist (30%)
  - medical laboratory technician (30%)
  - cardiovascular technologist/sonographer (30%)
  - medical assistant (29%)
  - magnetic resonance imaging technician (24%)
  - optician (23%)
  - dietitian (21%)

- The majority (63%) of allied health professionals receive their education at community colleges.

- An allied health professional who has achieved certification has many career advantages over one who has not. A certified professional is more marketable as a job applicant, is more likely to find a position at a nationally recognized or well-established healthcare facility, has a better opportunity to expand his or her scope of practice, and has the potential to earn a higher salary.

"I love being a physical therapist because of the positive impact I can make on the health and well-being of my patients. I have the opportunity to learn about my patients' lives, recognize what motivates them, discover their physical limitations, and design a rehabilitation program to get them back to the activities they desire. I also enjoy my role as a patient educator. Equipping patients with the knowledge and techniques they need to restore their mobility and manage their conditions promotes their independence as well as their quality of life."

—**David Filzen**, PT, CSCS
Physical Therapist

Learning Objectives

1 Differentiate between a health professional and an allied health professional.

2 List the two types of allied health professionals and their distinct roles in healthcare delivery.

3 Discover the various career positions that fall under the allied health umbrella.

4 Describe the personal qualities of a successful allied health professional.

5 State the education, training, and legal requirements of an allied health professional.

6 Define *scope of practice* and examine the general clinical and nonclinical responsibilities of an allied health professional.

7 Define *accreditation* and identify some of the major accreditation bodies in allied health.

8 Identify the factors that contribute to the growth of the allied health field.

Healthcare delivery has evolved tremendously in recent years. The traditional role of the physician as the authoritarian figure ordering and dispensing treatments and medications to a passive patient has changed. Today's patients are well versed in health topics because of easy accessibility to online information. As a result, they are taking more responsibility for their own health and wellness and are playing an active role in decisions regarding their treatments. This change can certainly be seen in the rising popularity of the patient portal, a web-based site that gives patients access to their health record, and the patient health record, a digital tool that allows patients to manage their health information.

The setting and delivery of healthcare services have also changed. Today, there is a decided shift from acute care services delivered in a medical facility, such as a hospital, to ambulatory care services delivered in urgent care, surgical, imaging, and other outpatient facilities. These ambulatory facilities provide services such as patient diagnosis, treatment, observation, and rehabilitation.

There has also been a paradigm shift in the delivery of health care by personnel, with a greater emphasis on the overall health and well-being of a patient and a team approach to patient care. As an allied health professional, you are part of this healthcare team and must have a good understanding of your role and responsibilities in this patient-centered approach.

Healthcare Team

Today's healthcare practices demand a vast body of knowledge and specialized skills that no one individual can possibly possess. To meet these expectations, healthcare professionals often implement a team approach to patient care, in which each specialist lends his or

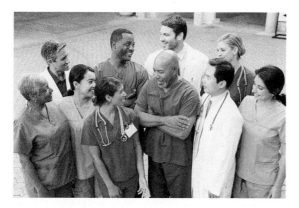

According to Dr. Kyu Rhee, former director of the Office of Innovation and Program Coordination at the National Institutes of Health, "A health care team is like a sports team. . . . It is essential to know the roles and responsibilities of each of the players and to have trust in one another. It is vital to have that team learn together and practice together so that when the game truly matters they can each play their best with trust and understanding leading to more positive outcomes."

her expertise to achieve patient treatment goals. This collaboration requires that specialists have a working knowledge of the following areas:

- other healthcare specialties and their roles in patient care
- the legal parameters of their position for the state in which they practice
- the scope of their position in the workplace setting
- health information technology systems
- pharmacology

Health Professionals and Allied Health Professionals

The **healthcare team** includes both health professionals and allied health professionals. A **health professional** is an individual who has been educated, trained, and state licensed to diagnose and/or treat the medical problems of patients whom they see on a routine basis. Health professionals include physicians, doctors of osteopathy, podiatrists, dentists, pharmacists, chiropractors, physician assistants, and nurse practitioners.

An **allied health professional** is an individual who has been educated, trained, and licensed and/or certified to provide a range of diagnostic, technical, therapeutic, and direct and indirect patient-care services. He or she also provides support services that are critical to other health professionals. According to the **Association of Schools of Allied Health Professions (ASAHP)**, an allied health professional "delivers services involving the identification, evaluation and prevention of diseases and disorders, dietary and nutrition services, and rehabilitation and health systems management."

Both health professionals and allied health professionals work in tandem to maintain the highest possible standards of professionalism in their communications, behaviors, and ethics to ensure patient safety and optimal patient outcomes. Research has also shown that a healthcare team approach results in lower **morbidity rates** (rates of disease incidence or prevalence in patients), lower **mortality rates** (death rates among patients), fewer patient hospitalizations, and lower healthcare costs.

Allied Health Professionals

In the United States, there are nearly 5 million allied health professionals, comprising nearly 60% of the healthcare work force. These professionals work in more than 200 distinct specialties in every part of the healthcare system—from large healthcare facilities such as hospitals and ambulatory clinics that support an extensive, diverse workforce to small specialty clinics that employ a select number of professionals. In these facilities, they work in nearly all departments, including radiology, cardiology, and surgery. Allied health personnel are also employed by laboratories, schools, creative arts studios, counseling centers, pharmaceutical and medical-equipment companies, and health technology firms.

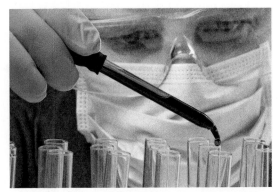

A medical laboratory technician works in a laboratory and often runs tests on patients' blood samples.

Types of Allied Health Professionals

Allied health professionals fall into two distinct categories: (1) technicians and assistants, and (2) technologists and therapists. **Allied health technicians and assistants** perform procedures and tasks behind the scenes under the guidance of technologists. Their post-secondary coursework is completed within a two-year period. The careers open to technicians and assistants are found in many specialties, such as medical laboratory technicians, occupational therapy assistants, pharmacy technicians, radiologic technicians, electrocardiography technicians, and ophthalmic assistants.

In the Know

According to the US Bureau of Labor Statistics (2014), almost half of the fastest-growing occupations are in allied health. These positions include personal care aides, home health aides, diagnostic medical sonographers, occupational therapy assistants and aides, physical therapy assistants and aides, and genetic counselors.

Allied health technologists and therapists are more involved in a patient's primary care and, therefore, require more intensive education and hands-on training. Individuals in these positions are responsible for assessment, diagnosis, creation of treatment plans, and evaluation of patients. Consequently, it is their obligation to implement safe, appropriate treatment plans and to monitor any potential adverse effects. In the allied health field, examples of technologists and therapists include neurodiagnostic technologists, nuclear medicine technologists, and physical therapists.

To view a listing of the many positions that are considered part of the allied health field, see Table 4.1.

Checkpoint 4.1

Take a moment to review what you have learned so far and answer these questions.

1. How do allied health professionals differ from health professionals?
2. What are the workplace settings that employ allied health professionals?
3. What are the two types of allied health professionals?

TABLE 4.1 | Allied Health Specialties

The allied health workforce comprises more than 200 specialties. Below is a sampling of some of these positions.

allergy technician
anesthesia technician
anesthesiologist assistant
apheresis technician
art therapist
athletic trainer
audiologist

behavioral health technician
behavioral specialist
blood bank technology specialist

cardiopulmonary rehabilitation
   specialist
cardiovascular and vascular
   interventional (CVI) technologist
cardiovascular perfusionist
cardiovascular technologist
case manager
certified bone densitometry
   technologist (CBDT)
certified clinical nutritionist
chemotherapy technician
clinical dietitian specialist
clinical immunology technologist
clinical laboratory scientist/
   technologist
clinical social worker
community health worker
computed tomography (CT)
   technician
cosmetic laser technician
cytogenetics technologist
cytotechnologist

dance therapist
dementia care specialist
dental assistant
dental hygienist
dermatology technician
diabetes educator
diagnostic medical scientist
diagnostic medical sonographer
dietitian

electrocardiogram (ECG) technician
electrologist
electrophysiology technician
emergency medical technician (EMT)
emergency room (ER) technician
endoscopy technician
environmental health officer/public
   health inspector

esthetician
exercise physiologist

genetic counselor

hand therapist
healthcare documentation
   specialist
healthcare language interpreter
health information administrator
health information technician
histotechnologist
HIV/AIDS counselor
home care assistant/aide
hospital occupational health and
   safety officer

intravenous (IV) pharmacy
   technician

kinesiotherapist

lactation consultant
laser hair removal technician
low vision therapist

magnetic resonance imaging (MRI)
   technician
marriage and family counselor/
   therapist
massage therapist
medical assistant
medical billing and coding
   specialist
medical dosimetrist
medical laboratory technician
medical laboratory technologist
medical office assistant
medical receptionist
medical transcriptionist
mental health counselor
music therapist

neurodiagnostic technologist
nuclear medicine technologist
nursing assistant

obstetric (OB) technician
occupational safety and health
   technician
occupational therapist
operating room (OR) technician
ophthalmic assistant

ophthalmic dispensing optician
ophthalmic laboratory technologist
ophthalmic laser technician
ophthalmic medical technologist
orientation and mobility (O&M)
   specialist
orthoptist
orthotist

pediatric occupational therapist
perioperative blood management
   technologist
pharmacy technician
phlebotomist
physical rehabilitation counselor
physical therapist (PT)
physical therapy (PT) assistant
positron emission tomography
   (PET) scan technician
prosthetist

quality control coordinator

radiation therapist
radiologic technologist
recreational therapist
registered dietetic technician
registered dietitian
registered nerve conduction
   studies technologist (RNCST)
renal dialysis technician
renal registered dietitian
renal social worker
research laboratory technician
respiratory therapist

social worker
sterile-processing technician
substance abuse counselor
surgical neurophysiologist for
   intraoperative neurophysiology
   monitoring
surgical technologist

urinalysis technician

weight consultant

Personal Qualities of Allied Health Professionals

Successful allied health professionals must possess a wide range of knowledge and skills and certain personal characteristics. They should have good critical thinking skills; a high degree of professionalism; effective communication skills; an aptitude for technology; and an awareness of and sensitivity to cultural and linguistic diversity.

Critical Thinking Skills

Critical thinking skills are important for all healthcare professionals. **Critical thinking** involves analyzing, evaluating, and applying information gathered through observation, experience, reflection, and reasoning to guide an individual's beliefs or actions. For allied health professionals, having expertise and knowledge is not enough. They must also use skills such as clarity, accuracy, consistency, relevance, sound reasoning, and fairness to solve problems and devise solutions. Healthcare personnel are required to think on their feet and address issues in the best interests of each patient. Oftentimes, the approach or solution must be initiated quickly and decisively.

Critical thinking also involves **self-direction**. For example, during a clinical visit, a medical assistant must anticipate the needs of the physician or other health professional by following a systematic approach when treating a patient who has diabetes. The medical assistant knows to ask the patient to remove his or her shoes so that a foot examination can be performed. In addition, the medical assistant follows a standard protocol of performing a finger stick to test the patient's blood glucose levels, preparing the blood sample for the laboratory, and arranging for the preparation and administration of medications. The medical assistant also gauges the patient's knowledge and ability to perform self-care measures in managing diabetes and provides support and informational materials as needed. Finally, the medical assistant ensures that the patient's medical record is updated accordingly. Performing these tasks allows the medical assistant to deliver a health status update to the health professional.

Developing critical thinking skills is a lifelong endeavor that must be practiced and nurtured. Allied health personnel can improve their critical thinking through observation of how other professionals handle certain situations, participation in preceptorships (see the "Preceptorship" section later in this chapter), and—simply—experience.

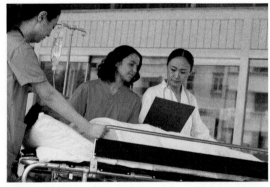

For emergency medical technicians, critical thinking and collaboration skills are put to the test during the golden hour, or the one-hour period following a traumatic injury in which prompt medical treatment may mean the difference between life and death.

Professionalism

Although allied health professionals have diverse roles in the healthcare setting, professionalism is one quality they have in common. **Professionalism** is defined as the conduct, aims (aspirations and intentions), and qualities that characterize a professional person. Appearance, attitude, work ethic, personal conduct, and ethics are all components of professional behavior.

Appearance

Allied health personnel work with other health professionals as well as patients, families, and caregivers. Therefore, projecting a professional appearance is important. All allied health personnel should check the **Policy & Procedures (P&P) manual** of their facility regarding personal appearance guidelines. These guidelines address clothing, jewelry, make-up, perfume, facial piercings, visible tattoos, and hair color. Healthcare facilities base their appearance guidelines on the regulations established by the Occupational Safety and Health Administration (OSHA). OSHA regulations protect both healthcare personnel and patients from the transmission of pathogens and exposure to hazardous drugs and chemicals.

Certain allied health positions have specific attire and appearance guidelines. Social workers, for example, may wear professional work attire. Operating room technicians, on the other hand, are required to wear **scrubs**. Chemotherapy and sterile compounding technicians must don **personal protective equipment (PPE)** and are not permitted to wear cosmetics, hair spray, perfume, artificial nails, or nail polish while performing their tasks. These substances can flake and compromise the aseptic environment. Chemotherapy and sterile compounding technicians must also remove any jewelry because these items can harbor microorganisms.

Commonsense guidelines dictate clean, neat clothing; close-toed shoes with nonskid soles; simple jewelry that does not impede work tasks; clean, modestly manicured nails; and light and natural make-up. In addition, many healthcare facilities prohibit the use of perfumes and colognes, which can trigger an allergic or respiratory reaction in some patients. Therefore, it is wise to avoid the use of any fragrance in the workplace. Clothing that emits a cigarette smell can also be a health hazard. Known as *third-hand smoke*, the residual contamination contained in a smoker's clothing is particularly harmful to infants and children and is offensive to others. Allied health workers must be cognizant of these odors when providing patient services.

Finally, allied health professionals should check their facility's P&P manual regarding the use of a photo identification (ID) badge. More than a dozen states have enacted legislation requiring all healthcare personnel to wear easily visible photo ID badges that state their name, title, hospital department, and license number (if applicable). With the movement toward a healthcare team approach to treating patients, the need for photo ID badges is becoming more apparent. These badges help patients and their families or caregivers identify the positions and/or licenses of the individuals who are providing patient care services. Requiring healthcare staff to wear photo ID badges also has the added benefit of increasing security in the workplace setting.

Work Wise

Prior to attending a job interview, an allied health professional should follow the appearance protocol that is common among healthcare facilities: good hygiene, including clean hair and nails; clean and well-fitting work attire; natural hair color (no brightly colored hair tints); close-toed shoes; and no visible tattoos or body piercings. "Dressing the part" during an interview increases an allied health professional's likelihood of getting the job.

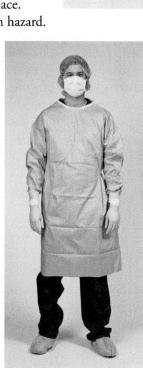

Allied health personnel, such as sterile compounding technicians, must don PPE to perform sterile compounding tasks. PPE includes clean shoe covers; a hair cover; a facemask; a clean, disposable gown; and sterile, powder-free gloves.

Attitude

Attitude is the overall emotional stance or disposition that a person adopts toward his or her duties, workplace personnel, and interactions with others. For allied health professionals, adopting a positive, caring attitude toward patients and their families or caregivers is important to establishing a trusting relationship. The ability to show compassion, actively listen to patients' concerns, and empathize with their conditions is also an important facet of healthcare provision.

Courteous words and phrases should also be used in every patient interaction. Allied health professionals should greet patients by name and exchange pleasantries before getting to the task at hand. Being respectful toward patients also means showing them dignity, paying attention to their needs, and recognizing that they are autonomous and have a voice in their health care.

Respect must also be shown to all employees who work in a healthcare facility because each individual has an important job to do that contributes to the overall care provided to a patient. The use of good manners and common courtesy will ensure professionalism in all interactions.

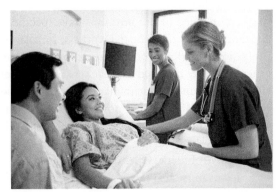

Showing compassion and listening to a patient's concerns are important qualities for an allied health professional to possess.

Work Ethic

A strong **work ethic** is mandatory for members of a healthcare team. Allied health professionals can project a strong work ethic by being punctual and reliable, demonstrating productivity, being detail-oriented, and showing commitment to a job well done. All health professionals have an absolute duty to provide the highest standard of care for their patients, which means that every individual must be able to trust their teammates to be present, on time, and engaged in the task at hand.

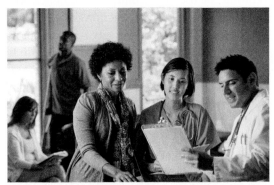

Healthcare team members must collaborate with the patient and with each other to devise a treatment plan that provides the optimal patient outcome.

Personal Code of Conduct and Ethics

Adopting a **personal code of conduct** based on high professional standards is an important quality for all healthcare professionals. Appropriate workplace behavior demands that an individual's personal life does not interfere with his or her work performance. An allied health professional must remain focused on delivering the highest standard of care to all patients. In light of that, personal phone calls, texting, and other non–work-related activities should be conducted during breaks to avoid lapses in concentration. These types of activities can be detrimental to the health and safety of patients.

Healthcare professionals must also follow a code of ethics that guides their behavior in the workplace. **Ethics** is the study of standards of conduct and moral judgment that outline the rights and wrongs of human conduct and behavior. In health care, ethical codes are based on the belief that a relationship of trust exists between a health professional or allied health professional and a patient. Consequently, it is important to put the good of the patient above any other consideration.

Ethics also plays a role in the protection of patient health information (see the section titled "Protection of Personal and Private Health Information" later in this chapter). Allied health personnel have a legal *and* ethical responsibility to maintain the security and privacy of a patient's sensitive medical information.

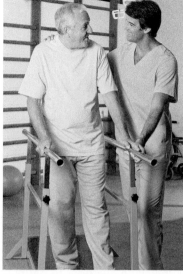

A healthcare professional should follow a high standard of professional conduct when interacting with a patient.

Work Wise

Healthcare personnel use several theoretical models as guideposts in ethical dilemmas. One model in particular—Dr. Bernard Lo's Clinical Model—focuses specifically on the dilemmas faced in the clinical arena. Other possible models for ethical guidance include the Seven-Step Decision Model (from *Ethics and the University* by Michael Davis) and The Five P's of Ethical Power (from *The Power of Ethical Management* by Kenneth Blanchard and Norman Vincent Peale). Allied health professionals may want to review these resources before entering clinical practice.

Kolb's Learning Styles

If you like outside-the-box learning activities and group work, as Divergers and Convergers do, develop a video that highlights attributes of professionalism. Some possible topics to cover in the video include appearance, attitude, work ethic, personal conduct, and ethics. Show your video in class and invite feedback on the presentation.

Communication Skills

Research shows that clear communication between healthcare professionals and patients is directly linked to greater patient satisfaction, improved patient adherence to medical advice and treatment plans, better clinical outcomes, and the adoption of preventive health behaviors. Clarity in communication is critical to patient safety as well. With that in mind, allied health professionals need to hone their verbal and written communication skills to ensure that these objectives are met.

Verbal Communication

Effective **verbal communication** in the clinical setting has four key elements: using precise language, actively listening, clarifying information through restatement, and establishing rapport and trust. During patient interactions, healthcare professionals should establish eye contact with the patient, speak at a moderate pace, and use precise language. They should also ensure that no physical barriers (such as computers or furniture) detract from the openness of the verbal interaction.

When gathering information from a patient, such as a health history, healthcare personnel should avoid asking close-ended questions that require a yes-or-no answer—for example, "Do you have regular headaches?" Rather, they should ask open-ended questions

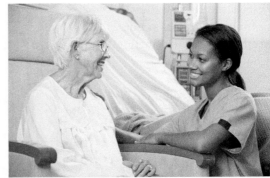

Maintaining eye contact during a patient interaction is important to establishing a trusting relationship.

that allow the patient to share more information about their allergies, past medical conditions, and treatments—for example, "Can you please describe your headache pain and how often you have headaches?" Allied health professionals should also ask follow-up questions to clarify issues and should summarize or restate parts of the conversation to confirm information.

At the heart of verbal communication is, of course, active listening. Allied health personnel must convey through nonverbal cues and body language that they are actively listening to a patient. Such **nonverbal communication** includes establishing eye contact, keeping an open posture, and leaning in toward the patient during the conversation. They should also acknowledge the patient's health concerns and feelings and provide feedback within the limitations of their position.

Written Communication

Allied health professionals must have good **written communication** skills as well, for they use these skills in their daily tasks. Whether completing medical record documentation; writing e-mail correspondence, memos, or letters; or taking phone messages, individuals must write clearly, accurately, and legibly. To ensure accuracy and promote professionalism, allied health professionals should proofread all written communications.

Technology Skills

Technology skills are utilized in every area of health care. Consequently, allied health professionals must have a good understanding of computers and computer applications as well as accurate data entry skills. Desktop computers, laptops, and tablets are commonly used in the workplace setting for patient documentation, electronic mail (e-mail), electronic prescribing (e-prescribing), and procedure and laboratory orders.

Many healthcare facilities are now using **electronic health records (EHRs)** to improve healthcare delivery. EHRs replace traditional paper medical records and allow patients' health information to be stored electronically and accessed by healthcare practitioners both inside and outside the facility. For healthcare professionals, the use of EHRs improves documentation, streamlines the workflow process, allows for immediate and improved access to patient information, and enhances communication among healthcare team members. For patients, the use of EHRs allows for continuity of care, improved outcomes, and the ability to manage some of their own health information with the **patient portal** that interfaces with the EHR system (see Figure 4.1).

FIGURE 4.1 Patient Portal

A patient portal interfaces with an EHR system and allows access to schedule an appointment, send a message, update health information, view laboratory results, and request prescription refills.

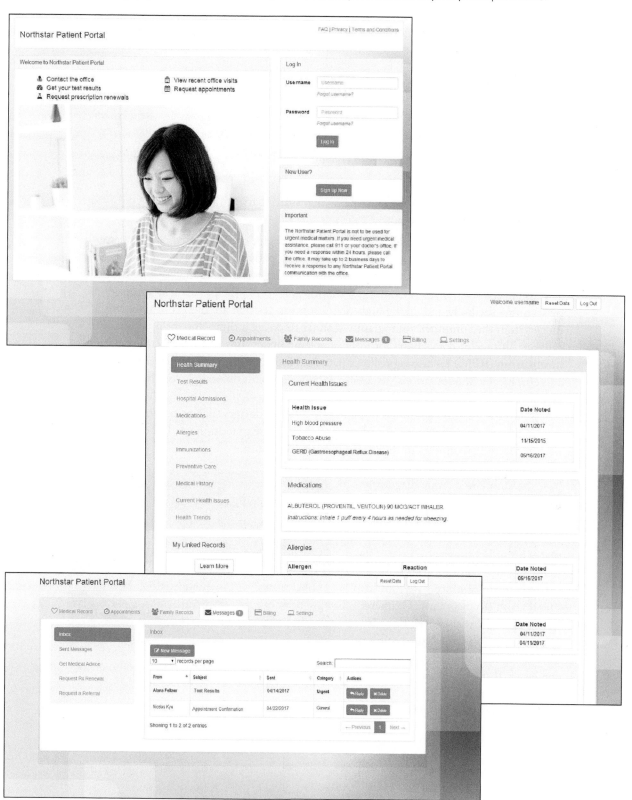

In addition to the EHR system, hospitals deploy several other types of information systems that health professionals and allied health professionals use to input, retrieve, and store information, including the following:

- *clinical decision support system (CDSS)*, which provides healthcare personnel with different tools—for example, computerized alerts, patient data reports, and clinical guidelines—to assist in decision-making

- *computerized provider order entry (CPOE)*, which allows healthcare prescribers to enter orders or instructions for a patient's treatment regimen

- *laboratory information system (LIS)* or *laboratory information management system (LIMS)*, which streamlines the laboratory workflow process

- *pharmacy information system (PIS)*, which streamlines the pharmacy workflow process

- *radiology information system (RIS)*, which stores patient radiologic data and images for radiology departments

Advances in technology have also allowed for integration of telemedicine, Bluetooth technology, and smartphone applications to assist in patient care.

Telemedicine uses computers and telecommunications lines to deliver health care at a distance, For example, Virtobot is a robotic system that helps perform autopsies by scanning the body and taking high-definition images that are then combined with images from the computed tomography scanner to create a three-dimensional image of a cadaver. This technology allows for forensic telemedicine consultations. **Remote patient monitoring (RPM) technology** allows patients who have high medical needs (geriatric and chronically ill populations) to send clinical data such as blood glucose levels to their physicians via a telehealth computer system.

Bluetooth technology allows implantable medical devices such as pacemakers and insulin pumps to send clinical data directly to healthcare practitioners. The device or a nearby controller connects to the Internet using Bluetooth.

Smartphone applications (apps) have the ability to capture diagnostic information. For example, AliveCor Mobile ECG heart app allows patients to detect heart arrhythmia. The patient places his or her fingers over the sensors, which communicate with a smartphone to produce a rhythm strip. The iHealth Wireless Pulse Oximeter allows a patient with a sleep disorder to wear a fingertip sensor linked to his or her smartphone that records blood oxygen levels. If the blood oxygen level is low, the patient may have sleep apnea. This device is also used by athletes to measure their pulse rate.

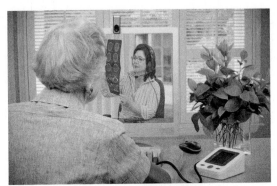

Telemedicine allows a patient to send a blood pressure measurement and pulse rate to his or her physician via a telecommunications line.

Awareness of and Sensitivity to Cultural and Linguistic Diversity

Regardless of healthcare specialty, all health and allied health professionals will interact with individuals from cultural and linguistic backgrounds that are different from their own. These individuals may be patients, family members or caregivers, or other healthcare personnel.

Differences in culture and language affect the ability to communicate effectively. Consequently, all healthcare professionals must achieve **cultural and linguistic competence**, or the adoption of attitudes and behaviors that enable personnel to deliver healthcare services tailored to the social, cultural, and linguistic needs of patients.

The importance of cultural and linguistic competence has increased in recent decades, as more than 20 million people in the United States now require language assistance to receive health care. In fact, Washington, California, Connecticut, New Jersey, and New Mexico have legislation in place that requires cultural- and linguistic-competence training for healthcare professionals. Many other states have this type of legislation pending as well. To achieve cultural and linguistic competence, healthcare personnel must do the following:

- educate themselves on the beliefs and practices of various cultures (including their own)

- treat patients with respect as defined by patients and their families

- communicate appropriately to patients, families, caregivers, and coworkers

- provide the best possible health care to patients from all cultural backgrounds

Navigator

To assist in acquiring these competencies, the Navigator+ learning management system that accompanies this textbook provides many suggestions for working in multicultural healthcare environments. These tips are intended to help maximize communication and build trust between healthcare professionals and the patients they serve.

Allied health students have the opportunity to specialize in linguistic competency by pursuing a career as a **healthcare interpreter**. This individual facilitates the communication between patients with limited or no English language proficiency and healthcare personnel. Interpreters may provide a verbal translation of healthcare documents, conduct phone calls or video chats to assist health professionals, and serve as liaisons during patient intake and discharge meetings.

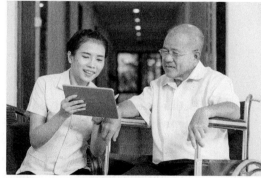

The Joint Commission requires hospitals to provide a healthcare interpreter for any patient who needs one.

 Checkpoint 4.2

Take a moment to review what you have learned so far and answer these questions.

1. What are the most important personal characteristics of an allied health professional? Name a minimum of three characteristics.

2. To present a professional appearance, what are some commonsense guidelines to follow?

3. What is the definition of *ethics*?

Educational, Training, and Legal Requirements of Allied Health Professionals

In the United States, more than 1,000 allied health programs enroll 30,000 students annually. These programs prepare students with the clinical and professional skills they need to be successful in allied health careers. Because each position has different educational, training, and legal requirements, allied health students must be sure to research the requirements for the state in which they plan to practice.

Educational Requirements

Because the allied health field encompasses many positions, the educational requirements differ widely. Technicians and assistants often must complete a two-year program at an accredited community college or technical school. Although this level of education is not required in many cases, career mobility will be very limited without it. The exact requirements for education depend on the regulations for the particular profession. Technologists and therapists are required to have at least a

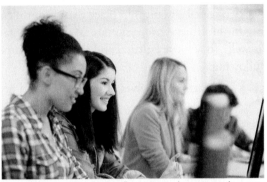

Formal education is the first step when pursuing an allied health career.

four-year degree from an accredited school in their particular field of study. They are also required to complete a certain number of hours of hands-on training before they can be fully licensed. This training—called a *preceptorship*, *practicum*, or *externship*—is discussed in detail later in this chapter.

Licensure, Registration, and Certification

Regulation of licensing and certification of the allied health professions takes place at the state level, rather than at the federal level. For any given allied health profession, there could be 50 different sets of rules and regulations governing it. However, there are usually more similarities than differences among states.

In addition, there is significant variation in the regulation of the various allied health professions even within a state. Some professions require licensure; others require registration or certification; still other professions are largely unregulated.

Licensure

Licensure is defined as the process by which the state board grants permission to an individual to engage in a given occupation upon finding that the applicant has attained the minimum degree of competency necessary to safeguard the public. Licensure is the strictest level of control, and frequently it requires a prescribed course of education from a certified educational institution as well as the successful completion of a licensure examination. Many states also require their licensed professionals to complete **continuing education** in their field in order to maintain a valid license.

Registration

The process of being enrolled on a list created by the state board that governs a particular occupation is known as **registration**. This list is used to safeguard the public. To qualify for registration, an allied health professional should be a graduate of an accredited institution, have completed the required number of clinical hours or work experience in the profession, and have met any other requirements his or her state requires. For example, a phlebotomy technician can qualify for the Registered Phlebotomy Technician certification examination by either graduating within the last 4 years from a phlebotomy program that includes at least 120 didactic clock hours (or as required by state law), or by completing at least 1,040 hours of work experience as a phlebotomy technician within the past 3 years, according to the American Medical Technologists certification agency. In addition, the applicant must have completed a minimum of 50 successful venipunctures and 10 successful skin punctures from human sources.

Certification

A **certification** is a recognition by a private board or professional organization that an individual has taken an assessment that demonstrates understanding of the qualifications of a particular profession. A less-stringent form of licensure, a certification indicates that a set of standards has been met. In some states, certification is voluntary; in other states, certification is part of the licensing process. For example, the requirements for a pharmacy technician vary from one state to the next. Many states require a certification, but not all states do. Some states require the successful completion of the Pharmacy Technician Certification Examination (PTCE) in order to obtain that certification. Some states require only completion of an accredited program, whereas others require only a high school education.

To demonstrate the variations in state laws for obtaining certification as a pharmacy technician, Table 4.2 provides the guidelines for certification of pharmacy technicians in three states: California, New York, and Texas.

In some programs, the level of certification and registration is one and the same. For example, a registered medical assistant (RMA) is registered with the American Medical Technologists, whereas a certified medical assistant (CMA) is certified through the American Association of Medical Assistants. The two credentials are recognized by employers as being equal.

TABLE 4.2 Certification Guidelines for Pharmacy Technicians in California, New York, and Texas

California	New York	Texas
• Pay the registration fee ($50) and submit an application to the state board of pharmacy • Hold a high school diploma or equivalent • Produce documents confirming identity • Produce a description of qualifications with supporting documentation • Undergo and pass a criminal background check	• No certification is required	• Complete the Texas application for registration • Pay the registration fee ($72 for a 2-year registration) • Have a high school diploma or equivalent • Pass the PTCE • Undergo and pass a criminal background check

Preceptorship

A **preceptorship** is required for allied health technologists and therapists who practice without supervision. To provide an authentic clinical experience, this hands-on training period pairs a student with an experienced practitioner (known as a **preceptor**) in a particular allied health field. A preceptorship is an opportunity for allied health students to apply what they have learned in the classroom to a clinical setting.

A preceptorship may take the form of an internship, externship, or residency, depending on the requirements of the profession. Typically, a preceptorship is required by a state law for licensure and takes place after the accredited coursework has been completed. For students, the mentoring experience provides them with valuable skills. It allows them to interact with patients and healthcare staff, use critical thinking skills, and complete real-world documentation. Preceptorships also help build confidence and reinforce the importance of good communication and professionalism skills in a career position.

For example, medical assistants who attend allied health programs accredited by the Commission on Accreditation of Allied Health Education Programs (CAAHEP) must participate in an unpaid, 160-hour preceptorship in an ambulatory care facility. For students who are pursuing a degree in physical therapy at a school accredited by the Commission on Accreditation in Physical Therapy Education (CAPTE), a minimum of 30 weeks of full-time clinical education is required.

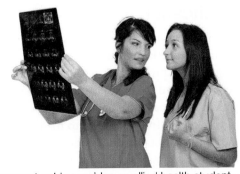

A preceptorship provides an allied health student—such as the magnetic resonance imaging intern (at right)—with real-world skills in a clinical setting.

 ## Checkpoint 4.3

Take a moment to review what you have learned so far and answer these questions.

1. What is the difference between *licensure* and *certification*?

2. What are the benefits of participating in a preceptorship?

Scope of Practice of Allied Health Professionals

Due to the variety of allied health positions, the roles and responsibilities of allied health professionals are diverse. Each particular profession has its own duties and scope of practice. The **scope of practice** defines the actions, procedures, and processes that a healthcare practitioner is allowed to perform based on federal, state, and local laws and regulations.

There are clear boundaries between the scope of practice of a health professional and that of an allied health professional. For example, a dental hygienist works as a member of a dental healthcare team to provide treatment, prevention, and education to patients. He or she updates the patient's health history; conducts radiographs, scaling, and polishing of teeth; provides fluoride treatments; performs patient teaching; and documents observations, patient complaints, and actions performed. However, the dentist diagnoses oral diseases, interprets radiographs and other diagnostic tests, creates a treatment plan, administers anesthetics, and performs oral surgeries.

Likewise, a medical assistant may prepare a written prescription for an ordering physician to sign or may be authorized to call in a telephone prescription to the pharmacy, but he or she cannot legally prescribe medications.

Consequently, all allied health personnel must do the following:

- understand the scope of practice for their specific allied health position and avoid performing any task for which they have insufficient educational or technical background

- be aware of the governing regulations concerning scope of practice for the state in which they practice and keep abreast of any changes in those regulations

- know their facility's P&P manual regarding scope of practice. An institution may *limit* the scope of practice for a particular position; however, the facility can never *exceed* the scope of practice for a particular position as defined by state law.

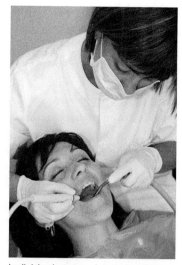

Individual states determine the scope of practice of a dental hygienist, including the services he or she is allowed to perform and the workplace settings in which to practice.

Ignorance of the law is not an acceptable defense when prohibited procedures are performed and/or when life-threatening critical errors occur as a result.

Professional Responsibilities

The professional responsibilities of allied health personnel involve clinical duties, non-clinical duties, or both. **Clinical duties** involve direct medical care of patients, whereas **nonclinical duties** consist of administrative tasks. Nonclinical duties are performed by all allied health professionals, with some personnel performing only these duties.

Clinical Duties

Some of the clinical duties of allied health professionals include interprofessional communication, direct patient care, clinical documentation, patient safety, protection of personal and private health information, and patient education.

Interprofessional Communication

As a member of a healthcare team, an allied health professional must learn to communicate effectively and accurately with other team members. The language used in the healthcare field is known as **medical terminology**. As mentioned in Chapter 1, the use of medical terminology dates back to the writings of Hippocrates and Galen, whose detailed classifications of disorders and their treatments influenced the lexicon of medical terms that are still in use today. It is not surprising then that 90% of these terms have Greek and Latin roots.

Most medical terms comprise word parts—a prefix, a root word or the combining form of a root word, and a suffix. A **root word** is just what the name implies: the word part that forms the basis—or *root*—of a term's meaning. Sometimes, a combining vowel is added to the root to connect it to a suffix or another root; this is called a **combining form**. A **prefix** is a word part that comes before the root or combining form and adds to or changes the meaning of the root. A **suffix** is a word part that follows the root and adds to or changes the meaning of the root. For example, the word parts *intra* (a prefix meaning "inside"), *muscul* (a root meaning "muscle"), and *ar* (a suffix meaning "pertaining to") combine to form the word *intramuscular*, which means "pertaining to the inside of a muscle." By building a vocabulary of these word parts, allied health professionals can master medical terminology. To help in this task, two features in this textbook, "Quick Study" and "Work Wise," focus on both verbal and written medical terminology that allied health professionals will encounter in the workplace. In addition, the Course Navigator learning management system that accompanies this textbook provides common root words associated with body systems, anatomy, and conditions.

COURSE NAVIGATOR

Allied health professionals must be able to recognize medical terms by sound and by sight. Precision in verbal and written communication is essential to preventing errors in patient care. Many words can have an entirely different meaning when they are mispronounced or misspelled. For example, confusing *hypotension* (low blood pressure) with *hypertension* (high blood pressure) could cause a medical error and perhaps endanger a patient. Great care must be taken to clearly pronounce medical terms, especially when speaking on the telephone, recording a voicemail message, or dictating for someone else to transcribe. In addition, allied health professionals must accurately record medical terminology in all communications with other healthcare workers and in patient documentation. Special attention must be paid to the names of medications because many drug names look and sound alike. For more information on the importance of precision in prescriptions and medication orders, see Chapter 5.

Healthcare professionals use medical terminology because it is an efficient method of communicating with each other across different medical settings, different medical specialties, and even across different languages. Use of this specialized language also ensures continuity of patient care and avoids medical and medication errors. By using the correct terminology, detailed information can be shared with just a few words.

Direct Patient Care

Allied health professionals deliver a variety of healthcare services to patients. Some individuals perform diagnostic tests that are used to guide a patient's treatment. For example, radiology technicians take X-rays; phlebotomy technicians take blood samples; medical laboratory technicians perform laboratory tests on tissue and fluid specimens; and electrocardiogram (ECG) technicians conduct cardiovascular tests to check for heart rhythm abnormalities. Other allied health professionals—for example, emergency medical technicians, pharmacy technicians, and renal dialysis technicians—prepare and/or administer medications. Still other allied health professionals, such as physical therapists, occupational therapists, exercise physiologists, and registered dietitians, provide restorative and rehabilitative care services that renew the health, well-being, and functioning of patients.

Medical assistants are unique in that they perform a broad range of healthcare services, depending on federal, state, and local laws. They may take vital signs and medical histories, assist a physician or other health professional during patient examinations,

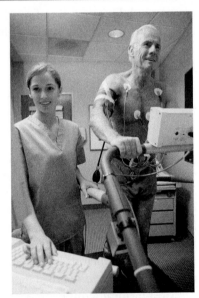

To perform a stress test, an ECG technician places electrodes on a patient's chest and asks the patient to walk on a treadmill. The electrodes are connected to a heart monitor that measures the heart's electrical activity.

collect and prepare laboratory specimens or arrange for laboratory services, administer immunizations, remove sutures, change dressings, and administer parenteral, oral, and topical medications.

Clinical Documentation

As a legal record of diagnosis and treatment, a patient's **medical record** is a conduit of information for members of a healthcare team. As such, accurate and truthful medical record documentation is the utmost personal responsibility of every allied health professional. With that in mind, all documentation should be recorded as soon as possible in order to capture the detailed information while it is still fresh in the mind of the healthcare professional.

As mentioned earlier, many healthcare facilities have implemented EHRs to maintain patients' health information. In some healthcare facilities, the EHR is linked to a **patient health record (PHR)**, a tool that enables a patient to plan and manage his or her own health information. A PHR provides a patient with a complete overview of his or her health history and current health status. With the advent of the **patient-centered approach** to health care, PHRs track and update healthcare information from any location, coordinate care among selected healthcare practitioners and facilities, avoid duplication of tests and procedures, and monitor prescriptions and allergies.

One aspect of the patient's medical record is the **medication profile**. Quite often, the allied health professional is responsible for updating the patient's medication profile. A complete list of all medications must be documented with each patient encounter to assist healthcare practitioners in safely and effectively providing treatment for the patient. When obtaining a **medication history**, allied health personnel must be sure to ask the right questions to obtain a complete list of every drug—both prescription and over-the-counter (OTC)—that the patient is taking. The use of alcohol, recreational drugs, and alternative medications such as herbal supplements must also be documented. The importance of having a thorough medication history cannot be overstated. Many patients are unaware of potentially serious drug interactions involving OTC drugs and may consider nonprescription drugs and vitamin supplements too insignificant to mention. In addition, all patients should be encouraged to use only one pharmacy when filling prescriptions so that pharmacy personnel can provide an additional check for safety.

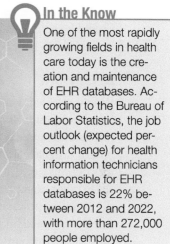

Accurate clinical documentation also dictates that an allied health professional inquire about drug allergies during each patient encounter. It cannot be assumed that the list of any allergies in the patient's medical record has not changed since the last visit. Allied health personnel should encourage the patient to report any allergic reaction he or she experienced since the last visit. An **allergic reaction** is a hypersensitivity reaction that may be mild or serious. Symptoms may include a skin rash, itching, hives, wheezing, difficulty breathing, or swelling of the eyes, lips, or tongue.

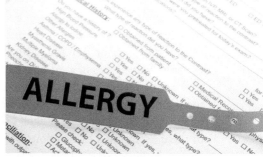

Allied health personnel must be sure to document a patient's allergies when updating a patient's medical record.

Finally, allied health professionals should ask the patient about any known food allergy or other type of allergy (such as latex). All allergies should be clearly documented in red ink (or font) in a conspicuous place in the patient's medical record.

Patient Safety

No matter what type of healthcare service is provided, an allied health professional must always consider **patient safety** in all aspects of patient care. Whenever a patient has an adverse reaction, has sustained an injury, or has been involved in a medication error, this event must be immediately documented and reported to the proper supervisor or to the attending physician. The patient should be observed and any reactions should be evaluated. Corrective steps should be performed as directed and documented. If a medication error has occurred, a staff meeting to discuss the case and evaluate the circumstances should be held as soon as possible so that steps can be taken to prevent similar incidents in the future. For additional information on medication safety, see Chapter 7.

Drug Handling and Storage

Patient safety also extends to the storage and special handling of medications. Allied health professionals should know which drugs require special handling. The storage instructions and any special handling directions for a drug can be found in that drug's official drug labeling information, which is often supplied with the drug. Special handling instructions can also be found on the website of the US Food and Drug Administration (FDA). For example, medications in the form of suspensions must be shaken twice in the handling process: The stock bottle of medication must be shaken by a pharmacy staff member prior to filling the patient's container, and the healthcare staff member or patient must shake the bottle prior to administration. This process is necessary because the contents of a suspension tend to settle to the bottom of the medication container. Failure to shake a suspension results in a variability in the dose of medication administered.

Another medication that requires special handling is nitroglycerin. Nitroglycerin tablets, which are used to treat angina, are stored in an amber-colored vial to shield the medication from sunlight, which degrades its potency. This vial has no safety cap, so that the patient can access the medication quickly when it is urgently needed.

Other oral dosage forms have special handling requirements as well. For example, the anticoagulant dabigatran (Pradaxa) is available in capsule form and must be stored in the container provided by the manufacturer to protect it from moisture. Because it decays rapidly, the drug must be discarded four months after the original container is opened.

Allied health professionals also need to know which drugs must be refrigerated and which drugs must be frozen. For example, blood products can be stored in the refrigerator or freezer, but insulin must be stored in the refrigerator only. Some types of eyedrops, such as the prostaglandin glaucoma treatment latanoprost (Xalatan), must also be refrigerated. Knowing the shelf life of these refrigerated medications is also important. For example, a vial of insulin, once opened, may be stored at room temperature for 28 to 30 days.

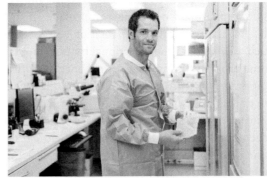

A blood bank technology specialist is responsible for testing blood and supervising the collection, separation, and storage of blood components, such as frozen plasma (shown here).

Protection of Personal and Private Health Information

The privacy of a patient's individually identifiable health information is protected by the **Health Insurance Portability and Accountability Act (HIPAA) of 1996**. A major goal of HIPAA is to ensure that each individual's **protected health information (PHI)** is properly secured while allowing the flow of health information needed to provide high-quality health care.

All of an individual's health information should be kept confidential, even the identity of an established patient. A form signed by the patient should be maintained in the patient's medical record. This form documents the patient's acknowledgment of the protection of his or her PHI provided by HIPAA. The patient may also give written permission authorizing other designated individuals access to his or her PHI. Allied health professionals must also exercise discretion when discussing any health information of an individual either with the patient or with another allied health professional or healthcare practitioner. These conversations must be discussed in a private setting and out of earshot of others.

Finally, allied health personnel should be aware that failure to adhere to HIPAA privacy regulations could result in costly fines, unemployment, and even imprisonment. The federal government may also impose certain obligations on a healthcare facility that is in violation of HIPAA regulations, such as staff training regarding privacy and confidentiality and audits of all releases of health information. (For more information on HIPAA, see Chapter 8.)

Patient Education

A key responsibility of allied health professionals is to assist in health literacy. As defined by the Patient Protection and Affordable Care Act of 2010, **health literacy** is "the degree to which an individual has the capacity to obtain, communicate, process, and understand basic health information and services to make appropriate health decisions." By sharing accurate and current information about treatments and medications with a patient or caregiver, allied health personnel can clarify any misunderstandings the patient or caregiver may have and encourage **patient adherence**, or the degree to which a patient follows medical advice. Optimal healthcare outcomes depend on patient adherence.

An allied health professional functions as a liaison between the prescriber and pharmacist and, as such, is entrusted to educate patients regarding the proper use of medications. Therefore, it is essential for all allied health personnel to have a working knowledge of commonly prescribed medications, OTC drugs, and herbal and alternative therapies. Patient education related to medication safety, including possible adverse reactions, must be documented. There can be legal consequences for the healthcare practitioner, pharmacist, or allied health professional who fails to provide and document patient education.

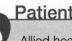

Patient Teaching

Allied health professionals should devote as much time as needed for patient teaching. Providing clear, precise instructions in a language that a patient can understand is critical. Using visuals and/or performing demonstrations are also effective strategies when giving instructions to a patient. After the patient-teaching session is finished, allied health professionals should ask the patient to restate the instructions or perform the procedure to verify understanding.

Allied health professionals must make special accommodations for patients with physical or mental disabilities to ensure that patient education is effective. Patients with visual impairment should have access to large-print or Braille materials. Patients who have hearing disabilities benefit from short, deliberate discourse and/or sign language. To accommodate patients with mental disabilities, healthcare personnel should include families and caregivers in patient education.

Finally, allied health professionals can direct patients to the websites of reputable organizations that can provide additional information about health and wellness topics:

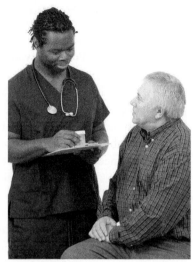

A key responsibility of an allied health professional is teaching a patient about each medication's dosage, side effects, contraindications, and cautions and considerations.

- US Food and Drug Administration (http://PharmEssAH.emcp.net/FDA)—for medication side effects, interactions, and contraindications

- Centers for Disease Control and Prevention (http://PharmEssAH.emcp.net/CDCvaccines)—for vaccine information and immunization schedules

- National Center for Complementary and Integrative Health (http://PharmEssAH.emcp.net/NIHsupplements)—for information regarding dietary and herbal supplements and their interactions with drugs

Nonclinical Duties

Some nonclinical duties performed by allied health professionals include the updating and filing of patient medical records, completion of insurance forms, patient billing and bookkeeping tasks, and inventory of supplies and equipment.

Updating and Filing of Patient Medical Records

Allied health professionals are responsible for updating the demographics, insurance data, and healthcare information for patients. Because most healthcare facilities have transitioned to electronic medical records (EMRs), the maintenance of these records involves data entry. For those facilities that still use the traditional paper medical records, allied health personnel are responsible for the updating and filing of the records. No matter what type of record is used, allied health personnel must receive training in the proper procedures for handling patient medical records and the importance of documentation accuracy.

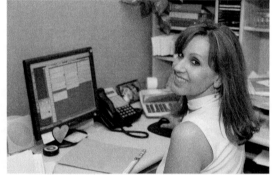

Among various other administrative tasks, a medical office assistant maintains patients' medical records.

Completion of Insurance Forms

Capturing of charges is a key responsibility of an allied health professional. Filling out the **super bill**, or **encounter form**, correctly with all healthcare procedures that were performed on the patient, as well as their corresponding codes, ensures that the appropriate charges are captured and billed to the patient's insurance company. These tasks are often performed by a medical billing and coding specialist. However, it is important for an allied health professional to understand how to complete an insurance form to ensure that there is no lost revenue due to missed charges.

Patient Billing and Bookkeeping Tasks

Proper billing and bookkeeping tasks have been simplified for allied health personnel due to the billing and bookkeeping software available to offices. Insurance claims may be filled out and submitted electronically, and insurance charges and reimbursement may be linked directly to a patient's chart, making bookkeeping more accurate. Payment needs to be entered into the patient's chart for correct posting to the patient's account. If there is a balance on the patient's account after the copayment and insurance payment, an allied health professional initiates the billing process. Outpatient facilities might contract a third party to handle all their billing and coding and insurance submission and reimbursement, whereas hospitals typically have a department designated to patient accounts.

Inventory of Supplies and Equipment

Facilities rely on allied health professionals to ensure that medical supplies are available for clinical procedures. Consequently, allied health personnel perform regular **inventory** checks to alert department managers or the central supply department when supplies need to be ordered. They also monitor the supplies in the patient examination rooms and replenish the stock as needed.

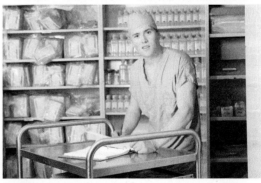

A sterile-processing technician manages the inventory of surgical supplies for a healthcare facility.

Kolb's Learning Styles

If you like to observe others (as Assimilators do) or apply what you learn from textbooks to real-life situations (as Convergers and Accommodators do), contact an allied health professional who works in a specialty that you are interested in pursuing as a career. Arrange a meeting with him or her to find out more about the clinical and nonclinical responsibilities that are inherent to the position.

Accreditation

Healthcare facilities and practitioners are regulated at the federal, state, and local levels on matters such as the provision of care, care settings, the licensing of health and allied health professionals, the privacy and security of patient information, and the protection of patients' rights. These organizations and practitioners are also subject to oversight by nongovernmental organizations through **accreditation** processes that monitor and evaluate performance based on best practices and other criteria. Some of these accreditation organizations include **The Joint Commission**, an agency that performs rigorous inspections of healthcare facilities to evaluate standard of care, and the **National Committee for Quality Assurance**, an organization that offers accreditation for health plans and provider organizations.

In addition to these organizations, certain professional agencies grant accreditation to healthcare programs that educate and train allied health professionals in general. Two examples of these accreditation agencies are the **Accrediting Bureau of Health Education Schools (ABHES)** and the **Commission on Accreditation of Allied Health Education Programs (CAAHEP)**. A discussion of these two organizations can be found in Chapter 8.

Other accrediting organizations in allied health are specific to the region and to a particular profession. The mission statements and policies of these organizations set standards; provide educational programs, resources, and training; and promote the professional development for their members. The primary way that these professional organizations help the allied health professions is through standardization of educational curriculum and training programs. Institutions that meet the standards set forth by the professional organization of a region—such as the New England Association of Schools and Colleges—are granted accreditation for the entire school (see Table 4.3). The professional organizations that are specific to an allied health profession—such as the Accreditation Council for Occupational Therapy Education—grant accreditation for individual programs (see Table 4.4). These organizations also provide information on the allied health specialty and its career path, education/training qualifications, and individual state practice requirements.

TABLE 4.3 Regional Accreditors

Regional Accreditor	Go To
Accrediting Commission for Schools: Western Association of Schools and Colleges	http://PharmEssAH.emcp.net/ACSWASC
Middle States Commission on Higher Education	http://PharmEssAH.emcp.net/MSCHE
New England Association of Schools and Colleges	http://PharmEssAH.emcp.net/NEASC
North Central Association of Colleges and Schools	http://PharmEssAH.emcp.net/NCA
Northwest Commission on Colleges and Universities	http://PharmEssAH.emcp.net/NWCCU
Southern Association of Colleges and Schools Commission on Colleges	http://PharmEssAH.emcp.net/SACSCOC

TABLE 4.4 Accreditation Organizations for Certain Allied Health Specialists

Allied Health Specialist	Accreditation Organization(s)
Allergy technician	AAAAI: American Academy of Allergy, Asthma & Immunology
Anesthesia technician	CAAHEP: Commission on Accreditation of Allied Health Education Programs
Anesthesiologist assistant	COA-NA: Council on Accreditation of Nurse Anesthesia Educational Programs
Athletic trainer	CAATE: Commission on Accreditation of Athletic Training Education
Audiologist	CAA: Council on Academic Accreditation in Audiology and Speech-Language Pathology of the American Speech-Language-Hearing Association (ASHA)
Blood bank technology specialist	AABB: American Association of Blood Banks
Cardiovascular sonographer	CAAHEP: Commission on Accreditation of Allied Health Education Programs
Cardiovascular technologist	CAAHEP: Commission on Accreditation of Allied Health Education Programs
Clinical diabetes educator	AADE: Diabetes Education Accreditation Program of the American Association of Diabetes Educators
Clinical immunology technologist	AAAAI: American Academy of Allergy, Asthma & Immunology
Computerized tomography (CT) technician	JRCERT: Joint Review Committee on Education in Radiologic Technology
Dental assistant	CODA: Commission on Dental Accreditation
Dental hygienist	CODA: Commission on Dental Accreditation
Diagnostic medical sonographer	CAAHEP: Commission on Accreditation of Allied Health Education Programs
Dietitian/nutritionist	CADE: Commission on Accreditation for Dietetics Education
Electrocardiogram (ECG) technician	CAAHEP: Commission on Accreditation of Allied Health Education Programs
Emergency medical technician (EMT)/paramedic	CAAHEP: Commission on Accreditation of Allied Health Education Programs
Genetic counselor	COAMFTE: Commission on Accreditation for Marriage and Family Therapy Education
Healthcare documentation specialist	CAHIIM: Commission on Accreditation for Health Informatics and Information Management Education
Healthcare language interpreter	CCHI: Certification Commission for Healthcare Interpreters
Health information technician	CAHIIM: Commission on Accreditation for Health Informatics and Information Management Education
Histotechnologist	NSH: National Society for Histotechnology
Intravenous (IV) technician	ACPE: Accreditation Council for Pharmacy Education
Lactation consultant	IBLCE: International Board of Lactation Consultant Examiners
Magnetic resonance imaging (MRI) technician	JRCERT: Joint Review Committee on Education in Radiologic Technology
Massage therapist	COMTA: Commission on Massage Therapy Accreditation
Medical assistant	ABHES: Accrediting Bureau of Health Education Schools CAAHEP: Commission on Accreditation of Allied Health Education Programs
Medical billing and coding specialist	AAPC: American Academy of Professional Coders AHIMA: American Health Information Management Association
Medical laboratory technician	ABHES: Accrediting Bureau of Health Education Schools NAACLS: National Accrediting Agency for Clinical Laboratory Sciences
Medical transcriptionist	AHDI: Association for Healthcare Documentation Integrity AHIMA: American Health Information Management Association
Nuclear medicine technologist	JRCERT: Joint Review Committee on Education in Radiologic Technology
Occupational therapist	ACOTE: Accreditation Council for Occupational Therapy Education
Occupational therapy assistant	ACOTE: Accreditation Council for Occupational Therapy Education

Allied Health Specialist	Accreditation Organization(s)
Orthotist/prosthetist	ABC: American Board for Certification in Orthotics, Prosthetics & Pedorthics
Perfusionist	ABCP: American Board of Cardiovascular Perfusion
Pharmacy technician	ACPE: Accreditation Council for Pharmacy Education
Phlebotomist	NAACLS: National Accrediting Agency for Clinical Laboratory Sciences
Physical therapist	CAPTE: Commission on Accreditation in Physical Therapy Education
Radiology technician	JRCERT: Joint Review Committee on Education in Radiologic Technology
Recreational therapist	CAAHEP: Commission on Accreditation of Allied Health Education Programs CARTE: Committee on Accreditation of Recreational Therapy Education
Rehabilitation counselor	CORE: Council on Rehabilitation Education
Respiratory therapist	CoARC: Commission on Accreditation for Respiratory Care
Surgical technician	ABHES: Accrediting Bureau of Health Education Schools CAAHEP: Commission on Accreditation of Allied Health Education Programs

Career Outlook for Allied Health Professionals

The demand for allied health professionals is growing rapidly. According to ASAHP, jobs in the industry will grow from 15.6 million in 2010 to 19.8 million by 2020. This growth can be attributed to a number of factors:

- technologic advances in health care
- new diagnostic and treatment methods that are providing opportunities for specialists
- changes in health information management
- expansion in healthcare coverage as a result of the Patient Protection and Affordable Care Act
- aging of the US population
- increased prevalence of chronic health conditions

Not only will the allied health workforce be expanding, but also the scope of practice of its members. Allied health professionals will play a larger role in patient care and education as healthcare delivery shifts to ambulatory and home-based settings. That increased responsibility underscores the importance of all allied health students to be educated, trained, and credentialed (having licensure, certification, and registration) before entering clinical practice and to actively participate in continuing education throughout their careers.

 ## Checkpoint 4.4

Take a moment to review what you have learned so far and answer these questions.

1. What clinical and nonclinical responsibilities are fulfilled by allied health professionals? Describe a minimum of three clinical duties and three nonclinical duties.

2. What types of information must an allied health professional obtain from a patient in order to have a thorough medication history?

3. What is *health literacy*?

Chapter Review

Chapter Summary

As healthcare services shift from acute care facilities, such as hospitals, to ambulatory or outpatient facilities, a healthcare team approach has become the norm. A healthcare team includes both health professionals and allied health professionals. A health professional is an individual who has been educated, trained, and state licensed to diagnose and/or treat the medical problems of patients. An allied health professional is an individual who has been educated, trained, and licensed and/or certified to provide a range of diagnostic, technical, therapeutic, and direct and indirect patient-care services. There are more than 200 allied health specialists, and they are employed in a variety of settings, including hospitals, ambulatory care facilities, clinics, laboratories, schools, creative arts studios, counseling centers, pharmaceutical and medical equipment companies, and health technology firms.

Allied health professionals fall into two distinct categories: (1) technicians and assistants, and (2) technologists and therapists. Allied health technicians and assistants typically attend two-year postsecondary programs and work under the guidance of technologists. Allied health technologists and therapists require more intensive education and hands-on training and are more involved in a patient's primary care.

Certain personal qualities lend themselves to success as an allied health professional. These qualities include good critical thinking skills, self-direction, a high standard of professionalism (evident in appearance, attitude, work ethic, and personal code of conduct and ethics), good verbal and written communication skills, an aptitude for technology, and an awareness of and sensitivity to cultural and linguistic diversity.

Educational, training, and legal requirements for allied health professionals typically include graduation from a two-year accredited community or technical school and the completion of a preceptorship. Licensing, registration, and certification requirements vary from state to state.

Although there is much variance among allied health professions, responsibilities often include both clinical and nonclinical duties. Clinical duties involve interprofessional communication, direct patient care, clinical documentation, patient safety, drug handling and storage, protection of personal and private health information, and patient education. Nonclinical duties include the updating and filing of patient medical records, completion of insurance forms, patient billing and bookkeeping tasks, and inventory of supplies and equipment.

Healthcare facilities and practitioners are regulated at the federal, state, and local levels on the provision of care, care settings, the licensing of health and allied health professionals, the privacy and security of patient information, and the protection of patients' rights. Accreditation of healthcare facilities may be granted by several nongovernmental agencies including The Joint Commission and the National Committee for Quality Assurance. Other accrediting organizations in allied health are specific to the region and to a particular profession.

Chapter Checkup

The Navigator+ learning management system that accompanies this textbook offers many opportunities to help you master chapter content, including end-of-chapter exercises, a glossary of key terms, flash cards, and additional interactive activities.

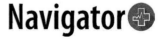

 Career Exploration

If you enjoyed learning about the allied health professions in this chapter, you may want to choose one of the positions in Table 4.1 to explore.

Prescriptions and Medication Orders

Pharm Facts

- According to the IMS Institute for Healthcare Informatics, US residents filled 4.3 billion prescriptions and spent $374 billion on medications in 2014.

- Approximately 35,000 abbreviations, acronyms, and symbols are used in pharmacy and medicine.

- Nearly 75% of individuals in the United States admit that they do not take their prescription drugs as directed. They provide the following reasons for their lack of medication therapy adherence:
  - They forgot to take the drug.
  - They did not fill the prescription they were given.
  - They stopped taking the drug before completing the regimen.
  - They took less than the recommended dosage to avoid side effects.
  - They took less than the recommended dosage to save money.

- According to CASAColumbia, an addiction-research organization, women are 50% more likely than men to obtain a controlled substance prescription from a physician's visit, despite being given the same diagnosis. Women are also more likely than men to become addicted to prescription drugs.

"Prior to my current role as an educator, I worked as a pharmacy technician. As a technician, I always had the mind-set that I was the "eyes and ears" of the pharmacist. I made sure that I was knowledgeable of the medication-filling process and potential drug interactions. Having that field experience underscored the importance of ensuring that students in my pharmacy technology program have the skill set to correctly interpret, process, and fill medication orders. As I look at my students from the time they start the program until their completion, I take pride in knowing that I have prepared them for success in the workplace setting."

—**Keith M. Binion**, BS, CPhT
Associate Dean of Pharmacy
Technology

Learning Objectives

1 Distinguish between a prescription and a medication order.

2 Identify the various types and components of prescriptions and medication orders.

3 Understand common medical abbreviations, acronyms, and symbols used in prescriptions and medication orders.

4 Identify the challenges of reading prescribers' orders.

5 Describe advantages and disadvantages of using a computerized provider order entry system.

6 Understand the information on a prescription medication label.

The prescribing, dispensing, and administration of medications are routine tasks in healthcare facilities. Although only health professionals such as physicians, dentists, physician assistants, nurse practitioners, and veterinarians can legally prescribe medications, allied health professionals are involved in the dispensing, administration, and documentation processes of prescription therapy. Depending on state practice regulations and institutional protocol, allied health professionals may be asked by physicians or other health professionals to call a pharmacy to order a new prescription for a patient or to request refills, or they may be asked to read a prescription or medication order and then administer a medication to a patient who is still in the practitioner's office. Under physicians' orders, allied health professionals may also be asked to dispense medication samples to patients during office visits. Still other allied health professionals may be involved in documenting the administration of drugs to patients.

In light of those responsibilities and in order to protect patient safety, all allied health professionals should be familiar with the types and components of prescriptions and medication orders, the lexicon of pharmacy terms and abbreviations, and the interpretation of drug labels.

Prescriptions

A **prescription** is an order of medication for a patient that is issued by a physician or another licensed healthcare prescriber, such as a nurse practitioner or a dentist, for a valid medical condition. Prescriptions are written for patients and are typically relayed from physicians' offices to pharmacies for dispensing to patients.

Types of Prescriptions

Health professionals use several different prescribing methods including written prescriptions, faxed prescriptions, telephone prescriptions, e-prescriptions, and controlled substance prescriptions.

Quick Study

The word *prescription* comes from the Latin word *praescriptus*, with the prefix *pre–* meaning "before" and the root word *script* meaning "written." Thus, the word *prescription* means "to write before," alluding to the fact that an order must be written down before a medication is prepared.

Written Prescription

A **written prescription** is recorded by a licensed health professional on a preprinted form bearing the name, address, and telephone and fax numbers of the prescriber; information about the patient; the date; and the medication prescribed. Sometimes, an allied health professional may complete the prescription for a prescriber, but only the prescriber can indicate through his or her signature that the prescription information is accurate and appropriate for the patient. A written prescription is typically given to the patient who then submits the form to a pharmacist for filling.

Faxed Prescription

A **faxed prescription** is written by a prescriber and then faxed to the appropriate pharmacy. This order contains the necessary demographic, prescriber, and medication information to fill the prescription. Faxed orders are entered into the patient's medication profile by a pharmacy technician and then verified by a pharmacist. Allied health professionals should be sure to place a faxed order into the patient's medical record.

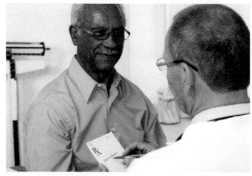

A physician or other healthcare practitioner who dispenses written prescriptions must prevent patient access to prescription pads. Easy access to prescription pads promotes drug diversion.

Telephone Prescription

A **telephone prescription** is phoned into a pharmacy. In most states, only a pharmacist may take verbal prescriptions over the telephone. Once the pharmacist transcribes the order into a written prescription and verifies its accuracy, a pharmacy technician can enter the information into the computerized patient profile.

E-prescription

An **electronic prescription (e-prescription)** is transmitted electronically from a prescriber to a pharmacy, typically via an examination room personal computer or from a handheld device such as a tablet or smartphone (see Figure 5.1). E-prescriptions have become the most common prescribing method for healthcare practitioners. For prescribers and healthcare personnel, e-prescriptions streamline the prescription-filling process, improve billing, minimize the potential for prescription forgeries, and reduce medication errors. For patients, e-prescriptions increase accuracy, improve safety, and decrease filling wait times.

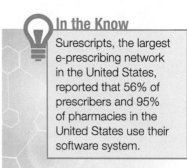

Controlled Substance Prescription

A **controlled substance prescription** must follow some specific regulations for delivery. Controlled substances in Schedules III–V are most frequently written, faxed, or communicated verbally. In most cases, prescriptions for Schedule II controlled substances are delivered as written prescriptions. There are a few exceptions. Schedule II prescriptions may be faxed for patients in hospice care or for patients who reside in long-term

FIGURE 5.1 E-prescription

A typical electronic health record (EHR) system has an e-prescription (e-Rx) feature that enables the system to electronically submit prescriptions to pharmacies. This figure shows the eRx screen in Paradigm Education Solutions' EHR Navigator.

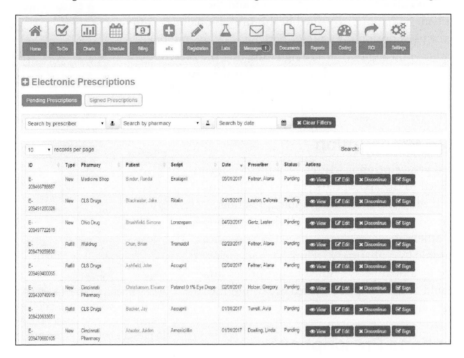

care facilities. In an emergency, a prescriber can call in a Schedule II prescription for any patient, as long as the prescriber follows up by sending a written prescription to the pharmacy within seven days. This seven-day period is allowed by federal law; however, some states have established a shorter period for a follow-up written prescription. Generally, these prescriptions provide only several days of a medication.

In the Know

Many states now require that prescriptions for controlled substances be written on tamper-resistant prescription pads (TRPPs) to eliminate forgeries. In addition, the Centers for Medicare & Medicaid Services require that all Medicaid prescriptions be written on TRPPs.

Federal law now also allows electronic transmission of controlled substance prescriptions (Schedules II–V). The law stipulates that electronically transmitted prescriptions for controlled substances are valid only if both the prescriber and the pharmacy that fills the prescription use software that is compliant with the security requirements outlined in the Electronic Prescriptions for Controlled Substances (EPCS) program of the US Drug Enforcement Administration (DEA). When such a prescription is transmitted, the pharmacist sees an EPCS logo appear on the computer screen that verifies the validity of the prescription. Some pharmacies and physicians' offices do not yet have the software required to transmit these prescriptions.

Components of a Prescription

Regardless of how prescriptions are transmitted, they must contain the same components (see Figure 5.2). Because allied health professionals may be involved in the interpretation, communication, or distribution of prescriptions, they must have a good understanding of these components.

FIGURE 5.2 Components of a Prescription

All prescriptions should be legible, written in ink (if handwritten), and include a leading zero before any number that is less than one (in this case, 0.5 mg). If appropriate, the prescription should also include the indication (in this case, *anxiety*).

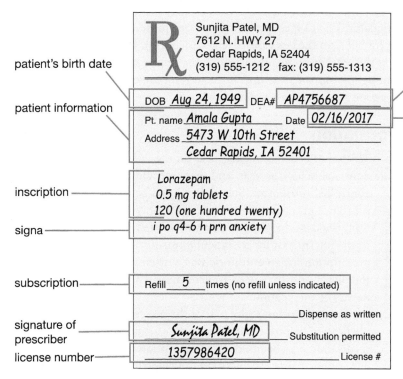

patient's birth date

patient information

Sunjita Patel, MD
7612 N. HWY 27
Cedar Rapids, IA 52404
(319) 555-1212   fax: (319) 555-1313

DOB _Aug 24, 1949_   DEA# _AP4756687_

Pt. name _Amala Gupta_   Date _02/16/2017_

Address _5473 W 10th Street_
Cedar Rapids, IA 52401

inscription

Lorazepam
0.5 mg tablets
120 (one hundred twenty)

signa

i po q4-6 h prn anxiety

subscription

Refill __5__ times (no refill unless indicated)

signature of prescriber

Sunjita Patel, MD

license number

1357986420

DEA number for controlled drug and insurance

date of prescription

Dispense as written

Substitution permitted

License #

Patient Information

A prescription must contain the patient's birth date, which is used by the pharmacy to distinguish between patients with the same name and to bill the patient's insurance provider. Knowing the patient's age also helps the pharmacist evaluate the appropriateness of the drug, its quantity, and the dosage form prescribed, thus minimizing medication errors. A prescription must also have the patient's first and last names (initials are not acceptable) as well as the patient's address and telephone number, which are needed for patient records.

Prescriber Information

The name, address, and telephone number of the prescriber should appear on a prescription but are not required. Other prescriber identification information, such as a **National Provider Identifier (NPI) number** and a **US Drug Enforcement Administration (DEA) number**, may also be included on a prescription. An NPI number is a 10-digit, unique identification number for healthcare providers. This number is required by the Health Insurance Portability and Accountability Act (HIPAA) for all administrative and financial healthcare transactions. A DEA number gives a prescriber the authority to write a prescription for a controlled substance; this number must appear on every

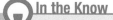

In the Know

The Rx symbol comes from the Latin word *recipere*, meaning "to take," and was first seen in the ancient manuscripts of the Roman Empire. Some theories claim that it refers to the Eye of Horus, an Egyptian symbol for protection and good health. Other theories state that the Rx symbol is derived from the ancient symbol for the Roman god Jupiter, upon whom early inhabitants called for protection from illness and disease. The written symbols for both the Eye of Horus and the god Jupiter bear a striking resemblance to the Rx symbol.

controlled substance prescription. Sometimes, the DEA number of the prescribing physician is handwritten (rather than preprinted) on a paper prescription to prevent forgeries.

The signature of the prescribing physician must be present on a prescription. For a paper prescription, the signature must be in ink. An electronic signature may be utilized on a faxed prescription for all medications except for controlled substances. In many states, a prescriber can use the signature line to specify that a pharmacy must dispense the brand-name version of a drug (rather than the less expensive generic form). In some states, there are two signature lines at the bottom of the prescription: one stating *dispense as written*, or *DAW*, and the other stating *substitution permitted*. If the *dispense as written* line is signed, then substitution of a generic equivalent is not permitted.

Medication Information

The date a prescription is written or ordered must appear on the document. Prescriptions for most medications are only usable for one year, and there are additional restrictions on controlled substances. Schedule III and Schedule IV controlled substance prescriptions are usable for only six months. In addition, the date the prescription was written may be important to the pharmacist for therapeutic reasons. For example, if the prescription for an antibiotic was written several weeks ago, the pharmacist may need to determine whether the patient still needs the medication.

The **inscription** is the part of the prescription that lists the medication prescribed, including the strength and amount. A medication may be listed on a prescription using a brand name or a generic name. As discussed in Chapter 2, a given drug (i.e., one with a particular generic name) may be marketed under various brand names. For example, Prinivil and Zestril are two brand names under which the generic drug lisinopril is marketed by pharmaceutical companies. Generic drugs are often less expensive than brand-name drugs and are often automatically substituted for brand-name drugs in the pharmacy software under regulations now existing in every state. If a prescription for a brand-name drug is filled with a generic equivalent, then the name, strength, and manufacturer of the generic substitution may be included on the dispensed medication container label.

Work Wise

If needed, an allied health professional can always look up a provider's NPI number on the NPI registry website at http://PharmEssAH .emcp.net/NPIRegistry.

Quick Study

The term *signa* comes from the Latin verb *signare*, meaning "to mark, write, or indicate." The signa is the section of the prescription that tells the patient how to use the medication.

The **signa** (commonly referred to as "the sig") is the part of the prescription that communicates the directions for use. This information is transferred from the prescription onto the label that is placed on the medication container for patient use.

The **subscription** is the part of the prescription that lists the instructions to the pharmacist about dispensing the medication, including compounding instructions, labeling instructions, information about the appropriateness of dispensing drug equivalents, and refill information. A **refill** is an approval by the prescriber to dispense the medication again without requiring a new prescription. If the refill section on the prescription is left blank, the prescription cannot be refilled. The words *no refill* (sometimes abbreviated *NR*) will appear on the medication container label, and *no refill* will be entered into the patient's record. Even if the refill blank on the prescription indicates a *prn* (or "as needed") order, unlimited duration is not allowed. Most pharmacies and state laws require at least yearly updates on *prn* (also written *PRN*) prescriptions. Some allied health professionals may be charged with processing patient refill requests, duties that would include obtaining signatures from prescribers and faxing the completed forms.

Medication Order

A **medication order**—also referred to as a *med order*, *medical order*, *physician order*, or *medication administration record (MAR)*—is a set of instructions given by a prescriber that specifies medications for an inpatient at a hospital or a resident of a long-term care facility. Medication orders are typically relayed within the healthcare facility to the on-site pharmacy.

Medication orders may be given verbally, written, or transmitted electronically. Written and electronic orders are generally preferred because there is a greater likelihood of medication errors when an order is given verbally. In many facilities, medication orders are entered directly into the computer by a prescriber. These orders communicate patient care directives to all members of the healthcare team. In addition to delivering instructions to the pharmacy, medication orders may also provide directions for laboratory, radiology, dietary, physical therapy, and other departments within a healthcare facility. However, some smaller facilities continue to house medication orders within paper medical records.

> **Work Wise**
>
> An allied health professional may be permitted to take a verbal medication order, depending on state regulations and the policies of the healthcare facility in which he or she practices. If so, it is best practice to read the verbal order back to the prescriber, spell out the name of the medication, and document the order in the patient's record immediately.

Types of Medication Orders

There are several types of medication orders, including an admission order, a daily order, a single order, a stat order, a PRN order, a standing order, and a discharge order. These orders are discussed in the following sections.

Admission Order

An **admission order** is written by a physician upon patient admission to a hospital (see Figure 5.3). The order may be written in an emergency department or in a patient's room. This type of medication order may contain drugs prescribed and taken before admission; suspected diagnoses; requests for laboratory tests or radiology examinations; instructions for the nursing staff; medication orders, including the notation of drug allergies; and a patient's dietary requirements.

Daily Order

A **daily order** is an order for a medication to be administered regularly following the same instructions until the prescriber stops the order (see Figure 5.4). Typically, a physician or other health professional examines a patient on a daily basis, but this frequency varies according to patient need. Critically ill patients may be examined several times a day. Patients may also be seen by numerous healthcare practitioners, according to their particular health issues. Every time a practitioner examines a patient, new orders, or changes to existing medication orders, may be written.

Single Order

A **single order** is a one-time order that is administered at a specified time. For example, an order for medication to be given to a patient before surgery or another medical procedure is considered a single order.

FIGURE 5.3 Admission Order

A physician typically creates an admission order after examining a newly admitted patient.

PHARMACY

B 427687

IN DOSAGE FORM AND THERAPEUTIC ACTIVITY MAY BE ADMINISTERED UNLESS CHECKED

Patient Information Below

START EACH NEW SERIES OF ORDERS BELOW

Check one: (FOR NEW PATIENTS OR CHANGE IN STATUS)

❑ OBSERVATION: short stay expected

❑ Admit – in patient; longer stay expected Height: 5′3″ Weight: 251

Diagnosis: (L) Leg DVT, Fe deficiency anemia

Activity: Bed rest c̄ bedside commode × 24° then ad lib

Diet: cardiac

Allergies: NKDA Reactions:

(1) Admit to Medicine – Dr. Galangal

(2) Condition – stable

(3) Vitals per routine

(4) Labs – PT/INR q AM – call c̄ results of PT/INR tonight
- guaiac stools × 3
- Fe/Ferritin next lab draw

(5) IV – HL flush q shift

NURSE'S SIGNATURE DATE TIME

ID#: S1008994566
Name: Hayashi, Amy
DOB: 08/24/1950
Room: 420
Dr.: Rashmi Galangal

PHARMACY

B 427687

START EACH NEW SERIES OF ORDERS BELOW

(6) Meds – Lovenox 1 mg/kg SQ q 12
- Coumadin 10 mg PO tonight × i dose
- Fe-Tinic 150 mg PO b.i.d.
- Vicodin 1–2 PO q6h prn
- Colace 100 mg PO b.i.d. – hold per loose stool
- LOC prn
- Benadryl 50 mg PO qHS prn insomnia

(7) Call per acute changes

(8) Nutrition consult re: vitamin K diet

Dr. Galangal

NURSE'S SIGNATURE DATE 11/16/2017 TIME

ID#: S1008994566
Name: Hayashi, Amy
DOB: 08/24/1950
Room: 420
Dr.: Rashmi Galangal

7ØØ781 (2-97)
H-NSO781B

MERCY HOSPITAL

PHYSICIAN'S INITIAL ORDERS SHEET

FIGURE 5.4 Daily Order

A physician creates a daily order following each patient examination, or to change orders or make new orders.

ID#: J1008912345 **Name:** Echeverria, Begonia **DOB:** 12/01/1939 **Room:** 804 **Dr.:** Yuka Sun, MD	**MEMORIAL HOSPITAL** **PHYSICIAN'S MEDICATION ORDER** BEAR DOWN ON HARD SURFACE WITH BALLPOINT PEN

↓ GENERIC EQUIVALENT IS AUTHORIZED UNLESS CHECKED IN THIS COLUMN

ALLERGY OR SENSITIVITY		DIAGNOSIS		COMPLETED OR DISCONTINUED		
TO Ø NONE KNOWN ☐ SIGNED:		S/p Hernia Repair				

DATE	TIME	ORDERS	PHYSICIAN'S SIG.	NAME	DATE	TIME
6/24	4 PM	Routine Orders				
		Height 5'7" Weight 186 lbs				
		Condition – stable				
		VS: q4° × 2, then q shift				
		Diet: Regular				
		D5 ½ NS w/20 mEq KCl/Liter				
		run at 100 ml/hr, DC when taking PO well				
		Meds:				
		meperidine 50 mg IM q3h prn pain				
		Vistaril 25 mg IM q3h prn pain				
		Halcion 0.25 mg PO q hs prn				
		LOC prn				
		cefazolin 1 gram IVPB q6h				
		Lance wound on foot in am				
		Call H.O. for: T > 101.5				
		BP > 180/100, or < 80/60				
			Yuka Sun, MD 06/24/2017			
		PHARMACY COPY				

Stat Order

A **stat order** is an emergency order that is typically called in or sent electronically to a pharmacy. This type of order must receive priority attention and, consequently, must be immediately input into a pharmacy database and filled. After a final verification from a pharmacist, the medication is then sent to a patient care unit by a pharmacist or pharmacy technician for patient administration.

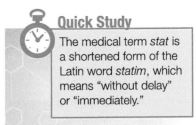

Quick Study

The medical term *stat* is a shortened form of the Latin word *statim*, which means "without delay" or "immediately."

PRN Order

A **PRN order** is an order for a specific amount of a medication to be administered on an "as needed" basis rather than at a regularly prescribed interval. Typically, this medication is administered to treat a specific sign or symptom, such as pain, anxiety, fever, or constipation. Whenever an "as needed" dose is administered, healthcare personnel must immediately document the date, the time given, and the reason that the medication was administered.

Standing Order

A **standing order** is a medication order in which the same set of medications and treatments applies for each patient who receives a similar treatment or surgery (see Figure 5.5). A physician or other prescriber may then sign this preprinted order or slightly modify the standing order by adding or deleting items before signing the form. For example, an orthopedic surgeon who specializes in knee replacement surgery may order the same medications, laboratory tests, and nursing directives for all patients having that procedure. Postoperative (postop) orders written after surgery are another example of standing orders.

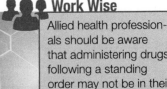

Work Wise

Allied health professionals should be aware that administering drugs following a standing order may not be in their scope of practice. Consequently, they should check the regulations for the state in which they practice to determine what duties they may legally perform.

Discharge Order

A **discharge order** is an order that provides take-home instructions for a patient who is being discharged from a hospital. This order includes all prescribed medications and dosages. Prescriptions are commonly written for a seven-day or one-month period or designed to last until the patient's follow-up visit with his or her healthcare practitioner.

Components of a Medication Order

Each medication order must contain the following components:

- date and time of order
- standard patient identification information (name of patient, identification number, room number, date of birth, gender, height, weight, and allergy information)
- names of medications
- dosages of medications
- routes of administration of medications

FIGURE 5.5 | Standing Order

A physician saves time and aids hospital efficiency and communication by using a preprinted standing order form.

ID#: M03822015669
Name: Cruz, Nestor
DOB: 05/11/1955
Room: 400
Dr.: Gary R. Smith, MD – Standing Orders

DR. GARY R. SMITH
STANDING ORDERS FOR POST-OP DISCECTOMY

1. VS q2h × 4, then q4h overnight.

2. Turn q2h.

3. May stand to void.

4. Bathroom privileges with assistance, if tolerated.

5. Ambulate with assistance ~~in A.M.,~~ if tolerated.

6. Heat lamp ~~back~~ 20 minutes q.i.d.

7. Reinforce dressing PRN.

8. Diet as tolerated after nausea subsides.

9. Percocet 5 mg/325 mg one or two q3h PRN pain.

10. M.S. 10 mg or 15 mg IM q3h PRN more severe pain.

11. Restoril 15 mg hs PRN sleep. MR × 1.

12. Tylenol 325 mg PO q4h PRN temperature elevation above 101 degrees.

13. Tigan 200 mg IM q6h PRN nausea.

14. Peri-Colace 1 capsule PO PRN or M.O.M. 30 cc PO PRN.

15. Laxative of choice.

16. Decadron 4 mg IV or PO q6h × 24 hrs. Then start Medrol Dosepak and label for home use.

17. ~~Tagamet 300 mg IV or PO b.i.d.~~

18. Intermittent cath. q 4–6h PRN.

19. R/L 90 cc q.h. DC after nausea subsides. × 1

20. *Resume home dosage of Prozac post nausea.*

21.

22.

23.

DOB: 05/11/55
5'6"
217#
NKDA
Rm 400

DATE: *August 21ˢᵗ, 2017*

SIGNATURE: *Gary R. Smith, MD*

Dr. Gary R. Smith, MD
711 W. 30th Street, Suite 200
Kalamazoo, MI 49001
Phone 269-555-0423
Fax 269-555-0566

- the time or frequency of administration (for example, *administer at 0800 hours*, or *administer at bedtime each night*, or *administer as needed for anxiety*)

- the signature of the prescriber

Like all components of a patient's medical chart, a medication order is considered **protected health information (PHI)**. Information may be viewed only by those departments that must see the data in order to correctly treat a patient. Examples of institutional departments permitted access to PHI include the nursing department, the pharmacy, and the laboratory. Authorized personnel must only access PHI in the course of performing their required job duties. For more information on PHI, see Chapter 8.

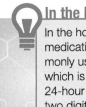

 Checkpoint **5.1**

Take a moment to review what you have learned so far and answer these questions.

1. What is the difference between a prescription and a medication order?

2. What part of a prescription communicates the instructions for use?

3. What type of medication order includes a standard set of medications and treatments that applies to each patient who receives a similar treatment or surgery?

4. What part of a prescription lists the medication prescribed, including the strength and amount?

Medical Abbreviations, Acronyms, and Symbols

To provide safe and effective health care, all allied health professionals must have a thorough understanding of medical abbreviations, acronyms, and symbols used on prescribers' orders. This knowledge is critical in medical practice, for any misinterpretation of abbreviations used on prescription or medication orders could result in a serious medication error such as administering the wrong drug or the wrong dose.

Medical abbreviations, acronyms, and symbols are used in both medicine and pharmacy to allow healthcare professionals to communicate with each other quickly, easily, and effectively. For example, it is faster and more convenient for a physician to write the abbreviation *TPN* on a medication order than to record the words *total parenteral nutrition*. Although learning these common abbreviations can be a challenging task, the importance of knowing this specialized "language" cannot be overstated.

Common Medical Abbreviations

Abbreviations refer to many components of health care. For example, abbreviations may indicate specific patient care facilities, units, or departments (e.g., *NICU* for "neonatal intensive care unit") or the titles of healthcare team members (e.g., *RN* for "registered nurse"). Abbreviations also refer to specific medical diagnoses and conditions, procedures, treatments, patient activities, equipment and supplies, and tests. Some examples of abbreviations include *COPD* for "chronic obstructive pulmonary disease," *ECG* for "electrocardiogram," *OOB* for "out of bed," and *NC* for "nasal cannula." In fact, most of the hundreds of laboratory and diagnostic procedures and tests performed in a medical setting have corresponding abbreviations that are used more frequently than the longer words to which they refer. For example, individuals with no training or knowledge specific to the medical field may be familiar with the term *MRI*, but few of those same people know that *MRI* is an abbreviation for "magnetic resonance imaging."

In the Know

The Institute for Safe Medication Practices (ISMP) and The Joint Commission have separately compiled a list of error-prone abbreviations to help healthcare personnel avoid dangerous documentation. Allied health professionals are encouraged to review ISMP's List of Error-Prone Abbreviations, Symbols, and Dose Designations (http://PharmEssAH.emcp.net/ErrorProneAbbrev) and The Joint Commission's Official "Do Not Use" List of Abbreviations (http://PharmEssAH.emcp.net/DoNotUse List). For more information about error-prone abbreviations, see Chapter 7.

Common Pharmacy Abbreviations

Abbreviations are also prevalent in pharmacy practice. They are typically seen on prescriptions and medication orders. Many of these abbreviations are derived from their Latin roots and refer to dosing intervals or routes of administration. For example, *q.i.d.* comes from the Latin words *quater in die*, meaning "four times a day"; *PO* is from the Latin words *per os*, meaning "by mouth"; and *prn* comes from the Latin words *pro re nata*, meaning "as necessary." Knowing these important abbreviations ensures the correct administration directives for medications.

Common Pharmacy Symbols

In addition to knowing pharmacy abbreviations, allied health professionals must also recognize and understand a number of symbols specific to pharmacy practice. Symbols such as ↑ and ↓ are frequently placed on medication orders to indicate "increase" and "decrease," respectively. For example, a physician may order a change in an intravenous flow rate to increase the dose of a medication, such as ↑ *normal saline to 150 mL per hour*. Another common symbol is the Greek delta symbol (Δ), which is used to indicate a desired change. For example, the medication order *famotidine Δ from 20 mg IV to 40 mg PO* communicates that the prescriber wants to change the dosage and the route of administration from intravenous (IV) to oral (PO).

Because symbols are drawn by hand, and handwriting may be poor or at least vary significantly among personnel, symbols can be misinterpreted easily. Therefore, allied health professionals should take extra care when using or interpreting pharmacy symbols. Computer-generated symbols are preferred over handwritten symbols, whenever possible.

Navigator

To help you recognize and interpret common pharmacy abbreviations and acronyms used on prescriptions and medication orders, refer to Table 5.1. For a more complete list of medical abbreviations, acronyms, and symbols, see the Navigator+ learning management system that accompanies this textbook.

TABLE 5.1 Common Prescription Abbreviations

Category	Abbreviation	Meaning
Amount	cc *	cubic centimeter (mL)
	g	gram
	gr	grain
	gtt	drop
	mg	milligram
	mL	milliliter
	qs	a sufficient quantity
	tbsp	tablespoonful
	tsp	teaspoonful
Dosage form	cap	capsule
	MDI	metered-dose inhaler
	sol	solution
	supp	suppository
	susp	suspension
	tab	tablet
	ung	ointment
Time of administration	ac	before meals
	am	morning, before noon
	bid	twice a day
	hs *	at bedtime
	pc	after meals
	pm	evening, after noon
	prn	as needed
	q6h	every 6 hours
	qd *	daily
	qid	four times a day
	tid	three times a day
	tiw *	three times a week
Site of administration	ad *	right ear
	as *	left ear
	au *	each ear
	od *	right eye
	os *	left eye
	ou *	each eye
	po	mouth (oral)
	pr	rectum
	sl	sublingual (under the tongue)
	top	topical (skin)
	vag	vagina

* These abbreviations, although commonly utilized by practitioners, are easily misread. Consequently, the abbreviations have been designated as *dangerous* by the Institute for Safe Medication Practices (ISMP).

Kolb's Learning Styles

If you are an Assimilator who enjoys learning by abstract conceptualization and reflective observation, you might find that making charts that visually organize information is especially useful. Try reorganizing the list of common abbreviations related to different sites of administration (see Table 5.1) in a diagram shaped like the human body. This activity will help you memorize the information in a way that will be useful in practice.

Challenges of Reading Prescribers' Orders

An allied health professional must ensure that a prescription is clearly written before giving the prescription to a patient or sending the prescription to a pharmacy. Any questions should be brought to the attention of a nurse or pharmacist, who will contact the prescriber for clarification. The same rule applies to a medication order: If any part of a medication order is unclear or undecipherable, an allied health professional must get clarification prior to preparing or administering the drug. This verification process helps to prevent medication errors and avoids unnecessary delays in dispensing medications to patients.

Handwritten Orders

Handwritten prescriptions and medication orders can be difficult to read because of poor penmanship and the use of medical abbreviations (see Figure 5.6). Other challenges allied health professionals may encounter when reading prescription or medication orders include the following:

- Many drugs have similar names, such as clonidine and Klonopin. These medications are referred to as *look-alike, sound-alike drugs*. (For more information on look-alike, sound-alike drugs, see Chapter 7.)

- A physician may refer to a drug using a brand name even though that brand name is no longer commonly stocked. For example, prescribers regularly refer to the diuretic furosemide by its brand name, Lasix.

- Prescribers may use abbreviations that are easily confused with other abbreviations. For example, the abbreviation *IU* (international unit) is not commonly used because it can be confused with the abbreviation *IV* (intravenous). In addition, prescribers sometimes use problematic abbreviations for drug names. For example, the abbreviations *MS* and *MSO_4* commonly mean "morphine sulfate" (a powerful pain medication) but can be confused with the abbreviation for magnesium sulfate, *$MgSO_4$* (a laxative).

- Drug names that end in the letter *L* can lead to dosage mistakes if adequate space is not left between the end of the drug name and the beginning of the dose. For example, if the writing is sloppy, *Tegretol 200 mg* could be mistakenly read as *Tegretol 1200 mg*.

- Dosing errors could also occur if the numerical dose and the unit of measure run together. For example, if *10 mg* is written as *10mg* and the penmanship is poor, the *m* could be mistaken for a zero: *100 g* or *100 mg*. The prescriber would need to be queried or, worse, the patient could end up with a much higher dose than intended.

FIGURE 5.6 Hard-to-Read Prescription

This prescription is for morphine sulfate (MS) 60 mg, but it is unclear if the prescriber is ordering MS ER (extended release) or MS IR (immediate release).

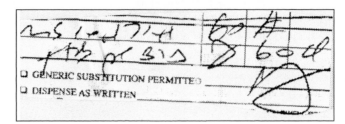

Orders that are communicated verbally have additional problems due to variations in the pronunciation of drug names, and differences in dialects and accents. For example, it is not difficult to mishear "15 mg" as "50 mg." For that reason, allied health professionals must always verify verbal orders before preparing or dispensing medication.

While working in the practice setting, allied health professionals will most likely encounter illegible handwriting on a prescriber's order. In such a situation, the first step they should take is to draw on their own knowledge of drug names and the standard dosing of drugs to try to make sense of what is written. The next step they should take is to show the illegible handwriting to a more experienced healthcare practitioner to see if he or she can offer assistance. If uncertainty remains after completing those two steps, allied health professionals should have a nurse or pharmacist call the prescriber to get the order clarified. Asking questions and implementing a verification process ensure the health and safety of patients.

Computerized Provider Order Entry Systems

Work Wise

Approximately 39% of medication errors occur during the prescribing of a medication. A computerized provider order entry system can help reduce medication errors associated with poor handwriting and inaccurate transcription.

The implementation of **computerized provider order entry (CPOE)** systems in healthcare facilities has enhanced the communication among healthcare personnel. As a result, patient care and safety have improved significantly. A CPOE system is patient management software that allows licensed prescribers to enter instructions for the treatment of patients within an inpatient or ambulatory care setting. This system replaces the traditional means of writing patient orders, such as handwritten medication orders, faxed orders, and so on. Prescribers use computers or mobile devices to access a CPOE system, which interfaces with an electronic health record (EHR).

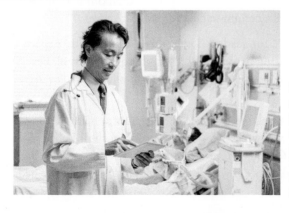

Often, a CPOE system has a clinical-decision support system that allows a prescriber to not only enter a patient's medication order but to also check for drug-drug interactions and drug allergies. This integrated system can help reduce medication errors during the prescribing phase of the prescription process.

Advantages of CPOE Systems

CPOE systems are designed to help prescribers communicate medication orders more quickly and clearly, and to decrease medication errors. Electronic order entry eliminates poor handwriting, decreases the number of spelling errors, and places restrictions on the use of nonstandard abbreviations. Other benefits of using CPOE systems include the following:

- immediate access to patients' medical records
- streamlined workflow processes
- improved documentation
- enhanced coordination of patient care

The economic stimulus program known as the American Recovery and Reinvestment Act (ARRA) of 2009 included funding to accelerate the adoption of CPOE programs. This program offered financial incentives for healthcare institutions that adopted EHR technology and used it to demonstrate meaningful improvements in healthcare delivery. A recent study by the Institute for Healthcare Improvement found that 34% of hospitals had already implemented CPOE. Those facilities that did not adopt EHRs and demonstrate meaningful use by the established deadline (2015) now receive lower reimbursement rates from Medicare and Medicaid.

Disadvantages of CPOE Systems

The initial implementation of a CPOE system is a costly and time-consuming process. In addition to the maintenance of the technology, expenses are incurred from the training of healthcare personnel. A CPOE system does not eliminate human error either. A prescriber could select the incorrect drug from a drop-down menu of medications or select the wrong dosage and wrong frequency.

 Checkpoint **5.2**

Take a moment to review what you have learned so far and answer these questions.

1. What is an example of an abbreviation that indicates a site or route of administration?
2. What is the abbreviation for *every six hours*?
3. How would you translate the following abbreviated instructions: *Take 10 mg po bid*?
4. What are two advantages of CPOE systems?

Prescription Medication Labels

Allied health professionals may need to help patients with their prescription therapy. For example, they may need to read the medication directions for them, show them how to order medication refills, or show them how to determine if their prescriptions are expired. Many patients do not realize that all of this information is right there on the medication container label. With that in mind, allied health personnel need to be familiar with reading and interpreting drug labels.

Patient Teaching

Allied health professionals should be sure that patients know where the Rx number is located on a medication container label. Automated pharmacy phone answering services often ask callers to enter the Rx number, and being aware of this number speeds up the process of ordering refills.

Information on a Medication Container Label

A **medication container label** is a label stating the dosage directions from the prescriber and is affixed to the container of the dispensed medication. The dosing directions are written in plain language, translated from the medical abbreviations the prescriber wrote on the prescription pad (see Figure 5.7). In addition to the dosage directions, the label customarily contains the date; the name, address, and telephone number of the pharmacy; the Rx number; the patient's name; the number of refills; the prescriber's name; the drug name; and the name of the drug's manufacturer. However, this label information may vary somewhat, depending on the laws and regulations of a given state.

Medication container labels for Schedule II–V drugs must feature a symbol that denotes the controlled substance schedule (typically, the symbols are CII, CIII, CIV, and CV, and are in a red font). Controlled substance prescription labels must also contain the transfer warning "Caution: Federal law prohibits the transfer of this drug to any person other than the patient for whom it was prescribed." It is common practice for this statement to be placed in small print on all medication container labels. Some states require veterinary labels to carry the name and address of the animal owner and the species of the animal.

FIGURE 5.7 Prescription and Label Comparison

The original prescription (on the left) contains the information that should be included on the label. The medication container label (on the right) transcribes the instructions for the patient.

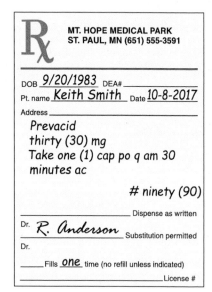

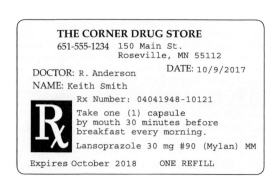

Auxiliary Labels

In addition to the main label, a medication container may feature an auxiliary label (see Figure 5.8). An **auxiliary label** is a small, colorful label that is added to a dispensed medication to supplement the directions on the medication container label. The application of these auxiliary labels is restricted to the professional judgment of the pharmacist. Auxiliary labels may address how to take the medication (e.g., *Take with food or fluids*), how to store the medication (e.g., *Refrigerate the medication* or *Store the medication away from sunlight*), or how to handle the medication (e.g., *Shake well before using* or *For topical use only*). Auxiliary labels may also warn patients about possible side effects (e.g., *Medication may cause drowsiness*) or drug interactions (e.g., *Do not take medication with antacids*). Allied health professionals should be sure that patients understand the purpose of auxiliary labels on their medications.

FIGURE 5.8 | Auxiliary Labels

Auxiliary labels on prescription medications help with safe administration of drugs and improved patient adherence and patient outcomes.

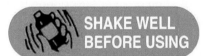
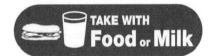

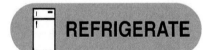
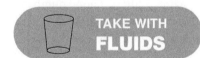

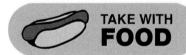
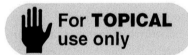

 Checkpoint 5.3

Take a moment to review what you have learned so far and answer these questions.

1. What information is included on a medication container label?

2. What is the purpose of an auxiliary label on a medication container? How does this label help to improve patient outcomes?

Chapter Review

Chapter Summary

Because allied health professionals are involved in the dispensing, administration, and documentation of prescription therapy, they need to be familiar with prescriptions and medication orders.

A prescription is relayed from an outpatient healthcare facility such as a medical office to a pharmacy for patient dispensing. Types of prescriptions include written prescriptions, fax orders, telephone orders, e-prescriptions, and controlled substance prescriptions. Controlled substances in Schedules II–V may be written, faxed, communicated verbally, or transmitted electronically between prescribers and pharmacies that have the required special software. The components of a prescription include a patient information section (patient's name, birth date, address, and phone number); a prescriber information section (prescriber's name, address, phone number, NPI number, DEA number, and signature); and a medication information section (inscription, signa, and subscription).

A medication order is relayed within an inpatient healthcare facility such as an institutional or hospital setting to the on-site pharmacy. Medication orders may be written, transmitted electronically, or delivered verbally. There are several types of medication orders, including admission orders, daily orders, single orders, stat orders, PRN orders, standing orders, and discharge orders. Components of a medication order include the date and time of the order, standard patient identification information, names of medications, dosages of medications, routes of administration of medications, the time or frequency of administration, and the signature of the prescriber.

Allied health professionals must have a thorough understanding of medical abbreviations, acronyms, and symbols used on prescribers'

orders. This knowledge is critical to patient safety and to the prevention of medication errors. Allied health personnel should also know which abbreviations should not be used in any type of medical documentation. Both The Joint Commission and the ISMP publish lists of abbreviations that healthcare professionals should avoid using.

When reading prescribers' orders, allied health professionals may encounter some challenges, including deciphering poor penmanship, understanding abbreviations, and distinguishing between look-alike, sound-alike drugs. If any part of a medication order or prescription is unclear or indecipherable, the allied health professional must ask a nurse or other health professional for clarification of the order. A CPOE system decreases these challenges and helps prescribers communicate medication orders more clearly. Adoption of this technology has resulted in reduced medication errors.

Because patients need to have an understanding of the information on a prescription medication label, allied health personnel must be familiar with the types of information found on this label so that they can perform patient teaching. A label for a prescription medication container includes the date; the name, address, and phone number of the pharmacy; the Rx number; the patient's name; the number of refills; the prescriber's name; the drug name; and the name of the drug manufacturer. Labels for controlled substance containers must also feature a symbol denoting the controlled substance schedule and should have the transfer warning. Auxiliary labels are also affixed to medication labels and provide additional information on how to take the medication, how to store the medication, or how to handle the medication. These labels also provide warnings about side effects.

Chapter Checkup

The Navigator+ learning management system that accompanies this textbook offers many opportunities to help you master chapter content, including end-of-chapter exercises, a glossary of key terms, flash cards, and additional interactive activities.

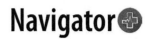

Career Exploration

If you enjoyed learning about prescriptions, medication orders, and medical abbreviations in this chapter, you may want to explore the following career options:

- chemotherapy technician
- emergency medical technician (EMT)/paramedic
- healthcare documentation specialist
- health information technician
- intravenous (IV) pharmacy technician
- medical assistant
- medical transcriptionist
- pharmacy technician
- physical therapist
- renal dialysis technician
- respiratory therapist

6 Pharmacy Measurements and Calculations

Pharm Facts

- A *hand* (also known as a *handbreadth*) is an ancient English unit of measurement based on the average breadth of an adult male hand: 4 inches (10.16 cm). This measurement is used to measure the height of horses from the ground to the withers (top of the shoulder).

- The metric system is widely used in global sport competitions. A balance beam is 10 centimeters wide, or about half the length of a dinner fork; the diameter of a basketball net is 45 centimeters, or twice the diameter of a basketball; the height of a diving platform, 10 meters, is approximately the height of a three-story building; a 5K race is 5 kilometers, which is equivalent to running the length of 54 football fields laid end to end.

- The 24-hour day can be traced back to ancient Egyptians, who established a 10-hour daytime and added 2 hours for twilight, 1 hour at both the beginning and end of the daytime period. Nighttime was 12 hours and was based on observations of the stars.

- The unit of measurement known as a *yard* comes from the Saxon word *gird*, meaning the circumference of an individual's waist. This measurement was taken from the sash that Saxon kings wore around their waists.

- A *jiffy* is actually a unit of time measurement and is equal to the time it takes for light to travel 1 centimeter—33. 3 picoseconds. A picosecond is one-trillionth of a second.

"I have always loved math for its logic and precision. As a pharmacy technician, I use math all day, every day—for calculating dosages, dilutions, and days' supply; for compounding unusual percentage strengths from the solutions the pharmacy has on hand; and for choosing the most economical option among multiple drug and healthcare products. Strong math skills are critical for ensuring that patients are safe and for keeping the pharmacy running smoothly."

—**Becky LaBrum**, PhD, CPhT
Pharmacy Technician

Learning Objectives

1 Understand fractions, decimals, ratios, percentages, and proportions, and be able to convert between these different types of numbers.

2 Perform basic mathematical operations (addition, subtraction, multiplication, division) with fractions and decimal numbers.

3 Develop a familiarity with the different number systems and measurement systems that are currently used in medicine and pharmacy.

4 Be able to perform conversions of values from other measurement systems to the metric system.

5 Use the ratio-proportion method and the dimensional analysis method to perform simple pharmacy calculations.

Mastering the fundamentals of math—such as Arabic numbers and Roman numerals, fractions, decimals, and percentages—and having a good understanding of the metric system are important skills when working in a healthcare setting. Whether calculating a medication dosage, checking the storage temperature of insulin, taking vital signs, or measuring a patient's height and weight, allied health professionals must be able to work with numbers and units of measurement confidently and accurately. Individuals who prepare and administer medications must have a mastery of math fundamentals and metric conversions to provide safe and effective care to patients.

With that in mind, this chapter reviews number systems and basic math skills and discusses systems of measurement including the apothecary system, avoirdupois system, household measurement system, and metric system. In addition, this chapter presents some strategies for calculating doses using the ratio-proportion and dimensional analysis methods.

Number Systems

Two types of number systems are used in pharmacy calculations: Roman numerals and Arabic numbers. The Roman numeral system uses letters to represent quantities or amounts, whereas the Arabic number system uses numbers, fractions, and decimals (see Table 6.1). The Arabic system is more commonly used in the healthcare setting.

Roman Numeral System

The **Roman numeral system** can be traced back to ancient Rome and includes seven main symbols: I (equal to 1), V (equal to 5), X (equal to 10), L (equal to 50), C (equal to 100), D (equal to 500), and M (equal to 1,000). This number system is based on a particular set of rules:

- A numeral cannot be used more than three times in a row. For example, the number 3 is represented in the Roman numeral system as III. The number 4 is not IIII but rather IV—which leads to the next principle in this numeral system.

- If a letter is placed *before* a letter of greater value, the letter is subtracted to determine the number. In addition to the Roman numeral IV (mentioned above), other examples that demonstrate this rule include Roman numerals IX (9), XL (40), and XC (90).

- If one or more letters are placed *after* a letter of greater value, the letters are added together to determine the number. For example, XV (15) + I (1) + I (1) + I (1) = XVIII (18).

Roman numerals are expressed as either capital letters or as lowercase letters— for example, I, II, III, IV, V, or i, ii, iii, iv, v. The most frequently used numerals in medicine and pharmacy are the uppercase I, V, and X, which represent 1, 5, and 10, respectively. For example, tablet quantities of a narcotic prescription may be written in uppercase letters, such as XXX, indicating 30 tablets.

TABLE 6.1 Relationship between Roman Numerals and Arabic Numbers

Roman Numeral	Arabic Number
I (i)	1
II (ii)	2
III (iii)	3
IV (iv)	4
V (v)	5
VI (vi)	6
VII (vii)	7
VIII (viii)	8
IX (ix)	9
X (x)	10
XI (xi)	11
XL (xl)	40
XLI (xli)	41
L (l)	50
LI (li)	51
XC (xc)	90
XCI (xci)	91
XCIX (xcix)	99
C (c)	100
CD (cd)	400
CDXCIX (cdxcix)	499
D (d)	500
DI (di)	501
CMXCIX (cmxcix)	999
M (m)	1,000
MI (mi)	1,001

Lowercase Roman numerals—for example, i, ii, and iii—are also used occasionally in pharmacy practice. These numerals are commonly seen on prescriptions using apothecary measures, and they follow—rather than precede—the unit of measurement. For example, *aspirin gr vi* means "six grains of aspirin." Lowercase Roman numerals are also sometimes used to express other quantities, such as volume (*tbsp iii*, meaning "3 tablespoonfuls"). To prevent errors in interpretation, a line may be drawn above the lowercase Roman numeral, with a dot above the line (for example, *i̇, i̇i, i̇ii*). Still, pharmacy practices are moving toward phasing out the use of Roman numerals in medication prescriptions and orders due to the risk for misinterpretation.

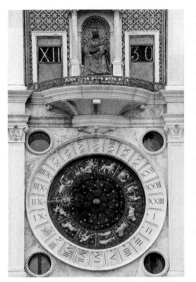

St. Mark's Clocktower in Venice, Italy, dates back to the fifteenth century. This ancient astronomical clock shows the 24 hours of the day (written in Roman numerals on the clock's face) and the 12 signs of the zodiac. At a later date, the Roman numerals (representing the hours) and the Arabic numbers (representing the minutes) were added above the clock.

Arabic Number System

The **Arabic number system** has its roots in India. This system spread to the Arab culture around 800 CE and eventually arrived in Europe. The Arabic number system—formally called the *Hindu-Arabic numeral system*—consists of 10 digits: 0, 1, 2, 3, 4, 5, 6, 7, 8, and 9. When these digits are combined, they represent every possible number. Today, this system is used worldwide, and most medication prescriptions and orders use Arabic numbers to represent dosages.

Number Sense and Mathematical Operations

Working in a healthcare setting often requires individuals to have **number sense**, or the ability to know what numbers and symbols mean, understand how numbers relate to one another, and apply their knowledge of numbers to real-world settings. Understanding fractions, decimals, ratios, percentages, and proportions and knowing how to manipulate these numbers in mathematical operations and conversions are critical skills, especially in the preparation, filling, and administration of medications.

Fractions

A **fraction** is a number that indicates the relationship of a part, or portion, to its whole. A **simple fraction** consists of two numbers: a **numerator**, or the number on the top that tells the "part" or number of pieces in the fractional portion, and a **denominator**, or the number on the bottom that tells the "whole" or the total number of pieces:

$$\frac{1}{8} \quad \begin{array}{l} \text{numerator} \\ \text{denominator} \end{array}$$

FIGURE 6.1 Fractions of the Whole Pie

If a whole pie represents eight slices or ⅛, then three slices is ⅜ and one slice is ⅛.

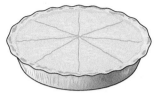 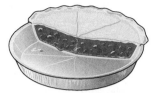 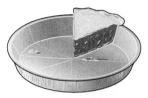

8 slices = 1 whole pie = $\dfrac{8}{8}$ of the whole pie   3 slices = $\dfrac{3}{8}$ of the whole pie   1 slice = $\dfrac{1}{8}$ of the whole pie

For example, a pie might be divided into eight slices, each one of which is a fraction, or ⅛ of the whole pie (see Figure 6.1). In this example, *1* is one slice of the pie, and *8* is the number of slices in the whole pie.

A simple fraction indicates two mathematical expressions: a division expression and a ratio. The **fraction bar**, or the line between the numerator and the denominator, indicates division. For example, the fraction ⅔ is a shorthand way of writing 6 divided by 3, which equals 2. A fraction can also be a way of writing a ratio, or the proportion of one element to another, such as 6 parts of an ingredient to 3 parts. (For more information on ratios and proportions, see the sections titled "Ratios" and "Proportions" later in this chapter.)

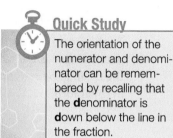

Quick Study

The orientation of the numerator and denominator can be remembered by recalling that the **d**enominator is **d**own below the line in the fraction.

Recognizing Types of Fractions

There are several types of fractions:

- A fraction with a value less than 1 (numerator smaller than denominator) is called a **proper fraction**. The fractions ¼, ⅔, ⅞, and ⁹⁄₁₀ are all examples of proper fractions.

- A fraction with a value greater than 1 (numerator greater than denominator) is called an **improper fraction**. The fractions 3/2, 7/5, 9/6, and ¹⁵⁄₈ are all examples of improper fractions.

- A **mixed number** consists of a whole number and a fraction and can be converted to an improper fraction by multiplying the whole number by the denominator and adding the numerator:

$$5\frac{1}{2} = \frac{(5 \times 2) + 1}{2} = \frac{11}{2}$$

- A fraction in which the numerator, the denominator, or both the numerator and denominator are fractions is called a **complex fraction**:

$$\frac{\frac{3}{4}}{25}$$

$$\frac{\frac{1}{4}}{2}$$

$$\frac{\frac{1}{4}}{\frac{1}{8}}$$

Comparing Fraction Size

When medications are dosed using fractions, it is important to recognize which strengths are largest and smallest. When fractions that have the same numerator are compared, the fraction with the smallest denominator will have the largest value. For example, nitroglycerin tablets—a medication used to treat chest pain—comes in $\frac{1}{100}$ grain, $\frac{1}{150}$ grain, and $\frac{1}{200}$ grain tablets. The $\frac{1}{100}$ grain tablet is the largest dose.

If fractions have the same denominator, the fraction with the largest numerator will have the largest value. For example, some tablets may be prescribed in a fractional quantity such as $\frac{1}{4}$ tablet or $\frac{3}{4}$ tablet. The $\frac{3}{4}$ tablet is the larger dose.

Expressing Fractions as Decimals

As the section on decimals later in this chapter will explain, in decimal fractions, the denominator is not written but is represented by the location of the number in relation to the decimal point. For now, it is sufficient to know that any fraction may be expressed in decimal form by dividing the numerator by the denominator. For example, $\frac{1}{2} = 1 \div 2 = 0.5$, and $\frac{3}{4} = 3 \div 4 = 0.75$.

Adding and Subtracting Fractions

When adding or subtracting fractions with unlike denominators, it is necessary to create a **common denominator**, a number into which each of the unlike denominators can be divided evenly. Think of it as making both fractions into the same size of "pie." Creating a common denominator requires transforming each fraction by multiplying it by a form of 1 that represents one entire "pie." Multiplying a number by 1 does not change the value of the number ($5 \times 1 = 5$). Therefore, multiplying a fraction by a fraction that equals 1 (such as $\frac{5}{5}$) does not change the value of the fraction. For a summary of the steps for finding a common denominator, see Table 6.2.

TABLE 6.2	Steps for Finding a Common Denominator

Step 1. Examine each denominator in the given fractions for its divisors, or factors:

$$\frac{1}{15} = \frac{1}{3 \times 5} \qquad \frac{5}{6} = \frac{5}{2 \times 3} \qquad \frac{11}{36} = \frac{11}{2 \times 2 \times 3 \times 3}$$

Step 2. See what factors any of the denominators have in common:

$$\frac{1}{15} = \frac{1}{3 \times 5} \text{ has a 3 in its denominator.}$$

$$\frac{5}{6} = \frac{5}{2 \times 3} \text{ and } \frac{11}{36} = \frac{11}{2 \times 2 \times 3 \times 3} \text{ both have 2 and 3 in their denominators.}$$

Step 3. Form a common denominator by multiplying all the factors that occur in all of the denominators. If a factor occurs more than once, multiply all the instances it occurs and use the resulting number for each denominator:

$$\text{Common denominator} = 5 \times 2 \times 2 \times 3 \times 3$$
$$= 5 \times 4 \times 9$$
$$= 180$$

Note: The product of all of the original denominators is $15 \times 6 \times 36 = 3{,}240$.

When adding fractions with like denominators, such as $\frac{3}{8} + \frac{5}{8}$, you simply add the numerators together and keep the common denominator:

$$\frac{3}{8} + \frac{5}{8} = \frac{8}{8} = 1$$

When adding fractions with unlike denominators, such as $\frac{1}{2} + \frac{3}{5}$, you would find the lowest number that can be divided evenly by both of the denominators, 2 and 5, and that number is 10.

To convert $\frac{1}{2}$ to tenths, multiply $\frac{1}{2}$ by $\frac{5}{5}$. To multiply fractions, you multiply the numerators (1×5) and the denominators (2×5), which results in the product $\frac{5}{10}$:

$$\frac{1}{2} = \frac{1}{2} \times \frac{5}{5} = \frac{5}{10}$$

To convert $\frac{3}{5}$ to tenths, multiply $\frac{3}{5}$ by $\frac{2}{2}$, which equals $\frac{6}{10}$:

$$\frac{3}{5} = \frac{3}{5} \times \frac{2}{2} = \frac{6}{10}$$

Then add $\frac{5}{10} + \frac{6}{10}$, which equals $\frac{11}{10}$ or $1\frac{1}{10}$:

$$\frac{5}{10} + \frac{6}{10} = \frac{11}{10} = 1\frac{1}{10}$$

After two fractions have been converted to a common denominator and added together, it may be necessary to reduce the resulting fraction to its **lowest terms**. This operation requires dividing both the numerator and denominator of the fraction by a common factor:

$$\frac{3 \div 3}{27 \div 3} = \frac{1}{9}$$

When subtracting fractions that have the same denominator, subtract the numerators and place the resulting number over the common denominator. It may be necessary to reduce the answer to its lowest terms. For example, $\frac{5}{6} - \frac{3}{6} = \frac{2}{6}$. Reducing the fraction to its lowest terms, the answer is $\frac{1}{3}$.

When subtracting fractions that have different denominators, find the lowest common denominator, convert to fractions with the same denominator, subtract the numerators, and place the resulting number over the denominator. It may be necessary to reduce the answer to its lowest terms:

$$\frac{3}{4} - \frac{2}{3}$$

The common denominator is 12. Convert the fractions and then subtract:

$$\frac{3}{4} = \frac{9}{12}$$

$$\frac{2}{3} = \frac{8}{12}$$

$$\frac{9}{12} - \frac{8}{12} = \frac{1}{12}$$

In this case, the fraction cannot be reduced further.

Quick Study

When working with fractions, allied health professionals should always include the units after the number.

Multiplying and Dividing Fractions

As mentioned earlier, the basic step in multiplying fractions is to multiply numerators by numerators and denominators by denominators; then reduce the product to its lowest terms:

$$\frac{2}{5} \times \frac{5}{9} = \frac{10}{45}$$

$$\frac{10}{45} = \frac{2}{9}$$

Before multiplying mixed numbers (e.g., 5 ¾), you need to convert each mixed number to an improper fraction by multiplying the whole number by the denominator and adding that product to the numerator. Then reduce the resulting fraction to its lowest terms:

$$5\frac{3}{7} \times 2\frac{1}{8}$$

$$5\frac{3}{7} = \frac{(5 \times 7) + 3}{7} = \frac{38}{7} \qquad 2\frac{1}{8} = \frac{(2 \times 8) + 1}{8} = \frac{17}{8}$$

$$\frac{38}{7} \times \frac{17}{8} = \frac{646}{56}$$

$$\frac{646}{56} = \frac{323}{28} = 11\frac{15}{28}$$

To divide fractions, you multiply the first fraction by the **reciprocal** of the second fraction. (To find the reciprocal, you flip the second fraction.) Then reduce the resulting fraction to its lowest terms:

$$\frac{1}{2} \div \frac{3}{4} = \frac{1}{2} \times \frac{4}{3} = \frac{4}{6} \text{ reduced to } \frac{2}{3}$$

To divide mixed numbers, you need to convert each mixed number to an improper fraction by multiplying the whole number by the denominator and adding that product to the numerator. Then multiply by the inverse of the second or reciprocal fraction:

$$9\frac{1}{4} \div 2\frac{1}{3}$$

$$9\frac{1}{4} = \frac{(9 \times 4) + 1}{4} = \frac{37}{4} \qquad 2\frac{1}{3} = \frac{(2 \times 3) + 1}{3} = \frac{7}{3}$$

$$\frac{37}{4} \div \frac{7}{3} = \frac{37}{4} \times \frac{3}{7} = \frac{111}{28} = 3\frac{27}{28}$$

To review the guidelines for multiplying and dividing fractions, see Tables 6.3 and 6.4.

TABLE 6.3 Guidelines for Multiplying Fractions

1. Multiplying the numerator by a whole number increases the value of a fraction:

$$\frac{1}{4} \times \frac{2}{1} = \frac{1 \times 2}{4 \times 1} = \frac{2}{4} = \frac{1}{2}$$

2. Multiplying the denominator by a whole number decreases the value of a fraction:

$$\frac{1}{4} \times \frac{1}{2} = \frac{1 \times 1}{4 \times 2} = \frac{1}{8}$$

3. The value of a fraction is not altered by multiplying or dividing both the numerator and the denominator by the same number:

$$\frac{1}{4} \times \frac{4}{4} = \frac{1 \times 4}{4 \times 4} = \frac{4}{16} = \frac{1}{4}$$

TABLE 6.4 Guidelines for Dividing Fractions

1. Dividing the denominator by a number is the same as multiplying the numerator by that number:

$$\frac{3}{\frac{20}{5}} = \frac{3}{4} \qquad 3 \times \frac{5}{20} = \frac{15}{20} = \frac{3}{4}$$

2. Dividing the numerator by a number is the same as multiplying the denominator by that number:

$$\frac{\frac{6}{3}}{4} = \frac{2}{4} = \frac{1}{2} \qquad \frac{6}{3 \times 4} = \frac{6}{12} = \frac{1}{2}$$

1₂³ By the Numbers

Take a moment to practice multiplying and dividing fractions by solving the following problems. For additional practice problems, refer to the Navigator+ learning management system that accompanies this textbook.

1. $\frac{8}{9} \times \frac{4}{6}$

2. $\frac{7}{5} \times 1\frac{3}{4}$

3. $\frac{10}{3} \div \frac{9}{5}$

4. $3\frac{4}{5} \div \frac{2}{3}$

Navigator

Answers: (1) 16/27 (2) 2 9/20 (3) 1 23/27 (4) 5 7/10

Decimals

A fraction in which the denominator is 10 or some multiple of 10 is a decimal fraction or, more simply, a **decimal**. In a decimal, the denominator is not written but is represented by the location of the number in relation to the decimal point. The **decimal point** represents the center. Numbers written to the right of the decimal point are decimal fractions with a multiple of 10—for example, tenths, hundredths, thousandths, and so on. These numbers have a value of less than 1. Numbers written to the left of the decimal point have a value of 1 or greater (whole numbers). To visualize decimal units and values, see Figure 6.2.

If a decimal is less than 1, with no numbers to the left of the decimal point, a zero is placed to the left of the decimal point. This zero is known as a **leading zero**. Healthcare personnel must consistently use leading zeros in the practice setting because their placement helps avoid medication errors.

An understanding of decimals is crucial to pharmacy calculations because most medication orders are written in decimals. Remember, numbers to the left of the decimal point are whole numbers; numbers to the right of the decimal point are decimal fractions (parts of a whole).

Quick Study

The word *decimal* comes from the Latin root word *decimus*, which means "tenth."

FIGURE 6.2 Decimal Units and Values

Every digit in a decimal has a place value, which is counted from the decimal point.

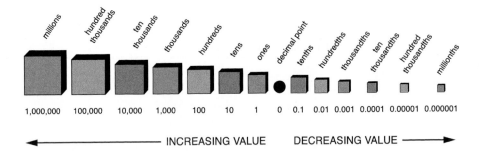

INCREASING VALUE   DECREASING VALUE

Expressing Decimals as Fractions

To express a decimal number as a fraction, remove the decimal point and use the remaining number as a numerator. To obtain the denominator, count the number of places to the right of the decimal point, and use Table 6.5 to find the corresponding multiple of 10 to put in the denominator:

$$2.33 = \frac{233}{100} \qquad 0.1234 = \frac{1{,}234}{10{,}000} \qquad 0.00367 = \frac{367}{100{,}000}$$

TABLE 6.5 Decimals and Equivalent Decimal Fractions

$1 = \frac{1}{1}$	$0.01 = \frac{1}{100}$	$0.0001 = \frac{1}{10{,}000}$
$0.1 = \frac{1}{10}$	$0.001 = \frac{1}{1{,}000}$	$0.00001 = \frac{1}{100{,}000}$

Adding and Subtracting Decimals

When adding decimals, place the numbers in columns so that the decimal points are aligned directly under each other:

$$
\begin{array}{r}
20.4 \\
+21.8 \\
\hline
42.2
\end{array}
\qquad
\begin{array}{r}
11.2 \\
13.6 \\
+16.0 \\
\hline
40.8
\end{array}
$$

You may need to add zeros after the decimal point to correctly align the decimal points:

$$
\begin{array}{r}
15.36 \\
+3.8
\end{array}
\qquad
\begin{array}{r}
15.36 \\
+3.80 \\
\hline
19.16
\end{array}
$$

To subtract decimals, place the numbers in columns so that the decimal points are aligned directly under each other:

$$
\begin{array}{r}
84.57 \\
-27.91 \\
\hline
56.66
\end{array}
$$

1 2 3 By the Numbers

Take a moment to practice adding and subtracting decimals by solving the following problems. For additional practice problems, refer to the Navigator+ learning management system that accompanies this textbook.

1. 4.56 + 6.87

2. 5.321 + 15.1

3. 19.32 – 14.689

4. 1.2 – 0.3

Navigator

Answers: (1) 11.43 (2) 20.421 (3) 4.631 (4) 0.9

Multiplying and Dividing Decimals

Unlike adding and subtracting decimals, the multiplication of decimals does not require you to align the decimal points. You simply multiply decimals the same way that you multiply whole numbers; then place the decimal point in the correct place:

$$
\begin{array}{r}
1.23 \\
\times 2.3 \\
\hline
369 \\
+2460 \\
\hline
2829
\end{array}
\quad \text{(A zero is added to align the columns.)}
$$

The final step is to position the decimal point in the correct place. To do this, count the number of digits to the right of the decimal point in both of the numbers that were multiplied. (For this example, that number is *3*.) Move the decimal point in the answer to the problem that number of positions to the left:

$$2.829$$

To divide decimals, you need to change both the **divisor** (the number doing the dividing or the denominator) and the **dividend** (the number being divided or the numerator) to whole numbers. After that step, you divide the numbers by following the same procedure you would use to divide whole numbers.

Work Wise

Healthcare personnel should always use a calculator when dividing decimals.

To change the decimals to whole numbers, move their decimal points the same number of places to the right. If the divisor and the dividend have a different number of digits after the decimal point, choose the one that has more digits and move its decimal point a sufficient number of places to make it a whole number. Then move the decimal point in the other number the same number of places, adding a zero at the end if necessary.

In the example below, the divisor (3.625) has more digits after the decimal point than the dividend (1.45); therefore, you would move the decimal point in the divisor three places to the right to make it a whole number. Then move the decimal point in the dividend the same number of places, adding a zero at the end:

$$1.45 \div 3.625$$

$$\frac{1.45}{3.625} = \frac{1450}{3625} = 0.4$$

In the example below, the dividend (1.617) has more digits after the decimal point than the divisor (2.31). Therefore, you would move the decimal point in the dividend three places to the right to make it a whole number. Then you would move the decimal point in the divisor three places to the right as well:

$$1.617 \div 2.31$$

$$\frac{1.617}{2.31} = \frac{1617}{2310} = 0.7$$

Rounding Decimals

Rounding decimals is essential for daily use of mathematical operations. The purpose of rounding is to keep the number you are working with to a manageable size. It is important to recognize, however, that rounding will affect the accuracy to which a medication can be measured. In some cases, it may be appropriate to calculate a dose to the nearest whole milliliter and, in other cases, to round to the nearest tenth or hundredth of a milliliter. Depending on the drug and strength prescribed, it may not be possible to accurately measure a very small quantity such as a hundredth of a milliliter.

When numbers with decimals are used to calculate a volumetric dose, a number with multiple digits beyond the decimal often results. It is not practical to retain all of these numbers, as a dose cannot be accurately measured beyond the hundredths or thousandths place for most medications. Frequently, the dose is rounded to the nearest tenth. It is common practice to round the weight of a dose to the hundredths or thousandths place, or as accurate as the particular measuring device (or medication) will permit.

To round off an answer to the nearest tenth, carry the division out two places, to the hundredths place. If the number in the hundredths place is 5 or greater, add 1 to the tenths place number. If the number in the hundredths place is less than 5, round the number down by omitting the digit in the hundredths place:

5.65 becomes 5.7

4.24 becomes 4.2

The same procedure may be used when rounding to the nearest hundredths place or thousandths place:

3.8421 = 3.84 (hundredths place)

41.2674 = 41.27 (hundredths place)

0.3928 = 0.393 (thousandths place)

4.1111 = 4.111 (thousandths place)

As mentioned earlier, when rounding numbers used in pharmacy calculations, it is common to round off to the nearest tenth. However, there are times when a dose is very small and rounding to the nearest hundredth or thousandth may be more appropriate:

The exact dose calculated is 0.08752 g

Rounded to the nearest tenth: 0.1 g

Rounded to the nearest hundredth: 0.09 g

Rounded to the nearest thousandth: 0.088 g

When a number that has been rounded to the tenths place is multiplied or divided by a number that was rounded to the hundredths or thousandths place, the answer must be rounded back to the tenths place. The reason is that the answer can only be accurate to the place to which the highest rounding was made in the original numbers:

1.23 g × 4.6 g = 5.658 g

It must be rounded off to the tenths place because rounding to the hundredths place would overstate the accuracy of the number: 5.7 g.

Ratios

As mentioned earlier in this chapter, a **ratio** is a numerical representation of the relationship between two parts of a whole. Ratios are written with a colon (:) between the numbers, which may read as *to*. The ratio 1:2 means that the second part has twice the value (e.g., size, number, weight, volume) of the first part. Ratios may also be written as fractions, and it is the ratio in fraction form that is most useful to healthcare personnel:

1:2	is read as	1 part to 2 parts	and may also be written as ½
3:4	is read as	3 parts to 4 parts	and may also be written as ¾
1:20	is read as	1 part to 20 parts	and may also be written as ¹⁄₂₀
1:10	is read as	1 part to 10 parts	and may also be written as ¹⁄₁₀

With medications, a ratio is used to express the weight or strength of a drug per dose or volumetric measurement. Ratios are commonly used to express concentrations of a drug in solution. For example, a 1:100 concentration of a drug means that there is 1 part of the drug to 100 parts of the solution. Ratios are typically written as the amount of drug per dose or unit of diluent (e.g., *1 g: 100 mL*).

Converting a Ratio to a Percent

To express a ratio as a percent, designate the first number of the ratio as the numerator and the second number of the ratio as the denominator. Multiply the fraction by 100 and add a percent sign after the number:

$$5{:}1 = \frac{5}{1} \times 100 = \frac{500}{1} = 500\%$$

$$1{:}5 = \frac{1}{5} \times 100 = \frac{100}{5} = 20\%$$

$$1{:}2 = \frac{1}{2} \times 100 = \frac{100}{2} = 50\%$$

Percents

Percent expresses the number of parts compared with a total of 100 parts. The word *percent* comes from the Latin term *per centum*, meaning "by the hundred." Therefore, percent literally means "per 100." Percent is represented by the symbol %. For example, if a test has 100 questions and you receive a score of 89%, you got 89 of the 100 questions correct.

A percent can be written as a fraction, decimal, or ratio. Being able to convert between ratios, percents, and decimals is an important skill in the healthcare setting. To visualize these equivalent values, refer to Table 6.6.

TABLE 6.6 Equivalent Values

Percent	Fraction	Decimal	Ratio
45%	$\dfrac{45}{100}$	0.45	45:100
0.5%	$\dfrac{0.5}{100}$	0.005	0.5:100

Percent strengths are often used to describe intravenous (IV) solutions and topically applied drugs. The higher the percentage of dissolved substances (in a solute or a topical drug), the greater the strength of the medication. Both of the following examples may be expressed as 1:100, $\frac{1}{100}$, or 0.01:

- A 1% solution contains 1 g of drug per 100 mL of fluid.

- A 1% hydrocortisone cream contains 1 g of hydrocortisone per 100 g of cream.

By multiplying the first number in the ratio (the solute) while keeping the second number unchanged, you can increase the strength. Conversely, by dividing the first number in the ratio while keeping the second number unchanged, you can decrease the strength.

Converting a Percent to a Ratio

To convert a percent to a ratio, first change the percent to a fraction by dividing it by 100; then reduce the fraction to its lowest terms. Express this fraction as a ratio by making the numerator the first number of the ratio and the denominator the second number of the ratio:

$$2\% = 2 \div 100 = \frac{2}{100} = \frac{1}{50} = 1:50$$

$$10\% = 10 \div 100 = \frac{10}{100} = \frac{1}{10} = 1:10$$

$$75\% = 75 \div 100 = \frac{75}{100} = \frac{3}{4} = 3:4$$

Converting a Percent to a Decimal

To convert a percent to a decimal, drop the percent symbol and divide the number by 100. Dividing a number by 100 is equivalent to moving the decimal point two places to the left and inserting zeros if necessary:

$$4\% = 4 \div 100 = 0.04$$

$$15\% = 15 \div 100 = 0.15$$

$$200\% = 200 \div 100 = 2$$

Proportions

A **proportion** is an expression of equality between two ratios. This expression can by written three ways: using an equal sign between the ratios, using a double colon (::) between the ratios, or writing the ratios as fractions, as shown below:

$$3{:}4 = 15{:}20 \qquad 3{:}4 :: 15{:}20 \qquad \frac{3}{4} = \frac{15}{20}$$

Two ratios that have the same value, such as ¾ and ¹⁵⁄₂₀, are said to be **equivalent ratios**, also known as **proportional ratios**. A proportion can be visualized by thinking of two triangles that resemble one another in shape but are different sizes (see Figure 6.3).

FIGURE 6.3 | **Triangles with Proportional Ratios**

These two triangles have equal proportions because ¹⁵/₂₀ can be reduced to its lowest terms: ³/₄.

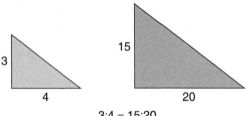

$$3{:}4 = 15{:}20$$

In a proportion, the first and fourth, or outside, numbers are called the **extremes**. The second and third, or inside, numbers are called the **means**:

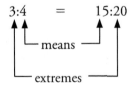

The product of the means must always equal the product of the extremes in a proportion. You can check the accuracy of a proportion by using this formula:

$$a:b = c:d$$

$$b \times c = a \times d$$

If a proportion is expressed as a relationship between fractions, then the numerator of the first fraction multiplied by the denominator of the second fraction is equal to the denominator of the first fraction multiplied by the numerator of the second fraction:

$$\frac{a}{b} = \frac{c}{d}$$

$$a \times d = b \times c$$

 By the Numbers

Take a moment to practice converting ratios and percents and determining the accuracy of proportions by solving the following problems. For additional practice problems, refer to the Navigator+ learning management system that accompanies this textbook.

1. Express the ratio 4:5 as a percentage.

2. Express the ratio 2:3 as a percentage.

3. Convert 23% to a decimal.

4. Convert 56.78% to a decimal.

5. Determine whether the following two ratios are equivalent: ⅔ = ⅝.

6. Determine whether the following two ratios are equivalent: ³⁄₁₈ = ⅙.

Navigator

Answers: (1) 80% **(2)** 67% **(3)** 0.23 **(4)** 0.5678 **(5)** not equivalent **(6)** equivalent

Checkpoint 6.1

Take a moment to review what you have learned so far and answer these questions.

1. Which number in a fraction is the denominator?

2. Why is the Roman numeral IX equal to 9, not 11?

3. Describe how you divide the fraction ⅚ by the fraction ⅔.

Systems of Measurement

In addition to having number sense, you must also have an understanding of the different systems of measurement that you may encounter in the healthcare setting. **Systems of measurement** are collections of units of measurement that are used to determine such quantities as volume, weight, distance, area, temperature, and time.

Units of measurement are one of humankind's oldest tools. To measure length, ancient Egyptians created a unit called the *cubit*, which was equal to the length of a forearm from the elbow to the tip of the middle finger. Ancient Roman cultures created the *mille passus*, a unit of length equal to 1,000 paces (in which each pace was the length of 5 human feet). Many early inhabitants measured the weight of lighter objects using items such as stones, seeds, and grains as reference points. To measure heavier items, they filled large ceramic vessels with water. This measurement of mass was called a *talent*, and—depending on the culture—the unit's equivalency fluctuated. The Greek talent weighed 57 pounds; the Egyptian talent weighed 60 pounds; and the Roman talent weighed 71 pounds. By nature, these common units of measurement were *inconsistent* and *imprecise*—two terms that run counter to scientific disciplines such as chemistry, medicine, and pharmacy.

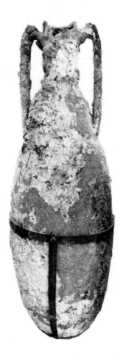

This ancient clay vessel, known as an *amphora*, was found in the Mediterranean Sea. The vessel was used for liquid storage; the weight of the water it contained represented a unit of measurement known as a talent.

The need for standardized units of measurement among these various sciences resulted in the establishment of three different systems of pharmaceutical measurement over the centuries: the apothecary system, the avoirdupois system, and the household system. Although some measurements of these systems are still used occasionally in medicine and pharmacy, the metric system has become the standard for the prescribing, preparation, and administration of medications. In fact, many pharmacy computer systems are programmed to accept only amounts given in metric units.

Apothecary System

The **apothecary system of measurement** is one of the oldest systems of measurement still in use today. Its roots can be traced back to medieval Europe where it was the primary system of measurement used by physicians, apothecaries, and scientists to prepare medicinal compounds. Based on the classical weight system developed by the Romans, this system of measurement includes units such as minims, fluid drams, scruples, drams, grains, ounces, and pounds. Many of these units of measurement are represented by unusual symbols (see Table 6.7).

The weight units of measurement in the apothecary system are the **scruple** (roughly equivalent to 1.3 g), the **dram** (roughly equivalent to 3.9 g), the ounce, and the pound. The scruple and the dram are rarely used today and could lead to medication errors if put

TABLE 6.7 | Apothecary System Symbols

Volume		Weight	
Unit of Measurement	Symbol	Unit of Measurement	Symbol
minim	♏	grain	gr
fluid dram	f ʒ	scruple	Ɔ
fluid ounce	f ℥	dram	ʒ
pint	pt	ounce	℥
quart	qt	pound	lb or #
gallon	gal		

into practice. Two other weight measurements—the ounce and the pound—continue to be used in pharmacy practice, although their equivalencies have changed since the inception of the apothecary system.

Another weight unit in the apothecary system is the **grain**, a measurement that is based on the weight of a single seed of wheat or barley. This dry weight measure has been used by nearly every culture in recorded history. Today, the grain is the most commonly encountered *nonmetric* unit in pharmacy practice. A common example of the use of the grain unit of measurement in modern-day pharmacy can be seen in aspirin and acetaminophen products, which are sometimes labeled as 5 grains (5 gr), an amount equivalent to approximately 325 mg. Phenobarbital is another example of a medication that is commercially available in grains: ¼ grain (16.2 mg), ½ grain (32.4 mg), and 1 grain (64.8 mg). In addition, thyroid medications are often prescribed as ¼ grain (15 mg), ½ grain (30 mg), or 1 grain (60 mg).

The volume units of measurement in the apothecary system include the minim, fluid dram, fluid ounce, pint, quart, and gallon. Although some of these measurements have survived over the centuries with changes to their equivalencies (e.g., the fluid ounce, pint, quart, and gallon), other measurements (e.g., the *minim* [roughly equivalent to .06 mL] and the *fluid dram* [about 3.7 mL]) are not used in medical and pharmacy practice today.

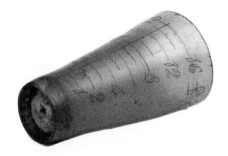

This eighteenth-century apothecary measurement device is made from a horn. The device is graduated with two scales that have been etched by hand. One scale indicates 0 to 16 fluid ounces; the other scale, indicated by the numbers 0 to 2, is equivalent to tablespoonfuls.

Avoirdupois System

The **avoirdupois system of measurement** originated in France and was eventually adopted by England in 1300CE as a standard for commerce. The name of the system comes from the French term *aveir de peis*, or "goods of weight," which referred to products sold in bulk that had to be weighed to determine their value. The avoirdupois system includes such common units of measurement as feet and miles as well as grains, ounces, and pounds. These units are shared with the apothecary system; however, their equivalencies are not the same. The avoirdupois system has since been replaced by the metric system and is no longer used in trade or pharmacy.

Household System

The **household system of measurement** is based on the apothecary system and was established to help patients take their medications at home. Like the apothecary and avoirdupois systems, this system includes such common units of measurement as the ounce and pound but also includes several liquid units that are still used in the food industry, some areas of pharmacy, and households today. These units include the drop, teaspoon, tablespoon, and cup (see Table 6.8). Other household measurement units, such as the hogshead and the jigger, have become obsolete in pharmacy practice. The household system will not need to be known or used for pharmaceutical calculations, but it is helpful to see how these measurements compare with metric measurements as some over-the-counter (OTC) medications use the household system for dosages.

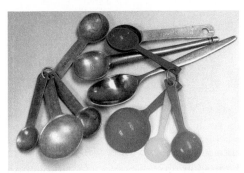

The volume held by a household teaspoon may vary, but a true teaspoon equals 5 mL.

TABLE 6.8 Household Measurement Equivalents

Volume		Weight	
3 teaspoonfuls (tsp)	= 1 tablespoonful (tbsp)	1 pound (lb)	= 16 ounces (oz)
2 tablespoonfuls (tbsp)	= 1 fluid ounce (fl oz)		
8 fluid ounces (fl oz)	= 1 cup		
2 cups	= 1 pint (pt)		
2 pints (pt)	= 1 quart (qt)		
4 quarts (qt)	= 1 gallon (gal)		

Kolb's Learning Styles

If you like gathering and organizing information, as Divergers and Assimilators do, create a series of flash cards for the household units of measurement. Record the measurement units for weights and volumes on one side of a card and their metric equivalents on the other side of the card. Choose a partner and help each other with the memorization of these conversions.

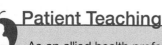
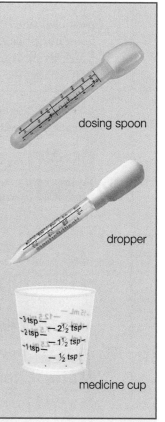
Metric System

The **metric system of measurement** was introduced in France in 1799 in response to the need for a standardized system of measurement that could be used internationally. The main advantage of the metric system is that it uses a group of **basic units of measurement** (such as *meter, liter,* and *gram*) in conjunction with a set of prefixes (such as *deci–, centi–,* and *milli–*) that represent multiples of ten. The **prefixes**, or syllables placed at the beginnings of words, are used to modify all of the base units of measurement in the system, which means that an individual only needs to know a few terms to be able to understand many measurements.

Over the next two centuries, the metric system was gradually adopted by countries around the world, and today it standardizes and simplifies international commerce and communication, especially in the areas of science and technology. The United States is one of three countries that do not use the metric system as its standard system of measurement. However, the United States has adopted this international system in two specific fields: medicine and pharmacy.

The modern metric system makes use of the standardized units of the **Système International (SI)**, adopted by agreement of governments worldwide in 1960. SI is a decimal system, with the prefixes denoting powers of 10 (see Table 6.9). In prescriptions using the metric system, numbers are also expressed as decimals rather than as fractions. To convert from one metric unit to another while performing calculations, healthcare personnel simply move the decimal point. As mentioned earlier, by moving the decimal point one place to the right, an individual is multiplying by 10, thus making the number larger. By moving the decimal point one place to the left, an individual is dividing by 10, thus making the number smaller. For that reason, an error of a single decimal place is an error by a factor of 10. Therefore, prescribers and other medical personnel must exercise due diligence when recording, interpreting, and measuring medication dosages containing decimals, for even minor typographical errors can lead to serious medication errors.

TABLE 6.9 Système International Prefixes

Prefix	Symbol	Meaning
micro–	mc	one-millionth (basic unit $\times$ 10^{-6}, or unit $\times$ 0.000001)
milli–	m	one-thousandth (basic unit $\times$ 10^{-3}, or unit $\times$ 0.001)
centi–	c	one-hundredth (basic unit $\times$ 10^{-2}, or unit $\times$ 0.01)
deci–	d	one-tenth (basic unit $\times$ 10^{-1}, or unit $\times$ 0.1)
hecto–	h	one hundred times (basic unit $\times$ 10^{2}, or unit $\times$ 100)
kilo–	k	one thousand times (basic unit $\times$ 10^{3}, or unit $\times$ 1,000)

Meter, Liter, and Gram

As mentioned earlier, the three basic units in the SI system are the meter, liter, and gram. Each of these basic units has its own abbreviation, and the same abbreviation is used for both single and plural measurements—for example, 1 mL, 3 mL; 1 g, 3 g (see Table 6.10). The liter and the gram are the metric units most commonly used in medicine and pharmacy. Consequently, allied health professionals must be familiar with these basic units of measurement.

TABLE 6.10 Common Metric Units

Measurement Unit	Equivalent
Length: Meter	
1 meter (m)	100 centimeters (cm)
1 centimeter (cm)	0.01 m; 10 millimeters (mm)
1 millimeter (mm)	0.001 m; 1,000 micrometers, or microns (mcm)
Volume: Liter	
1 liter (L)	1,000 milliliters (mL)
1 milliliter (mL)	0.001 L; 1,000 microliters (mcL)
Weight: Gram	
1 gram (g)	1,000 milligrams (mg)
1 milligram (mg)	1,000 micrograms (mcg); one-thousandth of a gram (g)
1 kilogram (kg)	1,000 grams (g)

As previously discussed, prefixes can be added to these basic metric units to specify a particular unit of measurement. For example, the prefix *milli–* (meaning ¹⁄₁,₀₀₀) can be added to the basic metric unit *liter* to form a new unit: milliliter, or one-thousandth of a liter. Being able to convert between basic units of measurement and their derivations is an important skill to learn, for conversions are performed every day by personnel in a healthcare setting. The most common metric calculations in medicine involve conversions to and from grams, milligrams, and kilograms and to and from milliliters and liters. Table 6.11 shows how to easily perform these conversions.

Meter

The **meter** is the unit used for measuring length, distance, area, and volume and is equivalent to approximately three feet. This unit of measurement has limited applications in a healthcare setting; however, a patient's height may be recorded in meters or centimeters in the medical chart.

Liter

The **liter** is the unit used for measuring the **volume** of liquid medications as well as liquids for oral and parenteral solutions. One liter is equivalent to 1,000 milliliters (abbreviated as mL), which means that there are 1,000 mL in every liter. Allied health personnel will frequently see the measurement *milliliters* used in the healthcare setting. For this reason, they should know how to convert liters to milliliters and vice versa. To review the conversion formulas associated with the liter, refer to Table 6.11.

Extremely small volumes are measured in **microliters (mcL)**, which have a volume of one-millionth of a liter. To convert a liter to a microliter, you multiply by 1,000,000 or move the decimal point six places to the right. To convert a microliter to a liter, you divide by 1,000,000 or move the decimal point six places to the left. For example, 17 L equals 17,000,000 mcL, and 500,000 mcL equals .5 L.

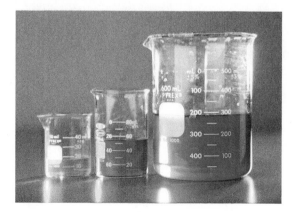

Liquid volumes are expressed in milliliters (which is the preferred unit) or in cubic centimeters. To measure the volumes of nonsterile liquids, volumetric flasks of varying sizes, such as the ones pictured here, are used.

TABLE 6.11 Common Metric Conversions

Conversion	Instruction	Example
kilograms (kg) to grams (g)	multiply by 1,000 (move decimal point three places to the right)	6.25 kg = 6,250 g
grams (g) to milligrams (mg)	multiply by 1,000 (move decimal point three places to the right)	3.56 g = 3,560 mg
milligrams (mg) to grams (g)	multiply by 0.001 (move decimal point three places to the left)	120 mg = 0.120 g
liters (L) to milliliters (mL)	multiply by 1,000 (move decimal point three places to the right)	2.5 L = 2,500 mL
milliliters (mL) to liters (L)	multiply by 0.001 (move decimal point three places to the left)	238 mL = 0.238 L

Gram

The **gram** is the unit used for (1) measuring the amount of medication in a solid dosage form, (2) indicating the amount of solid medication in a solution, and (3) expressing the weight of an object or a person. A medication dose is commonly expressed in milligrams (mg). The weight of an individual is frequently expressed in kilograms (kg). To review the conversion formulas associated with the gram, see Table 6.11.

Extremely small volumes are measured in **micrograms (mcg)**, which have a volume of one-millionth of a gram. To convert a gram to a microgram, you multiply by 1,000,000 or move the decimal point six places to the right. To convert a microgram to a gram, you divide by 1,000,000 or move the decimal point six places to the left. Some medications, such as levothyroxine (a medication used to treat hypothyroidism), are measured in micrograms.

By the Numbers

Take a moment to practice common metric conversions by solving the following problems. For additional practice problems, refer to the Navigator+ learning management system that accompanies this textbook.

1. Convert 6.234 L to milliliters.

2. Convert 155 mL to liters.

3. Convert 4.25 g to milligrams.

4. Convert 18,000,024 mg to kilograms.

Navigator

Answers: **(1)** 6,234 mL **(2)** 0.155 L **(3)** 4,250 mg **(4)** 18.000024 kg

Conversions between Measurement Systems

Prior to the nineteenth century, one challenge for medical practitioners was the lack of standard equivalencies among these three measurement systems. Depending on which system they used, practitioners were dispensing widely differing doses. For example, a pound in the apothecary system is equivalent to 12 ounces, whereas a pound in the avoirdupois and household systems is equivalent to 16 ounces. An apothecary ounce is 31.1 g, but an avoirdupois ounce is 28.35 g. These discrepancies often resulted in medication errors. To understand the variances among the apothecary, avoirdupois, and household units of measurement and their metric equivalents, see Tables 6.12, 6.13, and 6.14.

TABLE 6.12 Apothecary System

Measurement Unit	Equivalent within System	Metric Equivalent
Volume		
1 minim ($\mathfrak{m}$)	–	0.06 mL
16.23 $\mathfrak{m}$	–	1 mL
1 fluid dram (f 3)	60 $\mathfrak{m}$	5 mL (3.75 mL)*
1 f 3 (fluid ounce)	6 f 3	30 mL (29.57 mL)†
1 pint (pt)	16 f 3	480 mL
1 quart (qt)	2 pt or 32 f 3	960 mL
1 gallon (gal)	4 qt or 8 pt	3,840 mL
Weight		
1 grain (gr)	–	65 mg††
15.432 gr	–	1 g
1 scruple (Э)	20 gr	1.3 g
1 dram (3)	3 Э or 60 gr	3.9 g
1 ounce (3)	8 3 or 480 gr	30 g (31.1 g)
1 pound (#)	12 3 or 5,760 gr	373.2 g

* In reality, 1 f 3 contains 3.75 mL; however, that number is usually rounded up to 5 mL or 1 tsp.
† In reality, 1 f 3 contains 29.57 mL; however, that number is usually rounded up to 30 mL.
†† Many manufacturers use 60 mg instead of 65 mg as the equivalent for 1 gr.

TABLE 6.13 Avoirdupois System

Measurement Unit	Equivalent within System	Metric Equivalent
1 grain (gr)	–	65 mg
1 ounce (oz)	437.5 gr	30 g (28.35 g)*
1 pound (lb)	16 oz or 7,000 gr	454 g

* An avoirdupois ounce actually contains 28.34952 g; however, that number is usually rounded up to 30 g. It is common practice to use 454 g as the equivalent for a pound (28.35 g × 16 oz/lb = 453.6 g/lb, rounded to 454 g/lb) rather than 480 g (30 g X 16 oz/lb = 480 g/lb).

TABLE 6.14 Household System

Measurement Unit	Equivalent within System	Metric Equivalent
Volume		
1 teaspoonful (tsp)	–	5 mL
1 tablespoonful (tbsp)	3 tsp	15 mL
1 fluid ounce (fl oz)	2 tbsp	30 mL (29.57 mL)*
1 cup	8 fl oz	240 mL
1 pint (pt)	2 cups	480 mL
1 quart (qt)	2 pt	960 mL
1 gallon (gal)	4 qt	3,840 mL
Weight		
1 ounce (oz)	–	30 g
1 pound (lb)	–	454 g
2.2 lb	–	1 kg

* Technically, 1 fl oz (household unit of measurement) contains less than 30 mL; however, 30 mL is usually used.

Kolb's Learning Styles

If you are an Assimilator who enjoys learning by abstract conceptualization and reflective observation, try making a chart that compares the units of different measurement systems by weight, volume, and distance.

Checkpoint 6.2

Take a moment to review what you have learned so far and answer these questions.

1. How many grams are equivalent to 1 oz in the avoirdupois measurement system?

2. What unit of volume is equivalent to 1 cc?

3. What unit might be used to measure a drug dissolved in a liquid solution? (*Hint:* It is a ratio of the amount of drug to the amount of solution.)

Other Measurement Systems

In addition to learning the different measurement systems used in the healthcare setting, allied health professionals should also have an understanding of two other measurement systems: temperature and time.

Temperature

For allied health professionals, having an understanding of temperature scales is important. For example, pharmacy technicians may be asked to monitor the refrigerator and freezer temperatures of stored medications, or medical assistants may be involved in patient teaching regarding the conversion between Fahrenheit and Celsius temperatures.

Fahrenheit Temperature Scale

Daniel Fahrenheit, a German physicist, invented a temperature scale in 1724. The **Fahrenheit temperature scale** uses 32° F as the temperature at which water freezes to ice and 212° F as the temperature at which water boils. The difference between these two extremes is 180° F.

Today, the United States is one of the few countries in the world that uses the Fahrenheit temperature scale as its standard. Its citizens are used to seeing Fahrenheit temperatures on thermometers, thermostats, manufacturers' tags on winter apparel, and meteorologic forecasts.

Celsius Temperature Scale

Around 1742, Anders Celsius, a Swedish astronomer, suggested a thermometer with a difference of 100 degrees between freezing and boiling. He used 0° C as the freezing point and 100° C as the boiling point. The **Celsius temperature scale** is commonly used in Europe and globally in science. In addition, Celsius is often the scale used in healthcare settings.

Temperature Equivalencies

Storing unstable drugs at proper temperatures and maintaining refrigerator and freezer equipment at the appropriate temperatures may be tasks assigned to an allied health professional. Many of the new and expensive biologic medications must be kept refrigerated. For example, etanercept (Enbrel), an injectable medication that is used for rheumatoid arthritis and psoriasis, must be stored at 2° C to 8° C. The storage temperature requirements for any drug are given in Celsius on the manufacturers' drug package inserts. It is important to be able to convert those values to Fahrenheit as needed.

Table 6.15 shows the temperature equivalencies between these two scales. Every 5° C change in temperature is equivalent to a 9° F change.

TABLE 6.15 Temperature Equivalencies between Celsius and Fahrenheit

Celsius	Fahrenheit
0° C	32° F
5° C	41° F
10° C	50° F
15° C	59° F
20° C	68° F
37° C	98.6° F

In addition to using Table 6.15, here are several mathematical methods of converting from Fahrenheit to Celsius and vice versa. If you begin with a Fahrenheit measurement and want to convert it to a Celsius measurement, you use the following equation:

$$(° F – 32°) ÷ 1.8 = ° C$$

For example, if you want to convert 70° F to degrees Celsius, you would do the following:

$$(70° F – 32°) ÷ 1.8 = ° C$$

$$38° ÷ 1.8 = 21.1° C$$

$$21.1° C, \text{ rounded down to } 21° C, \text{ so } 70° F = \text{approximately } 21° C$$

If you begin with Celsius reading and need to convert it to Fahrenheit, you use the following equation:

$$(° C × 1.8) + 32° = ° F$$

For example, if you want to convert 30° C to degrees Fahrenheit, you would do the following:

$$(30° C × 1.8) + 32° = ° F$$

$$54° + 32° = 86° F$$

$$30° C = 86° F$$

Time

Standard time, also known as *civilian time*, is a system of time that relates to the natural day and is based on a 12-hour format. This system uses the designations of "a.m." and "p.m." and is a standard that is used by places within a similar longitude or geographical region. The United States and Canada are the only two countries who have adopted standard time as their official time standard; the remaining countries around the world have adopted the 24-hour time system as their official time clock.

24-Hour Time System

The **24-hour time system**, also known as *military time*, is based on a 24-hour clock, with a day running from midnight to midnight. The 24-hour system uses the numbers 0 through 24 to represent the 24-hour day. As mentioned in Chapter 5, this system uses four digits: The first two digits represent the number of hours past midnight; the last two digits represent the number of minutes past the hour (see Table 6.16). The start of each day is represented by 0000, and midnight is designated as 2400. (Be aware that some facilities use 0000 to refer to midnight.)

TABLE 6.16 | Standard Time and 24-Hour Time Equivalents

Standard Time	24-Hour Time	Standard Time	24-Hour Time
1:00 a.m.	0100 hours	1:00 p.m.	1300 hours
2:00 a.m.	0200 hours	2:00 p.m.	1400 hours
3:00 a.m.	0300 hours	3:00 p.m.	1500 hours
4:00 a.m.	0400 hours	4:00 p.m.	1600 hours
5:00 a.m.	0500 hours	5:00 p.m.	1700 hours
6:00 a.m.	0600 hours	6:00 p.m.	1800 hours
7:00 a.m.	0700 hours	7:00 p.m.	1900 hours
8:00 a.m.	0800 hours	8:00 p.m.	2000 hours
9:00 a.m.	0900 hours	9:00 p.m.	2100 hours
10:00 a.m.	1000 hours	10:00 p.m.	2200 hours
11:00 a.m.	1100 hours	11:00 p.m.	2300 hours
12:00 p.m.	1200 hours	12:00 a.m.	2400 hours

The 24-hour system was originally adopted by military personnel to avoid confusion between *a.m.* and *p.m.* Today, the 24-hour system has been adopted in the healthcare setting for the same reason. The use of 24-hour time allows personnel to document what time a medication is administered, what time a patient event occurs, or what time an IV medication runs out. Consequently, this precision results in fewer medication errors.

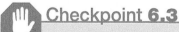

By the Numbers

Take a moment to practice temperature and time conversions by solving the following problems. For additional practice problems, refer to the Navigator+ learning management system that accompanies this textbook.

1. Convert 68° F to ° C.

2. Convert 38° C to ° F.

3. Convert 0845 to standard time.

4. Convert 3:26 p.m. to 24-hour time.

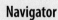

Navigator

Answers: (1) 20° C **(2)** 100.4° F **(3)** 8:45 a.m. **(4)** 1526

Checkpoint 6.3

Take a moment to review what you have learned so far and answer these questions.

1. Which countries use 24-hour time as their standard time system?

2. Which temperature scale has a 100-degree difference between the temperature of freezing water and boiling water?

3. What time system is used in hospitals?

Common Calculation Methods

In medical and pharmacy practice, several problem-solving approaches are used to calculate medication doses, IV flow rates and IV drip rates, and desired medication strengths. These approaches include the following:

- ratio-proportion method
- dimensional analysis method
- dilution method
- alligation method

Navigator

Allied health professionals who routinely perform dosage calculations typically use the ratio-proportion method. However, individuals who work in sterile compounding also need to know the dilution and alligation methods. To learn more about the dilution and alligation methods, refer to the Navigator+ learning management system that accompanies this textbook.

Ratio-Proportion Method

The **ratio-proportion method** is one of the most frequently used methods for calculating drug doses in the healthcare setting due to its straightforward approach. This method can be used to convert a quantity from one measurement system to another (e.g., pounds to kilograms), to calculate a specific dose, or to find out how much of a certain drug or medical supply a patient will need per month.

The ratio-proportion method can be used any time one ratio is complete and the other ratio has a missing component, or unknown quantity. When setting up ratios in the proportion, it is important that (1) the numbers remain in the correct position in the ratio; (2) the numbers in both numerators have the same units; and (3) the numbers in both denominators have the same units. Table 6.17 lists the rules for using the ratio-proportion method, and Table 6.18 outlines the steps for using this approach. Using that information, you can solve for the unknown quantity or *x*:

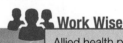

Quick Study

Ratios of drugs are usually written as the amount of drug per dose or unit. For example, ibuprofen for children is available as a liquid containing 100 mg of ibuprofen per 5 mL of solution.

Work Wise

Allied health professionals may hear other healthcare staff members refer to the ratio-proportion method by its technique: "cross multiply and divide."

$$\frac{x}{35} = \frac{2}{7}$$

$$x \times 7 = 35 \times 2$$

$$7x = 70$$

To isolate *x*, divide both sides by 7:

$$\frac{7x}{7} = \frac{70}{7}$$

$$x = 10$$

TABLE 6.17	Rules for Using the Ratio-Proportion Method
Rule 1.	Three of the four amounts must be known.
Rule 2.	The numerators must have the same unit of measurement.
Rule 3.	The denominators must have the same unit of measurement.

TABLE 6.18	Steps for Solving for *x* in the Ratio-Proportion Method
Step 1.	Create the proportion by placing the ratios in fraction form so that the *x* is in the upper left corner.
Step 2.	Check that the unit of measurement in the numerators is the same, and the unit of measurement in the denominators is the same.
Step 3.	Solve for *x* by using the "cross multiply and divide" method. Remember that, in an equation, a number within parentheses is multiplied by the number that precedes it. For example: $$2\,(3) = 2 \times 3$$

Conversion within the Same Measurement System

At times, you may need to convert quantities within the same measurement system—most likely, the metric system. For that reason, you need to memorize the metric values provided in Table 6.10 and be at ease with converting these values, as demonstrated in Table 6.11. Use these tables to help you solve the following problems using the ratio-proportion method:

Example 1 A prescriber has written an order for the thyroid medication levothyroxine in milligrams (mg), but the drug is available in tablet sizes measured in micrograms (mcg). Use the ratio-proportion method to convert 0.088 mg to micrograms.

According to Table 6.10, 1 mg is equal to 1,000 mcg.

$$\frac{x\ \text{mcg}}{0.088\ \text{mg}} = \frac{1,000\ \text{mcg}}{1\ \text{mg}}$$

$$x\ \text{mcg}\,(1\ \text{mg}) = 1,000\ \text{mcg}\,(0.088\ \text{mg})$$

$$\frac{x\ \text{mcg}\,(1\ \text{mg})}{1\ \text{mg}} = \frac{1,000\ \text{mcg}\,(0.088\ \text{mg})}{1\ \text{mg}}$$

$$x\ \text{mcg} = 88\ \text{mcg}$$

Example 2 A solution is to be used to fill hypodermic syringes each containing 60 mL. There are 3 L of the solution available. How many hypodermic syringes can be filled with the available solution?

According to Table 6.10, 1 L is equal to 1,000 mL. The available supply of solution is therefore:

$$3 \times 1,000\ \text{mL} = 3,000\ \text{mL}$$

Determine the number of syringes by using the ratio-proportion method:

$$\frac{x \text{ syringes}}{3{,}000 \text{ mL}} = \frac{1 \text{ syringe}}{60 \text{ mL}}$$

$$60 \text{ mL } (x \text{ syringes}) = 3{,}000 \text{ mL } (1 \text{ syringe})$$

$$\frac{60 \text{ mL } (x \text{ syringes})}{60 \text{ mL}} = \frac{3{,}000 \text{ mL } (1 \text{ syringe})}{60 \text{ mL}}$$

$$x \text{ syringes} = 50 \text{ syringes}$$

Therefore, 50 hypodermic syringes can be filled.

Conversion of One Measurement System to Another

Other situations in the healthcare setting call for conversion of quantities between different measurement systems. When possible, convert to the metric system because it is the preferred system. For the following example, refer to Table 6.14:

Example 3 How many milliliters are there in 1 gal, 12 fl oz?

According to the values found in Table 6.14, 3,840 mL are found in 1 gal. In addition, because 1 fl oz contains 30 mL, you can use the ratio-proportion method to calculate the amount of milliliters in 12 fl oz as follows:

$$\frac{x \text{ mL}}{12 \text{ fl oz}} = \frac{30 \text{ mL}}{1 \text{ fl oz}}$$

$$x \text{ mL } (1 \text{ fl oz}) = 30 \text{ mL } (12 \text{ fl oz})$$

$$\frac{x \text{ mL } (1 \text{ fl oz})}{1 \text{ fl oz}} = \frac{30 \text{ mL } (12 \text{ fl oz})}{1 \text{ fl oz}}$$

$$x \text{ mL} = 360 \text{ mL}$$

Add the two values:

$$3{,}840 \text{ mL} + 360 \text{ mL} = 4{,}200 \text{ mL}$$

Therefore, 4,200 mL = 1 gal, 12 fl oz.

Example 4 A patient weighs 44 lb. What is the patient's weight in kilograms?

According to the values found in Table 6.14, 1 kg equals 2.2 lb. Using the ratio-proportion method, solve the problem:

$$\frac{x \text{ kg}}{44 \text{ lb}} = \frac{1 \text{ kg}}{2.2 \text{ lb}}$$

$$x \text{ kg } (2.2 \text{ lb}) = 1 \text{ kg } (44 \text{ lb})$$

$$\frac{x \text{ kg } (2.2 \text{ lb})}{2.2 \text{ lb}} = \frac{1 \text{ kg } (44 \text{ lb})}{2.2 \text{ lb}}$$

$$x \text{ kg} = 20 \text{ kg}$$

Therefore, the patient weighs 20 kg.

Example 5 You are to dispense 300 mL of a liquid medication. If the dose is 2 tsp, how many doses will there be in the final preparation?

Step 1. Begin solving this problem by converting to a common unit of measurement using conversion values in Table 6.14:

$$1 \text{ dose} = 2 \text{ tsp}; \; 2 \text{ tsp} \times \frac{5 \text{ mL}}{1 \text{ tsp}} = 10 \text{ mL}$$

Step 2. Using these converted measurements, the solution can be determined using the ratio-proportion method:

$$\frac{x \text{ doses}}{300 \text{ mL}} = \frac{1 \text{ dose}}{10 \text{ mL}}$$

$$x \text{ doses } (10 \text{ mL}) = 1 \text{ dose } (300 \text{ mL})$$

$$\frac{x \text{ doses } (10 \text{ mL})}{10 \text{ mL}} = \frac{1 \text{ dose } (300 \text{ mL})}{10 \text{ mL}}$$

$$x \text{ doses} = 30 \text{ doses}$$

Calculation of a Specific Dose

The ratio-proportion method is frequently used to calculate specific dosages:

Example 6 Gentamicin is available as 20 mg/2 mL. The medication order calls for 50 mg. How many milliliters should you prepare?

$$\frac{x \text{ mL}}{50 \text{ mg}} = \frac{2 \text{ mL}}{20 \text{ mg}}$$

$$x \text{ mL } (20 \text{ mg}) = 2 \text{ mL } (50 \text{ mg})$$

$$\frac{x \text{ mL } (20 \text{ mg})}{20 \text{ mg}} = \frac{2 \text{ mL } (50 \text{ mg})}{20 \text{ mg}}$$

$$x \text{ mL} = 5 \text{ mL}$$

Example 7 A physician has prescribed diazepam for a patient. You have a vial of diazepam 5 mg/mL available. How many milligrams should be dispensed to the patient if the prescription is for 4 mL?

$$\frac{x \text{ mg}}{4 \text{ mL}} = \frac{5 \text{ mg}}{1 \text{ mL}}$$

$$x \text{ mg } (1 \text{ mL}) = 5 \text{ mg } (4 \text{ mL})$$

$$\frac{x \text{ mg } (1 \text{ mL})}{1 \text{ mL}} = \frac{5 \text{ mg } (4 \text{ mL})}{1 \text{ mL}}$$

$$x \text{ mg} = 20 \text{ mg}$$

Example 8 A dose of 30 mg of lamivudine oral solution is ordered. The drug is available in a 5 mg/mL oral solution. How many milliliters are needed to provide the ordered dose?

$$\frac{x \text{ mL}}{30 \text{ mg}} = \frac{1 \text{ mL}}{5 \text{ mg}}$$

$$x \text{ mL } (5 \text{ mg}) = 1 \text{ mL } (30 \text{ mg})$$

$$\frac{x \text{ mL } (5 \text{ mg})}{5 \text{ mg}} = \frac{1 \text{ mL } (30 \text{ mg})}{5 \text{ mg}}$$

$$x \text{ mL} = 6 \text{ mL}$$

Supplies in a Clinical Setting

You may be asked to order office supplies for a clinical facility or medical supplies for a particular patient. With that in mind, the ratio-proportion method is a simple method to use to determine quantity.

Example 9 File folders for your clinical facility cost $7.40 per box of 100 folders. Your budget allows you to spend $15.00. How many boxes can you buy if the boxes cannot be broken?

$$\frac{x \text{ folders}}{\$15.00} = \frac{100 \text{ folders}}{\$7.40}$$

$$x \text{ folders } (\$7.40) = 100 \text{ folders } (\$15.00)$$

$$\frac{x \text{ folders } (\$7.40)}{\$7.40} = \frac{100 \text{ folders } (\$15.00)}{\$7.40}$$

$$x \text{ folders} = 202.7 \text{ folders}$$

You can buy 2 boxes of 100 folders with a budget of $15.00.

123 By the Numbers

Take a moment to practice the ratio-proportion method by solving the following problems. For additional practice problems, refer to the Navigator+ learning management system that accompanies this textbook.

1. The antibiotic cefdinir is available as a 125 mg/5 mL solution. The patient needs a dose of 300 mg twice a day. How many milliliters is the medication dose?

2. The antidepressant fluoxetine is available in liquid form at a concentration of 20 mg/5 mL. A patient requires a daily dose of 30 mg. How many milliliters is the daily dose?

3. A patient requires 20 g of lactulose every 8 hours. The lactulose is provided in a 10 g/15 mL solution. How many milliliters of solution does the **Navigator** patient need per dose?

Answers: (1) 12 mL **(2)** 7.5 mL **(3)** 30 mL

Dimensional Analysis Method

Dimensional analysis is another problem-solving method that medical, pharmacy, and some allied health professionals use, particularly for simple dosage calculations. This method is based on the principle that any number can be multiplied by 1 without changing its value. This process helps to break down mathematical problems and assist in conversion to desired units of measurement. Unlike the ratio-proportion method, the dimensional analysis method is not based on a set formula.

The dimensional analysis method can be used for simple conversions between metric units:

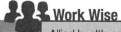

Work Wise

Allied health professionals may hear some healthcare staff members refer to the dimensional analysis method by its technique: "calculation by cancellation."

Example 10 Convert 486 mg to grams.

$$486 \text{ mg} \times \frac{1 \text{ g}}{1{,}000 \text{ mg}} = 0.486 \text{ g}$$

Because 1,000 mg equals 1 g, multiplying a number by 1 g/1,000 mg is the same as multiplying by 1.

Example 11 Convert 4.5 L to milliliters.

$$4.5 \text{ L} \times \frac{1{,}000 \text{ mL}}{1 \text{ L}} = 4{,}500 \text{ mL}$$

Example 12 Convert 240 mL to liters.

$$240 \text{ mL} \times \frac{1 \text{ L}}{1{,}000 \text{ mL}} = 0.24 \text{ L}$$

The dimensional analysis method can also be used to solve a pharmacy calculation problem.

Example 13 A patient is to take 7 mL of amoxicillin 250 mg/5 mL. How many milligrams are present in one dose?

$$7 \text{ mL} \times \frac{250 \text{ mg}}{5 \text{ mL}} = 350 \text{ mg}$$

Example 14 How many milligrams of medication are in 1 tbsp of clarithromycin that contains 125 mg/tsp?

Convert both volumes to the metric system using the following values from Table 6.14:

$$1 \text{ tbsp} = 15 \text{ mL}$$

$$1 \text{ tsp} = 5 \text{ mL}$$

Then plug these metric units into the calculation:

$$15 \text{ mL} \times \frac{125 \text{ mg}}{5 \text{ mL}} = 375 \text{ mg}$$

Take a moment to practice the dimensional analysis method by solving the following problems. For additional practice problems, refer to the Navigator+ learning management system that accompanies this textbook.

1. The long-acting insulin Lantus is available in prefilled pens (Lantus Solostar). If a patient injects 25 units per day, how many units does the patient use in 30 days?

2. A child who weighs 22 lb needs to receive 30 mg/kg a day of amoxicillin for an infection. How many milligrams of amoxicillin does the child need to receive per day? (To convert pounds to kilograms, the formula is 1 kg = 2.2 lb.)

Answers: (1) 750 units **(2)** 300 mg of amoxicillin per day

Navigator

Specialized Calculation Methods

Special dosing calculations are frequently used when determining medication doses for pediatric patients. These calculations use weight measurements or body surface measurements to determine proper dosages.

Weight-Based Calculations

The pediatric patient population requires customized doses because children weigh significantly less than normal adult patients, and manufacturers' dosing guidelines are generally designed for adult patients. In addition, the body systems of pediatric patients may not metabolize or eliminate a drug at the same rate as adults' body systems would do. (For additional information on the unique characteristics of the pediatric patient population, see Chapter 28.) Consequently, for some drugs, drug manufacturers offer weight-based prescribing guidelines. Dosing instructions are typically given in milligrams of drug per kilograms of body weight. Although allied health professionals do not perform weight-based calculations, they should have a general understanding of how these dose calculations are executed.

Example 15 A patient weighs 60 kg and is to receive a dose of 15 mg/kg. What will the patient's dose be?

To determine the dose, you can use either the ratio-proportion method or the dimensional analysis method.

Using the ratio-proportion method:

$$\frac{x \text{ mg}}{60 \text{ kg}} = \frac{15 \text{ mg}}{1 \text{ kg}}$$

$$x \text{ mg } (1 \text{ kg}) = 15 \text{ mg } (60 \text{ kg})$$

$$\frac{x \text{ mg } (1 \text{ kg})}{1 \text{ kg}} = \frac{15 \text{ mg } (60 \text{ kg})}{1 \text{ kg}}$$

$$x \text{ mg} = 900 \text{ mg}$$

Using the dimensional analysis method:

$$60 \text{ kg} \times \frac{15 \text{ mg}}{1 \text{ kg}} = 900 \text{ mg}$$

Body Surface Area Calculations

Body surface area (BSA) is a measurement that is based on weight and height variables and is expressed as meters squared (m^2). BSA is usually estimated using a **nomogram**, or a chart that is used to compare the height and weight of a patient in order to determine the patient's BSA. The BSA is then used to calculate the patient's dose. Table 6.19 outlines the steps for using a nomogram, and Figures 6.4 and 6.5 are nomograms used for estimating BSA of children and adults.

Nomograms are frequently used by physicians, pharmacists, nurse practitioners, physician assistants, and other health professionals who work in specialty areas such as pediatrics and chemotherapy. Nomograms are also used to calculate the doses and dosing intervals of specific drugs such as the class of IV antibiotics called aminoglycosides.

Although allied health personnel do not perform BSA calculations, they should be familiar with this specialized calculation method.

TABLE 6.19	Steps for Reading a Nomogram for Estimating BSA
Step 1.	Mark the patient's height on the left column.
Step 2.	Mark the patient's weight (mass) on the right column.
Step 3.	Draw a line or place a straight-edge ruler on the two marks.
Step 4.	Read the BSA by noting where the straight edge crosses the center column. When the straight edge crosses between two numbers, the BSA should be estimated to the nearest one-half unit.

 Checkpoint 6.4

Take a moment to review what you have learned so far and answer these questions.

1. What is a nomogram?

2. What patient population is most likely to need weight-based dosing?

3. List the three rules for using the ratio-proportion method.

FIGURE 6.4 | Nomogram for Estimating Body Surface Area of Children

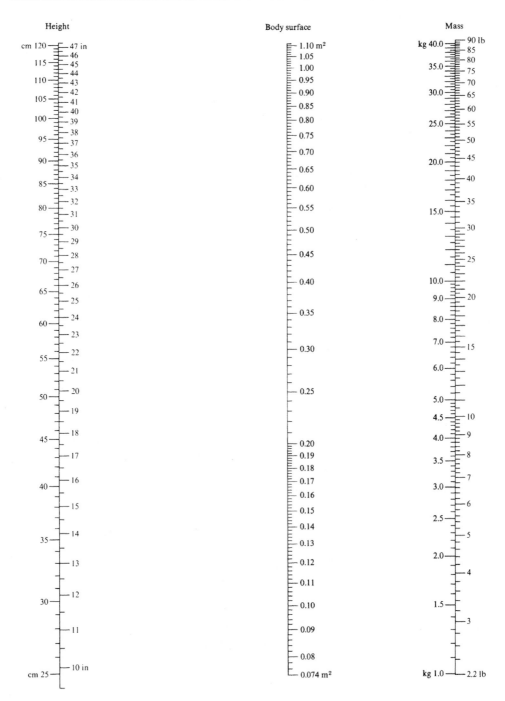

FIGURE 6.5 | Nomogram for Estimating Body Surface Area of Adults

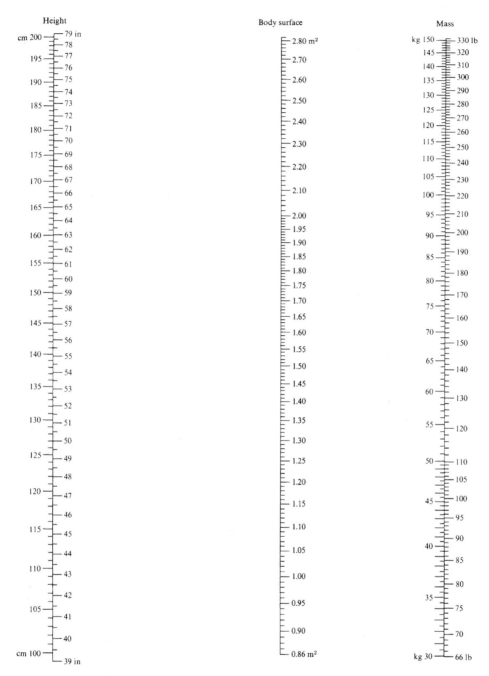

Chapter Review

Chapter Summary

Two types of number systems are used in pharmacy calculations: Roman numerals and Arabic numbers. The Roman numeral system uses letters to represent quantities or amounts. This system includes seven main symbols: I (equal to 1), V (equal to 5), X (equal to 10), L (equal to 50), C (equal to 100), D (equal to 500), and M (equal to 1,000). The Arabic number system consists of 10 digits: 0, 1, 2, 3, 4, 5, 6, 7, 8, and 9.

Working in a healthcare setting often requires individuals to have number sense and to apply their knowledge of numbers to real-world settings. Understanding fractions, decimals, ratios, percentages, and proportions and knowing how to manipulate these numbers in mathematical operations and conversions are critical skills.

A fraction is a number that indicates the relationship of a part, or portion, to its whole. A simple fraction consists of two numbers: a numerator and a denominator. The fraction bar, or the line between the numerator and the denominator, indicates division.

There are several types of fractions. For example, a fraction with a value less than 1 (numerator smaller than denominator) is called a *proper fraction*. Another type of fraction is an *improper fraction*, or a fraction with a value greater than 1 (numerator greater than denominator). A *mixed number* consists of a whole number and a fraction and can be converted to an improper fraction by multiplying the whole number by the denominator and adding the numerator. Finally, a fraction in which there is a fraction in the numerator, the denominator, or both the numerator and denominator is called a *complex fraction*.

When adding or subtracting fractions with unlike denominators, it is necessary to create a common denominator, a number into which each of the unlike denominators can be divided evenly. Creating a common denominator requires transforming each fraction by multiplying it by a form of 1. After two fractions have been converted to a common denominator and added together, it may be necessary to reduce the fraction to its lowest terms. This operation requires dividing both the numerator and denominator of the fraction by a common factor.

The basic step in multiplying fractions is to multiply numerators by numerators and denominators by denominators; then reduce the product to its lowest terms. Before multiplying mixed numbers, you need to convert each mixed number to an improper fraction by multiplying the whole number by the denominator and adding the product to the numerator. To divide fractions, you multiply the first fraction by the reciprocal of the second fraction. To divide mixed numbers, you need to convert each mixed number to an improper fraction by multiplying the whole number by the denominator and adding the product to the numerator. Then multiply the first fraction by the reciprocal of the second fraction.

A fraction in which the denominator is 10 or some multiple of 10 is a *decimal fraction* or, more simply, a *decimal*. The decimal point represents the center. Digits written to the right of the decimal point are decimal fractions with a multiple of 10—for example, tenths, hundredths, thousandths, and so on. These numbers have a value of less than 1. Digits written to the left of the decimal point have a value of 1 or greater (whole numbers). If a decimal number is less than 1, with no numbers to the left of the decimal point, a leading zero is placed to the left of the decimal point.

When adding or subtracting decimals, place the numbers in columns so that the decimal points are aligned directly under each other. You may need to add zeros after the decimal point to correctly align the decimal points.

The multiplication of decimals does not require you to align the decimal points. You simply multiply decimals the same way that you multiply whole numbers, and after multiplying, make sure that you position the decimal point in the correct place. Healthcare personnel should always use a calculator when dividing decimal numbers.

Rounding numbers is essential for daily use of mathematical operations. The purpose of rounding is to keep the number you are working with to a manageable size. Rounding will affect the accuracy to which a medication can be measured. To round an answer to the nearest tenth, carry the division out two places, to the hundredths place. If the number in the hundredths place is 5 or greater, add 1 to the tenths place number. If the number in the hundredths place is less than 5, round the number down by omitting the digit in the hundredths place.

A ratio is a numerical representation of the relationship between two parts of a whole. Ratios are written with a colon between the numbers. The ratio 1:2 means that the second part has twice the value of the first part. A ratio is used to express the weight or strength of a drug per volumetric measurement. Ratios are also commonly used to express concentrations of a drug in a solution. To express a ratio as a percent, designate the first number of the ratio as the numerator and the second number as the denominator. Multiply the fraction by 100 and add a percent sign after the number.

Percent expresses the number of parts compared with a total of 100 parts. A percent can be written as a ratio, a fraction, or a decimal. Being able to convert between ratios, percents, and decimals is an important skill in the healthcare setting. Percent strengths are often used to describe IV solutions and topically applied drugs. To convert a percent to a ratio, first change it to a fraction by dividing it by 100; then reduce the fraction to its lowest terms. Express this fraction as a ratio by making the numerator the first number of the ratio and the denominator the second number of the ratio.

A proportion is an expression of equality between two ratios. This expression can by written three ways: using an equal sign between the ratios, using a double colon between the ratios, or writing the ratios as fractions. Two ratios that have the same value, such as ¾ and ¹⁵⁄₂₀, are said to be equivalent, or proportional, ratios. In a proportion, the first and fourth, or outside, numbers are called the *extremes*. The second and third, or inside, numbers are called the *means*.

The need for standardized units of measurement among the various sciences resulted in the establishment of the apothecary system, the avoirdupois system, and the household system.

The apothecary system of measurement is one of the oldest systems of measurement still in use today. This system of measurement includes units such as minims, fluid drams, scruples, drams, grains, ounces, and pounds. The avoirdupois system includes such common units of measurement as feet and miles as well as grains, ounces, and pounds. These units are shared with the apothecary system; however, their values are not the same. The household system of measurement is based on the apothecary system and is used to help patients take their medications at home. Like the apothecary and avoirdupois systems, this system includes such common units of measurement as the ounce, pound, drop, teaspoon, tablespoon, and cup. The metric system of measurement uses a group of basic units of measure (such as meter, liter, and gram) in conjunction with a set of prefixes (such as *deci–*, *centi–*, and *milli–*) that represent multiples of ten.

Allied health professionals should also have an understanding of two other measurement systems: temperature and time. The Fahrenheit temperature scale uses 32° F as the temperature at which water freezes to ice and 212° F as the temperature at which water boils. The difference between these two extremes is 180° F. The Celsius temperature scale uses 0° C as the freezing point and 100° C as the boiling point. The difference between these two extremes is 100° C.

Standard time is a system of time based on a 12-hour format. This system uses the designations of "a.m." and "p.m." and is a standard that is used by places within a similar longitude or geographical region. The 24-hour time system, also known as *military time*, is based on a 24-hour clock, with a day running from midnight to midnight. The 24-hour system uses the numbers 0 through 24 to represent the 24-hour day. Today, the 24-hour system has been adopted in the healthcare setting.

In medical and pharmacy practice, several problem-solving approaches are used to calculate medication dosages, IV flow rates and IV drip rates, and desired medication strengths. These approaches include the ratio-proportion, dimensional analysis, dilution, and alligation methods.

The ratio-proportion method can be used to convert a quantity from one measurement system to another (e.g., pounds to kilograms), to calculate a specific dose, or to find out how much of a certain drug or medical supply a patient will need per month. The ratio-proportion method can be used any time one ratio is complete and the other ratio has a missing component, or unknown quantity.

Dimensional analysis is another problem-solving method based on the principle that any number can be multiplied by 1 without changing its value. This method can be used for simple conversions between metric units and can also be used to solve a pharmacy calculation problem.

Two other calculation methods—dilution and alligation—are used by sterile compounding personnel. In addition, special dosing calculations are frequently used when determining medication doses for pediatric patients. These calculations use weight measurements or body surface measurements to determine proper dosages. BSA is a measurement that is based on weight and height variables and is expressed as meters squared (m^2). BSA is usually estimated using a nomogram, or a chart that is used to compare the height and weight (mass) of a patient in order to determine the patient's BSA.

Chapter Checkup

The Navigator+ learning management system that accompanies this textbook offers many opportunities to help you master chapter content, including end-of-chapter exercises, a glossary of key terms, flash cards, and additional interactive activities.

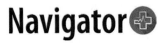

Career Exploration

If you enjoyed learning about pharmacy measurements and calculations in this chapter, you may want to explore the following career options:

- chemotherapy technician
- emergency medical technician (EMT)/paramedic
- intravenous (IV) technician
- medical assistant
- pharmacy technician

Medication Safety

Pharm Facts

- Between 50% and 75% of patients do not take prescription medications as directed, leaving themselves vulnerable for a medication error.

- The Food and Drug Administration has received almost 30,000 medication error reports since 1992.

- According to the American Association of Poison Control Centers, more than 3.1 million calls were made to the 51 poison control centers in the United States in 2013.

- The Latin expression *Primum non nocere*—translated as "First, do no harm"—has been the mantra of healthcare practitioners for more than a century. The expression was first used by Thomas Sydenham, a seventeenth-century English physician. The expression became well-known at the start of the twentieth century as pharmacology and health care became more regulated. Today, most healthcare personnel in the United States know this guiding principle from their clinical studies and use it as a reminder that the well-being of a patient is paramount when making medical treatment decisions.

"Knowledge of drugs, their uses, and their standard dosing can make a critical difference in medication safety. As a pharmacy technician working in a neonatal ICU, I discovered a medication error during our daily medication reconciliation procedure. A neonate born from an HIV-positive mother was prescribed zidovudine or AZT to decrease the chance of developing HIV. However, acyclovir was dispensed in error. Because of the high dose of acyclovir, I recognized the error, which allowed me to change the outcome of the patient's quality of life."

—**Veronica Velasquez**, BA, CPhT, PhTR
Pharmacy Technician

Learning Objectives

1 Define *medical error* and *medication error*.

2 Understand the extent of medical and medication errors and their effects on patient health and safety.

3 Identify the five major categories of medication errors.

4 Understand the three types of failures that cause medication errors.

5 Understand the responsibilities of patients, healthcare workers, and organizations in the prevention of medication errors.

6 Discuss the innovative designs, automation technologies, and strategies that are making a positive impact on medication safety.

7 Identify the common systems available for reporting medication errors.

Preventable medical errors are the third leading cause of death in the United States, according to a 2013 report in the *Journal of Patient Safety*. To be specific, an estimated 400,000 individuals die every year from errors in their healthcare treatment in US hospitals. This statistic has soared since the 1999 publication *To Err is Human* was released from the Institute of Medicine, or IOM (http://PharmEssAH.emcp.net/MedicalErrors). In that report, the IOM concluded that approximately 100,000 patients were the victims of preventable adverse events and that "the majority of medical errors do not result from individual recklessness or the actions of a particular group. . . . More commonly, errors are caused by faulty systems, processes, and conditions that lead people to make mistakes or fail to prevent them."

This spike in preventable hospital deaths has facilities examining their staff training and current policies and procedures to effect change and to ensure the health and well-being of their patients. Ensuring patient safety has an additional benefit: lowering the cost of health care. According to a study published in the *Journal of Health Care Finance*, the economic impact of medical errors is estimated to be close to $1 trillion, which takes into account the "lost human potential and contributions." Because government and private insurers no longer reimburse hospitals for the hospital costs associated with preventable medical errors, healthcare facilities assume a huge financial burden from these medical mistakes.

This chapter specifically examines one common type of medical error: the medication error. Some of the topics addressed include the types of medication errors; the strategies that healthcare professionals can implement to prevent these errors, including safety and disposal procedures; and the innovative designs and automation technologies that are making a positive impact on medication safety.

Medical Errors

A **medical error** is any circumstance, action, inaction, or decision related to health care that contributes to an unintended health result. A medical error can be as simple as a laboratory test blood sample drawn at the wrong time that returns an inaccurate result or an infection from improper technique, or it can be as serious as a major surgical error that ends in death. A majority of what is known about medical errors comes from information collected in the hospital setting; however, hospital data make up only part of a much larger picture. Generally, medical errors are difficult to define because the circumstances that can cause them are infinite.

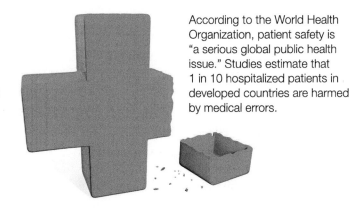

According to the World Health Organization, patient safety is "a serious global public health issue." Studies estimate that 1 in 10 hospitalized patients in developed countries are harmed by medical errors.

Scope and Impact of Medical Errors

As the third leading cause of death in the United States (behind heart disease and cancer), there are more deaths from preventable medical errors than from diabetes, Alzheimer's disease, pneumonia, influenza, or kidney disease. Any preventable medical error can also result in a serious physical injury. The number of medical-related lawsuits provides a sense of the real scope of medical errors in the United States. As mentioned earlier in the chapter, one of the most common types of medical error is a medication error.

Medication Errors

The National Coordinating Council for Medication Error Reporting and Prevention (NCC MERP) defines a **medication error** as "any preventable event that may cause or lead to inappropriate medication use or patient harm while the medication is in the control of the healthcare professional, patient, or consumer. Such events may be related to professional practice, health care products, procedures, and systems, including prescribing; order communication; product labeling, packaging, and nomenclature; compounding; dispensing; distribution; administration; education; monitoring; and use."

Scope and Impact of Medication Errors

Medication errors include prescribing, dispensing, or administering the wrong drug; administering a drug to the wrong patient; administering the wrong dose of a medication; and using the wrong route of administration during drug delivery. The information about the effect of medication errors comes mainly from studies done in the hospital setting and is most likely underreported and underestimated. According to the IOM, more than 1.5 million preventable medication errors cause harm in the United States every year.

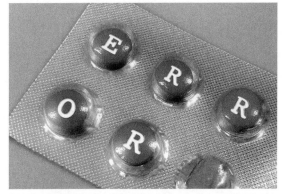

Deaths from medication-related errors are estimated at about 7,000 annually in the United States, or 19 deaths a day.

Types of Medication Errors

An exact list of medication errors is difficult to create because the possible causes of such missteps can often be too numerous to count. However, categorizing errors into types or groups often aids in the identification and prevention of future problems. Classic examples are grouped into the following five major categories:

- An **omission error** occurs when a prescribed dose is due, but not administered.

- A **wrong-dose error** occurs when a dose is either above or below the correct amount by more than 5%. An example of this type of error would be administering an injection of a premeasured pediatric dose to an adult patient.

- An **extra-dose error** occurs when a patient receives more doses than were ordered by the physician or other prescriber. For example, a patient who is self-administering insulin may misread the graduation marks on a syringe and fill the syringe with a higher dose than what is prescribed.

- A **wrong-dosage-form error** occurs when the dose formulation given to the patient does not match the prescriber's order. Examples include a drug given by mouth for a drug ordered as an intramuscular (IM) injection, an IM-prescribed drug given subcutaneously, or an immediate-release drug dispensed instead of a controlled-release or extended-release drug.

- A **wrong-time error** occurs when any drug is given 30 minutes or more before or after it was ordered to be administered, up to the time of the next dose. This type of error does not apply to drugs that are administered PRN (i.e., as needed). A wrong-time error is a common medication error in hospitals and nursing homes due to staffing shortages.

Reasons for Medication Errors

Medication errors can also be categorized according to what caused the failure of the desired result. The purpose of defining errors in this way is to identify clearly what the error was, where it took place, and—through closer examination—what specifically caused it (i.e., the *why*). Such analysis identifies ways to eliminate or reduce future mistakes. Most situations fall into one of three basic classes of failure: organizational failure, human failure, and technical failure.

Organizational Failure

An **organizational failure** occurs because of a deficiency in organizational rules, policies, or procedures. An example of this type of failure includes a policy or rule requiring the preparing or admixing of parenteral medications, such as chemotherapy drugs, in an inappropriate setting without proper environmental controls or equipment. Another example of an organizational failure would be an inadequate drug administration procedure in the Policy & Procedures (P&P) manual of a long-term care facility, which contributed to a patient medication error.

Prevention of Organizational Failure

The responsibility for organizational failure lies with the healthcare facility. To prevent medication errors, administrators and staff members need to evaluate the organizational

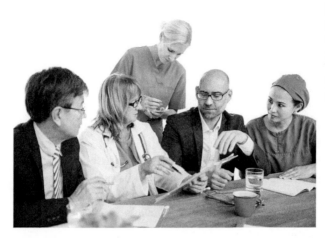

In a hospital setting, the Pharmacy and Therapeutics Committee reviews medication guidelines and monitors medication error reports. This committee typically includes hospital administrators and members of the healthcare staff.

structure and workflow of the facility for potential areas that put their patients at risk for medication errors.

Organizational Policies and Procedures

Each healthcare organization should have a P&P manual that specifies standard work and defines best practices for the facility, including practices designed to minimize the risk of medication errors. This manual is required by several accreditation and licensing organizations including The Joint Commission and state licensing boards. Healthcare organizations should also conduct periodic evaluations of current medication handling procedures.

Personnel Management

Organizations can also strive to decrease the likelihood of medication errors through personnel management: by selecting job candidates carefully, by training new hires thoroughly, and by providing ongoing safety training to all employees. Healthcare organizations can also decrease the likelihood of medication errors by ensuring that staffing levels are adequate. Overworked employees who feel pressured to work quickly are more likely to make medication errors.

Up-to-Date Technology

Healthcare organizations can also use technology to decrease medical errors. The implementation of bar-coding systems, electronic medical records, and electronic prescribing can help reduce medication errors. These technologies are discussed in detail later in this chapter.

Work Environment

The physical setting can certainly contribute to the overall safety of any healthcare environment. Healthcare facilities should provide adequate space, ventilation, and lighting, and they should maintain an appropriate temperature and level of cleanliness in all work areas. These factors are important to the safe preparation and handling of medications. In addition, facilities should encourage healthcare personnel to keep noise and distractions to a minimal level.

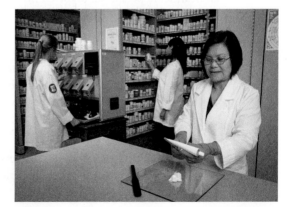

A hospital pharmacy should be clean, well lit, and organized to allow the safe preparation of medications.

Human Failure

A **human failure** occurs at an individual level. This type of failure can be made by either a patient or a healthcare worker.

Patient Failure

Patients in the outpatient setting may contribute to medication errors by **nonadherence**, or a failure to follow their prescribed drug therapy as instructed. The reasons behind this nonadherence vary and may include the cost of the medication or the transportation to acquire the medication; a misunderstanding of instructions, perhaps because of language or cultural barriers; and the practice of **polypharmacy**, or the simultaneous use of multiple drugs. Some behaviors that patients exhibit include the following:

- forgetting to take a dose or doses
- taking too many doses
- dosing at the wrong time
- not getting a prescription filled or refilled in a timely manner
- not following directions for dose administration
- terminating the drug regimen too soon

As a result, a medication does not work well, does not work at all (due to a **subtherapeutic dose**), or may cause harm (due to an adverse drug reaction or even a toxic dose). Not taking prescribed medication could also result in the progression of a chronic disease. In fact, more than 50% of patients taking essential long-term medication no longer take their medication after one year.

Patient Responsibilities in Medication Error Prevention

Patients can help prevent medication errors by taking an active role in their own health care. To do this, patients should be candid with their healthcare practitioners about all of the medications and supplements they are currently taking and should maintain an up-to-date list of these products. Patients should also make sure they understand the uses of the drugs they are prescribed, and accurately follow the dosage instructions.

Honest Communication

To ensure an optimal outcome, patients must establish honest, open communication with all healthcare personnel involved in their care. That honest communication begins at the initial interview. Patients must provide healthcare practitioners with accurate medication information, including all prescription medications, over-the-counter drugs, and alternative therapies they are taking, as well as information about allergies. This data must be documented in the patient record. Establishing a trusting environment also encourages patients to ask questions if some part of a prescribed drug regimen remains unclear and to report any adverse effects once therapy has begun.

An Understanding of Drug Therapy

All patients must have a complete understanding of their prescribed drug therapy. Table 7.1 lists the 10 pieces of information all patients must know about their medications.

TABLE 7.1 Medication Information Patients Must Know

1. Purpose of the medication, including whether the prescription is in addition to or replaces a current medication
2. Generic and brand names of the medication
3. Appearance of the medication
4. Correct dose and dosage (frequency) of the medication
5. Best time to take a dose, including the actions to take if they miss a dose
6. Duration of treatment
7. Medications or foods that interact with the prescribed medication
8. Common side effects of the medication and how to handle them
9. Special precautions necessary for the drug therapy
10. Proper storage of the medication

Adherence to Instructions

Patients must follow their medication regimen exactly as prescribed to achieve the desired effect. Skipping doses or stopping the therapy before the end date may result in inadequate treatment of a condition or disorder. For those patients who are taking a number of drugs, using a pill container helps keep the individual therapy regimens organized, thus allowing increased adherence to drug therapy.

Safe Handling of Medications

The safe handling of medications is also an important responsibility of patients. Proper disposal of expired drugs, unused medications, and syringes prevents accidental harm to other individuals and to the environment.

Drug Disposal Many individuals do not realize that, like foods, drugs have expiration dates. A drug's **expiration date** is the date after which a drug should not be used. The drug's manufacturer puts the expiration date on the medication container. Allied health professionals should show patients where expiration dates are located on the containers and should explain to them that most drugs lose some efficacy after they pass their expiration dates. With that in mind, any unused drugs in a prescription bottle

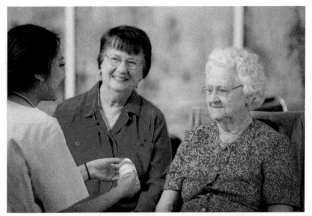

A patient who is taking multiple medications may be confused by his or her drug regimen. Having a family member or caregiver present during the medication discussion may reduce the possibility of medication errors.

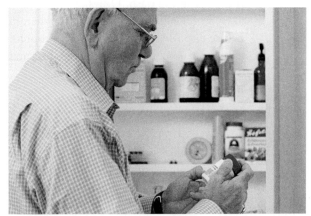

An individual should periodically check for expired medications in his or her medicine cabinet at home.

In the Know

should be disposed of one year after purchase. Patients should be reminded to keep track of their medications and to make a habit of periodically removing all unwanted or expired medications from their medicine cabinets.

Safe disposal of unwanted medications reduces the likelihood of accidental poisonings at home. In addition, the removal of leftover drugs from the house once they are no longer needed is also a way to prevent the misuse of medications, which is a growing problem in the United States. The US Food and Drug Administration (FDA) recommends that patients participate in medication take-back initiatives for their drug disposal. These programs are operated by pharmacies and allow individuals to deposit their unwanted medications in a locked bin in a participating pharmacy. The unwanted drugs are then collected and incinerated at a central location. However, patients should be aware that these programs do not accept controlled substances; unwanted or leftover controlled substances should be disposed of at a police station.

In addition, the Drug Enforcement Administration (DEA) coordinates a Prescription Drug Take-Back Day on a designated day each year. For more information on this national program, visit http://PharmEssAH .emcp.net/DrugTakeback.

Lastly, some municipalities and counties accept unwanted medications at recycling centers, police stations, or city halls. To learn more, consult the website of your county or state health department.

If a medication disposal initiative is not being conducted in their area, patients can mix their medications with kitty litter or coffee grounds in a sealed plastic container and place the container in the trash. Drugs disposed of this way are less likely to leach into the water supply than flushed medications. Before disposing of the empty drug containers, patients should remove or obscure any identifying information on the medication labels to protect their privacy.

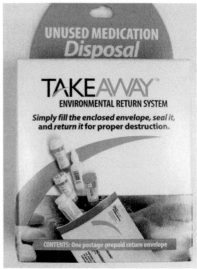

The Takeaway Environmental Return System is an example of a program whereby an individual may dispose of unwanted medications (except scheduled drugs) through the US Postal Service (USPS).

Drug Alert

Patients should be aware that the FDA has created a list of medications that should be flushed down the toilet rather than disposed of in the trash. For these medications, the danger of having access to these medications outweighs the environmental concerns. To view this list, visit http://PharmEssAH.emcp.net /FlushingMeds.

Sharps Disposal Besides medications, the proper disposal of all **sharps** (needles, lancets, scalpel blades, and so on) is a growing safety concern, as more patients every year are self-administering injections at home. In addition to self-injecting insulin, blood thinners, and migraine medications, many patients are using the new injectable treatments for hepatitis C, rheumatoid arthritis, psoriasis, and multiple sclerosis. Unfortunately, this increased patient use of sharps has resulted in an increase in improper waste disposal. In fact, up to 7.8 billion needles and syringes are disposed of each year, and most of these sharps are from insulin-dependent patients.

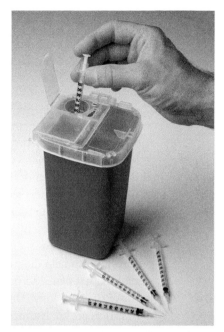

Because proper disposal of sharps protects others from the risk of injury or infection, healthcare personnel should encourage patients to purchase a puncture-resistant, plastic sharps container to collect these items. A sturdy plastic container with a lid such as a bleach bottle or laundry detergent bottle can also serve as a sharps container, but the user should make sure to write "Sharps—Do Not Recycle" on the outside of such a container and tape the lid securely shut prior to disposal.

Whether in a healthcare setting or place of residence, the proper disposal of syringes in a sharps container is important to minimize the transmission of infectious diseases.

Once full, a sharps container should be sealed by the patient and returned to a physician's office, hospital, pharmacy, or public health department. Some facilities may charge a small disposal fee, and not all facilities accept sharps. In some towns, a filled, sealed sharps container marked "Sharps—Do Not Recycle" can be dropped off at the local garbage transfer station. Healthcare staff members should instruct patients to check the website of their local public health department to find information on sharps disposal in their area. It is crucial for patients to understand that they should never put syringes in the trash. Doing so puts sanitation workers at risk of puncture wounds and serious infections, such as hepatitis C.

Patch Disposal An increasing number of patients are receiving their medications through a transdermal patch. Some of these medications include hormone treatments, smoking cessation treatments, antinausea medications, and pain medications. Consequently, patients who wear these patches must understand the importance of proper patch disposal. Healthcare practitioners should instruct patients to fold the patch in half so that the sticky side adheres to itself and then discard the patch into a trash container. Following these guidelines ensures that the patch will not stick to anyone who comes in contact with the trash and subsequently release medication into that individual's skin.

Drug Alert

Allied health personnel should be aware that the FDA recommends that certain transdermal patches be flushed down the toilet and not disposed of in a trash container. One of these transdermal patches is the potent narcotic fentanyl (Duragesic). Young children who have come in contact with fentanyl patches disposed of in the trash have become seriously ill, and several children have died from this accidental exposure.

Healthcare Worker Failure

Allied health professionals must put safety first. Because the effects of potential medication errors on patients cannot be predicted, all healthcare personnel must focus on treating the patient and ensuring the best possible outcome by the safest possible means.

Causes of Medication Errors

A medication error by preparers and handlers of medications has many causes. Using some of the basic principles of root-cause analysis, an individual can examine his or her own workflow to determine the potential for error and the type of failure that the potential error may involve. **Root-cause analysis** is a logical and systematic process used to help identify what, how, and why something happened to prevent recurrence and improve patient safety. Three of the most common causes are an assumption error, a selection error, and a capture error.

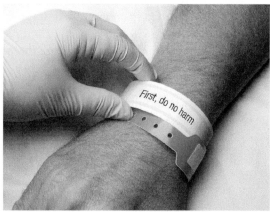

All healthcare professionals must make a commitment to "first, do no harm." Safety must always be a priority in patient care.

Assumption Error

An **assumption error** occurs when an essential piece of information cannot be verified; therefore, an assumption is made. An example of an assumption error that an allied health professional might make is misreading a poorly written abbreviation, drug name, or directions on a prescription or medication order.

Selection Error

A **selection error** occurs when two or more options exist and the wrong option is chosen. An example of a selection error that a pharmacy technician might make is mistakenly using a look-alike, sound-alike drug instead of the prescribed drug, or choosing an immediate-release formulation instead of an extended-release drug. Similar manufacturer labels can also lead to a mistaken medication selection.

Capture Error

A **capture error** occurs when a more practiced behavior automatically takes the place of a less familiar, intended one. In other words, focus on a task is diverted elsewhere, and the distraction prevents the person from detecting an error or causes an error to be made. A capture error might occur when taking a phone call in the middle of filling a prescription or medication order and, as a result, dispensing the wrong number of tablets (i.e., the correct number was not double-checked at the conclusion of the phone call), or inadvertently overriding a drug interaction alert because of a distraction. An error could also occur if a phone call interrupted a staff member who was preparing medications for patients in a long-term care facility (i.e., the arrangement of items on the medication cart could get mixed up, or a drug could be omitted).

Prevention of Medication Errors

Dispensing medications is a labor-intensive process with more than 10 discrete steps required from prescriber order entry to nurse administration at the patient's bedside. For large hospitals that administer more than 10,000 individual doses to patients each day (with 10 steps for each of these doses), the possibility of medication errors is obvious.

Learning to prevent medication errors means carefully examining potential points of failure and using all available resources to verify information or decisions. There is no acceptable rate for medication errors, and each step in prescribing, order processing, filling, and administering medication orders should be reviewed with a 100% error-free goal in mind. To that end, it is helpful to know the problematic areas in the medication-use process:

- *Prescribing*—Approximately 39% of medication errors occur during the prescribing of a medication. Prescribers inadvertently order the incorrect drug or dosage or overlook drug-drug or drug-allergy interactions.

- *Order Processing*—The processing of a medication order accounts for approximately 12% of medication errors. During this stage of the medication-use process, common errors include misinterpretation of handwriting or abbreviations, incorrect data entry of medication labels, and failure to crosscheck drug and label information.

- *Filling*—Approximately 11% of medication errors occur during the filling process. During this stage, common errors include incorrect pharmacy calculations, incorrect drug selection, and nonsterile preparation practices.

- *Administering*—The administration of medication orders accounts for approximately 38% of medication errors. During this phase of the medication-use process, common errors involve failure to ensure the six "rights" of correct drug administration (see Figure 7.1).

FIGURE 7.1 **Six "Rights" of Correct Drug Administration**

During medication administration, healthcare personnel must verify that the *right drug* in the *right strength* is being given by the *right route* to the *right patient* at the *right time*. They must also record this action by performing the *right documentation*. Failure to ensure the six "rights" can result in a medication error.

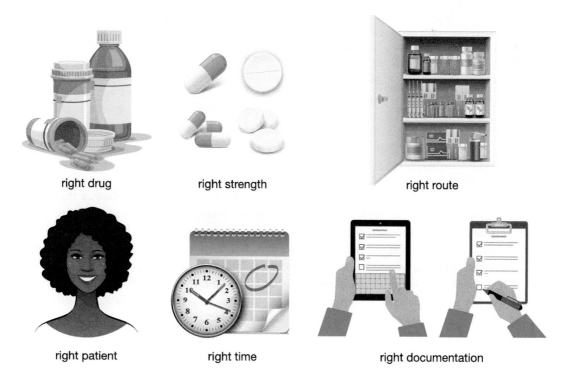

right drug   right strength   right route

right patient   right time   right documentation

Healthcare Worker Responsibilities in Medication Error Prevention

By following some basic safe-practice guidelines, healthcare professionals can work together to create a larger margin of safety.

In the Know

Actor Dennis Quaid has been an outspoken patient safety advocate after his newborn twins nearly died from an accidental overdose of heparin, a blood thinner, in 2007. The twins were administered a 10,000-unit dose of heparin—twice—during treatment of a staphylococcal infection. That dose is 1,000 times the correct dose. The packaging of the heparin dose used to treat young children (a 10-unit dose called Hep-Lock) was remarkably similar to the packaging of an adult heparin dose. The packaging has since been changed by the manufacturer to avoid this selection error, and the hospital where the medication error occurred has implemented new technologies, such as bar-code scanners and electronic health records, to improve patient safety.

Patient Awareness

Healthcare personnel must recognize that each patient's physiologic response to a medication is unique and somewhat unpredictable. The speed at which a body can process medication varies tremendously. Kidney function, in particular, can have a significant impact on a drug's effect. For that reason, healthcare professionals must pay special attention to two population groups that are particularly at risk for medication errors: children (younger than age 6) and the elderly (age 65 and older). Neonates, premature infants, and older adults have diminished kidney function and, therefore, an increased susceptibility to medication errors and adverse reactions. In some cases, a drug may be contraindicated or a dosage may need to be decreased by 25%–50% or more. If a medication dose is not lowered, then the drug could accumulate to toxic levels. Other vulnerable patient populations with decreased kidney function include patients with diabetes, high blood pressure, and chronic renal failure. Consequently, kidney function is one of many factors that the pharmacist must consider before approving and verifying a prescription or medication order.

Record-Keeping Responsibilities

Allied health professionals can help prevent errors by recording accurate information in the patient's medical profile. Each time a healthcare worker enters data about a patient, he or she should verify that the data are being entered for the correct patient by matching the patient's name *and* the patient's date of birth.

Healthcare personnel should also encourage patients to share complete information about their medications and allergies to medications. The list needs to include all prescription drugs as well as all over-the-counter (OTC) drugs, herbal preparations, supplements, and alternative therapies because there are some significant drug interactions between prescription drugs and other types of drugs and therapies.

Finally, healthcare workers should follow best practices and standardize their documentation of measurements and abbreviations. When recording measurements, they should always use metric measurements, even for height and weight. For decimal values that are less than zero, they should use a leading zero (e.g., 0.3) in order to prevent errors. Healthcare professionals should also avoid the use of abbreviations that are easily confused. For example, they should avoid using *QID* (four times a day), which can easily be misread as *QD* (once a day). Avoiding error-prone abbreviations is one of The Joint Commission's safety recommendations, which is discussed in more detail later in this chapter.

Drug Literacy

By having a basic knowledge of drugs, allied health professionals can help safeguard patients from medication errors. Healthcare workers should know the high-alert drugs, or the drugs that are most often involved in medication errors. They should also know which drugs are commonly confused, either because they look alike or because they sound alike. Finally, healthcare workers should also know if a given drug has a black box warning, which is an FDA-mandated special safety alert on the package insert that describes a serious adverse effect. For more information about these drug literacy topics, refer to the section titled "Medication Safety Initiatives" later in this chapter.

Patient Education

Patients and their caregivers must have the basic knowledge needed to handle, administer, and support safe medication use. Educating patients about proper medication use allows allied health personnel to monitor for potential errors or patient misunderstandings.

To begin this discussion, healthcare personnel should ensure that patients understand the 10 key pieces of information about every medication taken (see Table 7.1). Other discussion topics should include how to read medication labels and how to use medication devices—such as inhalers, insulin pumps, and blood glucose meters—safely and effectively. Patients may have questions about the auxiliary labels on their medications, so allied health professionals should be prepared to explain the meanings of some of the symbols found on these labels (for example, a label with a picture of a hamburger means "take with food"). All patients should be strongly encouraged to use only one pharmacy to lower the risks of serious medication errors.

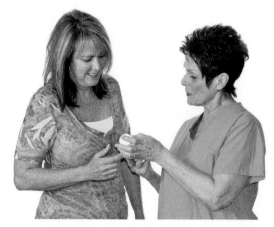

Healthcare staff members should also encourage patients to become informed about their conditions, to discuss any questions that they may have about their medications with their prescribers and pharmacists, and to invite a trusted friend or caregiver to accompany them on their medication-related appointments. Encouraging these practices empowers patients to be advocates for their own health and safety.

To reduce the risk of a medication error, a healthcare staff member must discuss all medications with a patient. Having the patient repeat the information back to the healthcare worker ensures patient comprehension.

Safe Handling of Medications

In the medical-practice setting, the proper disposal of all sharps is critical not only to the safety of individuals but also to the prevention of transmission of communicable diseases such as hepatitis or human immunodeficiency virus (HIV). Disposal of needles and syringes in a sharps container is mandatory. The sharps container should be placed in a secure location in the facility, away from children and, when full, should be sealed, labeled, and disposed of according to the facility's protocol.

Personal Prevention Strategies

Allied health professionals must take care of themselves as well as their patients. Although refusing to work a long shift or overtime is not always a realistic option, healthcare professionals can heed the recommendations of the Healthcare Provider Service Organization to help combat fatigue and, therefore, prevent medication errors. Allied health professionals should be mindful of the following lifestyle recommendations:

- *Get enough sleep.* Experts say that seven to nine hours of sleep a night is best for adults. Avoid staying up until you cannot keep your eyes open any longer; as soon as you feel sleepy, turn out the lights and turn in.

- *Exercise regularly.* You may feel more tired at first, but regular exercise should eventually help boost your energy level. Plan to do your workout several hours before bedtime so that you are not keyed up when it is time to sleep.

- *Take breaks at work.* Even when things are busy, take breaks to relax and revitalize yourself, even if it means going outside to clear your head for a couple of minutes. You will not be much help if you cannot think clearly.

- *Be wise about food.* Eat a well-balanced diet for optimal energy. Pack healthy snacks, stay hydrated, and avoid sugar-laden snacks as well as fatty, fried, or spicy foods.

- *Avoid excessive alcohol.* A nightcap at home may relax you at first, but as the alcohol wears off, it disrupts your normal sleep patterns.

- *Cut the caffeine.* Coffee, tea, and other drinks that contain caffeine do not prevent fatigue; they just hide it. Limit your caffeine intake, especially near bedtime.

If you feel tired on the job, then do not be afraid to ask for help, such as having a colleague double-check

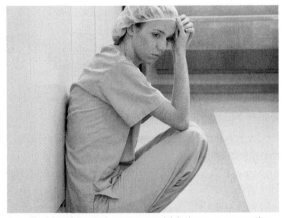

An allied health worker can avoid fatigue, a causative factor of medication errors, by taking breaks at work to clear the head and refocus on the task at hand.

your filling or dosage calculations. If you are fatigued and assigned to distribute medications to patients on a floor, you might want to have a colleague double-check your medication cart before you start your rounds.

Technical Failure

A **technical failure** results from equipment problems. This type of failure may result from either of these situations:

- a design defect in a medical device, such as a metal hip replacement joint that releases metallic debris from wear and tear

- the use of malfunctioning equipment, such as the incorrect preparation of a total parenteral nutrition (TPN) solution due to a malfunction of the automated compounding device (ACD) or an intravenous (IV) solution being dispensed at the wrong rate because of a malfunction in an IV pump

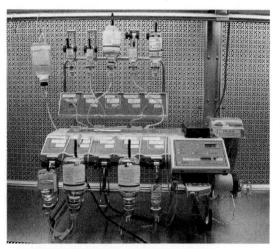

An ACD can add up to 15 ingredients to a patient's TPN solution. Therefore, both the pharmacy technician preparing the medication and his or her supervising pharmacist must continually monitor the accuracy of this device to avoid medication errors.

 Checkpoint **7.1**

Take a moment to review what you have learned so far and answer these questions.

1. What are the five major categories of medication errors?

2. What key pieces of information should a patient know about each medication he or she takes? Provide a minimum of three examples.

3. How can the work environment increase the likelihood of medication errors?

Medication Safety Measures

Measures to promote medication safety date back to 1970 with the passing of the Poison Prevention Packaging Act. Since that time, drug manufacturers and healthcare organizations have minimized the possibility of medication errors through a variety of innovations. These methods include the use of child-resistant containers; preprinted prescription forms; improved package, label, and medication designs; black box warnings for consumers and healthcare practitioners; and automation such as electronic prescribing (e-prescribing), bar-coding technology, and integrated systems.

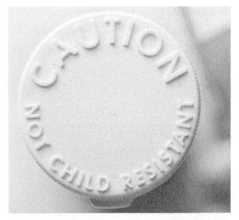 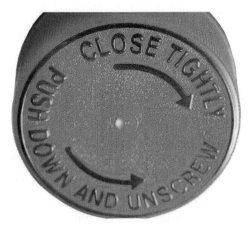

Unless specifically requested by the patient, medications are dispensed in child-resistant containers to prevent accidental poisoning.

Child-Resistant Containers

To prevent accidental childhood poisonings from prescription and nonprescription products, the Poison Prevention Packaging Act was passed in 1970. This act, enforced by the Consumer Product Safety Commission, required that most OTC and prescription drugs be packaged in a **child-resistant container** that cannot be opened by 80% of children younger than age 5 but can be opened by 90% of adults. The law also stipulated that a pharmacist or pharmacy technician, upon request from a patient, may dispense a drug in a non–child-resistant container. In fact, the patient—not the prescriber—could make a blanket request that all drugs be dispensed to him or her in non–child-resistant containers.

Today, this blanket request is often made by older patients and those with severe rheumatoid arthritis and is typically documented in the patient database. Medications that are commonly dispensed in non–child-resistant containers include the antibiotic azithromycin (or Z-Pak), Medrol Dosepak, birth control pills, sublingual nitroglycerin tablets, and metered-dose inhalers. For patients who request these containers, pharmacy personnel should remind them at medication pickup to place these non–child-resistant containers out of reach before young children visit their homes.

Work Wise

The lid on a child-resistant container is commonly referred to as a *safety cap*.

Preprinted Prescription Forms

Some healthcare prescribers whose specialties involve commonly prescribed medical treatments take advantage of preprinted prescription forms. These forms list all medications, doses, dosage intervals, nursing orders, and other treatments commonly prescribed for a particular procedure or disorder. The prescriber simply circles the necessary treatments or modifies the form by adding or deleting information. He or she then signs the form. Using preprinted prescription forms minimizes transcription or illegible prescription medication errors. This preprinted form is commonly used by optometrists and endocrinologists who prescribe a limited number of drugs or medical supplies for their patients.

Package, Label, and Medication Designs

To improve medication safety, drug manufacturers and pharmacies have developed several innovations in packaging, labeling, and product designs.

Package Design

An innovative package design by Target pharmacies has helped their customers manage their medications more safely. The ClearRx design uses color-coded rings to help patients identify medications intended for them, as opposed to those intended for other family members. In addition, the medication container label is larger and more prominently displayed. A consumer survey indicated a strong preference (85%) for the ClearRx design over conventional labels and medication containers. Consumers felt that the new design improved safety and provided an easier-to-read label featuring better-organized warnings in larger type.

ClearRx won the Gold award from NCC MERP in 2010 in the category, "Solution to a Consumer Problem." That solution includes clear labeling, large font size, an easy-to-use dispenser, and a label magnifier for visually impaired individuals.

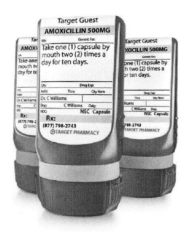

The Target ClearRx packaging is designed to help patients manage their medications by providing information in a clear, easy-to-read format.

Label Design

Pharmaceutical manufacturers are adopting innovations in labeling that should minimize medication errors with their products. Some manufacturers have implemented **tall-man lettering**, also known as *mixed-case lettering*, on their medication labels to help health-care professionals distinguish the names of two similar medications. For example, the medication labels for hydroxyzine and hydralazine, two products that look and sound similar and are available in similar doses, use tall-man lettering: hydrOXYzine and hydrALAZINE. Other drug companies have added warning statements on the stock labels of high-risk medications to help reduce medication errors. Still other manufacturers have printed the middle three- or four-digit product code of the **national drug code (NDC) number** in either a larger font or in boldface type to minimize selection errors.

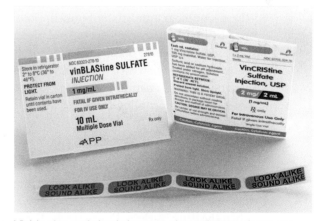

Vinblastine and vincristine, two chemotherapy drugs, are often printed in tall-man lettering on manufacturer-labeled vials to avoid a mix-up of these two look-alike, sound-alike drugs.

Medication Design

Many companies are manufacturing formulations with unique colors, shapes, or markings to assist in distinguishing between doses or competitor products. For some products, the markings on the tablet or capsule verify the dose. For other products, different doses of the same medication will have different colors and tablet or capsule identification on the stock bottle.

Black Box Warnings on Package Inserts

If a drug has a potential for a very serious adverse reaction, the FDA may require that the manufacturer include a **black box warning** describing that problem on the package insert for the drug. By mandating a black box warning, the FDA ensures that the information about this potential problem is prominently displayed on the first page of the package insert, so that healthcare practitioners will be more likely to read it. For example, the diabetes drug pioglitazone has a black box warning that states the drug may cause or exacerbate heart failure. The labels for fluoroquinolone antibiotics such as ciprofloxacin have a black box warning alerting healthcare personnel that the drugs are associated with an increased risk of tendonitis and tendon rupture in patients of all ages. Finally, many antidepressant drugs, including fluoxetine, bupropion, and duloxetine, have black box warnings that state that the use of these drugs may cause an increased risk of suicidal thinking and behavior in children, adolescents, and young adults.

Use of Automation

The use of automation in the practice setting has had a significant impact on patient safety. E-prescribing, bar-coding technology, and the use of an integrated, automated system have reduced human error, particularly in the medication process. In the hospital setting, automated dispensing cabinets have added a layer of safety to the medication-dispensing process as well.

Electronic Prescribing

The electronic transmission of prescriptions or **e-prescribing** continues to be increasingly used by healthcare prescribers to send prescriptions to the pharmacy (see Figure 7.2). E-prescribing, which is also known as computerized provider order entry (CPOE), minimizes the risk of potential medication errors due to a prescriber's handwriting, misinterpretation of abbreviations, and illegible faxes. The use of e-prescribing also decreases the potential for prescription forgeries.

Bar-Coding Technology

Many pharmacies use **bar-coding technology** throughout the medication-filling process. The prescription information is entered into the computerized system and verified by the pharmacist; the pharmacy technician then scans the selected stock bottle's NDC number when the drug is selected from stock. The computer automatically compares the scanned bar code against the verified prescription information. If the prescription does not match the NDC of the selected medication, the system indicates that an incorrect selection has been made. This technology minimizes the chances of selecting the incorrect drug or dose when filling a prescription.

FIGURE 7.2 e-Prescription

Use of an e-prescription (depicted as a screenshot below) greatly minimizes transcription errors, thus improving the safety and accuracy of processing prescriptions.

```
-----------------------------------------------------------------------
!!! -- START SECURED ELECTRONIC PRESCRIPTION TRANSMISSION -- !!!
-----------------------------------------------------------------------
FROM THE OFFICES OF PHIL JACKSON, MD; ETHEL JACOBSON, MD;
                    PETER JARKOWSKI, PA; EUGENE JOHNSON, DO

OFFICE ADDRESS:          67 EAST ELM
                         CEDAR RAPIDS, IA 52411
OFFICE TELEPHONE:        (319) 555-1212   TRANSMIT DATE: FEB 20, 2017
OFFICE FAX:              (319) 555-1313   WRITTEN DATE:  FEB 20, 2017
-----------------------------------------------------------------------
TRANSMITTED TO           THE CORNER DRUG STORE
PHARMACY ADDRESS:        875 PARADIGM WAY
                         CEDAR RAPIDS, IA 52410
PHARMACY TELEPHONE:      (319) 555-1414
-----------------------------------------------------------------------
PATIENT NAME:            JEFFREY KLEIN     D.O.B.: OCT 18, 1979
PATIENT ADDRESS:         1157 NORTH PLAZA AVE
                         CEDAR RAPIDS, IA 52411
-----------------------------------------------------------------------
PRESCRIBED MEDICATION:   FLUOXETINE 20 MG
SIGNA:                   i PO QD
DISPENSE QUANTITY:       30
REFILL(S):               3
-----------------------------------------------------------------------
PHYSICIAN SIGNATURE:     [[ ELECTRONIC SIGNATURE ON FILE ]]
                         [[ FOR DR. ETHEL JACOBSON ]]
-----------------------------------------------------------------------
!!! -- END SECURED ELECTRONIC PRESCRIPTION TRANSMISSION -- !!!
-----------------------------------------------------------------------
```

Integrated, Automated System

Moving from a paper-based system to an integrated, automated system has improved efficiency and allows resources in the hospital to be redeployed to increase patient safety and improve the quality of patient care. The use of **electronic health records (EHRs)** has allowed healthcare practitioners faster and more efficient access to patient information than was possible with paper charts.

Automation in the computer order entry, filling, preparation, and administration of medications has dramatically reduced medication errors by more than 50% in several hospital studies. The prescriber inputs the medication order directly from a handheld personal digital assistant or smartphone. The order is then sent electronically to the pharmacy where it is double-checked for accuracy by the pharmacist. The order is filled by the technician (or robot), checked by the technician and pharmacist, and sent to the nursing unit. The medication is then administered to the patient by the nurse who matches the bar

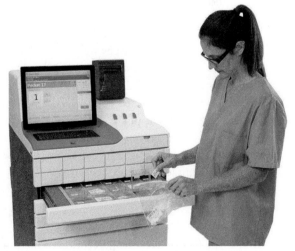

An automated medication-dispensing cabinet can be interfaced with bar-coding technology, allowing the tracking of dispensed medication. The use of this technology has helped to reduce the risk of medication errors.

code of the medication with the bar code on the patient wristband. With an **electronic medication administration record (eMAR)**, the administration of a medication is documented electronically by the nurse rather than on paper. The eMAR can minimize medication errors in both hospitals and nursing homes. The IOM encourages the adoption of automation technologies for all medication orders in all hospitals as soon as possible.

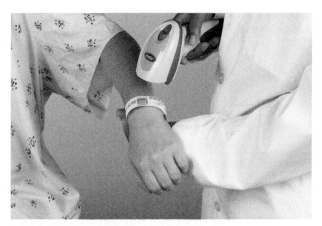

Bar-coding and scanning technology ensure that the correct patient is receiving the correct medication.

Checkpoint 7.2

Take a moment to review what you have learned so far and answer these questions.

1. What safety initiative resulted from the Poison Prevention Packaging Act of 1970?

2. What is the purpose of tall-man lettering?

3. How is automation used to protect patient safety?

Medication Error Discovery

Medication errors can be detected in a variety of ways: by direct observation of an error, by chart review, or as a result of a patient complaint. The task of error reporting is most often performed by the pharmacist; however, allied health professionals are an integral part of the process of error identification, documentation, and prevention. An understanding of the *what, when, where,* and *why* of error reporting is important for allied health professionals, as well as for pharmacists.

The pharmacist is also typically responsible for the delicate task of informing the patient that a medication error has taken place. The circumstances leading to the error should be explained completely and honestly. Patients should understand the nature of the error, what (if any) effects the error may have, and how he or she can become actively involved in preventing errors in the future. If the medication error will lead to a side effect or adverse drug reaction or affect the disease or illness being treated, the pharmacist must also contact the prescriber.

Medication Error Reporting Systems

The first steps in the prevention of medication errors are the identification of the problem and the collection of information. After all, what is not known cannot be fixed. Fear of punishment is always a concern when an error arises; as a result, healthcare professionals may decide not to report an error at all, leaving the door open for the same error to occur again. For this reason, anonymous or no-fault systems of reporting have been established, such as the Medication Error Reporting Program of the Institute for Safe Medication Practices. The focus of no-fault reporting is on fixing the problem rather than on assigning blame. Other medication error reporting systems, such as the FDA's MedWatch program, are aimed at collecting information about drug safety concerns. These two programs as well as other medication safety initiatives are discussed in detail below. In reality, however, most medication errors are reported internally by the pharmacist and analyzed within the organization rather than reported to a centralized national database.

State Boards of Pharmacy

Several efforts have been made to create a safe and comfortable atmosphere for individuals to report medication errors. Many states have mandatory error-reporting systems, but most officials admit that medication errors are still underreported, mostly because of fear of punishment and liability. State boards of pharmacy do not punish pharmacists for errors, as long as a good-faith effort was made to fill the prescription correctly. States such as Florida, Texas, and California have worked to reduce the fear of reporting by passing new regulations that allow pharmacists to document errors and error-prone systems without fear of punishment. Pharmacists in these states, however, need to indicate the steps that are being taken to eliminate weaknesses that might allow such errors to continue.

Many states regulate, require, or recommend a continuous quality improvement program to detect, document, and assess medication errors to determine the causes and to develop an appropriate response to prevent future errors. In addition, many state legislatures have proposed new laws that protect error reports from subpoena. These error reports must be separate from medical records because all medical records can be subpoenaed, including prescription records.

FDA's MedWatch

The FDA receives reports from consumers and healthcare professionals about medication errors and adverse events through its online reporting system, which is known as **MedWatch**. The collected data are compiled into the FDA Adverse Event Reporting System (FAERS). The FDA uses the data to monitor for new safety concerns about drugs. In some cases, potential adverse reactions to a drug may not fully be understood until a drug becomes available on the market and is used by a large number of people. When safety concerns do arise, the FDA can order further studies on a drug or take regulatory action to protect public safety. For example, the FDA can add warnings to a drug's labeling information, restrict the use of the drug, or even remove a drug from the market. The MedWatch system gathers a huge amount of data about adverse drug reactions: The system received more than 50,000 reports during one quarter of 2013.

The Joint Commission's Sentinel Event Policy

To contribute to error-reporting efforts, The Joint Commission has a centralized site through which hospitals and other healthcare organizations may channel information safely. This well-established site enacts The Joint Commission's **Sentinel Event Policy**. A **sentinel event** is an unexpected occurrence involving death, serious physical or psychological injury, or the potential for such occurrences to happen. When a sentinel event is reported, the organization (i.e., hospital, pharmacy,

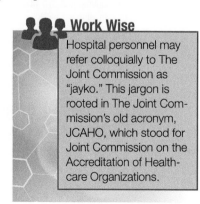

Work Wise

Hospital personnel may refer colloquially to The Joint Commission as "jayko." This jargon is rooted in The Joint Commission's old acronym, JCAHO, which stood for Joint Commission on the Accreditation of Healthcare Organizations.

or managed-care company) is expected to analyze the cause of the error (i.e., perform a root-cause analysis), take action to correct the cause, monitor the changes made, and determine whether the cause of the error has been eliminated. More than 10,000 sentinel events have been reported to The Joint Commission since 1996.

ISMP's Medication Errors Reporting Program

The **Institute for Safe Medication Practices (ISMP)** is a nonprofit healthcare agency whose mission is to understand the causes of medication errors and to communicate time-critical error-reduction strategies to the healthcare community, policymakers, and the public. The ISMP does not set standards but focuses on expert analysis and scientific studies to reduce medication errors.

The ISMP provides a national voluntary program called the **Medication Errors Reporting Program (ISMP MERP)**. ISMP is a federally certified patient safety organization that provides legal protection and confidentiality for submitted patient safety data and error reports. This program is designed to allow healthcare professionals to report medication errors directly. The ISMP shares all information and error-prevention strategies with the FDA.

According to the program, medication errors include the following:

- incorrect drug, strength, or dose
- wrong patient
- confusion over look-alike and sound-alike drugs or similar packaging
- incorrect route of drug administration
- calculation or preparation errors
- misuse of medical equipment (e.g., infusion pumps, automated controllers, etc.)
- errors in prescribing, transcribing, dispensing, administering, or monitoring medications

Reports can be completed online. See Table 7.2 for the type of information collected.

TABLE 7.2 Error Report of an ISMP MERP

1. Describe the error or preventable adverse drug reaction. What went wrong?
2. Was this an actual medication error (that reached the patient), or are you expressing concern about a potential error that was discovered before it reached the patient?
3. If an actual medication error occurred, what was the patient outcome?
4. Specify the practice site (e.g., hospital, private office, retail pharmacy, drug company, long-term care facility, etc.).
5. What are the generic names of all products involved?
6. What are the brand names of all products involved?
7. Describe the dosage form, concentration or strength, and so forth.
8. How was the error discovered or intercepted?
9. Please state your recommendations for error prevention.

Medication Safety Initiatives

Several organizations have developed medication safety initiatives to make healthcare personnel aware of error-prone areas in the medication-use process. Awareness of these troublesome areas helps to improve patient safety.

ISMP Initiatives

To alert healthcare personnel to the potential dangers of handling certain medications, the ISMP has created several valuable resources. These resources include compilations of high-alert medications, look-alike and sound-alike drugs, and medical abbreviations to avoid in healthcare communications.

High-Alert Medications

The ISMP publishes a list of **high-alert medications** that bear a heightened risk of causing significant patient harm when used in error in the hospital and community pharmacy settings. High-alert medications are potentially toxic and require additional safeguards to avoid the risk of medication errors. These medications include chemotherapy agents, digoxin, amiodarone, and warfarin. Due to potential drops in the blood glucose levels of diabetic patients, insulins and oral hypoglycemics should also be carefully monitored. The ISMP's high-alert medications are divided into two lists: ISMP *List of High-Alert Medications in Acute Care Settings* (http://PharmEssAH.emcp.net/AcuteCareHighAlert) and ISMP *List of High-Alert Medications in Community/Ambulatory Healthcare* (http://PharmEssAH.emcp.net/CommunityHighAlert). These lists are periodically updated by the ISMP.

List of Confused Drug Names

The ISMP also publishes a list of common look-alike and sound-alike drugs that often contribute to medication errors. This list, known as the ISMP's *List of Confused Drug Names* (http://PharmEssAH.emcp.net/ConfusedDrugs), offers hundreds of drug names that are easily confused—for example, Klonopin vs. clonidine. Klonopin is used to treat anxiety and calm seizures, whereas clonidine is used to lower blood pressure. If these medications are not spelled out or verified during a verbal prescription order, an error could occur. The ISMP stresses awareness of such drugs, promotes adding a medical indication for each drug, and encourages e-prescribing to avoid any ambiguity inherent to handwritten prescriptions.

List of Error-Prone Abbreviations, Symbols, and Dose Designations

The ISMP has compiled a list of error-prone abbreviations to help healthcare personnel avoid dangerous documentation. These abbreviations and other shorthand communication methods have been identified as the cause of many medication errors and should never be used in healthcare practice. Students are encouraged to review the ISMP's *List of Error-Prone Abbreviations, Symbols, and Dose Designations* (http://PharmEssAH .emcp.net/ErrorProneAbbrev).

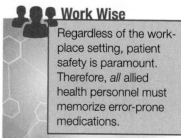

Work Wise

Regardless of the workplace setting, patient safety is paramount. Therefore, *all* allied health personnel must memorize error-prone medications.

Other Initiatives

The ISMP has sponsored national forums on medication errors, recommended the addition of labeling or special hazard warnings on potentially toxic drugs, and encouraged revisions of potentially dangerous prescription writing practices. For example, the ISMP first promoted the now-common practice of using the **leading zero** in pharmacy calculations, that is, if a dose is less than 1 mg, a zero should be placed to the left of the decimal point to prevent confusion. A dose written with a naked decimal point (*.5 mg*) is more easily confused with *5 mg* than a dose written with a leading zero (*0.5 mg*).

The ISMP is also active in disseminating information to healthcare professionals and consumers—such as e-mail newsletters, journal articles, and video training exercises—and has FDA safety alerts posted on its website.

The Joint Commission Initiatives

Because accreditation of hospitals is dependent on demonstrating an effective medical and medication error reporting system, The Joint Commission has worked alongside other healthcare organizations to establish safety initiatives for hospitals. The commission has also worked with hospitals to improve their medication safety procedures and with consumers to become their own healthcare advocates.

Accreditation and Medication Safety Standards

Accreditation of hospitals is dependent on demonstrating an effective medical and medication error reporting system. The Joint Commission supports the recommendations of the ISMP: (1) the elimination of certain abbreviations and (2) the education of healthcare professionals regarding frequently confused drug names to minimize errors. For example, units of insulin should always be spelled out so that a sloppily written *8U* is not confused with *80 units* of insulin—a 10-fold dosing error that could cause a dangerous reduction in a patient's blood glucose level (see Figure 7.3). Healthcare personnel should also use the abbreviation *mL* rather than the abbreviation *cc*. The latter abbreviation is frequently misinterpreted.

During an accreditation visit, The Joint Commission is most interested in documenting measurable changes in the implemented safety program of a healthcare facility. The organization may recommend a safety program to improve communications with physicians and nurses in the ordering, preparation, and dispensing of medications in an effort to minimize medication errors. The Joint Commission may also suggest an implementation of policies prohibiting the use of unapproved or "do not use" abbreviations or requiring computer checks and balances with look-alike, sound-alike drugs to ensure that the right drug, in the right dose, is given to the right patient. These safety-related standards

---

FIGURE 7.3 **Sample of Error-Prone Abbreviations in a Prescription**

This handwritten prescription contains the abbreviations *QID* and *Sub-Q*, two abbreviations that are listed on the ISMP's *List of Error-Prone Abbreviations*. In addition, the Lantus (insulin) dose can easily be misread: Is it *8 units* or *80 units*?

are based on the assumption that, if a preventable medication error occurs, investigating the cause and making necessary corrections in policy or procedure are much more important than assigning blame to an individual. When the cause of the error is identified, a repeat medication error may be prevented in the future. The Joint Commission standards also require that the hospital outlines its responsibility to advise a patient about any adverse outcomes of the error.

SPEAK UP Program

In concert with the Centers for Medicare & Medicaid Services, The Joint Commission has also developed an educational series of written brochures and videos as part of its **SPEAK UP** program (http://PharmEssAH.emcp.net/SpeakUp). This program is designed to encourage consumers to take a more active role in their health care and to minimize misunderstandings that may lead to medication errors. SPEAK UP is an acronym that stands for the following:

Speak up if you have questions or concerns. If you still do not understand, ask again. It is your body, and you have a right to know.

Pay attention to the care you get. Always make sure you are getting the right treatments and medications from the right healthcare professionals. Do not assume anything.

Educate yourself about your illness. Learn about the medical tests you get and your treatment plan.

Ask a trusted family member or friend to be your advocate (adviser or supporter).

Know what medications you take and why you take them. Medication errors are the most common healthcare mistakes.

Use a hospital, clinic, surgery center, or other type of healthcare organization that has been carefully checked out. For example, The Joint Commission visits hospitals to see if the facilities are meeting the organization's quality standards.

Participate in all decisions about your treatment. You are the center of the healthcare team.

AAPCC Initiatives

The **American Association of Poison Control Centers (AAPCC)** supports a network of 55 poison control centers all over the country. These **poison control centers** are available by phone 24 hours a day to provide information about exposures to poisonous, hazardous, or toxic substances at no cost. The centers are staffed by pharmacists, physicians, nurses, and poison information providers who are toxicology experts. They field calls from both consumers and healthcare professionals and provide information in both emergency and nonemergency situations. For details on the poison control center in your area, call the national hotline at 1-800-222-1222 or consult the American Association of Poison Control Centers on the Internet (http://PharmEssAH.emcp.net/AAPCC).

National Poison Data System

The AAPCC also maintains the National Poison Data System (NPDS), which is the only comprehensive poisoning exposure surveillance database in the United States. This database provides a real-time snapshot of poisoning patterns across the country and is updated every eight minutes.

Paradigm Shift in Healthcare Practice

In recent years, there has been a paradigm shift: The standard approach to medication errors has moved away from assigning blame and toward investigating root causes and preventing future errors. Newer initiatives emphasize the importance of a team approach to tackling medication safety problems.

TeamSTEPPS is a recent medication safety initiative of the US Department of Health & Human Services Agency for Healthcare Research and Quality. It is a team-based approach to improving patient care and safeguarding patients against medical errors. The theory is that when interdisciplinary teams in hospitals work together effectively, they can resolve conflicts, improve information sharing, and eliminate barriers to quality and safety. To learn more about TeamSTEPPS and access their training materials, visit http://PharmEssAH.emcp.net/TeamSTEPPS.

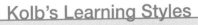

Kolb's Learning Styles

If you enjoy thinking to yourself as you learn new information, as Convergers do, you might enjoy this exercise for learning about medication errors. Take a look at the FDA's list of most common medication errors by visiting http://PharmEssAH.emcp.net/MedErrors. Write out that list and reflect on how a healthcare staff member could help protect patients from those types of errors.

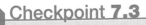

Checkpoint 7.3

Take a moment to review what you have learned so far and answer these questions.

1. What is a sentinel event?

2. What is an example of a high-alert medication?

3. What is the mission of the Institute for Safe Medication Practices?

Chapter Review

Chapter Summary

Preventable medical errors are the third leading cause of death in the United States. Organizational failures, human failures, and technical failures can all lead to medication errors. Root-cause analysis is a logical and systematic process used to help identify what, how, and why something happened to prevent recurrence. Using some of the basic principles of root-cause analysis, a person can examine his or her own workflow to determine the potential for error and the type of failure that the potential error may involve. Three of the most common causes are an assumption error, a selection error, and a capture error.

It can be useful to think of medication safety in terms of a patient's "bill of rights." There are six "rights": giving the *right drug* in the *right strength* via the *right route* to the *right patient* at the *right time*—and completing the *right documentation* after the drug administration. Patients should have

a complete understanding of their prescribed drug therapies to help protect them from medication errors.

Many efforts have been made by pharmaceutical manufacturers and healthcare facilities to minimize the possibility of medication errors. These include e-prescribing, using preprinted prescribing forms, improving packaging design, and using bar-coding technology to improve patient safety.

Fear of punishment is always a concern when an error arises; as a result, healthcare professionals may decide not to report an error at all, leaving the door open for the same error to occur again. For this reason, anonymous or no-fault systems of reporting have been established. The FDA collects adverse drug event reports through the MedWatch program, and ISMP provides a national voluntary program called the Medication Errors Reporting Program (MERP).

Chapter Checkup

The Navigator+ learning management system that accompanies this textbook offers many opportunities to help you master chapter content, including end-of-chapter exercises, a glossary of key terms, flash cards, and additional interactive activities.

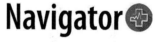

Career Exploration

If you enjoyed learning about medication safety in this chapter, you may want to explore the following career options:

- eMAR implementation consultant
- environmental health officer/public health inspector
- emergency medical technician (EMT)/paramedic
- healthcare documentation specialist
- health information administrator
- health information technician
- hospital occupational health and safety officer
- medical assistant
- pharmacy technician

8 Pharmacy Laws and Regulations

Pharm Facts

- The Occupational Safety and Health Administration (OSHA) monitors the safety of eight million workplaces in the United States.

- Twice a year since 2010, the Drug Enforcement Administration (DEA)—in cooperation with law enforcement agencies around the country—sponsors National Prescription Drug Take-Back Day. On that day, individuals are given the opportunity to dispose of unwanted prescription drugs at a secure disposal site. In 2014, the DEA collected 309 tons of prescription pills.

- Since the Controlled Substances Act was enacted in 1970, approximately 160 substances have been added, removed, or transferred from one schedule to another.

- More than 50% of adults in the United States take dietary supplements—particularly vitamins and minerals—to improve health and wellness. However, the majority of these individuals do not disclose complete information about their supplement use to healthcare professionals.

"As a pharmacy technician, I need to have a complete understanding of which tasks I can legally perform in the pharmacy and which tasks require the clinical judgment of a pharmacist. Working outside of my scope of practice could result in patient harm or death. As the role of the pharmacy technician continues to expand, I also must keep apprised of any changing legal responsibilities in the pharmacy workplace. Keeping current in pharmacy law provides me with a sense of comfort as I perform my daily tasks and protects both me and my patients."

—**Laurisa McKissack**, MBA, CPhT, RPT
Pharmacy Technician

In the United States, the laws related to drug approvals and pharmacy practice are generally stricter than those in other countries. For example, in some countries you may be able to get many medications, including antibiotics, without a prescription. To healthcare personnel in the United States, such lax drug control seems astonishing in light of the distinct possibility of inappropriate use, adverse reactions, and interactions with other drugs. Issues related to the stringent US drug laws and regulations continue to be debated publicly because of the ongoing illegal importation of drugs from Canada and Mexico by many individuals. However, the tight drug controls in the United States have safeguarded the health of its citizens for many decades.

This chapter provides a brief overview of pharmacy laws and regulations, medication and pharmacy regulatory agencies, standards and accreditation organizations, legal and ethical duties connected to medication preparation and administration, and guidelines for the handling and storage of controlled substances and hazardous drugs.

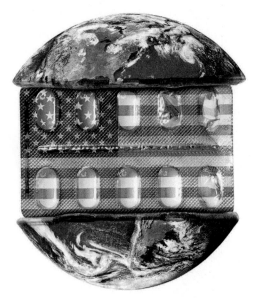

Unlike most other countries, the United States has strict federal and state laws, regulations, and professional standards for drug control.

Healthcare Laws and Regulations

A **law** is a rule that is passed and enforced by the legislative branch of government. Collectively, laws are a system of rules that reflect the society and culture from which they arise. Laws offer a minimum level of acceptable standards. The US Congress and state legislatures represent citizens in the passage and enforcement of laws that are designed to protect the public. Violations in laws may result in damages, fines, probation, loss of licensure, or—in extreme cases—incarceration.

In the past century, the federal government has passed a number of laws specific to the healthcare industry including the Pure Food and Drug Act of 1906; the Federal Food, Drug, and Cosmetic Act of 1938; the Controlled Substances Act of 1970; the Poison Prevention Packaging Act of 1970; the Health Insurance Portability and Accountability Act (HIPAA) of 1996; the Medicare Prescription Drug, Improvement, and Modernization Act (MMA) of 2003; and the Patient Protection and Affordable Care Act of 2010. To review these key pieces of healthcare legislation, refer to Table 8.1.

A **regulation** is a written rule and procedure that exists to carry out a law of the federal or state government. For example, at the federal level, the US Food and Drug Administration and the Drug Enforcement Administration regulate drugs. The federal programs of Medicare and Medicaid also have regulations that healthcare professionals must follow when processing prescriptions for elderly, low-income, and disabled patients.

Aside from federal regulations, each state's board of health has regulations that must be followed with regard to the distribution and administration of medications within that state. When there is a conflict between a state and a federal law or regulation, the more stringent law or regulation always applies.

State governments also establish the licensure, registration, and certification requirements for allied health professionals. These requirements vary from state to state. For more information on these requirements for allied health professionals, refer to Chapter 4.

Regulatory Agencies

A **regulatory agency** is a government organization that was created to implement and enforce a specific set of laws. For example, the Centers for Medicare & Medicaid Services (CMS) implemented the Medicare Prescription Drug, Improvement, and Modernization Act of 2003, which added an outpatient drug benefit to Medicare. Allied health professionals who are involved in billing for a medical practice may need to learn about the CMS rules regarding prescriptions, such as which medications are covered by Medicare and what quantities are allowed per month. Some of the other federal and state agencies involved in the regulation of drugs include the following:

- US Food and Drug Administration (FDA)
- Drug Enforcement Administration (DEA)
- Occupational Safety and Health Administration (OSHA)
- Federal Trade Commission (FTC), with authority over business practices including direct-to-consumer drug advertising
- state health and welfare agencies with personnel budgets for the provision of drugs needed by low-income or disabled individuals, such as Medicaid

TABLE 8.1 | Significant Federal Healthcare Legislation

Legislation	Description
Pure Food and Drug Act of 1906	To combat real-life abuses in drug formulation, labeling, and market claims, the US Congress passed the first of a series of landmark twentieth-century laws to regulate the development, compounding, distribution, storage, and dispensing of drugs. The purpose of the Pure Food and Drug Act of 1906 was to prohibit the interstate transportation or sale of adulterated and misbranded food and drugs. This act required that product labels not contain false information about a drug's strength and purity. In response to these mounting concerns, the manufacturer of Coca-Cola changed its product's key ingredient—from cocaine to caffeine—during the early development of this legislation. The act, although amended, proved unenforceable, and new legislation was later required.
Federal Food, Drug, and Cosmetic (FD&C) Act of 1938	A poisoning incident in 1937, in which a sulfa drug product caused the deaths of more than 100 individuals, led to the passage of the Federal Food, Drug, and Cosmetic (FD&C) Act of 1938. This legislation created the US Food and Drug Administration (FDA) and required pharmaceutical manufacturers to file a new drug application (NDA) with each new drug to obtain FDA approval before marketing. Manufacturers needed to prove that the product was safe for use by humans. Unfortunately, this act required only that drugs be safe for human consumption, not that they be effective or useful for the purpose for which they were sold.
Controlled Substances Act (CSA) of 1970	The Controlled Substances Act (CSA) of 1970 was created to combat and control drug abuse and to supersede previous federal laws regarding drug abuse. The act classified drugs with potential for abuse as *controlled substances,* or drugs that have a risk for abuse and physical or psychological dependence. The controlled substances were then ranked into five categories, or *schedules.* Schedule I drugs are not commercially available or legally dispensed in the United States due to their high potential for abuse and addiction. Schedule II drugs are the most highly regulated drug category and have no refills. Schedule III, IV, and V drugs have less abuse and addiction potential than Schedule II drugs but have quantity and time limits on refills.
Poison Prevention Packaging Act of 1970	To prevent accidental childhood poisonings from prescription and nonprescription products, the Poison Prevention Packaging Act was passed in 1970. This act, enforced by the Consumer Product Safety Commission, required that most over-the-counter (OTC) and prescription drugs be packaged in a child-resistant container that cannot be opened by 80% of children under age five but can be opened by 90% of adults. The law also stipulated that a pharmacist or pharmacy technician, upon request from a patient, may dispense a drug in a non–child-resistant container. Today, this request is often made by older patients and those with severe rheumatoid arthritis. Medications that are commonly dispensed in non–child-resistant containers include the antibiotic azithromycin (or Z-Pak), methylprednisolone (Medrol Dosepak), birth control pills, sublingual nitroglycerin tablets, and metered-dose inhalers.
Health Insurance Portability and Accountability Act (HIPAA) of 1996	HIPAA placed safeguards to protect patient confidentiality and used the term *protected health information (PHI)* to describe a patient's private medical information. The law requires that every healthcare facility have a written policy on patient confidentiality that must be provided to patients as a handout. HIPAA also gave patients the right to access their own medical records, with some exceptions. In addition, HIPAA placed limits on how much of a patient's PHI may be shared. Healthcare personnel are legally bound to disclose only the minimum amount of PHI required for the intended purpose.
Medicare Prescription Drug, Improvement, and Modernization Act (MMA) of 2003	The Medicare Prescription Drug, Improvement, and Modernization Act (MMA) of 2003, better known as Medicare Part D, became effective January 1, 2006; MMA provides prescription drug coverage to patients who are eligible for Medicare benefits. This voluntary insurance program requires patient co-payments but offers coverage for certain medications—especially for those patients with economic hardships or those needing high-cost medications. Through this program, patients are required to pay an extra premium, in addition to their Medicare premium, and may be subject to a deductible (depending on insurance selected) before benefits are realized.
Patient Protection and Affordable Care Act of 2010	The Patient Protection and Affordable Care Act of 2010 expanded health insurance coverage for Americans by providing tax credits for low- and middle-income individuals so that they could purchase insurance through the newly formed Health Insurance Marketplace. The law also required that all healthcare insurance plans cover some basic preventive care, such as vaccines, contraception, and well-child examinations. The act makes medications that senior citizens receive through the Medicare Part D prescription drug program more affordable by gradually closing the coverage gaps in those plans (also known as "donut holes"), with a total phaseout of such gaps planned by 2020. The law has prohibited insurance companies from denying patients coverage because of their medical history and from placing annual or lifetime limits on most patient benefits. Annual and lifetime limits had been a significant problem for patients with chronic conditions and catastrophic health events.

Brief descriptions of the regulatory agencies you are most likely to encounter in the course of your work as an allied health professional are discussed below.

FDA

The **US Food and Drug Administration (FDA)** is a federal government agency that is part of the US Department of Health & Human Services (see Figure 8.1). This agency provides regulations on the drug approval process, generic drug substitution, patient counseling, and adverse reaction reporting systems. The FDA has the primary responsibility and authority to enforce the law; however, the FDA has no legal authority over the practice of pharmacy in each state.

The FDA has several divisions; however, those individuals working with medications, especially in pharmacies, are most affected by its **Center for Drug Evaluation and Research (CDER)**. CDER is primarily involved in the following tasks:

- new drug development and review
- generic drug review
- over-the-counter (OTC) drug review
- postdrug approval activities

| FIGURE 8.1 | Logo of the US Food and Drug Administration |

In addition to drugs, the FDA regulates most food products (except meat and poultry), medical devices, cosmetics, and animal feed.

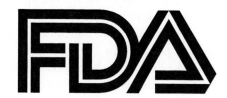

Drug Approval Process

The FDA has the ability to create and enforce regulations that will assist in providing the public with safe drug products. To that end, the agency requires that each new prescription drug undergo three phases of testing on human subjects before it can be approved for sale. Once the drug has been approved, the FDA grants the drug's manufacturer a 20-year patent, which usually starts well before the drug receives this final approval. A patent ensures the manufacturer that the drug cannot be manufactured in its generic form by another company until the patent expires. The duration of exclusivity is longer for some drugs, such as drugs that treat rare disease states (known as **orphan drugs**). For more information on drug development, see Chapter 2.

Drug Safety

As a **watchdog agency** for public safety, the FDA issues drug recalls as needed and enforces the packaging, labeling, advertising, and marketing guidelines for medications. For example, a manufacturer may not make speculative or false claims about the potential of the product, and it must also disclose the side effects, adverse reactions, and contraindications for each medication. OTC medications also undergo scrutiny by the FDA. The labels of OTC products must conform to a preferred format to make all of the information "understandable and readable" to laypersons.

As mentioned earlier, manufacturers must disclose the potential adverse reactions associated with use of their products. Sometimes, however, a patient may experience an unexpected, adverse reaction to a product and report the incident to a healthcare staff member. Oftentimes that staff member is an allied health professional. Consequently, allied health professionals must be familiar with MedWatch, an adverse reaction reporting system set up by the FDA. To learn more about the MedWatch program and how to report adverse reactions, refer to Chapter 7.

Dietary Supplement Monitoring

The FDA does not regulate dietary supplements as tightly as it regulates prescription drugs and OTC medications. The term **dietary supplement** refers to vitamins as well as herbal products such as ginger root and St. John's wort. The manufacturers of supplements are not required to prove the efficacy of their products. The FDA may only review "false claims" in advertisements for supplements and monitor the safety of the products.

Manufacturers of these dietary supplements are not permitted to make claims about curing or treating ailments; they may state only that the products are supplements to support health. If the FDA wants to remove a dietary supplement from the market for safety reasons, it may do so. For example, the drug ephedra, or its herbal equivalent *ma huang*, was at one time an ingredient in many weight-loss products. In 2004, the FDA removed the drug from the market because of reports of serious adverse reactions and some deaths. Still, dietary supplements are gaining popularity among consumers who are seeking alternative therapies. To instill confidence in their supplement selections, many consumers rely on a mark displayed on the supplements' labels. This mark, called a USP Verified Mark, indicates that the product has met the standards of the US Pharmacopeial Convention (USP). For more information on this program, refer to the "Standards Organizations" section later in this chapter.

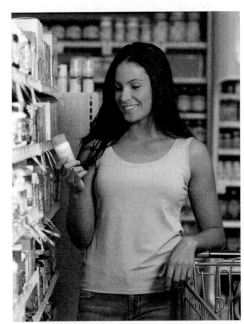

The FDA requires that all OTC medications containing acetaminophen have the active ingredient prominently displayed on the label as well as a warning about the potential for liver toxicity.

Drug Alert

In the 1950s and 1960s, thalidomide was prescribed to women in Europe, Japan, and Australia as a treatment for morning sickness. However, this drug had tragic results for the offspring of these mothers. In the ensuing years, approximately 10,000 children were born with severe birth defects, such as shortened or missing limbs. Thalidomide was not available for sale in the United States until 1998, when the FDA approved it specifically as a treatment for leprosy and multiple myeloma. Because of its teratogenic effects, thalidomide can be obtained only through a restricted distribution program that requires women of childbearing age to take monthly pregnancy tests and avoid pregnancy by using two reliable forms of birth control.

DEA

The **Drug Enforcement Administration (DEA)** is the primary agency responsible for enforcing the laws regarding both legal and illegal addictive substances (see Figure 8.2). Although this agency directs most of its funds and personnel toward the illegal trafficking of drugs, it is also responsible for supervising the legal use of narcotics and other **controlled substances**.

Every individual, institution, or business involved with the manufacture, distribution, dispensing, research, instructional activities, detoxification programs, importing, exporting, or compounding of controlled substances must be registered with the DEA. The DEA issues a license to medical practitioners that enables them to write prescriptions for scheduled drugs (or controlled substances) and to each individual pharmacy to order scheduled drugs from wholesalers. A hospital will register with coverage for both inpatient and outpatient dispensing. Registrations vary from one to three years in length.

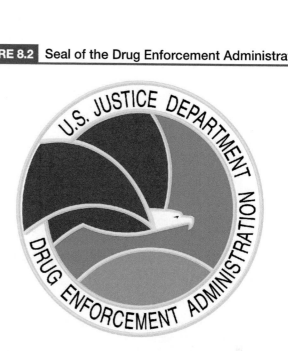

FIGURE 8.2 Seal of the Drug Enforcement Administration

Controlled Substances

Medications that have potential for abuse and dependence are categorized by the DEA as **scheduled drugs**. Through the **Controlled Substances Act (CSA) of 1970**, these drugs are placed in one of five schedules based on their degree of potential for abuse and addiction (http://PharmEssAH.emcp.net/CSAschedules). Schedule I substances are illegal and available only for research or experimental purposes, whereas Schedule II–V substances can be legally dispensed, with restrictions on numbers of refills and quantities (see Table 8.2). Dispensing procedures and inventory control measures for controlled substances are strictly regulated at both the federal and state levels. Schedule II drugs have the most stringent restrictions due to their high potential for abuse.

Allied health professionals should know which prescription drugs are controlled substances and should learn the restrictions placed on those drugs. For example, it may be useful to know that there are no refills allowed on prescriptions for Schedule II controlled substances such as morphine or methylphenidate. Consequently, each time a patient runs out of a Schedule II medication, the prescriber needs to write a new prescription. This process takes more time than a refill request for a medication that is not controlled. An allied health professional assigned the task of helping a patient with medication refills should allow at least an extra 48 hours when ordering additional Schedule II medication.

Work Wise

Schedule II controlled substances are commonly referred to as "C-2s" in the medical community. Each stock bottle of a controlled substance features a C followed by the number of its assigned schedule: C-2.

TABLE 8.2 | Schedules of Controlled Substances

Schedule	Description	Examples	Restrictions
I	Drugs with no accepted medical use having the highest potential for abuse/dependence. Illegal to possess, except for a few substances that can be used for research purposes (special registration and restrictions apply).	Lysergic acid diethylamide (LSD), marijuana (cannabis),* opium derivatives such as heroin, peyote, phencyclidine (PCP)	**Greatest**
II	Drugs with current accepted medical use having high potential for abuse. May lead to high risk of physiologic and psychological dependence.	Codeine, depressants (pentobarbital, secobarbital), fentanyl, hydromorphone, meperidine, methadone, morphine, oxycodone, stimulants (amphetamines such as methylphenidate [Ritalin])	
III	Drugs with accepted medical use having some potential for abuse. May lead to moderate physiologic but high psychological dependence.	Anabolic steroids, barbiturates, codeine combination products (e.g., codeine/acetaminophen), dronabinol	
IV	Drugs with accepted medical use having lower potential for abuse. May lead to low physiologic but moderate psychological dependence.	Appetite suppressants (phentermine), benzodiazepines, phenobarbital, sleep aids (eszopiclone, zaleplon, zolpidem)	
V	Drugs with accepted medical use with low potential for abuse. May lead to limited physiologic or psychological dependence.	Codeine combination products in oral liquid forms (mostly cough syrups)	**Least**

* Although the use of marijuana is illegal according to federal law, many states now have laws that allow its use for medical purposes. A few states have also legalized marijuana's recreational use.

In addition to the restrictions instituted by the DEA on these controlled substances, the sale of drugs considered precursors for making crystal methamphetamine is also limited in pharmacies. Pseudoephedrine and phenylpropanolamine are included in these restrictions. These medications have legitimate medical uses and, when used properly, do not cause abuse or dependence. They can be used, however, in making methamphetamine (a highly addictive and abused drug). Therefore,

In the Know

The weight-loss drug sibutramine (Meridia) was categorized as a Schedule IV controlled substance when it was introduced in 1997, but the manufacturer voluntarily withdrew it from the US market in 2010 because of the drug's cardiovascular risks.

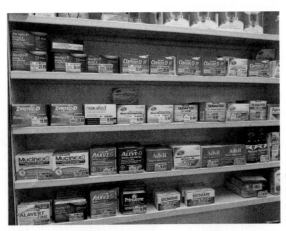

OTC products that contain pseudoephedrine must be stored in the prescription area of a pharmacy and require certain conditions for patient distribution.

the sale of these drugs in most states is limited to patients older than age 18. Pseudoephedrine and phenylpropanolamine must be stored behind the counter in the pharmacy.

Inspection of all medical facilities, including pharmacies, is also a function of the DEA and is usually limited to facilities where suspicious activity has been detected. The DEA works closely with the state drug and narcotic agencies that are responsible for annual physical inspections and local investigation of unsafe prescribing, dispensing, or forging of controlled drug prescriptions. The DEA has established an audit trail to allow the agency to track the flow of narcotics from manufacturer to warehouse to pharmacy to patient. Special forms and procedures must be completed and documented in all medical facilities for both the ordering and the disposal of narcotic drugs. Many pharmacies maintain a perpetual inventory record (or tablet-by-tablet records) for complete accountability of narcotic drugs.

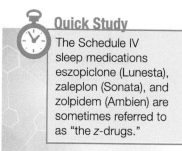

Quick Study

The Schedule IV sleep medications eszopiclone (Lunesta), zaleplon (Sonata), and zolpidem (Ambien) are sometimes referred to as "the z-drugs."

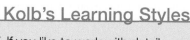

Kolb's Learning Styles

If you like to work with details, as Assimilators do, or enjoy thinking to yourself as you learn new information, as Convergers do, you might enjoy this exercise for learning about controlled substances. Take a look at the list of most commonly prescribed drugs in the United States. (This list can be accessed via Navigator+ that accompanies this textbook.) Then use a reputable drug information resource to look up which drugs are controlled substances. You might find it interesting to see how many prescriptions for controlled substances are dispensed in the United States every year.

Navigator

Prescribers of Controlled Substances

As mentioned earlier, all practitioners who prescribe controlled substances must register with the DEA. These practitioners are authorized to prescribe controlled substances by the jurisdiction in which they are licensed. Examples of practitioners include physicians, physician assistants, nurse practitioners (advanced practice registered nurses [APRNs] or doctors of nursing practice [DNPs]), dentists, veterinarians, and podiatrists. Prescribing privileges for controlled substances also depend on state laws and regulations. For instance, physician assistants and nurse practitioners can prescribe controlled substances in some states but not in others. Although state regulations and procedures may vary, for a physician assistant, an APRN, or a DNP to write prescriptions for Schedule III, IV, or V drugs, a written protocol signed by a delegating physician and approved by the state medical board may be required.

The prescription for a controlled substance must be written for a legitimate medical purpose in the course of the practitioner's professional practice activities. For example, a dentist may write a narcotic prescription for dental pain but not for back pain or cancer-related pain. A prescription for a controlled substance from a foreign physician cannot be filled in the United States because the prescriber must be licensed with the DEA.

Controlled substances in Schedules III–V may only be written, faxed, or communicated verbally. In most cases, prescriptions for Schedule II controlled substances may only be delivered as written prescriptions. There are a few exceptions to this rule: In an emergency situation, a prescriber can call in a prescription for a Schedule II controlled substance, as long as the prescriber follows up by sending a written prescription to the pharmacy within seven days. Generally these prescriptions are only for several days of a medication. The other exception is prescriptions for patients in hospice care: For those patients, prescriptions for Schedule II medications may be faxed.

OSHA

The **Occupational Safety and Health Administration (OSHA)** is an agency of the US Department of Labor. Its primary mission is to ensure the safety and health of America's workers by setting and enforcing regulations and standards; providing training, outreach, and education; establishing partnerships; and encouraging continual improvement in workplace safety and health. OSHA uses its resources to stimulate management commitment and employee participation in comprehensive workplace safety and health programs. In hospitals, home health care, and compounding pharmacies that prepare hazardous substances, OSHA is responsible for overseeing policies and procedures to protect personnel from inadvertent needle sticks and other unnecessary drug exposures. Allied health professionals who have concerns about safety in their workplace can report those concerns to OSHA. The agency will then investigate the complaints and may fine the healthcare facility. OSHA will also instruct the facility to correct the hazards.

 ## Checkpoint 8.1

Take a moment to review what you have learned so far and answer these questions.

1. What are the responsibilities of the FDA, DEA, and OSHA?

2. Can you name an example of a controlled substance in each of the following schedules: II, III, and IV?

3. Does pseudoephedrine require a prescription? Why is it more tightly controlled than other cold medicines?

Healthcare Standards

A **standard** is a set of criteria used to measure product quality or professional performance against a norm. Standards exist for both drug products and dietary supplements. Standards are also created to set expectations for professional training programs and individual professional behaviors.

Standards Organizations

Various professional organizations advocate the establishment of high standards of practice in order to advance the healthcare profession. Two professional organizations that provide standards in the healthcare industry are the US Pharmacopeial Convention and The Joint Commission.

USP

The **US Pharmacopeial Convention (USP)**, with input from scientists, sets standards or criteria for drug quality that must be met by pharmaceutical companies before their new products are submitted to the FDA. The USP also sets national standards for all pharmacies preparing sterile and nonsterile products. USP Chapter <795> covers procedures for making nonsterile preparations such as ointments, and USP Chapter <797> covers the procedures for sterile preparations such as injectable solutions.

In addition, USP works with governments, manufacturers, and practitioners worldwide to set public health standards for dietary supplements. The USP Verified Mark on a dietary supplement label tells consumers that the quality of the product has been verified under the USP's rigorous USP Dietary Supplement Verification Program. The program sets the following guidelines for a dietary supplement:

- The ingredients must be listed on its label, in the declared amounts.

- The supplement must not contain harmful levels of specified contaminants.

- The product must break down and release ingredients into the body within a specified period.

- The supplement has been made according to current FDA **good manufacturing practices (GMPs)**.

The Joint Commission

The Joint Commission ensures a high standard of care in hospitals and other healthcare facilities through a rigorous inspection in its accreditation process. Receiving accreditation from The Joint Commission is the healthcare equivalent of getting the Good Housekeeping Seal of Approval. Although accreditation is voluntary under the law, many insurance carriers require it for reimbursement when providing services for its members. Therefore, all hospitals and healthcare systems seek accreditation from The Joint Commission so they can request and receive reimbursement from insurance carriers.

Accreditation Standards

Accreditation is a process whereby a professional organization grants recognition to a healthcare institution or program for meeting established standards or criteria. As mentioned earlier, accreditation by The Joint Commission is paramount to hospitals. Accreditation of healthcare programs in educational institutions is critical to providing patients with safe and effective care.

Accreditation Organizations

Certain professional agencies grant accreditation to healthcare programs that fulfill predetermined standards. Two of these groups in the allied health arena include the Accrediting Bureau of Health Education Schools (ABHES) and the Commission on Accreditation of Allied Health Education Programs (CAAHEP). To learn more about ABHES, CAAHEP, and other specialized accreditation bodies, see Chapter 4.

ABHES

The **Accrediting Bureau of Health Education Schools (ABHES)** is a private, nonprofit, independent accrediting agency formed in 1968 to ensure the quality of the health education programs that train many medical assistants and other allied health professionals. To earn accreditation from ABHES, a college must show that its curriculum matches current standards. For example, ABHES requires that programs in medical assisting include an externship (experience at a work site) and that the coursework covers medical terminology, pharmacology, the collection of specimens, and many other topics. After earning initial accreditation, a college must also undergo an annual review process. This process ensures that health education programs cover similar core subject matter and are designed to prepare allied health students for their future workplace positions.

CAAHEP

Formed in 1994, the **Commission on Accreditation of Allied Health Education Programs (CAAHEP)** accredits medical assistant training programs and programs in 25 other health science occupations including anesthesiology assistants, lactation consultants, and emergency medical technicians. CAAHEP guidelines for medical assistant programs require that students gain 160 supervised contact hours in an ambulatory healthcare setting during their training. Some of the topics that must be covered in the curriculum of accredited programs include anatomy and physiology, medications, applied mathematics, applied microbiology, communication skills, safety, and ethics.

Checkpoint 8.2

Take a moment to review what you have learned so far and answer these questions.

1. What organization sets the standards for the compounding of sterile and nonsterile medications?

2. What does an accrediting agency do for a college that trains allied health professionals?

Legal Responsibilities of Allied Health Professionals

Like all healthcare workers, allied health professionals are legally obligated to operate within their scope of practice and to respect the privacy of patient medical information. For those allied health professionals who administer drugs, national standards dictate that they must accurately document every dose they administer and follow additional special regulations regarding controlled substances.

Knowing Your Scope of Practice

Allied health professionals in different fields fulfill distinct roles and responsibilities. Each allied health specialty has its own **scope of practice**, which is the set of procedures, actions, and processes that individuals are allowed to perform based on their specific training. For example, medical assistants may administer oral medications and some parenteral medications. To be specific, a medical assistant can give patients pills and liquid oral medications as well as inject intradermal, intramuscular, or subcutaneous

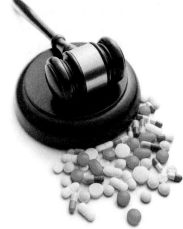

The many regulations governing the manufacturing, prescribing, and dispensing of prescription drugs were written to protect public safety.

medications, but, depending upon local laws, he or she may not be allowed to inject medications into a vein. It is your legal obligation as a healthcare professional to learn the scope of your practice and stay within the limits of that practice. In each state, the scope of practice of each licensed health profession is defined by the state's board of health. These regulations are designed to protect patient safety.

Kolb's Learning Styles

Accommodators and Convergers may enjoy learning about the scope of practice for various healthcare professionals by conducting interviews. Locate several allied health professionals, such as a medical assistant, pharmacy technician, or clinical laboratory technologist, and arrange to interview them about what tasks they are allowed and not allowed to do in their jobs. The information gathered from these interviews will put the scope of practice of these professions into context.

Protecting Patient Confidentiality

All healthcare professionals must understand the importance of maintaining patient confidentiality. **Confidentiality** may be defined as keeping privileged information about a patient from being disclosed without his or her consent. If a patient cannot trust healthcare professionals with health-related information, then both trust and a good patient may be lost. With that in mind, allied health professionals need to be aware of discussing sensitive medical issues in a public setting. They should also keep patient communications about medications at a quiet level of discussion. Outside of the immediate workplace, such as in the lunch break room, allied health professionals must avoid any discussion of patients, their medications, or any other protected health information.

Computer screens should be obscured so as to not be visible to the public or unauthorized personnel. When using the telephone, allied health professionals should not use a speakerphone when talking with a patient about his or her medications and should not leave a message for a patient that divulges any medical or drug information.

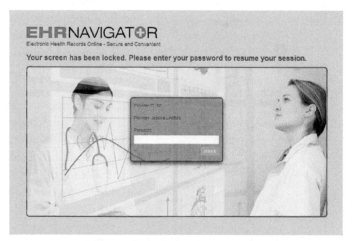

An electronic health record (EHR) system should be put in hibernation mode when the user steps away from the computer workstation. This precaution protects against disclosure of PHI.

HIPAA and Patient Privacy

The **Health Insurance Portability and Accountability Act (HIPAA) of 1996** placed safeguards to protect patient confidentiality and used the term **protected health information (PHI)** to describe a patient's private medical information. The law requires that every healthcare facility have a written policy on patient confidentiality that must be provided to patients as a handout. Healthcare personnel should record the acknowledged patient receipt of this handout in the patient's profile.

HIPAA also gave patients the right to access their own medical records, with some exceptions. Patients can request a copy of their medical records and medical billing information from a healthcare provider or health plan. The provider is not allowed to withhold copies of those records, even if the patient still owes medical bills. The provider is allowed to charge the patient a reasonable fee for copying and mailing the records. The exceptions to this rule include psychotherapy notes and information compiled for legal proceedings.

In addition, HIPAA placed limits on how much of a patient's PHI may be shared. There is no restriction on the sharing of information among different healthcare practitioners who are treating the same patient, but there are restrictions on most other disclosures of medical information. For example, the billing department for the healthcare facility may occasionally need some information about a patient's care in order to complete the required paperwork. The general rule for the sharing of PHI is as follows: Healthcare personnel are legally bound to disclose only the minimum amount of PHI required for the intended purpose. Breaking HIPAA rules about the confidentiality of patient health information is a serious violation that could result in the loss of employment and legal penalties including fines and imprisonment.

Documentation and Handling of Medications

Prescription drug documentation is regulated by federal and state laws. In addition, each hospital or healthcare facility may have internal rules governing how drugs are handled, stored, and tracked. Allied health personnel who administer medications in an inpatient care setting must document the event in the patient's chart. If a patient refuses a drug dose or vomits immediately after the dose, healthcare personnel must document that incident as well.

There are additional legal documentation requirements for controlled substances (Schedule II–V drugs), especially Schedule II drugs, because of the high potential for abuse of these drugs. According to federal law, each prescription for a Schedule II drug must be recorded in a special logbook before being dispensed. This logbook tracks the controlled substance inventory. In larger healthcare facilities, the pharmacy or nursing staff is responsible for this record keeping. Allied health professionals who handle controlled substances must follow the record-keeping guidelines of their state's statutes.

Work Wise

As an allied health professional, you should know which drugs are considered controlled substances and have a heightened awareness of the most tightly controlled Schedule II drugs (C-2s). To help you memorize controlled substances, start by making one list of Schedule II drugs and one list of Schedule III–V drugs.

Ordering Scheduled Drugs

All drugs, including Schedule III–V drugs, are ordered using an invoice. Schedule II medications, on the other hand, must be ordered from suppliers using the Federal Triplicate Order (DEA Form 222). One copy of the form goes to the DEA; the second copy of the form goes to the supplier; and the third copy is retained by the purchaser, which is typically a pharmacy. Records of the suppliers' invoices and a logbook of the administration of the medications must be kept for two years.

When controlled medications are received, they must be recorded on a special inventory form. Two employees then sign the receipt, which should show the exact amount of stock medication received. An inventory is required by the DEA every two years and should include the following:

- name and quantity of each controlled substance
- name, address, and DEA number of the physician
- date and time of the inventory process
- signature of (preferably two) persons taking the inventory

Storing Scheduled Drugs

In any healthcare facility, controlled substances must be kept in a securely locked, substantially constructed cabinet. In addition to the procedures dictated by federal regulations, healthcare facilities may have additional procedures designed to ensure close tracking of controlled medications. Make sure that you know and follow the regulations concerning controlled substances that are discussed in your facility's **Policy & Procedures (P&P) manual**.

Tracking Scheduled Drugs

Allied health professionals should also be aware of how much effort pharmacy professionals devote to tracking the inventory of controlled substances and preventing the diversion of those drugs. Pharmacy technicians routinely count the tablets of a controlled substance prescription twice, to ensure the accuracy of their count, and then the pharmacist typically counts the same bottle a third time.

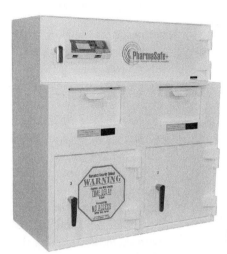

Authorized users of this PharmaSafe+™ narcotics safe open the locker using a thumbprint and access code; the cabinet maintains an electronic log of who accesses it.

Each filled prescription for a Schedule II controlled medication is recorded in a logbook that serves as a perpetual inventory. Pharmacy professionals ensure that the inventory level of the drug is accurate each time such a prescription is dispensed.

In the pharmacy, the records related to Schedule II prescriptions are kept separate from those for all other prescriptions. Records for Schedule III–V prescriptions are also kept separate from regular prescription medications. This filing system makes it easier for inspectors from the DEA or other government agencies to quickly access the records they need.

Disposing of Scheduled Drugs

If a tablet of a Schedule II controlled substance breaks or is past its expiration date, it cannot simply be thrown away. A form must be filled out, and the damaged or expired drug must be transferred to a DEA-registered reverse distributor, which then destroys the unused medication. A list of reverse distributors can be obtained from any DEA diversion field office (http://PharmEssAH.emcp.net/DEAdiversion).

Handling Hazardous Drugs

Some drugs require special handling because they are considered hazardous. The national standards for compounding sterile medications, USP Chapter <797>, includes special safety rules that workers should follow when preparing **hazardous drugs** such as chemotherapy agents, and OSHA regulates what should be done in the case of a hazardous medication spill or other accidental exposure. Drugs are classified as *hazardous* if low doses can cause cancer, birth defects, infertility, genotoxicity (cell mutations), or organ toxicity. Some of the drugs used for cancer chemotherapy, antiviral drugs, hormones, and some bioengineered drugs are considered hazardous. The special handling instructions and directions for proper disposal of a hazardous drug are described in the drug's official labeling information. An up-to-date list of hazardous drugs from the Centers for Disease Control and Prevention (CDC) can be found at http://PharmEssAH.emcp.net/HazDrug.

Professional Ethics

Ethics is the study of standards of conduct and moral judgment that outline the rights and wrongs of human conduct and character. Ethics is a process for reflection and analysis of behavior when the proper course of action is unclear. It is the basis on which to make judgments. Particular individuals, groups, and professions have their own specialized codes of ethics. For example, the American Association of Medical Assistants (AAMA) has its own code of ethics that outlines the principles of medical assistant practice (see Figure 8.3). It is not necessarily inherent to religious belief; those who subscribe to no religion can also have a sense of right and wrong conduct.

The most important aspect of studying ethics is to internalize a framework or set of guidelines based on high professional standards that guide your decision-making and actions. Be aware of a variety of situations you may encounter while working in the healthcare field, and discuss with your colleagues how to react and behave when faced with them. By thinking through your ethical choices ahead of time, you can avoid the paralyzing quandary when being confronted with questionable circumstances and not knowing what to do. Laws and regulations governing the practice of medicine do not always dictate the proper behavior in every situation.

FIGURE 8.3 | **AAMA's Medical Assisting Code of Ethics**

The Medical Assisting Code of Ethics establishes a code of conduct and professional ethics for the medical assisting field.

Render service with full respect for the dignity of humanity.

Respect confidential information obtained through employment unless legally authorized or required by responsible performance of duty to divulge such information.

Uphold the honor and high principles of the profession and accept its disciplines.

Seek to continually improve the knowledge and skills of medical assistants for the benefit of patients and professional colleagues.

Participate in additional service activities aimed toward improving the health and well-being of the community.

 Checkpoint 8.3

Take a moment to review what you have learned so far and answer these questions.

1. What is the role of ethics in health care?

2. How can allied health professionals help protect patient confidentiality?

3. What form must be used when ordering Schedule II drugs?

Chapter Review

Chapter Summary

The tight drug controls in the United States have safeguarded the health of its citizens for many decades. A law is a rule that is passed and enforced by the legislative branch of government. A regulation is a written rule and procedure that exists to carry out a law of the federal or state government.

The FDA regulates the drug approval process, generic drug substitution, patient counseling, and adverse reaction reporting systems. The DEA regulates controlled substances, which are substances that have a potential for abuse and dependence. These drugs are placed in one of five schedules, based on their degree of potential for abuse. Schedule I drugs, such as heroin, are illegal. Among the other controlled substances, drugs in Schedule II have the most stringent restrictions. Pharmacy personnel must carefully track the

inventory of controlled substances and prevent the diversion of these drugs.

Allied health professionals are legally obligated to operate within their scope of practice and respect the privacy of patient medical information. If their specific job responsibilities call for administering drugs, they must accurately document every dose they administer and follow additional special regulations regarding controlled substances and the handling of hazardous drugs such as chemotherapy.

Finally, allied health professionals must uphold high professional standards that guide decision-making and actions in the healthcare setting. Thinking through possible ethical dilemmas ahead of time helps individuals determine the proper course of action to take when responding to similar situations in the workplace.

Chapter Checkup

The Navigator+ learning management system that accompanies this textbook offers many opportunities to help you master chapter content, including end-of-chapter exercises, a glossary of key terms, flash cards, and additional interactive activities.

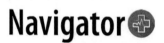

Navigator

Career Exploration

If you enjoyed learning about pharmacy laws and regulations in this chapter, you may want to explore the following career options:

- healthcare documentation specialist
- health information technician
- medical assistant
- pharmacy technician

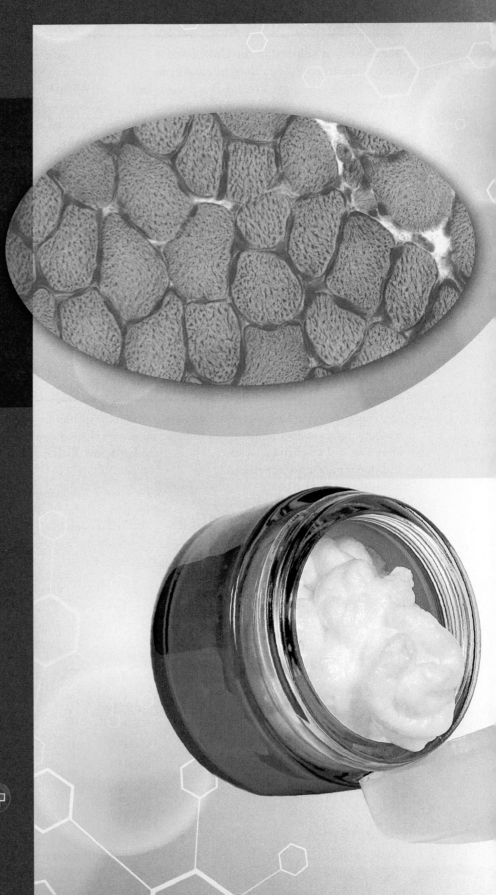

UNIT

3

Navigator✛

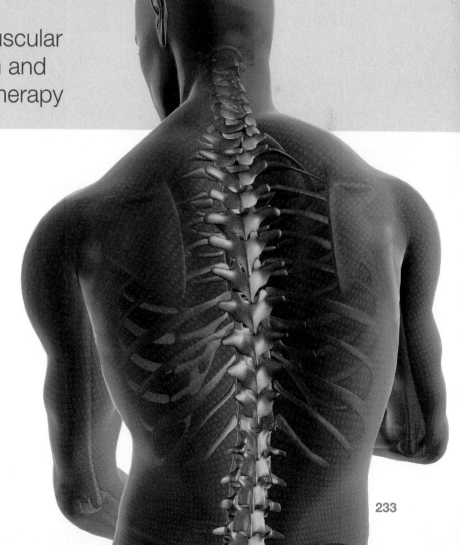

Pharmacotherapy for the Integumentary, Skeletal, and Muscular Systems

The Integumentary System and Drug Therapy

Pharm Facts

- The skin is the largest organ in the human body, encompassing 25 square feet in an adult.

- The thinnest area of skin is on the eyelids; the thickest area of skin is on the soles of the feet.

- Nineteen million skin cells make up every inch of the body.

- Approximately 30,000 to 40,000 skin cells are shed every day.

- Hair is one of the fastest-growing parts of the body. It grows about six inches a year, with male hair growing faster than female hair.

- The scalp contains approximately 100,000 hair follicles.

- Fingernails grow almost three times faster than toenails. The growth rate depends on an individual's age, overall health, and handedness (nails on the dominant hand grow faster).

"I always knew I wanted to work in health care. I chose to become a medical assistant because of the direct patient-care responsibilities and the variety of specialties in which to practice. One specialty area that I have worked in is dermatology. A medical assistant in a dermatologist's office works closely with the physician by providing direct patient care, assisting in minor surgical procedures, and providing administrative support. My hands-on experience in dermatology also broadened my knowledge about the integumentary system, such as how the skin reflects an individual's overall health. No matter what specialty area you would like to pursue as a medical assistant, you will find the position to be rewarding."

—**Stephanie Bernard**, MBA, NCMA
Medical Assistant

Learning Objectives

1 Understand the basic anatomy and physiology of the integumentary system.

2 Describe the common conditions that affect the integumentary system.

3 Explain the therapeutic and adverse effects of prescription medications and nonprescription medications commonly used to treat diseases of the integumentary system.

4 Identify the generic names, brand names, indications, dosage ranges, side effects, contraindications, and cautions and considerations associated with the drugs commonly used to treat diseases of the integumentary system.

5 Identify common herbal and alternative therapies that are related to the integumentary system.

After describing the normal structure and function of the integumentary system, this chapter presents the most common pathologic skin conditions for which drug therapy is needed. Many of these skin conditions can be self-treated, so proper patient education is important. Such conditions include acne; burns, wounds, and ulcers; hair loss; dermatitis; and skin damage due to sun exposure. Skin infections caused by bacteria, fungi, viruses, and parasitic insects are also covered. Some adverse and allergic reactions to drug therapy manifest as skin problems. Drug allergy rashes and photosensitivity are two examples of these side effects. Signs and symptoms of these problems must be recognized early so that patients can seek proper medical care.

Anatomy and Physiology of the Skin

The **integumentary system** refers to the tissue that covers the body and includes skin, nails, and hair. This system protects the body from exposure to harmful pathogens and harsh substances and helps to regulate body temperature. Accounting for 16% of body weight, the **skin** is the largest organ. The skin has three layers: the epidermis, dermis, and subcutaneous tissue (see Figure 9.1).

Epidermis

The **epidermis**, the outermost layer, is made up of dead and dried cells generated from the underlying layer, the dermis. This layer is thicker over the surface of the palms of the hands and soles of the feet and contains no blood vessels. Its cells are filled with a tough protein called **keratin**, which helps gives the skin its water-resistant property. A callus is a thickened area of the epidermis. Calluses form on the skin in areas where the skin frequently or continually comes into contact with objects, such as shoes, clothing, or pencils and pens. Typically, calluses are harmless and can be easily removed when necessary. The epidermis also contains **melanocytes** that provide skin pigmentation.

FIGURE 9.1 Normal Skin Structure

Collagen, a material used cosmetically to plump up lips and facial features, is part of the dermis.

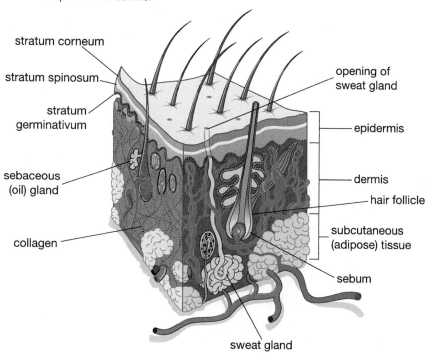

stratum corneum
stratum spinosum
stratum germinativum
sebaceous (oil) gland
collagen
opening of sweat gland
epidermis
dermis
hair follicle
subcutaneous (adipose) tissue
sebum
sweat gland

Dermis

The **dermis** comprises the living, functioning layer of skin where **hair follicles** and **nail beds** form, arteries and veins circulate blood, and nerves provide sensation. The dermis contains sweat, sebaceous, and ceruminous glands. **Sweat glands** are found all over the body and produce watery secretions, including pheromones and other odorous material. **Sebaceous glands** secrete oil for hair and skin lubrication. **Ceruminous glands** in the ear canal release waxy material called **cerumen**.

Subcutaneous Tissue

The **subcutaneous tissue** is the innermost layer and connects the dermis to underlying organs and tissues. This layer is composed of elastic fibers, also called **fascia**, and a layer of fat cells, also called **adipose tissue**. The thickness of the subcutaneous layer varies depending on the region of the body. Female breast tissue arises from the subcutaneous layer.

Common Skin Disorders

Acne, sunburn, and skin rashes are common skin conditions. Most medications for skin conditions are applied topically and are available over the counter. Self-treatment is the norm for most minor skin conditions, but a few of them can be dangerous if not recognized and examined by a healthcare practitioner for proper diagnosis. Dermatitis, eczema, psoriasis, and skin infections are conditions for which prescription drug therapy is often needed.

Aging, Sun Exposure, and Skin Cancer

Natural skin aging involves loss of **collagen** and **elastin** in the dermis. With loss of integrity of these fibrous structures, fine lines and wrinkles form. Over time, sebaceous glands produce less oil, leading to dryness. Subcutaneous tissue shrinks, skin thins, and sagging occurs as gravity pulls on dermal tissue, which is less elastic and pliable. This **intrinsic aging** process cannot be stopped, but good skin care can delay its effects.

Extrinsic aging is caused by external factors such as sun exposure (which accelerates the loss of collagen and elastin), air pollutants, smoking, and skin irritation. **Lesions**, or injuries to the skin, are caused by external factors, genetic predisposition, or a combination of the two. Skin is constantly exposed to sunlight and the oxidizing chemicals that cause deoxyribonucleic acid (DNA) mutation. DNA damage not only results in benign tumors, such as moles and skin tags, but can also cause precancerous conditions such as **actinic keratosis** and skin cancer including **squamous cell carcinoma**, **basal cell carcinoma**, and **melanoma**. Squamous and basal cell carcinomas grow slowly. Malignant melanoma, however, grows quickly and should be diagnosed and treated early to prevent it from spreading and becoming life-threatening.

Signs and symptoms of skin cancer are categorized into the "**ABCDEs**." When patches of skin—for example, moles—appear to have any of the following characteristics, a patient should be evaluated medically:

- **A**symmetry (one half unlike the other half)
- **B**order irregularity (edges are jagged)
- **C**olor variation (patches of tan, brown, black, red, and/or white)
- **D**iameter (larger than 6 mm, or the top of a pencil eraser)
- **E**volution (change in the size, shape, symptoms, surface, or color of a mole)

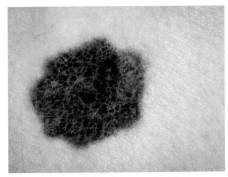

This mole has several characteristics of skin cancer: asymmetry, border irregularity, color variation, and a diameter greater than 6 mm.

Additional characteristics of worrisome skin lesions include a mole that is inflamed, bleeding, and crusting, and/or a mole that is tingling, itchy, or painful. Patients who notice any of these characteristics should alert their healthcare practitioners right away.

Drug Regimens and Treatments

Drug therapy can be used to limit **sun exposure** and prevent damage caused by **ultraviolet (UV) radiation**. It can also be used to treat damage once it has occurred. Because UV radiation has been strongly linked to skin cancer, treating damage once it has occurred is not as effective as limiting sun exposure in the first place. Sunscreens are over-the-counter (OTC) products. Medications to treat skin damage such as actinic keratosis, or for skin cancer itself, are usually applied in a physician's office by trained personnel.

Sunscreens

Sunscreens are products that limit skin exposure to UV radiation. UV radiation is divided into two types: UVA, which produces tanning (but can burn with prolonged exposure), and UVB, which leads to burning.

Sunscreens use chemicals to partially block harmful UV radiation. Many sunscreens are aimed at reducing UVB rays while allowing UVA rays to continue tanning the skin; however, some products block both UVA and UVB rays. Patients should be sure to read the product labeling for details. A variety of active ingredients can be found in these OTC lotions, creams, sprays, and gels. Although, for practical purposes, not all of these ingredients can be listed here, one ingredient that is commonly known is para-aminobenzoic acid (PABA). Because PABA can be allergenic, many products are now available without this ingredient. A telltale sign of a PABA allergy is a rash at the application site. If a rash appears, the patient should check the product's label for the presence of PABA and should switch products if that ingredient is listed on the label.

The **sun protection factor (SPF)** estimates the amount of resistance to burning that a product provides. In effect, the SPF number estimates how much longer a person can be in the sun and receive the same amount of radiation effects. For instance, an SPF of 8 generally means a patient can spend eight times longer in the sun than the typical time it would take to burn. Table 9.1 shows which factor is recommended for someone with each type of skin and burning tendency. Patient skin type is based on unprotected exposure to sun for 45 to 60 minutes. SPF ratings measure UVB blocking activity primarily, so patients should be aware that they are still at risk for exposure to harmful UVA radiation even when using a product with a high SPF.

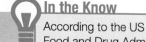

In the Know

According to the US Food and Drug Administration, a manufacturer can no longer label or advertise its sunscreen product as a "sunblock." Identifying the product as such indicates that its application provides an individual with 100% protection against harmful UVA rays—and that claim is simply not true. No sunscreen product can provide 100% protection. Accurate labeling of sunscreen products has become even more important as the rates of skin cancer continue to rise.

TABLE 9.1 Recommended Sunscreen Product Guide

Patient Skin Type	Minimum Suggested SPF Product
Always burns, rarely tans	20–30
Burns easily, tans minimally	12–20
Burns moderately, tans gradually	8–12
Burns minimally, tans well	4–8
Rarely burns, tans profusely	2–4
Never burns, deeply pigmented	None needed

Drug Alert

It is common for sunscreen users to apply less than the recommended amount (often using only one-third as much as they should). Therefore, many dermatologists recommend using sunscreen products with a minimum SPF of 15 or greater year-round.

Side Effects Sunscreens are usually safe for self-application and rarely cause side effects. If patients experience irritation or a rash, they should stop using the product, wash it off, and seek care from their healthcare practitioners. Some patients are allergic to PABA, in particular.

Contraindications Few contraindications exist for sunscreens. People who are allergic to parabens should not use a sunscreen containing PABA.

➕ *Note: Allied health professionals should be aware that an allergy to a particular drug contraindicates its use. This warning applies to all Contraindications sections in this chapter.*

Cautions and Considerations Patients should avoid contact of sunscreen products with the eyes. If contact occurs, flush the eyes generously with water and seek medical care. Likewise, sunscreens should not be applied to open cuts or wounds, as severe irritation and burning can occur. If contact occurs, wash the area thoroughly with water.

Spray products can be inhaled during application. Therefore, until the US Food and Drug Administration (FDA) completes an analysis it began in 2011 on the potential risks of spray sunscreens, it is advised that these products should generally not be used by or on children. If a child inhales and encounters breathing difficulty, urgent medical care should be sought.

Acne and Dandruff

In the United States, **acne** is the most common skin condition for which treatment, either over the counter or prescription, is sought. Acne is initiated by the overproduction of **sebum**, which is produced from glands around hair follicles. Such overproduction is most often stimulated by the hormonal changes encountered during puberty. **Pimples**, **blackheads**, and **whiteheads** appear as pores and follicles clogged with oily material, dead skin cells, and dirt from the skin's surface. Mild forms of acne can be treated with OTC products. However, acne in its most severe forms, such as **nodular acne** or **acne vulgaris**, can cause deep cysts that permanently damage the dermal layer. Visible scars and pockmarks can form. Prescription drug therapy is needed to treat moderate-to-severe acne.

Rosacea is categorized as acne (and is also called *adult acne*) but arises from a different physiologic process. Rosacea is a chronic inflammatory disorder seen in adults and characterized by redness, visible surface blood vessels, and raised bumps or pustules on the face and cheeks. Exposure to sunlight, stress, or extreme temperatures, as well as consuming alcoholic beverages or spicy foods, can worsen this condition.

Dandruff is a malfunction of the oil-producing glands around hair follicles on the scalp. Cell proliferation in the scalp is also accelerated. Overproduction of sebum and cells results in layers of epidermis sticking together and flaking off as they dry. Specks of skin become visible in the hair and on the scalp. Although unsightly, dandruff is not harmful.

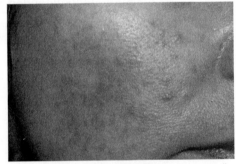

Rosacea, a chronic inflammatory skin condition, can be triggered by stress, temperature changes, and diet (especially the consumption of red wine and chocolate).

Drug Regimens and Treatments

First-line treatment for mild-to-moderate acne is to cleanse the affected area twice a day. Although this cleansing will not eliminate acne, it can help prevent new blackheads and pimples from forming. Mild soap or cleanser is used twice a day to remove excess oil, dirt, and dead skin cells that build up and clog pores.

Treatment of repeated acne lesions starts with OTC products, such as benzoyl peroxide. Moderate-to-severe acne requires the use of prescription products, starting with topical agents and progressing to oral agents when needed. Oral agents include anti-biotics such as erythromycin, tetracycline, doxycycline, minocycline, and clindamycin (see Chapter 23). Some women may use oral contraceptives to decrease acne (see Chapter 21). Metronidazole and azelaic acid are also used to treat rosacea. Because the use of oral agents is associated with more side effects, these medications are reserved for patients who do not gain adequate control with topical treatments.

Topical Acne Agents

Topical acne agents are used alone to treat mild acne and may be used in combination with oral agents to treat moderate-to-severe acne. Benzoyl peroxide and salicylic acid are the main-stays of treatment for mild acne. If they do not work, prescription topical agents are used.

Benzoyl peroxide is a bleaching agent that promotes cell turnover in follicles. It produces oxygen, which is toxic to the bacteria that cause pimples. Benzoyl peroxide is available in both OTC and prescription strengths. **Salicylic acid** is a **keratolytic** agent that breaks down and peels off dead skin cells, thereby preventing them from clogging pores. Both of these active ingredients can be found in numerous facial cleansers, washes, and masks in a variety of strengths (see Table 9.2).

TABLE 9.2 Common Topical Acne Products

Generic (Brand)	Dosage Form	Route of Administration
OTC Products		
Benzoyl peroxide (Benzac, Brevoxyl, Clearasil, Desquam-X, NeoBenz, Neutrogena, Oxy, PanOxyl, Triaz, ZoDerm)	Bar, cleanser, cream, gel, liquid	Topical
Salicylic acid (Clearasil, Fostex, Neutrogena, Oxy, PROPA pH, Sal-Clens, Stridex)	Cleanser, cream, lotion, pads, stick	Topical
Prescription Products		
Azelaic acid (Azelex, Finacea)	Cream, gel	Topical
Benzoyl peroxide (Benzac, Brevoxyl, NeoBenz, PanOxyl, Triaz, ZoDerm)	Bar, cleanser, cream, gel, liquid, lotion	Topical
Clindamycin (Cleocin T, Clindagel, ClindaMax, Clindets, Evoclin)	Foam, gel, lotion, topical solution	Topical
Erythromycin (Akne-Mycin, Emgel, Eryderm, Ery Pads)	Gel, ointment, pads, solution	Topical
Metronidazole (MetroCream, MetroGel, MetroLotion)	Cream, gel, lotion	Topical

Side Effects Common side effects of topical acne products include dryness, redness, burning, and flaking or peeling skin. Moisturizers can be applied to control these side effects. In general, less frequent use of these acne products is recommended if side effects are bothersome.

Contraindications Acne products should not be used on moles, warts, or areas of skin that are infected, red, or irritated. In addition, topical acne products should not be used to treat infants or patients with impaired circulation because their skin is more fragile.

Cautions and Considerations All of these products are for external use only. Some of the topical antibiotic products are flammable. Products should be kept away from intense heat.

Retinoids

Vitamin A derivatives including **retinoids** (see Table 9.3) work by increasing cell turnover in follicles, which pushes clogged material out of the pores. In acne vulgaris, retinoids alter cell development and inflammatory processes to reduce swelling and redness.

Retinoids are used to treat moderate-to-severe acne and to reduce the appearance of fine lines and wrinkles that accompany aging. Acitretin is used exclusively for psoriasis. Because of severe side effects and toxicities, oral retinoid agents are reserved for use in the most severe forms of acne or psoriasis.

TABLE 9.3 | Retinoid Agents

Generic (Brand)	Dosage Form	Route of Administration
Acitretin (Soriatane)	Capsule	Oral
Adapalene (Differin)	Cream, gel, lotion	Topical
Alitretinoin (Panretin)	Gel	Topical
Isotretinoin (Amnesteem, Claravis)	Capsule	Oral
Tazarotene (Avage, Tazorac)	Cream, gel	Topical
Tretinoin (Atralin, Avita, Renova, Retin-A)	Cream, gel	Topical

Side Effects Common side effects of topical retinoid agents include burning, peeling, dry skin, redness, and itching. Sensitive skin may be especially prone to these effects. If these effects are severe or bothersome, the patient should stop using the product. In addition, retinoids also should not be used along with topical antibiotics such as tetracycline because the antibiotics can increase these side effects.

Oral agents, such as isotretinoin, have systemic side effects that can include depression, psychosis, pancreatitis, high triglyceride levels, and hepatotoxicity. Patients who already have these conditions should not take isotretinoin. Patients must be monitored closely for mental status changes, and regular laboratory blood tests must be drawn to watch for pancreas or liver problems.

Contraindications Retinoids should not be used by patients with liver or kidney impairment. Due to side effects, they should be used with caution in patients with depression or hypertriglyceridemia. Isotretinoin cannot be used by women who are or might become pregnant. Severe birth defects are highly likely if a woman becomes pregnant while taking isotretinoin.

Cautions and Considerations As with all acne products, retinoids should not be used on areas of skin that are infected, red, or irritated. Care should also be taken to avoid applying these products close to the eyes or around the mouth. Because isotretinoin is contraindicated in pregnancy and harmful to a developing fetus, this drug is dispensed through a special distribution program approved by the FDA. This program, **iPLEDGE**,

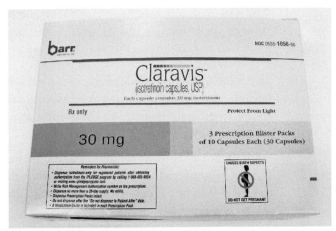

Claravis, a brand of isotretinoin, is distributed through the iPLEDGE program because of its harmful effects to a developing fetus.

requires pharmacies, wholesalers, and patients to be annually enrolled and certified to participate. Women with childbearing potential must agree to use effective contraception and submit to regular pregnancy tests as part of the program. Anyone taking isotretinoin should not donate blood for up to one month after taking it so that blood product recipients are not exposed. More information about this program is available by researching the iPLEDGE program online (http://PharmEssAH.emcp.net/ipledge) or by calling the toll-free phone number listed on its website.

Patient Teaching

Allied health professionals should be aware that the use of retinoids to minimize the signs of aging is considered by many insurance companies to be a cosmetic rather than a therapeutic indication. Consequently, these companies deny insurance coverage for the cost of these medications. It can be helpful to warn patients that these products can be costly before they have their prescriptions filled.

Dandruff Products

The active ingredients used most in dandruff products are **selenium sulfide** and **pyrithione zinc**. Both are available over the counter in shampoo, such as Head & Shoulders and Selsun Blue. These products are used once a day or on a regular basis to control dandruff. **Coal tar** shampoos including Neutrogena T/Gel are also available over the counter but tend to be used in severe cases. Coal tar is safe, but its use can be messy and odorous, and most patients find long-term use unpleasant. Nizoral shampoo is available in OTC and prescription strengths. It contains ketoconazole, which is typically considered an antifungal agent. All of these active ingredients work by slowing cell and oil production, which results in reduced skin flaking. In addition, these products have antipruritic properties that reduce the itching associated with dry, flaking skin.

Side Effects Side effects of dandruff products are rare and mild. However, possible effects include contact dermatitis, photosensitivity, and aggravation of preexisting skin conditions such as acne or psoriasis. If such effects occur, the patient should stop using the product and these effects will subside.

Contraindications No contraindications exist for these products.

Cautions and Considerations If dandruff and scalp itching continue with repeated use of these products, patients should seek medical advice to see if there is an alternative cause.

Checkpoint 9.1

Take a moment to review what you have learned so far and answer these questions.

1. How should SPF ratings guide the choice of sunscreens?

2. What are the active ingredients in OTC acne products?

3. What prescription drug products are used to treat acne?

Skin Infections

Fungal skin infections are commonly caused by **dermatophytes** and *Candida albicans*, a yeast. These organisms infect skin, nail beds, and even mucous membranes such as those inside the mouth. **Tinea** is a dermatophyte that causes **ringworm**, **athlete's foot**, and **jock itch**. Fungal infections affecting the skin, along with their corresponding antifungal medications, are covered in Chapter 23.

Few viruses affect the skin, but the herpes virus family causes many skin problems. **Herpes simplex virus type 1 (HSV-1)** causes cold sores, and **herpes zoster**, or the chicken pox virus, causes shingles (see Chapter 23). **Shingles** is an inflammation and reemergence of a systemic viral infection, but it affects nerve pathways near the skin and manifests as painful skin lesions.

Patient Teaching

Remind patients that the occurrence of shingles can be prevented or reduced in severity with administration of a vaccine, Zostavax. This vaccine is indicated for patients who are 50 years or older.

Genital herpes is a sexually transmitted infection that manifests as small, painful vesicles on the skin (see Chapter 21). Many different viruses cause warts on the skin. Most are harmless, but **human papillomavirus (HPV)** is particularly problematic. HPV causes genital warts and has been linked to cervical cancer in women (see Chapter 21).

Bacterial skin infections most frequently involve *Staphylococcus aureus*, which is considered normal flora and is not generally harmful unless overgrowth occurs or it is introduced internally through a cut or sore. Methicillin-resistant *Staphylococcus aureus* (MRSA), a particularly difficult-to-treat organism when introduced internally, is often found on the skin. Therefore, systemic antibiotics are given prior to surgery to prevent infection from an incision through the skin. **Impetigo** is another example of a skin infection caused by *S. aureus*. Impetigo typically occurs in children and is characterized by pus-filled blisters that break to form a yellow crust.

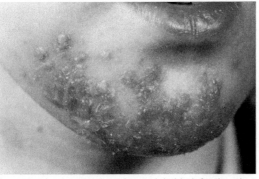

Impetigo is a contagious bacterial skin infection that presents as blisters or sores around the nose and mouth.

Drug Regimens and Treatments

When an infection is localized to the superficial layers of the skin, treatment with topical agents is appropriate. When skin infections become severe and spread to other soft tissues, systemic agents are needed (see Chapter 23).

Topical Antibiotics

Generic names for **topical antibiotic agents** differ from names of oral antibiotics, so familiarity with oral antibiotics does not automatically confer knowledge of topical products. Topical antibiotics are used to treat local skin infections such as cuts or scrapes, impetigo, and diaper rash. Mupirocin is used most often for treatment of impetigo, and topical metronidazole is commonly used to treat rosacea. These agents work by a variety of mechanisms, depending on their drug class (see Table 9.4).

TABLE 9.4 Common Topical Antibiotics

Generic (Brand)	Dosage Form	Dispensing Status
Bacitracin	Ointment	OTC
Bacitracin/neomycin/polymyxin B (triple antibiotic ointment)	Ointment	OTC
Clindamycin (Cleocin T, ClindaMax)	Foam, gel, lotion, solution	Rx
Erythromycin (Eryderm, Erygel, Ery Pads)	Gel, ointment, pledgets, solution	Rx
Metronidazole (MetroCream, Metrogel, MetroLotion, Noritate, Rosadan)	Cream, gel, lotion	Rx
Mupirocin (Bactroban)	Cream, ointment	Rx
Neomycin, polymyxin B (Neosporin)	Ointment, solution for irrigation	OTC
Retapamulin (Altabax)	Ointment	Rx

Side Effects Side effects of topical antibiotic products include burning, stinging, pain, skin rash, dry skin, swelling, and redness. Headache, runny nose, respiratory congestion, and sore throat can occur if products are applied near the nose.

Contraindications Patients with allergies to any of these antibiotics should not use any of these topical anti-infective products. Remember, when a patient is allergic to one antibiotic, they are allergic to all antibiotics in the same drug class. Patients can check with their pharmacists if they are not sure whether an allergy should prevent them from using one of these medications.

Cautions and Considerations These products are for external use only and should be kept away from the eyes and other mucous membranes during application. They should not be applied over large areas of skin because systemic absorption can occur.

Lice and Scabies Infestation

Two types of parasitic insects—lice and scabies—use the human body as a host. Another type of parasite, bedbugs, also feed by biting humans, but they do not live on the human body as lice and scabies do.

Lice feed on human blood, which causes intense itching. The normal life cycle for lice is 40 to 45 days. They lay eggs (nits) on hair follicles next to the skin, which hatch in about eight days. Three different species of lice affect humans: head lice, body lice, and pubic lice. **Head lice** are passed from person to person through direct contact or by sharing hats, hairbrushes or combs, clothing, or sometimes bedding. Children tend to get head lice most often because they play in close contact with each other and share personal items frequently. **Body lice** live and lay eggs in the seams of clothing. They are only on the body when feeding. The main symptom is severe itching, especially at night. Redness and sores appear in the armpits, waist, and other areas where seams of clothing rub against the skin. **Pubic lice** ("crabs") are very small and are typically passed through sexual contact. Symptoms include intense itching that may resemble dermatitis.

Scabies are insects that burrow into the epidermal layer of the skin and feed on cellular material there. Scabies are very small and difficult to see, but the burrows they make into the skin are visible as grayish-white wavy lines that are slightly raised. As they burrow, they secrete substances that disintegrate skin cells. The intense itching the host experiences is most likely from the fecal pellets the scabies leave behind. Scabies are spread through skin-to-skin contact or by sharing a bed (even without sexual contact). They are more common in urban, crowded areas where hygiene is not ideal.

Bedbugs are flat, oval-shaped insects that are about the size of an apple seed. They feed on human blood at night and can be found in beds, bedding, carpet, areas around the bed, and clothing. They can also inhabit furniture and closets. They are passed through exposure to infested furniture, bedding, or clothing and can spread from one room to another if not controlled. They are active at night and bite through the skin to extract blood for feeding. Bites may or may not be itchy at first, but itching gets worse over time. Bedbugs can get into very tight spaces (the width of a credit card) and will hide in crevices and cracks in mattresses, box springs, carpet, sheets, and other areas where humans sleep. They can live up to a year without feeding and can be difficult to get rid of when encountered.

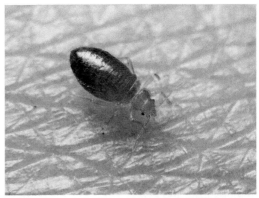

This bedbug is engorged after biting its sleeping victim and sucking the blood. The residual bite marks appear as small, flat or raised red bumps on the victim's skin.

Drug Regimens and Treatments

Table 9.5 shows common products used to treat lice and scabies. Allied health professionals should be aware that many patients are embarrassed about these infestations because they carry a stigma. With that in mind, be sensitive to patients' concerns, but also be forthright with accurate information so that patients can use the appropriate treatments with success.

TABLE 9.5 Common Lice and Scabies Products

Generic (Brand)	Dosage Form	Route of Administration
Lindane	Lotion, shampoo	Topical
Malathion (Ovide)	Lotion	Topical
Permethrin (Acticin, Elimite, Nix)	Cream, lotion	Topical
Pyrethrin (Pronto, Rid, Tisit)	Gel, lotion, mousse, shampoo	Topical

In addition to treating an infestation of lice and scabies with drugs, patients should wash all clothing, underwear, pajamas, pillows, towels, and bed linens in hot water. Hair should be combed with a fine-tooth comb to remove dead lice and nits. Stuffed animal toys may be washed or enclosed in airtight bags or containers for four weeks. Rooms should be thoroughly vacuumed. Hairbrushes, combs, and other personal items that could contain insects should be washed in hot water or treated with a pediculicide (discussed in the following section).

Other than topical anti-itch products, medications are not used to treat bedbugs. Instead, the bugs themselves must be killed and removed. Bedding and clothing should be washed in hot water and dried on the highest dryer heat setting. Mattresses should be scrubbed and vacuumed (especially cracks and seams) frequently for up to a year. Infested mattresses or furniture should be encased in tightly woven zippered covers for at least a year or disposed of entirely. Chemical extermination is usually necessary for eradicating bedbugs.

Pediculicides and Scabicides

In conjunction with the washing regimen described, treating lice and scabies involves applying a drug that kills insects. **Pediculicides** kill lice, and **scabicides** are used against scabies. These products have activity that is similar to insecticides such as dichloro-diphenyl-trichloroethane, or DDT. They impair the central nervous system (CNS) of insects, thereby causing seizure and death. These agents are used to treat infestations but should not be used to prevent them.

Pediculicides and scabicides are spread on the hair or body, left on for a specified period, and then washed off. For head lice, the product is applied to the hair and scalp, allowed to remain for 10 minutes, and then rinsed off. Repeat treatment is recommended in one week to kill newly hatched lice. For body lice, the patient must first bathe from the neck down, and then the product is applied and allowed to remain on the skin overnight. Treatment is repeated, if needed, in one week. For pubic lice, the product is applied from the thighs to the trunk of the body and allowed to remain on the skin overnight. Treatment is repeated, if needed, in one week. For scabies, the product is applied to the skin from the neck down, allowed to remain on the skin overnight, and then washed off. Repeat treatment is rarely needed.

Pyrethrin and **permethrin** are considered first-line therapies because they are available over the counter. Pyrethrin is used, however, only for head lice. Permethrin, depending on the formulation, can be used for either lice or scabies and has residual activity for up to 14 days. Neither of these products kills both the lice and nits, so repeat application is often needed in seven days.

Malathion is a prescription product used to treat head lice. This product kills both the adult lice and the nits. To use malathion, apply the lotion to dry hair until fully wetted and then leave it on the hair to dry naturally for 8 to 12 hours. Afterward, the hair can be shampooed and all nits removed with a fine-tooth comb. If lice are present in seven days, repeat this procedure.

Lindane lotion is used for scabies, and the shampoo is used for lice. Lindane has significant CNS toxicities and can cause seizures, so it is limited to prescription use only. It should be used only with great caution to treat children or infants. Patients must follow instructions closely and avoid getting the lotion in the eyes or on mucous membranes. Lindane should be washed off in 8 to 12 hours. Repeat applications can cause dermatitis, so reapplication is not recommended. Patients or caregivers applying lindane should wear gloves or wash their hands thoroughly after application.

Side Effects Side effects of pyrethrin and permethrin include mild itching, burning, tingling, numbness, and skin rash in the area of application. These agents can also cause headache, dizziness, diarrhea, nausea, and vomiting. Side effects can be avoided or lessened by using only the recommended amount for only the period indicated on the package.

Side effects of lindane are significant and possibly life-threatening, so patients must follow application instructions carefully. Seizures and even death have occurred from lindane use, usually when used incorrectly. Patients should not use more than two ounces, as prescribed, and should wash the product off in 8 to 12 hours to reduce systemic absorption. Additional side effects include dermatitis, itching, headache, pain, and hair loss. Other OTC products should be tried first, if at all possible, to avoid these potential, toxic effects.

Contraindications Malathion and lindane should not be used on children younger than six years old and on patients with seizure disorders. Lindane should also not be used on any skin that is irritated or has a rash. Systemic absorption could occur if applied to such areas.

Cautions and Considerations All pediculicide products are for external use only. In case of contact with the eyes, patients should flush their eyes with a generous amount of water. Ingestion is very dangerous, especially for lindane. Ingestion is considered a poisoning situation. If lindane is swallowed, patients should call a poison control center.

Kolb's Learning Styles

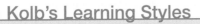

If you like active experimentation (as Accommodators do), try this homework. Look up the websites for Nix and Rid lice treatments. Investigate the information provided, and then find a classmate with whom you can discuss your findings. What are the advantages and disadvantages of these products? What other non-drug therapy measures are necessary to eliminate head lice?

Hair Loss

Two major types of **hair loss** include androgenic alopecia and alopecia areata. **Androgenic alopecia** is more common, affecting both men and women, even though it is often referred to as male-pattern baldness. It is genetically related and hormonally mediated. Hair follicles shrink and produce finer hair. **Alopecia areata** is a chronic inflammatory disorder affecting hair follicles and may cause areas of complete hair loss. It can affect nail beds as well.

In the Know

Minoxidil was originally developed as an anti-hypertensive. However, it was found to have a serious side effect: orthostatic hypotension, or a sudden drop in blood pressure upon standing. Although this side effect made minoxidil less than effective for treating hypertension, another one of its side effects—excessive body hair growth—made minoxidil effective for male-pattern baldness.

Drug Regimens and Treatments

Androgenic alopecia is usually treated with minoxidil or finasteride. Treatment for alopecia areata includes potent topical corticosteroids (see Table 9.6).

Drugs for Hair Loss

Minoxidil (Rogaine) treats hair loss by improving bloodflow to the scalp and stimulating resting hair follicles. Applied to the scalp twice a day, minoxidil is available over the counter as a 2% or 5% strength solution or foam. Although men can use either strength, the 2% strength is recommended for women. Hair regrowth, should it occur, takes four months or longer to become noticeable. Patients should apply only a small amount

(1–2 mL); using more product does not improve results. Patients should wash their hands after each application.

In addition to minoxidil, treatment for hair loss may include finasteride (Propecia). Finasteride works by inhibiting 5-alpha reductase, thereby reducing the breakdown of testosterone. Type I 5-alpha reductase is found in sebaceous glands, so inhibition can have effects on hair growth. Finasteride also inhibits type II 5-alpha reductase, a substance found primarily in the prostate and testicles. Consequently, finasteride is also used to treat prostate enlargement.

Side Effects Side effects of minoxidil are rare but can include dermatitis, redness, itching, skin flaking, and possibly worsening of hair loss. If any of these effects occur, the patient should stop using the treatment and seek medical care if effects are severe.

Contraindications Finasteride is contraindicated in women because it affects testosterone production and may affect a developing fetus if the patient is pregnant.

Cautions and Considerations Patients should be aware that minoxidil does not work for everyone. If no hair regrowth is seen after four to six months, patients should talk with their healthcare practitioners about alternative treatments. In addition, once treatment is stopped, hair regrowth will stop and newly grown hair will be shed within a few months.

 Checkpoint 9.2

Take a moment to review what you have learned so far and answer these questions.

1. What prescription topical antibiotics are used to treat skin infections?

2. What products are used to treat lice and scabies and how are they different from each other?

3. What drugs can be used to treat hair loss?

Dermatitis, Eczema, and Psoriasis

Dermatitis is **pruritic** (itchy), inflamed skin that can be caused by a variety of factors. The most severe cases can result in blisters and oozing erosions on the skin, but typical symptoms include areas of redness, dry flaky skin, raised or bumpy skin, and pruritus. Types of dermatitis include contact dermatitis, seborrheic dermatitis, diaper rash, and atopic dermatitis.

Contact dermatitis occurs in response to exposure to irritants or allergenic substances. Rash appears wherever skin has come into contact with the offending substance, such as soaps or detergents. Poison ivy, poison oak, and other plants can cause redness, itching, rash, and blisters when their oils come into contact with the skin.

Seborrheic dermatitis, also called **cradle cap**, is a greasy, scaly area on the skin that sometimes appears red, brown, or yellow. It usually occurs in infants and in areas where

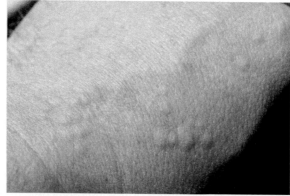

Irritant contact dermatitis is often caused by these common substances: soaps, cosmetics, rubbing alcohol, bleach, and solvents.

sebaceous follicles are concentrated, such as the scalp, ears, upper trunk, eyebrows, and around the nose. In adult men, it can occur in the beard area.

Another skin rash common in infants is **diaper rash**. This acute and easily treated condition occurs most frequently in children who are not yet toilet trained, but it can also occur in adults who must wear incontinence pads. When skin remains wet for long periods, tissue breakdown allows bacteria on the surface to gain entry to deeper tissues. Diaper rash products are used for irritation and redness when skin comes into frequent contact with urine and/or feces. These products contain a variety of ingredients that combine to promote healing, protect skin from further insult, and prevent infection. Common ingredients include the following:

- balsam of Peru for wound healing and tissue repair
- camphor or menthol to provide local anesthetic action to relieve pain and itching
- eucalyptol (eucalyptus oil) for antimicrobial activity
- talc or kaolin for moisture absorption
- zinc oxide, a drying agent

These agents should be used as soon as redness appears in order to protect the skin from further damage and prevent infection from bacteria or fungi.

 ## Patient Teaching

If you work with expectant mothers, you might recommend that they purchase a good diaper rash product with the listed ingredients prior to giving birth. Having a product available is important because diaper rash comes on quickly. Delaying treatment of the rash can make the condition worse.

 ## Kolb's Learning Styles

Divergers and Accommodators are people oriented. If you possess this quality, find a classmate or friend with young children. Interview the person about his or her preferred diaper rash product. Ask the interviewee to explain the application of the product as well as other products that he or she has tried. This activity will provide you with real-world context for the active ingredients in diaper rash products.

Atopic dermatitis, also called **eczema**, is a chronic condition that usually first occurs in childhood and can continue into adulthood. Atopic dermatitis is not well understood but has an immunologic component, in that patients tend to have elevated levels of immunoglobulin E (IgE) in their blood. Patients with atopic dermatitis have a greater tendency to develop asthma or hay fever sometime in life. Eczema appears as dry, flaky, red skin that is very itchy. Patients sometimes scratch enough to cause secondary skin infections. Unlike other

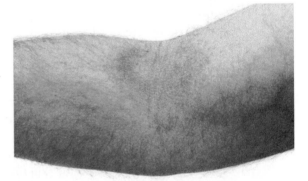

Atopic dermatitis typically appears on the face, hands, feet, behind the knees, or on the inside of elbows (as shown here) and has periods of flare-up and remission.

types of dermatitis that are usually curable, atopic dermatitis is a chronic condition. Periods of severe symptoms (exacerbation) can cycle with periods of remission. Common triggers for exacerbations include stress, exposure to skin irritants, and food allergies.

Psoriasis is an immunologic condition affecting T-cell activity in the skin. It manifests on the skin as well-defined plaques (patches) that are raised, silvery or white, flaky, and pruritic. The plaques can appear anywhere on the body and may be very small or quite large and painful. Like eczema, psoriasis is characterized by periods of exacerbation that cycle with periods of remission. Stress and exposure to environmental factors that dry out skin can trigger exacerbation.

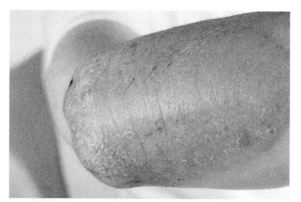

Psoriasis changes the life cycle of skin cells, which results in the buildup of these cells and the subsequent formation of white or silvery patches on the epidermis.

Drug Regimens and Treatments

Corticosteroids are usually first-line therapy for dermatitis and eczema. Therapy starts with topical medications but may include oral corticosteroids if severe. Seborrheic dermatitis can be treated with attention to good hygiene and topical antihistamines, anti-inflammatory agents, and moisturizing creams. Eczema treatment involves constant maintenance of skin condition with moisturizers to prevent exacerbations, along with topical corticosteroids for flare-ups. If the affected skin becomes infected, topical antibiotics may be used.

Psoriasis can be difficult to treat and does not always respond well to drug therapy. Like dermatitis and eczema, corticosteroids are the first-line treatment for psoriasis. Immunosuppressants and immunomodulators are sometimes required. Immunosuppressants used to treat psoriasis include azathioprine, cyclosporine, and methotrexate. Immunomodulators used include biologic therapies such as adalimumab (Humira) and etanercept (Enbrel). Biologic agents (also called *tumor necrosis factor alpha [TNF-alpha] inhibitors*) are a costly but effective treatment for severe psoriasis. (For more information on biologic therapies, see Chapter 24.)

Topical Corticosteroids

Anti-inflammatory agents that work by inhibiting redness, swelling, itching, and pain in the dermal layer of the skin, **topical corticosteroids** are used to treat contact dermatitis, eczema, psoriasis, and allergic reactions. A thin layer of medication is applied to affected skin for a limited period. Because corticosteroids can penetrate the skin and be absorbed systemically, they should be used sparingly. Systemic absorption can cause **hypothalamus-pituitary-adrenal (HPA) axis suppression**, which is associated with appetite changes, weight gain, fat redistribution, fluid retention, and insomnia.

Treatment with topical corticosteroids starts with OTC-strength products, such as 0.5% or 1% hydrocortisone. Both strengths are usually effective for treatment of poison ivy and diaper rash (the lower strength should be used for infants and children). Combination products that contain an antifungal along with a corticosteroid can be useful for treating severe diaper rash.

Corticosteroid products vary in potency, depending on the formulation (see Tables 9.6 and 9.7). Ointments are typically more potent than creams. Ointments are most appropriate for treating dry, scaly lesions, whereas creams are most effective for treating moist or oozing lesions. When using gels, patients should follow package and prescription instructions. Creams, gels, and ointments are not interchangeable and should not be substituted for each other.

Drug Alert

Hydrocortisone acetate is a low-potency corticosteroid, whereas hydrocortisone valerate is a high-potency corticosteroid. Be careful to ensure that orders do not confuse these two different products. High-potency corticosteroids should be used for a limited period because they can cause thinning skin. In addition, high-potency topical corticosteroids that are spread over a large enough area of skin can cause systemic absorption and other unwanted side effects.

Side Effects Common side effects of topical corticosteroids include burning, itching, dryness, excessive hair growth, dermatitis, acne, hypopigmentation, and thinning of the skin. Use of the least amount over the smallest area for the shortest length of time possible is recommended to minimize these effects.

Quick Study

Make your own flash cards to study the topical corticosteroids. Use color coding to differentiate low to very high potency—for example, green for low potency, yellow for high potency, and red for very high potency.

Contraindications Topical corticosteroids have no contraindications.

Cautions and Considerations Occlusive wound dressings should not be applied over topical corticosteroid products, especially the high-potency ones. To reduce the potential for systemic absorption and HPA axis suppression, super-potent corticosteroid products are restricted in the length of treatment or total amount used. These agents should not be used for longer than two consecutive weeks. The total amount used in one week should not exceed 45–50 g, and these products should not be applied close to the eyes or mucous membranes.

Calcineurin Inhibitors

These medications are immunomodulators that work by inhibiting T-cell activation, which prevents release of chemical mediators that promote inflammation. **Calcineurin inhibitors**, such as pimecrolimus (Elidel) and tacrolimus (Prograf, Protopic), are used to treat severe eczema, especially when topical corticosteroids have not been effective. These agents are available in the following forms: capsule, cream, ointment, and solution.

Side Effects Common side effects of calcineurin inhibitors include burning, itching, tingling, acne, and redness at the site of application. Other effects include headache, muscle aches and pains, sinusitis, and flulike symptoms. To minimize these effects, these agents should be used sparingly for a short treatment period.

Contraindications No contraindications exist for calcineurin inhibitors.

Cautions and Considerations Calcineurin inhibitors have been associated with increased occurrence of cancer (skin cancer and lymphoma). Topical application is less likely to

TABLE 9.6 | Common Topical Corticosteroids

Generic (Brand)	Dosage Form	Dispensing Status	Strength
Low-to-Medium Potency			
Alclometasone (Aclovate)	Cream, ointment	Rx	0.05%
Hydrocortisone (Cortaid, Cortizone 10, Dermolate, Hydro-SKIN, Procort, Scalpicin)	Cream, gel, liquid, lotion, ointment, spray, stick	OTC	0.5%, 1%
Hydrocortisone (Acticort, Ala-Cort, Cetacort, Cort-Dome, Eldecort, Hi-Cor, Hycort, Hydrocort, Hytone, LactiCare, Penecort, Synacort, Texacort)	Cream, liquid, lotion, ointment, solution	Rx	1%, 2.5%
Hydrocortisone acetate (Cortaid, Cortef, Corticaine, Gyne-cort, Lanacort, Tucks)	Cream, ointment	OTC, Rx	0.5%, 1%
Hydrocortisone butyrate (Locoid)	Cream, lotion, ointment, solution	Rx	0.1%
Hydrocortisone probutate (Pandel)	Cream	Rx	0.1%
Prednicarbate (Dermatop)	Cream, ointment	Rx	0.1%
High Potency			
Betamethasone dipropionate (Diprosone, Maxivate)	Aerosol, cream, lotion, ointment	Rx	0.05%, 0.1%
Betamethasone valerate (Beta-Val, Luxiq, Psorion)	Cream, foam, lotion, ointment	Rx	0.05%, 0.1%
Clocortolone (Cloderm)	Cream	Rx	0.1%
Desoximetasone (Topicort)	Cream, gel, ointment	Rx	0.05%, 0.25%
Fluocinolone acetonide (Capex, Derma-Smoothe, Synalar)	Cream, oil, ointment, shampoo, solution	Rx	0.01%, 0.025%
Fluocinonide (Lidex, Vanos)	Cream, gel, ointment, solution	Rx	0.05%, 0.1%
Fluticasone (Cutivate)	Cream, lotion, ointment	Rx	0.05%
Halcinonide (Halog)	Cream, ointment, solution	Rx	0.1%
Hydrocortisone valerate (Westcort)	Cream, ointment	Rx	0.2%
Mometasone (Elocon)	Cream, lotion, ointment, solution	Rx	0.1%
Triamcinolone (Flutex, Kenalog, Kenonel)	Aerosol, cream, lotion, ointment	Rx	0.025%, 0.1%, 0.5%
Very High or Super Potency			
Amcinonide	Cream, lotion, ointment	Rx	0.1%
Betamethasone dipropionate, augmented (Diprolene)	Cream, gel, lotion, ointment	Rx	0.05%
Clobetasol propionate (Clobex, Cormax, Olux, Temovate)	Cream, foam, gel, lotion, ointment, shampoo, solution, spray	Rx	0.05%
Desonide (DesOwen, LoKara, Verdeso)	Cream, foam, gel, lotion, ointment	Rx	0.05%
Halobetasol propionate (Ultravate)	Cream, ointment	Rx	0.05%

TABLE 9.7 | Combination Antifungal and Corticosteroid Products

Generic (Brand)	Dosage Form	Dispensing Status	Strength
Clotrimazole and betamethasone (Lotrisone)	Cream, lotion	Rx	0.05%, 1%
Triamcinolone and nystatin (Mycogen, Mycolog, Myconel, Myco-Triacet, Nystatin, Tri-Statin)	Cream, ointment	Rx	0.1%, 100,000 units/g

cause malignancy, but patients must be informed of this risk. Use of calcineurin inhibitors, even topical application, can cause alcohol intolerance. Facial flushing can occur when drinking alcohol and using these medications.

Vitamin D Analogs

A synthetic form of vitamin D, **calcipotriene** (Dovonex, Taclonex) regulates cell growth and development of skin cells. In psoriasis, skin cells reproduce abnormally and rapidly to form plaques. Vitamin D naturally regulates this cell process. Calcipotriene is a **vitamin D analog** used to treat psoriasis. Some dosage forms that can be used on the scalp are effective for treating psoriatic lesions in the hair when other creams and ointments are too greasy and thick for such use. Vitamin D analogs are available in several forms including cream, foam, ointment, and solution.

In the Know

Vitamin D is converted to its active form in the skin with exposure to sunlight. Patients who live in areas where sun is scarce are commonly found to be deficient in vitamin D. For example, many patients in the Pacific Northwest region of the United States are prescribed vitamin D supplements to combat deficiency due to a lack of sunlight exposure.

Side Effects Common side effects of calcipotriene include burning, itching, and redness at the site of application. Less common effects include inflamed hair follicles (folliculitis), skin irritation, change in skin color at the site of application, and thinning of the skin. Patients who experience these problems should stop using calcipotriene and contact their healthcare practitioners.

Contraindications Patients who have hypercalcemia, vitamin D toxicity, or acute psoriasis should not use calcipotriene.

Cautions and Considerations Vitamin D analogs can cause alterations in calcium metabolism, so patients who have had problems with too much calcium in the blood (such as a history of kidney stones) should not use them without medical supervision. Periodic blood tests may be performed to monitor calcium levels.

Calamine

Mild itching from insect bites, rashes, hives, poison ivy or poison oak, and other allergic reactions can be relieved with **calamine**. It works through a counterirritant action that involves evaporation and cooling, which soothe the itchy sensation. Many calamine products also contain zinc oxide, an ingredient with antiseptic properties that protect against infection from repeated scratching.

Side Effects Calamine can be used frequently and has few side effects.

Contraindications Calamine should not be used on broken or blistered skin. It is also not recommended for children younger than two years old.

Cautions and Considerations If itching and rash are not relieved within a few days of using calamine, patients should see their healthcare practitioners. Stronger prescription products may be needed, or there may be an underlying problem that requires medical treatment.

Decubitus Ulcers

Decubitus ulcers, also called **pressure sores**, are severe wounds that involve tissue damage through the epidermal and dermal layers. Decubitus ulcers are caused by constant pressure applied to an area of skin, usually from lying in one position for a long period. Such ulcers are referred to as **bedsores** because they are prominent in patients who are bedridden. The ulcers tend to appear in areas where skin covers bony protrusions that receive constant pressure when a patient is lying or sitting, or from frequent friction and rubbing on sheets, casts, or braces. This pressure and friction cut off bloodflow to dermal layers, thereby allowing necrosis (decay) to begin. Areas most affected are the coccyx (tail-bone), heels, hips, spine, and elbows. Patients who have mobility problems, such as those confined to beds or wheelchairs, are most at risk. Decubitus ulcers are categorized into stages, depending on the depth of tissue damage. Wounds that are not cared for progress in severity.

Because decubitus ulcers can be hard to treat, healthcare personnel must try to prevent their occurrence through aggressive nursing care. This care involves turning and repositioning immobile patients every two hours and applying skin protection to high-risk areas. Two hours is the maximum amount of time that tissue can withstand constant pressure before breakdown and damage occur. Special air beds that minimize pressure points can be used for patients at high risk. Maintaining good hydration and nutrition also helps. Once an ulcer has developed, treatment involves wound cleaning and removal of necrotic (dead) tissue while the wound heals on its own. This process is known as **debridement**. Decubitus ulcers, especially deep ones, can take significant time to heal.

Drug Regimens and Treatments

Drugs are not usually used to treat decubitus ulcers directly. Usually, treatment involves cleaning, disinfecting, using a wound vacuum-assisted closure (VAC), and protecting wounds while they heal. Good nutrition including vitamins is helpful to provide the body with substances needed to grow new skin tissue.

Debridement

As mentioned earlier, severe decubitus ulcers are treated using debridement, a procedure that removes dead, crusted, or contaminated tissue around a wound to promote healing. This procedure leaves a clean edge around the wound so that healing progresses with less scarring. Debridement can be painful, so pain medication is usually administered prior to the procedure. Sometimes, general anesthesia is used to allow the patient to sleep through the debridement of a large wound area.

Positioning

Patients who are bedridden must be repositioned in bed every two hours to prevent tissue decomposition and death that cause decubitus ulcers. This physical measure is used to prevent new wounds from developing and existing wounds from getting worse. Patients who are unable to move on their own in bed will require 24-hour care so that they can be moved from side to side in different positions every two hours.

Burns

Burns are caused by heat and thermal injury or by electrical and chemical sources. When burn wounds are extensive, treatment and prognosis depend on the severity and percentage of body surface area affected. Surface area affected is estimated by dividing the body into major sections, each representing approximately 9% of the total surface area (see Figure 9.2). Severity of burns is categorized by how deeply the tissue damage penetrates the skin layers (see Table 9.8). Treatment at a burn center is needed for third-degree burns over a significant portion of the body. Prognosis for survival gets worse as a greater percentage of body surface area is affected. Patients with burns on 80% or more of their bodies are not likely to survive long term.

FIGURE 9.2 **Estimating Body Surface Area for Burns**

Estimating body surface area in this manner is referred to as the "rule of 9s," whereby values of 9% are assigned to specific regions.

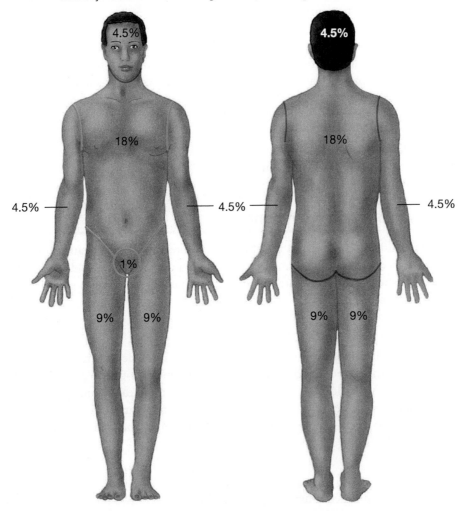

TABLE 9.8 **Burn-Wound Staging**

Degree	Damage
First-degree burn (superficial)	Surface epidermal layers damaged, causing redness and possibly peeling, but no blisters or scarring.
Second-degree burn (partial thickness)	Epidermal and dermal skin layers damaged, causing redness, blisters, swelling, and pain. Scarring is possible.
Third-degree burn (full thickness)	Destruction of epidermal and dermal layers, with possible damage to tissue underneath. Permanent scarring is problematic. Pain may not be present immediately because sensory nerve endings are typically damaged or destroyed. Management requires medical treatment.

Drug Regimens and Treatments

Treatment for burns begins nonpharmacologically with cooling, cleaning, and debridement. Ice should never be applied directly to a burn as it could cause additional damage. Burns can be cleaned and treated with cool water, a mixture of refrigerated and room temperature saline, or water-soaked gauze pads cooled in the refrigerator. Once wounds are cooled and cleaned, debridement may be necessary. Blisters should be left alone to heal; they should not be popped or drained. Once proper wound care is applied, pain can be managed with analgesics (see Chapter 25). Burn wounds are susceptible to infection. Nonsuperficial burn wounds will need topical anti-infective prophylaxis.

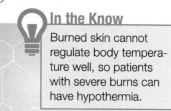

In the Know

Burned skin cannot regulate body temperature well, so patients with severe burns can have hypothermia.

Silver Sulfadiazine

In addition to other topical antibiotics, **silver sulfadiazine** is sometimes used to protect nonsuperficial wounds from bacterial infection. It is applied once or twice a day in a thick layer and left in place as healing occurs.

Side Effects Side effects of silver sulfadiazine include skin discoloration, rash, and a burning sensation.

Contraindications Pregnant women and infants in the first two months of life should not use this product.

Cautions and Considerations Patients who are allergic to sulfonamides can have an allergic reaction to silver sulfadiazine, so careful consideration must be given before its use. Tissue necrosis (death) in the area of application has occurred, so careful wound care and monitoring are necessary. Silver sulfadiazine does not protect against fungal organisms, so the wound should be monitored for development of a fungal infection.

Checkpoint 9.3

Take a moment to review what you have learned so far and answer these questions.

1. What is the difference between dermatitis, eczema, and psoriasis?
2. What medications are used to treat both dermatitis and eczema?
3. How are decubitus ulcers and burn wounds treated?

Adverse Drug Reactions Affecting the Skin

A few of the most common reactions to medication manifest on the skin, so it is useful to be familiar with drug-induced skin problems. Skin rash is the most prominent sign of allergy. However, just because a patient has received prescriptions in the past with no allergies documented does not mean that he or she has not developed a new allergy since that time. Healthcare professionals must diligently ask about and document any drug allergies (and the nature of the symptoms) so that patient safety is maintained.

Photosensitivity

A frequent side effect of many drug therapies is photosensitivity. **Photosensitivity** is an excessive response to solar exposure, wherein skin easily burns after a short time in the sun. Patients taking drugs with this side effect may find they get sunburned more quickly or more severely than usual. Education should be provided so that patients can take the necessary precautions to avoid severe sunburns. Sunscreen and clothing should be used to protect skin from sun exposure when drugs that cause photosensitivity are in use. Drugs that are most associated with this reaction are shown in Table 9.9.

TABLE 9.9 Drugs Most Commonly Associated with Photosensitivity

Drug Class	Drug Examples
Angiotensin-converting enzyme (ACE) inhibitors	All agents
Antibiotics	Griseofulvin, quinolones, sulfas, tetracyclines
Antidepressants	Clomipramine, maprotiline, sertraline, tricyclic antidepressants (TCAs)
Antihistamines	Cyproheptadine, diphenhydramine
Antipsychotics	Haloperidol, phenothiazines
Cardiovascular drugs	Amiodarone, diltiazem, quinidine, simvastatin, sotalol
Chemotherapeutic agents	Dacarbazine, 5-fluorouracil (5-FU), fluorouracil, methotrexate, procarbazine, vinblastine
Diuretics	Acetazolamide, furosemide, metolazone, thiazides
Hypoglycemics	Sulfonylureas
Nonsteroidal anti-inflammatory drugs (NSAIDs)	All agents

Drug-Allergy Rashes

Rashes from **drug allergies** present as **urticaria (hives)** and pruritus, or as a diffuse redness on the trunk of the body that may not be pruritic. The reaction typically appears soon after a new medication is started, but occasionally it can occur after a drug has been taken for a while. Patients should inform their prescribers and pharmacists if they get either of these types of rash while taking any drug therapy. Allergic reactions can progress in severity and become life-threatening if the patient continues to take the drug. **Anaphylaxis** is a severe and potentially fatal reaction to drug therapy, causing airway swelling and affecting one's ability to breathe (see Chapter 24). Therefore, the offending drug should be discontinued immediately, and proper documentation of the allergy should be made in the patient's medical record. Antihistamines, corticosteroids, and even epinephrine are used to treat allergic reactions to drugs.

One rare but potentially life-threatening skin reaction is **Stevens-Johnson syndrome**. This drug reaction begins as a localized rash, which, if not treated, can progress to

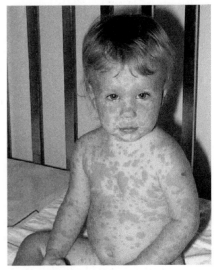

The reaction from Stevens-Johnson syndrome starts as a diffuse red rash that, if left untreated, spreads deeper, causing the dermis to slough off.

a generalized condition in which layers of skin slough off, exposing vulnerable tissues beneath. If skin integrity is lost over a large enough area of the body, severe infection and temperature regulation problems can ensue. Although this reaction is rare, it tends to occur with specific drug therapies such as antiepileptic agents, penicillin, and some antibiotics including sulfonamides and tetracyclines. If caught early and use of the offending drug is discontinued, this syndrome can be treated without life-threatening consequences.

Heparin-induced thrombocytopenia (HIT) is an allergic reaction to the anticoagulant heparin that can be life-threatening. This reaction involves a severe and dangerous drop in platelet count in the blood, which can put a patient at risk for bleeding. The reaction first appears as a diffuse red, pruritic rash on the trunk and/or upper legs after a patient receives the anticoagulant drug heparin. Heparin should be stopped immediately and alternative anticoagulation started. Heparin is used frequently in hospitals to keep intravenous lines open and to treat various clotting disorders encountered in the inpatient setting. Special attention should be given to recognizing and documenting HIT.

Drug Alert

If you notice any kind of rash on the torso or upper legs of a patient who is taking heparin, notify his or her healthcare practitioner right away. This rash may be a sign of HIT and, if so, heparin therapy should be discontinued immediately.

Herbal and Alternative Therapies

Numerous herbal and natural substances are added to topical skin care products and cosmetics. Many natural substances, such as **lanolin**, **cocoa butter**, and **vegetable or seed oils**, are added as moisturizers to creams and lotions. These substances work in conjunction with the base vehicle to promote moisture in the epidermis. They supply added oils and cover the skin, thereby preventing moisture evaporation. Together, these actions keep skin hydrated and soft. **Vitamins A**, **D**, and **E** are emollients added to moisturizers to promote skin health and healing.

Aloe vera is another frequent ingredient in skin care products. It contains a variety of active compounds that have several proven healing and anti-inflammatory properties. When used in concentrated form on a regular basis, aloe vera has been an effective treatment for mild psoriasis and burn-wound healing. To have significant effects, it needs to be applied three times a day for up to four weeks. Concentrations of aloe vera in many lotions and oils may not be sufficient to produce measurable effects beyond moisturizing.

Checkpoint 9.4

Take a moment to review what you have learned so far and answer these questions.

1. What skin rashes/conditions are actually allergic reactions to drug therapy?
2. What drugs can cause photosensitivity?
3. What herbal therapy can be used for the treatment of burns?

Chapter Review

Chapter Summary

The skin, the largest body organ, is made up of three layers: epidermis, dermis, and subcutaneous tissue. The dermis comprises the living layer where most glands, hair follicles, blood vessels, and nerves are located.

Skin damage can arise from sun exposure, natural aging, wounds, burns, and infections. Damage from wounds and burns is staged, based on the layer of skin affected. Sunscreens are applied to reduce the risk of sunburn.

Acne is probably the most common skin condition for which drug therapy is sought. Acne is caused by the overproduction of sebum produced from glands around hair follicles, which clogs pores and forms blackheads, pimples, and even cysts. In addition to skin cleansing twice a day, OTC topical agents and retinoids are used to promote clearing and reduce bacterial buildup in pores. Topical antibiotics are used to treat acne as well as skin infections such as impetigo. Pediculicides are used to treat head, body, and pubic lice.

Contact dermatitis occurs when skin comes in contact with an allergen or irritant. Atopic dermatitis is eczema, an inflammatory condition that causes dry skin, scaling, and itching. Psoriasis is an immunologic condition that causes scaly patches on the skin that are pruritic and painful. Topical corticosteroids and calcineurin inhibitors are used to treat dermatitis and eczema, and vitamin D analogs are used for psoriasis. Some drug reactions—for example, drug allergies, photosensitivity, and Stevens-Johnson syndrome—manifest on the skin.

Chapter Checkup

The Navigator+ learning management system that accompanies this textbook offers many opportunities to help you master chapter content, including end-of-chapter exercises, a glossary of key terms, flash cards, and additional interactive activities.

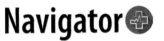

Career Exploration

If you enjoyed learning about the integumentary system in this chapter, you may want to explore the following career options:

- cosmetic laser technician
- dermatology technician/assistant
- electrologist
- esthetician
- laser hair removal technician
- massage therapist
- medical assistant
- pharmacy technician

10 The Skeletal System and Drug Therapy

Pharm Facts

- Surprisingly, a baby has more bones (approximately 300) than an adult (exactly 206). Why? As babies and children grow, multiple bones—particularly in the skull and spine—fuse together to form single bones, thus reducing the number of bones in the body.

- The foot contains 26 of the 206 bones in the body; the hand and the wrist contain 54 bones.

- When you crack your knuckles or any other joint, you stretch the joint capsule where two bones meet. This movement releases dissolved gases (bubbles) in the synovial fluid of the joint, creating a popping sound.

- Located deep inside the ear, the stirrup bone is the size of a grain of rice, making it the smallest bone in the human body.

- At least one human bone is stronger than steel. Engineering studies have shown that, ounce for ounce, the human thighbone (femur) has a greater pressure tolerance and bearing strength than a cast steel rod of equivalent size.

- The hyoid bone, which is located in the neck, is unique in that it is not connected to any other bone in the human body.

"My job as a radiologic technologist requires a good understanding of the skeletal system. Some of the key responsibilities that I have include taking X-rays of bones and assisting physicians with joint injections. I enjoy the variety of tasks associated with this position, as well as the flexibility to work in a variety of settings: clinics, surgical sites, and hospitals. I also enjoy working closely with other healthcare practitioners to provide patients with the best possible care. Radiologic technology is a great career for anyone interested in a challenging yet rewarding position in health care."

—**Tara Lothspeich**, RT (R)(CT)
Radiologic Technologist

Learning Objectives

1 Understand the basic anatomy and physiology of the skeletal system.

2 Describe the common conditions that affect the skeletal system.

3 Explain the therapeutic effects of prescription medications and non-prescription medications commonly used to treat diseases and disorders of the skeletal system.

4 Identify the generic names, brand names, indications, dosage ranges, side effects, contraindications, and cautions and considerations associated with the drugs commonly used to treat diseases and disorders of the skeletal system.

5 Identify common herbal and alternative therapies that are related to the skeletal system.

onditions of the **skeletal system**, such as arthritis or osteoporosis, are quite common. As the average age of the US population increases, the number of individuals with these skeletal system conditions is growing. In fact, arthritis is now the leading cause of disability in the United States, according to the Centers for Disease Control and Prevention (CDC). Consequently, medications used to treat arthritis appear in the top 50 most commonly prescribed drugs in the United States. Osteoporosis is also on the rise as the population ages. The National Institutes of Health (NIH) states that in the over-50 patient population, 50% of women and 25% of men will break a bone as a result of osteoporosis. Because of the strong correlation between aging and skeletal system conditions, advertisers in all forms of media (print, television, and digital) have targeted this age-group by marketing drug treatments for arthritis and osteoporosis.

This chapter provides an overview of the basic anatomy and physiology of the skeletal system. Joint function and bone homeostasis are important concepts to learn because the drugs used to treat skeletal system disorders target these areas. The different types of arthritis are explained, with a focus on osteoarthritis and rheumatoid arthritis. The treatment approach differs for these distinct physiologic processes. Acute and chronic drug treatments for gout and the risk factors, prevention strategies, and treatments for osteoporosis are also addressed. Finally, common dietary supplements that augment the skeletal system, such as glucosamine and chondroitin, are discussed.

Anatomy and Physiology of Bones and Joints

Bones serve multiple functions beyond the most obvious, that is, providing structure and support for the body (see Figure 10.1). Without bones to attach to and pull on, muscles would have a difficult time moving parts of the body effectively. Some bones, including the ribs and pelvis, do not produce movement but instead provide protection for delicate organs. Long bones, such as the femur, contain a substance called *marrow*, which is the birthplace for blood cells. Consequently, bones are important for the normal functioning of multiple body systems.

All bones store calcium and maintain its balance in the body in a constant process of buildup and breakdown called **bone remodeling**. **Osteoclasts** break down bone tissue

FIGURE 10.1 Anatomy of the Skeletal System

Bones are grouped into two categories: appendicular, which includes the bones in the extremities, and axial, which includes the skull, spine, and thorax (ribs).

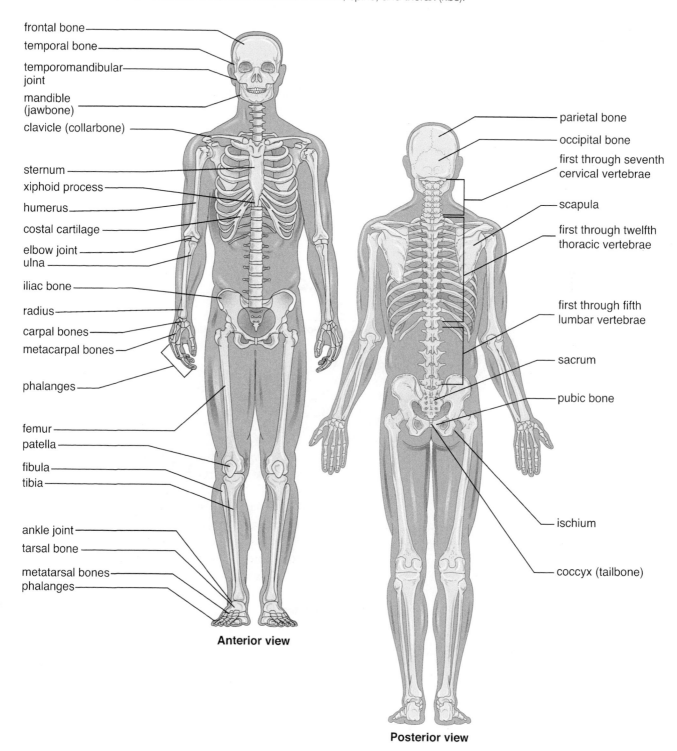

frontal bone

temporal bone

temporomandibular joint

mandible (jawbone)

clavicle (collarbone)

sternum

xiphoid process

humerus

costal cartilage

elbow joint

ulna

iliac bone

radius

carpal bones

metacarpal bones

phalanges

femur

patella

fibula

tibia

ankle joint

tarsal bone

metatarsal bones

phalanges

Anterior view

parietal bone

occipital bone

first through seventh cervical vertebrae

scapula

first through twelfth thoracic vertebrae

first through fifth lumbar vertebrae

sacrum

pubic bone

ischium

coccyx (tailbone)

Posterior view

Quick Study

To remember the difference between an osteoclast and an osteoblast, break the words into their root words: *osteo* meaning "bone"; *clast* meaning "to break"; *blast* meaning "forming or immature."

and release calcium into the bloodstream. **Osteoblasts** take calcium from the blood to build bone tissue (see Figure 10.2). Bones grow and increase in density at the greatest rate during childhood and continue to build into the thirties. After that time, a gradual decrease in **bone density** occurs, with the greatest decline later in life, especially for women after menopause. Estrogen is a strong supporter of osteoblast activity that promotes bone density maintenance. After menopause, a woman's estrogen level decreases dramatically, which leads to a natural decline in bone density.

Articulations, the **joints** between bones, are necessary for fluid and efficient movements. As shown in Figure 10.3, the ends of bones are coated with **cartilage** and cushioned from friction by the **synovial membrane** and **synovial fluid**.

FIGURE 10.2 Microscopic View of Bone

Osteoclasts and osteoblasts provide bone remodeling, a continual process that grows and repairs bone.

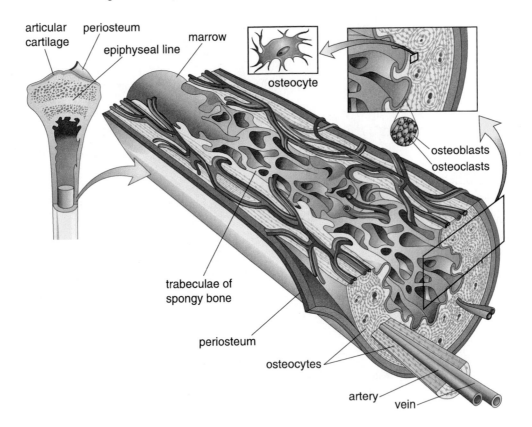

articular cartilage • periosteum • epiphyseal line • marrow • osteocyte • osteoblasts • osteoclasts • trabeculae of spongy bone • periosteum • osteocytes • artery • vein

FIGURE 10.3 Anatomy of a Joint

Although the joint shown here moves like a hinge (as do knees and elbows), other joints have different mechanisms such as a ball-and-socket movement (the shoulders and hips) and a pivot movement (the neck).

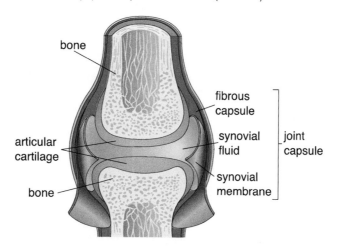

 Checkpoint 10.1

Take a moment to review what you have learned so far and answer these questions.

1. What are four different functions of bones?

2. What happens to bone density after menopause (when women's estrogen levels decrease dramatically)?

Common Skeletal System Disorders

As mentioned in the opening of this chapter, the most common disorders of the skeletal system are arthritis (which affects the joints) and osteoporosis (which affects the bones). In addition to treating these disorders with medications, prescribers may also recommend other types of therapy performed by allied health professionals such as physical therapists, occupational therapists, and exercise physiologists.

Arthritis

Arthritis, or inflammation of a joint, is the most common joint disorder, affecting millions of individuals. This disorder causes persistent pain and diminished joint function for patients. Drug therapy is used to treat the three main types of arthritis: osteoarthritis, rheumatoid arthritis, and gouty arthritis.

Osteoarthritis

Osteoarthritis (OA) occurs more frequently than the other types of arthritis and is caused by the wear and tear on joints that come with age. In fact, its onset is usually after age 40. The cartilage that normally coats the ends of bones inside joints erodes, resulting in painful rubbing. The large joints (for example, the knees, shoulders, and hips) are affected first because the majority of body weight and force is placed on these joints (see Figure 10.4). Fingers and hands can also be affected because they get daily stress throughout life. OA does not necessarily affect the joints on both sides of the body equally; in other words, this disorder is not symmetric. Although morning stiffness is prominent, it fades within an hour and is relieved by activity.

FIGURE 10.4 Osteoarthritis of the Knee Joint

Osteoarthritis, which commonly affects the knee joint, may result in a total knee replacement if pain or stiffness does not improve with other treatments such as medication or physical therapy.

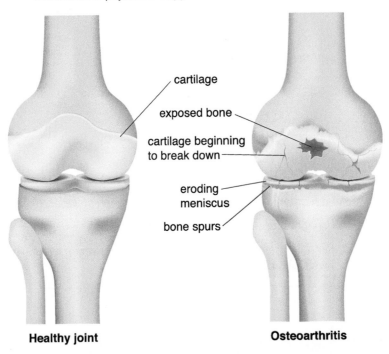

cartilage

exposed bone

cartilage beginning to break down

eroding meniscus

bone spurs

Healthy joint

Osteoarthritis

Drug Regimens and Treatments

Drug therapy for OA is aimed at the reduction of symptoms and the prevention of disability. If OA is severe enough, surgery or joint replacement is performed. Nonpharmacologic therapy for arthritis includes cold packs, hot packs, and massage. Resting the affected joint(s) is usually helpful, but prolonged immobility is not recommended because it will worsen arthritis symptoms.

Acetaminophen

The drug of choice for noninflammatory OA is **acetaminophen** because it treats pain but does not have as many side effects as do other agents. Acetaminophen is advantageous because of its relative safety and efficacy. Many patients do not take acetaminophen for arthritis, even though it is considered the drug of choice, because it must be taken multiple times a day to maintain pain control. Arthritis can become so severe that acetaminophen no longer manages the pain.

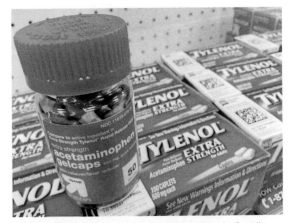

Tylenol, a brand name of acetaminophen, is first-line therapy for pain relief of noninflammatory OA.

Side Effects Acetaminophen is generally well tolerated; in rare cases, an allergic reaction may occur. Liver disorders may also be associated with acetaminophen use. Signs and symptoms of these disorders may include dark-colored urine, fatigue, loss of appetite, stomach pain, light-colored stools, or yellow skin or eyes. The risk of liver problems increases when the dose of acetaminophen exceeds therapeutic recommendations.

Other acetaminophen-related side effects include hives and itching. A serious skin reaction called **Stevens-Johnson syndrome** may occur, which presents as redness, swelling, blisters, sores, or peeling of the skin. Stevens-Johnson syndrome is a medical emergency, and patients who have these symptoms must seek treatment immediately.

Contraindications Patients who have severe liver impairment or severe active liver disease should avoid acetaminophen use.

 Note: *Allied health professionals should be aware that an allergy to a particular drug contraindicates its use. This warning applies to all Contraindications sections in this chapter.*

Cautions and Considerations An acute overdose of acetaminophen or doses greater than 4,000 mg a day may cause liver toxicity. Long-term daily use of this medication may lead to liver damage in some patients. Use caution with concomitant acetaminophen and ethanol (drinking alcohol) use. Acetaminophen should be used cautiously in patients with alcoholic liver disease or patients who consume three or more alcoholic drinks each day.

Drug Alert

Acetaminophen is a component of hundreds of prescription and nonprescription medications. When used correctly, acetaminophen is remarkably safe. However, when taken at doses above recommended levels, acetaminophen may cause serious liver damage. In fact, acetaminophen poisoning has become the most common cause of acute liver failure in the United States.

NSAIDs

The class of drugs known as **nonsteroidal anti-inflammatory drugs (NSAIDs)** blocks pain by inhibiting **cyclooxygenase-1 (COX-1)** and **cyclooxygenase-2 (COX-2)**. Cyclooxygenase is an enzyme that converts arachidonic acid to prostaglandins (see Figure 10.5). **Prostaglandins** are produced in response to various stimuli. They promote inflammation and connect to pain receptors to trigger the pain response.

NSAIDs are often used as first-line therapy in patients with inflammatory OA. In noninflammatory OA, NSAIDs are used when patients experience inadequate pain reduction with acetaminophen. Other indications for the use of NSAIDs include inflammation associated with injury, dysmenorrhea (painful menstrual cycle), and fever.

NSAID therapy is ideally kept as short as possible to address immediate needs. In arthritis, however, long-term therapy is needed to control chronic pain. Table 10.1 lists commonly used NSAIDs and dosage information.

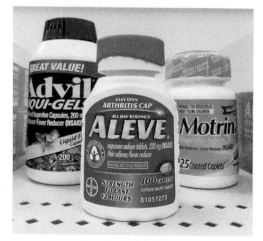

NSAIDs such as naproxen sodium (Aleve) and ibuprofen (Advil, Motrin) are often used to manage the pain associated with inflammatory OA.

FIGURE 10.5 Pain Pathway

In addition to promoting inflammation and triggering the pain response, prostaglandins stimulate fever in the central nervous system. Consequently, some NSAIDs such as ibuprofen are used as antipyretics, or agents that treat fever.

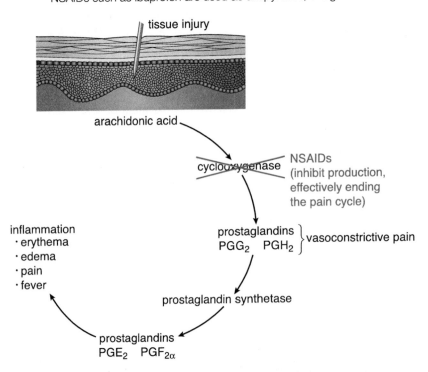

tissue injury

arachidonic acid

cyclooxygenase — NSAIDs (inhibit production, effectively ending the pain cycle)

prostaglandins PGG$_2$ PGH$_2$ } vasoconstrictive pain

prostaglandin synthetase

prostaglandins PGE$_2$ PGF$_{2\alpha}$

inflammation
· erythema
· edema
· pain
· fever

TABLE 10.1 Commonly Used NSAIDs for Treatment of Osteoarthritis

Generic (Brand)	Dosage Form	Dispensing Status	Route of Administration	Common Dosage
Diclofenac (Voltaren)	Capsule, tablet, topical gel	Rx	Oral, topical	PO: 100–200 mg a day Topical: 2–4 g every 6 hr
Etodolac (Lodine)	Capsule, tablet	Rx	Oral	600–1,000 mg a day
Ibuprofen (Advil, Motrin)	Capsule, chewable tablet, oral drops, oral suspension, tablet	OTC, Rx	Oral	OTC: 200 mg taken 3 or 4 times a day Rx: 400–800 mg taken 3 or 4 times a day
Indomethacin (Indocin)	Capsule, injection, oral suspension, suppository	Rx	Oral, rectal	PO: 50–200 mg a day Rectal: 50–200 mg a day
Ketoprofen	Capsule	Rx	Oral	200–300 mg a day
Ketorolac (Toradol)	Injection, tablet	Rx	IM, IV, oral	IM/IV: 30–60 mg every 4–6 hr* PO: 10–20 mg every 4–6 hr but not to exceed 40 mg in 24 hr*
Meloxicam (Mobic)	Oral suspension, tablet	Rx	Oral	7.5–15 mg a day
Nabumetone (Relafen)	Tablet	Rx	Oral	1,000–2,000 mg a day
Naproxen (Aleve, Naprosyn)	Capsule, oral suspension, tablet	OTC, Rx	Oral	250–550 mg twice a day
Oxaprozin (Daypro)	Tablet	Rx	Oral	600–1,200 mg a day
Piroxicam (Feldene)	Capsule	Rx	Oral	20 mg a day
Sulindac (Clinoril)	Tablet	Rx	Oral	150–200 mg a day

* Ketorolac is meant for short-term use only (5 days maximum).

Side Effects NSAIDs block the production of prostaglandin, a substance that protects the stomach and intestines from erosion caused by gastric acid. Therefore, these medications have a harmful effect on the lining of the stomach and intestines when taken in high doses or over a long period. Gastrointestinal (GI) side effects may include indigestion, heartburn, abdominal pain, bleeding, and even ulcers. To avoid these adverse effects, patients should be advised to take NSAIDs with food and to alert their healthcare practitioners if any of these signs of GI bleeding occur: abdominal pain, heartburn, blood in the stool, or black or tarry stools. Patients who have GI bleeding while taking NSAIDs can become mildly anemic.

Other side effects of NSAIDs can include headache, diarrhea, nausea, constipation, and, occasionally, dizziness and drowsiness. These effects are usually mild and dose dependent.

Patients who take NSAIDs on a long-term basis, such as patients with OA, should be monitored by their healthcare practitioners.

Contraindications All NSAIDs that appear in Table 10.1 are contraindicated for perioperative pain during coronary artery bypass graft (CABG) surgery. NSAID use is also contraindicated if an individual has asthma, hives, or other allergic reactions after taking aspirin or other NSAIDs. For example, if an individual experienced hives and asthma with ibuprofen use, all other NSAIDs would also be contraindicated, due to concerns about cross-sensitivity.

Some NSAIDs have unique contraindications. Indomethacin suppositories should not be used in people with inflammation of the rectal lining or recent rectal bleeding. Ketorolac use is contraindicated in patients with peptic ulcer disease, a history of GI bleeding or perforation, advanced kidney disease or risk of kidney failure, suspected or confirmed cerebral bleeding, or a high risk of bleeding. Ketorolac should also not be used in combination with aspirin or other NSAIDs, probenecid, or pentoxifylline. In addition, ketorolac should not be given by epidural or intrathecal administration and should not be used during labor and delivery (see Figure 10.6).

Name Exchange

A commonly used NSAID that is available by prescription and over the counter is ibuprofen. You may be more familiar with ibuprofen's brand names, Advil and Motrin.

FIGURE 10.6	Ketorolac Injection

The medication label pictured below is for ketorolac injection, an NSAID that is commonly used to treat the moderate-to-severe pain associated with OA. Injectable-product labels often differ in appearance from oral-product labels. The label includes the drug name, the concentration, a description of the appropriate route of administration, volume, lot and expiration date, and bar code.

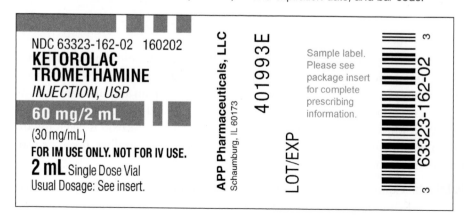

NDC 63323-162-02   160202
KETOROLAC TROMETHAMINE
INJECTION, USP
60 mg/2 mL
(30 mg/mL)
FOR IM USE ONLY. NOT FOR IV USE.
2 mL Single Dose Vial
Usual Dosage: See insert.

APP Pharmaceuticals, LLC
Schaumburg, IL 60173

401993E

LOT/EXP

Sample label. Please see package insert for complete prescribing information.

63323-162-02

Cautions and Considerations NSAIDs have been associated with an increased risk of cardiovascular events, such as heart attack and stroke. NSAID use in patients with cardiovascular disease or risk factors for cardiovascular disease and heart failure must be evaluated carefully by a healthcare practitioner.

NSAIDs may increase the risk for GI bleeding, especially in older adults. The use of NSAIDs in patients with a history of GI disease, smoking, alcohol use, or concurrent use of other medications that contribute to bleeding should be carefully evaluated by a medical professional.

NSAIDs can cause kidney problems and fluid accumulation, especially if the patient becomes dehydrated. Patients should drink plenty of water and immediately report any edema (swelling) or difficulty urinating. NSAIDs interact with a few medications, some of which can add to potential kidney problems. Taking NSAIDs with diuretics or methotrexate can increase the risk of kidney damage. Warfarin (Coumadin) and cyclosporine can interact with NSAIDs as well. Prescribers and pharmacists can help determine whether a patient should continue taking these medications with NSAIDs.

There are many over-the-counter (OTC) products that contain NSAIDs, and healthcare practitioners should help patients avoid duplication of therapy. Patients should not take aspirin with other NSAIDs because aspirin will decrease the effectiveness of NSAIDs by competing for similar sites of action. If a patient using NSAIDs also requires an OTC analgesic or fever reducer, he or she should use acetaminophen instead.

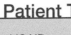

Patient Teaching

NSAIDs, even OTC products, need to be administered with caution. To ensure your patients are using NSAIDs safely, tell patients to follow these instructions:

- Drink plenty of water before and after NSAID use.

- Take NSAIDs with food.

Kolb's Learning Styles

If you prefer active, hands-on learning, as Convergers do, you may enjoy taking a trip to the local pharmacy to check the OTC products for OA. You will likely find acetaminophen and a variety of NSAIDs. At the pharmacy, make a list of the various names and doses of products available.

COX-2 Inhibitors

Celecoxib (Celebrex) is an NSAID and is the only COX-2 inhibitor available in the United States. It works by selectively inhibiting cyclooxygenase-2 (COX-2), an enzyme that promotes production of the prostaglandins that cause pain and inflammation but not those prostaglandins that protect the GI lining. NSAIDs and aspirin block both COX-1 and COX-2, which arrests prostaglandins in the GI lining. Celecoxib is taken for arthritis pain and other pain in patients with a history of ulcers or GI bleeding. It can be taken on a short-term or long-term basis.

Side Effects Common side effects of celecoxib are headache, abdominal pain, heartburn, and nausea. Reminding patients to take celecoxib with food can reduce these effects.

Occasionally, upper respiratory tract infections can occur. Although COX-2 inhibitors do not ordinarily cause GI irritation and bleeding to the extent that NSAIDs or aspirin do, they occasionally produce such effects. Patients should report blood in the stool, black or tarry stools, and abdominal pain to their healthcare practitioners, because these signs indicate GI bleeding and irritation.

Contraindications As with the NSAIDs discussed previously, celecoxib should not be used for treatment of perioperative pain related to CABG surgery. Allergy to sulfonamides, aspirin, or other NSAIDs contraindicates celecoxib use.

Cautions and Considerations Other COX-2 inhibitor agents were removed from the market in the United States because of adverse effects involving heart problems and death from cardiac complications. Some patients recall the news coverage of this event and are hesitant to take a COX-2 inhibitor. Celecoxib has not been associated with such effects, but patients should work with their prescribers to monitor health conditions.

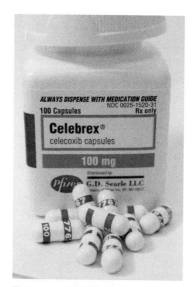

The drug insert for Celebrex contains a black box warning alerting prescribers to the potential cardiovascular risks associated with COX-2 inhibitors. Consequently, prescribers must closely monitor patients using this drug for any adverse cardiovascular effects.

Rheumatoid Arthritis

Rheumatoid arthritis (RA) is an entirely different disease from OA. RA involves an abnormal process in which the immune system destroys the synovial membrane of the joint, producing inflammation. Small joints, such as those in the fingers, wrists, and elbows, are affected first. Usually symmetry is present. Signs of RA are morning pain and stiffness that last longer than an hour and are not relieved by activity. The resulting deformation of the joints can be disabling. Four main laboratory tests are used to help diagnose RA: rheumatoid factor (RF), anti-cyclic citrullinated peptide (anti-CCP) antibodies, erythrocyte sedimentation rate (ESR), and C-reactive protein (CRP). The disease is not curable but can be slowed with medication.

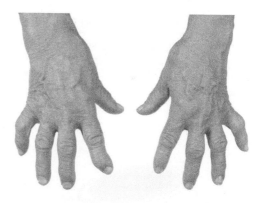

RA typically affects the small joints of the fingers and may result in deformity.

Drug Regimens and Treatments

The goal of drug therapy in RA is to maintain mobility and delay disability for as long as possible. Medication cannot cure RA, but it can improve pain symptoms, increase function, and slow the disease progression that eventually erodes and distorts joints. Some of the drugs used to treat RA, such as NSAIDs, are used to treat symptoms, whereas other drugs actually modify the course and progression of the disease.

Work Wise

A new diagnosis of RA can be emotionally and psychologically taxing for patients. As an allied health professional, you have the opportunity to make a positive and lasting impact on your patients. Remember to smile when appropriate and show respect and empathy.

DMARDs

In treating RA, **disease-modifying antirheumatic drugs (DMARDs)** are used to improve functional status by slowing the disease progression. They do this through a variety of mechanisms, depending on the agent selected. Many DMARDs work by inhibiting the immune system to slow down the destruction of joint tissue.

DMARDs are taken on a regular basis to maintain disease and symptom control. If one agent does not generate a response, others are tried or combinations of multiple DMARDs are used. They work best when started within the first three months after RA diagnosis. Disease remission can sometimes be achieved. At a minimum, early therapy slows the joint destruction that creates disability. Azathioprine (Imuran) and cyclosporine (Neoral, Sandimmune) have two approved uses according to the US Food and Drug Administration (FDA): as immunosuppressants after organ transplantation and as DMARDs for RA. The injectable **biologic response modifiers**, including etanercept (Enbrel), infliximab (Remicade), adalimumab (Humira), and anakinra (Kineret), are made through recombinant DNA technology and work by inhibiting either interleukin-1 (IL-1) or tumor necrosis factors (TNFs), two substances that cause inflammation and joint damage. See Table 10.2 for a list of commonly used DMARDs.

Quick Study

The names of the DMARDs can be difficult to learn. It may be helpful for you to remember that many of the generic names of the biologic DMARDs end with *–mab*. This ending is an abbreviation for **m**ono-clonal **a**nti**b**ody, which is a laboratory-produced molecule designed to mimic the antibodies in humans.

TABLE 10.2 Commonly Used DMARDs

Generic (Brand)	Dosage Form	Route of Administration	Common Dosage	Side Effects
Auranofin (Ridaura)	Capsule	Oral	3 mg 1–2 times a day	Diarrhea, nausea, vomiting, abdominal pain, anorexia, indigestion, gas, constipation, itching, rash, hair loss, photosensitivity, blood disorders, kidney and liver damage, lung problems (serious but rare)
Azathioprine (Imuran)	Tablet	Oral	1 mg/kg a day initially, then may increase or decrease based on patient response	Malaise, nausea, vomiting, leukopenia, neoplasia, thrombocytopenia, liver toxicity, increased susceptibility to infection, myalgia, fever
Cyclophosphamide (Cytoxan)	Injection, tablet	IV, oral	1–2 mg/kg a day	Anorexia, nausea, vomiting, hair loss, blood disorders, kidney damage, infertility, fluid imbalance, secondary malignancy (cancer), heart problems, lung problems (serious but rare)
Cyclosporine (Neoral, Sandimmune)	Injection, tablet	IV, oral	2.5 mg/kg, divided twice a day	Nausea, diarrhea, hypertension, edema, headache, paresthesia, hypertrichosis, hirsutism, increased serum triglycerides, female genital tract disease, gingival hyperplasia, abdominal distress, dyspepsia, urinary tract infection, increased susceptibility to infection, viral infection, tremor, leg cramps, kidney insufficiency, upper respiratory tract infection

TABLE 10.2 Commonly Used DMARDs *(continued)*

Generic (Brand)	Dosage Form	Route of Administration	Common Dosage	Side Effects
Hydroxychloroquine (Plaquenil)	Tablet	Oral	200–300 mg a day	Nausea, vomiting, abdominal pain, diarrhea, anorexia, headache, dizziness, confusion, seizures, blurred vision or vision changes, allergy, skin rash, muscle weakness/pain, anemia, blood disorders, hearing loss, heart problems
Leflunomide (Arava)	Tablet	Oral	100 mg a day for 3 days, then 10–30 mg once a week	Headache, dizziness, diarrhea, abdominal pain, indigestion, weight loss, liver problems, peripheral neuropathy (nerve pain), hair loss, high blood pressure, anemia, blood disorders, lung disease
Methotrexate (Rheumatrex)	Injection, tablet	IM, IV, oral, sub-Q	7.5–15 mg a week	Mouth sores, nausea, vomiting, abdominal distress, anemia and blood disorders, liver and kidney damage, Stevens-Johnson syndrome, eye irritation, heart problems
Sulfasalazine (Azulfidine)	Tablet	Oral	500 mg twice a day, then increase to 1 g twice a day	Anorexia, diarrhea, abdominal pain, indigestion, headache, nausea/vomiting, colitis, blood disorders, rash, Stevens-Johnson syndrome, liver and kidney problems, hair loss, male infertility
Biologic Response Modifiers				
Adalimumab (Humira)	Injection	Sub-Q	40 mg every 2 weeks	Headache, nausea, vomiting, flulike symptoms, rash, itching, heart problems, anemia and blood disorders, secondary malignancy, nephrotic syndrome, confusion, tremor, reactivation of hepatitis B
Anakinra (Kineret)	Injection	Sub-Q	100 mg a day	Headache, nausea, vomiting, diarrhea, redness and pain at injection site, flulike symptoms, blood disorders
Certolizumab (Cimzia)	Injection	Sub-Q	400 mg every 2–4 weeks	Headache, runny nose, upper respiratory tract and urinary tract infections, rash, heart failure, high blood pressure, back pain
Etanercept (Enbrel)	Injection	Sub-Q	25 mg twice a week or 50 mg every 7 days	Pain, itching, and swelling at injection site; headache; nausea; vomiting; hair loss; cough; dizziness; abdominal pain; rash; indigestion; swelling; mouth sores; blood disorders; secondary lymphoma; Stevens-Johnson syndrome; seizures; heart problems; pancreatitis; difficulty breathing
Golimumab (Simponi)	Injection	Sub-Q	50 mg once a month	Upper respiratory tract infections, runny nose, fever/chills, dizziness, redness at injection site
Infliximab (Remicade)	Injection	IV	3 mg/kg at 0, 2, and 6 weeks, then every 8 weeks	Nausea, vomiting, headache, diarrhea, abdominal pain, cough, indigestion, fatigue, back pain, fever/chills, chest pain, flushing, dizziness, heart failure, nerve problems, seizures, Stevens-Johnson syndrome

Side Effects Side effects for DMARDs vary among agents (see Table 10.2). In many cases, these effects mimic those of chemotherapy: diarrhea, hair loss, liver damage, and bone marrow suppression. Several of these effects can have severe consequences and become barriers to treatment. Patients must work closely with their healthcare practitioners to manage such effects. At times, patients will have to stop one drug and try another simply because of the side effects.

Sometimes these agents (especially auranofin) can cause severe diarrhea, which is treated with antidiarrheal agents. Patients should be instructed to purchase an OTC antidiarrheal product when getting a new prescription for auranofin, so that they are prepared if diarrhea occurs.

Many of the DMARDs can cause kidney damage. Patients are instructed to drink plenty of water to counteract this effect.

Contraindications There are multiple contraindications for DMARDs. Auranofin is contraindicated in patients with a history of severe toxicity from gold compounds. Cyclophosphamide should not be used in patients with urinary flow obstruction. Hydroxychloroquine is contraindicated in individuals with hypersensitivities to 4-aminoquinoline derivatives or retinal or visual field changes attributable to 4-aminoquinolines. Hydroxychloroquine also should not be used on a long-term basis in children. Leflunomide is contraindicated in pregnancy. Methotrexate is contraindicated in breast-feeding, pregnancy, alcoholism, alcoholic liver disease or other chronic liver disease, immunosuppressed states, and preexisting blood dyscrasias. Sulfasalazine should be avoided in patients with a hypersensitivity to sulfa drugs or salicylates and in patients who have an intestinal or urinary obstruction or porphyria.

Adalimumab, certolizumab, and golimumab do not have any manufacturer-reported contraindications. Anakinra is contraindicated in patients with a hypersensitivity to *Escherichia coli*–derived proteins. The main contraindication of etanercept is sepsis. Infliximab should be avoided in patients with a hypersensitivity to murine (mouse family) proteins.

Cautions and Considerations Liver, kidney, and blood problems caused by many of the DMARDs can be serious. Laboratory tests should be conducted periodically to gauge these effects.

Because many DMARDs are immunosuppressants, they can increase a patient's risk of getting infections. In fact, increased incidence of infection is common with the biologic response modifiers. Patients may be instructed to avoid people who are ill and follow special precautions to prevent infection. An individual's tuberculosis status should be ascertained prior to the use of immunosuppressant therapy. When infection and illness occur, patients on these drugs should seek medical attention.

Work Wise

You may have noticed that many biologic response modifiers are delivered via subcutaneous (sub-Q) injection. If you are certified or trained in injection technique, include this certification or training on your résumé and highlight this skill when communicating with potential employers during the interview process. Injection skills may make you a more marketable job candidate.

Gouty Arthritis

Gouty arthritis, commonly known as *gout*, is a condition in which excessive uric acid accumulates in the blood. As a result, urate crystals form in the synovial fluid and irritate the joints. Usually, joint pain and swelling first occur in the big toe. Other joints may also be affected, especially in the elbows and ankles. If the condition is allowed to continue, urate crystals may eventually cause kidney damage. Medications that predispose an individual to gout include diuretics, salicylates, nicotinic acid (niacin), ethanol, and cytotoxic agents

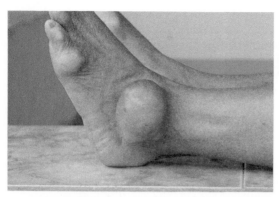

Gouty arthritis typically causes swelling of a patient's ankle or toe joints. Gout often has a familial link, so allied health personnel should note any family history of the disease.

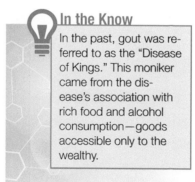

such as those used for cancer treatment. Certain foods rich in the amino acid purine, such as red meat, are also implicated in gout. An acute gout attack is treated with drug therapy. Chronic preventive therapy is warranted if a patient has a particularly severe gout attack or more than two to three attacks in one year.

Drug Regimens and Treatments

Treatment during an **acute gout attack** differs from **preventive (prophylactic) gout treatment** (see Table 10.3). If a patient has a particularly severe attack or repeated gout exacerbations within a year, chronic low-dose therapy will be used to prevent future attacks. Medications for gout work by lowering uric acid levels in the bloodstream and reducing inflammation within the joints, which is caused by urate crystal formation.

NSAIDs

Potent oral NSAIDs, such as naproxen or indomethacin, are frequently used to treat acute gout attacks. They may help with bothersome symptoms such as pain and swelling.

Colchicine

Colchicine can be used to treat an acute gout attack and to reduce the frequency of recurrent episodes of gouty arthritis. When used for preventive gout treatment, therapy is often short term due to potentially toxic side effects. Colchicine's exact mechanism is not completely known, but it is thought to work as an anti-inflammatory and may decrease uric acid deposition.

Triamcinolone

Triamcinolone injection is a corticosteroid administered directly into the joint to relieve pain and swelling during acute gout attacks. Triamcinolone injections generally relieve symptoms quickly—within one day—and typically last for a few days to several weeks.

Prednisone

Oral **prednisone**, a corticosteroid, may be used to reduce pain associated with acute gout attacks.

Allopurinol

Allopurinol is often used for preventive gout treatment and is usually one of the top 200 drugs dispensed in pharmacies. Allopurinol works by inhibiting the production of uric acid. It is classified as a xanthine oxidase inhibitor.

TABLE 10.3 | Gout Agents

Generic (Brand)	Dosage Form	Route of Administration	Common Dosage	Side Effects
Acute Treatment				
Colchicine	Tablet	Oral	0.6–1.2 mg initially, then 0.6 mg hr or 1.2 mg every 2 hr (maximum: 8 mg)	Diarrhea, nausea, vomiting
Triamcinolone (Aristospan)	Injection	Intra-articular	20–40 mg injected into joint	Skin rash, fluid retention, allergic reaction, pain, redness, swelling in joint where injected
Preventive (Prophylactic) Treatment				
Allopurinol	Tablet	Oral	200–600 mg a day	Skin rash, nausea, diarrhea
Colchicine	Tablet	Oral	0.6 mg twice a day	Diarrhea, nausea, vomiting, blood disorders
Febuxostat (Uloric)	Tablet	Oral	80–120 mg a day	Diarrhea, headache, angioedema
Probenecid	Tablet	Oral	250 mg twice a day for 1 week, then 600 mg twice a day for 2 weeks; increase 500 mg/day every other week until 3,000 mg a day	Nausea, vomiting, anorexia

Febuxostat

Febuxostat works by inhibiting uric acid production. Like allopurinol, it is classified as a xanthine oxidase inhibitor. Febuxostat is used for chronic management of high uric acid levels in patients with gout.

Probenecid

Probenecid is used for preventive gout treatment in patients with relatively low kidney uric acid excretion. It works by inhibiting the renal reabsorption of uric acid and therefore promotes uric acid excretion.

Side Effects Common side effects for gout agents are listed in Table 10.3. If a patient experiences diarrhea when taking colchicine, he or she should stop taking it and contact a doctor about alternative therapy. For an acute attack, colchicine may be given until the patient has diarrhea and then stopped. When taking probenecid, patients should drink plenty of water because this drug can be harmful to the kidneys.

Contraindications Colchicine use is contraindicated in patients with kidney or liver impairment. Colchicine also should not be used in combination with drugs that may slow the drug's clearance from the body, such as P-glycoprotein inhibitors or strong cytochrome P-450 (CYP) 3A4 inhibitors. Allopurinol and intra-articular triamcinolone have very few contraindications. Febuxostat should not be used concurrently with azathioprine or mercaptopurine. Probenecid use is contraindicated with aspirin therapy (small-dose or large-dose), blood dyscrasias, and uric acid kidney stones. Probenecid should not be used in children less than two years of age, and therapy should not be initiated during an acute gout attack.

Cautions and Considerations Colchicine should be used with caution in older adults, and dosage adjustments should be considered. Clearance of colchicine is decreased in patients with liver or kidney impairment.

Allopurinol, febuxostat, and probenecid use has been associated with severe hypersensitivity reactions and should be discontinued if signs are present. Allopurinol should be used with caution in patients with kidney impairment due to an increased risk of hypersensitivity reactions. Liver failure has been reported with febuxostat use. Febuxostat should also be used with caution in patients with severe hypersensitivity reactions to allopurinol. Patients with decreased kidney function may not find probenecid to be effective.

Checkpoint 10.2

Take a moment to review what you have learned so far and answer these questions.

1. What medications are used to treat OA?

2. When is acetaminophen contraindicated?

3. What medications are used to treat RA? List a minimum of three drugs.

4. What medications are used to treat gouty arthritis? List a minimum of three drugs.

Osteoporosis

Osteoporosis is a reduction in bone density that results in weakened bones and fractures. Although a decline in bone density is expected later in life, osteoporosis occurs when this decline accelerates beyond the normal rate. This condition causes fractures in the hips, spine, and wrists, which cause pain and debilitation. **Hip fractures** can be life-threatening because the subsequent hip replacement surgery, recovery, and potential complications are often dramatic. Older patients may never return to normal function after a hip fracture.

Risk Factors

Individuals at risk for developing osteoporosis typically have one or more of these characteristics:

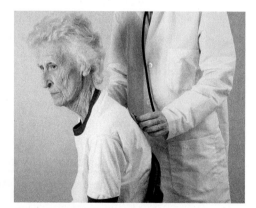

- female gender (90% of patients)

- Caucasian or Asian ethnicity

- family history of osteoporosis

- small body frame

- smoking

- heavy caffeine intake

- poor nutrition (i.e., low calcium intake)

A Caucasian woman who has a small body frame is at risk for developing osteoporosis in her later years.

The risk for osteoporosis can be assessed using a **bone mineral density (BMD)** machine. This machine uses X-ray and ultrasound technology to determine bone density measurements. Typically, the heel bone is measured because it is a good estimate of hip and spine bone density. The result of a BMD screening yields a **T-score**, which is an estimate of risk, not a diagnosis. Armed with such information, patients can make changes in their lives, such as adding weight-bearing exercises, eating foods high in calcium, quitting smoking, and decreasing caffeine intake, which are all ways to increase bone density. If a diagnosis of osteoporosis is made by a healthcare practitioner, drug therapy may be prescribed.

Drug Regimens and Treatments

It would seem to make sense that supplementing estrogen in women whose levels are declining would stave off drastic drops in bone mineral density. However, the increased risk of heart disease, cancer, and stroke associated with estrogen replacement products has been found to outweigh this benefit. Consequently, **hormone replacement therapy (HRT)** with estrogen has fallen out of favor as a treatment for osteoporosis. HRT does continue to be used for perimenopausal symptoms such as hot flashes but is taken at the lowest dose for the shortest time possible with the sole goal of alleviating menopausal symptoms.

Calcium and Vitamin D

Normal, healthy adults should get around 1,000 mg of calcium a day to maintain bone strength. Patients with osteoporosis, individuals over age 65, and women after menopause should get 1,200–1,500 mg of calcium a day. This daily total can be obtained from diet and dietary supplement products. When diet alone does not provide enough calcium, a variety of calcium-containing products are available in several dosage forms. Only 500–600 mg of calcium is absorbed at a time, so the total daily requirement must be given in divided doses.

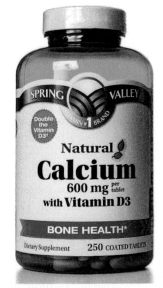

When patients take prescription drugs for osteoporosis, they should also take **calcium** and **vitamin D**. Without calcium, osteoblasts cannot build more bone. Vitamin D improves calcium absorption from the GI tract. Therefore, calcium and vitamin D supplementation helps other osteoporosis agents work more effectively. Supplementation of calcium and vitamin D is also useful for patients with **osteopenia** (bone weakening), who are at high risk for developing osteoporosis.

The exact amount of calcium absorbed varies among calcium salts (see Table 10.4). Only **elemental calcium** (dissociated calcium ions) gets absorbed into the bloodstream.

Calcium supplements are often recommended for postmenopausal women to maintain bone health.

Often, vitamin D comes as a combination product with calcium. Vitamin D can be found in fish and is added to milk and breakfast cereals. Exposure to sunlight activates

TABLE 10.4   Calcium Salts and Elemental Absorption

Salt	Brand Name	Elemental Calcium Absorbed
Calcium acetate	Calphron, Eliphos, PhosLo	~25%
Calcium carbonate	Caltrate, Os Cal, Tums	~40%
Calcium citrate	Cal-Cee, Cal-Citrate, Citracal	~21%
Calcium glubionate	Calcionate	~7%
Calcium gluconate	Cal-G	~9%
Calcium lactate	Cal-Lac	~13%
Calcium phosphate, tribasic	Citracal Gummies, Posture	~38%

vitamin D in the skin, converting it to a form that can be used by the body. Published recommended requirements for vitamin D are 400 international units (IUs) a day, but many clinicians prescribe up to 50,000 IUs a week to replenish and maintain vitamin D stores. One microgram (mcg) of vitamin D equals one IU.

Side Effects Common side effects of calcium supplements are nausea, vomiting, and constipation. Taking calcium with food helps alleviate these problems.

Common side effects of vitamin D supplements are nausea, vomiting, and edema (swelling). These effects are usually mild. Occasionally, fever, chills, flulike symptoms, light-headedness, and pneumonia can occur. If patients experience any of these effects, they should stop taking vitamin D and talk with their healthcare practitioners. Because vitamin D is a fat-soluble vitamin, excessive amounts can accumulate and lead to a condition called hypervitaminosis D, which is commonly known as vitamin D toxicity. **Vitamin D toxicity** manifests as confusion, increased thirst, increased urination, anorexia, vomiting, and muscle weakness.

Contraindications There are no listed contraindications for calcium supplements.

Cautions and Considerations Taking too much calcium can lead to kidney stones, which are usually caused by crystallization of excess calcium in the urine. Patients with a history of kidney stones should not take calcium supplements.

Calcium supplements should not be taken at the same time as quinolone antibiotics, tetracyclines, or iron supplements. Calcium binds to these other drugs and keeps them from being absorbed. Patients should avoid taking these drugs within two hours of taking a calcium supplement. Calcium has also been found to decrease the effects of verapamil, a medication used to treat high blood pressure and angina. Patients should speak with their prescribers if they would like to take a calcium supplement while taking verapamil.

Taking too much vitamin D can lead to hypercalcemia and kidney problems. Patients should follow labeling closely to avoid taking more than recommended. Patients with prior kidney problems should talk with their clinicians before taking vitamin D.

Bisphosphonates

Bisphosphonates inhibit osteoclasts from removing calcium from bone tissue. These medications prevent bone breakdown so that stronger bones are maintained. Over time, bone density can be maintained and, hopefully, fractures can be prevented. Bisphosphonates are used primarily for osteoporosis but can treat Paget's disease (a chronic disorder that results in weakened bones, fractures, and arthritis). Sometimes, bisphosphonates are used in bone and spinal injury cases to promote bone regrowth and strengthening. Depending on the product chosen, bisphosphonates can be taken orally on a daily, weekly, or monthly basis. They can even be administered intravenously (IV) every month, three months, or annually. The variety of dosage regimens allows prescribers to individualize drug therapy.

Side Effects Side effects of bisphosphonates can include headache, nausea, vomiting, diarrhea, constipation, abdominal pain, indigestion, and esophagitis. Taking oral dosage forms with a full glass of water and remaining upright afterward can reduce side effects such as reflux and esophageal issues. Other side effects include insomnia and anemia, for which patients must seek medical advice to manage. A less common yet severe side effect is osteonecrosis (bone tissue death) of the jaw. The IV dosage forms can cause fever, so acetaminophen is given.

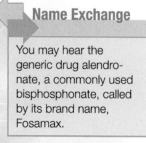

Name Exchange

You may hear the generic drug alendronate, a commonly used bisphosphonate, called by its brand name, Fosamax.

Contraindications Bisphosphonates are contraindicated in the case of hypersensitivity to other bisphosphonates. For example, if a patient has a hypersensitivity to alendronate, the use of all other bisphosphonates is contraindicated.

Specific bisphosphonates have unique contraindications. Alendronate, ibandronate, and risedronate are contraindicated in patients with hypocalcemia, abnormalities of the esophagus, and an inability to stand or sit upright for at least 30 minutes. The effervescent tablets and oral solution of alendronate are contraindicated in patients at increased risk for aspiration. Zoledronic acid should not be used in patients with hypocalcemia and kidney dysfunction.

Cautions and Considerations Oral bisphosphonates are poorly absorbed from the GI tract and are adversely affected by food. Therefore, they must be taken on an empty stomach (preferably first thing in the morning) with water. After taking a bisphosphonate, patients should wait at least 30 minutes before eating. Bisphosphonates are also highly irritating to the GI tract, so they must be taken with a full glass of water to ensure that they do not become lodged in the esophagus. Patients must remain upright for at least 30 minutes after medication administration to prevent reflux. In most cases, bisphosphonate infusions are administered in a physician's office or clinic. Table 10.5 lists agents for treating osteoporosis and dosage information.

> **Quick Study**
>
> Almost all of the bisphosphonate agents used to treat osteoporosis end with the suffix *–ate*. The exception to this rule is zoledronic acid, which is a bisphosphonate derivative.

TABLE 10.5 Osteoporosis Agents

Generic (Brand)	Dosage Form	Route of Administration	Common Dosage
Bisphosphonates			
Alendronate (Fosamax)	Oral solution, tablet	Oral	5–10 mg a day 70 mg once a week
Ibandronate (Boniva)	Injection, tablet	IV, oral	PO: 2.5 mg a day or 150 mg once a month IV: 3 mg infused every 3 months
Pamidronate (Aredia)	Injection	IV	30 mg infused every 4 weeks
Risedronate (Actonel)	Tablet	Oral	35 mg once a week 75 mg on 2 consecutive days once a month
Zoledronic acid (Reclast)	Injection	IV	5 mg infused once a year
Selective Estrogen Receptor Modulator (SERM)			
Raloxifene (Evista)	Tablet	Oral	60 mg a day
Other Osteoporosis Agents			
Calcitonin (Miacalcin)	Nasal spray	Nasal	1 spray a day, alternate nostrils
Denosumab (Prolia, Xgeva)	Injection	Sub-Q	60 mg every 6 months
Teriparatide (Forteo)	Injection	Sub-Q	20 mcg a day

Kolb's Learning Styles

Divergers and Accommodators are people oriented. If you possess this quality, find a friend or family member with osteoporosis and ask about the drug therapy he or she is using. Pay attention to what your interviewee shares: medication name, dosage, side effects, and administration technique. This activity will provide you with real-world context for the treatment of osteoporosis.

SERMs

Selective estrogen receptor modulators (SERMs) work as estrogen receptors by mimicking the beneficial effects of estrogen on bone mineral density. However, they do not increase the risk of breast or uterine cancer the way regular estrogen can. In fact, they can improve cholesterol levels, although they are not used for hyperlipidemia. While there are multiple SERMs on the market, raloxifene (Evista) is the one indicated to treat osteoporosis (see Table 10.5).

Side Effects Common side effects of SERMs are hot flashes, headache, diarrhea, joint pain, leg cramps, and flulike symptoms. The most serious side effect is deep-vein thrombosis or blood clots.

Contraindications Raloxifene is contraindicated in patients who have a history of or current venous thromboembolic disorders (including deep-vein thrombosis and pulmonary embolism). This medication should not be taken by women who are pregnant or could become pregnant or by women who are breast-feeding.

Cautions and Considerations Raloxifene should not be taken if prolonged immobility is anticipated because the drug carries an increased risk of thromboembolic events. If patients using SERMs experience pain, swelling, or bruising in one leg or difficulty breathing, they should seek medical care immediately.

Other Osteoporosis Agents

There are several other medications used for osteoporosis in addition to those previously mentioned. These medications include calcitonin, denosumab, and teriparatide (see Table 10.5). Calcitonin is a peptide found in the body that binds to osteoclasts and inhibits bone resorption. Denosumab is a bone-modifying agent that works to decrease osteoclast formation. Teriparatide supplements the body's production of **parathyroid hormone**, which regulates calcium-phosphate balance and stimulates new bone growth. It is used in patients with especially severe osteoporosis as a short-term therapy.

Side Effects Calcitonin is administered nasally, and the most common side effect is a runny nose. Side effects such as dermatitis, eczema, and skin rash are reported with denosumab use. Teriparatide use is associated with hypercalcemia and dizziness.

Contraindications There are no contraindications to calcitonin and teriparatide use. Denosumab is contraindicated in pregnancy and preexisting hypocalcemia.

Cautions and Considerations Calcitonin is derived from salmon; therefore, there is a risk for hypersensitivity reactions in patients with fish allergies. In addition, there is concern over an increased risk of cancer development with long-term use of calcitonin.

Bone fractures have been reported with denosumab use. Consider discontinuing use if severe dermatologic symptoms occur.

Use teriparatide with caution in patients who have an increased risk for dizziness or falling. Teriparatide has been associated with osteosarcoma, so patients with Paget's disease or with an increased risk for bone cancer should not use teriparatide. In addition, patients must be taught how to use the injector device, and teriparatide must be kept in the refrigerator.

 ## Checkpoint 10.3

Take a moment to review what you have learned so far and answer these questions.

1. What are the main side effects of calcium supplementation?
2. How do bisphosphonates work for osteoporosis treatment?

Herbal and Alternative Therapies

Glucosamine is used by some individuals to improve pain and stiffness from OA. This supplement is derived from the exoskeleton of shellfish and is thought to slow joint degeneration. If patients want to take glucosamine, typical dosing is 1,500 mg a day (given in divided doses, 500 mg three times a day). Side effects are usually mild and include nausea, heartburn, diarrhea, and constipation. Taking glucosamine with food can decrease these effects. Although glucosamine has not proven to be harmful in studies, it is recommended that patients with shellfish allergies avoid taking it.

Chondroitin is taken by some individuals in combination with glucosamine for hip and knee OA. However, studies do not clearly show that chondroitin taken with glucosamine is effective for OA. Chondroitin is derived from shark cartilage and bovine (cow) sources and is thought to work by inhibiting an enzyme that promotes inflammation. If patients want to take chondroitin, typical dosing is 200–400 mg two or three times a day. Common side effects tend to be mild and include nausea, heartburn, diarrhea, and constipation. Rare side effects include eyelid swelling, lower limb swelling, hair loss, and allergic reaction. If patients experience any of these effects, they should stop taking chondroitin.

Chapter Review

Chapter Summary

Bones support the body frame and maintain calcium balance. Bone density builds early in life but drops off with increasing age.

Osteoarthritis (OA) is common and is caused by age and joint stress over time. Acetaminophen is considered the first-line choice of therapy for non-inflammatory OA. For patients with inadequate response to acetaminophen or those with inflammatory OA, nonsteroidal anti-inflammatory drugs (NSAIDs) may be used on a long-term basis to control pain symptoms. Glucosamine and chondroitin are two natural products also used for OA.

Rheumatoid arthritis is an abnormal immune process in which joint tissue is inflamed and damaged. The pain and resulting joint deformation can be disabling to patients. Disease-modifying antirheumatic drugs (DMARDs), in addition to NSAIDs for analgesia, are used to slow the destructive immune process and improve function. These drugs have many side effects and are difficult for patients to take but can keep patients from becoming disabled.

Gout is a joint disorder resembling arthritis, in which uric acid accumulates in the bloodstream, causing urate crystals to form in joint spaces. Drugs such as colchicine and allopurinol are used to treat this condition.

Osteoporosis occurs when bone density drops below the average level. Several drugs are now available to treat and prevent osteoporosis and the bone fractures it causes. The most frequently used medications for osteoporosis are bisphosphonates and selective estrogen receptor modulators (SERMs). A variety of dosage forms are available, from monthly oral therapy to annual infusions. Consequently, patients have many choices. Patients with osteoporosis should also take calcium and vitamin D to promote bone strength.

Chapter Checkup

The Navigator+ learning management system that accompanies this textbook offers many opportunities to help you master chapter content, including end-of-chapter exercises, a glossary of key terms, flash cards, and additional interactive activities.

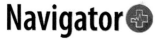

Career Exploration

If you enjoyed learning about the skeletal system in this chapter, you may want to explore the following career options:

- certified bone densitometry technologist (CBDT)
- certified clinical nutritionist
- computed tomography (CT) technician
- magnetic resonance imaging (MRI) technician
- massage therapist
- medical assistant
- pharmacy technician
- positron emission tomography (PET) scan technician
- radiologic technologist
- registered dietitian

11

The Muscular System and Drug Therapy

Pharm Facts

- The muscular system accounts for approximately 40% of an average individual's body weight.

- According to the Library of Congress, the heart is the hardest-working muscle; the masseter (jaw muscle) is the strongest muscle; and the gluteus maximus is the largest muscle.

- While many scientists agree that smiling requires fewer muscles than frowning, the actual number involved remains up for grabs (depending on how one defines *smile*). It is true, however, that human beings tend to mirror each other's expressions, so smiling can be contagious.

- Muscles can only contract, or pull; they cannot push. So, when you exert a pushing movement, such as pushing open a door, some of the muscles in your body are actually pulling to allow that movement to occur.

- Taking just one step uses 200 muscles.

- One type of muscle in the body, known as smooth muscle, is responsible for involuntary motor activity such as breathing and digesting food.

" *Your tools are your hands.* That has been my motto since I decided to become an occupational therapist specializing in hand therapy. Working in a private orthopedic clinic, I treat a variety of diagnoses including acute injuries, such as bone fractures; crush injuries; and cumulative trauma conditions, such as tennis elbow and carpal tunnel syndrome. It is so rewarding for me to educate patients on their exercise programs or teach them alternative ways to perform their daily activities so that they can be as independent as possible. "

—**Sally Nguyen**, MS, OTR/L, CHT
Hand Therapist

1   Understand the basic anatomy and physiology of the muscular system.

2   Describe the common conditions that affect the muscular system.

3   Explain the therapeutic effects of prescription medications and nonprescription medications commonly used to treat disorders of the muscular system.

4   Identify the generic names, brand names, indications, dosage ranges, side effects, contraindications, and cautions and considerations associated with the drugs commonly used to treat muscular disorders.

5   Identify common herbal and alternative therapies that are related to the muscular system.

Muscles allow us to move and react to the environment. Everything from running and jumping to smiling and sitting upright requires muscle tone and movement. Unfortunately, muscle injuries are also a common part of life. Neck strains, back problems, and other traumas frequently necessitate prescriptions for muscle relaxants, making these agents some of the most commonly ordered prescriptions in the United States.

This chapter begins with an overview of the types and functions of muscles and specific muscle names and locations. Knowledge of specific muscle locations is essential to the proper administration of intramuscular drug therapy, such as vaccines. Drugs prescribed to treat muscle spasm are discussed. These medications are commonly prescribed for lower back and sports injuries. One muscle relaxant, botulinum toxin (Botox), has been popularized in the media for its cosmetic use. Finally, this chapter addresses drug therapy for certain muscular disorders such as fibromyalgia, myasthenia gravis, poliomyelitis, and muscular dystrophy.

Anatomy and Physiology of the Muscular System

The **muscular system** is comprised of more than 600 muscles that make up approximately 40%–50% of an individual's body weight. This system is responsible for movement, posture, strength, and—to a great extent—body heat.

Types of Muscle

The muscular system is divided into three types of muscle: skeletal, cardiac, and smooth (see Figure 11.1 for a comparison).

Skeletal muscle is connected to bones and joints by tendons. This **striated** type of muscle facilitates voluntary movement, such as walking, clapping, and chewing. Bodybuilding and performance training in sports focus on developing and enhancing skeletal muscle.

Cardiac muscle is found only in the heart. This striated type of muscle is involuntarily controlled by the autonomic nervous system. Cardiac muscle cells are specifically designed for the pumping and squeezing action required for each heartbeat. Cardiovascular activities such as aerobics and jogging exercise the cardiac muscle by raising the heart rate.

Smooth muscle can be found in the stomach, intestines, bladder, uterus, blood vessel walls, and other hollow organs. This nonstriated type of muscle is designed for **peristalsis**, a kind of movement that pushes material through tubes and other openings, such as when food progresses through the intestines or blood flows through the vasculature. These muscles are involuntarily controlled by the autonomic nervous system (see Chapter 12).

Muscle Contraction

The **neuromuscular junction** (see Figure 11.2) is where nerve cells interface with muscle cells to initiate muscle contraction. **Acetylcholine (ACh)** is a neurotransmitter that is

FIGURE 11.1   Types of Muscle Tissue

Under the microscope, both cardiac and skeletal muscles appear to have stripes called *striations*.

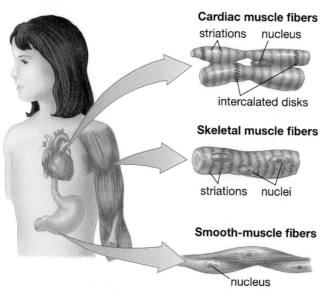

FIGURE 11.2   Neuromuscular Junction

The energy needed for muscle contraction comes from breaking the chemical bond that holds a phosphate functional group to adenosine triphosphate (ATP) molecules inside of muscle cells.

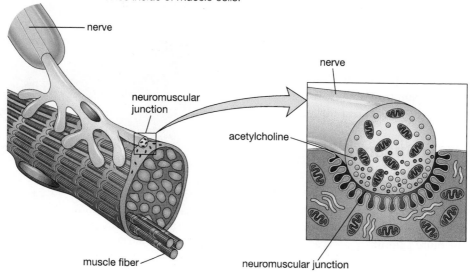

released from the nerve cell, travels across the neuromuscular junction (the tiny space between the nerve cell and the muscle cell), and stimulates muscle cell receptors to cause cell membrane depolarization. **Depolarization** changes the balance of positive and negative electrical charges along the membrane surface and opens ion channels, allowing sodium (Na^+) to enter the cells. **Sodium influx** causes the release of the **intracellular calcium stores** that stimulate muscle-fiber contraction. **Muscle fibers** contract and shorten the muscle, which in turn pulls on attached bones and joints, thereby creating movement. Muscle contraction stops when ACh is deactivated in the neuromuscular junction by the enzyme **acetylcholinesterase**.

Muscles and Drug Therapy

The muscles most relevant to the study of drug therapy are those that are commonly injured and those that are used for intramuscular drug administration (see Figure 11.3). **Intramuscular (IM) injections** are administered to adults in the **deltoid muscle** (in volumes up to 2.5 mL) of the upper arm and the **gluteus medius** (in volumes up to 5 mL) of the buttocks. In children, injections are often given in the **vastus lateralis**, a muscle in the quadriceps group of the legs. Read the labeling and dosing instructions when administering injections to children. The volume injected is often cut in half for children.

Checkpoint 11.1

Take a moment to review what you have learned so far and answer these questions.

1. What are the differences among skeletal, cardiac, and smooth muscle?

2. What process in the neuromuscular junction causes a muscle to move?

3. What muscles are most frequently used as IM injection sites for medications?

Common Muscular System Disorders

Disorders of the muscular system are relatively uncommon. Some of these disorders include myasthenia gravis, poliomyelitis, and rhabdomyolysis. These conditions are discussed later in this section. **Muscle injuries**, however, are frequently encountered at all ages. In fact, according to the US Department of Labor, more than a million workers have back injuries every year. A majority of these injuries involve lower back muscle strain and are the result of lifting. Damage to these muscle cells causes muscle spasm and inflammation. Fortunately, lower back pain from muscle spasm requires only short-term treatment 90% of the time.

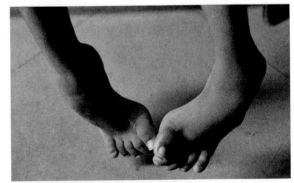

Muscle spasticity causes increased tension in a muscle and is often seen in patients with cerebral palsy.

Muscle Spasm

A **muscle spasm**, also known as a *cramp*, is an involuntary contraction of muscle fibers. Until repair and healing of damaged muscle cells occurs, muscle spasms and inflammation can be quite painful.

FIGURE 11.3 Anatomy of the Muscular System

Muscles commonly injured or strained tend to be those of the lower back (latissimus dorsi), head and neck (trapezius), and legs (hamstring group, quadriceps group, and soleus).

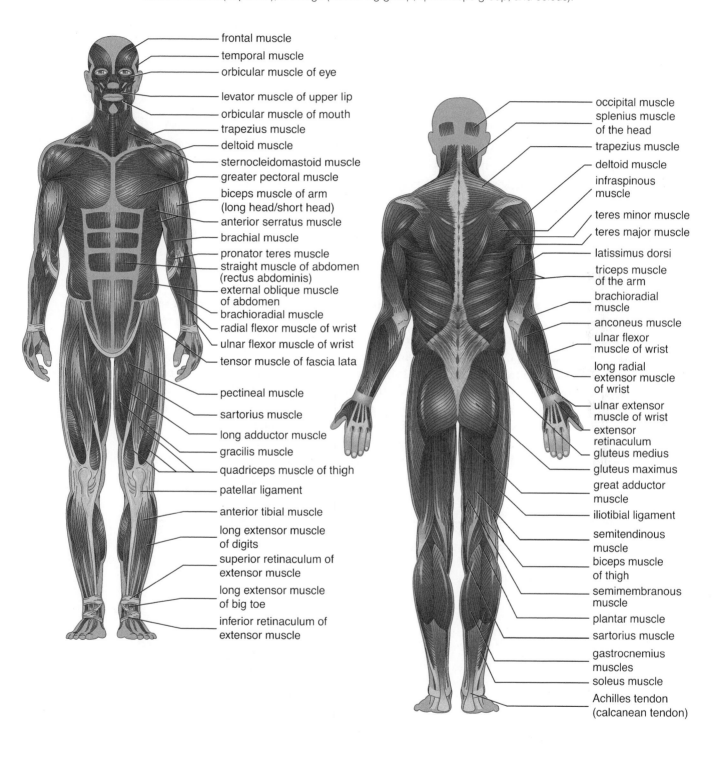

frontal muscle
temporal muscle
orbicular muscle of eye
levator muscle of upper lip
orbicular muscle of mouth
trapezius muscle
deltoid muscle
sternocleidomastoid muscle
greater pectoral muscle
biceps muscle of arm
(long head/short head)
anterior serratus muscle
brachial muscle
pronator teres muscle
straight muscle of abdomen
(rectus abdominis)
external oblique muscle
of abdomen
brachioradial muscle
radial flexor muscle of wrist
ulnar flexor muscle of wrist
tensor muscle of fascia lata

pectineal muscle
sartorius muscle
long adductor muscle
gracilis muscle
quadriceps muscle of thigh
patellar ligament
anterior tibial muscle
long extensor muscle
of digits
superior retinaculum of
extensor muscle
long extensor muscle
of big toe
inferior retinaculum of
extensor muscle

occipital muscle
splenius muscle
of the head
trapezius muscle
deltoid muscle
infraspinous
muscle
teres minor muscle
teres major muscle
latissimus dorsi
triceps muscle
of the arm
brachioradial
muscle
anconeus muscle
ulnar flexor
muscle of wrist
long radial
extensor muscle
of wrist
ulnar extensor
muscle of wrist
extensor
retinaculum
gluteus medius
gluteus maximus
great adductor
muscle
iliotibial ligament
semitendinous
muscle
biceps muscle
of thigh
semimembranous
muscle
plantar muscle
sartorius muscle
gastrocnemius
muscles
soleus muscle
Achilles tendon
(calcanean tendon)

Although muscle spasm is a common condition, muscle spasticity—a look-alike, sound-alike condition—is not. In **muscle spasticity**, the muscles become rigid and difficult to control for coordinated movement. This disorder can be caused by brain damage, spinal cord injury, multiple sclerosis, cerebral palsy, or **malignant hyperthermia**, a rare but serious side effect of anesthesia. In malignant hyperthermia, muscles become rigid and body heat rises to life-threatening levels.

Kolb's Learning Styles

Learners who prefer interpersonal activities and fieldwork when applying new concepts to real-life situations (as Accommodators and Convergers do) may enjoy interviewing a pharmacist about handling prescriptions for muscle relaxants. Because some agents have the potential for addiction, how does the pharmacist assess prescriptions for fraud and abuse? How does the pharmacist counsel patients who are taking these medications?

Drug Regimens and Treatments

Nondrug therapy to treat muscle spasms involves immobilization of the affected area, physical therapy, heat and cold packs, ultrasound, and massage. Patients may be referred to physical therapists for these treatment modalities.

Drug therapy, on the other hand, includes the use of muscle relaxants that block and slow muscle contraction (see Figure 11.4). The most commonly used muscle relaxants block brain and spinal cord nerve signals that control muscle contraction. These drugs are **central nervous system (CNS) depressants**. The exact mechanism or site of action within the CNS for these centrally acting drugs is unknown and probably varies among agents. All agents are generally sedating: They slow reflexes and relax muscle spasms. Some drugs are also used as anticonvulsants and antianxiety agents due to their depressive effects on the CNS (see Chapters 12 and 13).

FIGURE 11.4 Muscle Control and Relaxation

Muscle relaxants work by (1) slowing CNS signal conduction, (2) preventing intracellular calcium release, or (3) inhibiting ACh at the neuromuscular junction.

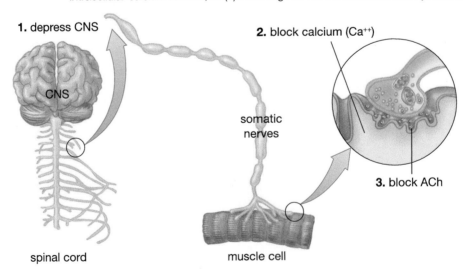

1. depress CNS

CNS

2. block calcium (Ca⁺⁺)

somatic nerves

3. block ACh

spinal cord

muscle cell

Centrally Acting Muscle Relaxants

Muscle spasms related to acute injury are frequently treated with **centrally acting muscle relaxants**. These drugs are used primarily for this condition and are usually prescribed for a defined period (days to weeks) until pain relief and healing occur. On the other hand, some drugs—such as baclofen and tizanidine—are used for long-term treatment of muscle spasm. Centrally acting muscle relaxants are often used in conjunction with over-the-counter (OTC) and prescription-strength anti-inflammatory drugs, such as ibuprofen, to control pain and inflammation associated with injuries (see Table 11.1 for descriptions of these drugs).

Side Effects Sedation is the most common side effect of centrally acting muscle relaxants. Patients may complain of drowsiness, dizziness, fatigue, confusion, impaired judgment, and altered coordination. Other side effects include headache, nausea, vomiting, dry mouth, blurred vision, and constipation. Taking these drugs with food can help to reduce nausea and vomiting.

TABLE 11.1 Centrally Acting Muscle Relaxants

Generic (Brand)	Dosage Form	Route of Administration	Common Dosage
Baclofen (Lioresal)	Intrathecal (IT) solution, tablet	IT, oral	IT: 90–800 mcg/day via continuous infusion pump PO: 20–80 mg/day in divided doses 3–4 times a day
Carisoprodol (Soma)	Tablet	Oral	250–350 mg 3 times a day and at bedtime
Chlorzoxazone (Parafon Forte)	Tablet	Oral	250–750 mg 3–4 times a day
Cyclobenzaprine hydrochloride (Flexeril)	Extended-release (ER) capsule, tablet	Oral	ER capsule: 15–30 mg a day Tablet: 5–10 mg 3 times a day
Metaxalone (Skelaxin)	Tablet	Oral	800 mg 3 times a day
Methocarbamol (Robaxin)	Injectable solution, tablet	IM, IV, oral	IM/IV: 1,000 mg (maximum infusion rate of 300 mg/min), may be repeated every 8 hr as needed PO: 750–1,500 mg 3–4 times a day
Orphenadrine citrate (Norflex)	ER tablet, injectable solution, tablet	IM, IV, oral	IM/IV: 60 mg, may be repeated every 12 hr as needed PO: 100 mg 2 times a day in the morning and evening
Tizanidine (Zanaflex)	Capsule, tablet	Oral	4–8 mg every 6–8 hr

 Drug Alert

The names of some muscle relaxants are similar to other drug names, creating the potential for mix-ups. For example, tizanidine looks and sounds like tiagabine (generic name for Gabitril), an antiseizure drug. Storing drugs with similar names apart from each other and always double-checking the drug label with the order can help to reduce such errors.

Contraindications Centrally acting muscle relaxants are contraindicated in patients with serious gastrointestinal (GI) problems such as a bleeding ulcer or bowel obstruction. They also should not be used in patients with aspirin-induced asthma or porphyria (a disorder of enzyme production and heme regulation in the blood), or in children immediately after surgery.

✚ *Note: Allied health professionals should be aware that an allergy to a particular drug contraindicates its use. This warning applies to all Contraindications sections in this chapter.*

Cautions and Considerations Because these drugs cause sedation and possible changes in mental function, patients who are taking these medications should avoid driving, operating machinery, and making important decisions. In addition, patients should not drink alcohol while taking these medications. Patients who are taking other drugs that also cause CNS depression (such as opioids or other narcotic pain drugs, antihistamines, or other controlled substances) should be careful about taking muscle relaxants. Patients taking antidepressants or antipsychotic medications should be monitored closely if they are taking muscle relaxants.

Certain centrally acting muscle relaxants (cyclobenzaprine and tizanidine) interact with monoamine oxidase inhibitors (MAOIs) and should not be taken in conjunction with them (see Chapters 12 and 13). Patients should also be warned that methocarbamol can turn urine brown, black, or green. This side effect can be alarming to patients but is harmless. In addition, patients should be directed to swallow orphenadrine whole rather than chew it. Finally, if a skin rash or yellowing of the eyes occurs, patients should be referred to their healthcare practitioners immediately because these signs may indicate an allergic reaction or liver dysfunction.

Tolerance and **dependence** can occur when systemic muscle relaxants are taken long term. Due to euphoria-like symptoms caused by these agents, abuse and addiction can be an issue, and patients must be monitored as with all controlled substances. Many of these drugs can cause hallucinations and other withdrawal symptoms if their use is discontinued abruptly. Instead, doses should be tapered if the patient has been taking the medication for longer than a couple of weeks.

One particular muscle relaxant that requires heightened monitoring for abuse and addiction is carisoprodol (Soma). After absorption into the bloodstream, this drug is metabolized by the liver to meprobamate, an antianxiety medication that is a controlled substance with a high risk for abuse. Consequently, patients taking carisoprodol experience some of the euphoric effects that occur with meprobamate. Because of its potential for abuse, carisoprodol is now a Schedule IV controlled substance (as is meprobamate). This change in classification has placed limits on the prescribing and dispensing of carisoprodol, making it more difficult to obtain.

Although rare, centrally acting muscle relaxants can cause serious changes in heart function and blood pressure. Consequently, patients with heart conditions, high blood pressure, or clotting disorders should be monitored closely when taking these medications or should avoid taking them entirely.

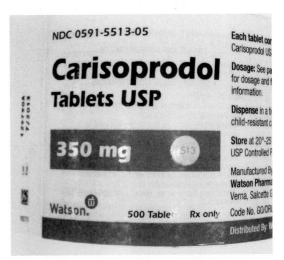

Carisoprodol, a Schedule IV drug, is one of the most commonly abused prescription drugs according to the Drug Enforcement Administration.

Locally Acting Muscle Relaxants

Botulinum toxin (Botox) is an example of a **locally acting muscle relaxant**. This agent works by blocking release of ACh into the neuromuscular junction. Although botulinum toxin is approved for a few select conditions (e.g., migraine headache, muscle spasticity, and **hyperhidrosis** [excess sweating]), the most widespread use of this drug is for the reduction of facial lines and wrinkles. It is administered as a subdermal injection in doses individualized to the patient. Once injected, localized muscle paralysis occurs, making small lines and wrinkles in the skin less apparent. The effect lasts for weeks to months, after which normal function and contractility return. To maintain the cosmetic effect indefinitely, repeated injections are needed. When Botox is administered as a **cosmetic treatment**, it is rarely covered by health insurance.

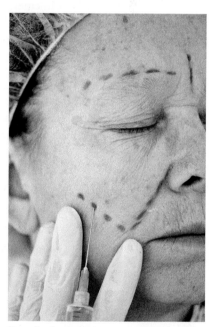

Despite the long-term, exorbitant costs, Botox injections are the most common type of cosmetic procedure performed in the United States.

Side Effects Side effects from prepared products containing botulinum toxin (such as Botox) are rare but can include dry mouth; headache; neck or back pain; pain, itching, or bruising at the injection site; upper respiratory tract infection; fever; and flulike symptoms. Less common but more serious side effects include allergic reaction, chest pain, difficulty swallowing, difficulty breathing, and heart attack or arrhythmias. These effects are more likely at high doses and when the drug is used to treat conditions not based on cosmetic preferences. If these effects occur, patients should seek medical attention. If muscle weakness or paralysis occurs in a larger area than the local area where the drug was administered or affects the ability to swallow, see, breathe, or otherwise move, medical attention should be obtained immediately.

Contraindications Botulinum toxin (Botox) should not be used in patients who have any infection near where the injection site would be or in those patients who have developed an infection at the site of a previous injection.

Cautions and Considerations Botox should be used with caution in patients with muscle dysfunction such as cerebral palsy, muscle spasm, or dystonia. Patients who have hyperhidrosis should avoid using deodorant for 24 hours prior to injection and avoid situations that cause sweating for 30 minutes prior to injection.

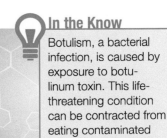

Direct-Acting Muscle Relaxants

One **direct-acting muscle relaxant** that works by blocking the intracellular release of calcium and weakening muscle contractility is **dantrolene** (Dantrium). Dantrolene is used to treat muscle spasticity resulting from spinal cord injury or cerebral palsy. It is the drug of choice for treatment of malignant hyperthermia, an emergency situation that occurs in some individuals when they are administered general anesthesia. Injectable dantrolene is typically kept in emergency drug kits in areas where anesthesia is administered. Dantrolene is available in both intravenous (IV) and oral forms, but, in an emergency, it is administered intravenously and is commonly dosed at 2.5 mg/kg.

Side Effects Common side effects of dantrolene are drowsiness, dizziness, fatigue, confusion, impaired judgment, and altered coordination. If diarrhea develops, patients should consult their healthcare practitioners because this side effect can sometimes become severe. Dantrolene can cause photosensitivity. With long-term use, dantrolene can be toxic to the liver, so special monitoring with periodic liver function tests is required.

Drug Alert

Dantrolene tends to have a short shelf life, so it is important to regularly verify the expiration date of this drug in emergency drug kits. Having a set schedule (every six months) for checking all drugs in an emergency kit or crash cart for expiration dates is essential. An emergency situation is not the time to find out that the supply of dantrolene is no longer effective.

Contraindications Dantrolene should not be used in patients with liver disease. Alert the patient's healthcare practitioner if you encounter such a situation.

Cautions and Considerations Dantrolene should be used with great caution in patients with lung disease. In addition, dantrolene should be used with particular caution in women and patients over 35 years old because these patients seem to have a greater likelihood of drug-induced liver disease.

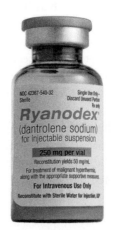

Ryanodex® (dantrolene sodium) for injectable suspension is indicated for the treatment of malignant hyperthermia in conjunction with appropriate supportive measures, and for the prevention of malignant hyperthermia in patients at high risk.

Neuromuscular Blocking Agents

In all cases, **neuromuscular blocking agents** (see Table 11.2) cause temporary paralysis. These agents are used with anesthesia for short-term muscle relaxation during endotracheal intubation, mechanical respiration, and surgical procedures. Under no circumstance should these drugs be prescribed in the outpatient setting or for anyone not on a ventilator.

TABLE 11.2 Neuromuscular Blocking Agents

Generic (Brand)	Dosage Form	Route of Administration
Short-Acting Agent (onset of action: immediate; duration of action: seconds to minutes)		
Succinylcholine (Anectine, Quelicin)	Injectable and IV solution	IM, IV
Intermediate-Acting Agents (onset of action: a few minutes; duration of action: 30–40 minutes)		
Atracurium	IV solution	IV
Cisatracurium (Nimbex)	IV solution	IV
Rocuronium (Zemuron)	IV solution	IV
Vecuronium	IV powder for solution	IV
Long-Acting Agent (onset of action: a few minutes; duration of action: 60–100 minutes)		
Pancuronium	IV solution	IV

Neuromuscular blockers work by competitively blocking ACh receptors or inhibiting breakdown of ACh, thereby allowing the muscle to continuously contract until fatigue and paralysis occur. Drug choice among these agents depends on the length of the procedure (a few minutes to hours) or the desired period of time for ventilation (days or longer).

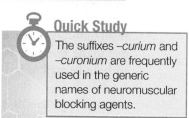

Quick Study

The suffixes *–curium* and *–curonium* are frequently used in the generic names of neuromuscular blocking agents.

Side Effects Low blood pressure and respiratory depression are the most common side effects of neuromuscular blocking agents. Blood pressure and respiratory rate are monitored closely whenever these agents are used.

Contraindications Neuromuscular blocking agents have no contraindications.

Cautions and Considerations Cardiac arrest and changes in cardiac function have occurred in patients, especially children, treated with these agents. These drugs must be dosed individually. Special care must be taken to ensure that these drugs be given for intubation or to ventilated patients only. Neuromuscular blocking agents paralyze all muscles, including those that control respiration.

 Checkpoint **11.2**

Take a moment to review what you have learned so far and answer these questions.

1. What drugs are prescribed to treat muscle spasms due to injury and lower back pain?

2. What are the indications for the use of dantrolene?

3. How are neuromuscular blocking agents used?

Kolb's Learning Styles

Action and goal-oriented learners (like Accommodators and Convergers) might enjoy looking ahead to Chapter 25: "Drugs for Pain and Anesthesia" and thinking about analgesics used in combination with the muscle relaxants from this chapter. Which combinations seem appropriate and which do not? Have you or a family member ever taken medication for a muscle injury? What combination of drugs was prescribed?

Other Muscular System Disorders

Although they are relatively rare, a few other conditions that affect muscle function should be mentioned. These conditions represent a collection of autoimmune, infectious, and other disease processes.

Myasthenia Gravis

Myasthenia gravis is a condition in which an autoimmune process attacks and destroys ACh receptors on muscle cells in the neuromuscular junction. It is a progressive disease that begins with muscle weakness in the face and neck and eventually impairs movement in all limbs. A person in myasthenic crisis is in danger of dying from respiratory failure due to the weakness of the respiratory muscles. Although myasthenia gravis is disabling and can be fatal, this disease can be managed with current drug therapies.

Drug Regimens and Treatments

Drugs for myasthenia gravis include anticholinesterase inhibitors that enhance muscle strength and immunosuppressants that slow the progression of the disorder (see Table 11.3). Choice of therapy is highly individualized and depends on the patient's age and the severity of disease.

TABLE 11.3 Drugs for Myasthenia Gravis

Generic (Brand)	Dosage Form	Route of Administration
Anticholinesterase Inhibitors		
Neostigmine (Prostigmin)	IV solution, tablet	IV, oral
Pyridostigmine (Mestinon)	Syrup, tablet	Oral
Immunosuppressants		
Azathioprine (Imuran)	IV solution, tablet	IV, oral
Cyclosporine (Gengraf, Neoral, Sandimmune)	Capsule, IV solution, oral solution	IV, oral

Anticholinesterase Inhibitors

Neostigmine (Prostigmin) and pyridostigmine (Mestinon) work by inhibiting acetylcholinesterase, the enzyme that breaks down ACh in the neuromuscular junction. In effect, this process increases the amount of ACh available for muscular function. Anticholinesterase inhibitors must be taken around the clock to maintain muscle function, so multiple daily doses are needed. Neostigmine and pyridostigmine can also be used to reverse neuromuscular blockade after surgery.

Side Effects If too much of an anticholinesterase agent is taken, toxicity can result, which can cause extreme muscle weakness and difficulty breathing. If such symptoms occur, patients should seek medical attention immediately.

Contraindications Patients who have peritonitis (infection of the abdomen) or a GI obstruction should not take these medications. These agents are also contraindicated in patients with asthma or other breathing problems.

Cautions and Considerations Anticholinesterase inhibitors should be used with caution in patients with cardiac arrhythmias, asthma, or seizure disorders such as epilepsy.

Immunosuppressants

Azathioprine (Imuran) and cyclosporine (Gengraf, Neoral, Sandimmune) are the immunosuppressants used most frequently in the treatment of myasthenia gravis. These agents work by inhibiting the immune system's production of antibodies that attack muscle cells. Adjunct therapy may include corticosteroids, which also suppress the immune system when used in high doses. For more detailed information on immunosuppressant therapy, see Chapter 24.

Side Effects Common side effects, especially in patients first starting these medications, include nausea, vomiting, and diarrhea. Some blood disorders (anemia and low platelets) have been associated with use of these immunosuppressants. Blood tests are used to monitor for this side effect.

Contraindications Patients with uncontrolled high blood pressure or malignancy should not take these medications. In addition, patients with poor renal function or hepatic function along with psoriasis or rheumatoid arthritis should not take cyclosporine.

Cautions and Considerations Immunosuppressants make patients more prone to infections, so good infection control measures should be implemented to avoid illness. In addition, immunosuppressants can increase the risk of developing some cancers such as lymphoma. Patients should be aware of this risk and undergo regular cancer screening as appropriate.

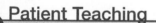 Patient Teaching

> Patients who are immunocompromised should limit exposure to common sources of infectious organisms such as raw fruits and vegetables, fresh flowers, and tap water. Even stethoscopes, if not cleaned with alcohol, can introduce infection in someone without a fully functioning immune system. Many people do not realize the risk certain items can pose.

Poliomyelitis

Poliomyelitis, commonly referred to as **polio**, is an infection of the nerves that control the muscular system. This disorder is nearly eradicated in the United States and in other developed countries due to the administration of the polio vaccine. However, polio remains a significant health threat in underdeveloped areas of the African, Asian, and South American continents where the vaccine is not readily available.

Drug Regimens and Treatments

Treatment of polio is difficult as there is no cure. The likelihood of encountering active polio cases is very low unless you travel to affected countries or regularly treat patients from those countries.

Polio Vaccine

Preventive therapy in the form of vaccination is the most effective approach. The polio vaccine is given to children in four doses at the following ages: 2 months, 4 months, 6 to 18 months, and 4 to 6 years. Polio is a required vaccination series for all children entering kindergarten in the United States.

Most health systems require healthcare workers to show documentation of polio vaccination, among other immunizations, upon employment. Because these vaccinations are administered to children, it can be difficult for adults to locate this documentation. Routine vaccination for adults in the United States is not recommended by the Centers for Disease Control and Prevention (CDC) because the likelihood of encountering the disease is so low. However, if an adult who is not vaccinated is exposed to polio while traveling or caring for patients with polio, he or she should get the polio vaccine as soon as possible.

Side Effects As with all immunizations, the most frequent side effects include redness and soreness at the injection site. Children can sometimes have an upset stomach, irritability, crying, fever, and fatigue in the first 48 hours after the injection. Few long-term adverse effects are associated with the polio vaccine. Those suspecting an adverse effect should report it to the **Vaccine Adverse Event Reporting System (VAERS)**, a national vaccine-safety surveillance system operated by the US Food and Drug Administration (FDA) and the CDC to collect and analyze information on adverse effects that occur after immunization. Healthcare professionals should also report such effects to the vaccine's manufacturer. Parents with concerns that their child has experienced potential adverse effects should contact the **National Vaccine Injury Compensation Program (VICP)**, which is part of the Health Resources and Services Administration of the US Department of Health & Human Services.

Contraindications Patients with an allergy to any component of the vaccine, yeast, polymyxin B, or neomycin should not receive this vaccine. Patients who have encephalopathy or neurologic disorders, or who have had a seizure in the past seven days, should not receive this vaccine. Immunocompromised patients should also not receive this vaccine.

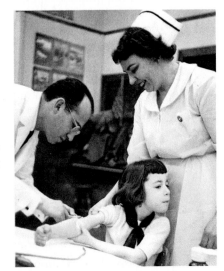

Two years before the polio vaccine was developed by Jonas Salk (left), approximately 50,000 cases of polio occurred.

Cautions and Considerations The polio vaccine is recommended for all children entering kindergarten. As mentioned previously, the CDC recommends that adults in the United States who have not been vaccinated should not receive the vaccine unless they are traveling to a country where polio is present. Many insurance companies deny coverage of the polio vaccine when given to an adult because it is not considered to be medically necessary. This restriction makes it difficult for adult patients to obtain the polio vaccine.

Rhabdomyolysis

Rhabdomyolysis is a syndrome in which muscle breakdown occurs and toxic cell contents are released into the bloodstream. This syndrome is a rare but serious side effect of the cholesterol-lowering class of drugs called statins. Symptoms may be silent but can include muscle aches and pain, red- to brown-colored urine, and muscle weakness. Laboratory tests are used to detect muscle enzymes (creatine kinase [CK], also known as creatine phosphokinase [CPK]) in the blood when rhabdomyolysis is suspected. Patients taking statins are monitored closely for rhabdomyolysis because the condition can lead to acute kidney failure. Patients taking statins should report any unexplained muscle pain or weakness to their healthcare practitioners.

 Checkpoint 11.3

Take a moment to review what you have learned so far and answer these questions.

1. What drugs are used to treat myasthenia gravis?
2. What are the recommended polio vaccine guidelines for children and adults in the United States?
3. What is rhabdomyolysis?

Herbal and Alternative Therapies

Few herbal and natural products are used for treating muscular conditions. However, several herbal therapies taken for other problems can interact with prescription muscle relaxants. St. John's wort, valerian, and kava are examples of products taken for depression and insomnia that could intensify the CNS depression resulting from the use of muscle relaxants. If you encounter patients using such products along with their prescription muscle relaxants, alert their healthcare practitioners.

Spinal realignment performed by a chiropractor has been found to relieve muscle pain and injury. Acupuncture and acupressure have also been used with some success to treat neuromuscular pain. Patients interested in **chiropractic therapy** or **acupuncture therapy** should check with their health insurance providers about coverage of this service. Many health insurance programs now include it.

Work Wise

To avoid a potential drug interaction, allied health personnel should be sure to ask patients about their use of OTC, herbal, and natural remedies when taking medication histories.

Chapter Review

Chapter Summary

The muscular system contains three types of muscle: skeletal, cardiac, and smooth muscle. Acetylcholine, or ACh, is a neurotransmitter that travels across the neuromuscular junction to stimulate muscle-fiber contraction. Muscle contraction is also dependent on sodium influx and calcium release within the muscle cell.

Most muscle relaxants are used for muscle injury and spasm. Centrally acting muscle relaxants are dispensed frequently to treat muscle spasm. They work by suppressing the CNS, which controls muscle contraction. These drugs tend to cause sedation. Locally acting muscle relaxants work by blocking the release of ACh into the neuromuscular junction. One locally acting relaxant is botulinum toxin (Botox). This expensive cosmetic agent is frequently administered by local injection to relax muscles in the face and reduce wrinkles. Direct-acting muscle relaxants are used primar-

ily to treat muscle spasticity due to spinal cord injury or cerebral palsy. They work by inhibiting intracellular calcium release. Because the names of some muscle relaxants are similar to the names of other unrelated drugs, special precautions should be taken to prevent medication errors, including verification of the medication labels.

Neuromuscular blocking agents are used during intubation and ventilation to temporarily relax and paralyze muscles for specialized procedures.

Few herbal products are used to treat muscle spasm directly, but some herbal products interact with prescription muscle relaxants, including St. John's wort, valerian, and kava. Consequently, patients should be warned about concurrent use of herbal products with muscle relaxants. Chiropractic and acupuncture therapies have been found to be effective in treating muscle pain and injury.

Chapter Checkup

The Navigator+ learning management system that accompanies this textbook offers many opportunities to help you master chapter content, including end-of-chapter exercises, a glossary of key terms, flash cards, and additional interactive activities.

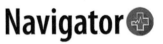

Career Exploration

If you enjoyed learning about the muscular system in this chapter, you may want to explore the following career options:

- athletic trainer
- computed tomography (CT) technician
- dance therapist
- exercise physiologist
- hand therapist
- kinesiotherapist
- magnetic resonance imaging (MRI) technician
- massage therapist

- medical assistant
- orientation and mobility (O&M) specialist
- orthotist
- pharmacy technician
- physical rehabilitation counselor
- physical therapist (PT)
- physical therapist (PT) assistant
- prosthetist
- recreational therapist

UNIT 4

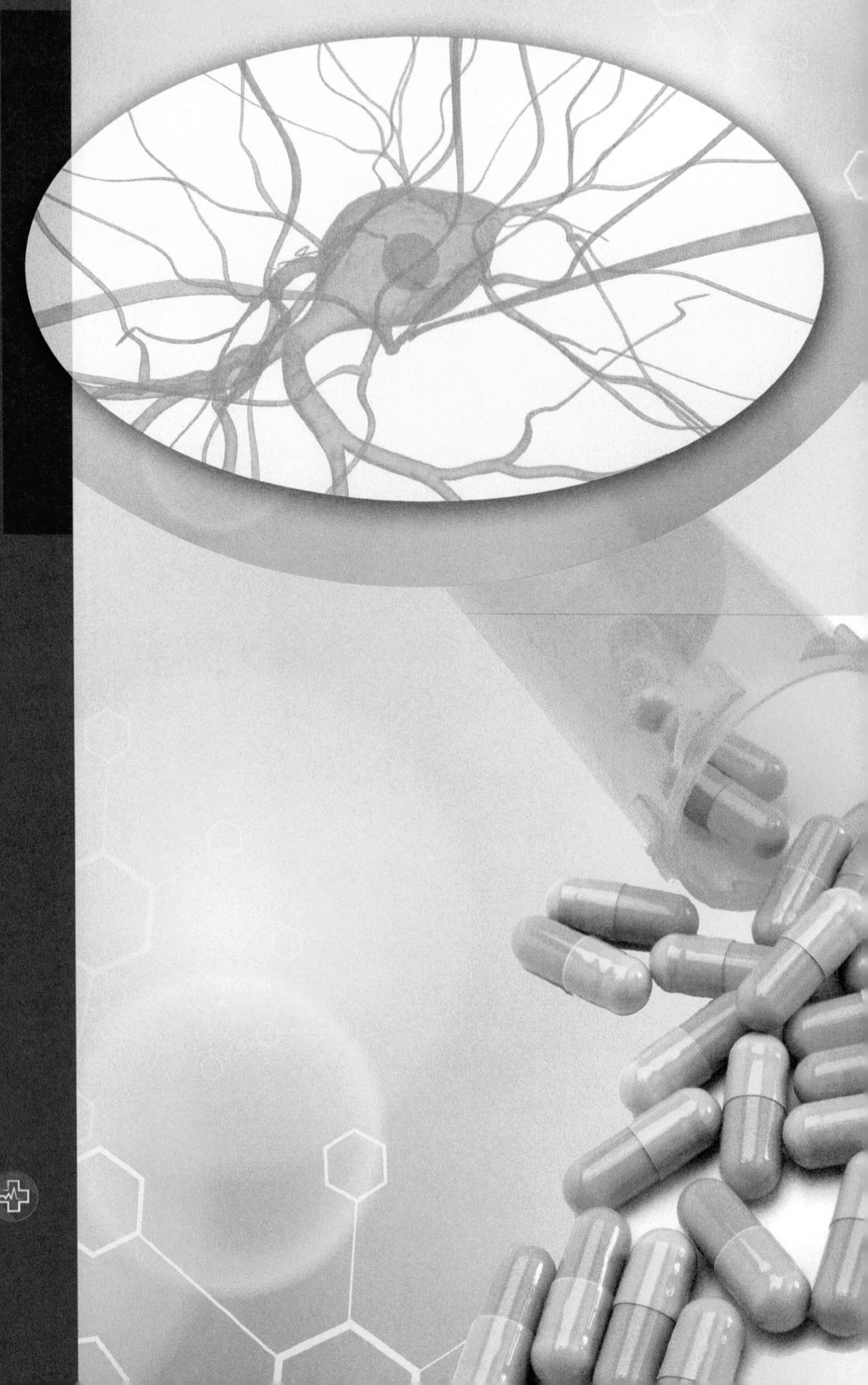

Navigator

Pharmacotherapy for the Nervous and Sensory Systems

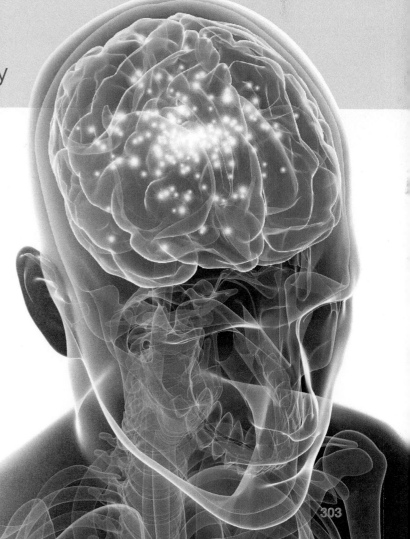

12

The Nervous System and Drug Therapy

Pharm Facts

- Eating chocolate activates neurotransmitters in the brain to release serotonin. These elevated levels of serotonin make a person feel relaxed and happy.

- The human brain has more than 100 billion neurons. If these neurons were lined up, that line would stretch 600 miles.

- Only 4% of brain cells are actually used, while the rest are kept in reserve.

- The neurons in a developing fetus grow at a rate of 250,000 neurons a minute.

- Although the human brain only accounts for 2% of a person's body weight, this organ consumes 20% of the oxygen and calories received.

"As a nerve conduction study technologist, I perform the first part of an electromyography (EMG) test, which is used to diagnose carpal tunnel syndrome, amyotrophic lateral sclerosis, and myasthenia gravis. During the performance of nerve conduction studies, I am responsible for documenting, evaluating, and calculating electrical impulses directly recorded from the peripheral sensory and motor nerves. The second part of the test is performed by a specially trained EMG physician who analyzes the electrical activity of the different muscle groups. This technologist/physician partnership has fostered my lifelong learning in the challenging and rewarding field of neurodiagnostics."

—**Peggy J. Neal**, AS, R.NCS.T., CNCT
Nerve Conduction Study Technologist

Learning Objectives

1   Describe the basic anatomy and physiology of the nervous system.

2   Understand the common conditions that affect the nervous system.

3   Explain the therapeutic effects of prescription medications, nonprescription medications, and alternative therapies commonly used to treat diseases of the nervous system.

4   Identify the generic names, brand names, indications, dosage ranges, side effects, contraindications, and cautions and considerations associated with the drugs commonly used to treat nervous system disorders.

5   Identify common herbal and alternative therapies that are related to the nervous system.

This chapter provides an overview of the anatomy and physiology of the nervous system as well as common disorders that affect the central and autonomic nervous systems. Central nervous system conditions such as Parkinson's disease, Alzheimer's disease, and attention-deficit/hyperactivity disorder (ADHD) are discussed. These well-known disorders have been portrayed dramatically in film and television and continue to be the focus of scientific research and media attention. Parkinson's disease is not curable, but various choices for drug therapy can mean the difference between being active and being bedridden. Alzheimer's disease is increasingly encountered as the US population ages, but few drugs treat it effectively. On the other hand, there are several drug regimens known to be effective for treatment of ADHD, but successful treatment requires a unified approach involving both pharmacotherapy and behavioral therapy.

Few disorders of the autonomic nervous system exist, but drug therapy used to treat other conditions sometimes has an effect on this system, which controls heart rate, blood pressure, breathing, pupil dilation, and digestion. It is important to be familiar with these agents because they are used to treat common conditions such as high blood pressure and glaucoma and because many of them cause anticholinergic side effects (dry mouth, blurred vision, constipation, and difficulty urinating). Therefore, you should understand the effects of drug activity on the autonomic nervous system because you will encounter such medications regularly.

Anatomy and Physiology of the Nervous System

The **nervous system** senses and interprets an individual's surroundings and controls his or her vital body functions (see Figure 12.1). The nervous system is divided into the central nervous system and the peripheral nervous system. The **central nervous system (CNS)**, which includes the brain and spinal cord, is responsible for processing information received from the body. The **peripheral nervous system**, which is made up of all nerves outside the brain and spinal cord, is responsible for bringing signals to the CNS for interpretation. Signals from the brain are then conducted back through the peripheral nervous system to direct movement and other responses. The peripheral nervous system is further divided into the somatic and automatic nervous systems. The **somatic nervous system** controls intentional, voluntary movement. The **autonomic nervous system** controls involuntary and automatic body functions, such as heart rate, respiration, and digestion. The autonomic system is further divided into the **sympathetic nervous system** (which uses adrenergic receptors and some cholinergic receptors) and the **parasympathetic nervous system** (which uses cholinergic receptors only).

FIGURE 12.1 Anatomy of the Nervous System

Peripheral nerves branch out from the spinal cord to all parts of the body.

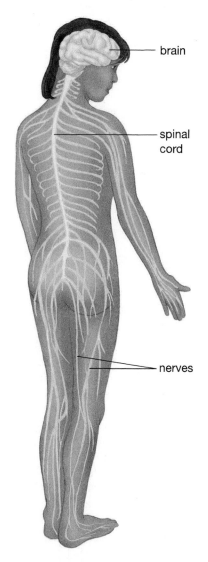

Structures and Functions of the Brain

The brain is divided into sections, and each section is responsible for different functions. The **cerebrum**, including the **cerebral cortex**, performs higher cognitive functions, such as thinking and memory (see Figure 12.2). The **cerebellum** coordinates movement and balance. The **pons** and **medulla** in the **brain stem** regulate autonomic and reflex functions of the body. In the middle of the brain are the **thalamus** and **hypothalamus**, which control various functions, including hormone regulation and body temperature.

FIGURE 12.2 Anatomy of the Brain

The cerebrum and cerebral cortex perform higher cognitive functions, and the cerebellum coordinates movement.

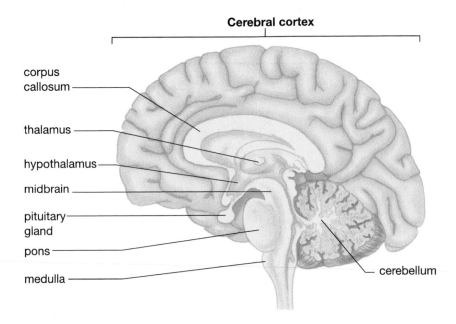

Cell Structure of the CNS

The cell structure along the border of the CNS is different from elsewhere in the body. Oxygen, carbon dioxide, small molecules (e.g., glucose), and small, lipid-soluble drugs pass easily from the blood to the CNS tissue; however, larger, water-soluble molecules, including drugs and most pathogens, do not easily enter the brain or spinal cord. The barrier surrounding the CNS tissue, called the **blood-brain barrier (BBB)**, protects this delicate tissue from potentially harmful chemicals. This barrier must be overcome, however, when drug therapy enters the CNS to exert its action.

Neurotransmission

Neurotransmitters are chemicals that carry signals from one nerve cell to the next or from a nerve cell to a muscle cell (see Table 12.1). These chemicals are released from the end of one nerve, cross the **synaptic space** between cells, and connect to receptors on the adjoining cell so that the signal is passed. This process is known as **neurotransmission** (see Figure 12.3).

Altered production, release, or metabolic breakdown of neurotransmitters appears to be at the core of many nervous system conditions. Deficiencies in certain neurotransmitters are assumed to underlie or contribute to mood disorders, such as depression, and psychiatric problems, such as schizophrenia and bipolar disorder (see Chapter 13). In fact, most drugs that treat these conditions supplement, mimic, or block the actions of specific neurotransmitters.

Individual nerve cells consist of a **cell body**, where the nucleus resides, and other cell parts. **Dendrites** bring signals into the cell body. **Axons** carry signals away from the nucleus to neighboring cells. **Schwann cells** in the peripheral nervous system and oligodendrocytes in the CNS form a **myelin sheath** that surrounds and protects axons. Without this sheath, signal conduction from cell to cell is not well-coordinated and becomes sporadic. Sporadic nerve conduction makes coordinated muscle movement, including walking and talking, difficult. Destruction of this myelin sheath occurs in diseases such as multiple sclerosis.

TABLE 12.1 Neurotransmitters and Their Actions

Neurotransmitter	Action
Acetylcholine (ACh)	Used in the parasympathetic nervous system and between nerves and skeletal muscle. Acts on receptors in smooth muscle to control blood pressure and digestion, in cardiac muscle to control heart rate, and in exocrine glands.
Dopamine (DA)	Used primarily in the CNS to control mood and coordinated movement.
Epinephrine	Used in the sympathetic nervous system. Acts on receptors to regulate cardiac function and bronchodilation. Also called adrenaline.
Gamma-aminobutyric acid (GABA)	Used in the brain to regulate signal delivery.
Norepinephrine	Used in the CNS and the sympathetic nervous system. In the brain, involved in mood and emotions. In the periphery, acts on receptors to control blood pressure, cardiac function, and digestion.
Serotonin (5-HT)	Used in the peripheral nervous system and the CNS. In the periphery, acts on receptors in smooth muscle (blood vessels and the lining of the gastrointestinal tract). In the brain, involved in mood and emotions.

FIGURE 12.3 Neurotransmission

Nerve signals are carried from cell to cell by neurotransmitters.

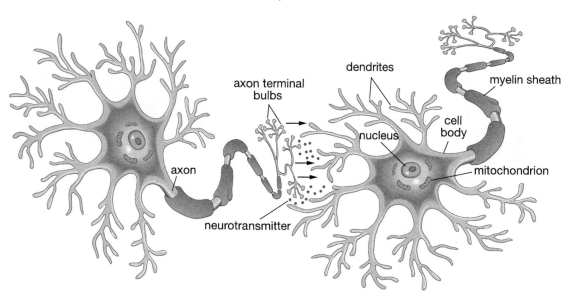

Checkpoint 12.1

Take a moment to review what you have learned so far and answer these questions.

1. What are the parts of the brain and their unique functions?

2. How is a nerve signal transmitted from nerve cell to nerve cell?

3. What are the specific neurotransmitters and their functions?

Common Nervous System Disorders

Parkinson's disease and Alzheimer's disease are disorders associated with age. Seizure disorders and ADHD can be seen in patients of any age but are most commonly seen in children. These disorders are not related but are grouped here because they all occur in the brain. Drug therapy and treatment vary significantly across these disorders.

Seizure Disorders

Seizures (convulsions) are uncoordinated bursts of neuronal activity that result in brain dysfunction. Depending on the extent of the seizure and the area of the brain affected, symptoms can be as mild as staring or twitching to as severe as a total loss of consciousness and whole-body convulsions. **Epilepsy** is a chronic seizure disorder that causes a variety of different types of seizures (see Table 12.2). All patients with epilepsy have seizures, but not all patients with seizures have epilepsy. Although only 1%–2% of US residents have epilepsy, almost 1 in 10 individuals will have a single, unprovoked seizure within his or her lifetime. Common causes for seizure include these conditions:

- alcohol or drug withdrawal
- brain tumors or scar tissue
- electric shock
- head injury or trauma
- high fever
- hypocalcemia (low calcium in the blood)
- hypoglycemia or hyperglycemia (low or high blood glucose)
- hyponatremia (low sodium in the blood)
- infection (e.g., meningitis)
- stroke

In the Know

One of the nondrug therapy options for patients with seizure disorders is the use of a seizure-alert dog. Such canines are trained to recognize the warning signs of an impending seizure and to alert their owners or seek assistance. For children, such assistance dogs provide social and emotional support to reduce stress and the occurrence of seizures.

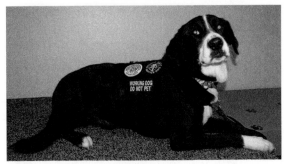

A seizure-alert dog is trained to detect signs of an impending seizure, including changes in an individual's respiratory rate, body scent, or behavior.

Sometimes, drug therapy can reduce the seizure threshold in the brain. If drug therapy is combined with one of the other causes listed previously, a seizure can occur more easily. The most common type of seizure is a **partial seizure**, in which a localized area of the brain is affected. The patient usually does not lose consciousness. Instead, a defined area of the body is affected. A partial seizure may manifest as twitching or muscle tightness in a specific area of the body; some patients may, at the same time, experience visual disturbances or hallucinations. Even so, a patient can usually communicate during a partial seizure. A **generalized seizure** does not occur as often but tends to be the type of seizure that is dramatized in movies and other media. During a generalized seizure, loss of consciousness usually occurs. Afterward, the patient experiences a period of memory loss, confusion, and tiredness that may last for a few minutes or up to a few hours (see Figure 12.4).

TABLE 12.2 Types of Seizures

Partial	
Simple	Localized area of the body is affected in movement. May result in twitching, tightness, or contortion of specific body parts. No loss of consciousness.
Complex	Localized area of the body is affected in movement. May result in twitching, tightness, or contortion of specific body parts. Impaired consciousness may occur, but not complete loss.
Generalized	
Absence (petit mal)	Begins with interruption of normal activity, such as blank stare, rolling or blinking eyes, uncontrolled facial movements, or arm/leg jerking. No whole-body convulsions occur. Attacks are short (≈30 seconds) but occur frequently, usually multiple times a day. Common in children with epilepsy and can progress to tonic-clonic seizures later in life.
Tonic-clonic (grand mal)	Tonic phase happens first: The body goes rigid, and the patient usually falls down. Clonic phase happens next: Whole body convulsions occur and may be accompanied by altered breathing rhythm, loss of bladder control, and excessive salivation.
Atonic	Sudden loss of muscle tone and consciousness. Appears as if the patient has fainted.
Myoclonic	Sudden massive muscle jerks, which may throw the patient down or wake him or her from sleeping. Consciousness is often not lost.
Status epilepticus	Continuous tonic-clonic convulsions with or without loss of consciousness for at least 30 minutes. Usually characterized by high fever and a lack of oxygen severe enough to cause brain damage or death. This type of seizure is a medical emergency because 10% of patients die, regardless of treatment.

FIGURE 12.4 Partial and Generalized Seizure Activity

A partial seizure and a generalized seizure affect brain activity differently, as shown on the simulated EEGs.

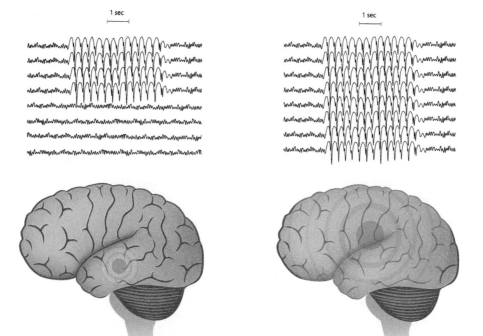

Partial seizure   Generalized seizure

Drug Regimens and Treatments

Drugs used to treat seizure disorders are called **anticonvulsants**. They vary in their mechanisms of action and can work via multiple mechanisms at once. Therefore, these agents are covered together as one group in this chapter. Drug therapy must be individualized for each patient. Monotherapy with one drug is tried first, and other agents may be added to control seizures. Combination therapy (using two or more drugs from different classes) is common among patients with severe forms of epilepsy. It can take up to a month to see the full benefit from these drugs.

Antiepileptic Drugs

Collectively, **antiepileptic drugs (AEDs)** affect the movement of sodium, calcium, or chloride ions across the nerve cell membrane in some way. This effect slows the transmission of erratic nerve impulses because membranes are less excitable. **Glutamate** is an excitatory neurotransmitter that affects sodium and calcium influx; **gamma-aminobutyric acid (GABA)** is an inhibitory neurotransmitter that affects chloride influx. Some anticonvulsants work directly on ion channels, whereas others inhibit glutamate or enhance GABA. Some AEDs work in multiple ways. For instance, topiramate blocks sodium channels, inhibits glutamate, and enhances GABA, all at the same time. For difficult-to-manage epilepsy, combinations of AEDs may be necessary to achieve and maintain control of seizures.

Treatment for **status epilepticus**, an emergency situation, includes one of two benzodiazepines (diazepam or lorazepam [see Chapter 13]) plus phenytoin or fosphenytoin. Phenobarbital may also be used. This drug combination may be stored in crash cart kits (container carrying medication for use in emergency resuscitations).

Several AEDs have other uses. Some of these uses include migraine headaches and mood regulation in patients with bipolar disorder. Valproic acid, gabapentin, and topiramate are sometimes used for migraine prevention. In addition, gabapentin is frequently used to treat nerve pain related to diabetic neuropathy, nerve injury (such as back and spinal cord injuries), and shingles. The dosing range varies widely for these conditions and must be individualized for each patient. (To review all commonly used AEDs, see Table 12.3.)

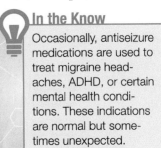

In the Know

Occasionally, antiseizure medications are used to treat migraine headaches, ADHD, or certain mental health conditions. These indications are normal but sometimes unexpected.

Side Effects Many side effects of AEDs (as listed in Table 12.3) are dose-dependent, so blood levels are monitored for highest (peak) and lowest (trough) concentrations. Dosing AEDs is highly individualized because some AEDs have nonlinear pharmacokinetics. For example, phenytoin undergoes what is called **Michaelis-Menten pharmacokinetics**: A patient's metabolism becomes saturated with the drug to a point after which even slight dose increases result in dramatic elevations in blood concentrations. Severe toxicity and side effects necessitate close monitoring of drug concentrations with blood tests.

Many AEDs cause drowsiness, dizziness, and confusion. These effects improve with time, but when patients first start taking these medications, they should be careful when driving or making important decisions.

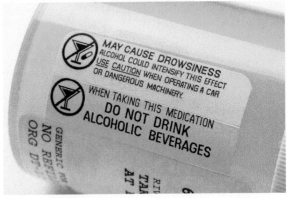

AEDs are dispensed in vials with auxiliary warning labels. These labels remind patients about the side effects of the medications.

TABLE 12.3 Commonly Used AEDs

Generic (Brand)	Dosage Form	Route of Administration	Common Use(s)	Side Effects
Sodium-Channel Blockers				
Carbamazepine (Tegretol)	Capsule, suspension, tablet	Oral	Tonic-clonic, partial seizure (no effect on absence seizure)	Dizziness, drowsiness, nausea, unsteadiness, vomiting, abnormal vision, hyponatremia, hepato-toxicity, arrhythmias, increased suicide risk
Eslicarbazepine (Aptiom)	Tablet	Oral	Partial seizure	Dizziness, drowsiness, headache, tiredness, nausea, blurred or double vision
Ethotoin (Peganone)	Tablet	Oral	Tonic-clonic, partial seizure	Diarrhea, nausea, dizziness, fatigue, headache, insomnia, double vision
Fosphenytoin (Cerebyx)	Injection	IM, IV	Status epilepticus (short-term use until phenytoin can be given)	Dizziness, itching, numbness, headache, tired-ness, decreased movement, hypotension, cardio-vascular collapse (rare but serious)
Lacosamide (Vimpat)	Solution, tablet	IV, oral	Partial seizure	Dizziness, fatigue, headache, nausea, tremors, slurred speech, blurred or double vision
Oxcarbazepine (Trileptal)	Suspension, tablet	Oral	Partial seizure (alternative uses: bipolar disorder, diabetic neuropathy, neuralgia)	Abdominal pain, headache, trouble walking, abnormal or double vision, difficulty moving, dizziness, fatigue, nausea, tremors, vomiting, hyponatremia
Phenytoin (Dilantin)	Capsule, injection, suspension, tablet	IV, oral	Tonic-clonic, partial seizure, status epilepticus	Decreased coordination/movement, mental confusion, slurred speech, dizziness, headache, insomnia, twitches, nervousness, hepatotoxicity, gingival hyperplasia, hair growth
Vigabatrin (Sabril)	Tablet	Oral	Partial seizure	Fatigue, headache, confusion, poor coordination, memory loss, tremors, weight gain, blurred vision, depression
Calcium-Channel Blockers				
Ethosuximide (Zarontin)	Capsule, syrup	Oral	Absence seizure	Drowsiness, headache, dizziness, hiccups, aggression, fatigue, difficulty moving, loss of appetite, upset stomach, diarrhea, nightmares
Valproate sodium (Depakote)	Capsule, injection, syrup, tablet	IV, oral	Partial and absence seizures, tonic-clonic (alternative use: bipolar disorder)	Dizziness, headache, nausea, vomiting, tremors, diarrhea, tiredness, weight gain, hair loss, hepato-toxicity
Valproic acid (Depakene)	Capsule, injection, syrup, tablet	IV, oral	Partial and absence seizures	Dizziness, headache, nausea, vomiting, tremors, diarrhea, tiredness, hair loss, hepatotoxicity
Zonisamide (Zonegran)	Capsule	Oral	Partial seizure (alternative uses: binge-eating disorder, obesity)	Tiredness, dizziness, loss of appetite, headache, nausea, irritability, difficulty thinking, sulfa allergy, kidney stones
GABA Enhancers				
Gabapentin (Neurontin)	Capsule, oral solution, tablet	Oral	Partial seizure (alternative uses: diabetic neuropathy, neuralgia, shingles, fibromyalgia, hot flashes, hiccups, restless legs syndrome, others)	Dizziness, drowsiness, tiredness, nausea, vomiting, diarrhea, dry mouth, swelling in legs/arms, abnormal thinking, difficulty moving, weight gain

TABLE 12.3 **Commonly Used AEDs** *(continued)*

Generic (Brand)	Dosage Form	Route of Administration	Common Use(s)	Side Effects
GABA Enhancers (continued)				
Phenobarbital (Luminal)	Capsule, elixir, injection, tablet	IV, oral	Tonic-clonic, status epilepticus (alternative use: sedative for anxiety and insomnia)	Tiredness, drowsiness, hepatotoxicity, aggression or mood changes, hypotension
Pregabalin (Lyrica)	Capsule, oral solution	Oral	Partial seizure, neuropathic pain, fibromyalgia	Dizziness, drowsiness, dry mouth, blurred vision, fluid retention, weight gain
Primidone (Mysoline)	Tablet	Oral	Tonic-clonic seizure (alternative use: tremors)	Difficulty moving, dizziness, nausea, loss of appetite, vomiting, fatigue, mood changes, impotence, double vision
Tiagabine (Gabitril)	Tablet	Oral	Partial seizure (alternative use: bipolar disorder)	Dizziness, tiredness, nausea, nervousness, tremors, abdominal pain, abnormal thinking, depression
Glutamate Inhibitors				
Felbamate (Felbatol)	Suspension, tablet	Oral	Tonic-clonic, partial seizure	Insomnia, loss of appetite, weight loss, nausea, vomiting, headache, dizziness, tiredness, acne, rash, constipation, diarrhea
Lamotrigine (Lamictal)	Tablet	Oral	Tonic-clonic, partial seizure (alternative use: bipolar disorder)	Rash, decreased coordination/movement, dizziness, headache, insomnia, tiredness, rash, nausea, vomiting, blurred or double vision
Perampanel (Fycompa)	Tablet	Oral	Partial seizure	Fatigue, sleepiness, dizziness, irritability, nausea, weight gain, aggression, anger, anxiety, hostility, confusion, suicidal thoughts
Topiramate (Topamax)	Capsule, tablet	Oral	Tonic-clonic, partial seizure (alternative use: migraine)	Dizziness, numbness, memory problems, depression, kidney stones, insomnia, nausea, tiredness, loss of appetite, weight loss
Unknown Mechanism				
Levetiracetam (Keppra)	Injection, oral solution, tablet	IV, oral	Partial seizure	Dizziness, tiredness, lack of energy, depression, behavioral changes and/or psychosis

Patients should also avoid drinking alcohol when taking these drugs because alcohol creates additive effects when mixed with AEDs.

Rarely, some of these medications can alter mental status to cause thoughts of suicide, aggression, hostility, and psychosis. Any change in a patient's behavior or mental status is reason to contact the patient's healthcare practitioner immediately.

Many patients are concerned about the dulling effect these medications can have on their ability to think. This effect is a common reason for discontinuing treatment with an AED. This issue is especially sensitive for children in school trying to learn and keep up with classmates.

Several AEDs can cause rare but serious side effects such as Stevens-Johnson syndrome (a severe and sometimes fatal rash) and blood abnormalities. Patients should be advised to alert their prescribers if any type of rash appears. Blood tests are taken periodically to check for abnormalities in blood cells.

Phenytoin and ethotoin can cause **gingival hyperplasia**, which is an overgrowth of gum tissue in the mouth. Therefore, patients should maintain good oral hygiene when using these drugs.

Topiramate and zonisamide can cause kidney stones, so patients should drink plenty of fluids to avoid this effect. Vigabatrin can cause permanent vision loss (tunnel vision), so it is reserved for instances when other drug therapies have failed to work.

Contraindications The sodium-channel blockers have multiple contraindications. Carbamazepine use is contraindicated in bone marrow depression; with or within 14 days of monoamine oxidase inhibitor use; and with concurrent use of nefazodone. Use of delavirdine or nonnucleoside reverse transcriptase inhibitors is contraindicated with carbamazepine, phenytoin, and fosphenytoin drug therapy. Fosphenytoin and phenytoin should be avoided in patients who have a variety of cardiac issues (including sinus bradycardia, sinoatrial block, second- and third-degree atrioventricular [AV] block, and Adams-Stokes syndrome), an occurrence of rash during treatment, and treatment of absence seizures. Use of lacosamide is contraindicated in patients with liver abnormalities and blood disorders.

Many of the sodium-channel blockers have contraindications related to hypersensitivity. Eslicarbazepine is contraindicated in patients with oxcarbazepine hypersensitivity. Fosphenytoin and phenytoin should be avoided in patients with a hypersensitivity to hydantoins. Oxcarbazepine and vigabatrin do not have contraindications.

In addition, many of the calcium-channel blockers have contraindications related to hypersensitivity. Ethosuximide is contraindicated in patients with a history of sensitivity to succinimides. Valproate and valproic acid should not be used in patients with divalproex or divalproex derivative hypersensitivity, liver disease, urea cycle disorders, and mitochondrial disorders. Zonisamide use should be avoided in patients with sulfonamide hypersensitivity.

Gabapentin and pregabalin do not have contraindications. Phenobarbital should not be used in patients with liver impairment, shortness of breath or airway obstruction, porphyria, and sedative addiction. Primidone use is contraindicated in porphyria. Tiagabine has no contraindications.

Felbamate use should be avoided in patients with carbamate sensitivity, a history of blood dyscrasia, or liver impairment. Topiramate in the extended-release formula is contraindicated in patients with recent alcohol use and in those with metabolic acidosis who are also taking metformin. Lamotrigine and immediate-release topiramate have no contraindications. Levetiracetam also has no contraindications.

➕ *Note: Allied health professionals should be aware that an allergy to a particular drug contraindicates its use. This warning applies to all Contraindications sections in this chapter.*

Cautions and Considerations Abrupt withdrawal of AEDs should always be avoided because sudden discontinuation may trigger seizures. The dose should be slowly tapered if a patient needs to stop taking an anticonvulsant.

Several anticonvulsants are harmful to a developing fetus if taken while the patient is pregnant. However, seizures can also pose life-threatening effects for the mother and baby. Anticonvulsants are selected carefully for pregnant women.

Phenytoin is highly bound to protein in the bloodstream, and it interacts with many other medications that are also bound to protein. All alerts for drug interactions should be taken seriously, and the pharmacist must evaluate each one carefully. Phenytoin can adhere to nasogastric tubing. If it is given through a tube into the stomach, it must be mixed well with normal saline and separated by two hours from feedings given through the same tube. Intravenous (IV) phenytoin should be mixed or prepared using only normal saline. Suspensions of phenytoin must be shaken well—as should any medication in suspension form.

Patient Teaching

The extended-release form of carbamazepine works as an osmotic pump and leaves an empty pill casing in the stool. Tell patients that they should not be alarmed by the appearance of this "ghost tablet" in their stool. Explain to them that the drug is released while going through the gastrointestinal system.

Kolb's Learning Styles

To become familiar with the many side effects of AEDs, make a list of the effects from Table 12.3 that would pose a personal barrier for you. Which effects would you consider intolerable or would affect your ability to remain adherent to therapy? If you enjoy details and working alone (as Assimilators do), make a list of the AEDs associated with each side effect you find particularly difficult. If you enjoy reflection (as Divergers do), think about which AEDs are associated with these particularly difficult side effects and discuss your thoughts with a classmate.

Valproate and valproic acid tablets should be swallowed whole, not crushed or chewed. (Chewing can interfere with the extended-release properties of some dosage forms.) They should not be taken with aspirin or carbonated beverages. Aspirin competes with valproic acid for protein-binding sites, and carbonated beverages can break down valproic acid before absorption can occur. Ethosuximide, however, works best when taken with food.

Phenobarbital and primidone are controlled substances. With the use of these drugs, patients can develop tolerance. Consequently, special storage and handling requirements are needed. Some pharmacies require double and triple counting of controlled substances. In addition, refills are limited on controlled substances.

Parkinson's Disease

Parkinson's disease (PD) was first described by James Parkinson in 1817. The condition is characterized by tremors, muscle rigidity, difficulty moving, and balance problems. It can be quite debilitating and is most common among elderly patients. In fact, 1% of people in the United States over the age of 60 have PD; however, this disease

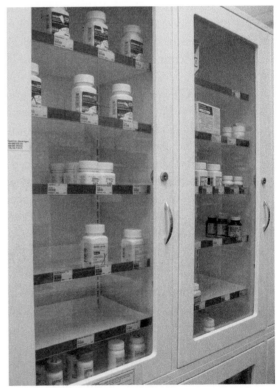

Certain AEDs—such as phenobarbital and primidone—are controlled substances and must be secured in a locked cabinet.

can also develop in the fourth decade of life. PD is a CNS disorder in which cells are lost in the **substantia nigra**, a region in the midbrain (see Figure 12.5). These cells produce dopamine, a neurotransmitter used in initiating and coordinating muscle movement. Most

FIGURE 12.5 | Substantia Nigra in the Midbrain

In PD, the damaged or destroyed cells in the substantia nigra result in an interruption of nerve impulses to the part of the brain that controls movement.

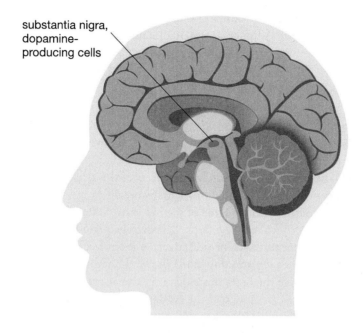

substantia nigra, dopamine-producing cells

patients with PD lean forward and walk with a shuffling gait; they are also somewhat off-balance. Tremors and an inability to move make activities of daily life difficult. The disease is progressive and has no cure. Drug therapy can relieve symptoms, thereby allowing patients freedom to move instead of being wheelchair bound.

Other symptoms associated with PD include anxiety, depression, fatigue, slow thinking, dementia, fragmented sleep, and hallucinations. Abnormalities of the autonomic nervous system can cause night sweats, orthostatic hypotension (low blood pressure on standing), sexual dysfunction, and constipation. Some patients also experience tingling sensations, lack of energy, loss of sense of smell, and diffuse pain. PD is a major reason for nursing home admissions.

Some drugs cause symptoms that mimic Parkinson's disease. Usually these parkinsonian effects are reversible on discontinuation of the medications. Occasionally, these effects are permanent. Drugs that can cause these symptoms include the following:

In the Know

Michael J. Fox, a popular television and film actor, announced he had Parkinson's disease in his thirties. Since then, Fox has raised awareness of the disease through his speaking engagements and fundraising efforts.

- amoxapine
- antipsychotic agents
- lithium
- metoclopramide
- phenothiazine antiemetics
- pimozide
- selective serotonin reuptake inhibitors (SSRIs)

Patients with movement problems should have their drug regimens evaluated. If a drug can be eliminated, parkinsonian symptoms may disappear.

Drug Regimens and Treatments

As PD progresses from early symptoms to advanced disease, the approach to drug therapy changes. Initial therapy starts with one drug, such as an anticholinergic agent or a dopaminergic agent such as levodopa. Eventually, adjunct (add-on) therapy is used to improve symptom control. Adjunct treatments include catechol-O-methyltransferase (COMT) inhibitors, selegiline, apomorphine, and amantadine. Surgical options are available, but the risks associated with brain surgery limit its use to the most severely affected patients.

Dopamine Agonists

Dopamine agonists are the mainstay of treatment for PD. **Levodopa** is widely recognized as the most effective treatment for PD because it significantly improves movement and restores normal function. Unfortunately, the effects of this drug (that is, its ability to provide movement control, or "on" time to patients) wear off over time. Dopamine agonists offer another alternative without some of the movement effects that levodopa causes, but they are not always as effective as levodopa. The average period for which a dopaminergic drug will work without significant side effects is about five years.

This group of drugs either replaces dopamine or mimics its action in the brain. In effect, these agents either give the brain more dopamine or provide a drug that has the same action. Dopamine itself cannot cross the BBB, so its prodrug, levodopa, is given. Once levodopa enters the brain, it is broken down into dopamine. Carbidopa is usually given in combination with levodopa (see Table 12.4) because it slows the breakdown of levodopa before it reaches the CNS, allowing more of the drug to enter the brain. Apomorphine is a self-injected agent used for acute treatment of intermittent "off" time, or the inability to move. Despite its name, apomorphine is not an opioid drug. It should not be used regularly; instead, it is saved for when levodopa wears off more quickly than anticipated. Apomorphine boosts the effects of levodopa until the next dose can be taken. If repeated doses of apomorphine are needed, adjustments in other therapies should be made to avoid frequent "off" times.

TABLE 12.4 Dopamine Agonists and Levodopa/Carbidopa

Generic (Brand)	Dosage Form	Route of Administration	Common Dosage
Apomorphine (Apokyn)	Injection	Sub-Q injection	2–6 mg
Bromocriptine (Parlodel)	Capsule, tablet	Oral	2.5–100 mg a day
Levodopa/carbidopa (Sinemet)	Tablet	Oral	Levodopa: 400–1,600 mg a day Carbidopa: 70–100 mg a day
Pramipexole (Mirapex)	Tablet	Oral	0.375–4.5 mg a day
Ropinirole (Requip)	Tablet	Oral	Extended release: 2–24 mg a day Immediate release: 0.75–3 mg a day

Side Effects Common side effects of dopamine agonists include dizziness, constipation, nausea, insomnia, daytime sleepiness, "sleep attacks," yawning, hallucinations, and mood elevations that increase risk-taking behavior, such as gambling. Taking these medications with food can alleviate upset stomach, but other side effects are difficult to treat.

Daytime sleepiness and "sleep attacks" may impair a patient's ability to drive or participate in daily activities. Patients should also avoid drinking alcohol because it will intensify these effects. Dopamine agonists should be used with caution in patients with preexisting sleep disorders.

Common side effects of levodopa/carbidopa include nausea and **dyskinesias**, which are abnormal, involuntary writhing movements of the arms, legs, neck, and mouth. Dyskinesias are associated with peak concentrations of levodopa in the bloodstream. They tend to occur 60 to 90 minutes after taking a dose. The only way to alleviate dyskinesias is to lower the dose or add adjunct drug therapy. Taking levodopa with food can help with nausea.

Bromocriptine is associated with soft tissue fibrosis, which can affect the heart valves and lung function. Thus, this drug is not used very often. Apomorphine can cause significant drops in blood pressure. Patients with orthostatic hypotension should not use this agent. A test dose may be given in a physician's office to see how the drug will affect a patient's blood pressure before self-injection at home.

Contraindications Apomorphine should not be administered intravenously, and its use is contraindicated in patients taking a serotonin (5-HT) antagonist. Bromocriptine should be avoided in patients with a hypersensitivity to ergot alkaloids. Use of levodopa/carbidopa is contraindicated in patients with narrow-angle glaucoma, recent monoamine oxidase inhibitor use, and melanoma or undiagnosed skin lesions. Pramipexole and ropinirole do not have contraindications.

Cautions and Considerations Apomorphine should not be taken along with antiemetic agents such as ondansetron, granisetron, or alosetron. If a patient complains of nausea and drug treatment is needed, other antiemetic medications should be used.

Apomorphine comes in a self-injector pen. The pharmacist needs to teach the patient how to use the pen if he or she has not been instructed already. Ampules and cartridges for the injector can be stored at room temperature. If syringes are prefilled with apomorphine, they can be stored in the refrigerator for one day.

Anticholinergics and Amantadine

These agents are used early in PD to treat mild symptoms (primarily tremors). They are used later in the disease progression as adjunct therapy for the movement side effects caused by levodopa. By blocking muscarinic receptors in the brain, **anticholinergics** help balance cholinergic activity and reduce tremors. **Amantadine**, an antiviral drug used for influenza, inhibits the reuptake of dopamine into presynaptic nerve endings. This inhibition allows more dopamine to accumulate in the synaptic cleft and stimulate more dopamine receptors. (See Table 12.5 for information on these drugs.)

TABLE 12.5 Anticholinergics and Amantadine

Generic (Brand)	Dosage Form	Route of Administration	Common Dosage
Amantadine (Symmetrel)	Capsule, syrup, tablet	Oral	200–400 mg a day
Anticholinergics			
Benztropine (Cogentin)	Injection, tablet	IM, IV, oral	1–2 mg a day
Trihexyphenidyl (Trihexy)	Elixir, tablet	Oral	6–15 mg a day

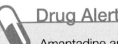

Drug Alert

Amantadine and amiodarone are considered look-alike drugs. When viewing a medication order, be vigilant for this potential medication mix-up. Amiodarone is used to treat cardiac arrhythmia, not PD.

Side Effects The use of amantadine can lead to orthostatic hypotension and peripheral edema; CNS effects such as agitation and anxiety; and gastrointestinal (GI) effects such as loss of appetite, constipation, and dry mouth. Amantadine also can cause the skin condition *livedo reticularis*. Common side effects of anticholinergics are anxiety, confusion/memory impairment, drowsiness, dry nose and mouth, blurred vision, constipation, rapid heartbeat, and difficulty urinating. These drugs also decrease sweating, making body heat regulation a potential problem. Heatstroke can occur easily.

Contraindications Benztropine use should be avoided in children younger than three years old. Amantadine and trihexyphenidyl do not have contraindications.

Cautions and Considerations Because these agents can cause drowsiness and confusion, patients should avoid alcohol, which can intensify these effects. Patients may also be advised to drink plenty of fluids and eat foods high in fiber to counteract the constipation these agents can cause.

COMT Inhibitors

As an adjunct therapy, **COMT inhibitors**, such as entacapone and tolcapone, help when levodopa starts to wear off at the end of each dosing interval. Typically, one of these agents (see Table 12.6) is given with each dose of levodopa to increase the amount of "on" time by one to two hours each day. Usually, the levodopa dose is decreased by approximately 100 mg a day when one of these drugs is added. This class of drug works by blocking an enzyme that metabolizes dopamine. COMT inhibitors boost the effects of levodopa and dopamine by allowing dopamine to remain present longer.

TABLE 12.6 COMT Inhibitors

Generic (Brand)	Dosage Form	Route of Administration	Common Dosage
Entacapone (Comtan)	Tablet	Oral	200–1,600 mg a day
Tolcapone (Tasmar)	Tablet	Oral	100–200 mg a day

Side Effects Common side effects of entacapone include worsening of dyskinesias, nausea, diarrhea, and abdominal pain. Orthostatic hypotension can also occur. Patients should rise slowly from a sitting position. They should take care in driving until they know how this drug will affect them. These effects may decrease over time.

Common side effects of tolcapone include orthostatic hypotension, dizziness, fainting, fatigue, strange dreams, headache, hallucination, stomach pain, loss of appetite, diarrhea, constipation, and nausea and vomiting. This medication has also been associated with movement disorders and muscle cramps. All of these effects must be monitored by a healthcare practitioner, so regular physician visits are essential.

Contraindications Entacapone does not have contraindications. Tolcapone is contraindicated in patients with liver disease.

Cautions and Considerations Entacapone can cause urine discoloration (urine may appear red, brown, or black), so warn patients of this sometimes alarming but harmless effect. Tolcapone can cause liver damage, so this medication should be used only when other drug therapies for PD fail.

MAOIs

Mild dopamine-boosting drugs that are used early on in disease progression or as adjunct therapy in advanced PD are **monoamine oxidase inhibitors (MAOIs)**. Rasagiline is often used for mild PD symptoms. Selegiline is usually used as adjunct therapy when levodopa begins wearing off. (See Table 12.7 for information on these drugs.) These agents block MAO, an enzyme that breaks down dopamine in neurons.

TABLE 12.7 **MAOIs**

Generic (Brand)	Dosage Form	Route of Administration	Common Dosage
Rasagiline (Azilect)	Tablet	Oral	0.5–1 mg a day
Selegiline (Eldepryl, Emsam, Zelapar)	Capsule, tablet, transdermal patch	Oral, transdermal	2.5–5 mg twice a day

Side Effects Common side effects of MAOIs include insomnia, confusion, hallucinations, euphoria, dizziness, and orthostatic hypotension. If a second dose is prescribed, patients should take it early in the afternoon to avoid insomnia. Rasagiline does not produce as much insomnia, so it is a good alternative to selegiline.

Contraindications Rasagiline should be avoided with concurrent use of other MAOIs, meperidine, methadone, tramadol, cyclobenzaprine, dextromethorphan, or St. John's wort. Selegiline should not be used with meperidine. Patients using the oral disintegrating tablet form of selegiline should not concurrently use dextromethorphan, methadone, tramadol, or other MAOIs. The transdermal form of selegiline is contraindicated in pheochromocytoma; concomitant use of bupropion, serotonin reuptake inhibitors, tricyclic antidepressants, tramadol, propoxyphene, methadone, dextromethorphan, St. John's wort, mirtazapine, cyclobenzaprine, oral selegiline and other MAOIs, carbamazepine, and oxcarbazepine; elective surgery requiring general anesthesia; use of sympathomimetics; foods high in tyramine (see "Cautions and Considerations" below); and supplements containing tyrosine, phenylalanine, tryptophan, or caffeine.

Cautions and Considerations MAOIs block the metabolism of **tyramine**, a substance in many aged and pickled foods. If tyramine concentrations rise high enough in the blood, they can raise the blood pressure to dangerous levels. Therefore, patients should be instructed to limit their intake of the following tyramine-rich foods and beverages:

- aged cheese
- beef
- beer
- peppers
- red wine
- sauerkraut
- sausage

Take a moment to review what you have learned so far and answer these questions.

1. What are the classes of drugs used to treat epilepsy and other seizure disorders?

2. What drugs are used to treat PD?

3. How are the various drugs prescribed to treat PD used together?

Dementia and Alzheimer's Disease

Alzheimer's disease is a form of **dementia** that affects more than 5 million people in the United States. Up to 250,000 people are diagnosed each year, and an individual's risk of developing Alzheimer's disease doubles for every 5 years over age 65. No clear cause of Alzheimer's disease has been identified, so it is diagnosed by ruling out all other causes of dementia.

 In the Know

Initial research has shown that individuals with high cholesterol levels seem to be at a greater risk for developing Alzheimer's disease. The use of "statins," a common class of drugs used to treat high cholesterol, has been linked to reduced dementia.

Alzheimer's disease is a degenerative brain disorder leading to loss of memory, intellect, judgment, orientation, and speech. Losing these higher brain functions causes patients with this disease to wander, become irritable or hostile, and experience changes in personality. Depression and anxiety are common in patients with Alzheimer's disease. Eventually, patients reach a "failure to thrive" level that causes death. This disease has no cure and poses difficult challenges to family members as they care for their loved ones.

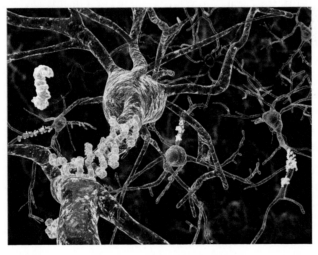

A hallmark of Alzheimer's disease, amyloid plaques (the white structures in this image) form between the neurons of the brain, damaging brain cells.

Drug Regimens and Treatments

Drug therapy for Alzheimer's disease does not alter the disease's progression. The goal of drug therapy is to maintain cognitive function and awareness for as long as possible. Unfortunately, few drugs are available to treat Alzheimer's disease (see Table 12.8).

TABLE 12.8 Alzheimer's Disease Drugs

Generic (Brand)	Dosage Form	Route of Administration	Common Dosage
Memantine (Namenda)	Oral solution, tablet	Oral	5–20 mg a day
Cholinesterase Inhibitors			
Donepezil (Aricept)	Tablet	Oral	5–23 mg a day
Galantamine (Razadyne)	Capsule, oral solution, tablet	Oral	8–24 mg a day
Rivastigmine (Exelon)	Capsule, oral solution, transdermal patch	Oral, transdermal	3–12 mg a day

Cholinesterase Inhibitors and Memantine

Cholinesterase inhibitors and memantine are used to treat mild symptoms early in disease progression and will not work once severe memory and functional loss have occurred. These agents work by inhibiting enzymes that break down **acetylcholine (ACh)**, a neurotransmitter thought to be deficient in early Alzheimer's disease. Later in the course of the disease, antidepressants can be used to treat depression, and benzodiazepines can be used to treat anxiety and sleep problems. Hallucinations may be treated with antipsychotic medications such as haloperidol.

Side Effects Common side effects of cholinesterase inhibitors include nausea, vomiting, agitation, rash, loss of appetite, weight loss, and confusion. These effects can be significant, so doses must be started low and increased slowly. If these effects do not ease with time or are particularly bothersome, the drug should be discontinued.

Some common side effects of memantine include dizziness, headache, sleepiness, constipation, vomiting, confusion, high blood pressure, and skin rash. If the patient experiences difficulty breathing, he or she should seek medical care immediately.

Contraindications Donepezil is contraindicated in patients with piperidine hypersensitivity. Contraindications to rivastigmine include hypersensitivity to related compounds and a history of application-site reaction to rivastigmine patch use. Memantine and galantamine do not have contraindications.

Cautions and Considerations Donepezil can interact with nonsteroidal anti-inflammatory drugs (NSAIDs), theophylline, and nicotine (through smoking). These substances should be avoided while taking donepezil. Patients with cardiac disease, liver problems, or PD should not take donepezil.

Memantine should be used with caution in patients with the following conditions: seizure disorder, heart disease, kidney disease, or liver disease.

ADHD

Attention-deficit/hyperactivity disorder (ADHD) has received a lot of media attention and carries with it many misconceptions about diagnosis and treatment. The condition is characterized by inattention, impulsivity, and hyperactivity. To be diagnosed with ADHD, an individual must exhibit six or more symptoms of inattention and six or more symptoms of hyperactivity/impulsivity that impair daily life in at least two settings for at least six months. Although many think environment and stressors cause someone to have ADHD, research has shown that these factors merely exacerbate the condition rather than cause it.

Some estimate that 3%–10% of school-aged children have some aspect of the disorder, whereas 5% of adults have ADHD. Onset occurs by age three and is more prevalent in boys. Although hyperactivity symptoms decline with age, the inattention and impulsivity can persist into adulthood for half of those who have this condition. Usually symptoms improve after puberty when the frontal lobe of the brain fully matures. Several other disorders can coexist with ADHD. Most often these disorders include learning disabilities and sometimes depression or anxiety. Proper diagnosis and assistance with any learning disabilities that may be present are important steps to take in helping children with ADHD perform in school. Counseling and behavioral strategies can help develop good coping mechanisms. When inadequate treatment and poor coping mechanisms occur, adults with ADHD can sometimes have problems with substance abuse. Therefore, ADHD and its coexisting conditions can be a difficult mix to treat effectively.

Drug Regimens and Treatments

Controversy around the use and misuse of drugs to treat ADHD has been a public argument. Some believe that ADHD is overdiagnosed and overmedicated. However, studies have shown drug therapy to be effective, if approached appropriately. The best results occur when drugs are used in conjunction with counseling or behavioral therapy. A dual approach also helps identify and treat coexisting conditions. Drug therapy for ADHD includes CNS stimulants as well as nonstimulant drugs. These medications have risks and should, consequently, be used judiciously.

CNS Stimulants

The first-line drug therapy for children and adults with ADHD is the use of **CNS stimulants**. These agents work best when used in conjunction with behavioral therapy. Dosing starts low and is increased until optimal improvement in symptoms is seen without side effects. Immediate-release products are usually tried first. The first dose is given before school (for children); if a second dose is needed, it will be given after school. (See Table 12.9 for more specific dosing information.) If longer effects are needed, extended-release products are used. Transdermal patches are applied in the morning, worn for nine hours, and then removed.

TABLE 12.9 Drugs for ADHD

Generic (Brand)	Dosage Form	Route of Administration	Common Dosage
Stimulants (Schedule II drugs)			
Amphetamine salts (Adderall, Adderall XR)	Capsule, tablet	Oral	5–40 mg a day
Dexmethylphenidate (Focalin, Focalin XR)	Capsule, tablet	Oral	5–40 mg a day
Dextroamphetamine (Dexedrine, ProCentra, Zenzedi)	Capsule, oral solution, tablet	Oral	5–40 mg a day
Methylphenidate extended-release (Concerta, Daytrana, Methylin, Quillivant XR, Ritalin LA or SR)	Capsule, oral solution, suspension, tablet, transdermal patch	Oral, transdermal	54–72 mg a day
Methylphenidate immediate-release (Ritalin)	Tablet	Oral	2 mg/kg/day or 60 mg
Nonstimulants (noncontrolled drugs)			
Atomoxetine (Strattera)	Capsule	Oral	40–100 mg a day

CNS stimulants work by enhancing the release and blocking the reuptake of dopamine and norepinephrine in presynaptic nerve cells. Increasing the levels of these neurotransmitters enhances executive functions, increases inhibition, improves attention, and allows for better focus. In effect, boosting these neurotransmitters dampens the "noise" patients with ADHD experience with thought and allows them to focus and concentrate. CNS stimulants can also help with self-control, aggression, and productivity. However, these agents may not help with reading skills, social skills, or academic achievement.

Drug Alert

Adderall, an ADHD drug, looks and sounds a lot like Inderal, a blood pressure medication. Likewise, atomoxetine, another ADHD drug, looks similar to atorvastatin, a high cholesterol medication. Be careful not to get these medications mixed up.

Side Effects Common side effects of CNS stimulants include headache, stomachache, loss of appetite, weight loss, insomnia, and irritability. Growth suppression in children has also been found to occur, so it is recommended that the prescriber monitor patient height and weight every three to six months. To minimize these effects, children are given a therapeutic holiday, where the drug is stopped when school is not in session. Although rare, liver dysfunction can occur with these agents. The drug should be stopped immediately if a patient develops jaundice, or yellowing of the eyes and skin.

Contraindications All stimulant and nonstimulant drugs used to treat ADHD mentioned in this chapter are contraindicated with or within 14 days of the use of MAOIs. Amphetamine salts, dextroamphetamine, and methylphenidate are contraindicated in patients with cardiovascular disease, high blood pressure, hyperthyroidism, glaucoma, and agitated states, and in patients with a history of drug abuse. Contraindications to dexmethylphenidate include high levels of anxiety, tension, and agitation; glaucoma; and motor tics or a diagnosis of Tourette's syndrome.

Drug Alert

Ritalin and all stimulant medications for ADHD are prescription drug therapies that have the potential for abuse. As cousins of methamphetamine, their action can mimic "speed." Individuals should never take these medications to improve performance or to stay awake for studying. The potential for addiction is real and dangerous.

Cautions and Considerations Rare but serious (even fatal) cardiac abnormalities have occurred with the use of CNS stimulants. Adderall XR should not be used in patients with cardiac abnormalities. All CNS stimulants are controlled substances (Schedule II) and have abuse and addiction potential. Therefore, no refills are allowed, and limited supplies can be given at a time.

Nonstimulant Drugs

Nonstimulant drugs are also used to treat ADHD. Atomoxetine (Strattera) is a good choice for addressing ADHD in a patient who has substance abuse problems because it does not have potential for abuse and, therefore, is not a controlled substance. Atomoxetine works by potentiating norepinephrine and/or dopamine in the brain, which, alone or in combination with CNS stimulants, helps patients increase their focus and curb their impulsivity. A typical dose is 100 mg a day. Patients should be aware that it can take up to two to four weeks to experience the full effect. Other nonstimulant agents, including antidepressants such as bupropion, desipramine, nortriptyline, and venlafaxine, may also be used (see Chapter 13). Clonidine and guanfacine are used when a patient has tics or insomnia as part of ADHD.

Side Effects Common side effects with atomoxetine are nausea, heartburn, fatigue, and decreased appetite.

Contraindications Atomoxetine should be avoided in patients with narrow-angle glaucoma, pheochromocytoma, and heart disorders.

Cautions and Considerations Atomoxetine can cause severe liver injury; therefore, laboratory tests will be conducted and results monitored for patients taking this medication. Patients with preexisting liver problems should avoid atomoxetine, if possible. Finally, atomoxetine has been associated with increased suicidal thoughts. Children and adolescents who are prescribed atomoxetine should be monitored closely. Patients with depression may not be good candidates for this drug therapy.

 ### Checkpoint 12.3

Take a moment to review what you have learned so far and answer these questions.

1. What cholinesterase inhibitors are used to treat Alzheimer's disease?
2. What symptoms are used to diagnose and monitor ADHD?
3. What drugs are used to treat ADHD?

Autonomic Nervous System

As mentioned earlier in this chapter, the autonomic nervous system controls involuntary and automatic body functions. This system is divided into the sympathetic nervous system and the parasympathetic nervous system. In a general sense, sympathetic and parasympathetic nerve stimulation have opposite effects on body functions (see Figure 12.6).

FIGURE 12.6 Autonomic Nervous System Anatomy and Effects

The autonomic nervous system regulates sweating (among other responses), which is decreased with parasympathetic activity and increased with sympathetic activity.

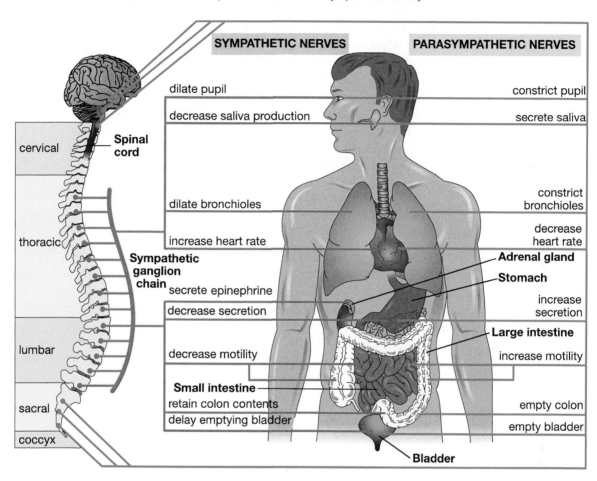

Sympathetic Nervous System

The sympathetic nervous system is responsible for a set of responses to stressful stimuli, which are collectively called the **"fight-or-flight" response**. This response occurs when an individual is confronted with a scary or surprising situation. The **adrenergic receptors** of the **sympathetic nerves** release the neurotransmitter **norepinephrine**, also known as *noradrenaline*, as part of this "fight-or-flight" response. (The one exception to the release of norepinephrine occurs at the sweat glands, where acetylcholine [ACh] is the neurotransmitter.) In addition, the adrenal medulla, a component of the autonomic nervous system, releases the hormone epinephrine into the bloodstream during the "fight-or-flight" response. These physiologic processes cause the heart and respiration rates to increase and the pupils to dilate in anticipation of the need to physically fight or flee immediately. Blood pressure also rises to increase circulation for a burst of activity.

Types of Adrenergic Receptors

Two subsets of adrenergic receptors include alpha receptors and beta receptors. Both subsets are activated by norepinephrine and epinephrine in the sympathetic part of the autonomic nervous system. **Alpha receptors** are found in the blood vessels and in the

GI tract. When stimulated, they constrict blood vessels, raising blood pressure. When they are blocked by drugs, blood pressure lowers. Consequently, alpha receptor blockers can be used to treat hypertension.

Beta receptors are divided into two types: beta-1 receptors and beta-2 receptors. **Beta-1 receptors** are found mostly within the heart. When stimulated, they increase heart rate and contraction force. When beta-1 receptors are blocked with drug therapy, heart rate slows and the demand for oxygen within the heart decreases. Beta-blocking medications decrease contractility in the heart, thus lowering blood pressure. **Beta-2 receptors** are found in the smooth muscle of arteries and bronchioles in the lungs and also in other tissues. When stimulated, these receptors cause blood vessels and bronchioles to dilate.

Sometimes, the goal of drug therapy is to stimulate both alpha and beta receptors. During cardiac arrest, severe shock, or anaphylactic reactions, it is necessary to increase heart rate, raise blood pressure, or dilate airways. Adrenergic agonist agents are used to exert these effects in urgent situations.

Parasympathetic Nervous System

The parasympathetic nervous system regulates restful body functions. When a person is relaxed or resting, his or her heart rate and breathing slow, digestion occurs, and the bladder and rectum are able to relax and release their contents. These functions are not desired during a frightening situation. **Parasympathetic nerves** have **cholinergic receptors**, and their primary neurotransmitter is ACh.

Drugs that Affect the Autonomic Nervous System

Most drugs that affect the autonomic nervous system are used to control blood pressure, heart rate, and benign prostatic hyperplasia (BPH). **Adrenergic inhibitors** block alpha and beta receptors; **adrenergic agonists** stimulate these receptors. Sometimes, these medications and their indications can be confusing to understand. Once you know what happens when alpha and beta receptors are stimulated, you can reason what happens when they are blocked and predict why specific agents are chosen. In many ways, blocking sympathetic action appears to cause parasympathetic effects.

Adrenergic Inhibitors

Because alpha and beta receptors are found in the blood vessels and heart, respectively, stimulating these receptors causes an increased heart rate, vasoconstriction, and elevated blood pressure. Activating alpha receptors also delays bladder emptying. Blocking these receptors with drugs causes an opposite reaction—a slowed heart rate and lowered blood pressure.

Alpha Blockers

The class of drugs known as **alpha blockers** is used primarily to treat hypertension (HTN). These drugs are especially useful in men who also have BPH, a condition in which the prostate enlarges with age.

Because alpha blockers delay bladder emptying, they are used to relieve urinary urgency and frequency associated with BPH (see Table 12.10).

Side Effects Common side effects seen with alpha blockers include headache, dizziness, nausea, and fatigue. Patients should avoid driving until they know how tired these medications can make them. Fortunately, these effects usually improve over time, as a patient gets used to the medication.

TABLE 12.10 Alpha Blockers

Generic (Brand)	Dosage Form	Route of Administration	Common Dosage
Doxazosin (Cardura)	Tablet	Oral	BPH: 1–8 mg a day HTN: 1–16 mg a day
Prazosin (Minipress)	Capsule	Oral	HTN: 2–20 mg a day, taken in divided doses
Terazosin (Hytrin)	Capsule, tablet	Oral	BPH: 1–10 mg a day HTN: 1–20 mg a day

Although rare, male patients have also experienced priapism (erection lasting longer than four hours) while taking alpha blockers. If this side effect occurs, patients should seek medical help right away because this condition can cause permanent impotence if left untreated.

Contraindications There are no contraindications to the alpha blockers listed in Table 12.10.

Cautions and Considerations Patients should be warned of significant hypotension and heart palpitations that can occur with the first few doses of these agents. Some physicians recommend that the first dose be taken in the office, with medical monitoring available. Symptoms of this effect are dizziness, light-headedness, and fainting. Patients should work with family members or others who can monitor them as they begin taking one of these medications. They should not drive or undertake hazardous tasks for 12 to 24 hours after taking their first dose. Drinking alcohol or taking verapamil can intensify the hypotensive effects and should be avoided when possible. If these symptoms occur, the patient should lie down until the symptoms pass and notify a physician. Doses can be adjusted slowly to minimize or avoid this effect.

Beta Blockers

Beta blockers are a class of drugs used to treat hypertension, **angina** (chest pain), and arrhythmias (see Table 12.11). In fact, beta blockers make up the entire **Class II of antiarrhythmic agents** (see Chapter 15). The volume of published research that supports their use and their low cost makes them an attractive and frequent choice for treating high blood pressure. Beta blockers are also recommended for heart attack patients because these agents reduce oxygen demands and stress on the heart. This benefit has been found to help prevent subsequent heart attacks. **Cardioselective beta blockers** (e.g., atenolol, esmolol, bisoprolol, betaxolol, and metoprolol) inhibit only beta-1 receptors in the heart. They are useful in treating angina and certain arrhythmias without causing bronchoconstriction. Another, less common use for beta blockers is as prophylaxis against migraine headache and mild anxiety. Ophthalmic formulation beta blockers are used to treat glaucoma (see Chapter 14).

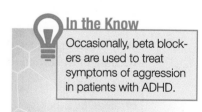

In the Know

Occasionally, beta blockers are used to treat symptoms of aggression in patients with ADHD.

Side Effects Common side effects for beta blockers include headache, dizziness, light-headedness, nausea, and fatigue/weakness. Patients should avoid driving until they know how these medications affect them. Fortunately, these effects generally improve over time as a patient gets used to the medication. This class of drugs has been associated with an increased incidence of depression. Patients who complain of depressive symptoms should be referred to their physicians for appropriate evaluation.

TABLE 12.11 Beta Blockers

Generic (Brand)	Dosage Form	Route of Administration	Common Dosage
Acebutolol (Sectral)	Capsule	Oral	400–800 mg a day
Atenolol (Tenormin)	Tablet	Oral	50–100 mg a day
Betaxolol (Kerlone)	Tablet	Oral	10–20 mg a day
Bisoprolol (Zebeta)	Tablet	Oral	5–20 mg a day
Carteolol (Cartrol)	Tablet	Oral	2.5–5 mg a day
Carvedilol (Coreg)	Capsule, tablet	Oral	Capsule: 10–80 mg once a day Tablet: 6.25–25 mg twice a day
Esmolol (Brevibloc)	Injection	IV	Varies depending on patient weight Infused over 1–4 min
Metoprolol (Lopressor, Toprol)	Injection, tablet	IV, oral	IV: 5 mg bolus every 2–5 min for 3 doses, then switch to oral Succinate oral: 50–100 mg a day Tartrate oral: 100–450 mg a day
Nadolol (Corgard)	Tablet	Oral	40–320 mg a day
Nebivolol (Bystolic)	Tablet	Oral	5–40 mg a day
Penbutolol (Levatol)	Tablet	Oral	20–80 mg a day
Pindolol (Visken)	Tablet	Oral	10–60 mg a day in divided doses
Propranolol (Inderal)	Capsule, injection, oral solution, tablet	IV, oral	Dose and frequency vary depending on indication/use
Sotalol (Betapace)	Tablet	Oral	80–160 mg twice a day
Timolol (Blocadren)	Tablet	Oral	10–40 mg twice a day

Beta blockers can sometimes slow the heart rate too much and exacerbate cardiac conditions such as angina, arrhythmia, and heart failure. Patients who experience difficulty breathing (especially with physical activity or when lying down), night coughing, or swelling of the extremities should seek medical attention right away.

Contraindications Beta blockers are contraindicated in bradycardia (slow heart rate), cardiogenic shock, and heart block. Specific beta blockers may have additional contraindications. For example, atenolol should not be used in patients with pulmonary edema or in pregnancy. Carteolol, carvedilol, propranolol, sotalol, and timolol are contraindicated in lung disorders such as asthma and chronic obstructive pulmonary disease (COPD). Carvedilol and nebivolol should not be used in patients with liver impairment. Sotalol should be avoided in patients with prolonged QT interval, kidney dysfunction, and low potassium levels.

Quick Study

As you can see in Table 12.11, many of the generic names of beta blockers end in –olol.

Cautions and Considerations Beta blockers can inhibit beta-1 receptors (which are located in the heart) and beta-2 receptors (which are found in the airways of the lungs). If beta-2 receptors are blocked, airways constrict and blood pressure lowers. This effect can be harmful to patients with impaired respiratory function—for example, those with asthma or COPD. For these individuals, care must be taken to choose drugs that selectively block beta-1 receptors only. Beta blockers that can be used by patients with asthma or COPD include metoprolol, acebutolol, betaxolol, bisoprolol, and atenolol.

Patient Teaching

Patients with diabetes should use beta blockers with caution. These drugs can inhibit the usual signs and symptoms of a reaction to low blood glucose. The only symptom of low blood glucose that a patient taking a beta blocker may have is sweating. Make sure patients with diabetes understand to look for this symptom as their clue that their blood glucose is dropping.

Abrupt withdrawal from a beta blocker can cause severe cardiac problems, such as heart attack, angina, or arrhythmia. Thus, patients should not stop taking a beta blocker suddenly. If a change in medication is made, the dose will be decreased slowly until the agent is discontinued.

Metoprolol works best when taken with food, thus decreasing the likelihood of upset stomach. Sotalol and propranolol can be taken without regard to food.

Over-the-counter decongestants are vasoconstrictors that can raise blood pressure. Patients taking beta blockers for high blood pressure should avoid taking oral decongestants.

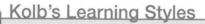

Kolb's Learning Styles

If you are a visual learner or enjoy learning in a group atmosphere (as Accommodators do), you might find that creating a graphic organizer of the adrenergic drugs and then using the graphic to quiz your classmates is a good way to learn this classification of drugs. For this activity, draw three circles: one for alpha receptors, one for beta-1 receptors, and one for beta-2 receptors. On scrap paper, write down all generic and brand-name drugs for alpha blockers, beta blockers, and adrenergic agonists. Then cut out each drug name individually. Work with a classmate to put each drug name into its appropriate circle and explain your reasoning out loud. Does a drug go in the beta-2 receptor circle because it stimulates or blocks receptor activity? Which drugs could be put into multiple circles? Explain why.

Adrenergic Agonists

Adrenergic agonists stimulate the autonomic nervous system to produce sympathetic activity, such as increased heart rate, bronchodilation, and elevated blood pressure. Depending on how they are used, these drugs can stimulate the heart to start beating again, open airways that are constricted, raise blood pressure when large amounts of blood have been lost, and constrict blood vessels to treat the swelling that occurs during sinus infections and severe allergic reactions.

Sympathomimetics and Vasopressors

Adrenergic agonists are sympathomimetics in that they mimic the effect of stimulating the sympathetic nervous system. Therefore, they are used in respiratory distress, allergic reactions, and sinus congestion. Ophthalmic versions of these agents are used to treat glaucoma.

Many adrenergic agonists also have vasopressor action, which increases the heart rate and blood pressure. They are used for cardiac arrest and shock situations. Dosing ranges vary, depending on how and why they are used (see Table 12.12).

Epinephrine is used as a sympathomimetic agent in severe allergic reactions. It opens airways to assist in breathing and constricts blood vessels to treat swelling during anaphylactic reactions. Patients with life-threatening allergies (such as to peanuts or bee stings) can keep a prefilled autoinjector with this medication on hand for when they are exposed and begin to have allergy symptoms. Epinephrine is used for anaphylactic reactions, during which swelling and closure of airways is possible, but not for simple skin rashes, hives, or itching allergies.

Epinephrine and phenylephrine are used topically in the nose as decongestants to reduce sinus swelling during respiratory infections (see Chapter 17). Ephedrine is used as an IV medication during surgery to support blood pressure and respiration.

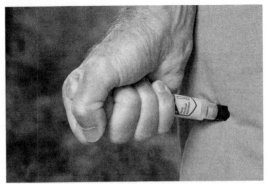

In an emergency, the EpiPen autoinjector allows the user to push the tip of the pen through clothing and inject the epinephrine into the upper thigh.

TABLE 12.12 Adrenergic Agonists

Generic (Brand)	Dosage Form	Route of Administration	Common Use(s)
Dobutamine	Injection	IV	Cardiac stimulation during cardiac arrest, shock, or surgery
Dopamine	Injection	IV	Cardiac stimulation during cardiac arrest or shock
Ephedrine	Capsule, injection	Oral, IV	Bronchodilation for asthma
Epinephrine (Adrenaline, EpiPen, Primatene)	Inhalation, nasal aerosol, solution for injection	Inhalation, IV, nasal, sub-Q	Bronchodilation for asthma Cardiac stimulation during cardiac arrest Anaphylactic reactions Nasal decongestant
Isoproterenol (Isuprel)	Injection	IV	Cardiac stimulation during cardiac arrest or shock Bronchospasm during anesthesia
Midodrine (ProAmatine)	Tablet	Oral	Orthostatic hypotension
Norepinephrine (Levophed)	Injection	IV	Restoration of blood pressure during cardiac arrest or shock
Phenylephrine (Anu-Med, Neofrin, Neo-Synephrine, Sudogest PE)	Liquid solution, nasal solution, ophthalmic solution, rectal cream/ointment, tablet	Nasal, oral, topical	Glaucoma, hemorrhoids, nasal congestion, pupil dilation

 Drug Alert

Dobutamine and dopamine are two adrenergic agonists that have look-alike, sound-alike names. Therefore, be sure to select the correct drug. Remember to verify the drug's expiration date as well. You don't want to find out in an emergency situation that your available drug stock is no longer effective.

Side Effects Common side effects of adrenergic agonists include headache, excitability, rapid heart rate, restlessness, and insomnia. A rare side effect is a drug-induced arrhythmia. Consequently, these medications are used only when needed.

Contraindications Dobutamine is contraindicated in patients with idiopathic hypertrophic subaortic stenosis. Dopamine should be avoided in patients with a hypersensitivity to sulfites, pheochromocytoma, and ventricular fibrillation. Ephedrine should be avoided in patients with glaucoma. Isoproterenol should be avoided in patients with chest pain and certain heart arrhythmias. Contraindications to midodrine include heart disease, kidney failure, urinary retention, pheochromocytoma, and high blood pressure when lying down. Norepinephrine is contraindicated in patients with a hypersensitivity to bisulfites or low blood pressure. There are no contraindications to epinephrine use.

Cautions and Considerations Adrenergic agonists are mostly handled by clinical staff members in the emergency department or critical care unit. These agents are often mixed as needed in the unit for cardiac code situations. Allied health professionals who work with these agents should be aware that they are mixed in dextrose solution, not normal saline. Some may be stocked in the emergency drug kits that are required to be on hand.

Epinephrine in the autoinjector form is increasingly prescribed and dispensed in an outpatient setting. The pharmacist will need to counsel patients or their caregivers on how to inject this medication in times of severe allergic reaction. It should be injected into the thigh, not the buttocks. The autoinjector contains only one dose, so a refill will be needed once it is used. When dispensing, healthcare personnel should alert patients or caregivers to the expiration date. If a patient does not use the medication by the expiration date, he or she should return the device for a refill. That way, the device is ready if needed.

 Checkpoint 12.4

Take a moment to review what you have learned so far and answer these questions.

1. How do alpha blockers and beta blockers differ in action?

2. What specific disorders are treated by alpha blockers and beta blockers?

3. What are the common side effects of beta blockers?

Drugs that Affect the Parasympathetic System

Drugs that block cholinergic activity in the parasympathetic nervous system may produce **anticholinergic side effects** in patients. These side effects include dry mouth, dry eyes, constipation, urinary retention, and elevated blood pressure. Depending on a patient's medical condition, these effects could be problematic. For instance, patients with urinary difficulty (e.g., BPH) or bowel problems (e.g., irritable bowel syndrome or constipation) should not use drugs with anticholinergic side effects.

Opioid pain medications (see Chapter 25) and bladder spasticity agents (see Chapter 22) are drugs that cause significant anticholinergic side effects—constipation and dry mouth, respectively. These side effects are the basis for many drug-disease interactions.

Herbal and Alternative Therapies

Ginkgo biloba may have a modest benefit for patients with early Alzheimer's disease, but serious side effects (e.g., bleeding, seizures, and coma) have occurred with its use. Results of studies are inconclusive and do not necessarily show dramatic improvement in memory or thinking. It is questionable whether taking ginkgo biloba actually prevents Alzheimer's disease, although many patients take it for this purpose. If patients choose to take ginkgo biloba, they should clearly realize the risks and benefits.

Typical doses are 120–720 mg ginkgo extract, and commercially available products vary in their content. Ginkgo biloba has antiplatelet effects that affect bleeding. Patients taking warfarin or aspirin for coagulation effects should not use ginkgo biloba without medical supervision. This supplement also interacts with several other prescription medications, particularly anticonvulsants. Therefore, patients who take other prescription medications should discuss taking ginkgo biloba with their prescribers and pharmacists before doing so.

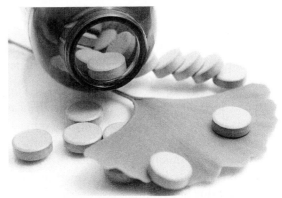

One of the oldest types of trees in the world, the gingko bilboa produces fan-shaped leaves that are used to make tablets, capsules, and teas.

Dietary supplements that contain **ephedra**, also called **ma huang**, were banned from sale in the United States in April 2004. This plant (*Ephedra sinica*) contains ephedra alkaloids (like ephedrine), which boost physical activity, suppress appetite, and promote weight loss. Ephedra can also cause heart palpitations, tremors, and insomnia. Deaths from cardiac arrest have occurred as a result of using this dietary supplement.

Chapter Review

Chapter Summary

The nervous system is categorized into the central nervous system and the peripheral nervous system as well as the autonomic and somatic nervous systems. Certain disorders are associated with different parts of the nervous system.

CNS disorders include PD, Alzheimer's disease, and ADHD. Seizure disorders are CNS conditions in which signals in the brain become sporadic. Seizures vary in their presentation, and a variety of antiepileptic drugs are used to control them. Side effect profiles are considerable for antiepileptic drugs. PD is a deficiency of dopamine in the brain and usually occurs with increasing age. Drugs used to treat PD include dopamine agonists, anticholinergics, and COMT inhibitors. Alzheimer's disease is a type of dementia. Cholinesterase inhibitors and memantine are drugs that can be used to enhance cognitive function early in the disease, but their effects are usually short-lived. ADHD is usually diagnosed during childhood and involves symptoms of inattention, impulsivity, and hyperactivity. CNS stimulants are used to control brain activity and allow patients to focus and learn. These agents are controlled substances requiring special handling.

The autonomic nervous system controls functions of the body typically considered to be reflexive or automatic. This system is divided into sympathetic and parasympathetic actions. Sympathetic actions are associated with increased heart rate, bronchodilation, elevated blood pressure, and pupil dilation. Parasympathetic actions include promoting digestion, urination, and relaxation. The drugs that affect the sympathetic nervous system, alpha and beta blockers, are usually prescribed to control blood pressure, heart rate, and airway openness. Adrenergic agonists (such as dobutamine and isoproterenol) trigger sympathetic action and are used to stimulate the heart in cardiac arrest or shock situations. Epinephrine is used in anaphylactic reactions to open airways and relieve severe swelling. When parasympathetic activity is inhibited, anticholinergic effects including constipation and dry mouth can occur. Many drugs have these side effects.

Ginkgo biloba is used to treat memory loss and may be helpful in Alzheimer's disease. Ephedra (ma huang) is an herbal product that has sympathomimetic activity and was banned from sale in the United States. It was used for weight loss, but it caused severe cardiac problems and even death in some patients.

Chapter Checkup

The Navigator+ learning management system that accompanies this textbook offers many opportunities to help you master chapter content, including end-of-chapter exercises, a glossary of key terms, flash cards, and additional interactive activities.

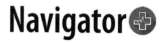

Navigator

Career Exploration

If you enjoyed learning about the nervous system in this chapter, you may want to explore the following career options:

- computed tomography (CT) technician
- dementia care specialist
- magnetic resonance imaging (MRI) technician
- medical assistant
- neurodiagnostic technologist
- nuclear medicine technologist
- pharmacy technician
- positron emissions tomography (PET) scan technician
- registered nerve conduction studies technologist (RNCST)
- surgical neurophysiologist for intra-operative neurophysiology monitoring

CHAPTER

13

The Nervous System and Drug Therapy for Psychiatric and Mood Disorders

Pharm Facts

- Researchers in Sweden have determined that highly creative individuals are more likely to have mental health disorders. In fact, the works of several famous artists—including Vincent van Gogh's *Starry Night*, Edvard Munch's *The Scream*, and Pablo Picasso's *The Old Guitarist*—reflect the artists' bouts with severe depression.

- Although the statistics on insomnia vary widely, the condition is quite common. A recent survey of primary care patients reported that 69% had insomnia.

- Affecting 18% of the US population, anxiety is the most common mental illness. However, only one-third of those affected seek treatment.

- According to the National Alliance on Mental Illness, one-half of chronic mental health disorders begin by age 14.

- Seasonal affective disorder, a type of depression, affects approximately 5% of the US population during the fall and winter months,when natural light wanes. Affected individuals have increased melatonin levels in their bloodstream and are treated with light therapy to reduce these levels.

"I have always been curious about the functions of sleep—an activity that accounts for approximately one-third of an individual's life span. From my research in sleep and circadian physiology, I have learned that there is a vast number of health and safety consequences related to insufficient sleep and circadian misalignment. Sleep can be just as important as good nutrition and physical activity. Although neurocognitive consequences of insufficient sleep are well documented, continued research is needed to fully understand the relationship between sleep and circadian disorders and an individual's overall health and well-being."

—**Tina M. Burke**, PhD, CPhT
Pharmacy Technician Program Director/Faculty

Learning Objectives

1   Understand the basic anatomy and physiology of neurotransmission as it relates to psychiatric and mood disorders.

2   Describe the most common psychiatric and mood disorders.

3   Explain the therapeutic effects of prescription medications and non-prescription medications commonly used to treat psychiatric and mood disorders.

4   Identify the generic names, brand names, indications, dosage ranges, side effects, contraindications, and cautions and considerations associated with the drugs commonly used to treat psychiatric and mood disorders.

5   Identify common herbal and alternative therapies that are related to the treatment of psychiatric and mood disorders.

Psychiatrists, psychologists, and counselors are not the only healthcare professionals who see and treat patients with mental illness. Healthcare professionals in all settings encounter medications used to treat psychiatric and mood disorders on a regular basis. Managing these patients requires special care and sensitivity.

This chapter begins with a description of how neurotransmitters work and how deficiencies in these neurotransmitters can result in mental illness. Next, specific disorders—including depression, anxiety, bipolar disorder, and schizophrenia—are described. Drug therapies used in the treatment of these various conditions include selective serotonin reuptake inhibitors (SSRIs), sedatives, and atypical antipsychotic agents. Insomnia, a sleep disturbance, is also addressed in this chapter. Similar drug classes are used to treat both insomnia and anxiety.

Anatomy and Physiology of Neurotransmission

As you recall from Chapter 12, **neurotransmitters** are chemicals that are responsible for transmitting signals from nerve cell to nerve cell within the brain. Neurotransmitters such as **serotonin**, **norepinephrine**, and **dopamine** are released from one cell, cross the **synaptic cleft** between cells, and connect with receptors on the membranes of adjacent cells to create **signal conduction** (see Figure 13.1). Neurotransmitters are then either taken back up into the presynaptic nerve cell (a process called **reuptake**) or broken down by metabolic enzymes while in the cleft. **Monoamine oxidase** is one enzyme that breaks down neurotransmitters in neurons.

Disorders affecting mood and mental function are related to deficiency or dysfunction of neurotransmitters, although research is ongoing to elucidate brain pathophysiology. For instance, depression is related to a deficiency or dysfunction of neurotransmitters such as serotonin and norepinephrine. Psychoses, including schizophrenia, are connected to an overabundance of the neurotransmitter dopamine. Drug therapy is used to manipulate levels of neurotransmitters by either mimicking their actions or altering the processes that eliminate them from the synaptic cleft.

FIGURE 13.1 Signal Conduction across the Synaptic Cleft

Blocking the breakdown or reuptake of neurotransmitters allows them to remain in the synaptic cleft longer and activate more receptors.

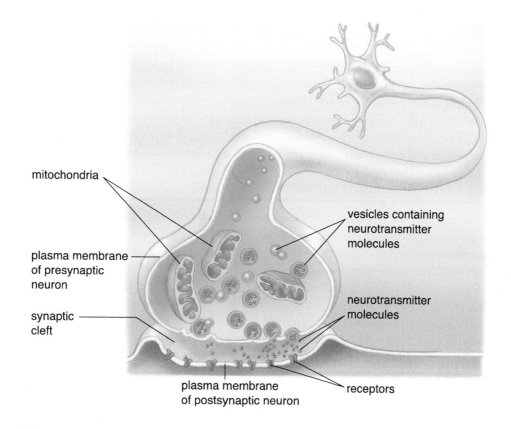

mitochondria

vesicles containing neurotransmitter molecules

plasma membrane of presynaptic neuron

neurotransmitter molecules

synaptic cleft

plasma membrane of postsynaptic neuron

receptors

Common Psychiatric and Mood Disorders

Mental health conditions such as depression, anxiety, bipolar disorder, and schizophrenia can be difficult to diagnose properly and often occur together in various combinations in the same patient. For instance, an individual with anxiety can often have symptoms of depression. A patient with bipolar disorder usually has some component of depressive symptoms but can also have symptoms of mania or even overt psychosis during an exacerbation. Sometimes, multiple medications are needed to manage symptoms. Therefore, managing these conditions with medications can be complex and requires good communication among the patient, family or caregivers, prescribers, and the pharmacist.

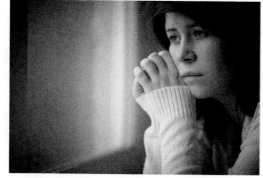

According to the World Health Organization, more than 350 million individuals worldwide have depression—the majority of whom are women.

Depression

Depression is a leading health concern; treatment for this condition accounts for several of the top 50 prescription medications in the United States. Depression can result from external (exogenous) sources, such as a response to the death of a loved one, or have internal (endogenous) origins that lack logical, observable reasons for occurrence. In both cases, counseling can be helpful and necessary. **Endogenous depression** is more likely to require drug therapy to control. Neurotransmitters involved in mood include norepinephrine, serotonin, and dopamine. Signs of depression include crying (often without obvious cause), loss of interest in life or social activities, increased focus on death, and significant weight loss or gain. Symptoms that patients express are low self-esteem, pessimism, sleep disturbances (insomnia or hypersomnia), loss of energy and ability to think, feelings of worthlessness and guilt, confusion, poor memory, and thoughts of **suicide**.

Drug Regimens and Treatments

Drug therapy for depression includes selective serotonin reuptake inhibitors (SSRIs), serotonin-norepinephrine reuptake inhibitors (SNRIs), tricyclic antidepressants (TCAs), monoamine oxidase inhibitors (MAOIs), bupropion, and trazodone (see Figure 13.2). It may take three to six weeks for a patient to experience the full effects of one of these antidepressants. Therefore, a genuine drug therapy trial should last at least three to four weeks, and doses should be changed only once a month (absent serious or intolerable side effects) under the guidance of the prescriber. Patients should understand that changes in mood and relief from symptoms do not occur immediately.

Teens and young adults are at an increased risk for suicide, especially when starting therapy with an antidepressant. Such patients should be monitored closely for worsening symptoms of depression, suicidal thoughts, and unusual behaviors. Families and caregivers of these young patients should communicate with their prescribers as therapy begins and is adjusted appropriately.

Antidepressants should not be stopped abruptly. Patients may experience worsened depression symptoms if they stop taking an antidepressant without gradually decreasing the dose. Some agents are associated with acute withdrawal symptoms when stopped abruptly. If patients want to stop therapy, they should talk with their prescribers to determine an appropriate plan.

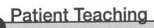 Patient Teaching

> Patients would like it if antidepressants worked immediately, but it is important for them and their caregivers to realize that it takes three to six weeks for these medications to achieve full effect. Encourage them to be patient and to give the drugs time to work. Antidepressants will help with sleep problems within a week or so, but the other psychiatric effects take longer to achieve full efficacy.

SSRIs and SNRIs

First-line therapy for depression includes **selective serotonin reuptake inhibitors (SSRIs)** and **serotonin-norepinephrine reuptake inhibitors (SNRIs)**. These medications are listed in Table 13.1. SSRIs block serotonin reuptake into the presynaptic neuron, and SNRIs block reuptake of both serotonin and norepinephrine.

FIGURE 13.2 Prozac and Cymbalta Medication Labels

Fluoxetine (Prozac), an SSRI, and duloxetine (Cymbalta), an SNRI, are two well-known medications used to treat depression.

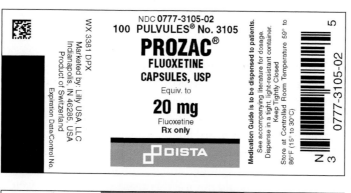

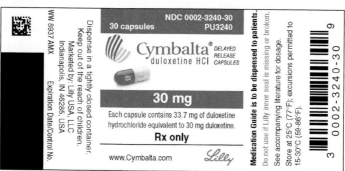

TABLE 13.1 Common SNRIs and SSRIs

Generic (Brand)	Dosage Form	Route of Administration	Common Dosage
SNRIs			
Desvenlafaxine (Pristiq)	Tablet	Oral	50 mg a day
Duloxetine (Cymbalta)	Capsule	Oral	20–60 mg a day
Levomilnacipran (Fetzima)	Capsule	Oral	20–120 mg a day
Venlafaxine (Effexor)	Capsule, tablet	Oral	75–375 mg a day
SSRIs			
Citalopram (Celexa)	Oral solution, tablet	Oral	10–40 mg a day
Escitalopram (Lexapro)	Oral solution, tablet	Oral	5–20 mg a day
Fluoxetine (Prozac, Sarafem)	Capsule, oral solution, tablet	Oral	10–80 mg a day
Fluvoxamine (Luvox)	Capsule, tablet	Oral	25–150 mg a day
Paroxetine (Paxil)	Capsule, suspension, tablet	Oral	10–60 mg a day
Sertraline (Zoloft)	Oral concentrate, tablet	Oral	50–200 mg a day

SSRIs are also used to treat obsessive-compulsive disorder and premenstrual dysphoric disorder. **Obsessive-compulsive disorder (OCD)** is a form of anxiety wherein obsessive thoughts intrude on daily consciousness and impair function. Patients engage in repetitive behaviors, such as hand washing and counting, in an attempt to relieve fears and anxiety.

Premenstrual dysphoric disorder (PMDD) is marked by emotional and behavioral changes during the second half of a woman's menstrual cycle. Although some symptoms are similar to premenstrual syndrome (PMS), PMDD is more severe and life altering.

SSRIs may also be used to treat posttraumatic stress disorder (PTSD), fibromyalgia, anxiety, and panic disorder. Duloxetine is indicated for depression and is also often used to treat nerve pain.

Side Effects SNRIs are commonly associated with nausea, vomiting, insomnia, agitation, and drowsiness. Common side effects of SSRIs include nausea, vomiting, dry mouth, drowsiness, insomnia, headache, and diarrhea. These side effects can subside over time, but if bothersome, a different agent may be prescribed. Most of these agents can also cause sexual dysfunction, including decreased libido, inability to achieve orgasm, or impaired ejaculation. In fact, sexual dysfunction is a frequent reason that patients stop therapy.

Fluoxetine can also cause weight loss and is sometimes used to treat eating disorders, including bulimia. Patients should not use this agent simply to lose weight.

Contraindications SNRIs and SSRIs are contraindicated with the use of MAOIs intended to treat psychiatric disorders. SNRIs and SSRIs should not be started in patients who are receiving linezolid or intravenous (IV) methylene blue. Desvenlafaxine is contraindicated in patients with a hypersensitivity to venlafaxine. Levomilnacipran is contraindicated in patients with a hypersensitivity to milnacipran and in those individuals with narrow-angle glaucoma. Pimozide use is contraindicated with SSRIs. Fluoxetine, fluvoxamine, and sertraline should not be used with thioridazine. Fluvoxamine use is contraindicated with alosetron, ramelteon, and tizanidine.

➕ *Note: Allied health professionals should be aware that an allergy to a particular drug contraindicates its use. This warning applies to all Contraindications sections in this chapter.*

Cautions and Considerations SNRIs and SSRIs have been associated with an increased risk of suicide in the first few weeks of therapy, especially in pediatric and adolescent patients. Patients should be monitored closely, particularly until the drug's full effects are experienced. Patients should be offered counseling and psychotherapy in addition to medication.

Because SSRIs increase serotonin levels, they increase the risk for **serotonin syndrome**, a potentially fatal medical condition. This syndrome occurs when too much serotonin is present, causing changes in cardiovascular function and even heart attack, in severe cases. The risk for serotonin syndrome is particularly high for patients taking more than one antidepressant or taking St. John's wort, an herbal product sold to treat depression. If patients experience the combination of a racing heart rate, fever, high blood pressure, and headache, which may be signs of serotonin syndrome, they should seek immediate medical attention.

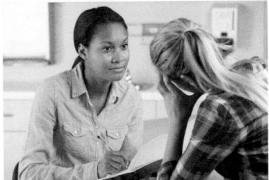

Teenagers who are taking antidepressants must be monitored closely by healthcare professionals for signs of suicidal thoughts or worsening depression.

TCAs

Tricyclic antidepressants (TCAs) get their name from their chemical structure, which contains three rings. TCAs block reuptake of norepinephrine and/or serotonin. TCAs are sometimes prescribed for insomnia because their primary side effect is drowsiness.

Consequently, they can be an effective choice for therapy when a patient's depression symptoms include insomnia. TCAs are also used to treat nerve pain and to prevent migraine headaches. A tetracyclic agent is also included in this class. As the name indicates, tetracyclic agents have a fourth ring in their chemical structure. Drug activity and properties are similar for tricyclic and tetracyclic agents (see Table 13.2 for dosage information on tricyclic and tetracyclic agents). Prior to the availability of SSRIs, TCAs were the most widely prescribed class of antidepressants.

TABLE 13.2 Common TCAs

Generic (Brand)	Dosage Form	Route of Administration	Common Dosage
Tricyclic Agents			
Amitriptyline (Elavil)	Tablet	Oral	30–300 mg a day
Clomipramine (Anafranil)	Capsule	Oral	25–75 mg a day
Desipramine (Norpramin)	Tablet	Oral	75–200 mg a day
Doxepin (Silenor)	Capsule, oral solution, tablet	Oral	25–150 mg a day
Imipramine (Tofranil)	Capsule, tablet	Oral	75–200 mg a day
Nortriptyline (Aventyl, Pamelor)	Capsule, oral solution	Oral	25–100 mg a day
Tetracyclic Agent			
Mirtazapine (Remeron)	Oral disintegrating tablet, tablet	Oral	15–45 mg a day

Side Effects The most common side effect of TCAs is drowsiness, so patients should take these drugs at bedtime. Other common side effects include anticholinergic effects (e.g., dry mouth, blurred vision, constipation, and urinary retention). Some of these agents can cause **priapism**, an erection lasting longer than four hours. If priapism occurs, the patient should seek medical attention immediately.

Contraindications TCAs should not be used with MAOIs because serotonin syndrome could develop. If a TCA is not working and an MAOI must be tried, the TCA must be discontinued for two weeks prior to initiation of an MAOI. This time in between therapies is called a **washout period**.

Amitriptyline, clomipramine, desipramine, and imipramine are contraindicated in the phase immediately after a heart attack. Clomipramine, desipramine, imipramine, and mirtazapine are contraindicated in patients using linezolid or IV methylene blue. Doxepin should not be used in patients with glaucoma or urinary retention.

Cautions and Considerations TCAs can cause cardiotoxicity and heart arrhythmias. Patients with preexisting heart conditions or who have recently had a heart attack should exercise caution when taking TCAs. These drugs can also cause orthostatic hypotension (a drop in blood pressure on sitting or standing up). Patients should take care to change positions slowly—that is, from a supine position to a seated position, or from a seated position to a standing position.

TCAs can lower the seizure threshold, so most patients with seizure disorders should not take these drugs. Because these agents can also cause liver toxicity, patients with liver problems should be cautious when taking TCAs. Periodic blood tests are required to monitor liver function.

An overdose of TCAs can be fatal, so prescriptions written for a large supply of medication all at once can be dangerous. Pharmacists may be resistant to filling such prescriptions for patients at risk for suicide. Be aware that many prescribers are also wary of warning patients that an overdose could be lethal because that message could suggest a pathway to suicide. It is important for healthcare prescribers to assess a patient's risk for suicide when prescribing these antidepressants.

MAOIs

Monoamine oxidase inhibitors (MAOIs) are not used as often as they once were. Other drug therapies with fewer side effects and drug interactions are available, so MAOIs are reserved as a last resort to treat intractable depression symptoms. MAOIs work by inhibiting one of the primary enzymes that metabolizes neurotransmitters, which results in increased neurotransmitter levels in the synaptic cleft. (See Table 13.3 for common dosage information.)

TABLE 13.3 **Common MAOIs**

Generic (Brand)	Dosage Form	Route of Administration	Common Dosage
Isocarboxazid (Marplan)	Tablet	Oral	10–60 mg a day
Phenelzine (Nardil)	Tablet	Oral	45–90 mg a day
Tranylcypromine (Parnate)	Tablet	Oral	30–60 mg a day

Side Effects MAOIs can cause heart palpitations and orthostatic hypotension. Patients should take care to change positions slowly—that is, from a supine position to a seated position, or from a seated position to a standing position. Other side effects include dizziness, headache, tremors, insomnia, anxiety, restlessness, agitation, and anticholinergic effects (e.g., dry mouth, blurred vision, constipation, and urinary retention). These side effects frequently cause patients to discontinue therapy.

Contraindications MAOIs have many contraindications. These agents should not be used in patients with cardiovascular disease, cerebrovascular defect, a history of headache or liver disease, pheochromocytoma, or severe kidney impairment. In addition, MAOIs are contraindicated with the use of antihistamines, blood pressure medications, bupropion, buspirone, caffeine (excessive use), depressants (such as alcohol), dextromethorphan, diuretics, general anesthesia, meperidine, other MAOIs or TCAs, carbamazepine, SNRIs, SSRIs, spinal anesthesia, sympathomimetics, and foods high in tyramine content.

Cautions and Considerations These agents interact with numerous other drugs. When patients are taking an MAOI, they should work closely with their physicians and pharmacists to manage any additional prescription or over-the-counter (OTC) medications they want to take.

MAOIs also interact with **tyramine**, a substance found in aged and pickled foods. This interaction causes serotonin syndrome, a life-threatening condition involving a rapid heart rate, high blood pressure, headache, and fever. Patients who take MAOIs should avoid consuming foods and beverages containing tyramine such as aged cheeses, beer, wine, and sauerkraut and other pickled foods.

Bupropion

The antidepressant **bupropion** blocks the reuptake of dopamine primarily, but it also weakly blocks the reuptake of serotonin and norepinephrine. In addition to treating depression, bupropion is used as adjunct therapy for **smoking cessation** and anxiety. The bupropion generic product and the brand-name versions Wellbutrin and Zyban are all produced as tablets for oral administration, with a common dosage of 300 mg a day.

Side Effects Bupropion can cause headache, agitation, weight loss, and insomnia. Taking doses early in the day can help with insomnia.

Contraindications Bupropion is contraindicated in patients with seizures and in individuals who have a history of anorexia or bulimia. This drug is also contraindicated in patients who are undergoing abrupt discontinuation of ethanol or sedatives, using MAOIs, or using linezolid or IV methylene blue. The Aplenzin form of bupropion should not be used in conditions that increase seizure risk.

Cautions and Considerations Patients who have been prescribed this medication should not take it with alcohol or other drugs that cause central nervous system (CNS) depression (such as opiate pain medications). The extended-release tablets should not be chewed or crushed.

Trazodone

Trazodone (Oleptro) is a widely used antidepressant, but its mechanism of action is not fully understood. It may affect serotonin reuptake. Trazodone is used to treat depression with insomnia because its predominant side effect is drowsiness. This medication is often used for neuralgic pain and sometimes anxiety that affects sleep. In addition, this medication is used in alcohol- and cocaine-withdrawal regimens. Doses typically range from 50–300 mg a day.

> **Work Wise**
>
> It is best to treat patients with psychiatric disorders just the same as you would any other patient: with empathy and respect. Try not to overreact to unusual behaviors.

Side Effects Common side effects are often associated with trazodone's sedative effect, which is usually a desired effect, but can cause confusion, dizziness, headache, fatigue, blurred vision, and muscle aches and pains. Patients should talk with their prescribers if these effects are bothersome. Trazodone can also cause anger or hostility, fainting, or nervousness. Patients should stop taking trazodone and contact their prescribers right away if any of these side effects occur.

Contraindications Trazodone is contraindicated in patients using MAOIs. In addition, trazodone should not be given to a patient receiving linezolid or IV methylene blue.

Cautions and Considerations If trazodone is to be used in combination with other antidepressants such as SNRIs, SSRIs, TCAs, or MAOIs, the patient should be monitored closely for symptoms of serotonin syndrome. Therapy should be stopped immediately if any of the following symptoms occur, especially if in combination: fever, agitation, hallucinations, racing heart rate, flushing, tremors, diarrhea, or nausea and vomiting. Trazodone has been associated with a serious and potentially fatal cardiac arrhythmia called **torsades de pointes**. Patients with a history of heart disease should be cautious about taking trazodone. Trazodone has also been associated with lowering blood pressure and subsequent fainting. Therefore, it should be used with caution in combination with antihypertensive medications.

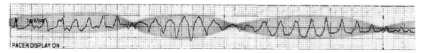

Torsades de pointes is a French term meaning "twisting of the points," as shown by the loops (not points) on this electrocardiography (ECG) strip. The outline of the arrhythmia on an ECG strip resembles a twisted party streamer, as shown by the green shading. Similar to ventricular fibrillation, *torsades de pointes* can be fatal.

Trazodone can interact with many other medications and OTC products:

- alcohol
- antidepressants (SNRIs, SSRIs, TCAs, and MAOIs)
- antifungals (itraconazole, ketoconazole)
- carbamazepine
- ginkgo biloba
- macrolide antibiotics (clarithromycin or erythromycin)
- phenytoin
- warfarin

Consequently, patients should check with their prescribers and pharmacists before taking these products in combination with trazodone.

Kolb's Learning Styles

If you are a learner who prefers to work with concrete information and details, as Assimilators and Convergers do, you may find creating a table of antidepressants useful. Make one column for each major drug class of antidepressants. Include a row for the mechanism of action and list the neurotransmitter(s) on which each class works. List all generic and brand drug names under each class; then use this table as a reference for studying and memorizing.

Checkpoint 13.1

Take a moment to review what you have learned so far and answer these questions.

1. What classes of drugs are used to manage depression?
2. Which drugs inhibit the reuptake of serotonin?
3. What are the side effects of TCAs?

Anxiety

Anxiety is associated with the abnormal function of the neurotransmitters that regulate brain activity, mood, and the fear response. The brain has natural benzodiazepine receptors that help regulate neurotransmitters. Serotonin and norepinephrine are also involved.

Anxiety is a constellation of symptoms categorized into two main types: panic disorder and generalized anxiety disorder. Other types, including phobic disorders and OCD, are treated with similar drugs.

Panic disorder is characterized by symptoms such as chest pain, difficulty breathing, palpitations, dizziness, sweating, a choking sensation, trembling, and unrealistic feelings of doom. These feelings and symptoms occur in the absence of typical stimuli such as physical activity, life-threatening situations, or fearful events. The onset of these symptoms is sudden and quick, often described as an "attack." A formal diagnosis of panic disorder is made when a patient experiences at least three panic attacks in three weeks.

Generalized anxiety disorder is defined as excessive worry that causes significant distress or disturbance to work or social functioning and that continues for at least six months. Symptoms of worry include restlessness, irritability, difficulty concentrating, muscle tension, sleep disturbances, and fatigue. Unlike panic disorder, these symptoms are constant and do not subside. They can become debilitating and interfere with a patient's normal life activities.

Posttraumatic stress disorder (PTSD) is a variation of anxiety. It is prevalent among military personnel returning from combat zones. PTSD occurs in response to a traumatic event after which a reexperiencing syndrome continues for at least a month. Reexperiencing symptoms include avoidance behavior in which the patient avoids thoughts, conversations, activities, people, or places he or she would normally enjoy. This behavior has a numbing effect, and the patient often displays a **flattened affect** (diminished facial expression, lack of appearance of emotion). Avoidance behavior is coupled with hyperarousal symptoms including sleep disturbances, an exaggerated startle reflex, irritability, outbursts, and difficulty concentrating. Treatment for PTSD is similar to that for other anxiety disorders in that both counseling and drug therapy are used to maintain control and normal function.

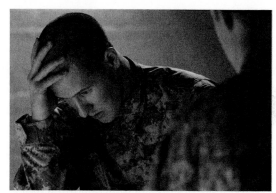

According to the Institute of Medicine, 8% of veterans from the US conflicts in Iraq and Afghanistan have PTSD.

Drug Regimens and Treatments

Anxiety often requires drug therapy, but counseling is useful to address contributing factors. A **hypnotic** is a term for a medication that is used to induce sleep. A **sedative** is used to diminish symptoms of anxiety and cause relaxation. For panic disorder, agents with sedative effects, such as benzodiazepines, may be useful for short-term treatment. For generalized anxiety disorder, benzodiazepines typically are necessary. SSRIs are often used to treat PTSD and generalized anxiety disorder.

Benzodiazepines

Commonly used drugs for generalized anxiety disorder are **benzodiazepines**. These agents are also used to treat panic disorder and PTSD. They are regularly used as preanesthetic medications to calm patients prior to procedures such as colonoscopy or surgery (see Chapter 25). Benzodiazepines are also part of the standard treatment for alcohol withdrawal symptoms and status epilepticus (see Chapter 12).

Benzodiazepines work by stimulating omega receptors in the CNS, thereby causing drowsiness and relaxation. When used to treat anxiety, benzodiazepines have a calming and sometimes euphoric effect. When used for sleep, they reduce the time it takes to fall asleep, decrease early morning wakening, and generally improve sleep quality (see Table 13.4 for dosage information).

TABLE 13.4 Common Benzodiazepines

Generic (Brand)	Dosage Form	Route of Administration	Common Dosage
Alprazolam (Xanax)	Oral disintegrating tablet, oral solution, tablet	Oral	1–6 mg a day
Chlordiazepoxide	Capsule	Oral	15–100 mg a day
Clonazepam (Klonopin)	Oral disintegrating tablet, tablet	Oral	0.5–20 mg a day
Clorazepate (Tranxene)	Tablet	Oral	15–60 mg a day
Diazepam (Valium)	Injection, oral solution, rectal gel, tablet	IM, IV, oral, rectal	IM, IV, PO: 4–40 mg a day Rectal: 0.2 mg/kg (20 mg a day max)
Lorazepam (Ativan)	Injection, oral solution, tablet	IM, IV, oral	IM, IV: dosing varies widely by indication PO: 1–10 mg a day
Oxazepam	Capsule	Oral	30–120 mg a day
Temazepam (Restoril)	Capsule	Oral	7.5–30 mg a day
Triazolam (Halcion)	Tablet	Oral	0.125–0.5 mg a day

Side Effects Common side effects of benzodiazepines include muscle weakness, impaired reflexes, and constipation. Patients may also experience difficulty waking up in the morning and residual drowsiness the following day. The pharmacy should affix an auxiliary warning label about drowsiness to each benzodiazepine prescription.

Other concerning effects include drowsiness, oversedation, and respiratory depression (slowed breathing). Patients should be informed of these effects and notify their physicians if they occur. In settings where patients taking benzodiazepines can be observed, such as an inpatient or long-term care facility, caregivers should monitor these patients for slowed breathing and excessive sleepiness. Patients should not drink alcohol or take other medications that cause sedation (e.g., opiate pain medications) because excessive sedation and drastically slowed breathing can occur. Breathing can slow to the point of causing death.

Contraindications Alprazolam is contraindicated in patients with narrow-angle glaucoma and in individuals taking ketoconazole or itraconazole. Clonazepam should not be used in patients with acute narrow-angle glaucoma or liver disease. Clorazepate is contraindicated in narrow-angle glaucoma. Contraindications to diazepam include myasthenia gravis, respiratory insufficiency, liver disease, sleep apnea, and acute narrow-angle glaucoma. Lorazepam is contraindicated in acute narrow-angle glaucoma, sleep apnea, and respiratory insufficiency. Temazepam contraindications include narrow-angle glaucoma and pregnancy. Triazolam is contraindicated in pregnancy and should not be used with itraconazole, ketoconazole, or nefazodone. Chlordiazepoxide and oxazepam do not have contraindications.

Cautions and Considerations All benzodiazepines have dependence and abuse potential. Consequently, they are considered Schedule IV controlled substances. Patients can become both physically and psychologically dependent on benzodiazepines, making it difficult to stop therapy. Patients should be aware of this potential and should understand that benzodiazepines should be used only for a short time. If used for longer than a couple of weeks, doses must be slowly tapered to avoid withdrawal symptoms. Because they are controlled substances, benzodiazepine prescriptions have a limited number of refills and may have specific storage requirements. You should be familiar with regulations and follow your facility's policies and procedures for dispensing benzodiazepines at your practice site.

Patients with heart conditions may not be able to take benzodiazepines and should be monitored closely. These medications can increase heart rate.

Drug Alert

Patients who consistently request refills of benzodiazepines a few days early could be exhibiting physical or psychological dependence. Alert the prescriber if you receive frequent refill authorization requests from the pharmacy as this could be a sign that dependence is developing. Some patients may need help to stop taking these drugs and may benefit from intervention.

Buspirone

A preferred antianxiety medication, **buspirone** works by blocking serotonin receptors in the brain. It is preferred because it is not a controlled substance and does not cause euphoria as do benzodiazepines. Buspirone is available as tablets for oral administration and is commonly dosed at 15–60 mg a day. Unlike benzodiazepines, which can be taken episodically, buspirone must be taken on a regular basis to be effective.

Side Effects Common side effects of buspirone include drowsiness, dizziness, headache, and nausea, all of which may decrease over time. More serious effects include hostility, depression, serotonin syndrome, and extrapyramidal symptoms such as tremors, muscular rigidity, difficulty initiating movement (akinesia), motor restlessness, and constant movement of the limbs. (To learn more about extrapyramidal symptoms, see the section titled "Typical Antipsychotics" later in this chapter.) Patients who experience these effects should see their healthcare practitioners right away.

Contraindications Buspirone does not have contraindications.

Cautions and Considerations Buspirone has been associated with depression and increased suicidal tendencies. Patients taking this medication should be monitored closely. Counseling should accompany buspirone therapy when warranted. Because buspirone interacts with MAOIs and may cause elevated blood pressure, concomitant use should be discouraged.

Insomnia

Insomnia is the inability to fall asleep (sleep latency) or stay asleep (sleep maintenance). It often is a symptom of depression, anxiety, and other mental disorders. Sometimes other medical conditions, such as gastric reflux disease, have an impact on the ability to sleep. Other disorders that affect sleep include obstructive sleep apnea, restless legs syndrome, and narcolepsy. However, insomnia is usually a reaction to a stressful situation and simply a disruption in the normal sleep cycle.

Drug Regimens and Treatments

Treatment for insomnia begins with identifying and eliminating external or medical causes, followed by implementing good **sleep hygiene** (bedtime habits that promote quality sleep). Drug therapy is a last resort for treatment of insomnia, and even then should be used on a short-term basis.

Drug therapy options begin with OTC antihistamines. Diphenhydramine and hydroxyzine cause drowsiness. These agents may be useful for individuals who need short-term assistance with falling asleep. However, they are not necessarily effective long-term treatment choices for insomnia. TCAs also cause drowsiness and are sometimes used for insomnia, especially if it accompanies depression.

Nonpharmacologic therapy for insomnia includes setting a consistent time for going to bed and waking, using the bedroom only for sleeping, increasing physical activity during the day but not close to bedtime, reducing alcohol and caffeine consumption and cigarette use, eliminating naps, and stopping medications that can affect sleep. If sleep problems continue for longer than two weeks, the patient should see a healthcare practitioner.

Sleep Aids

Ramelteon, a sleep aid, is a selective melatonin agonist that works by mimicking **melatonin**, one of the body's natural sleep/wake cycle hormones (see Figure 13.3). Eszopiclone, zaleplon, and zolpidem are sleep aids that are used exclusively for insomnia. They are shorter acting than are benzodiazepines and do not cause as much residual drowsiness the next day. In some cases, these agents can be taken in the middle of the night when frequent awakening is a problem (see Table 13.5).

Side Effects   Common side effects of eszopiclone, zaleplon, and zolpidem include headache, drowsiness, dry mouth, dizziness, nausea, hallucinations, and memory loss. These agents should be used only short term so that such effects do not pose a long-term problem. Some sleep aids can cause facial and tongue swelling and difficulty breathing. If patients experience swelling, they should seek medical attention right away. A warning label about drowsiness and caution when driving should be affixed to sleep aid containers. Although rare, sedatives can cause sleepwalking, and talking and eating while sleepwalking.

Contraindications   Ramelteon is contraindicated with concurrent use of fluvoxamine. The other sleep agents listed in Table 13.5 do not have contraindications.

FIGURE 13.3	Pineal Gland

The pineal gland, a small endocrine gland in the brain, produces melatonin, a hormone that affects the body's sleep/wake cycle. Low levels of this natural hormone can be supplemented with the use of ramelteon.

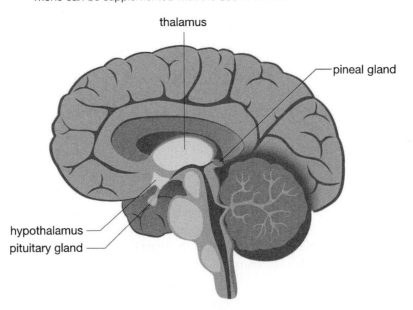

TABLE 13.5 | Common Prescription Sleep Aids

Generic (Brand)	Dosage Form	Route of Administration	Common Dosage	Dispensing Status
Eszopiclone (Lunesta)	Tablet	Oral	1–3 mg a day	Schedule IV
Ramelteon (Rozerem)	Tablet	Oral	8 mg 30 min prior to bedtime	Rx
Zaleplon (Sonata)	Capsule	Oral	5–20 mg a day	Schedule IV
Zolpidem (Ambien)	Oral solution, sublingual tablet, tablet	Oral	5–12.5 mg 30 min prior to bedtime	Schedule IV

Cautions and Considerations Like the benzodiazepines, eszopiclone, zaleplon, and zolpidem are controlled substances. They should be prescribed for two weeks or less due to their addictive properties. Ramelteon is not a controlled substance, but it should not be taken with or immediately following a high-fat meal. It interacts with many other prescription drugs that are metabolized through the liver; therefore, healthcare personnel should be sure to have a thorough medication history for all patients taking ramelteon. Patients with liver problems should discuss use of ramelteon with their healthcare practitioners before taking it.

Checkpoint 13.2

Take a moment to review what you have learned so far and answer these questions.

1. What drug classes are used to treat anxiety?

2. What drug classes are used to treat insomnia?

3. What are the brand names of the benzodiazepines?

4. What are the generic names of the prescription sleep aids?

Bipolar Disorder

Bipolar disorder is related to the dysfunction of neurotransmitters such as γ-aminobutyric acid (GABA), serotonin, and norepinephrine. This disorder is characterized by periods of depression alternating with periods of **mania**, during which the patient exhibits irritability, elevated mood, excessive involvement in work or other activities, grandiose ideas, racing thoughts, and a decreased need for sleep. Patients vary in how much they experience mania versus depression. Patients with bipolar disorder can struggle with psychotic features such as thought disorders, hallucinations, or delusions. For example, half of patients with bipolar disorder will have at least one psychotic feature at least once in their lifetime. Frequently, other psychiatric disorders coexist with bipolar disorder.

In the Know

Several famous performing artists who have been diagnosed with bipolar disorder have become advocates for individuals with this mental health condition. Carrie Fisher, Catherine Zeta-Jones, Patty Duke, Demi Lovato, and Britney Spears have all discussed their struggles with bipolar disorder. Other highly creative individuals are thought to have had this disorder, including famous authors Mark Twain and Virginia Woolf.

Acute bipolar mood episodes are treated based on presenting symptoms. Patients generally require maintenance treatment following remission of acute bipolar episodes. This treatment plan is necessary because recurrent bipolar episodes are associated with a greater number of suicide attempts, poorer social and occupational functioning, and potential treatment resistance. Maintenance therapy usually consists of agents that were successful in treatment of the acute episode.

Lithium is a commonly prescribed drug in the treatment of bipolar disorder. It works best when used in conjunction with psychotherapy, counseling, or cognitive behavioral therapy. Valproic acid (see Chapter 12) and lamotrigine, traditionally thought of as anticonvulsants, are also commonly used. Antidepressants and some antipsychotic medications can also be used in the treatment of bipolar disorder, but close monitoring is required.

Name Exchange

Lithium has been around for so long that it is typically referred to by its generic name rather than the brand name (Lithobid).

Lithium

Lithium works by altering sodium transport in nerve cells that affect neuronal metabolism in the brain, which has a mood-stabilizing effect. Lithium is available in tablet, capsule, and solution forms for oral administration and is commonly dosed at 900–1,800 mg a day. Several atypical antipsychotic agents may be used instead of lithium to treat bipolar disorder. In patients with bipolar disorder, mood stabilizer therapy must accompany antidepressants during depressive episodes.

Side Effects Common side effects that can occur when initiating therapy include dry mouth, thirst, fine hand tremor, and mild nausea. These effects usually subside with continued treatment. Patients taking lithium sometimes complain of fatigue, mental dullness, somnolence, and impotence. These side effects may be chronic; therefore, patients should discuss these effects with their prescribers before stopping therapy on their own. Symptoms associated with elevated levels of lithium in the blood include diarrhea, vomiting, muscular weakness, slowed heart rate, low blood pressure (which can result in fainting), blackouts, incontinence, frequent urination, confusion, and hallucinations. If any of these effects occur, patients should seek medical attention right away.

Contraindications Contraindications to lithium include severe cardiovascular or kidney disease, dehydration, and sodium depletion.

Cautions and Considerations Lithium can become toxic, even in doses at the upper end of the normal dosing range, so regular laboratory tests to check blood concentration levels are needed to appropriately dose and monitor therapy. Lithium should be used with caution in patients with kidney disease, cardiovascular disease, or dehydration, as these conditions could increase the risk of lithium toxicity. Patients taking diuretics or angiotensin-converting enzyme (ACE) inhibitors should be cautious when taking lithium, as these medications could also increase the risk of lithium toxicity. Patients taking nonsteroidal anti-inflammatory drugs (NSAIDs) or thyroid hormone with lithium should be monitored closely.

The National Alliance on Mental Illness (NAMI) has designated a lime green ribbon to promote mental health awareness. The organization is hoping to erase the stigma of mental health disorders by encouraging conversation about the topic.

Schizophrenia and Psychosis

The pathophysiology of **schizophrenia** is not fully understood. Although schizophrenia is related to an imbalance of various neurotransmitters, the processes associated with dopamine and serotonin have been studied the most. In general, schizophrenia comprises **positive symptoms** (including hallucinations and delusions) and **negative symptoms** (including withdrawal, ambivalence, behavior changes, memory loss, and confusion). Negative symptoms are associated with thought disorders in which the patient displays language and communication that is illogical, contradictory, irregular, distracting, and tangential. Onset of symptoms usually occurs in the teenage or early adult years. Most often, drug therapy is necessary for patients to maintain normal thought and function. Drugs are usually successful in treating positive symptoms but may not always completely eliminate negative symptoms.

A **psychosis** is a loss of connection with reality. Patients experiencing psychosis may have delusions, hallucinations, unusual behaviors, and disorganized thinking. Schizophrenia is one of a variety of psychotic disorders. A few of these related conditions include (1) **reactive psychosis**, which occurs briefly, lasting from only a few hours to just under a month, and then subsides; (2) **delusional disorder**, which is characterized by delusional (but not necessarily illogical) thoughts that last longer than a month but do not impair normal function; and (3) **schizophreniform disorder**, which involves symptoms that are similar to those of schizophrenia but occur for less than six months. Patients with dementia can also display psychotic symptoms. Psychosis can also be caused by drugs. When symptoms continue for more than six months and are not the result of illicit or prescription drug use, a formal diagnosis of schizophrenia is made.

Drug Regimens and Treatments

Drug therapy for schizophrenia is highly individualized and often requires changing therapies over time. Doses are slowly increased over weeks to months and then adjusted to achieve a balance between the control of symptoms and minimal side effects. Typical antipsychotics are discussed first in the following section because they have been available longer than have atypical agents. However, their side-effect profiles are problematic and often dose limiting. Usually, patients are given atypical agents first.

Typical Antipsychotics

The mechanisms of action of **typical antipsychotic agents** vary and are not fully understood. However, many drugs in this category are phenothiazines or thioxanthenes, which block dopamine. Blocking dopamine activity reduces abnormal thoughts and hallucinations but does not always affect other behavior characteristics of schizophrenia, such as withdrawal and ambivalence. Two antipsychotics have alternative uses: Haloperidol is used to treat Tourette's syndrome, and prochlorperazine is used in low doses to treat nausea and vomiting (see Table 13.6 for more information).

Many of these medications are used to treat agitation and delirium in patients who do not have schizophrenia. In these cases, lower doses are prescribed to minimize side effects. However, prescribers must be careful about giving these agents to elderly patients in long-term care. Dementia and its related effects, such as irritability, confusion, and delirium, are common in this patient population. Elderly patients taking antipsychotics (typical or atypical) are at an increased risk of mortality from cardiovascular and infectious events.

TABLE 13.6 Typical Antipsychotics

Generic (Brand)	Dosage Form	Route of Administration	Common Dosage
Chlorpromazine (Thorazine)	Capsule, injection, tablet	IM, IV, oral	IM: 200–800 mg a day IV: dosing varies by indication PO: 30–800 mg a day
Fluphenazine (Prolixin)	Injection, oral solution, tablet	IM, oral	IM: 12.5–25 mg every 2–4 weeks PO: 2.5–20 mg a day
Haloperidol (Haldol)	Injection, oral solution, tablet	IM, IV, oral	IM: 50–200 mg every 4 weeks IV: dosing varies by indication PO: 0.5–30 mg a day
Perphenazine (Trilafon)	Tablet	Oral	4–64 mg a day
Prochlorperazine (Compazine)	Capsule, injection, suppository, syrup, tablet	IM, IV, oral, rectal	IM: 10–40 mg a day IV: dosing varies by indication PO: 15–40 mg a day
Thioridazine	Tablet	Oral	100–800 mg a day
Trifluoperazine	Tablet	Oral	2–20 mg a day

Antipsychotics can cause excessive dizziness and drops in blood pressure and thus can increase the risk of falls. Reduced kidney and liver functions in elderly patients slow the elimination of these drugs. Thus, smaller doses are necessary, and patients must be monitored closely for falls. Laws and regulations govern the use of antipsychotic agents in long-term care settings and limit their use in patients who are simply wandering, calling out, or agitated. A true medical need, such as behavior that is harmful to the patient or to others, should be present for these agents to be used appropriately in elderly patients.

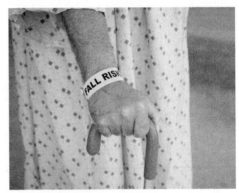

In some healthcare facilities, elderly patients taking antipsychotics are identified by a fall risk identification wristband.

Side Effects Common side effects of typical antipsychotics include sedation, dizziness, constipation, dry mouth, blurred vision, weight gain, photosensitivity, and changes in sexual desire or function. Taking these medications at bedtime can help with drowsiness, an effect that improves with time. Decreases in blood pressure, especially on standing or sitting up, can occur. Patients should rise slowly after sitting or lying down. Older patients should be especially careful until they know how these medications will affect them. An auxiliary label that warns patients about drowsiness should be affixed to an antipsychotic medication container.

Typical antipsychotics can cause **extrapyramidal symptoms (EPS)** or **EPS effects**. Such effects include tremors, muscular rigidity, and difficulty initiating movement (akinesia). Women tend to have motor restlessness and constant movement of the limbs. These unusual movements can make normal activities difficult and embarrassing. Because EPS effects occur mostly at higher doses, dose amounts are slowly increased. The intention of use of these agents is to gain relief from schizophrenia symptoms without causing significant EPS effects. To reduce EPS effects, patients are sometimes given benzodiazepines or anticholinergic drugs such as benztropine (Cogentin) or diphenhydramine.

Another concerning side effect is **tardive dyskinesia**. This late-onset effect causes uncontrollable tongue thrusting and lip smacking. This effect is not always dose dependent and can even show up months after discontinuing therapy with a typical antipsychotic. It is sometimes permanent, so typical antipsychotic agents are saved as second-line therapy for schizophrenia.

Contraindications The typical antipsychotics should not be used in patients with severe CNS depression or coma. Contraindications to fluphenazine use include brain damage and liver disease. Haloperidol is contraindicated in Parkinson's disease. Perphenazine and trifluoperazine should not be used in patients with bone marrow suppression or liver damage. Contraindications to prochlorperazine use include pediatric surgery and children younger than two years. Thioridazine should not be used in patients with heart disease or in combination with drugs that prolong the QT interval or drugs that inhibit thioridazine metabolism.

Cautions and Considerations Some typical antipsychotics can cause arrhythmias and alterations in heart function called QT-wave prolongation. These effects can be problematic for patients with heart disease or for those individuals who take other drugs that also have this effect. Close cardiac monitoring is necessary.

Patients with liver or kidney problems should avoid taking typical antipsychotics, if possible. Typical antipsychotics may also cause bone marrow suppression, a rare but serious effect that may result in underproduction of blood cells. Regular laboratory tests are necessary to monitor for this effect.

Patients should not drink alcohol while taking antipsychotic medications because excessive sedation and hallucinations can occur. The pharmacy should affix an auxiliary warning label about avoiding alcohol to the containers of these medications.

Atypical Antipsychotics

The mechanisms of action for **atypical antipsychotics** are not fully understood and vary among agents. Some block dopamine and others enhance it. Atypical antipsychotics are first-line therapy for schizophrenia and other psychoses. Each agent has a variable effectiveness for individual patients. If one agent does not work, others are tried until a medication and dosage is found to provide symptom control (see Table 13.7). Unlike typical antipsychotics, atypical antipsychotics may be effective for the negative symptoms of schizophrenia.

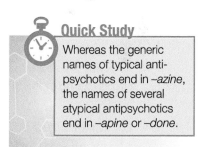

Quick Study

Whereas the generic names of typical antipsychotics end in –*azine*, the names of several atypical antipsychotics end in –*apine* or –*done*.

Side Effects Side effects are similar to those of typical antipsychotics, but their incidence is lower. Common side effects of atypical antipsychotics include drowsiness, headache, constipation, dry mouth, urinary incontinence or retention, rash, excitation, and, occasionally, frequent hiccups. Taking these medications at bedtime can help with drowsiness, an effect that gets better with time. Atypical antipsychotic agents can cause EPS effects, but to a much lesser extent than do typical antipsychotic agents. Quetiapine can increase a patient's risk for cataracts, so regular eye examinations are necessary.

Decreases in blood pressure, especially when changing to a standing or seated position, can also occur. Patients should rise slowly after sitting or lying down. Older patients should be especially careful until they know how these medications will affect them.

Significant weight gain occurs for many patients on these medications. This weight gain is often associated with high cholesterol levels and new-onset diabetes. Many patients on atypical antipsychotic agents will need medication for Type 2 diabetes.

TABLE 13.7 Atypical Antipsychotics

Generic (Brand)	Dosage Form	Route of Administration	Common Dosage
Aripiprazole (Abilify)	Injection, oral disintegrating tablet, oral solution, tablet	IM, oral	IM: 5.25–15 mg every 2 hr (30 mg a day max) PO: 10–30 mg a day
Clozapine (Clozaril)	Oral disintegrating tablet, oral suspension, tablet	Oral	25–500 mg a day
Olanzapine (Zydis, Zyprexa)	Injection, oral disintegrating tablet, tablet	IM, oral	IM: 150–300 mg every 2 weeks or 300–405 mg every 4 weeks PO: 5–20 mg a day
Paliperidone (Invega)	Injection, tablet	IM, oral	IM: 39–234 mg every 4 weeks PO: 6–12 mg a day
Quetiapine (Seroquel, Seroquel XR)	Tablet	Oral	300–800 mg a day
Risperidone (Risperdal)	Injection, oral disintegrating tablet, oral solution, tablet	IM, oral	IM: 25–50 mg every 1–2 weeks PO: 1–8 mg a day
Ziprasidone (Geodon)	Capsule, injection	IM, oral	IM: 10 mg every 2 hr or 20 mg every 4 hr (40 mg a day max) PO: 40–160 mg a day

Drug Alert

Zyprexa (an atypical antipsychotic agent) and Celexa (an SSRI) have sound-alike drug names. A mix-up with these drugs could produce undesirable consequences for a patient.

Some atypical antipsychotics can cause arrhythmias and QT-wave prolongation. These effects can be problematic in patients with heart disease. Close cardiac monitoring is necessary.

Contraindications Clozapine should not be used in patients with clozapine sensitivity or a history of clozapine-induced agranulocytosis or severe granulocytopenia. Paliperidone should not be used in patients with risperidone hypersensitivity. Contraindications to ziprasidone include a known history of QT prolongation, recent acute myocardial infarction (MI), uncompensated heart failure, and concurrent use of other drugs that prolong the QT interval (including amiodarone, arsenic trioxide, chlorpromazine, disopyramide, dofetilide, dolasetron, droperidol, gatifloxacin, halofantrine, ibutilide, levomethadyl, mefloquine, moxifloxacin, pentamidine, pimozide, procainamide, quinidine, sotalol, tacrolimus, or thioridazine). Aripiprazole, olanzapine, and risperidone do not have contraindications.

Drug Alert

Clozapine is associated with severe blood disorders affecting blood cell growth and development. Patients who are prescribed clozapine are required to have regular laboratory blood work.

Cautions and Considerations Atypical antipsychotics can lower the seizure threshold, so patients with seizure disorders must be monitored closely when taking these medications. Patients with liver or kidney problems should avoid taking atypical antipsychotics, if possible. Some atypical antipsychotics can cause bone marrow suppression, a rare but serious effect. Regular laboratory tests are necessary to check for this condition.

Atypical antipsychotics should be used with caution in elderly patients because excessive dizziness, drops in blood pressure, and sedation can cause falls. Elderly patients taking antipsychotics (typical or atypical) are at an increased risk of mortality from cardiovascular and infectious events. Due to reduced kidney and liver functions, elderly patients cannot effectively eliminate these medications. Smaller doses are necessary, and patients must be monitored closely for falls.

Because patients at any age who have schizophrenia or psychosis can have thought disorders, it is important for patients to be monitored closely and offered counseling or psychotherapy in addition to drug treatment.

Patients should not drink alcohol while taking atypical antipsychotic medications because excessive sedation and hallucinations can occur. The pharmacy should affix an auxiliary warning label about alcohol use to the containers of these medications.

Paliperidone comes in extended-release tablets only. Consequently, these tablets should not be chewed or crushed.

Kolb's Learning Styles

If you are a learner who enjoys group discussion and problem solving, as Accommodators and Divergers do, find a few classmates and name all of the side effects for typical and atypical antipsychotic agents. Have you ever witnessed these effects? Share which ones would be most concerning if you had to take one of these drugs yourself.

Checkpoint 13.3

Take a moment to review what you have learned so far and answer these questions.

1. What drug(s) are used to treat bipolar disorder?

2. What are the generic names of atypical antipsychotic medications used to manage schizophrenia?

3. What are the side effects of commonly used atypical antipsychotic medications?

Herbal and Alternative Therapies

Melatonin is used for sleep and insomnia disorders, as well as for benzodiazepine and nicotine withdrawal. It is used occasionally for a variety of other disorders including headache. Melatonin is a naturally produced hormone that helps regulate circadian rhythms (the sleep/wake cycle). People generally take 1–5 mg before bedtime to induce sleep. Common side effects include drowsiness, headache, and dizziness. Melatonin can also cause mild tremor, anxiety, abdominal cramps, irritability, confusion, nausea, and low blood pressure. Melatonin interacts with other medications; it should never be taken with CNS depressants, as excessive sedation could occur.

Kava is used to treat anxiety and insomnia. It has been found to be effective but dangerous. Kava can induce hepatotoxicity and liver failure, so patient self-treatment is not recommended. Kava lactone is the active ingredient and is thought to work by affecting GABA and dopamine in the brain. Other side effects include upset stomach, headache, dizziness, drowsiness, dry mouth, and EPS. Patients should also realize that herbal, dietary, and other supplements are not subject to standardization among manufacturers as are prescription and OTC drugs.

In the Know

Evidence of the healing properties of St. John's wort dates back to ancient Greek civilizations in which inhabitants would place the herb in their homes or at the base of statues of Greek gods to ward off evil spirits.

St. John's wort is taken orally for mild depression with some success. It has also been used to relieve the psychological symptoms of menopause when used with black cohosh (Remifemin). The active ingredient in St. John's wort is hypericin, which has activity similar to that of SSRIs. Common starting doses range from 300–400 mg three times a day. Maintenance doses are often lower and may range from 300–900 mg a day. Side effects include insomnia, vivid dreams, restlessness, anxiety, irritability, upset stomach, diarrhea, fatigue, dry mouth, dizziness, and headache. Usually these effects are mild. St. John's wort can cause photosensitivity, so proper skin protection should be used.

This herbal supplement should not be taken with other antidepressants because serotonin syndrome could develop. In addition, it should not be taken with CNS depressants, digoxin, phenytoin, or phenobarbital. St. John's wort can alter the effectiveness of these and other drugs, including warfarin and some HIV/AIDS drugs. Patients should discuss St. John's wort with their healthcare practitioners before taking it, and its usage should be documented in their medication histories.

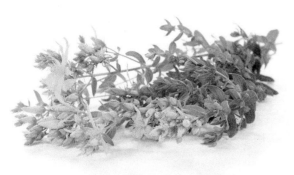

The leaves and yellow flowers of St. John's wort are used to make a medicinal supplement for the treatment of depression.

SAMe is used to treat mild depression and osteoarthritis. It may also be effective for fibromyalgia. SAMe is produced naturally in the body and supports neurotransmitter formation. It also has anti-inflammatory effects. For depression, dosing is 400–1,600 mg a day. For osteoarthritis, the dose is 200 mg three times a day. Common side effects include gas, nausea, vomiting, diarrhea, constipation, dry mouth, headache, mild insomnia, anorexia, sweating, dizziness, and nervousness. However, this product is usually well tolerated. SAMe should never be taken with other antidepressants.

Patients taking natural products for mood disorders or insomnia should discuss this therapy with their healthcare practitioners. Herbal and dietary supplements may not adequately treat symptoms of depression or insomnia. Patients who display symptoms of mental illness should be evaluated by a physician and should not be self-treated. Encourage patients to communicate with their healthcare practitioners.

Chapter Review

Chapter Summary

Mental illness is pervasive throughout the health-care system, and medications used for these conditions are frequently handled by allied health professionals. Depression is so common that drugs used to treat it are among the top 50 most commonly dispensed drugs in the United States. Medications used for depression primarily include SSRIs, TCAs, and MAOIs.

Anxiety is categorized into panic disorder and generalized anxiety disorder. Benzodiazepines, controlled substances with addiction and abuse potential, are used most often for anxiety. They can also be used for insomnia, but normally nonpharmacologic and OTC remedies are tried first.

Ramelteon is a prescription agent for insomnia that enhances melatonin. Other prescription sleep aids include eszopiclone, zaleplon, and zolpidem.

Lithium is the drug of choice for bipolar disorder. Drugs for schizophrenia and psychosis are categorized as typical and atypical antipsychotics. Usually, patients are given atypical agents first. Antipsychotic agents have significant side effects, such as EPS effects and tardive dyskinesia. Side effects must be managed in patients who need these valuable drugs for normal life function.

Natural products used for anxiety and insomnia include melatonin and kava. St. John's wort and SAMe are used to treat mild depression and should be documented in the patient's chart.

Chapter Checkup

The Navigator+ learning management system that accompanies this textbook offers many opportunities to help you master chapter content, including end-of-chapter exercises, a glossary of key terms, flash cards, and additional interactive activities.

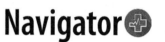 **Navigator**

 ## Career Exploration

If you enjoyed learning about psychiatric and mood disorders in this chapter, you may want to explore the following career options:

- art therapist
- behavioral health technician
- behavioral specialist
- case manager
- licensed clinical social worker
- marriage and family counselor/therapist
- medical assistant
- mental health counselor
- music therapist
- pharmacy technician
- social worker
- substance abuse counselor

CHAPTER

14

The Sensory System and Drug Therapy

Pharm Facts

- Even small, incidental noises can bother an individual who must remain focused while performing a task that requires manual dexterity, such as surgery. Unexpected sounds cause the pupils to dilate, temporarily changing an individual's focus and blurring his or her vision.

- Ever wonder why babies have such big eyes and older people seem to have large ears? The eyes remain the same size throughout your lifetime, but the nose and ears continue to grow—in fact, they never *stop* growing.

- Women who lived during the Roman Empire used the berry juice from the belladonna plant to achieve the desirable effect of dilated pupils—making the eyes appear large, limpid, and innocent. When repeated use of the drops led to blindness, the plant's name, *belladonna* (meaning "beautiful lady" in Italian), was more commonly known as *deadly nightshade*.

"As a certified ophthalmic medical technologist (COMT), my primary responsibility is to provide preliminary technical data to the ophthalmologist prior to examination of the patient's eyes. This career has been extremely rewarding for my skills have helped many patients live independent lives due to their improved vision. As the US population ages, there will be an increased demand for qualified ophthalmic medical technicians (OMTs) who can assess the ophthalmic needs of the geriatric population—presbyopia, cataracts, glaucoma, and macular degeneration—and allay their genuine concerns about becoming blind."

—**Sergina M. Flaherty**, COMT
Ophthalmic Technologist

Learning Objectives

1 Understand the basic anatomy and physiology of the eyes and the ears.

2 Describe the common conditions that affect the eyes and the ears.

3 Explain the therapeutic effects of prescription medications and non-prescription medications commonly used to treat diseases of the eyes and the ears.

4 Identify the generic names, brand names, indications, dosage ranges, side effects, contraindications, and cautions and considerations associated with the drugs commonly used to treat eye and ear disorders.

5 Identify common herbal and alternative therapies that are related to the sensory system—specifically, the eyes and the ears.

This chapter addresses two of the organs that are components of the sensory system: the eyes and the ears. The discussion includes the anatomy and physiology of the eyes and the ears as well as the conditions affecting these sensory organs, including glaucoma, conjunctivitis, ear infections, and ototoxicity.

The eyes and the ears are unique administration sites for drug therapies, requiring special instructions for use. Medications for these sensory organs are ordered as prescriptions and purchased over the counter regularly. Drug classes used to treat eye conditions include prostaglandin agonists, ophthalmic beta blockers, and ophthalmic alpha receptor agonists. Drug classes used to treat ear disorders include oral antibiotics, otic antibiotics and analgesics, drying agents, and earwax removers. Finally, this chapter addresses a few natural and herbal products used to treat eye and ear conditions.

Anatomy and Physiology of the Eyes and the Ears

The **sensory system** includes organs that produce the five senses: vision, hearing, smell, taste, and touch. Because the eyes and the ears are sites of administration for instilling medication, it is important to understand their structures and functions.

Structures and Functions of the Eye

The eyes are sensory organs specially designed to sense light and produce vision. Light enters the eye through the pupil and is focused by the lens (see Figure 14.1). The lens is located just behind the **pupil**, the black center of the eye. The **lens** of the eye acts like a lens in a camera, focusing light onto the back of the eye—the retina. The **iris**, which surrounds the pupil, determines eye color. The **sclera** is the outer coating of the eyeball, commonly referred to as the white of the eye.

Sight begins with light that travels through the lens to the retina in the back of the eye. In the **retina**, photoreceptor cells detect light and color. These rod- and cone-shaped sensory cells send signals via the optic nerve to the brain, where sight is ultimately perceived and interpreted (see Figure 14.2). **Rod cells** are sensitive to light in dimly lit conditions. They are responsible for night vision. Vitamin A deficiency can cause malfunctions in retinal rod cells, which then affects night vision. Rod cells are also considered responsible for black-and-white vision. **Cone cells** sense color and are responsible for day vision. **Color blindness** (usually a genetic trait that affects mostly male offspring) is a condition in which cone cells do not differentiate colors. The most common form of color blindness is being

Anatomy of the Eye

Drugs are used to treat problems in the conjunctiva, anterior chamber, retina, and macula.

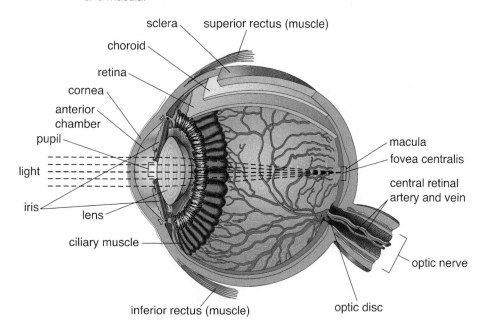

Anatomy of the Retina

Rod cells help individuals (and animals) see in the dark.

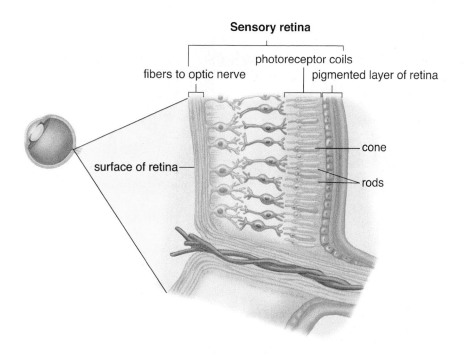

unable to differentiate red from green. Inside the **macula**, a yellowish spot near the center of the retina, is the focal point (fovea centralis) where light is concentrated for vision (see Figure 14.1). This part of the retina is rich in cone cells.

Other parts of the eye relevant to drug therapy include the cornea, anterior chamber, aqueous humor, ciliary muscle, and conjunctiva. The **cornea** covers the **anterior chamber**. The anterior chamber holds **aqueous humor**, a fluid that lubricates and protects the lens. **Vitreous humor** is the fluid inside the eye, behind the lens. The **ciliary muscle** holds the lens in place. The **conjunctiva** forms the mucous membranes of the socket that hold the eye in place.

Structures and Functions of the Ear

The **ears** are sensory organs designed to sense sound waves and produce hearing. As seen in Figure 14.3, the ear is divided into three parts: external, middle, and inner. The **external ear** captures **sound waves** and directs them through the **auditory canal** to the **tympanic membrane** (eardrum). **Cerumen** (earwax) is produced by follicles lining the auditory canal.

The eardrum separates the **middle ear** from the external ear. It vibrates in response to sound waves, causing the three bones (**malleus, incus,** and **stapes**) of the middle ear to move. The stapes in effect taps on the **oval window**, the entrance to the inner ear. The

---

FIGURE 14.3 Anatomy of the External, Middle, and Inner Ear

Ear "popping" created by yawning is the characteristic sound of fluid exchange in the eustachian tube.

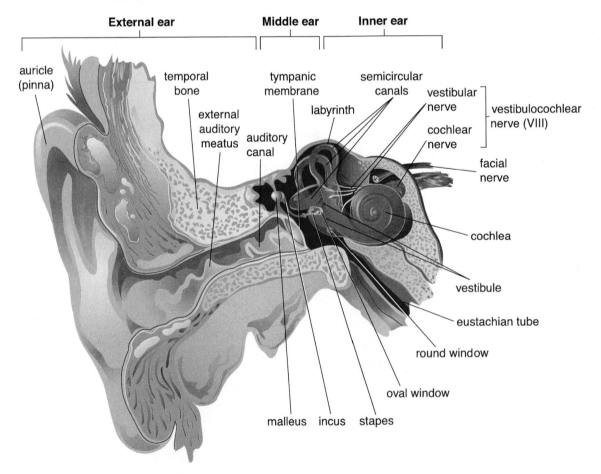

eustachian tube connects the middle ear to the throat to allow fluid to drain and to allow equalization of the pressure in the middle ear when atmospheric air pressure changes. The **inner ear** includes the semicircular canals and the cochlea. Fluid in the **cochlea** responds to the tapping on the oval window, producing pressure waves that flow through the spiral-shaped organ (see Figure 14.4). Sensory hairs line the surface of the cochlea in what is called the **organ of Corti**. Sound is perceived and interpreted when corresponding vibrations in these tiny hairs send signals via nerves to the brain. Damage to sensory hairs in the inner ear occurs naturally with age and exposure to loud noise. This kind of hearing loss is called **presbycusis**. The first sounds lost to perception are those produced by high-pitched sound waves.

Fluid in the **semicircular canals** maintains balance and orientation. The semicircular canals are arranged in a three-dimensional manner. Gravity pulls the fluid in these channels downward, signaling to the **vestibular nerves** when the body is vertical, horizontal, or upside down. **Vertigo** is a malfunction of these semicircular canals, resulting in balance problems and dizziness.

FIGURE 14.4 Sound Movement Through the Inner Ear

Strong waves from loud noises break off tiny hairs in the cochlea, causing hearing loss.

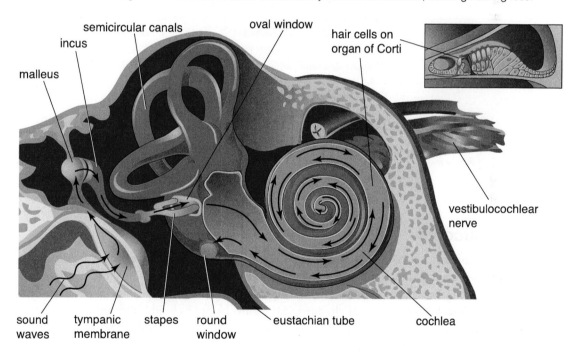

Checkpoint 14.1

Take a moment to review what you have learned so far and answer these questions.

1. What are the parts of the eye that are responsible for seeing colors and black-and-white images?

2. What are the structures of the middle ear?

3. What underlying factor causes presbycusis?

Common Eye Disorders

Some eye disorders require chronic (long-term) treatment, whereas others need only acute treatment (treatment for the duration of an infection, which is typically less than two weeks). For example, glaucoma and chronic dry eye are managed primarily with long-term or chronic use of medications. Conversely, conjunctivitis and cytomegalovirus require acute treatment to resolve these eye infections. Cytomegalovirus may also require long-term treatment in patients with immune deficiency. In addition, certain types of macular degeneration can now be treated chronically with injections of vascular endothelial growth factor (VEGF) inhibitors such as ranibizumab (Lucentis). However, certain conditions such as retinopathy cannot currently be treated with medications.

Allied health professionals—in particular, those who work in an ophthalmologist or optometrist office—should also be aware of several medications that are used during eye examinations and procedures. These products do not usually treat ophthalmic disorders and are rarely dispensed in pharmacies. Still, it can be useful to be familiar with them (see Table 14.1).

TABLE 14.1 Ophthalmic Products for Eye Examinations and Procedures

Drug Class	Generic (Brand)	Common Use
Mydriatics	Atropine ophthalmic (Atropine Care, Isopto Atropine) Cyclopentolate ophthalmic (Cyclogyl) Homatropine ophthalmic (Homatropaire, Isopto Homatropine) Scopolamine ophthalmic (Isopto Hyoscine) Tropicamide ophthalmic (Mydral, Mydriacyl)	Pupil dilation during eye examinations
Ophthalmic local anesthetics	Lidocaine ophthalmic (Akten) Proparacaine eyedrops (Alcaine, Parcaine) Tetracaine eyedrops (Altacaine, Tetcaine, TetraVisc, TetraVisc Forte)	Ocular surface analgesia during procedures

Glaucoma

Glaucoma is a condition in which abnormally high **intraocular pressure** pushes on the **optic nerve** and damages it. Glaucoma can lead to blindness if it is not treated. The increased pressure comes from either overproduction of aqueous humor or blockage of its outflow from the anterior chamber (see Figure 14.5). As fluid builds up in the anterior chamber, intraocular pressure increases, and pressure is applied to the optic nerve. **Open-angle glaucoma** is a slowly progressing, chronic condition managed with medication alone. **Narrow-angle glaucoma** is an acute condition that comes on quickly and is resolved with emergency surgery followed by drugs.

Drug Regimens and Treatments

The majority of eye conditions, especially glaucoma, are treated with topical agents administered directly in the eyes. Although oral medication administration may be more convenient for most patients, the undesirable systemic effects of oral therapy can pose problems. Ophthalmic agents generally limit drug therapy to local effects. To teach your patients how to administer **ophthalmic drops**, commonly known as *eyedrops*, refer to the following Patient Teaching feature box.

FIGURE 14.5 | Normal Aqueous Humor Flow and Glaucoma

In open-angle glaucoma, the trabecular meshwork becomes congested, restricting the flow of aqueous humor from the anterior chamber. In narrow-angle glaucoma, the canal of Schlemm is blocked completely, cutting off aqueous humor flow.

CROSS SECTIONS OF UPPER EYEBALL

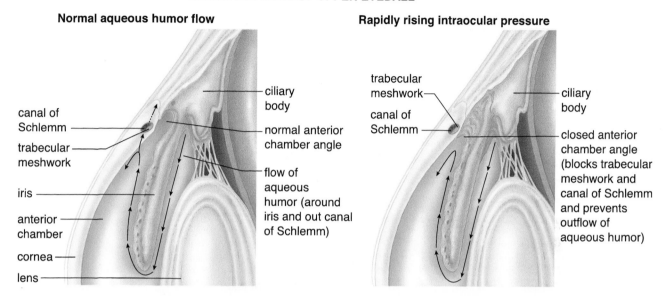

Normal aqueous humor flow — canal of Schlemm, trabecular meshwork, iris, anterior chamber, cornea, lens, ciliary body, normal anterior chamber angle, flow of aqueous humor (around iris and out canal of Schlemm)

Rapidly rising intraocular pressure — trabecular meshwork, canal of Schlemm, ciliary body, closed anterior chamber angle (blocks trabecular meshwork and canal of Schlemm and prevents outflow of aqueous humor)

Patient Teaching

Allied health professionals should remind patients that eyedrops are sterile medications. To ensure sterility of the medication, tell patients to keep the dropper bottle in a clean place and to avoid touching the tip of the drop applicator to surfaces, the fingers, or the eye itself. If the drop applicator accidentally touches a surface, instruct patients to use an alcohol swab to clean the applicator and let the alcohol evaporate before dispensing drops into the eye.

Prior to instilling eyedrops, patients who are contact lens wearers must remove their contacts and leave them out for at least 15 minutes after the procedure. If the medication is a suspension, patients should also shake the dropper bottle well before administering the eyedrops.

To instill the drops, advise the patient to lie down, pull the lower eyelid downward, and gently squeeze the container to allow the required number of drops to fall into the eye without touching the tip of the applicator to the eye, eyelid, eyelashes, or fingers.

Multiple drug classes are used to treat glaucoma (see Table 14.2). These include prostaglandin agonists, ophthalmic beta blockers, and ophthalmic alpha receptor agonists. (Oral dosage forms of beta blockers and alpha blockers are covered in Chapter 12.) Miotic eyedrops are also used to treat glaucoma.

TABLE 14.2 Ophthalmic Agents for Glaucoma

Generic (Brand)	Dosage Form
Prostaglandin Agonists	
Bimatoprost (Lumigan)	Ophthalmic solution
Latanoprost (Xalatan)	Ophthalmic solution
Tafluprost (Zioptan)	Ophthalmic solution
Travoprost (Travatan)	Ophthalmic solution
Unoprostone (Rescula)	Ophthalmic solution
Beta Blockers	
Betaxolol (Betoptic)	Ophthalmic solution and suspension
Carteolol	Ophthalmic solution
Levobunolol (Betagan)	Ophthalmic solution
Metipranolol (OptiPranolol)	Ophthalmic solution
Timolol (Timoptic)	Ophthalmic solution
Alpha Receptor Agonists	
Brimonidine (Alphagan P)	Ophthalmic solution
Miotics	
Carbachol (Miostat)	Ophthalmic solution
Echothiophate (Phospholine Iodide)	Ophthalmic powder for reconstitution
Pilocarpine (Isopto Carpine)	Ophthalmic gel and solution

Ophthalmic Glaucoma Agents

Ophthalmic glaucoma agents work by reducing aqueous humor production and, in some cases, enhancing its drainage from the anterior chamber. Miotic agents constrict the pupil slightly by contracting the ciliary muscle. This contraction enhances aqueous humor outflow. Beta blockers are first-line therapy for glaucoma and tend to be used most frequently.

Side Effects Glaucoma agents are usually well tolerated. Side effects include mild stinging, tearing, itchiness, and dryness of the eyes. These effects generally improve with time. Many glaucoma agents have the potential to cause systemic effects if enough medication is absorbed into the bloodstream. These effects are primarily associated with beta blockers and include slowed heartbeat, heart problems, insomnia, dizziness, vertigo, headache, tiredness, and difficulty breathing. If any of these effects occur, patients should contact their prescribers right away. A change in drug therapy may be needed.

Contraindications The prostaglandin agonists do not have contraindications.

Name Exchange

The prostaglandin agonist bimatoprost, which is used to treat glaucoma, is best known by its brand name, Lumigan.

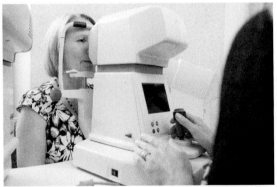

A tonometer measures an individual's intraocular fluid pressure. Normal intraocular fluid pressure is 12–22 mm Hg; patients with glaucoma typically exceed 22 mm Hg. However, many patients with glaucoma do not have elevated intraocular fluid pressure.

The beta blocker ophthalmic products are contraindicated in patients with heart problems including sinus bradycardia, heart block greater than first degree, cardiogenic shock, and uncompensated heart failure. Carteolol and levobunolol should not be used in patients with respiratory problems such as chronic obstructive pulmonary disease (COPD), bronchial asthma, and pulmonary edema.

The alpha receptor agonist brimonidine should not be used in children younger than two years of age.

In terms of the miotics ophthalmic products, carbachol use is contraindicated in acute iritis and acute inflammatory disease of the anterior eye chamber. Echothiophate should not be used in narrow-angle glaucoma and acute uveal inflammation. Acute inflammatory disease of the anterior chamber of the eye contraindicates pilocarpine use.

➕ *Note: Allied health professionals should be aware that an allergy to a particular drug contraindicates its use. This warning applies to all Contraindications sections in this chapter.*

Cautions and Considerations Patients with heart or thyroid problems should discuss their choices for glaucoma treatment with their prescribers before selecting and using these products. Specifically, the systemic effects of beta blockers can interfere with these conditions and the other drug therapies used to treat them.

Prostaglandin agonists have a unique effect in that they cause the iris of the eye to turn brown. Patients should be informed of this effect because their eye color will likely change.

Conjunctivitis

Conjunctivitis (commonly called "pinkeye") is an inflammation caused by viruses or bacteria in the mucous membranes surrounding the eye. Symptoms include redness of the sclera and the insides of the eyelids, itching, pain, tearing, and the release of exudate. This exudate can be white, yellow, or green. Treatment with antibiotics is relatively easy.

Newborns of mothers with untreated gonorrhea are at high risk for gonococcal conjunctivitis. Treatment for newborns suspected to be infected includes topical ophthalmic anti-infectives for prevention and systemic antibiotics. Pregnant women should be tested for gonorrhea and treated before giving birth, if possible.

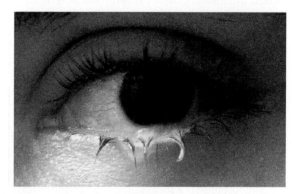

Viral and bacterial conjunctivitis typically begin in one eye and then spread to the other eye. This condition is extremely contagious, so patients should avoid sharing towels, washcloths, pillowcases, and blankets.

Drug Regimens and Treatments

The number of ophthalmic anti-infective agents is large and can be intimidating to learn. However, this extensive number of products ensures that proper treatment of eye infections can be achieved easily. Many of these medications are given as **ophthalmic ointments** (eye ointments) and, therefore, require patients to learn a specific administration technique. To teach your patients how to administer eye ointment, refer to the following Patient Teaching feature box.

Patient Teaching

Because the technique for applying eye ointment is not easy, allied health professionals should provide guidance to their patients. Remind patients that eye ointments must remain sterile and that the applicator tip of the container should not touch surfaces, the fingers, or the eye or eyelid itself. Also, instruct patients who are contact lens wearers to remove their contacts and leave them out for at least 15 minutes after the procedure.

To apply eye ointment, advise patients to pull the lower eyelid downward and squeeze a continuous ribbon of ointment (half-inch long) along the space between the eyeball and lower lid. The patient should then close the eye for a few minutes to allow the ointment to liquefy. Vision may be blurry for a few minutes until the ointment dissipates. Excess ointment can be gently wiped away. Instruct the patient to repeat the procedure in the other eye as prescribed.

ointment

Topical Anti-infectives

Topical anti-infectives for the eyes are chosen based on the type of infection and suspected organism. Unless the infection is systemic, topical ophthalmic agents are used (see Table 14.3).

Side Effects Common side effects of topically administered anti-infectives are few, and, if present, they are usually mild and tolerable (such as temporary eye irritation right after administering the medication). Although systemic absorption is typically low with these dosage forms, systemic side effects are possible. To learn more about the systemic side effects of anti-infectives, see Chapters 23 and 24.

Contraindications Tobramycin should not be used in patients with hypersensitivities to other aminoglycosides. Gentamicin does not have contraindications.

Ophthalmic erythromycin, a macrolide, does not have contraindications.

Sulfacetamide, a sulfonamide, is contraindicated in patients with a hypersensitivity to sulfonamides. Trimethoprim/polymyxin B does not have contraindications.

TABLE 14.3 Commonly Used Ophthalmic Anti-infectives

Generic (Brand)	Dosage Form	Route of Administration	Common Dosage
Aminoglycosides			
Gentamicin (Genoptic, Gentak)	Ointment, solution	Ophthalmic	Half-inch ribbon 2–3 times a day (ointment); 1–2 drops every 4 hr (solution)
Tobramycin (Tobrex)	Ointment, solution	Ophthalmic	Half-inch ribbon 2–6 times a day (ointment); 1–2 drops every 4 hr (solution)
Macrolides			
Erythromycin	Ointment	Ophthalmic	Half-inch ribbon 2–6 times a day
Sulfonamides			
Sulfacetamide (Bleph-10)	Solution	Ophthalmic	1–2 drops every 2–3 hr
Trimethoprim/polymyxin B (Polytrim)	Solution	Ophthalmic	1–2 drops every 4–6 hr
Quinolones			
Ciprofloxacin (Ciloxan)	Ointment, solution	Ophthalmic	Half-inch ribbon 2–3 times a day (ointment); 1–2 drops every 2–5 hr (solution)
Levofloxacin (Iquix, Quixin)	Solution	Ophthalmic	1–2 drops every 2–4 hr
Ofloxacin (Ocuflox)	Solution	Ophthalmic	1–2 drops every 2–4 hr or 4 times a day
Miscellaneous Combinations			
Gentamicin/prednisolone (Pred-G)	Ointment, suspension	Ophthalmic	Half-inch ribbon 1–3 times a day (ointment); 1 drop every 2–4 hr (suspension)
Neomycin/bacitracin/polymyxin B/hydrocortisone (Cortisporin)	Ointment	Ophthalmic	Half-inch ribbon every 3–4 hr
Neomycin/polymyxin B/dexamethasone (Maxitrol)	Ointment, suspension	Ophthalmic	Half-inch ribbon 3–4 times a day (ointment); 1–2 drops every 3–4 hr (suspension)
Sulfacetamide/fluorometholone (FML-S)	Solution	Ophthalmic	1–3 drops every 2–3 hr
Sulfacetamide/prednisolone (Blephamide)	Ointment, suspension	Ophthalmic	Half-inch ribbon 3–4 times a day (ointment); 2 drops every 4 hr (suspension)
Tobramycin/dexamethasone (TobraDex)	Ointment, suspension	Ophthalmic	Half-inch ribbon 3–4 times a day (ointment); 1–2 drops every 4–6 hr (suspension)

All of the miscellaneous combination products (see Table 14.3) that contain an aminoglycoside or steroid are contraindicated in patients with a hypersensitivity to aminoglycosides or corticosteroids. In addition, all of the miscellaneous combination products are contraindicated in viral disease of the cornea and conjunctiva and in mycobacterial or fungal infection of the eye.

Cautions and Considerations Anti-infectives are drugs to which many patients have allergies. Therefore, you should ask each patient about allergies and document them in the patient's medical record. Even topical anti-infective agents can cause serious allergic reactions, so updated allergy information is important for patient safety.

Ophthalmic Corticosteroids

Sometimes, **ophthalmic corticosteroids** (see Table 14.4) are useful for calming inflammation caused by an infection. These agents do not help cure the infection but can reduce pain, redness, and irritation. Patients should follow instructions for using ophthalmic drops and ointments and keep the product sterile to prevent reintroducing infection into the eye.

TABLE 14.4 Commonly Used Ophthalmic Corticosteroids

Generic (Brand)	Dosage Form	Route of Administration	Common Dosage
Dexamethasone (Maxidex, Ozurdex)	Solution, suspension	Ophthalmic	1–2 drops every 1–4 hr
Difluprednate (Durezol)	Emulsion	Ophthalmic	1 drop 2–4 times a day
Fluorometholone (Flarex, FML)	Ointment, suspension	Ophthalmic	Half-inch ribbon 1–3 times a day (ointment); 1 drop 2–4 times a day (suspension)
Loteprednol (Alrex, Lotemax)	Gel, ointment, suspension	Ophthalmic	1–2 drops 4 times a day (gel, ointment); 1 drop 4 times a day (suspension)
Prednisolone (Pred Forte, Pred Mild)	Solution, suspension	Ophthalmic	2 drops 4 times a day
Rimexolone (Vexol)	Suspension	Ophthalmic	1–2 drops every 2 hr or 4 times a day
Triamcinolone (Triesence)	Suspension for intravitreal injection	Ophthalmic	1–4 mg injected once, then as needed

Side Effects Common side effects of ophthalmic corticosteroids are few, and, if present, they are usually mild and tolerable. Although systemic absorption is typically low with these dosage forms, systemic side effects are possible. Such symptoms can include headache, dizziness, insomnia, and increased appetite. If these effects occur, patients should talk with their healthcare practitioners.

Contraindications Dexamethasone, difluprednate, fluorometholone, loteprednol, prednisolone, and rimexolone should not be used in patients with viral disease of the cornea and conjunctiva and in mycobacterial or fungal infection of the eye. Fluorometholone should not be used in patients with untreated eye infections. Prednisolone is contraindicated in patients with a hypersensitivity to corticosteroids, acute purulent ocular infections, and after uncomplicated removal of a superficial corneal foreign body. Rimexolone should not be used in patients with untreated pus-forming bacterial ocular infections. Triamcinolone should not be used in cerebral malaria, idiopathic thrombocytopenic purpura, and systemic fungal infections.

Cautions and Considerations Ophthalmic suspensions should be shaken well before administration to ensure proper dosage.

Checkpoint 14.2

Take a moment to review what you have learned so far and answer these questions.

1. What classes of drugs are used to treat glaucoma?

2. Which antibiotic drug classes are used to treat eye infections?

3. What conditions are treated with ophthalmic corticosteroids?

Cytomegalovirus Retinitis and Herpes

Cytomegalovirus (CMV) retinitis is a viral infection of the inner eye that occurs almost entirely in patients with human immunodeficiency virus (HIV)/acquired immune deficiency syndrome (AIDS). Most people are exposed to this virus early in life but do not develop an active infection because a normally functioning immune system easily defends against it. In immunocompromised patients, CMV retinitis becomes an active infection that can lead to blindness. It is most common in patients at the end stages of AIDS and those who have high virus counts in the bloodstream. CMV retinitis is difficult to cure.

Herpes zoster, the virus that causes chicken pox and shingles, and **herpes simplex**, the virus that causes cold sores, can cause various problems with the eyes and eyelids. Symptoms usually include eye pain and can include redness, cloudiness of the cornea, tearing, decreased vision, and aversion to bright light. Serious herpetic viral infections can cause blindness.

Drug Regimens and Treatments

Treatment of CMV retinitis involves chronic viral suppression with antiviral medication to control symptoms and preserve eyesight. Herpes treatment involves topical antiviral agents, which may be used in addition to systemic agents when necessary.

Antivirals for Ophthalmic Infections

Antiviral therapy works by suppressing viral DNA production. This effect stops the growth and proliferation of the infection. Antiviral agents do not cure the infection but can reduce it to a remission-like status when used properly (see Table 14.5).

TABLE 14.5 Ophthalmic Antivirals

Generic (Brand)	Dosage Form	Route of Administration	Common Dosage
Cidofovir (Vistide)	Solution	IV	5 mg/kg IV over an hour given every 1–2 weeks
Foscarnet (Foscavir)	Solution	IV	90 mg/kg IV every 12 or 24 hr
Ganciclovir (Zirgan)	Capsule, injection	Intravitreal, IV, oral	1 implant every 5–8 months; 5 mg/kg IV every 12–24 hr; 1,000 mg orally 3 times a day
Trifluridine (Viroptic)	Solution	Ophthalmic	1 drop every 2–4 hr
Valganciclovir (Valcyte)	Tablet	Oral	900 mg once or twice a day

Side Effects Eye irritation and decreased visual acuity have been reported with use of some antiviral agents. Intraocular pressure may decrease when cidofovir (Vistide) is given or increase when trifluridine (Viroptic) is given. Ophthalmic corticosteroids can be used to reduce eye irritation, but patients need to be monitored by their healthcare practitioners for the other effects. Laboratory tests are sometimes used in this monitoring.

Contraindications Cidofovir is contraindicated in patients with a severe hypersensitivity to probenecid or other sulfa-containing drugs, and in patients with decreased kidney function. Cidofovir should also not be used with or within seven days of the administration of nephrotoxic drugs and should not be administered via direct intraocular injection. Ganciclovir should not be used in patients with a hypersensitivity to acyclovir. Valganciclovir should not be used in patients with a hypersensitivity to ganciclovir. Foscarnet and trifluridine do not have contraindications.

Cautions and Considerations Antiviral medications should be used with caution in patients with poor kidney function. Staying properly hydrated can help to reduce the risk of nephrotoxicity, a condition that can cause kidney damage. Patients with seizure disorders should talk with their prescribers before using antiviral medications. Some antiviral medications can lower the seizure threshold, making seizures more common.

Eye Allergies

Exposure to allergens (including pollen, dust, smoke, and pollution) triggers the redness, itching, and tearing that are the symptoms of **eye allergies**. Allergies can also cause inflammations such as conjunctivitis.

Drug Regimens and Treatments

Drug therapy for eye allergies (see Table 14.6) includes **topical antihistamines, decongestants, mast cell stabilizers,** and **nonsteroidal anti-inflammatory drugs (NSAIDs)**. These agents reduce the redness and inflammation caused by eye allergies. Ophthalmic NSAIDs are also used for the pain associated with cataract surgery.

Side Effects Side effects of these ophthalmic agents, if present, are typically mild and tolerable. Mild stinging or burning immediately after instillation of the agent may occur. The time to maximum effect varies, depending on the specific agent.

Contraindications Ophthalmic cyclosporine does not have contraindications. The antihistamines listed in Table 14.5 do not have contraindications. Of the decongestants, naphazoline is the only one with contraindications (narrow-angle glaucoma or anatomically narrow angle). The mast cell stabilizers and the NSAIDs listed in Table 14.6 do not have contraindications.

Cautions and Considerations When used topically, decongestants can cause rebound congestion and eye redness if used for longer than three days. As a result, patients using decongestant eyedrops for longer than a few days at a time may have worsened allergy symptoms when they stop using them. This rebound swelling lasts a few days and then subsides.

   Antihistamines and NSAIDs can take a few days to provide relief of symptoms. Patients should be informed of the length of these delays, so that they do not get discouraged and quit their drug therapy before it starts to work.

TABLE 14.6 Ophthalmic Agents for Allergies and Chronic Dry Eye

Generic (Brand)	Dosage Form	Dispensing Status	Route of Administration	Common Dosage
Immunomodulator				
Cyclosporine (Restasis)	Emulsion	Rx	Ophthalmic	1 drop twice a day
Antihistamines				
Azelastine (Optivar)	Solution	Rx	Ophthalmic	1 drop twice a day
Emedastine (Emadine)	Solution	Rx	Ophthalmic	1 drop 4 times a day
Epinastine (Elestat)	Solution	Rx	Ophthalmic	1 drop twice a day
Ketotifen (Alaway, Zaditor)	Solution	OTC, Rx	Ophthalmic	1 drop every 8–12 hr
Olopatadine (Pataday, Patanol)	Solution	Rx	Ophthalmic	1–2 drops 2 times a day
Decongestants				
Naphazoline (AK-Con, Clear Eyes, Naphcon)	Solution	OTC, Rx	Ophthalmic	1–2 drops every 3–4 hr
Oxymetazoline (Visine LR)	Solution	OTC	Ophthalmic	1–2 drops every 6 hr
Phenylephrine (AK-Dilate, Altafrin, Neofrin, Relief)	Solution	OTC, Rx	Ophthalmic	1 drop up to 3 times a day
Tetrahydrozoline (Altazine, Murine, Opti-Clear, Visine)	Solution	OTC	Ophthalmic	1–2 drops 4 times a day
Mast Cell Stabilizers				
Cromolyn sodium (Crolom)	Solution	Rx	Ophthalmic	1–2 drops 4–6 times a day
Lodoxamide (Alomide)	Solution	Rx	Ophthalmic	1–2 drops 4 times a day
Nedocromil (Alocril)	Solution	Rx	Ophthalmic	1–2 drops twice a day
NSAIDs				
Bromfenac (Bromday, Prolensa)	Solution	Rx	Ophthalmic	1 drop twice a day
Diclofenac (Voltaren)	Solution	Rx	Ophthalmic	1–2 drops 4 times a day
Ketorolac (Acular)	Solution	Rx	Ophthalmic	1 drop 4 times a day
Nepafenac (Nevanac)	Suspension	Rx	Ophthalmic	1 drop 3 times a day

Chronic Dry Eye

Chronic dry eye is the inability to produce sufficient tears and lubrication for the eye. Chronic dry eye can be caused by hormonal changes (especially menopause) or auto-immune disorders that affect tear production such as Sjögren's syndrome, collagen vascular disease, rheumatoid arthritis, and lupus. Any condition that impedes proper closing of the eyes or impairs the blink reflex, such as a stroke, can also result in chronic dry eye. Environmental causes of chronic dry eye may include dry air from air conditioning or heat. Finally, chronic dry eye may be a side effect of some drugs with anticholinergic effects (see Chapter 12).

Drug therapy for chronic dry eye starts with **normal saline drops** or **artificial tears**. These products simply lubricate the eye by providing needed hydration. Eye lubricant products that are more viscous (thicker) are likely to provide longer-lasting relief from dry eye symptoms. (For example, a gel will last longer than a solution.) If sufficiently serious, the condition may be treated with topical cyclosporine, which directly reduces immune activity within the eye.

Side Effects Side effects of these ophthalmic agents are typically mild and tolerable. Mild stinging or burning immediately after application may occur. The time to maximum effect varies, depending on the specific agent.

Contraindications There are no contraindications to normal saline drops or artificial tears.

Cautions and Considerations Cyclosporine can take four weeks or more to reach full effect. Patients should be informed of the length of this delay, so that they do not get discouraged and quit therapy before it starts to work. Cyclosporine is available in single-use vials. Patients who choose to continue using artificial tears should separate their use of cyclosporine and artificial tears by at least 15 minutes in order to avoid diluting cyclosporine's effects.

Retinopathy and Macular Degeneration

Retinopathy refers to the destruction of the retina. It can be caused by a variety of conditions, and the most common is diabetes. In diabetic retinopathy, tiny blood vessels that supply the retina with blood are damaged, allowing minute hemorrhaging to occur. Diabetic retinopathy is a leading cause of blindness in the United States, but it can be prevented through proper treatment and control of blood glucose levels. If retinopathy is detected early, laser treatments can keep vision loss at bay.

Macular degeneration is generally associated with increasing age and is a painless condition that can go undetected until vision is significantly affected. The macula is responsible for central vision. **Central vision** is used for reading, driving, and focusing on others' faces. When the breakdown of tissue in this area occurs slowly with age, the condition is referred to as **dry macular degeneration**. Changes in sight include blurry vision and requiring more light to read. **Wet macular degeneration**, in which tissue breakdown occurs rapidly from fast blood vessel growth and rupture, is not associated with age. Vision changes are quick to develop and make straight lines appear wavy.

These two photos show the same image as seen by an individual with normal vision and by an individual with diabetic retinopathy.

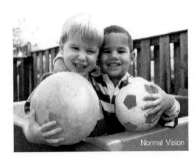

Normal Vision

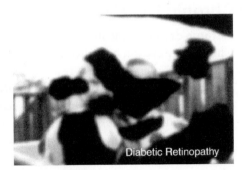

Diabetic Retinopathy

Patient Teaching

Healthcare professionals should remind patients with diabetes about the importance of annual eye examinations to prevent retinopathy and preserve eyesight. This eye examination must be conducted during pupil dilation for adequate visualization of the early stages of damage from retinopathy.

Drug Regimens and Treatments

Although there is no drug treatment for dry macular degeneration, wet macular degeneration can now be treated with injectable vascular endothelial growth factor (VEGF) inhibitors such as ranibizumab (Lucentis).

Checkpoint 14.3

Take a moment to review what you have learned so far and answer these questions.

1. What drug class is commonly used to treat CMV retinitis and herpes?
2. What drug classes are used to treat eye allergies?
3. What are four causative factors for chronic dry eye?

Common Ear Disorders

Infections make up the majority of ear disorders that require drug therapy. Oral drug therapy is usually necessary for middle ear infections (see Chapter 23). Antibiotic eardrops will not effectively treat an infection of the middle ear because medication applied to the external ear will not reach the intended site of action unless the tympanic membrane is ruptured.

Otitis Media

Middle ear infection (otitis media) is most common in children. Because the eustachian tube is more horizontal than vertical in children as compared with adults, fluid from the middle ear does not drain well, allowing bacteria and viruses to flourish. Most middle ear infections are viral and clear on their own. Often otitis media develops after a viral respiratory tract infection in which mucus and fluid build up and provide a growing medium for bacteria. Symptoms of an ear infection include ear pain, jaw pain, sinus pain, itching, and fever. Pain is often dramatic enough to cause patients (or their parents) to seek medical attention. Sometimes, congestion in the ear can cause fluid pressure on the semicircular canals and cause dizziness (vertigo).

Work Wise

Patients with ear infections may have difficulty hearing, so make sure to communicate clearly with such patients and provide them with written instructions when possible.

Drug Regimens and Treatments

To treat otitis media, healthcare practitioners prescribe oral antibiotics to eradicate the infection and topical analgesics to relieve the pain. To reduce antibiotic resistance, these practitioners attempt to be conservative when prescribing antibiotics for ear infections. Overuse of antibiotics can decrease their efficacy because bacteria constantly exposed to a given drug will develop resistance to that drug. Patients experiencing dizziness can use decongestants (discussed in Chapter 17) to reduce pressure in the middle ear.

 ## Drug Alert

Some physicians prescribe ophthalmic products to be used in the ear. For example, some antibiotics available as eyedrops are not available as eardrops, so an eyedrop may be prescribed for an ear infection. Although it may be appropriate for patients to use ophthalmic drops in the ears, they should not administer otic drops in the eyes. Unlike ophthalmic drops, otic drops are *not* sterile. In addition, instilling otic drops in the eyes can be painful and may even cause damage to the eyes.

Otic Antibiotics and Analgesics

There are not as many otic antibiotics as oral antibiotics. Otic antibiotics are usually used as adjunct therapy to oral antibiotics for severe ear infections in cases where the eardrum is ruptured or tubes have been surgically placed in the eardrum (see Table 14.7). Topical otic analgesics are used for patients with severe ear pain associated with infection. These products work by temporarily numbing the ear canal (see Table 14.8).

Side Effects The few side effects of otic agents are rarely experienced. Although systemic absorption is seldom seen with otic agents, allergic reactions are still possible. Be sure to update the patient's allergy profile each time new orders are written.

Contraindications The quinolone otic products are contraindicated in patients with a hypersensitivity to other quinolones. Ciprofloxacin/dexamethasone should not be used in patients with a quinolone or steroid hypersensitivity and viral infection of the external ear canal. Neomycin/polymyxin B/hydrocortisone should not be used in patients with viral infections, fungal diseases, or mycobacterial infections.

TABLE 14.7 Commonly Used Otic Antibiotics

Generic (Brand)	Dosage Form	Route of Administration	Common Dosage
Quinolones			
Ciprofloxacin (Cetraxal)	Solution	Otic	1 single-use container twice a day
Ofloxacin (Floxin Otic)	Solution	Otic	10 drops a day
Combinations			
Ciprofloxacin/dexamethasone (Ciprodex)	Solution	Otic	3–4 drops 2–4 times a day
Ciprofloxacin/hydrocortisone (Cipro HC)	Solution	Otic	3 drops twice a day
Neomycin/polymyxin B/hydrocortisone (Antibiotic Ear, Cortisporin)	Solution	Otic	3–4 drops 2–4 times a day

TABLE 14.8 Miscellaneous Otic Products

Generic (Brand)	Dosage Form	Route of Administration	Common Dosage
Drying Agents			
Acetic acid	Solution	Otic	5–10 drops 2–4 times a day
Isopropyl alcohol/glycerin (Auro-Dri, Ear Dry)	Solution	Otic	4–5 drops in each ear
Earwax Remover			
Carbamide peroxide (Debrox)	Solution	Otic	5–10 drops twice a day
Analgesic			
Antipyrine/benzocaine (Aurodex)	Solution	Otic	2–4 drops 4 times a day as needed

Cautions and Considerations Few problems are encountered with otic antibiotics. In severe cases, children can have conjunctivitis along with an ear infection. If both eyedrops and eardrops are prescribed, be sure to inform the patient about the difference between these medications.

Kolb's Learning Styles

Learners who like details and reflective learning, such as Assimilators, may find this exercise useful for putting ophthalmic and otic antibiotics into context. Compare the drugs listed in Tables 14.3 and 14.7 to the antibiotics covered in Chapter 23. Which antibiotics are available in oral, ophthalmic, and otic dosage forms? Which drug classes from Chapter 23 are represented in this chapter?

Otitis Externa

External ear infection (otitis externa) is an infection of the ear canal and involves bacteria or fungi that thrive in moist environments such as that found in cerumen (earwax). When cerumen builds up, hearing can become impaired and infection can follow. Regular swimmers have the highest propensity to develop external ear infections because pool water and moisture may not properly drain. For that reason, otitis externa is commonly known as *swimmer's ear*.

Drug Regimens and Treatments

Treating external ear infections calls for removing moisture, wax, and any bacteria present from the ear canal. Topical otic preparations are necessary, as oral administration would not reach the desired site of action. These preparations, commonly known as **eardrops**, are effective only for otitis externa. If an infection is in the middle ear or inner ear, medication applied to the external ear will not reach the

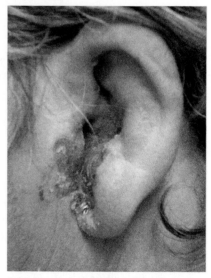

An external ear infection, also known as *swimmer's ear*, is often caused by water that is trapped in the ear after swimming. Signs and symptoms include itching, redness, and drainage from the ear.

intended site of action. Systemic absorption of otic preparations usually is not possible. To teach your patients how to administer eardrops, refer to the following Patient Teaching feature box and to Figure 14.6.

Patient Teaching

Eardrops are more likely than ophthalmic agents to come in suspensions as well as solutions. Allied health professionals should remind all patients to shake suspensions well before instilling the medications. Patients should also be instructed to avoid contaminating the dropper tip by touching it to surfaces, fingers, or the ears.

Special instructions should be given to patients who have tubes in their ears. This patient population should only instill suspensions and should be extra careful to keep otic preparations sterile to avoid introducing infection in the ears.

When administering eardrops to a patient, ask the patient to lie down with the affected ear directed upward. In children younger than three years old, pull the earlobe gently down and back. In older children and adults, pull the earlobe up and out. (This manipulation of the earlobe creates the best angle for administration.) Then gently squeeze the dropper bottle to instill the required number of drops into the ear canal.

FIGURE 14.6 | Administering Otic Drops

(a) Children ages three and older and adults should have the earlobe pulled up and back when otic medications are administered.

(b) Children under age three should have the earlobe pulled down and back.

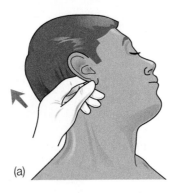 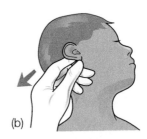

(a)   (b)

Drying Agents and Earwax Removers

Drying agents are used for treatment or prevention of otitis externa. Treatment may be given on a short-term basis for active infection or taken on a regular (even daily) basis to prevent potential infection. **Earwax removers** are used for patients with cerumen impaction. Earwax removers first loosen and dissolve cerumen, after which irrigation with warm water flushes it out. To become familiar with these two drug classes, refer to Table 14.7.

Side Effects Side effects from the instillation of otic drying agents and earwax removers are rare.

Contraindications Drying agents are contraindicated in patients with a perforated tympanic membrane. Carbamide peroxide is also contraindicated in patients with a perforated tympanic membrane as well as ear drainage, ear pain, or rash in the ear. Antipyrine/benzocaine should not be used in patients with a perforated tympanic membrane or with ear discharge.

Cautions and Considerations Other than the contraindications described previously, there are no other notable cautions and considerations associated with the use of otic drying agents and earwax removers.

Ototoxicity

Ototoxicity is damage to the ear caused by chemical or drug exposure. Several drugs can cause ototoxicity (see Table 14.9), and a few drugs, such as aminoglycosides, can cause hearing loss, although the loss is usually temporary if caught early. Symptoms can begin as ringing in the ears (tinnitus) and progress to noticeable hearing loss. Because these symptoms are unexpected among patients, allied health professionals should inform patients to contact their healthcare practitioners right away if these side effects occur.

TABLE 14.9 Drugs That Can Cause Ototoxicity
Aminoglycosides
Aspirin and salicylates
Benzodiazepines
Calcium-channel blockers
Cisplatin and some other chemotherapy agents
Erythromycin and macrolides
Furosemide
Neomycin
NSAIDs
Quinine
Some antiviral agents used in HIV/AIDS
Tricyclic antidepressants
Valproic acid

 Checkpoint 14.4

Take a moment to review what you have learned so far and answer these questions.

1. What drugs are used to treat otitis media and otitis externa?
2. What is another name for swimmer's ear?
3. What is ototoxicity?

Herbal and Alternative Therapies

Vitamin A, or **beta-carotene**, is essential for photoreceptor cell growth and regeneration. Deficiency in vitamin A can cause night blindness. Natural sources of vitamin A include carrots, potatoes, and peppers. Vitamin A, vitamin C, vitamin E, and zinc may slow disease progression of age-related macular degeneration. Ocuvite is a brand-name combination product made especially for this use. It is taken in doses of two tablets each morning and evening with food. This combination of vitamins does not cure or prevent macular degeneration. Patients who smoke or have a high risk of certain types of cancer may not be good candidates for therapy with this product. Patients should talk with their healthcare practitioners before starting to take any vitamin products to treat eye conditions.

Olive oil is an ingredient in some natural otic products used to soften earwax in order to remove it from the ears. Docusate sodium, a common stool softener, is combined with olive oil as a base and applied in the ear to soften earwax.

 In the Know

Beta-carotene is the yellowish-orange pigment found in nectarines, pumpkins, mangoes, and carrots. But did you know that flamingos get their characteristic color from beta-carotene? Their diet of blue-green algae and crustaceans is rich in beta-carotene.

Chapter Review

Chapter Summary

Eye conditions include glaucoma, conjunctivitis, CMV retinitis and herpes infections, eye allergies, chronic dry eye, retinopathy, and macular degeneration. The most common eye disorders for which drug therapy is used are glaucoma, bacterial infections, and viral infections. Topical prostaglandin agonists, beta blockers, alpha receptor agonists, and miotics are given as ophthalmic drops to treat glaucoma. Numerous antibiotics and antiviral medications are administered as eyedrops and ointments. Eyedrops must be kept sterile, so the applicator tip should not touch anything.

Applying eye ointments requires a technique that can take practice to learn and perform well.

Middle ear infections are the most common ear condition. Oral antibiotics are the prescribed drug therapy. Eardrops are used most often for external ear infections but can be used as adjunct treatment for middle ear infections in a few cases. Instilling eardrops in young children (younger than age three) requires the parent or caregiver to pull the patient's earlobe down and back; administering eardrops to older children and adults requires the patient or caregiver to pull the earlobe up and out.

Chapter Checkup

The Navigator+ learning management system that accompanies this textbook offers many opportunities to help you master chapter content, including end-of-chapter exercises, a glossary of key terms, flash cards, and additional interactive activities.

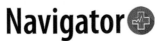

Career Exploration

If you enjoyed learning about the eyes and ears in this chapter, you may want to explore the following career options:

- audiologist
- low vision therapist
- medical assistant
- ophthalmic assistant
- ophthalmic dispensing optician
- ophthalmic laboratory technologist
- ophthalmic laser technician
- ophthalmic medical technologist
- orthoptist
- pharmacy technician

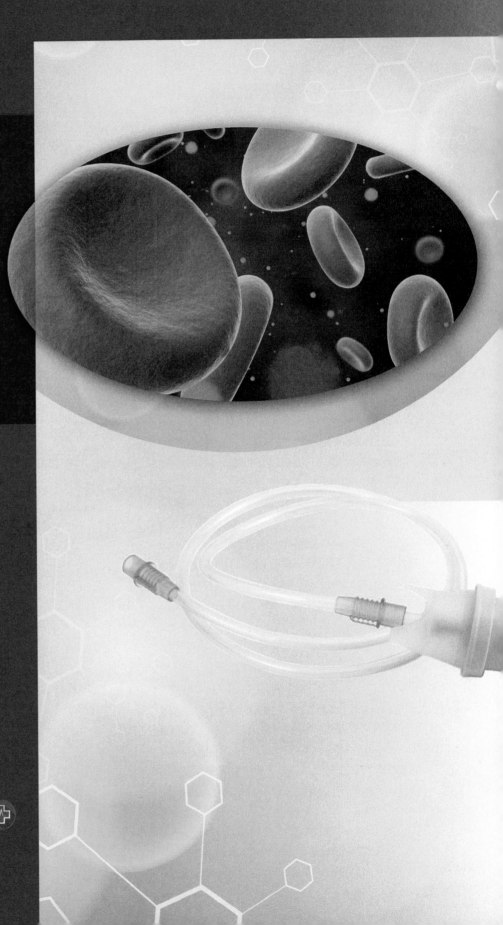

Navigator

Pharmacotherapy for the Cardiovascular and Respiratory Systems

15 The Cardiovascular System and Drug Therapy

Pharm Facts

- The heart beats, on average, 72 times a minute. So, if you do the math, the heart beats more than 100,000 times in a 24-hour period and almost 38 million times in a year.

- It takes only 20 seconds for blood to circulate through your entire body.

- If an individual's blood vessels were attached end-to-end, the vessels would extend 60,000 miles—a distance equivalent to circling Earth about two-and-a-half times.

- Your heart is actually a high-pressure pump, so strong it can squirt blood up to 30 feet.

- The commonly held belief that the heart is bright red is not quite accurate. The heart is really reddish-brown in color, and its outer surface has a yellowish tinge from fatty deposits.

"A cardiovascular perfusionist operates the heart-lung machine for patients undergoing surgery that requires cardiopulmonary bypass. It's multitasking taken to the next level, for I need to artificially mimic native cardiovascular work once the patient's heart is stopped. I'm responsible for the safe handling of the patient's blood through the circuit, which means that I must maintain adequate oxygenation of the blood and sufficient blood pressure/cardiac output for the patient. It truly feels like magic when the patient's heart resumes its independent functioning and the EKG converts from a straight line to a beating heart. If you're looking for a challenging job opportunity and want to be part of a multidisciplinary team in the cardiac operating room, cardiovascular perfusion is your calling. You will not regret it."

—**Bharat Datt**, Msc, CCP, CPC, FPP
Chief Cardiovascular Perfusionist

Learning Objectives

1 Understand the basic anatomy and physiology of the cardiovascular system.

2 Describe the common conditions that affect the cardiovascular system.

3 Explain the therapeutic and adverse effects of prescription medications and nonprescription medications commonly used to treat disorders of the cardiovascular system.

4 Identify the generic names, brand names, indications, dosage ranges, side effects, contraindications, and cautions and considerations associated with the drugs commonly used to treat disorders of the cardiovascular system.

5 Identify common herbal and alternative therapies that are related to the cardiovascular system.

The drugs used to prevent and treat cardiovascular disorders represent a large number of the total prescriptions dispensed nationally. In fact, most healthcare professionals will encounter high blood pressure medications on a daily basis. Be aware that the number of medications used for the cardiovascular system is large, and learning them can be a daunting task. Nonetheless, the frequency with which you will encounter such agents makes familiarity with these drugs imperative.

This chapter describes the function of the heart and blood vessels and then outlines the most common disorders affecting the cardiovascular system. These disorders include hypertension, arrhythmia, angina, and heart failure. The drug classes used most frequently for these conditions include beta blockers, angiotensin-converting enzyme (ACE) inhibitors, calcium-channel blockers, antiarrhythmic agents, digoxin, and nitroglycerin. Finally, this chapter also covers hyperlipidemia because this condition contributes to cardiovascular disease.

Anatomy and Physiology of the Cardiovascular System

The **cardiovascular system**, which includes the heart and blood vessels, circulates blood throughout the body, bringing needed oxygen and nutrients to tissues and carrying away carbon dioxide and toxic by-products. Without a properly functioning cardiovascular system, life is not sustainable. The heart pumps blood to the body through **arteries**, which carry blood away from the heart, and receives blood back from the tissues through **veins** (see Figure 15.1). In the **capillaries** (tiny blood vessels), critical fluids, gases, and nutrients are exchanged between the blood and body tissues. The heart also pumps blood through the lungs, where the blood is replenished with **oxygen** and releases **carbon dioxide**, which is then exhaled.

FIGURE 15.1 Bloodflow through the Circulatory System

Oxygenated blood is depicted in red, whereas blood returning from the body, in need of oxygen, is shown in blue.

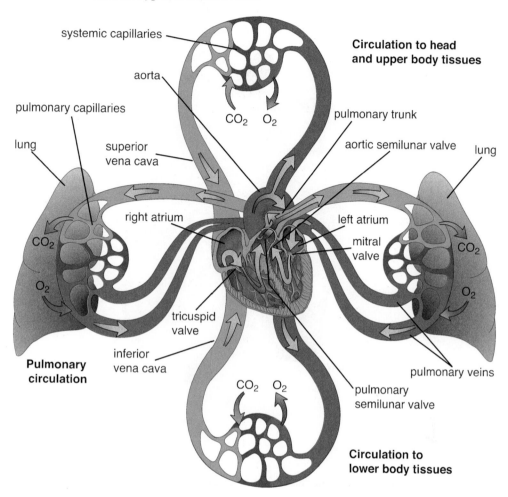

Cardiac Muscle Contraction and Relaxation

The heart is made of specialized **cardiac muscle fibers** that make up the heart's four chambers: the right and left **atria** and the right and left **ventricles**. Figure 15.2 shows the functional anatomy of the heart. The atria receive the blood that is brought to the heart, and the ventricles push blood out, either to the lungs or to other body tissues.

Systole refers to the period during which the heart is contracting and actively pumping blood. **Diastole** refers to the period when heart muscle relaxes, allowing blood to passively flow into the heart and fill the heart's chambers. Cardiac muscle contraction in the atria and ventricles is coordinated by special conduction fibers that carry electrical signals through the heart tissue (see Figure 15.3). These electrical signals control muscle contraction (systole) and relaxation (diastole) by depolarizing and repolarizing the surface of cardiac muscle cells. In effect, a wave of positive-to-negative electrical charges passes from cell to cell, causing them to contract in sequence. Potassium, sodium, and calcium ions, all positively charged, cross the cell membrane through tiny channels and create the waves of positive and negative charges.

FIGURE 15.2 Anatomy of the Heart

Blood is prevented from flowing backward within the heart by the one-way valves between the atria and ventricles. These valves snap shut in a coordinated, two-step process that creates an audible sound—the distinctive "lub-dub" of a heartbeat.

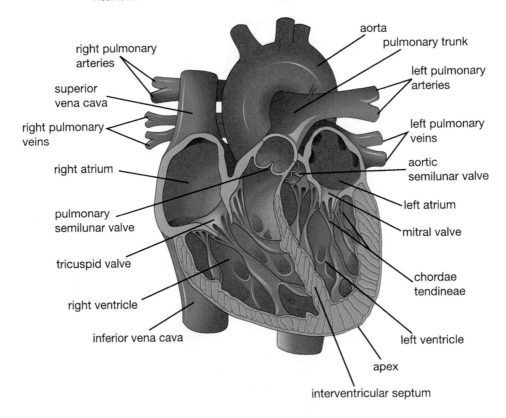

The heartbeat starts in the **sinoatrial (SA) node**, a bundle of conduction fibers in the right atrium and often called the heart's natural pacemaker. The electrical signal is carried through the atria and at the same time down to the **atrioventricular (AV) node**. After a delay, the signal travels through the **bundle of His**. At this point, the signal branches into the **Purkinje fibers**, which stretch into the ventricles to contract the lower—and largest—part of the heart. The signal travels down to the apex of the heart first, and then back up to the ventricular myocardium. The typical rate at which the SA node fires to initiate each heartbeat is 60 to 100 times per minute. **Heart rate (HR)** is reported in **beats per minute (BPM)** and is measured by taking a person's **pulse**. Easy places to feel a pulse include the carotid artery on the neck and the radial pulse on the thumb side of the wrist.

The electrical signal flowing through the heart is measured with an **electrocardiogram (ECG or EKG) machine**. This machine translates these signals into a wave line that is drawn onto paper or displayed on a screen (see Figure 15.3). Cardiologists look for abnormalities in the shape or size of these waves to diagnose heart dysfunction.

Work Wise

An allied health professional can become a Certified EKG Technician (CET) through the National Healthcareer Association (NHA). Benefits of obtaining an EKG technician certification may include more job opportunities, higher pay scale, added job security, and increased subject matter expertise.

Typically, an ECG has five deflections (spikes and dips), arbitrarily named *P to T waves*. Each section of the ECG is labeled and corresponds to action in a particular part of the heart. The PR interval corresponds to atrial function, and the QT interval refers to ventricular function. The P wave represents the depolarization of the atria; the QRS complex represents the depolarization of the ventricles; and the T wave represents the repolarization of the ventricles.

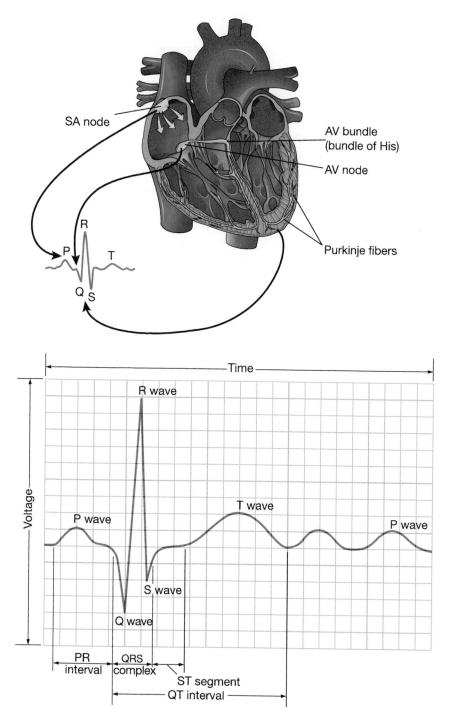

Blood Pressure

Blood pressure, the force of blood that fills the circulatory system, is maintained by complex feedback mechanisms. Figure 15.4 shows the variety of mechanisms that work together to properly balance blood pressure. In simple terms, blood pressure is a function of the following mechanisms:

- **capacitance**—the amount of blood held in the system

- **peripheral vascular resistance (PVR)**—the degree to which the blood vessels are constricted or relaxed

- **cardiac output (CO)**—the force and volume of blood coming from the heart

- **renin-angiotensin system**—the feedback mechanism that is regulated by the kidneys and that balances fluid volume and vessel constriction

If blood vessels are constricted, causing increased PVR, the heart has to work harder to maintain the same cardiac output to keep blood pressure stable. Therefore, **constriction** or **dilation** of blood vessels will raise or lower blood pressure, respectively. High blood pressure is often caused by elevated PVR. Stress on the heart from high blood pressure may cause cardiac disease. High blood pressure also affects vital organs and can eventually result in kidney failure and stroke. Sympathetic nerves in the autonomic nervous system (see Chapter 12) regulate this multifaceted system. Alterations in any one of these compensatory checks and balances can cause hypertension. Losing large amounts of blood lowers blood pressure to dangerous levels. If blood pressure falls low enough, the patient may go into shock, a condition during which vital organs are not perfused with blood and begin to shut down.

FIGURE 15.4 | Maintaining Blood Pressure

The sympathetic nerves of the central nervous system (CNS) regulate the multi-faceted system that maintains blood pressure.

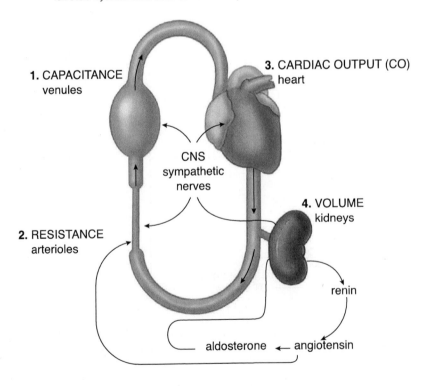

Blood Pressure Measurement

Blood pressure is measured with an instrument called a **sphygmomanometer** and a cuff that is wrapped around a patient's arm and inflated to apply pressure. The cuff briefly cuts off bloodflow through the brachial artery in the upper arm. Air is slowly released from the cuff, lowering the pressure to a point at which the blood begins flowing (with turbulence, however) through the artery again. This turbulent bloodflow is audible through a stethoscope placed over the brachial artery. When blood starts flowing again, the first or upper number reported in a blood pressure result is obtained. This number is called the systolic reading or the **systolic blood pressure (SBP)**. The diastolic reading or the **diastolic blood pressure (DBP)**, the lower number in a blood pressure result, is obtained at the point at which the cuff is loose enough that blood flows freely through the artery without turbulence. At this turbulence-free point, the pulsing sound heard through the stethoscope fades away and becomes silent. Therefore, when taking a reading, you listen first for the start of the sound (and note the systolic reading or SBP) and second for when the sound goes away (and note the diastolic reading or DBP). Ideal blood pressure is 120/80 mm Hg, but this number can be affected by recent stress, physical activity, caffeine intake, nicotine use, and various medical conditions. An athlete may have lower blood pressure readings than 120/80 mm Hg, which is normal as long as the patient is not experiencing symptoms of blood loss to the brain or other organs. Symptoms of blood loss include dizziness, nausea, or fatigue.

In the Know

The beating sounds you listen for when measuring blood pressure are called *Korotkoff sounds*. Korotkoff sounds are the arterial noises heard through a stethoscope when applied to the brachial artery. These sounds change as the blood pressure cuff undergoes inflation and deflation. Dr. Nicolai Korotkoff, a Russian physician, introduced the auscultation (or hearing) method of blood pressure measurement in 1905.

Kolb's Learning Styles

If you are a learner who prefers visual images and abstract thought, as Divergers do, you may find it helpful to superimpose a list of drugs and their dosage forms onto Figure 15.4. Under each of the four primary compensatory mechanisms for maintaining blood pressure, list the drugs that affect each one. To complete this list, think about a drug's mechanism of action.

Checkpoint 15.1

Take a moment to review what you have learned so far and answer these questions.

1. What roles do arteries, veins, and capillaries play in the cardiovascular system?

2. What part of the heart is considered the body's natural pacemaker?

3. What is the difference between systolic blood pressure and diastolic blood pressure?

Allied health professionals should discuss with their patients who have high blood pressure the importance of taking regular blood pressure readings. Recommend that patients use either a blood pressure machine at a store or an at-home blood pressure device to perform this task. At-home blood pressure devices are available as manual devices and digital devices and contain an inflatable cuff, a gauge, and—sometimes—a stethoscope. The manual device requires the user to inflate the cuff and use a stethoscope to listen to arterial sounds. The digital device contains a cuff that automatically inflates and that has a built-in sensor that records arterial sounds.

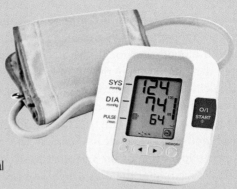

A digital blood pressure monitor allows patients to take their blood pressure readings at home.

Advise patients to wait a minimum of 30 minutes after exercising, smoking, bathing, or drinking alcohol before obtaining a blood pressure reading. Direct the patient to sit comfortably with his or her feet on the floor for several minutes prior to taking the reading. For a manual monitor, the patient should place the blood pressure cuff around the upper arm; for a digital device, the patient can place the cuff around the upper arm or around the wrist, depending on the model. A machine that measures blood pressure on the arm is preferable to one that measures blood pressure on the wrist. For the latter technique, the patient must have the wrist cuff at the level of the heart to produce accurate results. Finally, remind the patient to sit still during the blood pressure reading.

Common Cardiovascular System Disorders

Because **heart disease**, more formally known as **cardiovascular disease**, is the leading cause of death in the United States, many healthcare resources are devoted to its treatment. Unfortunately, it seems that everyone knows someone who has experienced a heart attack. But cardiovascular disease encompasses many conditions, not just heart attacks. Other conditions that are considered under the umbrella of cardiovascular disease include hypertension (high blood pressure), cardiac arrhythmias, angina, and heart failure.

Hypertension

Hypertension (HTN), or high blood pressure, is a silent killer that affects more than 50 million people in the United States. Patients cannot immediately feel the effects of hypertension, but damage to vital organs such as the heart, kidneys, eyes, and brain occurs when pressure is high for extended periods. Elevation in either systolic or diastolic blood pressure, or both, is considered hypertension. If blood pressure is especially high (greater than 180/110 mm Hg), urgent medical attention is needed. At that pressure, capillaries might burst and cause immediate stroke and blindness. Factors that contribute to high blood pressure include smoking, diabetes, kidney disease, age, family history, gender, and lifestyle (diet, lack of exercise, weight, and alcohol use). High blood pressure usually develops over time. Consequently, a single elevated reading is not sufficient to diagnose hypertension.

Drug Regimens and Treatments

Blood pressure goals are determined by the patient and his or her prescriber. The "2014 Evidence-Based Guideline for the Management of High Blood Pressure in Adults," published in the *Journal of the American Medical Association*, offers recommendations for the management of hypertension. The article suggests treating high blood pressure when it exceeds 150/90 for people age 60 and older and 140/90 for people younger than age 60. Patients with diabetes or kidney disease should begin treatment for high blood pressure when it exceeds 140/90 no matter what age they are. Some healthcare professionals use a staged system for diagnosing and treating high blood pressure:

- stage 1 hypertension =
  systolic blood pressure (SBP) ≥ 140 mm Hg; or
  diastolic blood pressure (DBP) ≥ 90 mm Hg

- stage 2 hypertension = SBP ≥ 160 mm Hg; or DBP ≥ 100 mm Hg

- hypertensive emergency = SBP ≥ 180 mm Hg; or DBP ≥ 110 mm Hg

Healthy lifestyle modifications, such as weight loss and regular exercise, are used to treat hypertension at all stages.

The "2014 Evidence-Based Guideline" also suggests that drug selection to treat hypertension should be based on patient-specific factors such as age, ethnicity, and the presence of diabetes and chronic kidney disease. Regardless of the drug choice, dosing strategies for antihypertensives are included in the article.

Because hypertension is a progressive condition that often worsens over time, patients may find themselves taking multiple medications to get their blood pressure under control. Eventually, blood pressure medications alter the compensatory systems that control blood pressure. Abruptly stopping therapy can cause an immediate rebound in blood pressure, putting a patient at risk for a hypertensive emergency.

Work Wise

For some patients, a visit to a physician's office can make them feel anxious, ill at ease, or uncomfortable. These heightened stress levels can abnormally elevate blood pressure readings—a reaction known as *white coat syndrome*. A skilled healthcare professional can help minimize this effect by making sure the patient is seated comfortably in a quiet room. If an uncomfortable procedure is scheduled and the patient seems anxious about it, perform the procedure early in the visit and wait until later to measure the patient's blood pressure.

Patient Teaching

Remind patients to refill their blood pressure medications regularly. They should not stop taking blood pressure medications suddenly if they run out, as this can cause a rapid rise in blood pressure that can be dangerous.

Also, tell patients that they should not stop taking their blood pressure medications because they feel their blood pressure is low enough. Remind them that these medications are controlling their blood pressure, not curing their hypertension.

ACE Inhibitors

This class of drugs is used for a variety of cardiac conditions: hypertension, angina, heart attack, heart failure, and kidney disease (see Table 15.1). Patients with diabetes may be prescribed **angiotensin-converting enzyme (ACE) inhibitors** to protect the kidneys from long-term damage. ACE inhibitors are said to be renal protective and are used even when blood pressure is not elevated. Consequently, you cannot assume that all patients with diabetes who take ACE inhibitors have hypertension.

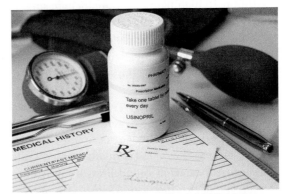

Lisinopril is a commonly prescribed ACE inhibitor used to treat hypertension.

ACE inhibitors regulate blood pressure through the renin-angiotensin system. **Renin**, an enzyme produced by the kidneys, is converted to **angiotensin I** in the bloodstream. Angiotensin I is, in turn, converted to **angiotensin II** by **angiotensin-converting enzyme (ACE)**. Angiotensin II is a potent vasoconstrictor; blocking its production usually allows blood vessels to relax, which lowers vascular resistance and overall blood pressure.

TABLE 15.1 **Common ACE Inhibitors**

Generic (Brand)	Dosage Form	Route of Administration	Common Dosage
Benazepril (Lotensin)	Tablet	Oral	5–40 mg a day
Captopril (Capoten)	Tablet	Oral	25–100 mg a day
Enalapril (Epaned, Vasotec)	Injectable solution, tablet	IV, oral	IV: 1.25 mg every 6 hr infused over 5 min PO: 5–20 mg a day
Fosinopril (Monopril)	Tablet	Oral	10–40 mg a day
Lisinopril (Prinivil, Zestril)	Tablet	Oral	5–40 mg a day
Moexipril (Univasc)	Tablet	Oral	7.5–30 mg a day
Perindopril (Aceon)	Tablet	Oral	4–16 mg a day
Quinapril (Accupril)	Tablet	Oral	10–80 mg a day
Ramipril (Altace)	Capsule	Oral	2.5–20 mg a day
Trandolapril (Mavik)	Tablet	Oral	1–4 mg a day

Side Effects Common side effects of ACE inhibitors include headache, dizziness, fatigue, mild diarrhea, and a dry, hacking cough. Dizziness occurs most frequently in patients taking ACE inhibitors for heart failure. A cough is a frequent but odd side effect that patients often do not associate with their blood pressure medication. The cough is caused by a buildup of a substance called bradykinin in the respiratory tract and is an unintended effect of ACE inhibitors. Pharmacists and other healthcare workers can help identify those patients with this annoying but harmless side effect. Unfortunately, if a patient experiences a cough with one ACE inhibitor, other ACE inhibitors will likely produce the same effect. The cough will resolve when the ACE inhibitor is discontinued.

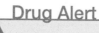
Angioedema is a rare but serious side effect of ACE inhibitors. It is an allergic-like reaction wherein swelling of the tongue and face are sufficiently severe to threaten breathing. If patients report slurred speech, difficulty swallowing, or an enlarged tongue, medical help should be sought immediately.

Quick Study

When you are studying cardiovascular drugs, remember that all of the generic names for ACE inhibitors end with –*pril*.

Contraindications ACE inhibitors should not be used in patients who have experienced angioedema with previous ACE inhibitor use. Other contraindications include idiopathic or hereditary angioedema and concomitant use with aliskiren in patients with diabetes mellitus.

Pregnant patients should not take ACE inhibitors because these agents can cause severe birth defects. Patients with a kidney condition called bilateral renal artery stenosis also should not take ACE inhibitors because the kidneys could shut down.

➕ *Note: Allied health professionals should be aware that an allergy to a particular drug contraindicates its use. This warning applies to all Contraindications sections in this chapter.*

Cautions and Considerations In rare instances, **hypotension**, or low blood pressure, can occur. For ACE inhibitors, hypotension can happen dramatically, sometimes on the first dose. Careful monitoring is necessary when a patient starts taking an ACE inhibitor. In some cases, the first dose may be given in the physician's office, so the patient's blood pressure can be monitored for drastic drops.

Elevated potassium levels (hyperkalemia) is another rare but serious effect. It tends to occur when patients are also taking potassium-sparing diuretics such as spironolactone. Periodic blood tests for potassium levels will be conducted. Patients who take diuretics along with an ACE inhibitor should be warned against taking potassium supplements.

Patients who have kidney problems (other than bilateral renal artery stenosis) can take ACE inhibitors, but doses are adjusted downward.

ARBs

Like ACE inhibitors, **angiotensin receptor blockers (ARBs)** are used to treat hypertension and heart failure. They are often used as an alternative choice when a patient cannot tolerate ACE inhibitors. Some ARBs can also be used for their renal protective effects in patients with diabetes (see Table 15.2).

Quick Study

All of the generic drug names for ARBs end with –*sartan*.

ARBs work by binding to the same receptors to which angiotensin II binds. Instead of stimulating vasoconstriction, as angiotensin II does, ARBs block these receptors, thereby preventing constriction and causing blood vessels to relax, which lowers blood pressure. ARBs do not cause bradykinin buildup as ACE inhibitors do, so coughing is not a typical side effect.

Side Effects Common side effects of ARBs include headache, dizziness, fatigue, and mild diarrhea. Dizziness occurs most frequently in patients who also have heart failure. Patients taking ARBs may also have more respiratory tract infections, but the reason for this side effect is unknown.

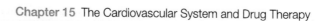

TABLE 15.2 Common ARBs

Generic (Brand)	Dosage Form	Route of Administration	Common Dosage
Azilsartan (Edarbi)	Tablet	Oral	40–80 mg a day
Candesartan (Atacand)	Tablet	Oral	8–32 mg once or twice a day
Eprosartan (Teveten)	Tablet	Oral	400–800 mg a day
Irbesartan (Avapro)	Tablet	Oral	150 mg a day
Losartan (Cozaar)	Tablet	Oral	25–100 mg a day
Olmesartan (Benicar)	Tablet	Oral	20–40 mg a day
Telmisartan (Micardis)	Tablet	Oral	20–80 mg a day
Valsartan (Diovan)	Tablet	Oral	80–320 mg a day

Contraindications ARBs are contraindicated in patients with diabetes mellitus who are taking aliskiren.

Cautions and Considerations Patients taking diuretics along with ARBs may experience hypotension. Patients should be careful about getting up too quickly from a sitting or lying position until they know how these drugs affect them. A drop in blood pressure upon sitting or standing is called *orthostatic hypotension*. Dizziness, fainting, and falling down may be signs of hypotension. Patients with kidney or liver impairment may need special dosing and monitoring if they are to take these medications.

Calcium-Channel Blockers

This drug class is used regularly to treat hypertension, heart failure, and arrhythmias. Because of adverse effects, **calcium-channel blockers** (see Table 15.3) are not usually the first therapeutic choice for high blood pressure. They can be useful when a patient has more than one cardiovascular condition necessitating drug therapy.

Calcium-channel blockers decrease blood pressure by preventing calcium from entering the smooth-muscle cells of arterial walls. When calcium cannot enter as usual, smooth-muscle cells relax to open up blood vessels and lower blood pressure.

TABLE 15.3 Common Calcium-Channel Blockers

Generic (Brand)	Dosage Form	Route of Administration	Common Dosage
Amlodipine (Norvasc)	Tablet	Oral	5–10 mg a day
Clevidipine (Cleviprex)	Emulsion	IV	16–21 mg/hr
Diltiazem (Cardizem, Dilacor)	Capsule, solution, tablet	IV, oral	IV: 20–25 mg infused over 2 min or 5–10 mg/hr continuous infusion × 24 hr PO: 180–240 mg a day
Felodipine	Tablet	Oral	2.5–10 mg a day
Isradipine	Capsule	Oral	5–20 mg a day
Nicardipine (Cardene)	Capsule, injectable solution	IV, oral	IV: 0.5–2.2 mg/hr continuous infusion PO: 20–40 mg three times a day
Nifedipine (Adalat, Procardia)	Capsule, tablet	Oral	30–120 mg a day
Nisoldipine (Sular)	Tablet	Oral	17–34 mg a day
Verapamil (Calan, Isoptin, Verelan)	Capsule, injection, tablet	IV, oral	IV: 5–10 mg infused over 2–3 min PO: 240–320 mg a day

Drug Alert

Two of the calcium-channel blockers are easily confused: nicardipine and nifedipine. Be sure your orders and drug supply match accordingly. The dosages are different for these two medications.

Side Effects Common side effects of calcium-channel blockers include headache, dizziness, fatigue, constipation, nausea, heartburn, and flushing. In most cases, these effects are mild. If patients cannot tolerate these effects, they should be referred to their healthcare prescribers for a change of medication.

Contraindications Clevidipine should not be used in patients with a hypersensitivity to soy or egg, or in patients who have high triglyceride levels, nephrosis, or severe aortic stenosis. Contraindications to diltiazem include sick sinus syndrome, second- or third-degree AV block, severe low blood pressure, acute heart attack, and pulmonary congestion. Felodipine and nisoldipine should not be used in patients with a hypersensitivity to other calcium-channel blockers. Nicardipine should not be used in patients with aortic stenosis. Nifedipine is contraindicated in patients with cardiogenic shock and acute heart attack. Contraindications to verapamil include severe left ventricular dysfunction, hypotension, cardiogenic shock, sick sinus syndrome, second- or third-degree AV block, Wolff-Parkinson-White syndrome, and Lown-Ganong-Levine syndrome. The intravenous (IV) form of verapamil is also contraindicated with concurrent use of beta blockers and in patients with ventricular tachycardia. Amlodipine and isradipine do not have contraindications.

Cautions and Considerations Some calcium-channel blockers cause fluid retention (edema) and heart palpitations. To balance the positive and negative effects on the heart, healthcare practitioners closely monitor patients taking this class of drugs.

Select calcium-channel blockers come in extended-release dosage forms that need to be taken just once a day. These products should be swallowed whole, not crushed or chewed. Crushing or chewing the medication ruins the release mechanism and could result in drastically lowered blood pressure because the entire large dose would be released at once.

Patients should be warned that some of the extended-release dosage forms (such as the oral form of verapamil) work by releasing the drug from a capsule or tablet called a **ghost pill** while in the digestive system. This ghost pill then moves through the gastrointestinal (GI) tract and appears in the patients' stool. Tell patients not to be alarmed by the appearance of this casing in their stool, and reassure them that the medication has been absorbed by the body.

Thiazide Diuretics

As a cornerstone of hypertension treatment, **thiazide diuretics** have been on the market for years. These diuretics are either the first or second choice for control of a patient's blood pressure. These drugs work by helping the kidneys eliminate sodium and fluid from the body, which decreases blood volume and lowers blood pressure.

Side Effects Side effects of thiazide diuretics at low doses are rare but can include hypotension, dizziness, headache, skin rash, hair loss (alopecia), upset stomach, diarrhea, and constipation. Getting up slowly from sitting or lying down can help with dizziness and drops in blood pressure.

Contraindications Thiazide diuretics are contra-indicated in patients with a hypersensitivity to sulfonamide-derived drugs and in patients who have anuria.

Cautions and Considerations Thiazide diuretics can deplete potassium levels in the body. Taking potassium supplements is sometimes necessary with these diuretics to maintain proper electrolyte balance. Patients should understand that taking these supplements is important because potassium is essential for good cardiac function.

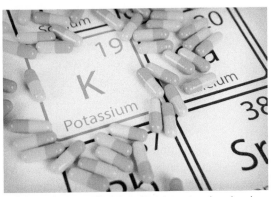

Because thiazide diuretics deplete potassium levels in the body, healthcare practitioners often concurrently prescribe potassium supplements to maintain electrolyte balance.

Thiazide diuretics can interact with alcohol to contribute to drops in blood pressure. Patients should use caution when drinking alcohol while taking these medications. Thiazide diuretics can also interact with diabetes medications because they can raise blood glucose levels. However, at low doses, this is not a concern. Thiazide diuretics interact with corticosteroids and lithium, so they should not be taken in conjunction with them.

Alpha Blockers and Beta Blockers

As explained in Chapter 12, alpha blockers and beta blockers are adrenergic inhibitors that control blood pressure by blocking certain adrenaline receptor types found in the body (see Table 15.4). **Alpha blockers** are especially useful for men with both high blood pressure and benign prostatic hyperplasia (BPH). **Beta blockers** have beneficial effects on the heart, especially after a heart attack. These drugs have been on the market for years, and most are inexpensive and available generically.

Side Effects Common side effects seen with alpha blockers include headache, dizziness, nausea, and fatigue. Patients should avoid driving until they know how these medications affect them. Fortunately, these effects typically improve over time, as a patient gets used to the medication. On rare occasions, male patients have also experienced priapism (erection lasting longer than four hours). If this condition occurs, the patient should seek medical help right away because priapism can cause permanent impotence if left untreated.

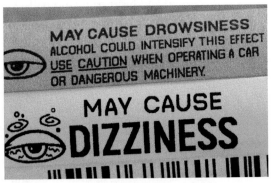

An alpha blocker or a beta blocker should have an auxiliary label affixed to the container that warns a patient about the possibility of dizziness as a side effect.

Common side effects of beta blockers include headache, dizziness, nausea, fatigue, and weakness. Patients should avoid driving until they know how these medications affect them. Fortunately, these effects generally improve over time. This class of drugs has been associated with an increased incidence of depression. Patients who complain of symptoms of depression should be referred to their healthcare prescribers for appropriate evaluation. Beta blockers can sometimes slow the heart rate too much and exacerbate cardiac conditions such as angina, arrhythmia, and heart failure. Patients who experience difficulty breathing (especially with physical activity or when lying down), night coughing, or swelling of the extremities should seek medical attention right away.

TABLE 15.4 Alpha Blockers and Beta Blockers

Generic (Brand)	Dosage Form	Route of Administration	Common Dosage
Alpha Blockers			
Doxazosin (Cardura)	Tablet	Oral	BPH: 1–2 mg a day HTN: 1–16 mg a day
Prazosin (Minipress)	Capsule	Oral	HTN: 2–20 mg a day, taken in divided doses
Terazosin (Hytrin)	Capsule, tablet	Oral	BPH: 1–10 mg once a day HTN: 1–5 mg a day
Beta-1 Selective Beta Blockers			
Acebutolol (Sectral)	Capsule	Oral	400–800 mg a day
Atenolol (Tenormin)	Tablet	Oral	50–100 mg a day
Betaxolol (Kerlone)	Tablet	Oral	10–20 mg a day
Bisoprolol (Zebeta)	Tablet	Oral	5–20 mg a day
Esmolol (Brevibloc)	Injection	IV	Varies depending on patient weight Infused over 1–4 min
Metoprolol (Lopressor, Toprol)	Injection, tablet	IV, oral	Succinate oral: 50–100 mg a day Tartrate oral: 100–450 mg a day
Nebivolol (Bystolic)	Tablet	Oral	5–40 mg a day
Nonselective Beta Blockers			
Nadolol (Corgard)	Tablet	Oral	40–320 mg a day
Propranolol (Inderal)	Capsule, injection, oral solution, tablet	IV, oral	Dose and frequency vary depending on indication/use
Sotalol (Betapace)	Tablet	Oral	80–160 mg twice a day
Timolol (Blocadren)	Tablet	Oral	10–40 mg twice a day

Contraindications Alpha blockers have no contraindications. Beta blockers are contraindicated in bradycardia (slow heart rate), cardiogenic shock, and heart block. Specific beta blockers may have additional contraindications. Atenolol should not be used in patients with pulmonary edema or in female patients who are pregnant. Propranolol, sotalol, and timolol are contraindicated in lung disorders such as asthma and chronic obstructive pulmonary disease (COPD). Nebivolol should not be used in patients with liver impairment. Sotalol should be avoided in patients with long QT syndrome, kidney dysfunction, and low potassium levels.

Cautions and Considerations Patients taking alpha blockers should be warned of significant hypotension and heart palpitations, which can occur with the first few doses of these agents. Symptoms of these effects are dizziness and fainting. Patients should work with family members or others who can monitor them as they begin taking one of these medications. They should not drive or undertake hazardous tasks for 12 to 24 hours after taking their first dose. Drinking alcohol or taking verapamil can intensify the hypotensive effects and should be avoided when possible. If these symptoms occur, the patient should lie down until the symptoms pass and notify a physician. Doses can be adjusted slowly to minimize or avoid this effect.

Blocking of beta-2 receptors constricts airways in the lungs in addition to lowering blood pressure. This effect can be harmful to patients with impaired respiratory function, for example, those with asthma or COPD. For these individuals, care must be taken to choose drugs that selectively block beta-1 receptors only. Beta blockers that can be used by patients with asthma or COPD include acebutolol, atenolol, betaxolol, bisoprolol, metoprolol, and nebivolol.

Abrupt withdrawal from a beta blocker can cause severe cardiac problems, such as heart attack, angina, or arrhythmia. Thus, patients should not stop taking a beta blocker suddenly. If a change in medication is made, the dose will be decreased slowly until it is discontinued.

Quick Study

A humorous way to recall generic names for beta blockers is to remember that they all end in –lol ("laughing out loud").

Patients with diabetes should use beta blockers with caution. These drugs can inhibit the usual signs and symptoms of a reaction to low blood glucose. The only symptom of low blood glucose that a patient taking a beta blocker may have is sweating. The pharmacist should counsel patients with diabetes who are taking beta blockers.

Over-the-counter (OTC) decongestants are vasoconstrictors that can raise blood pressure. Patients taking beta blockers for high blood pressure should avoid taking oral decongestants.

Patient Teaching

Metoprolol, a commonly used beta blocker, comes in various oral dosage forms. Metoprolol is available as tartrate or succinate salt forms. The tartrate form is an immediate-release tablet that is best taken with food. The succinate form is an extended-release tablet that can be taken with or without food. Be sure that your patients know which form of metoprolol they are taking.

Checkpoint 15.2

Take a moment to review what you have learned so far and answer these questions.

1. What are two recommendations based on the "2014 Evidence-Based Guideline for the Management of High Blood Pressure in Adults"?

2. What classes of drugs are used to treat high blood pressure?

3. Can you name a common side effect for each class of antihypertensive medications?

Cardiac Arrhythmias

Normal heart rhythm is called **sinus rhythm** because it originates from the SA node, or pacemaker, which is located in the left atrium (see Figure 15.3). Any deviation from sinus rhythm is considered an **arrhythmia**. Such deviations could be changes in the rate at which the heart beats or alterations in electrical conductivity through the heart. **Tachycardia** refers to an increased heart rate, whereas **bradycardia** is a decreased heart rate. Other terms, such as *flutter* and *fibrillation*, refer to changes in the way certain parts of the heart beat out of sync with each other. **Flutter** occurs when select portions (the atria, for example) are slightly out of sync with the rest of the heart. It is not necessarily life threatening. In contrast, **fibrillation** can be life threatening and occurs when large portions of the heart beat out of sequence. In ventricular fibrillation, no blood flows through the heart; therefore, the use of an electronic defibrillator to the chest is necessary to shock the heart components back into sequence. ECG readings are used to observe heart function and diagnose arrhythmias (see Figure 15.5). Symptoms of cardiac arrhythmias include palpitations, syncope (fainting), light-headedness, weakness, sweating, chest pain, and pallor (skin paleness).

FIGURE 15.5 Abnormal Heart Rhythms

A straight line (flat line) on the ECG means there is no heartbeat, signaling a cardiac arrest.

Arrhythmia	BPM	ECG Rhythm Strip
Sinus tachycardia	> 100	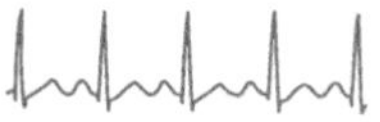
Ventricular tachycardia	150–250	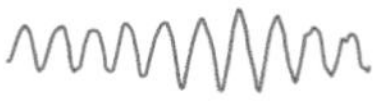
Bradycardia	< 60	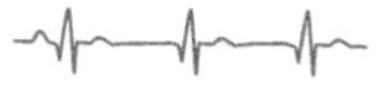
Atrial flutter	200–350	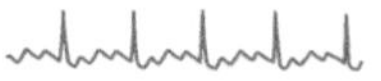
Atrial fibrillation	100–175	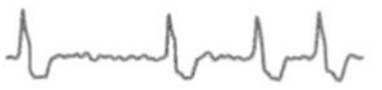
Premature atrial contraction	Varies	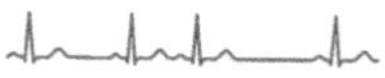
Premature ventricular contraction	Varies	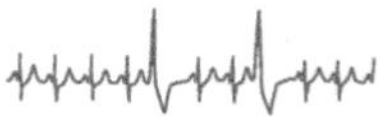
Ventricular fibrillation	Varies	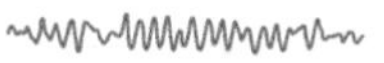
Absence of rhythm (asystole)	0	

Drug Regimens and Treatments

Treatment for arrhythmias attempts to restore normal sinus rhythm by changing the heart rate and conductivity. Antiarrhythmic drugs are categorized into classes by their mechanisms of action. These categories include other drug classes that have effects on heart rhythm. Such medications are chosen and dosed individually, based on desired patient results. Drug interactions can alter the effectiveness of these drugs (see Table 15.5).

TABLE 15.5 Antiarrhythmic Agents

Generic (Brand)	Dosage Form	Significant Drug Interactions	Side Effects	Special Notes
Class I (Membrane-Stabilizing Agents)				
Disopyramide (Norpace)	Capsule	Clarithromycin, erythromycin, fluoroquinolones	Hypotension, anticholinergic effects,* headache, gas, muscle aches/pains	Used only for life-threatening ventricular arrhythmias. Avoid use in patients with heart failure as can reduce heart rate too much.
Flecainide (Tambocor)	Tablet	Cisapride, ritonavir	Dizziness, shortness of breath, headache, nausea, fatigue, palpitations, tremor, angina	Used only for life-threatening ventricular arrhythmias. Avoid use in patients with heart failure as can reduce heart rate too much.
Lidocaine (Xylocaine)	IV	Anticonvulsants	Bradycardia, hypotension, dizziness, drowsiness, blurred vision, confusion	Used only for life-threatening ventricular arrhythmias. Often used to treat acute heart attack.

*Anticholinergic effects include blurred vision, dry mouth, constipation, and reduced urination.

TABLE 15.5   Antiarrhythmic Agents *(continued)*

Generic (Brand)	Dosage Form	Significant Drug Interactions	Side Effects	Special Notes
Mexiletine	Capsule	Caffeine, cimetidine, rifampin, theophylline	Palpitations, chest pain, dizziness, tremor, nervousness, insomnia, nausea, vomiting, blurred vision, headache, shortness of breath	Used only for life-threatening ventricular arrhythmias. Can cause leukopenia (low white blood cells) and agranulocytosis, a severe blood condition.
Procainamide	IV	Amiodarone, antiarrhythmics, cimetidine, fluoroquinolones, ranitidine, thioridazine, ziprasidone	Anorexia, nausea, vomiting, diarrhea, lupus-like syndrome	Used only for atrial arrhythmias. Can cause heart failure in patients with ventricular dysfunction. Can cause leukopenia (low white blood cells) and agranulocytosis, a severe blood condition.
Propafenone (Rythmol)	Capsule, tablet	Cimetidine, digoxin, ritonavir, selective serotonin reuptake inhibitors (SSRIs), theophylline	New arrhythmias, dizziness, nausea, vomiting	Used only for life-threatening ventricular arrhythmias.
Quinidine	IV, tablet	Amiodarone, antacids, cimetidine	Hypotension, anticholinergic effects,* headache, tinnitus, confusion, nausea	Gluconate, polyglyconate, and sulfate salts of quinidine contain varying amounts of active drug and are not interchangeable. Can cause thrombocytopenia, a life-threatening condition of low platelet production.
Class II (Beta Blockers)				
Acebutolol (Sectral)	Capsule	Reserpine	Dizziness, fatigue, headache, diarrhea, indigestion, nausea, gas	None
Esmolol (Brevibloc)	IV	Calcium-channel blockers, nonsteroidal anti-inflammatory drugs (NSAIDs), theophylline	Hypotension	None
Propranolol (Inderal)	Capsule, IV, oral liquid, tablet	Antacids, cimetidine, fluconazole, fluoroquinolones, haloperidol, phenytoin, ritonavir, rizatriptan, SSRIs, theophylline, zolmitriptan	Hypotension, dizziness, fatigue, lupus-like syndrome	None
Sotalol (Betapace)	Tablet	Antacids, antiarrhythmics, calcium-channel blockers, fluoroquinolones, reserpine, thioridazine, ziprasidone	New arrhythmias, bradycardia, chest pain, nausea, vomiting, fatigue, shortness of breath	Used only for life-threatening ventricular arrhythmias. Should not be used in patients with asthma.
Class III (Potassium-Channel Blockers)				
Amiodarone (Cordarone)	IV, tablet	Azole antifungals, cimetidine, fentanyl, fluoroquinolones, loratadine, macrolide antibiotics, other antiarrhythmics, statin antihyperlipidemics, warfarin	Fatigue, tremor, photosensitivity, anorexia, constipation, nausea, vomiting, blurred vision	Takes days to months for full effect. Must use glass bottle for IV solution. Can cause fatal toxicities to lungs, liver, and heart—use with caution.

*Anticholinergic effects include blurred vision, dry mouth, constipation, and reduced urination.

TABLE 15.5 Antiarrhythmic Agents *(continued)*

Generic (Brand)	Dosage Form	Significant Drug Interactions	Side Effects	Special Notes
Dofetilide (Tikosyn)	Capsule	Cimetidine, ketoconazole, trimethoprim, verapamil	New arrhythmias, headache, chest pain, dizziness, shortness of breath, nausea	Used in cardioversion procedures to restore normal rhythm.
Dronedarone (Multaq)	Tablet	Azole antifungals, cyclosporine, fentanyl, fluoroquinolones, other antiarrhythmics, statin antihyperlipidemics, warfarin	Dermatitis, fatigue, hypokalemia, kidney dysfunction, liver dysfunction, skin rash	Similar to amiodarone, but without the iodine. May increase risk of death in patients with symptomatic heart failure. May increase risk of death and stroke in patients with permanent atrial fibrillation.
Class IV (Calcium-Channel Blockers)				
Diltiazem (Cardizem, Dilacor)	Capsule, IV, tablet	Benzodiazepines, carbamazepine, cimetidine, rifampin	Hypotension, bradycardia, nausea, constipation, headache, dizziness, fatigue	Used only for atrial arrhythmia.
Verapamil (Calan, Covera, Isoptin, Verelan)	Capsule, IV, tablet	Alcohol, amiodarone, carbamazepine, cimetidine, grapefruit juice, macrolide antibiotics	Hypotension, bradycardia, nausea, constipation, headache, dizziness, fatigue, indigestion, increased infections	Used only for atrial arrhythmia.

Class I (Membrane-Stabilizing Agents)

This large group of drugs known as **membrane-stabilizing agents** (class I) includes a combination of medications from a few different drug classes that all happen to block sodium channels in cardiac muscle cells. By slowing the influx of sodium, a positively charged ion, the cell membrane becomes more stable and less able to depolarize. Thus, the electrical charge must be stronger to stimulate the cardiac muscle cells to contract and make the heart beat. This effect regulates heart rhythm because it decreases the incidence of abnormal beats.

Side Effects To learn the side effects of membrane-stabilizing agents, refer to Table 15.5.

Contraindications Disopyramide is contraindicated in patients with cardiogenic shock, preexisting second- or third-degree AV block, long QT syndrome, and sick sinus syndrome. Contraindications to flecainide include preexisting second- or third-degree AV block, cardiogenic shock, coronary artery disease, and concurrent use of ritonavir or amprenavir. Systemic lidocaine should be avoided in patients with Adams-Stokes syndrome; Wolff-Parkinson-White syndrome; or severe degrees of SA, AV, or intraventricular heart block. Some commercially available forms of premixed lidocaine for injection may include corn-derived products and, therefore, should be avoided in patients with corn hypersensitivity. Mexiletine is contraindicated in patients with cardiogenic shock and second- or third-degree AV block. Procainamide should not be used in patients with complete heart block, second-degree AV block, and torsades de pointes. Contraindications to propafenone include SA, AV, and intraventricular disorders; Brugada syndrome; sinus bradycardia; cardiogenic shock; uncompensated cardiac failure; marked hypotension, bronchospastic disorders, or severe pulmonary disease; and uncorrected electrolyte abnormalities. Quinidine should not be used in patients with thrombocytopenia, thrombocytopenic purpura, myasthenia gravis, heart block greater than first degree, or idiopathic conduction delays, or with concurrent use of quinolone antibiotics, cisapride, amprenavir, or ritonavir.

Cautions and Considerations Antiarrhythmic drugs should be used with caution. Please refer to Table 15.5 for more information.

Class II (Beta Blockers)

Some beta blockers inhibit beta-1 receptors on the heart (class II). They are used to treat arrhythmia because they inhibit sympathetic nervous system activity on the heart. Normally, sympathetic stimulation makes the heart beat harder and faster. By blocking this stimulation, conduction is slowed through the AV node. This effect slows the rate and force of heartbeats just enough to reduce arrhythmia.

Side Effects To learn the side effects of beta blockers, refer to Table 15.5.

Contraindications The beta blockers are contraindicated in bradycardia (slow heart rate), cardiogenic shock, and heart block. Esmolol should not be used in patients with decompensated heart failure and pulmonary hypertension. Propranolol should not be used in patients with bronchial asthma. Sotalol should not be used in patients with uncontrolled heart failure.

Cautions and Considerations Sotalol should be used with caution. Please refer to Table 15.5 for more information.

Class III (Potassium-Channel Blockers)

Another class of agents, **potassium-channel blockers** (class III), blocks potassium channels in cardiac muscle cells. Like class I antiarrhythmic agents, these drugs work by slowing the influx of a positively charged ion (i.e., potassium), which makes the cell membrane more stable and less able to depolarize. Consequently, the electrical charge must be stronger to make the heart beat. This effect regulates heart rhythm because it decreases the incidence of abnormal beats.

Side Effects To learn the side effects of potassium-channel blockers, refer to Table 15.5.

Contraindications Amiodarone (see Figure 15.6) is contraindicated in patients with a hypersensitivity to iodine, severe sinus-node dysfunction, second- and third-degree AV block, bradycardia, and cardiogenic shock. Contraindications to dofetilide include long

FIGURE 15.6 Amiodarone Medication Label

Amiodarone is available in oral and injectable formulations. Regardless of its route of administration, amiodarone has several contraindications and cautions.

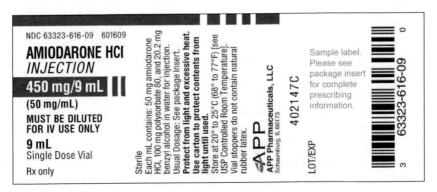

QT syndrome; kidney impairment; and concurrent use of verapamil, cimetidine, hydro-chlorothiazide, trimethoprim, itraconazole, ketoconazole, prochlorperazine, dolutegravir, or megestrol.

Cautions and Considerations Potassium-channel blockers have many cautions and considerations. Please refer to Table 15.5 for more information.

Drug Alert

Amiodarone contains two iodine atoms and may greatly increase a patient's daily iodine load. Increased iodine can lead to several problems, most notably hypo-thyroidism. It is estimated that one-third of patients taking amiodarone develop hypothyroidism. Patients should have their thyroid function assessed several weeks after starting amiodarone and every few months subsequently. Droneda-rone, a drug that is similar to amiodarone, does not contain iodine.

Class IV (Calcium-Channel Blockers)

Two calcium-channel blockers (class IV), diltiazem and verapamil, are used frequently for atrial fibrillation, a common but nonfatal heart arrhythmia. These agents block calcium, another positively charged ion, from entering cardiac muscle cells. This effect dilates cardiac arteries, providing better oxygen supply. The heart rate slows because the heart works more efficiently.

Side Effects To learn the side effects of calcium-channel blockers, refer to Table 15.5.

Contraindications Contraindications to diltiazem include sick sinus syndrome, second- or third-degree AV block, severe low blood pressure, acute heart attack, and pulmonary congestion. The IV form of verapamil is contraindicated in patients who are taking beta blockers and in those patients with ventricular tachycardia.

Cautions and Considerations Antiarrhythmic drugs should be used with caution. Please refer to Table 15.5 for more information.

Digoxin

This drug is not included in Table 15.5 because, although it is considered an antiarrhythmic drug, it is in a class by itself. Digoxin is especially useful for treating atrial fibrillation and flutter. It is not often used for other arrhythmias. Digoxin works by inhibiting sodium-potassium ATPase, an enzyme that regulates the influx of these ions in cardiac muscle cells. Digoxin alters SA node conductivity, conduction velocity through the heart, and rest time between beats. Digoxin also increases the force and velocity of muscle contraction, making the heart pump more efficiently.

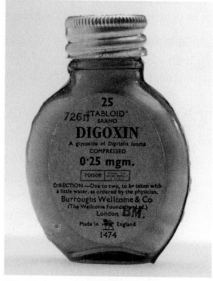

Digoxin is made from the extract of the foxglove plant, which has been used to treat heart ailments since the 1600s. The bottle shown here dates back to the turn of the twentieth century.

Side Effects Digoxin has a narrow **therapeutic window**. In other words, the amount needed to produce the desired effect is not much lower than the amount that causes toxicity. Side effects are not common when drug levels are maintained within the therapeutic range (see Table 15.6 for significant drug interactions). Patients must undergo regular laboratory testing to monitor the therapeutic effects and adjust the dosage accordingly. When toxicity occurs, patients should seek medical attention right away. Symptoms of digoxin toxicity include visual disturbances (seeing yellow or green halos around objects), headache, dizziness, confusion, nausea, and vomiting. Other side effects include gynecomastia (breast enlargement), anorexia, mental disturbances (anxiety, depression, delirium, hallucination), and heart block (extremely slow heartbeat). If these effects occur, the patient should discuss them with his or her prescriber.

TABLE 15.6 Digoxin

Generic (Brand)	Dosage Form	Significant Drug Interactions
Digoxin (Lanoxin)	Elixir, IV, tablet	IV calcium, succinylcholine, thyroid hormones (use with caution with beta agonists, beta blockers, calcium-channel blockers, diuretics)

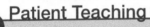

Patient Teaching

Because digoxin slows the heart rate, a patient taking this medication must be taught to take his or her pulse rate prior to taking the drug. Demonstrate how to take an accurate pulse rate, and tell the patient that if the pulse rate is below 60, he or she should not take the medication and should contact a physician for further instruction.

Contraindications Patients who have a hypersensitivity to digitalis, digoxin, or a diagnosis of ventricular fibrillation should not be given digoxin.

Cautions and Considerations While taking digoxin, patients should not change between the brand and generic versions of digoxin because even small differences in tablet strength among manufacturers can affect blood concentrations.

Kolb's Learning Styles

Just about all types of learners can benefit from creating their own flash cards to help them learn the generic names, brand names, and drug classes of cardiovascular medications. The process of creating the cards is, in itself, an exercise in categorizing and reviewing these drugs. If you are a visual learner, you may find it especially useful to create color-coded flash cards or use specific colors of ink to categorize the drugs into their classes.

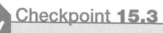
Take a moment to review what you have learned so far and answer these questions.

1. What drug classes are included in each of the classes (I–IV) of antiarrhythmic medications?
2. What commonly used drugs have interactions with antiarrhythmic agents?
3. What two arrhythmias are treated with the administration of digoxin?

Angina and Heart Attack

Angina pectoris, or simply angina, is chest pain caused by inadequate bloodflow to a portion of the heart (i.e., **myocardial ischemia**). Ischemia usually occurs as a result of a blockage in the coronary arteries that supply the heart with blood (see Figure 15.7). When one or more of these arteries become significantly blocked (usually by 70% or more), tissue damage in that area of the heart ensues, causing a heart attack. In angina, tissue damage is not extensive enough to be considered a heart attack but does cause recurring chest pain episodes.

Stable angina refers to a predictable pattern of chest pain and tightness that happens in response to specific triggers, such as exercise, physical pain, emotional stress, exposure to cold, or smoking. **Unstable angina** is chest pain and tightness that occurs with increasing frequency and less predictability. It occurs with less exertion or may be brought on by factors other than physical activity or stress. Unstable angina can be a warning that a heart attack is impending. **Variant angina** is another type of chest pain that involves spasm of the coronary blood vessels, rather than blockage.

FIGURE 15.7 | Coronary Arteries

Cardiac bypass surgery takes a vein from the leg and connects it to an artery in the heart to divert blood around a blockage in a coronary artery.

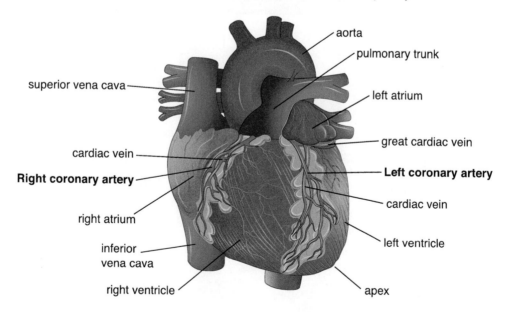

When heart muscle is deprived of oxygen long enough, cardiac muscle cells die (infarct) causing a **heart attack (myocardial infarction or MI)**. A heart attack is signaled by the following symptoms:

- tightness, heaviness, or squeezing sensation in the chest

- chest, neck, or jaw pain

- chest pain that radiates down the left arm

- indigestion or nausea

- a sense of impending doom

- weakness or fatigue

- sweating

If blockage in the coronary arteries is extensive, **cardiac catheterization** (a procedure to reopen blocked arteries) or **coronary bypass surgery** is performed. In coronary bypass surgery, a vessel from the leg is used to create an arterial bypass around a blockage in a coronary artery, thus restoring bloodflow to previously blocked-off heart tissue. Stents, supportive structures made of metal wire mesh, are also placed surgically to keep coronary arteries open (see Figure 15.8). If tissue damage becomes permanent, electrical conductivity in that part of the heart is affected, increasing the likelihood of a permanent arrhythmia.

| FIGURE 15.8 | Placement of a Stent in a Coronary Artery |

The placement of a stent in a coronary artery compresses plaque and thereby increases bloodflow through the artery.

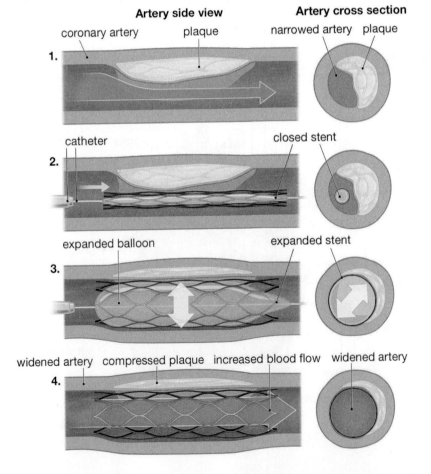

Cautions and Considerations Because short-acting forms are designed for immediate absorption, sublingual (under the tongue) and buccal (through the cheek) tablets should not be swallowed. Instead, they are placed in the mouth and allowed to dissolve. Long-acting oral forms are swallowed and should be taken on an empty stomach with a full glass of water.

If patients do not get relief from chest pain within 5 minutes of taking a dose of short-acting nitroglycerin, they can repeat one dose, and they should then call for emergency medical care (such as 911). If this second dose is needed, a patient could be experiencing a heart attack and should be medically evaluated immediately.

Sublingual nitroglycerin tablets must be kept in their original amber-colored container and protected from light, heat, and moisture. These tablets lose their effectiveness easily in warm and moist conditions. Once the bottle is opened, the tablets are only good for six months, and the date on which it was opened should be written on the container. After six months have passed, the patient should throw away any remaining tablets.

Patients taking nitrates should not take erectile dysfunction drugs (such as Viagra, Levitra, and Cialis). Erectile dysfunction agents also cause vasodilation, and additive effects between these drug classes could lower blood pressure to dangerous levels.

Tolerance to the beneficial effects of nitrates is an additional concern. Tolerance occurs after constant exposure to the drug, resulting in reduced effectiveness of the medication for the patient. Therefore, a drug-free period of at least eight hours a day (usually overnight) is necessary. For example, the transdermal nitrate patch should be removed before bedtime and left off overnight. A new patch should be applied in the morning.

 Patient Teaching

Patients who are prescribed nitroglycerin should carry it with them at all times. Ask patients each time you see them to show you their bottle. You can check the expiration date and remind them how to take the medication properly.

Other Drugs for Angina (ACE Inhibitors, Beta Blockers, and Calcium-Channel Blockers)

ACE inhibitors, beta blockers, and calcium-channel blockers are all used to treat angina and heart attack. In some cases, these agents are used during the acute heart attack itself, but usually they are used after one has occurred. These drugs have shown beneficial effects on heart tissue that has already experienced ischemia. They increase oxygen supply to cardiac tissue, increase pumping efficiency, and can reduce stress on a heart that has suffered an infarction.

Side Effects To review the side effects of ACE inhibitors, refer to the "ACE Inhibitors" section in this chapter. To review the side effects of calcium-channel blockers and beta blockers, refer to Table 15.5.

Contraindications ACE inhibitors should not be used in patients who experienced angioedema with previous ACE inhibitor use. Other contraindications include idiopathic or hereditary angioedema and concomitant use with aliskiren in patients with diabetes mellitus. The beta blockers are contraindicated in bradycardia (slow heart rate), cardiogenic shock, and heart block.

Calcium-channel blockers have a variety of contraindications. Contraindications to diltiazem include sick sinus syndrome, second- or third-degree AV block, severe low blood pressure, acute heart attack, and pulmonary congestion. The IV form of verapamil is contraindicated in patients who are taking beta blockers and in patients with ventricular tachycardia.

Cautions and Considerations To review the cautions and considerations of ACE inhibitors, refer to the "ACE Inhibitors" section in this chapter. To review the cautions and considerations of beta blockers and calcium-channel blockers, refer to Table 15.5.

Heart Failure

Over time, high blood pressure and coronary artery blockage can cause the heart to be overworked, which can result in enlargement and weakening. The heart is then no longer able to pump sufficiently to supply the body with oxygenated blood. **Heart failure** is characterized by weakness, fatigue, severe fluid retention, and difficulty breathing due to pulmonary edema (fluid accumulation in the lungs). Eventually, vital organs such as the heart, brain, kidneys, and liver shut down due to lack of blood supply, which explains why half of patients die within five years of experiencing heart failure. Hypertension and coronary artery disease are the primary causes of heart failure; other factors, including alcoholism, liver disease, kidney disease, valvular heart disease, anemia, and even drug therapy, can contribute to this condition.

Drug Regimens and Treatments

Drug therapies for heart failure have already been covered in this chapter in sections on hypertension and arrhythmias. Typically, diuretics, ACE inhibitors, and beta blockers are therapy mainstays. Some patients may also use vasodilators and digoxin. In most cases, the difference between using these drugs for heart failure and using them for other cardiovascular conditions, such as hypertension or angina, lies in dosing amounts and frequencies.

Loop Diuretics

Loop diuretics work primarily in the ascending loop of Henle and distal renal tubule, sites of water and sodium recovery. Loop diuretics inhibit reabsorption of sodium, chloride, and water, which leads to fast and profound diuresis (urine production). For this reason, loop diuretics are used to pull fluid from the body rapidly. This effect reduces swelling and fluid accumulation that happens when the heart cannot pump blood efficiently. Loop diuretics include bumetanide, ethacrynate, furosemide (see Figure 15.9), and torsemide. More information on loop diuretics can be found in Chapter 22.

Side Effects Side effects of loop diuretics are rare but can include dizziness, headache, skin rash, upset stomach, diarrhea, and constipation. Pulling fluid rapidly from the body can lower blood pressure. Getting up slowly from sitting or lying down can help with dizziness associated with drops in blood pressure.

Contraindications The loop diuretics should not be used in patients with anuria. Bumetanide should be avoided in patients with hepatic coma or in patients who have severe electrolyte depletion.

Cautions and Considerations Electrolyte balance, hydration, and kidney function must be monitored in patients taking loop diuretics. Patients may have to get blood tests to monitor these effects. To maintain electrolyte balance, patients often take potassium supplements with loop diuretics.

FIGURE 15.9 Furosemide Medication Label

Furosemide is a commonly used loop diuretic. You may see patients taking furosemide in its tablet form.

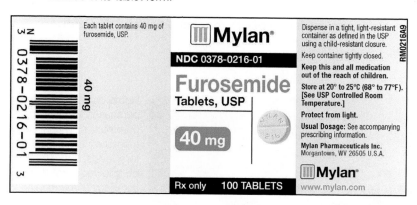

Kolb's Learning Styles

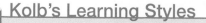

Try this exercise if you like working with details as Assimilators do. On a piece of paper, write the following terms in separate columns across the top of the paper: *high blood pressure, arrhythmia, angina, heart failure,* and *high cholesterol.* Under each column, list the drug classes used to treat it. Remember, some classes will be listed under multiple conditions. For each drug class, list as many generic drug names as you can remember. Write the brand name next to each generic drug name. Put a star next to the drugs that should be taken with food. Underline the drugs that expire six months after being opened. Circle the drugs that are usually stocked in a crash cart or emergency room drug kit. Try to do this exercise from memory first, and then refer to the text for answers.

Hyperlipidemia

Hyperlipidemia is a condition of elevated cholesterol, phospholipids, and/or triglycerides in the blood, resulting in cardiovascular disease and coronary artery blockage. **Cholesterol** itself is both made within the body and ingested with foods. Cholesterol is used to build cell membranes and form hormones. Eating foods high in fat and cholesterol can raise a person's blood cholesterol above normal levels. However, many people with hyperlipidemia also make too much cholesterol in their livers. In some individuals, a genetic factor causes high cholesterol that cannot be overcome by diet and exercise. An accumulation of cholesterol in the bloodstream leads to blockage of and dysfunction in blood vessel walls. These blockages cause angina and heart attacks.

In the bloodstream, cholesterol is packaged into multiple types of molecules: lipoproteins and triglycerides. **Low-density lipoproteins (LDLs)** are the worst type of cholesterol and contribute to artery blockages. **High-density lipoproteins (HDLs)** are the good kind of cholesterol; these molecules help to break up plaques and blockages in blood vessels. **Triglycerides**, another kind of lipid molecule, contribute to atherosclerosis (blocking and hardening of artery walls due to fat buildup). Hyperlipidemia exists when LDLs or triglycerides are elevated in the blood. Often, hyperlipidemia coexists with low HDL cholesterol levels. Treatment begins with reducing fat and cholesterol in the diet, but if this is unsuccessful, drug therapy is started.

Patients should be aware of abnormal blood lipid levels so that they can keep their cholesterol in check. With that in mind, share the following abnormal values with patients:

- Total cholesterol > 200 mg/dL

- LDL varies with patient-specific factors, but usually > 160 mg/dL

- HDL < 45 mg/dL

- Triglycerides >150 mg/dL

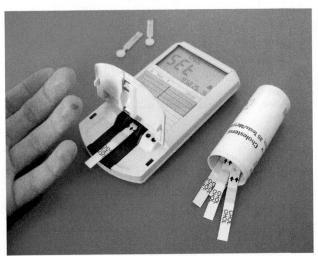

Home cholesterol kits can be purchased by individuals at retail pharmacies. These kits typically measure individuals' total cholesterol levels, and directions must be followed carefully to aid the accuracy of the readings.

Drug Regimens and Treatments

Lowering cholesterol (lipid) levels in the blood has been found to significantly reduce the risk of a heart attack. Once an individual has had one heart attack, the risk for subsequent heart attacks rises dramatically. Drugs for hyperlipidemia are used either to prevent a first heart attack (primary prevention) or to prevent subsequent attacks after an MI (secondary prevention).

Lipids can be tested by a finger-stick test. A special technique is needed to complete this test accurately, so proper training is recommended before performing it. Healthcare professionals generally do this, but at-home lipid-testing kits are available.

HMG-CoA Reductase Inhibitors (Statins)

The drug class **HMG-CoA reductase inhibitors**, or statins, lowers LDL cholesterol primarily and can have beneficial effects on other lipids as well (see Table 15.9). These medications are usually the first-line choice of therapy for hyperlipidemia. Statins reduce the amount of cholesterol made in the body by blocking an enzyme, **HMG-CoA reductase**, which is required for cholesterol production.

Side Effects Most side effects of statins are mild and tolerable. However, they can cause upset stomach and diarrhea, so patients may take them with food if needed. Muscle aches and weakness can also occur. Muscle breakdown (rhabdomyolysis) is a rare but serious side effect. Severe rhabdomyolysis may

Quick Study

HMG-CoA reductase inhibitors are often referred to as "statins" because the generic names of these drugs end with the suffix –statin.

cause permanent kidney failure. Patients should report any muscle aches or weakness to their healthcare practitioners to determine whether the symptom is simply due to muscle weakness or to actual muscle breakdown. Occasionally, statins cause liver toxicity, so patients should have liver function tests performed periodically.

Contraindications Statins are contraindicated in patients who have active liver disease or unexplained persistent elevations of serum transaminase. These medications are also contraindicated in patients who are pregnant, planning to get pregnant, or breast-feeding. Lovastatin and simvastatin should not be used in patients who are concomitantly using strong liver enzyme inhibitors such as clarithromycin, erythromycin, itraconazole, ketoconazole, nefazodone, posaconazole, voriconazole, and protease inhibitors. Pitavastatin should not be used in patients using cyclosporine.

TABLE 15.9 Common Antihyperlipidemic Drugs

Generic (Brand)	Dosage Form	Route of Administration	Common Dosage
Statins			
Atorvastatin (Lipitor)	Tablet	Oral	10–80 mg a day
Fluvastatin (Lescol)	Tablet	Oral	20–80 mg a day
Lovastatin (Mevacor)	Tablet	Oral	20–80 mg a day
Pitavastatin (Livalo)	Tablet	Oral	1–4 mg a day
Pravastatin (Pravachol)	Tablet	Oral	40–80 mg a day
Rosuvastatin (Crestor)	Tablet	Oral	5–40 mg a day
Simvastatin (Zocor)	Tablet	Oral	10–80 mg a day
Fibrates			
Fenofibrate (Antara, Lofibra, TriCor, Triglide)	Capsule, tablet	Oral	130–200 mg a day
Gemfibrozil (Lopid)	Tablet	Oral	600 mg twice a day, before morning and evening meals
Miscellaneous			
Ezetimibe (Zetia)	Tablet	Oral	10 mg a day
Ezetimibe + simvastatin (Vytorin)	Tablet	Oral	10 mg + 10 mg to 10 mg + 80 mg a day

Cautions and Considerations HMG-CoA reductase inhibitors work best when taken at night. Grapefruit juice alters the activity of statins, so patients should avoid drinking it when taking these medications. Certain statins have dangerous interactions with specific drugs, so allied health professionals should contact a pharmacist regarding any medication changes for patients who are taking statins.

Fibrates

Another class of drugs used daily to lower high cholesterol, especially elevated triglycerides, is **fibrates**. These drugs are also used as an alternative to statins when statins cannot be tolerated. Fibrate drugs, also called fibric acid derivatives, lower LDL cholesterol but are best at lowering triglycerides and increasing HDL cholesterol. Their exact mechanism of action is not well understood.

Side Effects Common side effects of fibrates include upset stomach, diarrhea, indigestion, and abdominal cramps. These effects improve over time and can be diminished by taking the medication with food.

Contraindications Fenofibrate and gemfibrozil are contraindicated in patients with active liver disease, severe kidney dysfunction, and gallbladder disease. Fenofibrate is contraindicated in breast-feeding. Gemfibrozil is contraindicated in patients using repaglinide.

Cautions and Considerations Patients with gallbladder problems probably should not take fibrates, and they should not be taken in combination with statins because rhabdomyolysis can occur.

Drug Alert

Allied health professionals may see patients who are prescribed more than one medication to treat high cholesterol. Statins are the most commonly used cholesterol medications. However, an adverse effect of statins is myopathy and muscle breakdown, or rhabdomyolysis. This risk is increased when statins are used in combination with fibrates. For example, the use of gemfibrozil with a statin increases the risk of myopathy and rhabdomyolysis to a greater extent than the use of fenofibrate without a statin. Consequently, allied health personnel should have a heightened awareness of this potential risk in their patients who are being treated for hyperlipidemia.

Ezetimibe

The oral drug **ezetimibe** inhibits cholesterol absorption from the GI tract. It works on all forms of cholesterol but may not significantly reduce lipid levels when large reductions are needed.

Side Effects Side effects, such as abdominal cramps and diarrhea, are usually mild, making this drug quite tolerable.

Contraindications Ezetimibe is contraindicated when used with a statin in patients with active liver disease. The combined ezetimibe/simvastatin product should not be used by patients who are pregnant or breast-feeding.

Cautions and Considerations Few problems are seen with this medication, as it is not systemically absorbed.

Niacin

Vitamin B$_3$ (nicotinic acid) is also known as **niacin**. This dietary supplement is available over the counter as well as via prescription (see Table 15.10). Niacin reduces triglycerides and LDL cholesterol while raising HDL cholesterol.

Side Effects The main side effect of niacin is vasodilation in the face and neck, which causes flushing (reddening) and itching. This effect can be uncomfortable and is a barrier for some patients. The flushing effect can be reduced by taking an aspirin 30 minutes prior

TABLE 15.10 | Niacin Products

Generic (Brand)	Dosage Form	Prescription Status	Common Dosage
Various products	Capsule, tablet	OTC	1–2 g, 2–3 times a day
Niacin (Niacor)	Tablet	Rx	250–750 mg a day
Niacin (Niaspan)	Tablet	Rx	250–750 mg at bedtime
Niacin (Slo-Niacin)	Tablet	OTC	250–750 mg a day

to the niacin dose. Sometimes taking niacin before bedtime will ensure that flushing, if it occurs, happens during sleep, and is more likely to go unnoticed. The prescription dosage forms are formulated specifically to release the drug slowly to reduce this side effect.

Contraindications Niacin should not be used in patients with active liver disease or persistent elevations in hepatic transaminases, active peptic ulcers, and arterial hemorrhage.

Cautions and Considerations Niacin taken in large doses can raise blood glucose levels. Patients who also have diabetes should be aware of this side effect. Dosages of their diabetes medications may need to be adjusted accordingly.

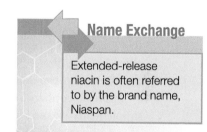

Name Exchange

Extended-release niacin is often referred to by the brand name, Niaspan.

Checkpoint 15.4

Take a moment to review what you have learned so far and answer these questions.

1. What drugs are commonly used for angina and chest pain?
2. What drugs are commonly used to treat heart failure?
3. What drugs are used to lower cholesterol?

Herbal and Alternative Therapies

Omega 3 fatty acids are polyunsaturated fatty acids (also called **DHA** and **EPA**) available in a variety of fish oil products. Patients can get DHA and EPA from eating fish or taking fish oil supplements. Fish oil is used frequently to treat high cholesterol, hypertension, and coronary artery disease. Although not as effective as prescription drugs to treat high triglycerides, fish oil supplements or increased dietary intake of fish has been found to lower triglycerides significantly. A variety of fish oil products are available; Lovaza (465 mg EPA and 375 mg DHA) is approved by the Food and Drug Administration (FDA) to treat hypertriglyceridemia. Consuming 1 g of fish oil a day or eating fish (3 ounces) twice a week has been found to prevent cardiovascular disease.

Plant sterol esters have been found to significantly lower LDL cholesterol and can be helpful adjuncts to diet and drug therapy for hyperlipidemia. **Beta-sitosterol** is a plant sterol similar in chemical structure to cholesterol. It is used in several food products (nutraceuticals), such as margarine and juice, for cardiovascular disease. The typical dosage of beta-sitosterol is 800 mg–6 g a day in divided doses with meals. It should not be taken with ezetimibe (Zetia) because this drug blocks sitosterol absorption and renders the dose ineffective.

Red yeast rice is a fermented rice product that is used in recipes and in medications to lower cholesterol and improve cardiovascular health. Red yeast rice is available in a capsule and tablet form and contains varying amounts of monacolins, agents with HMG-CoA reductase inhibitor activity. There are other ingredients in red yeast rice that may lower cholesterol, such as sterols, isoflavones, and monounsaturated fatty acids. Red yeast rice supplements are usually taken at a dosage of 1,800 mg a day, divided in two doses.

Alpha tocopherol (vitamin E) supplements are used for a variety of conditions, such as cardiovascular disease, cancer, and diabetic neuropathy. The effectiveness of vitamin

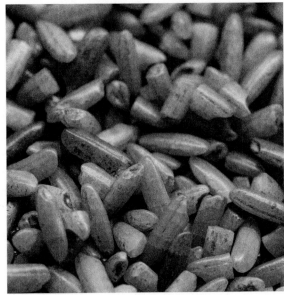

Red yeast rice is a fermented product that may be used to lower cholesterol.

E for these uses has not been proven; even so, many individuals take this antioxidant for better health. A total dosage of 400 IU a day has been found to be safe and possibly effective for selected conditions, whereas higher dosages can cause side effects and are associated with poor outcomes.

Garlic contains organosulfur compounds that have antihyperlipidemic, antihypertensive, and antifungal effects. A variety of garlic products and supplements is available, and garlic has been found to be possibly effective in treating atherosclerosis, hypertension, some cancers, and skin fungal infections. The garlic product must contain **allicin**, the odorous, active ingredient produced upon crushing garlic cloves. A dosing regimen of 600–1,200 mg a day, divided into three doses, has been used in clinical trials. One clove of fresh garlic a day has also been used. Patients taking warfarin, saquinavir (a drug used to treat human immunodeficiency virus), or other protease inhibitors should not take garlic.

Chapter Review

Chapter Summary

Cardiovascular disease is a frequent diagnosis in the United States and encompasses multiple conditions for which drugs are used. The most common conditions are hypertension, arrhythmias, angina, heart attack, and heart failure. Hyperlipidemia contributes to cardiovascular disease. In fact, drugs used to treat high cholesterol are on the list of the top 50 drugs dispensed.

ACE inhibitors, beta blockers, and calcium-channel blockers are used in almost all of these cardiovascular conditions. Consequently, they can be challenging to learn and remember.

Other classes covered are ARBs for hypertension, nitrates for angina, and antihyperlipidemic agents (statins and fibrates). The drugs used for heart arrhythmias are divided into four classes, all of which have complications to consider. Some have serious side effects and toxicities. Beta blockers and calcium-channel blockers are also used to treat arrhythmias.

Finally, a variety of dietary supplements are used for cardiovascular disease. Niacin, for which both OTC and prescription products are available, is prescribed frequently for high cholesterol.

Chapter Checkup

The Navigator+ learning management system that accompanies this textbook offers many opportunities to help you master chapter content, including end-of-chapter exercises, a glossary of key terms, flash cards, and additional interactive activities.

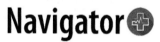

Career Exploration

If you enjoyed learning about the cardiovascular system in this chapter, you may want to explore the following career options:

- athletic trainer
- cardiac and vascular interventional (CVI) technologist
- cardiopulmonary rehabilitation specialist
- cardiovascular perfusionist
- cardiovascular technologist
- certified clinical nutritionist
- diagnostic medical sonographer
- electrocardiogram (ECG) technician

- electrophysiology technician
- emergency medical technician (EMT)/paramedic
- exercise physiologist
- medical assistant
- nuclear medicine technologist
- pharmacy technician
- registered dietitian

16 The Blood and Drug Therapy

Pharm Facts

- One pint of blood contains 2.4 trillion red blood cells.

- The red color of human blood comes from hemoglobin, a substance that turns red when it is oxygenated. However, not every animal has red blood. A crab has blue blood; a starfish has clear blood; and earthworms and leeches have green blood.

- At rest, the human body makes, on average, 17 million red blood cells every second. Under stress, the body can make four times that number.

- Humans have four different blood types: A, B, AB, and O. Animals also have blood types, including cats (3 major blood types), dogs (at least 6 major blood types), horses (7 major blood types), and cows (800 major blood types).

- Late in his life, George Washington received a bloodletting treatment to cure his bad cold. Unfortunately, the treatment was worse than the illness, and Washington died soon after the procedure, when more than half of his blood supply was drained.

"As a hematologist, I have spent many years studying the circulatory system. In fact, blood has a rich history that dates back to the ancient Greeks and their belief in the four humors of the body. Although balancing the humors through bloodletting proved to be a medically unsound practice, scientists would later discover the circulatory system and the role of blood transfusions in restoring health. Today, curative bone marrow transplants have saved many lives, and artificial blood holds much promise for those with blood disorders. It is extremely rewarding to be part of the exciting field of hematology."

—**Lisa J. Gunderson**, BS, ASCP
Cell Biologist/Hematologist

1   Understand the basic anatomy and physiology of the blood and the hematologic system.

2   Describe the common conditions that affect the blood and the hematologic system.

3   Explain the therapeutic effects of prescription medications and non-prescription medications commonly used to treat diseases of the blood and the hematologic system.

4   Identify the generic names, brand names, indications, dosage ranges, side effects, contraindications, and cautions and considerations associated with the drugs commonly used to treat diseases of the blood and the hematologic system.

5   Identify common herbal and alternative therapies that are related to the blood and the hematologic system.

T he blood is a hematologic system comprising a variety of blood cells suspended in plasma. These blood cells sustain life by circulating needed oxygen and other nutrients to cells and tissues of the body. Without constant bloodflow to essential organs including the brain, heart, lungs, and kidneys, life is not possible. To work properly, the blood must adequately perfuse body tissues, contain functional blood cells able to do their various tasks, and clot when injury or bleeding occurs.

This chapter describes the components of the hematologic system that make the blood and support its physiologic functions. You will also learn about the coagulation cascade, the process by which blood forms clots. Blood clotting is a necessary process. When clots form unnecessarily and cut off bloodflow, the results are stroke, heart attack, and pulmonary embolism (clot in the lungs). Stroke, clotting disorders, and hemophilia are discussed, as are iron deficiency and pernicious anemia.

Some of the medications used to treat blood conditions are inexpensive and used extensively, whereas others are rarely used and quite costly. In this chapter, anticoagulants such as warfarin (one of the top 100 drugs most widely prescribed) and heparin are discussed. Like all of the medications used to treat blood disorders, warfarin has special considerations for side effects and drug interactions. As the reports of medication errors with heparin have shown, attention to detail is imperative when handling this medication. Errors with use of these lifesaving therapies can have dire consequences. All allied health professionals must appreciate the sensitive nature of these hematologic agents and understand their special considerations in order to ensure patient safety.

Anatomy and Physiology of the Blood

The **blood** serves several functions besides supplying the cells of the body with oxygen and nutrients. It also carries the hormones and enzymes that control bodily functions and helps to regulate body temperature. The blood is made up of cells suspended in liquid plasma. Blood **plasma** contains water, **protein** (albumin and immunoglobulins), and various dissolved substances. Drug molecules are carried by the blood either as dissolved substances in plasma or as substances bound to proteins such as **albumin**.

Types of Blood Cells

Three types of cells are found in the blood: erythrocytes, leukocytes, and platelets or, also know as *thrombocytes* (see Figure 16.1).

FIGURE 16.1 | **Components of the Blood**

Red blood cells (RBCs, or *erythrocytes*) give blood its characteristic red color.

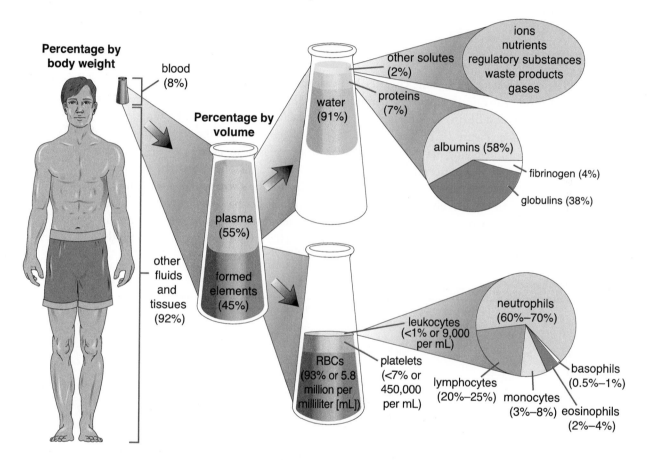

Erythrocytes

Erythrocytes, also known as **red blood cells (RBCs)**, contain iron and hemoglobin to which oxygen and carbon dioxide bind during transport. The main function of erythrocytes is to carry oxygen from the lungs to the body's tissues. Erythrocytes are formed in the bone marrow when molecules of iron attach to hemoglobin. Folate (also known as folic acid) and vitamin B_{12} also play key roles in the development of erythrocytes in the bone marrow. After production, erythrocytes are released into the bloodstream. This process, known as **erythropoiesis**, is stimulated by erythropoietin, a substance made by the kidneys.

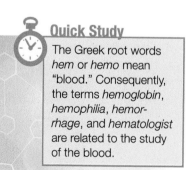

Quick Study

The Greek root words *hem* or *hemo* mean "blood." Consequently, the terms *hemoglobin, hemophilia, hemorrhage,* and *hematologist* are related to the study of the blood.

Leukocytes

Leukocytes, also known as **white blood cells (WBCs)**, are a central component of the immune system and are responsible for fighting disease. Leukocytes are formed in the bone marrow and are found in both blood and tissue, where they fight infections. The precise functions of the different types of leukocytes are discussed in Chapter 23.

Platelets

Platelets, or **thrombocytes**, are another type of blood cell. These cells are formed in the bone marrow and stored in the spleen. Platelets help the blood to clot during injury or bleeding by clumping together and adhering to surrounding tissue.

Coagulation Cascade

Platelets play a key role in the **coagulation cascade**, which is the process by which blood clots form. The cascade involves a complicated series of reactions that attract **thrombin**, **fibrinogen**, and **fibrin**, coagulation proteins that facilitate the growth of a functional blood clot (see Figure 16.2). The combination of platelet activity, the coagulation cascade, and reactions involving natural anticoagulants (tissue plasminogen activator [TPA] and proteins C and S) produces the body's ability to form and dissolve clots. The two pathways of the cascade, which stimulate blood clotting, are the **extrinsic pathway** and the **intrinsic pathway**. An abnormality in a single step of either pathway can affect coagulation and produce too much or too little clotting. These pathways converge with the use of **clotting factor X**, thrombin, and fibrin (see Figure 16.3). If a problem occurs with this common pathway, clotting is severely affected.

FIGURE 16.2 | **Formation of Blood Clots**

Tissue damage triggers the accumulation of platelets and activates clotting factors to start coagulation.

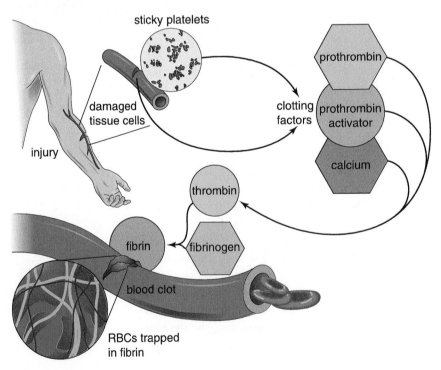

FIGURE 16.3 Coagulation Cascade

When one pathway malfunctions, usually the other pathway compensates.

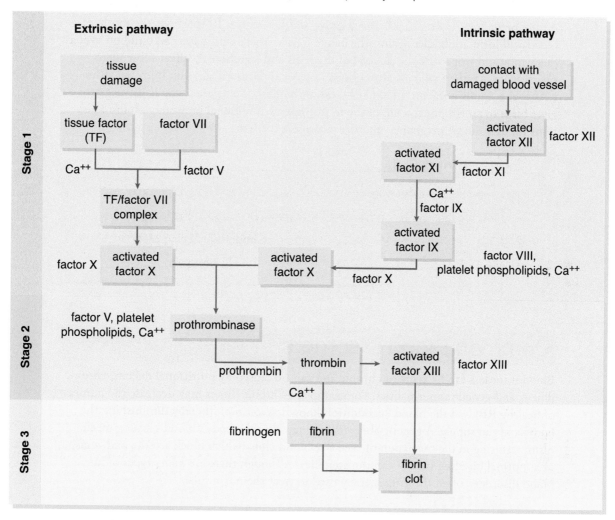

Blood Types

When clotting is unable to slow bleeding, blood loss can be life threatening and may require transfusion. Blood typing allows donor blood to be matched to a recipient for transfusion. Blood type is determined by specific antigen proteins on the surface of RBCs. If the blood that is given to a patient possesses surface antigens that are different from those present in the patient's own blood, antibodies form and cause RBCs to clump together. **Blood types** are categorized as A, B, AB, and O, such that AB has both kinds of antigens, and O has none. Blood type O is considered the universal donor because it is least likely to have antigens that can cause serious reactions during a transfusion. Blood type AB is considered the universal recipient because it already contains any antigens the donor blood could bring.

Rh Factor

The process of typing blood for a transfusion also includes another marker molecule on RBCs: the Rh factor. The **Rh factor** is a protein that may be present on RBCs. Those individuals who have the protein marker are considered Rh-positive; those individuals who are missing this marker are considered Rh-negative.

The presence of this marker and the antibodies made against it are most important during pregnancy. If a mother is Rh-negative and her fetus is Rh-positive, the mother's blood will form antibodies against the baby's RBCs. These antibodies can build up over a pregnancy and jeopardize the survival of the fetus and significantly affect subsequent pregnancies. Mothers who are Rh-negative receive an immunoglobulin injection (Rho-GAM) that inhibits the production of these antibodies. If a mother who is Rh-negative gives birth to an Rh-positive child, she must undergo additional immunoglobulin injections for each future pregnancy in order to protect the fetus.

 ## Checkpoint 16.1

Take a moment to review what you have learned so far and answer these questions.

1. What are the various components that make up blood in the body?
2. What is the Rh factor? Why is that protein so important during pregnancy?
3. What three substances facilitate the growth of a functional blood clot?

Common Blood Disorders

Blood disorders can be acute or chronic and can be caused by nutritional deficits, chronic illness, and genetic abnormalities. For example, a chronic illness may decrease the number of healthy RBCs in the blood (a condition known as *anemia*), thereby diminishing the body's oxygen supply. A genetic abnormality may alter the body's blood-clotting mechanism, resulting in the formation of excessive blood clots (which block arteries and veins) or abnormal bleeding (which can threaten life). Although there are many types of rare blood disorders, often the drug therapy used to treat them is similar.

Anemia

Anemia is characterized by a lower-than-normal number of healthy RBCs that contain functional hemoglobin in the blood. Many causes of anemia exist, but most can be categorized into one of several types: anemia caused by inadequate production of RBCs, by rapid destruction of RBCs, or by blood loss.

The inadequate production of RBCs is the most common cause of anemia. This predisposing factor is found in up to half of the patients admitted to an inpatient setting and is usually related to nutrition. As mentioned earlier, iron, folate, and vitamin B_{12} are essential nutrients for forming healthy, abundant RBCs.

Iron-deficiency anemia can happen relatively quickly, but replenishing these iron stores in the body can take several months. **Folate-deficiency anemia** is commonly seen in patients who are alcoholics because they tend to not get proper nutrition. A deficiency in vitamin B_{12}, called **pernicious anemia**, may take weeks or months to develop, but replenishing this vitamin takes only days or weeks.

Anemia of chronic disease is most often caused by chronic kidney disease. The kidneys produce erythropoietin, the substance that stimulates bone marrow to make RBCs.

Kidney disease reduces the kidneys' ability to make erythropoietin; therefore, erythropoiesis diminishes. In this type of anemia, simply providing more iron will not produce more RBCs. Erythropoietin must be given to increase RBC production. Erythropoietin may also be used for anemia related to cancer chemotherapy, which damages bone marrow and slows erythropoiesis.

The rapid destruction of RBCs is another cause of anemia. This type of anemia, known as **hemolytic anemia**, can be triggered by infection, malignancy, or drug therapy. Some of the drugs that can lead to hemolytic anemia include cephalosporins, dapsone, levodopa, levofloxacin, methyldopa, nitrofurantoin, nonsteroidal anti-inflammatory drugs (NSAIDs), penicillins, phenazopyridine, and quinidine.

Blood loss can also cause anemia. Rapid blood loss may lead to **rapid-onset anemia**. Some signs of rapid-onset anemia may include an accelerated heart rate, light-headedness, and breathlessness. Rapid-onset anemia may require a blood transfusion to treat the condition. Chronic blood loss may lead to **chronic anemia**. This type of anemia can be caused by stomach ulcers, for example. Chronic anemia produces fatigue, weakness, headache, vertigo, light-headedness, sensitivity to cold, pallor, and loss of skin tone. The treatment for chronic blood loss is to stop the bleeding at the source.

Finally, **sickle-cell anemia** is a genetic disorder that causes malformation of RBCs. The misshapen cells look like half-moon crescents or sickles because the hemoglobin within them is abnormal. These cells die quickly and cause organ damage by blocking bloodflow through small blood vessels. The condition causes pain throughout the body as well as several other life-threatening problems. (see Figure 16.4).

Work Wise

African-American patients are statistically more likely than other patients to have sickle-cell anemia, an inherited form of hemolytic anemia that causes periodic episodes of pain, frequent infections, delayed growth, vision problems, stroke, and other serious complications such as organ damage.

FIGURE 16.4 Sickle-Cell Anemia

Normal RBCs are disc shaped and move easily through the body's circulatory system. Sickle-shaped RBCs are sticky and tend to clump together in the bloodstream, causing bloodflow obstruction. This obstruction results in organ damage.

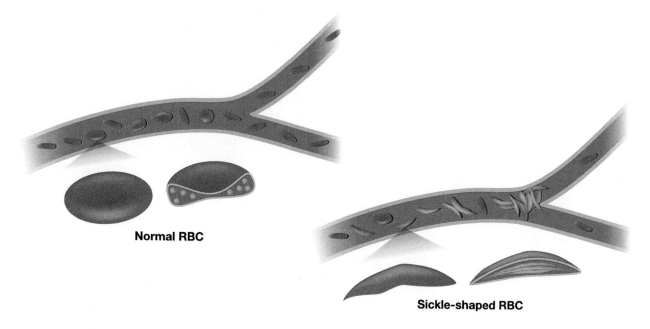

Normal RBC

Sickle-shaped RBC

Drug Regimens and Treatments

Drug therapy for anemia depends on the type of anemia present. **Hemoglobin (Hgb)** and **hematocrit (HCT)** are laboratory markers for the blood tests used to diagnose anemia. These blood tests measure hemoglobin and oxygen-carrying capacity in the blood. When these numbers are low, anemia is suspected. Other diagnostic measures and iron studies are used to determine the cause(s) of the anemia. If nutrient deficiency is the cause, simply replacing the appropriate missing nutrient usually corrects the anemia. If **hematopoiesis** is altered, administration of erythropoietin therapy will be necessary. For instance, patients with chronic renal failure do not make enough erythropoietin to support adequate hematopoiesis. Therefore, they may be given exogenous erythropoietin to treat their anemia. Sometimes, multiple factors contribute to anemia, making drug treatment more complicated.

Iron and Other Supplements

Iron, folic acid (folate), and vitamin B_{12} are used as supplements to treat anemia caused by nutrient deficiency (see Table 16.1).

Iron is used alone for iron-deficiency anemia or in combination with hematopoietic agents to treat anemia associated with chronic kidney disease. **Iron supplementation** can take up to six months to replenish iron stores and produce normal RBCs with adequate hemoglobin content.

Folic acid is used in low doses for prenatal supplementation to support fetal brain and spinal development. In fact, it is a recommended supplement for all women who are

TABLE 16.1 Commonly Used Supplements for Anemia

Generic (Brand)	Dosage Form	Route of Administration	Common Dosage
Cyanocobalamin (Nascobal, vitamin B_{12})	Injection, intranasal gel, tablet	IM, intranasal, oral, sub-Q injection	Injection: 100–1,000 mcg for 5 days, then weekly for 1 month, then monthly Intranasal: 500 mcg once a week for 5–10 days followed by injections PO: 1,000 mcg a day
Ferrous gluconate (Ferate, Fergon)	Tablet	Oral	100–200 mg elemental iron a day in divided doses
Ferrous gluconate complex (Ferrlecit)	Injection	IV	1 g in divided doses
Ferrous sulfate (Feosol, FeroSul, Slow Iron)	Capsule, elixir, syrup, oral drops, tablet	Oral	100–200 mg elemental iron a day in divided doses
Folic acid	Injection, tablet	IM, IV, oral, sub-Q injection	Maintenance: 400 mcg a day Deficiency: 1–5 mg a day Pregnancy: 0.4–0.8 mg a day (Oral dosing is preferred but IV can be used. Doses per day are the same regardless of route.)
Iron dextran (Dexferrum, INFeD)	Injection	IM, IV	Test dose first 25–100 mg a day
Iron sucrose (Venofer)	Injection	IV	20–100 mg a day

pregnant or planning to become pregnant because it decreases the occurrence or recurrence of neural tube defects. Folic acid in higher doses is also used to treat anemia caused by alcoholism because folic acid is frequently found to be deficient in these patients.

Vitamin B$_{12}$ is used to treat pernicious anemia and to prevent neuropathy and certain types of dementia. This vitamin builds and protects nerve tissue. Unlike the length of time needed for iron replacement, replenishing a deficiency of vitamin B$_{12}$ takes only days to weeks.

Side Effects Common side effects of iron supplementation include constipation, upset stomach, urine discoloration, and dark stools. Constipation can be relieved by drinking plenty of fluids, incorporating fiber into the diet, and taking a stool softener if needed. Most oral dosage forms are enteric coated to help with upset stomach, but if nausea occurs, taking iron with food may help. Common side effects of vitamin B$_{12}$ are itching, diarrhea, headache, and anxiety. These effects are usually mild and may improve over time.

Contraindications Vitamin B$_{12}$ should not be used in patients with a hypersensitivity to cobalt. Oral ferrous gluconate and ferrous sulfate are contraindicated in hemochromatosis and hemolytic anemia. Iron dextran is contraindicated in any anemia not associated with iron deficiency. Intravenous (IV) ferrous gluconate, IV iron sucrose, and oral folic acid do not have contraindications.

➕ ***Note:*** *Allied health professionals should be aware that an allergy to a particular drug contraindicates its use. This warning applies to all Contraindications sections in this chapter.*

Cautions and Considerations Oral iron supplements are enteric coated and should not be crushed or chewed. Most oral iron supplements are available over the counter, making them cost-effective and easily accessible. However, they can pose a poison risk to children. Iron overdose in children can be fatal, and doses do not have to be extremely large to cause significant problems. Patients should be instructed to keep iron supplements in childproof packaging and out of the reach of children.

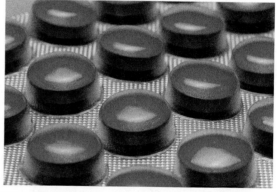

The shiny, enteric coating on iron tablets makes the pills resemble candy, which creates a potential poisoning hazard for children.

Iron supplements should not be taken with antacids or other acid-reducing medications because absorption of iron will be decreased. Iron supplements are sometimes given with vitamin C because it increases iron absorption. Iron supplements should not be taken with tetracycline or fluoroquinolones because iron binds to these antibiotics and reduces their effectiveness at fighting infection.

Iron dextran has been associated with severe allergic reactions; therefore, a test dose must be given first. Other IV forms of iron do not tend to cause this same allergic reaction, so they are used more often.

 Patient Teaching

Iron doses are based on the amount of elemental iron the product contains. The elemental iron content is different for various salts (e.g., gluconate, sulfate). Advise patients to stick with one product once they have started treatment.

Hematopoietic Agents

Two **hematopoietic agents**, **darbepoetin** and **erythropoietin**, are used to treat anemia associated with chronic kidney disease (see Table 16.2). They are sometimes used when cancer chemotherapy causes bone marrow suppression and affects blood cell production. Erythropoietin and darbepoetin should always be used in combination with iron supplements because they will deplete iron stores as RBC production increases. These agents work by supplementing the body's normal production of erythropoietin, which stimulates blood cell production in the bone marrow. It can take a few weeks for these agents to reach their full effect.

Work Wise

In the workplace, healthcare practitioners commonly refer to erythropoietin as *epo*.

TABLE 16.2 Commonly Used Hematopoietic Agents

Generic (Brand)	Dosage Form	Route of Administration	Common Dosage
Darbepoetin (Aranesp)	Injection	IV, sub-Q injection	100 mcg every week or 200 mcg every 2 weeks
Erythropoietin or epoetin alfa (Epogen, Procrit)	Injection	IV, sub-Q injection	40,000 units every week or 150 units/kg 3 times a week

Side Effects Common side effects of darbepoetin and erythropoietin include headache, fatigue, fever, muscle or joint pain, edema, diarrhea, nausea, and vomiting. These agents can also cause high blood pressure, clotting, and a rapid heart rate. Therefore, careful monitoring of blood pressure and cardiac function is necessary. Patients with uncontrolled high blood pressure may not be good candidates for hematopoietic therapy. Patients with a history of seizures need to inform their prescribers and pharmacists before using one of these agents because the risk of seizures is increased with the use of these drugs.

Contraindications Darbepoetin and epoetin alfa are contraindicated in uncontrolled high blood pressure and pure RBC aplasia. Multidose vials of epoetin alfa include benzyl alcohol and should not be used in neonates, infants, pregnant women, and nursing women. The use of hematopoietic agents in patients with hemoglobin levels greater than 11 g/dL increases the risk of serious cardiovascular events, thromboembolic events, stroke, and mortality. Therefore, these drugs should not be used in this patient population.

Cautions and Considerations Laboratory tests used to monitor hematopoietic therapy include complete blood count (CBC), a blood test that includes Hgb and HCT as well as information regarding WBC, RBC, and platelets. Other blood-work studies include **reticulocyte count**, which is a measure of newly formed RBCs released from the bone marrow to the bloodstream. In some settings, allied health professionals may help physicians or other healthcare practitioners retrieve these results. When monitoring darbepoetin and erythropoietin therapy, Hgb levels should not exceed 12 g/dL because increased cardiac and clotting problems can occur at high levels. (The normal range of Hgb levels in women is 12–15 g/dL; for men, this range is 13–18 g/dL.)

Darbepoetin and erythropoietin products should be refrigerated. They should not be shaken or diluted during preparation. Some erythropoietin products have a limited shelf life and must be discarded after 21 days if not used.

Darbepoetin should be protected from light; therefore, a special covering is sometimes placed over the IV bag.

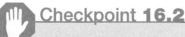
Take a moment to review what you have learned so far and answer these questions.

1. What are the types of anemia and their underlying causes?
2. What are the symptoms of anemia?
3. What drugs and supplements are used to treat anemia?

Stroke and Clotting Disorders

A common cause of death and disability around the world, **stroke**, or **cerebrovascular accident (CVA)**, is an interruption in oxygen supply to the brain. The brain is an oxygen-rich organ and requires a constant supply of oxygenated blood to keep brain tissue alive and functional. When oxygen cannot reach parts of the brain, it takes only minutes for a patient to lose consciousness and for tissue damage to occur. The brain is incapable of regeneration, so cell death is permanently disabling.

The two types of stroke are ischemic and hemorrhagic. An **ischemic stroke** results from an obstruction of bloodflow: A blood clot or cholesterol plaque occludes a blood vessel that supplies brain tissue. If the block in bloodflow is brief and causes only temporary dysfunction, it is called a **transient ischemic attack (TIA)**. A TIA is often a precursor to a stroke. Risk factors for ischemic stroke include high cholesterol, cardiac arrhythmia, coronary artery disease, prosthetic heart valve, diabetes, hypercoagulable states, obesity, and physical inactivity. These conditions increase the likelihood of blood clots forming and traveling to the brain.

A **hemorrhagic stroke** is a rupture in a blood vessel that supplies an area of the brain. Blood spills out of the ruptured vessel and then cannot reach the part of the brain that the vessel serves. Risk factors for hemorrhagic stroke are high blood pressure, cigarette smoking, and excessive alcohol intake. In these conditions, tiny vessels in the brain become weakened and form an **aneurysm**, a thin-walled protrusion in an artery wall that can easily burst. Other risk factors for any kind of stroke include diabetes, increased age, male gender, genetic predisposition, smoking, and prior CVA.

Clotting disorders involve both **hypercoagulation** (overproduction of blood clots) and **hemophilia** (inability to produce blood clots). Although many causes for clotting disorders exist, the majority are related to genetics. For instance, patients with hemophilia usually lack the genes that control the ability to produce specific clotting factors in the coagulation cascade. Type A hemophilia

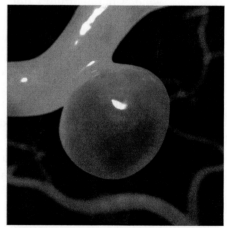

A cerebral aneurysm may leak or rupture, causing blood to flow into surrounding tissue. This event has dire consequences including permanent nerve damage, stroke, or, possibly, death.

is the inability to produce factor VIII, and Type B hemophilia is a deficiency in factor IX. Both hemophilia types are rare, particularly in females. Hemophilia predominantly affects only males directly, whereas females with hemophiliac genes are typically carriers. More common clotting disorders include deficiencies in von Willebrand factor, protein C, protein S, and factor V Leiden. Because many clotting factors are made in the liver, liver disease also affects coagulation.

In many cases, however, specific causes for coagulation abnormalities are not apparent. In **deep-vein thrombosis (DVT)**, a clot forms in an extremity such as the lower leg or calf. In **pulmonary embolism (PE)**, the clot is in the lungs. Most often, the clot forms elsewhere in the body and then breaks loose and travels to the lungs. These clotting problems are the result of hypercoagulation (excess clotting). Risk factors for DVT include age older than 40 years, estrogen therapy (such as birth control pills), smoking, obesity, surgery, trauma, prolonged immobility, hip replacement, and varicose veins. Physical inactivity has been found to increase the risk of DVT, as blood pools in the legs and then forms clots. Many patients in the inpatient setting who are immobile due to sickness will receive preventive anticoagulation therapy. Because it takes the body time to absorb a clot, treatment for DVT and PE will usually last for at least three to six months to prevent emboli as the body dissolves the clot.

When a clot occurs, the greatest concern (other than relieving pain and local tissue injury associated with an unwanted clot) is that a piece of the clot (called an **embolus**) will dislodge and travel to the heart, brain, or lungs. Occlusion of small vessels in one of these organs is a life-threatening emergency. Other conditions that can create a hypercoagulable state are pregnancy, severe infection, liver disease, and cancer.

Drug Regimens and Treatments

Because brain cell death is irreversible, most drug therapy for stroke is aimed at prevention rather than treatment after the fact. However, it is difficult to accurately predict a patient's risk for a stroke. Often, anticoagulation therapy starts only after someone has had a stroke or a TIA. Thrombolytic (fibrinolytic) therapies can be used to break up an ischemic clot if it caused a measurable neurologic deficit. However, there is a short window of opportunity from the time of the onset of symptoms to when thrombolytic therapy would no longer be effective. Proper diagnosis of the type of stroke and timing is necessary. Consequently, anticoagulation and antiplatelet therapies are used more often to prevent stroke rather than to break up a clot once it has already caused a stroke. Sometimes, patients who do not have a history of stroke but who do have multiple risk factors, such as diabetes and high cholesterol, will be prescribed low-dose aspirin therapy to reduce the risk of stroke and heart attack. Anticoagulants, antiplatelet drugs, and thrombolytic therapies are described later in this chapter.

Prevention and treatment of unwanted clots, whether the cause is a stroke or a clotting disorder, employs anticoagulants, antiplatelet agents, and thrombolytics. Patients taking such therapies should be monitored regularly by undergoing specific laboratory tests:

- **Partial thromboplastin time (PTT)** measures the function of the intrinsic and common pathways of the coagulation cascade. This marker monitors heparin therapy.

- **Prothrombin time (PT)** measures the function of the extrinsic and common pathways of the coagulation cascade. This measurement can vary, so reference ranges produced by the local laboratory must be used to interpret this test. This marker monitors warfarin therapy.

- **International normalized ratio (INR)** gives a reference for coagulation involving the extrinsic and common pathways of the coagulation cascade. It standardizes the PT to remove variability. This marker monitors warfarin therapy. INR can be tested using finger-stick technology so that results are available quickly for therapy decisions.

Anticoagulant Agents

Blood clots that have already formed can be treated with a choice of **anticoagulant agents**. These agents do not necessarily break down a clot that has already formed, but they halt growth and keep emboli from forming as the body reabsorbs the clot on its own.

Treatment usually starts with IV **heparin**. This medication is used for immediate, short-term anticoagulation treatment of blood clots. Heparin works by inhibiting clotting factors in the coagulation cascade and inactivating thrombin and factor Xa (which is also known as activated factor X). It also affects the platelets' ability to clump together. Heparin does not affect an existing clot but prevents emboli from forming while the body slowly dissolves and absorbs a clot. It is also used as a flushing agent to keep IV lines open and as a subcutaneous prophylactic in patients at high risk for developing clots. Heparin use is allowed during pregnancy because it does not cross the placental barrier.

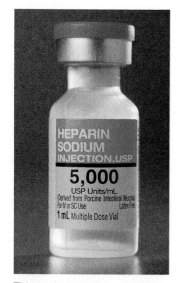

This sealed, sterile, multidose glass vial of heparin contains several doses of medication with a preservative.

Drug Alert

Heparin is available in many different concentrations (1–20,000 units/mL), so it is especially important to read the medication label and verify that the concentration is correct before administering a dose. A patient who receives too much heparin will experience excessive thinning of the blood, which can be deadly.

After heparin administration, therapy is often switched from heparin to a **low-molecular-weight heparin (LMWH)** product. An LMWH works similarly to heparin, but it affects factor Xa more than it affects thrombin. However, unlike heparin infusion, this product can be injected subcutaneously and it has a longer half-life than heparin does. For patients, an LMWH is more convenient to use because it can be given once or twice a day as a self-injection, which facilitates discharge from a hospital. LMWHs are the preferred anticoagulant for pregnant patients and are used as a bridge therapy from IV heparin to oral warfarin.

If patients cannot tolerate heparin or LMWH therapy, alternative anticoagulants are available. **Fondaparinux** works by selectively inhibiting factor Xa in the coagulation cascade. It is injected subcutaneously once a day. **Direct thrombin inhibitors** are administered via continuous infusion and work by inhibiting thrombin directly (see Table 16.3).

After initial treatment with heparin or LMWH, oral **warfarin** therapy can begin (see Table 16.4). Warfarin works by inhibiting the production of vitamin K–dependent clotting factors in the liver. This medication is used to treat conditions in which clot formation is a concern, such as heart valve disease, artificial heart valve placement, prior stroke, atrial fibrillation, DVT, PE, and heart attack. Because warfarin is used for long-term anticoagulation and requires five or more days for the onset of full effect, it cannot initially be used alone when treating a clot. Instead, it must be overlapped by at least five days with

TABLE 16.3 | Anticoagulants

Generic (Brand)	Dosage Form	Route of Administration	Common Dosage
Fondaparinux (Arixtra)	Injection	Sub-Q injection	2.5 mg once a day
Heparin or unfractionated heparin (UFH)	Injection	Continuous IV infusion, sub-Q injection	IV: doses are individualized but often in thousands of units per infusion Sub-Q: 3,000–5,000 units every 8–12 hr
Warfarin (Coumadin)	Tablet	Oral	2–10 mg a day (doses are individualized)
Direct Thrombin Inhibitors			
Argatroban	Injection	Continuous IV infusion	Doses are individualized, but 2 mcg/kg/min is common
Bivalirudin (Angiomax)	Injection	Continuous IV infusion	Doses individualized, but 1.75 mg/kg/hr is common
Dabigatran (Pradaxa)	Capsule	Oral	150 mg twice a day
LMWHs			
Dalteparin (Fragmin)	Injection	Sub-Q injection	200 units/kg/day given in doses twice a day
Enoxaparin (Lovenox)	Injection	Sub-Q injection	1–1.5 mg/kg/day given in doses once or twice a day
Tinzaparin (Innohep)	Injection	Sub-Q injection	175 units/kg/day given once a day

TABLE 16.4 | Warfarin Tablet Strength and Associated Color

For patient-safety reasons, all manufacturers of oral warfarin in the United States use the same color-coding that corresponds with tablet strength. Although the color of the tablet remains the same, the shape of the tablet varies according to the manufacturer. For example, the brand name Coumadin produces a round tablet, and the generic form of warfarin manufactured by Taro Pharmaceuticals produces an oval tablet.

Tablet Strength	Tablet Color
1 mg	Pink
2 mg	Lavender (light purple)
2.5 mg	Green
3 mg	Tan
4 mg	Blue
5 mg	Peach (light orange)
6 mg	Teal (blue green)
7.5 mg	Yellow
10 mg	White

either heparin or an LMWH. This duration of dual therapy may be more than five days, and the patient's warfarin dose is adjusted according to blood test results until the patient achieves the desired therapeutic range. When there is no immediate need to treat an acute clot, warfarin is given alone as a preventive therapy, and doses are adjusted to achieve the desired results.

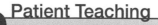

Patient Teaching

As an allied health professional, reinforce adherence to therapy and regular follow-up for patients who are receiving anticoagulation therapy. It is critical for patient safety that patients work with their healthcare practitioners to adjust doses properly. Patients who are taking warfarin initially require frequent blood tests, including an INR test every couple of days. Even after a patient has achieved a stable INR level, monthly INR tests are generally required.

In addition, encourage your patients who are prescribed warfarin to take their medication at the same time each day to maintain steady drug levels in the body. Advise these patients to also maintain a consistent diet because a change in the consumption of green, leafy vegetables can affect the efficacy of warfarin. Green, leafy vegetables such as spinach, kale, and broccoli contain high levels of vitamin K.

Side Effects Common side effects of heparin include bruising, bleeding due to excessive anticoagulation, and thrombocytopenia (low platelet count). **Heparin-induced thrombocytopenia (HIT)** is a rare but serious side effect that can be life threatening. It can only be fully detected by laboratory tests but often is preceded by a skin rash. Patients should report any signs of bleeding or skin rashes to their prescribers right away.

Common side effects of LMWHs include bruising, bleeding due to excessive anticoagulation, fever, pain at the injection site, and thrombocytopenia. Patients who have had HIT should not take LMWHs. Patients should report any signs of bleeding or skin rashes to their prescribers immediately.

Common side effects of fondaparinux include nausea, fever, anemia, and bleeding due to excessive anticoagulation. Patients should report any signs of bleeding to their prescribers and follow instructions regarding laboratory tests.

Common side effects of direct thrombin inhibitors include nausea, headache, back pain, and bleeding due to excessive anticoagulation. Patients should report any signs of bleeding to their prescribers and follow instructions regarding laboratory tests.

The most common side effects of warfarin include bleeding due to excessive anticoagulation, hair loss, skin lesions, and purple/blue toe syndrome (in which clots form in the toe, causing tissue death and even gangrene if not treated). Signs of bleeding include blood in the urine or stool; black, tarry stools; bleeding in the mouth or gums; unusual or unexplained bruising; vomiting blood (or material that resembles coffee grounds); and nosebleeds. If any of these side effects occur, patients should see their prescribers.

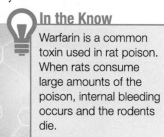

In the Know

Warfarin is a common toxin used in rat poison. When rats consume large amounts of the poison, internal bleeding occurs and the rodents die.

Contraindications Fondaparinux is contraindicated in severe kidney impairment, active major bleeding, bacterial endocarditis, and thrombocytopenia associated with a positive test for antiplatelet antibodies in the presence of fondaparinux.

Heparin should not be used in patients with severe thrombocytopenia or uncontrolled active bleeding (except when bleeding is due to disseminated intravascular coagulation [DIC]). Full-dose heparin should also be avoided when proper coagulation tests cannot be obtained.

Contraindications to warfarin include hemorrhagic tendencies, recent or potential surgery of the eye or central nervous system, major regional lumbar block anesthesia or traumatic surgery resulting in large open surfaces, blood dyscrasias, severe uncontrolled high blood pressure, pericarditis or pericardial effusion, bacterial endocarditis, eclampsia or preeclampsia, threatened abortion, and pregnancy. Warfarin should also not be used in patients with a high potential of medication nonadherence.

Argatroban and bivalirudin are contraindicated in patients with major bleeding. Dabigatran should not be used in active pathologic bleeding and patients with mechanical prosthetic heart valves.

LMWHs are contraindicated in patients with a history of HIT, a hypersensitivity to heparin or pork products, and active major bleeding. Dalteparin is contraindicated in patients with unstable angina, non–Q-wave myocardial infarction (MI), or prolonged venous thromboembolism prophylaxis undergoing epidural neuraxial anesthesia. Tinzaparin is contraindicated in acute or subacute endocarditis; hemophilia or major blood clotting disorders; acute cerebral insult or hemorrhagic cerebrovascular accidents without systemic emboli; uncontrolled severe high blood pressure; diabetic or hemorrhagic retinopathy; injury or surgery involving the brain, spinal cord, eyes, or ears; spinal or epidural anesthesia; and the use of multidose vials containing benzyl alcohol in children younger than two years of age, premature infants, and neonates.

Cautions and Considerations Heparin should not be given as an intramuscular (IM) injection because severe bruising can occur. LMWHs, fondaparinux, and direct thrombin inhibitors require dose adjustment in patients with impaired renal function and are contraindicated in some cases of severe kidney problems. Patients should inform their prescribers and pharmacists if they know they have kidney disease.

Warfarin is highly protein-bound and metabolized through the liver, so it interacts with many over-the-counter (OTC) and prescription drugs. The drug interactions with warfarin are too numerous to mention here, but some of the most common prescription drugs that interact with warfarin are listed in Table 16.5. Aspirin and NSAIDs affect clotting by changing platelet action, so they should not be taken with warfarin or other anticoagulants. (The risk is lower with some of the other anticoagulants, such as heparin and LMWHs.) If a patient must take NSAIDs, increased warfarin monitoring will be required.

TABLE 16.5 Drugs that Interact with Warfarin

Amiodarone	Lovastatin
Carbamazepine	Metronidazole
Cimetidine	Phenytoin
Fenofibrate	Rifampin
Fluconazole	Rosuvastatin
Fluoxetine	Simvastatin
Fluvastatin	Sulfamethoxazole
Gemfibrozil	Tamoxifen
Levothyroxine	Voriconazole

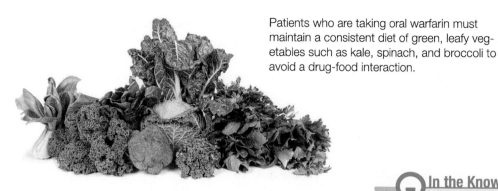

Patients who are taking oral warfarin must maintain a consistent diet of green, leafy vegetables such as kale, spinach, and broccoli to avoid a drug-food interaction.

Interactions that affect warfarin activity can be serious. A decrease in effectiveness can cause unwanted clots; an increase in effectiveness can cause bleeding. Either way, the results of these interactions can be life threatening. Patients should tell their prescribers and pharmacists about all medications they take so that potential interactions can be identified. Allied health professionals can help by obtaining a thorough medication history.

Warfarin is also affected by certain foods. Because it inhibits vitamin K–dependent clotting factors, changes in the amount of vitamin K a patient ingests can affect warfarin activity. All patients, especially those just starting warfarin therapy, should learn about food and drug interactions. Foods high in vitamin K (such as green, leafy vegetables) do not have to be avoided entirely. Patients should simply avoid varying the amount of these foods that they typically eat. Wide swings in the amount of vitamin K consumed will affect the activity of oral anticoagulants. Warfarin doses are adjusted according to each patient's typical daily food intake.

Alcohol increases warfarin's effects. Patients taking anticoagulant drugs should not drink excessive amounts of alcohol or bleeding could occur. Moderate alcohol intake (one to two drinks a day) does not affect anticoagulation therapy.

In the Know

Green, leafy vegetables such as kale, spinach, and collard greens have the highest vitamin K content, but many other vegetables also contain vitamin K. Patients taking warfarin should have access to a list that shows the vitamin K content of different foods, so that they can maintain a consistent intake of this vitamin. A good resource for food nutrient content is the Food-A-Pedia, published within the SuperTracker program offered by the United States Department of Agriculture (USDA). This resource can be accessed at http://PharmEssAH.emcp.net/foodapedia.

Patient Teaching

The serving size of different types of alcoholic beverages varies, so patients should be mindful of what one to two drinks a day will mean for them. Serving sizes are 5 to 6 ounces for wine, 8 to 12 ounces for beer, and 1.5 ounces for hard liquor.

Warfarin therapy requires frequent laboratory tests and close monitoring. For successful anticoagulation therapy, doses should be taken consistently, at the same time each day. Missed doses should be taken as soon as the patient remembers but should not overlap with subsequent doses. Missed doses should be reported to the prescriber or pharmacist who is adjusting doses.

Anticoagulants are considered high-risk medications for potential mistakes. These agents do not leave much room for error, and slight changes in doses (either underdosing or overdosing) can have life-threatening consequences. Healthcare personnel should never assume doses are correctly written as ordered. Use appropriate references to look up doses; double-check all calculations involved in ordering, preparing, and administering these products; and verify the medication label with the patient's prescription to avoid medication errors.

Kolb's Learning Styles

Opportunistic learners, like Accommodators, may find that looking through their own medicine cabinets is a useful way to become familiar with warfarin drug interactions. Using a reputable drug resource, look up the drugs you have at home and determine which ones interact with warfarin. Be aware that many patients who are taking warfarin have these same drugs in their medicine cabinets.

Anticoagulation Antagonists

Another class of drugs used to treat coagulation problems is **anticoagulation antagonists**, such as vitamin K and protamine (see Table 16.6). **Vitamin K** is used in the body to make clotting factors II, VII, IX, and X in the coagulation cascade as well as proteins C and S. It is used to reverse warfarin effects when signs of bleeding are present. If the INR results are elevated but signs of bleeding are not present, the patient may simply be instructed to skip a dose or two of warfarin. The pharmacist and prescriber should handle these decisions and adjustments directly with the patient. If bleeding is severe, the patient will be given fresh whole blood with clotting factors to stop blood loss.

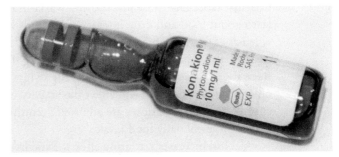

Phytonadione, a manufactured form of vitamin K, is used to treat bleeding disorders and vitamin K deficiencies.

TABLE 16.6 Anticoagulation Antagonists

Generic (Brand)	Dosage Form	Route of Administration	Common Dosage
Phytonadione or vitamin K (Mephyton)	Injection, tablet	IM, IV, oral, sub-Q	1–10 mg a dose
Protamine	Injection	IV	Based on degree of heparin reversal desired

Drug Alert

Oral vitamin K tablets are not the same as potassium supplements—although these supplements are abbreviated in prescription orders as *K*. It is crucial that you take extra care that these medications are not mixed up because such an error could be fatal.

Protamine is used to reverse heparin effects. It works by combining with heparin to form a complex that is no longer able to exert anticoagulation effects. It is used when a patient is hemorrhaging or has a high risk of hemorrhage.

Side Effects Common side effects of vitamin K include flushing, changes in taste sensation, dizziness, sweating, rapid pulse, and difficulty breathing. Pain at the injection site can also occur. Vitamin K should be administered under direct supervision to monitor for these effects and signs of **anaphylaxis** (severe allergic reaction).

Contraindications Phytonadione (or vitamin K) and protamine do not have contraindications.

Cautions and Considerations Vitamin K should be administered subcutaneously whenever possible. If IM or IV administration is unavoidable, the medication must be given very slowly (no faster than 1 mg a minute). Fatalities have occurred with more rapid administration of vitamin K. In addition, vitamin K should be mixed in preservative-free normal saline or dextrose 5% in water (D_5W).

Antiplatelet Agents

Medications known as **antiplatelet agents** are used to decrease the risk of stroke, DVT, and clotting associated with cardiovascular blockage (see Table 16.7). These agents are usually administered to patients who have already had a cardiovascular blockage in order to prevent further clotting.

Low-dose aspirin (81–325 mg a day) is used to prevent clots associated with stroke and heart attack. This dose of aspirin has antiplatelet effects but may not alleviate pain or fever. Aspirin can be used during a heart attack to keep clots from completely occluding blood vessels in the heart. Other uses for aspirin are covered in Chapter 25.

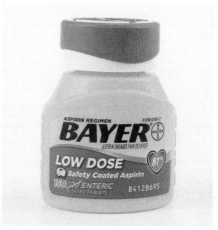

Millions of individuals in the United States take low-dose aspirin once a day to reduce their risk of a stroke or heart attack.

TABLE 16.7	Commonly Used Antiplatelet Agents

Generic (Brand)	Dosage Form	Route of Administration	Common Dosage
Aspirin	Chewable tablet, effervescent tablet, suppository, tablet	Oral, rectal	PO: 81–650 mg a day Rectal: 120–600 mg a day
Clopidogrel (Plavix)	Tablet	Oral	75 mg a day
Dipyridamole (Persantine)	Injection, tablet	IV, oral	IV: varies depending on patient weight PO: 75–100 mg 3–4 times a day
Pentoxifylline (Trental)	Tablet	Oral	400 mg 3 times a day
Ticlopidine	Tablet	Oral	250 mg twice a day with food

Side Effects Common side effects of aspirin, clopidogrel, and ticlopidine include bleeding due to excessive anticoagulation, upset stomach, headache, dizziness, and skin rash. Signs of bleeding include blood in the urine or stool; black, tarry stools; bleeding in the mouth or gums; unusual or unexplained bruising; vomiting blood (or material that resembles coffee grounds); and nosebleeds. If any of these effects occur, patients should see their prescribers. These agents should not be used in patients who are already at risk for bleeding, such as those about to have surgical procedures. Usually patients will be instructed to temporarily discontinue these drugs prior to their procedures.

Contraindications Aspirin is contraindicated in patients with a hypersensitivity to other salicylates or NSAIDs, and in patients with asthma, rhinitis, nasal polyps, or bleeding disorders. In addition, aspirin should not be used in children to treat viral infections due to a potential association with Reye syndrome. Clopidogrel should not be used in active pathologic bleeding such as peptic ulcer or intracranial hemorrhage. Pentoxifylline should not be used in patients with an intolerance to xanthines and in patients who have recent cerebral and/or retinal hemorrhage. Contraindications to ticlopidine include active bleeding, intracranial hemorrhage, severe liver impairment, and hematopoietic disorders. Dipyridamole does not have contraindications.

Cautions and Considerations Antiplatelet agents should be avoided or used with caution in patients with a history of ulcers due to an increased risk for hemorrhage. For this same reason, patients should not take NSAIDs along with antiplatelet or anticoagulation therapy. NSAIDs can affect platelet activity and increase bleeding risk.

Clopidogrel and ticlopidine can cause thrombocytopenia (low platelets) and neutropenia (low WBC count). CBC is used to monitor for drops in platelet or WBC counts. Liver function tests are usually tracked as well. Antiplatelet agents work best when taken with food.

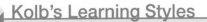

Kolb's Learning Styles

All learners can benefit from putting the drug therapies they handle into the context of patient care. Anticoagulants (see Table 16.3 and Table 16.7) are used to maintain a patient's INR within a specific range. Use any nursing handbook to look up the ranges for patients taking anticoagulation therapy for DVT treatment, atrial fibrillation, prosthetic heart valve, and cardiac stents. The goal of therapy is to elevate the INR just enough to prevent clot formation but not so much as to cause bleeding.

Thrombolytic Agents

When immediate return of bloodflow is crucial, **thrombolytic agents** are used to dissolve clots that have formed. Use of these medications is limited to select situations, including massive MI, stroke, and PE. These agents can yield dramatic lifesaving results but must be administered within hours to days of the event to be effective. Examples of thrombolytic agents are shown in Table 16.8.

Thrombolytic medications work through a variety of mechanisms, all of which break up clots that have already formed. Many work by dissolving fibrin (see Figure 16.5). Unlike the other medications discussed earlier in this chapter that prevent formation or further growth of clots, these drugs, in contrast, dissolve and shrink blood clots. However, their cost and potential serious side effects must be weighed along with their benefits.

TABLE 16.8 Commonly Used Thrombolytic Agents

Generic (Brand)	Dosage Form	Route of Administration	Common Dosage
Alteplase (Activase, TPA)	Powder for injection	IV	0.09–0.75 mg/kg over 30–60 min
Reteplase (Retavase)	Injection	IV	10 units over 2 min
Tenecteplase (TNKase)	Powder for injection	IV	Varies depending on patient weight

FIGURE 16.5 Formation of a Blood Clot

Fibrin, a fibrous protein, forms a network in which RBCs become entrapped, thereby forming a blood clot.

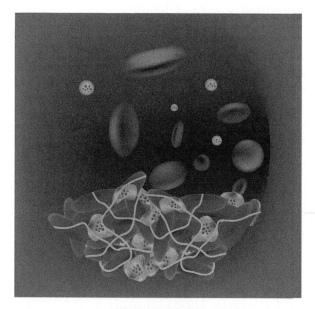

Thrombosis

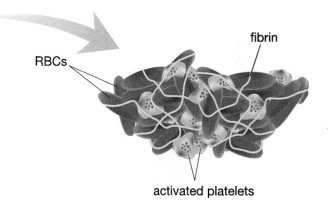

RBCs

fibrin

activated platelets

Side Effects Common side effects of thrombolytic medications include bleeding, bruising, slow heart rate, decreased blood pressure, arrhythmias, fever, and allergic reactions. These agents are administered in the inpatient setting, so the effects are monitored closely. Risk of severe bleeding is high, so use of these agents is limited to life-threatening situations.

Contraindications When used to dissolve clots in the body, thrombolytics are contraindicated in patients who have active bleeding or internal bleeding; a history of CVA; recent intracranial or intraspinal surgery or trauma; intracranial neoplasm, arteriovenous malformations, or aneurysm; known bleeding diathesis; severe uncontrolled high blood pressure; ischemic stroke within three months; prior intracranial hemorrhage; suspected aortic dissection; and significant closed head or facial trauma within the preceding three months. Alteplase can be used to restore central line catheter function. When used for this indication, there are no contraindications.

Cautions and Considerations Tenecteplase should not be shaken during **reconstitution** (the process of adding a diluent to a powdered medication to prepare a solution or suspension). It should be mixed with sterile water only, not dextrose solution, and allowed to sit for a few minutes. Reteplase must be refrigerated and protected from light.

Hemophilia Agents

Drugs for hemophilia replace specific missing clotting factors in patients with this condition. Replacing missing factor(s) allows the coagulation cascade to function and restores normal coagulation. These injectable **hemophilia agents** include factors VIIa, VIII, and IX, as well as von Willebrand factor.

Side Effects Side effects of hemophilia agents include allergic reactions, mild chills, nausea, and irritation at the injection site. Because these agents are derived from human blood products and plasma, infectious diseases can be passed to the recipient of these products. Pregnant patients or those with poor immune function must be aware of this risk.

Contraindications Factor VIIa does not have contraindications. Factor VIII is contraindicated in patients with a hypersensitivity to the drug. Factor IX (human-type) does not have contraindications, but recombinant factor IX is contraindicated in patients with a hypersensitivity to factor IX or any component of the formulation, and in patients with DIC or signs of fibrinolysis. The combination drug containing von Willebrand factor and factor VIII is contraindicated in patients with a history of anaphylaxis or severe systemic response to any of the components of the medication.

Cautions and Considerations Hemophilia agents are usually dispensed from a specialty pharmacy and are quite expensive. Due to their high cost, these medications are closely monitored by prescribers and by health insurance providers. Prevention of major bleeding events in patients with hemophilia is important for sustaining life as well as keeping costs of health care down. One hospitalization for a hemophilia-related bleeding event can cost millions of dollars.

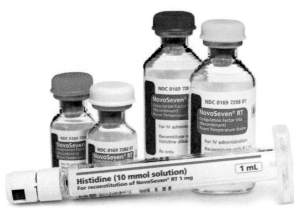

NovoSeven RT is used to prevent or treat bleeding in patients with hemophilia A or B, acquired hemophilia, or congenital factor VII deficiency.

© Novo Nordisk

Checkpoint 16.3

Take a moment to review what you have learned so far and answer these questions.

1. What is the difference between an ischemic stroke and a hemorrhagic stroke?

2. What categories of drug therapies are used to treat ischemic stroke?

3. What are the side effects of anticoagulants?

4. What agents are used to treat hemophilia?

Herbal and Alternative Therapies

Other than iron, folic acid, and vitamin B_{12} supplements, few herbal or dietary supplement products are used to treat blood disorders. **Vitamin C** is sometimes prescribed along with iron supplements to boost absorption. No other OTC products are available to treat coagulation and clotting disorders. Frequently, however, patients take herbal products that interact with drugs discussed in this chapter. For instance, anticoagulants (such as warfarin) and antiplatelet agents (such as aspirin and ticlopidine) interact with numerous herbal/dietary and nutritional supplement products, including cranberry juice, *dong quai*, Feverfew, ginger, garlic, ginkgo biloba, green tea, St. John's wort, and vitamin E.

Patient Teaching

You can help patients and practitioners detect drug–herbal/dietary supplement interactions by obtaining a thorough medication history from all patients who are taking anticoagulants, antiplatelet agents, and/or other drugs mentioned in this chapter. By asking about herbal and dietary supplement products specifically, you can remind patients to inform their healthcare practitioners when they take these products. Entering these medications into the patient's profile is an important step in checking for drug interactions.

Chapter Review

Chapter Summary

The blood contains plasma and three main types of blood cells: RBCs, WBCs, and platelets. RBCs contain hemoglobin, which carries oxygen to the body's tissues. Iron, folic acid, and vitamin B_{12} are essential building blocks of hemoglobin and RBCs. Anemia is a reduction in the number of healthy RBCs that contain functional hemoglobin. It can be caused by a deficiency in these nutrients or a reduction in hematopoiesis, the process whereby RBCs are produced. Drug therapy for anemia includes iron, folic acid, and vitamin B_{12} supplementation as well as hematopoietic agents such as epoetin alfa and darbepoetin.

Platelet activity and the coagulation cascade regulate the blood's ability to form clots. When the blood cannot clot, dangerous bleeding can occur. Hemophilia, a life-threatening bleeding condition, is a genetic disorder in which certain clotting factors are absent or deficient. Missing clotting factors are administered to prevent bleeding.

When the blood forms unwanted clots, bloodflow can be cut off to vital organs, including the brain, heart, and lungs. Clots cause stroke, heart attack, PE, and DVT. Anticoagulants and antiplatelet drug therapies are used frequently to prevent and treat such clots. These drugs have many drug interactions and side effects that must be monitored closely. Thrombolytic drugs can be used in certain situations to break down clots that have formed.

Chapter Checkup

The Navigator+ learning management system that accompanies this textbook offers many opportunities to help you master chapter content, including end-of-chapter exercises, a glossary of key terms, flash cards, and additional interactive activities.

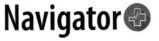

 ## Career Exploration

If you enjoyed learning about the blood and drug therapy in this chapter, you may want to explore the following career options:

- blood bank technology specialist
- medical assistant
- perioperative blood management technologist
- pharmacy technician
- phlebotomist

17

The Respiratory System and Drug Therapy

Pharm Facts

- The lungs of an average adult may not seem very large, but their surface area is similar to the size of a tennis court.

- Added end-to-end, the airways in the lungs of an average adult stretch about 1,500 miles, or about the distance from New York City to Dallas.

- If you live to be 80 years of age, you will take approximately 673 million breaths.

- Most individuals think that breathing involves lung inflation followed by chest expansion. Actually, the opposite is true. The diaphragm muscle pulls down and the intercostal muscles push out, creating a vacuum in the chest. The lungs expand to fill this vacuum.

- The left lung is slightly smaller than the right lung to make room for the heart, which is tilted slightly to the left.

- Every day, your nasal passages secrete about four cups of mucus, most of which you swallow without noticing.

"As a respiratory therapist, I work with patients who have pulmonary conditions that prevent them from breathing effortlessly. Anyone who has experienced the feeling of 'having the wind knocked out of you' or being desperate for air recognizes how difficult life must be for patients with respiratory problems. Respiratory therapists work in all areas of health care—from critical care to diagnostic labs. No matter the healthcare setting, all of us share a common goal: to bring breath and life to patients."

—**Chad Condren**, MBA, RRT
Respiratory Therapist

Diseases and conditions of the respiratory tract range from the common cold and seasonal allergies to asthma and tuberculosis. As an allied health professional, you will encounter patients with some type of respiratory disease on a regular basis. Being familiar with the drug therapies used to treat diseases of the respiratory tract will be helpful in your future practice.

This chapter covers the normal physiology of the respiratory system, followed by an explanation of the conditions that most often affect it. Conditions are discussed in the context of the upper and lower respiratory tracts. Such conditions include rhinitis, seasonal allergies, cough and cold, asthma, chronic obstructive pulmonary disease, and pneumonia. The chapter then briefly touches on tuberculosis and cystic fibrosis treatments. Finally, this chapter addresses the products used for smoking cessation.

Anatomy and Physiology of the Respiratory System

The respiratory tract is divided into the upper and lower tracts (see Figure 17.1). These tracts contain different structures and have varying physiologic functions. Different diseases and conditions tend to affect the upper and lower respiratory tracts, so distinct drug therapies may be used for each region.

Upper Respiratory Tract

The **upper respiratory tract** includes the **nasal passages**; **sinuses**; the **pharynx**, which is comprised of the **nasopharynx**, **oropharynx**, and **laryngopharynx**; and the **larynx** (voice box), where the **epiglottis** is located (see Figure 17.2). In the upper respiratory tract, the sinuses, throat, and nasal passages are common sites for viral and bacterial infections. The viruses responsible for the common cold typically cause symptoms that affect the upper respiratory tract, including coughing, sinus pain, and postnasal drainage. Inflammation associated with allergies also affects upper respiratory tissues, causing congestion and runny nose (rhinitis).

FIGURE 17.1 | Upper and Lower Respiratory Tracts

The epiglottis, a flap of tissue that covers the tracheal opening to the lungs when you swallow, is in effect the dividing line between the upper and lower respiratory tracts.

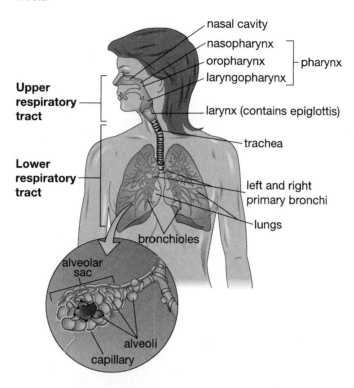

FIGURE 17.2 | Upper Respiratory Tract

The upper respiratory tract includes structures above the trachea.

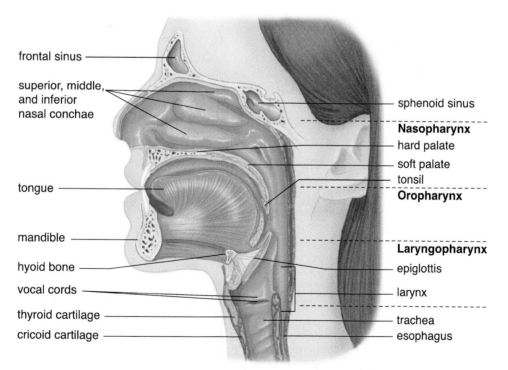

Lower Respiratory Tract

The **lower respiratory tract** includes the **trachea** (windpipe) and the **bronchi**, **bronchioles**, and **alveoli** of the **lungs**. When a person breathes, air is pulled into and pushed out of the lungs. This mechanical process facilitates the movement of oxygen into the lungs and the release of carbon dioxide. In the lungs, small sacs called *alveoli* fill with air and allow for gas exchange with the blood. The surface area of the alveoli is extremely large, and respiratory tissue is well supplied with blood vessels, allowing gases such as oxygen and carbon dioxide to move easily into and out of the bloodstream.

Inside the alveoli, oxygen moves into the blood, and carbon dioxide, a by-product of cellular function, leaves the blood. This **gas-exchange process** (see Figure 17.3) provides needed oxygen to the cells of the body to supply energy and to fuel cellular respiration. This process also helps maintain the acid-base balance in the blood.

FIGURE 17.3 | **Gas-Exchange Process**

Oxygen picked up in the lungs is carried by red blood cells to all the cells of the body, while carbon dioxide is returned to the lungs to be expelled during exhalation.

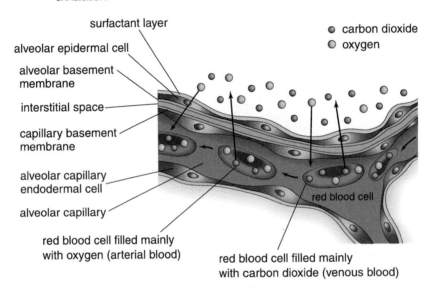

Checkpoint 17.1

Take a moment to review what you have learned so far and answer these questions.

1. What structures are included in the upper respiratory tract?

2. What structures are included in the lower respiratory tract?

3. Where does the gas-exchange process occur?

Common Upper Respiratory Tract Disorders

Upper respiratory conditions addressed in this chapter include the common cold and rhinitis, as well as their associated symptoms. These conditions are commonly diagnosed and treated in most practice settings.

Common Cold

The **common cold** is an infection of the upper respiratory tract and primarily affects the nose and throat. Common symptoms include runny nose, sore throat, cough, watery eyes, sneezing, and congestion. The common cold is the most prevalent viral infection, with more than 60 million cases in the United States annually. Many viruses have been associated with the common cold, with rhinovirus being the most common. The common cold has no cure or vaccine because there are too many virus strains (close to 250), and they quickly mutate.

Kolb's Learning Styles

Accommodators appreciate learning activities that apply new information to real life. Before you go through this section on cough and cold products, look in your medicine cabinet. What medications do you use when you have a stuffy or runny nose? What cough medicine works best for you? Make a list of the active ingredients in the products you use, and think about how they work as you learn about their mechanism of action, side effects, and other properties.

Drug Regimens and Treatments

Treatment for the common cold focuses on symptom relief. While the virus runs its course, antihistamines, decongestants, cough suppressants, and expectorants can be used to relieve runny nose, stuffy nose, coughing, and chest congestion. Many cough and cold products contain various combinations of antihistamines, decongestants, cough suppressants, and expectorants. These products also contain analgesics such as acetaminophen or ibuprofen. Patients sometimes do not realize which active ingredients they are receiving when they take a combination product. This uncertainty can lead to duplicate therapy and overdose if a patient takes more than one product. This confusion also leads to unnecessary treatment when a patient takes a combination product for multiple symptoms when all he or she really needs is just one active ingredient to treat one or two specific symptoms.

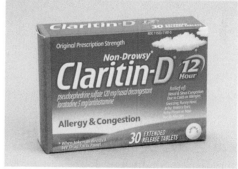

Claritin-D, an over-the-counter allergy and congestion product, contains a combination of loratadine (an antihistamine) and pseudoephedrine (a decongestant).

Patient Teaching

To help patients use cough and cold medications properly, remind them to use products that contain only those ingredients that treat their symptoms. Show patients how to read the labels of cough and cold products, so they can identify which active ingredients they contain. Individuals with high blood pressure should be especially careful about reading product labels because decongestants can raise blood pressure.

Antihistamines

This drug class is used for symptomatic relief from excess nasal secretions, itching, sneezing, and coughing. **Antihistamines** are also used to relieve the itching and redness resulting from allergic reactions (such as hives and rashes). Many antihistamines cause sedation, which is useful for mild insomnia and relaxation prior to anesthesia or other anxiety-producing procedures. However, the sedative effects of many antihistamines may cause problems for patients as they drive or perform other tasks that require mental alertness. In fact, the active ingredient in most over-the-counter (OTC) sleep aids is an antihistamine. First-generation antihistamines tend to cause the most sedation. Second-generation antihistamines do not cross the blood-brain barrier as readily; therefore, they cause less sedation. Antihistamines have also been used to treat motion sickness and Parkinson's disease.

Antihistamines work by blocking **histamine (H_1) receptors**, which reduce capillary dilation and leakage. Dosages for each agent vary widely based on patient age, dosage form, and reason for use (see Table 17.1).

TABLE 17.1 Commonly Used Antihistamines

Generic (Brand)	Dosage Form	Route of Administration	Common Dosage
First Generation			
Chlorpheniramine (Chlor-Trimeton)	Capsule, suspension, syrup, tablet	Oral	Varies by age
Clemastine (Tavist)	Syrup, tablet	Oral	Varies by age and use
Diphenhydramine (Benadryl)	Capsule, elixir, injection, liquid, oral strip, suspension, syrup, tablet	IM, IV, oral	Varies by age, dosage form, and use
Second Generation			
Cetirizine (Zyrtec)	Syrup, tablet	Oral	Varies by age and use
Desloratadine (Clarinex)	Syrup, tablet	Oral	Varies by age
Fexofenadine (Allegra)	Suspension, tablet	Oral	Varies by age
Loratadine (Claritin)	Syrup, tablet	Oral	Varies by age

Side Effects Side effects of antihistamines are drowsiness (most common in first-generation antihistamines), dry mouth, and urinary retention. Patients who take other medications that also cause drowsiness should take care with antihistamines because sedation could be excessive. For this same reason, patients should avoid drinking alcohol while taking antihistamines. Patients who have urination problems, including patients with prostate enlargement, should not use antihistamines because they can make urination even more difficult.

In some children, antihistamines have a paradoxical effect, causing excitation rather than drowsiness. Parents should be aware of this potential side effect.

Contraindications Contraindications to chlorpheniramine include narrow-angle glaucoma, bladder neck obstruction, prostate enlargement, acute asthma attacks, stenosing peptic ulcer, and pyloroduodenal obstruction. Clemastine is contraindicated in narrow-angle glaucoma. Diphenhydramine should not be used in patients with acute asthma, neonates or premature infants, or breast-feeding mothers. Cetirizine, desloratadine, fexofenadine, and loratadine do not have contraindications.

➕ *Note: Allied health professionals should be aware that an allergy to a particular drug contraindicates its use. This warning applies to all Contraindications sections in this chapter.*

Cautions and Considerations Patients who have high blood pressure or heart problems should talk with their prescribers before taking antihistamines. Antihistamines should usually not be given to infants or mothers who are breast-feeding. Patients with glaucoma or patients who are using monoamine oxidase inhibitors (MAOIs) generally should not take antihistamines.

Kolb's Learning Styles

If you are a reflective learner, as are Divergers and Assimilators, try this activity. Write down the brand names of cough and cold products you have taken in the past. Try to recall the generic drug names and symptoms treated by each product you list.

Decongestants

Decongestants are used to treat the upper respiratory congestion and pain caused by common colds, sinus infections, or allergies. These medications reduce sinus and nasal tissue swelling and allow for better drainage. They work by stimulating adrenergic receptors in nasal passages, which constricts blood vessels and reduces swelling. Some commonly used decongestants are listed in Table 17.2.

Doses for each agent vary widely according to the patient's age, dosage form, and reason for use. Product packaging should be consulted whenever possible to verify proper dosing for the age of the patient being treated.

TABLE 17.2 Commonly Used Decongestants

Generic (Brand)	Dosage Form	Route of Administration	Common Dosage
Phenylephrine (Neo-Synephrine, PediaCare, Sudafed PE, Triaminic)	Chewable tablet, nasal spray, oral liquid, oral strip, tablet	Nasal, oral	Varies by age and dosage form
Pseudoephedrine (Genaphed, Simply Stuffy, Sudafed, SudoGest, Zephrex)	Capsule, drops, oral liquid, suspension, syrup, tablet	Oral	Varies by age and dosage form

Side Effects Common side effects of decongestants include headache, dizziness, light-headedness, insomnia, nervousness, and nausea. These effects are usually mild, but if they persist or are severe, patients should contact their healthcare prescribers. Topical preparations can cause sneezing and nasal irritation but are less likely to cause systemic side effects.

Potentially serious effects include increased blood pressure and a fast or irregular heartbeat and occur most frequently with oral preparations. Patients with high blood pressure or heart problems should not use decongestants unless they talk with their prescribers first.

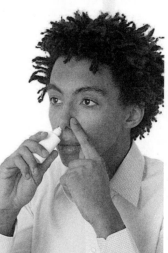

A patient should use a nasal spray for no longer than three consecutive days to avoid rebound congestion. Overuse of a nasal spray can also cause nasal passage damage and, in rare cases, septal perforation, in which the membrane dividing the nostrils develops a tear.

Contraindications Phenylephrine contraindications include high blood pressure and ventricular tachycardia. Pseudoephedrine should not be used with or within 14 days of MAOI therapy.

Cautions and Considerations When used topically for longer than three days, decongestants can cause rebound swelling and congestion. As a result, patients using decongestant nasal sprays for longer than a few days at a time may have worsened congestion when they stop using them. This rebound swelling lasts a few days and then subsides. Rebound congestion can make stopping decongestant use difficult because symptoms will seem to have returned and worsened. Consequently, patients may find themselves using such a product longer than is truly needed.

The decongestant **pseudoephedrine** is available over the counter, but purchases are restricted. Because these drugs can be used to prepare methamphetamine (crystal meth), a highly addictive and illegal drug, state and federal laws place limits on the quantities that can be purchased. Usually patients must be at least 18 years old, provide proof of age, and sign for the drug at the time of purchase.

Quick Study

Spend some time in the cough and cold aisle of a pharmacy near you. Familiarize yourself with the active ingredients of products available for purchase.

Cough Suppressants and Expectorants

When coughing is excessive and nonproductive (dry, hacking), **cough suppressants** are used. These agents suppress the cough reflex in the cough center of the medulla in the brain. The chemical structure of dextromethorphan is similar to that of codeine, but dextromethorphan does not have the pain-relieving or addictive properties of opiates. Hydrocodone and codeine are opiates that can be used to treat severe coughing at low doses because they too suppress the cough reflex. At higher doses, some of these products may treat pain.

Expectorants are used when a cough is productive (wet, mucus producing). They work by liquefying respiratory secretions to allow them to be cleared easily.

Dosages for each agent vary widely according to the patient's age, dosage form, and reason for use (see Table 17.3).

TABLE 17.3 | **Commonly Used Cough Medications**

Generic (Brand)	Dosage Form	Route of Administration	Common Dosage
Suppressants			
Codeine (many brands)	Capsule, oral solution, syrup, tablet	Oral	Varies by product and dosage form
Dextromethorphan (Delsym, PediaCare, Vicks 44, others)	Capsule, freezer pop, oral liquid, lozenge, oral strip, oral solution, suspension, syrup	Oral	Varies by age and dosage form
Hydrocodone (many brands)	Liquid, tablet	Oral	Varies by product and dosage form
Expectorant			
Guaifenesin (Mucinex, Robitussin, others)	Granules, oral liquid, syrup, tablet	Oral	Varies by age and dosage form

Side Effects Common side effects of cough suppressants include drowsiness, dizziness, and upset stomach. Patients should see how these agents affect them before driving. In addition, while taking cough suppressants, patients should avoid alcohol or other drugs that cause drowsiness. Additive effects can cause excessive drowsiness and dangerously slow breathing.

The side effects of guaifenesin are rare and mild when they occur and can include upset stomach and headache.

Contraindications Contraindications to codeine include respiratory depression, acute or severe asthma, presence of or suspicion for paralytic ileus, and postoperative pain management in children who have undergone tonsillectomy. Dextromethorphan should not be used with an MAOI or within two weeks of discontinuing an MAOI. Hydrocodone is contraindicated in paralytic ileus, respiratory depression, and acute and severe bronchial asthma. There are no contraindications associated with guaifenesin use.

Cautions and Considerations Codeine-derivative cough suppressants may be available over the counter but are restricted. Many states limit the quantities of these drugs that can be purchased at one time. Codeine and hydrocodone are classified as controlled substances and can only be acquired by prescription.

Rhinitis and Nasal Congestion

Rhinitis (runny nose) and **nasal congestion** have multiple causes. Acute rhinitis is most often caused by viral upper respiratory infection or the common cold. These causes are often self-limiting and treatment is usually symptom based. Of note, use of some medications such as angiotensin-converting enzyme (ACE) inhibitors, beta blockers, nonsteroidal anti-inflammatory drugs (NSAIDs), oral contraceptives, and topical decongestants is associated with acute rhinitis.

Chronic rhinitis is caused by allergic or nonallergic sources. Common allergens that trigger chronic rhinitis include dust, pollen, pet dander, and cigarette smoke. Cells in the respiratory tract release histamine and other inflammatory mediators in response to allergen exposure. **Histamine** dilates arterioles, allowing blood contents to leak into the local area. This process facilitates the movement of white blood cells (WBCs) to the affected area. (WBCs fight disease and foreign allergens.) Histamine also causes swelling, production of mucus, and soreness. Treatment of allergies includes the avoidance of allergens as well as the use of anti-inflammatory medication and antihistamines and decongestants (for symptomatic relief). Nonallergic causes of chronic rhinitis include anatomic abnormalities, irritant odors, temperature changes, and alcohol consumption.

Drug Regimens and Treatments

Treatment for rhinitis includes many of the same drugs used to treat symptoms of the common cold: antihistamines, decongestants, and cough remedies. Systemic antihistamines, nasal antihistamines, and nasal corticosteroids are used to treat symptoms including runny nose, watery and/or itchy eyes, and sneezing, whether the symptoms are caused by allergies or infection (see Table 17.1 for commonly used antihistamines). Decongestants may be used to treat allergies that are severe enough to cause nasal congestion (see Table 17.2 for commonly used decongestants). Decongestants are used more frequently when a cold produces symptoms of stuffy nose and sinus pain.

Nasal Corticosteroids and Antihistamines

Nasal allergy symptoms limited to the upper respiratory tract (i.e., nasal passages) are often treated with **topical nasal corticosteroids** and **topical nasal antihistamines** (see Table 17.4). Use of these agents during seasons when allergies are most likely reduces inflammation and allergy symptoms.

Patient Teaching

Nasal corticosteroids are administered intranasally. Use the following instructions to teach patients how to instill these medications:

1. Shake product well before use.

2. Clear nasal passages by either blowing the nose or using a saline irrigation system.

3. Sit in an upright position with the head tilted slightly forward.

4. Close one nostril by pressing it with a finger and insert the sprayer tip into the other nostril, with the tip pointing away from the nasal septum. Breathe in and depress the applicator to deliver a metered dose.

5. Breathe out from the mouth.

6. Repeat the procedure for the other nostril.

You may want to tell patients that it is not necessary to breathe in quickly or forcefully or to hold their breath. The site of action is in the nose, not deep in the sinuses or lungs. Warn patients that postnasal drip may occur and that they may taste the nasally administered medication. Finally, instruct them to avoid sneezing or blowing their nose just after using the spray.

TABLE 17.4 Commonly Used Nasal Antihistamines and Corticosteroids

Generic (Brand)	Dosage Form	Route of Administration	Common Dosage
Nasal Antihistamine			
Azelastine (Astelin, Astepro, Optivar)	Spray	Nasal	1 spray in each nostril twice a day
Nasal Corticosteroids			
Beclomethasone (Beconase AQ)	Spray	Nasal	1–2 sprays in each nostril twice a day
Budesonide (Rhinocort Aqua)	Spray	Nasal	2–4 sprays in each nostril once a day
Ciclesonide (Omnaris)	Spray	Nasal	2 sprays in each nostril once a day
Flunisolide	Spray	Nasal	1–2 sprays in each nostril 2–3 times a day
Fluticasone (Flonase, Veramyst)	Spray	Nasal	2 sprays in each nostril once a day
Mometasone (Nasonex)	Spray	Nasal	1–2 sprays in each nostril once a day
Triamcinolone (Nasacort AQ)	Spray	Nasal	1–2 sprays in each nostril once a day

Side Effects Common side effects of nasal allergy products include cough, sore throat, headache, and runny nose. Typically, these effects are mild and tolerable. Nosebleeds can also occur, especially in children. Patients who experience nosebleeds while taking one of these agents should speak with their healthcare prescribers.

Contraindications Flunisolide is contraindicated in infections of the nasal mucosa, such as bacterial or viral infections. The other nasal corticosteroids listed in Table 17.4 do not have contraindications.

Cautions and Considerations To ensure proper dosing, patients should shake these products well before administration. The pharmacy should affix an auxiliary warning label to the drug container to remind patients to shake the container prior to using the medication.

The spray application bottle should be primed when new and whenever it has not been used for a while. **Priming** a nasal spray means that the patient should pump the sprayer a few times away from the nose until an even amount of spray exits the applicator.

Checkpoint 17.2

Take a moment to review what you have learned so far and answer these questions.

1. What are the generic drug names for the first-generation and second-generation antihistamines?

2. What drugs are used to treat sinus congestion, runny nose, and cough?

Common Lower Respiratory Tract Disorders

Lower respiratory conditions addressed in this chapter include asthma, chronic obstructive pulmonary disease (COPD), pneumonia, tuberculosis, and cystic fibrosis. Asthma, COPD, and pneumonia are common conditions that affect millions of Americans each year. Tuberculosis and cystic fibrosis, although less common, are serious conditions that require special medical treatment.

Asthma

Asthma is an inflammatory disorder of the airways and causes coughing, wheezing, breathlessness, and chest tightness. Bronchioles constrict, mucous production increases, and lung tissue swells (see Figure 17.4), making normal breathing difficult. Asthma affects more than 25 million individuals in the United States. Seven million of these individuals are children. The number of people living with asthma in the United States has increased in the last 20 years. In fact, asthma accounts for thousands of emergency room visits, hospitalizations, and deaths each year.

Asthma is a chronic condition, which means that it is not curable. However, asthma is a reversible lung disease, in that it can improve or be controlled if a patient uses appropriate medications. If the patient regularly takes anti-inflammatory medication, lung function may return to normal.

In the Know

The Global Initiative for Asthma (GINA), in collaboration with healthcare organizations and asthma educators, organizes a special event each year called World Asthma Day. The purpose of World Asthma Day is to raise awareness about asthma and improve care throughout the world. The first World Asthma Day occurred in 1998 and was celebrated in 35 countries.

FIGURE 17.4 Asthmatic Lung

A lung with asthma in effect "overreacts" to produce excess mucus and swelling. The combination of excess mucus and bronchoconstriction makes airflow difficult.

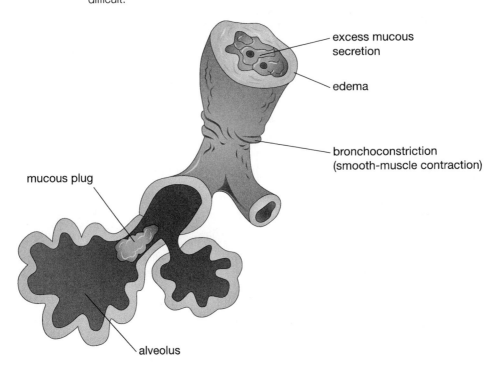

excess mucous secretion

edema

bronchoconstriction (smooth-muscle contraction)

mucous plug

alveolus

Asthma is episodic, meaning that times of poor airflow and difficulty with breathing alternate with times of normal function. Acute difficulty with breathing, known as an **asthma attack**, is characterized by hyperreactivity of the airways and **bronchospasm**, usually in response to allergens or irritants. Common triggers include smoke, dust, exercise, pet dander, cold weather, gastroesophageal reflux disease (GERD), and colds or flu. Other potential triggers can include medications, anxiety, laughing, and certain foods. Immediately after exposure to a trigger, mast cells in the lung tissue release histamine and other chemical mediators that cause bronchospasm and increase mucous production.

Asthma attacks make patients anxious and can be life-threatening when severe. Over time, continued release of histamine, bradykinins, prostaglandins, and leukotrienes causes tissues to inflame and airways to constrict and can result in permanent lung tissue damage. Fortunately, in many cases, breathing symptoms and airway constriction can be controlled with proper treatment. Without treatment, lung function can steadily decline.

Asthma is categorized into levels of severity (intermittent, mild, moderate, and severe) based on how patients' symptoms affect their ability to sleep at night, continue normal daily activities, and breathe freely. Objective **pulmonary function tests** can be done to assess asthma severity. In addition, if a patient is waking up at night more than twice a month due to asthmatic symptoms or is using relief medication such as an inhaler more than twice a week, asthma is considered "not controlled." Patients should understand that if their asthma is not controlled, they should seek medical treatment and be sure to adhere to prescribed medication schedules. Drug therapy for asthma includes long-term treatment to prevent exacerbations as well as **rescue therapies** to help once asthma attack symptoms have begun. Many patients need more than simple rescue therapies. Long-term, steady treatment can improve overall lung function, reduce exacerbations, and decrease the need for short-term relief therapies.

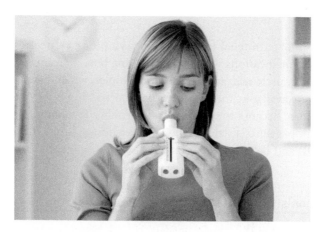

A peak flow meter allows an individual to monitor lung function daily. This information helps to establish treatment goals.

One way that patients can monitor their lung function at home is to use a **peak flow meter**. This small, portable device is sold in most pharmacies, and it measures the strength of airflow exiting the lungs. The patient takes a deep breath, seals the lips around the mouthpiece, and then blows into the device as fast and as forcefully as possible. The indicator moves in response to airflow, and a number is generated. Although this device is not diagnostic, it can provide a crude assessment of lung function if patients use it regularly and chart the results daily. The chart helps patients determine if their lung function is declining over time. In such cases, patients can work with their healthcare practitioners to prevent worsening lung function before the trend leads to a bigger problem and asthma attacks intensify. As an allied health professional, you might suggest that patients using multiple inhalers for asthma also use a peak flow meter regularly.

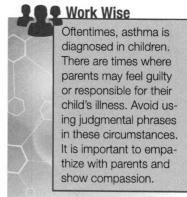

Work Wise

Oftentimes, asthma is diagnosed in children. There are times where parents may feel guilty or responsible for their child's illness. Avoid using judgmental phrases in these circumstances. It is important to empathize with parents and show compassion.

Drug Regimens and Treatments

The primary goals of treating asthma are to reduce acute and chronic troublesome symptoms, prevent exacerbations, and minimize hospitalizations or visits to the emergency room. Other goals of treatment are for asthmatic patients to be as physically active as they would like, and to sleep without interruption from asthmatic symptoms.

Drug therapy for asthma has two components: quick-relief medications and long-term persistent medications. **Quick-relief medications** are used intermittently and provide rapid relief, as needed, when asthma symptoms present or when an asthma attack occurs. **Long-term persistent medications** are used regularly to prevent asthma symptoms or attacks. Allied health professionals can help patients treat and prevent asthma attacks by promoting correct use of quick-relief medications and adherence to long-term persistent medications.

Asthma management is a stepwise process that generally begins with inhalers and proceeds to oral therapies. Typically, a quick-relief medication such as a short-acting beta agonist is first-line therapy. Long-term persistent medications (including inhaled corticosteroids, long-acting beta agonists, leukotriene inhibitors, mast cell stabilizers, phosphodiesterase inhibitors, and monoclonal antibodies) are added as asthma severity increases. Agents such as leukotriene inhibitors or mast cell stabilizers are effective for more severe cases. Healthcare professionals also recommend that patients with asthma get a flu shot every year because asthmatics are at an increased risk of flu-related complications such as pneumonia and other acute respiratory diseases.

Short-Acting Beta Agonists

Short-acting beta agonists provide short-term relief from breathing symptoms related to asthma and, sometimes, COPD. These medications work by stimulating beta-2 receptors in the lungs and by producing smooth-muscle relaxation in the bronchioles, which open airways. Although oral dosage forms are available, most patients use short-acting beta agonists by inhaling them into the lungs. Because their effects last for only a few hours, these agents may need to be used multiple times a day. Of the available dosage forms, the handheld metered-dose inhaler (MDI) and nebulizer solution are the most frequently prescribed (see Table 17.5).

TABLE 17.5 Common Short-Acting Beta Agonists

Generic (Brand)	Dosage Form	Route of Administration	Common Dosage
Albuterol (ProAir, Proventil, Ventolin, VoSpire ER)	Aerosol (MDI), nebulizer solution, syrup, tablet	Inhalation, oral	Inhalation: 2.5 mg 3–4 times a day via nebulizer MDI: 1–2 puffs 3–4 times a day PO: 2–4 mg 3–4 times a day
Levalbuterol (Xopenex)	Aerosol (MDI), nebulizer solution	Inhalation	Inhalation: 0.31–0.63 mg 3 times a day via nebulizer MDI: 2 puffs every 4–6 hr
Metaproterenol (Alupent)	Syrup, tablet	Oral	PO: 10–20 mg 3–4 times a day
Pirbuterol (Maxair)	Aerosol (MDI)	Inhalation	MDI: 2 puffs (400 mcg) every 4–6 hr

A **metered-dose inhaler (MDI)** is a handheld device that delivers medication through inhalation. In most cases, healthcare practitioners recommend that patients use a spacer along with an MDI to improve drug delivery to the lungs. A **spacer** suspends the medication mist in the air for a few seconds, allowing patients more time to coordinate the two required actions: breathing in and activating the inhaler.

Young children or elderly patients who find it difficult to use an inhaler will need to have nebulizer treatments. A **nebulizer** sends a stream of air through the drug solution, creating a fine mist that patients inhale by breathing normally through a mask for 10 to 15 minutes.

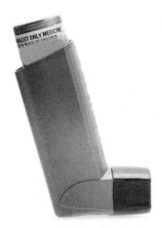

An MDI sprays a controlled amount of medication through the opening when the canister is pressed downward.

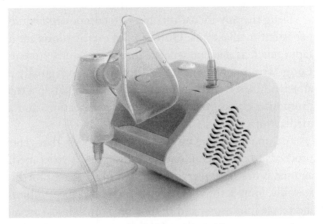

A nebulizer machine typically has clear tubing, a compartment to hold solution from single-dose vials, and an adjustable mask strap.

Side Effects Common side effects of short-acting beta agonists include dizziness, nervousness, heartburn, nausea, and tremors. These agents can also have cardiac effects including increased blood pressure and tachycardia. Patients with high blood pressure or heart problems should discuss the side effects of short-acting beta agonists with their healthcare practitioners before using them.

Contraindications Levalbuterol is contraindicated in patients with a hypersensitivity to albuterol. Albuterol, metaproterenol, and pirbuterol do not have contraindications.

Cautions and Considerations Short-acting beta agonists interact with beta blockers, which are frequently used by people with heart disease. Beta blockers inhibit the effect of these beta agonist drugs. Short-acting beta agonists and beta blockers should not be used together; if they must be, prescribers must carefully adjust the doses.

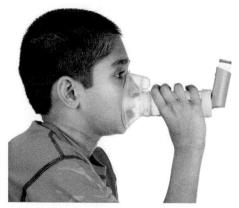

If a spacer is added to an MDI, the medication is more likely to penetrate deeper into the lung tissue than if the MDI is used alone. Spacers come with masks (often used in children, as pictured) and without masks.

MDIs should be shaken before each use. Pharmacists should teach patients how to use their inhalers properly with each new prescription and periodically for refills.

Patient Teaching

Most patients with asthma have prescriptions for MDIs. Although it may seem easy, the use of an MDI can be difficult and requires the proper technique to administer the medication effectively. Provide your patients with the following instructions on how to use an MDI with a spacer:

1. Inspect the MDI and prime the inhaler, if necessary.

2. Shake the MDI well.

3. Attach the MDI to the spacer.

4. Breathe out completely.

5. Put the mouthpiece of the spacer in your mouth and close your lips around the mouthpiece to form a tight seal.

6. Press down on the canister of the MDI.

7. Take a slow, deep breath and breathe in as much air as you comfortably can.

8. Remove the mouthpiece from your mouth and hold your breath for 10 seconds or as long as possible.

9. If another puff of the inhaler is needed, wait one minute (except during asthma exacerbations) and repeat. During an asthma exacerbation, you may repeat steps immediately.

10. Rinse the plastic portion of the inhaler as well as the spacer once a week and allow the devices to air-dry.

Corticosteroids

Used for long-term treatment and control of persistent asthma, corticosteroids are produced in oral, parenteral, and inhaled forms. **Oral corticosteroids** are used for short-term therapy only, and their systemic side effects may be problematic for patients. Sometimes oral agents may be needed initially to gain control during severe exacerbations of asthma or COPD. Generally, oral administration of corticosteroids is preferred to parenteral routes. There are instances, such as vomiting, when a patient cannot tolerate oral medications. In these situations, you may see patients receive intravenous or intramuscular corticosteroids (see Chapter 24).

Inhaled corticosteroids, however, are the preferred dosage form for respiratory disorders. Use of the inhalation route of administration results in less systemic absorption and fewer side effects than oral corticosteroid use. An inhaled corticosteroid works by decreasing the inflammation that contributes to bronchoconstriction and excess mucous production. Typically, this agent is added to a patient's regimen if the patient is using a short-acting beta agonist inhaler more than twice a week.

Inhaled corticosteroids can be used long term and are sometimes used for COPD. To be effective, they must be used on a regular basis rather than only when an asthma attack occurs. The purpose of these agents is to *prevent* frequent asthma attacks from occurring; they should not be used to *treat* an asthma attack after it has started. Common inhaled corticosteroids are listed in Table 17.6.

TABLE 17.6 Common Inhaled Corticosteroids

Generic (Brand)	Dosage Form	Common Dosage
Beclomethasone (QVAR)	Aerosol (MDI)	40–160 mcg twice a day
Budesonide (Pulmicort)	Powder for inhalation, suspension for inhalation	200–800 mcg twice a day
Flunisolide (AeroBid)	Aerosol (MDI)	80–160 mcg twice a day
Fluticasone (Flovent)	Aerosol (MDI), powder for inhalation	88–440 mcg twice a day
Mometasone (Asmanex)	Powder for inhalation	110–440 mcg 1–2 times a day
Triamcinolone (Azmacort)	Aerosol (MDI)	1–2 puffs 3–4 times a day
Combinations		
Budesonide/formoterol (Symbicort)	Aerosol (MDI)	2 inhalations twice a day
Fluticasone/salmeterol (Advair)	Aerosol (MDI), powder for inhalation	100 mcg/50 mcg to 500 mcg/50 mcg twice a day

Allied health professionals can help improve patient safety by monitoring patients to ensure proper inhaler use. In addition to an MDI, a **dry powder inhaler (DPI)** can also be used to administer an inhaled corticosteroid. A discus-shaped inhaler contains dry, powdered medication that is pulled into the lungs when an individual breathes in quickly and forcefully at the inhaler opening. Another DPI looks more like a conventional MDI, but capsules filled with powdered drug for inhalation are inserted, punctured, and administered.

As mentioned earlier, young children or elderly patients who find it difficult to use an MDI or who

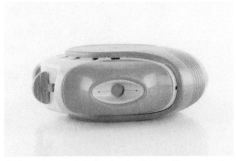

A dry powder inhaler looks like a discus and is actuated by breathing in deeply at the opening instead of pressing with the fingers.

cannot breathe in forcefully enough to use a dry powder inhaler will need to have nebulizer treatments.

Side Effects Common side effects of inhaled corticosteroids include dry mouth, headache, sore throat, hoarseness, coughing, and oral fungal infection (oral thrush). **Oral thrush** appears as a visible white coating on the inside of the mouth and tongue. Washing out the mouth after each inhalation decreases the incidence of oral thrush significantly and may decrease throat irritation. Using a spacer can also reduce symptoms of dry mouth, sore throat, and hoarseness.

Contraindications Inhaled corticosteroids are contraindicated during acute asthma episodes. Fluticasone and mometasone powder for inhalation contain lactose and should not be used in those patients with a hypersensitivity to milk proteins or lactose. The same applies for the combined product, fluticasone/salmeterol.

Cautions and Considerations MDIs should be shaken before each use. Dry powder inhalers should not be shaken prior to use. Patients should carefully follow instructions for puncturing the powder packet or capsule and then placing the device in the mouth before forceful inhalation. Allied health professionals should teach patients how to use their inhalers properly.

Drug Alert

DPIs are available in two types: a device that comes preloaded with medication or a device that needs to be loaded with medication. For the latter, the patient must obtain capsules containing powdered medication to load into the device. DPIs with medication preloaded include Advair Diskus, Anoro Ellipta, Pulmicort Flexhaler, Tudorza Pressair, and Asmanex Twisthaler. DPIs that require the loading of powdered medication include Foradil Aerolizer, Spiriva HandiHaler, and Arcapta Neohaler. Patients using DPIs should receive clear instructions and counseling on the appropriate use of the devices from pharmacists or other healthcare personnel.

Leukotriene Inhibitors

Used for long-term control of moderate-to-severe asthma, **leukotriene inhibitors** (see Table 17.7) are often prescribed when short-acting beta agonists and inhaled corticosteroids are not providing adequate control of breathing symptoms. **Leukotrienes** are inflammation mediators that cause mucous secretion and bronchoconstriction. Zileuton inhibits the enzyme involved in leukotriene synthesis, and zafirlukast and montelukast are leukotriene receptor blockers. Use of some leukotriene inhibitors is limited to children of specific ages. For example, zafirlukast can be used in children as young as five years old.

TABLE 17.7 Common Leukotriene Inhibitors

Generic (Brand)	Dosage Form	Route of Administration	Common Dosage
Montelukast (Singulair)	Chewable tablet, granules, tablet	Oral	4–10 mg once a day
Zafirlukast (Accolate)	Tablet	Oral	10–20 mg twice a day
Zileuton (Zyflo)	Tablet	Oral	600–1,200 mg twice a day

Side Effects The most common side effects of leukotriene inhibitors include nausea, sore throat, and sinusitis. Less common effects include diarrhea, stomach pain, and skin rash. These effects tend to be mild; if they become bothersome, patients should talk with their healthcare practitioners.

Contraindications Montelukast does not have contraindications. Zafirlukast and zileuton are contraindicated with liver impairment, and patients using either drug will need periodic liver tests.

Cautions and Considerations Leukotriene inhibitors are not to be used for reversal of bronchospasm in acute asthma attacks. Leukotriene inhibitors have been associated with liver problems, eosinophilia, vasculitis, and behavioral changes (such as unusual dreams, agitation, anxiety, and hallucinations).

Other Asthma Agents

If asthma is severe and difficult to control with beta agonists, corticosteroids, or leukotriene inhibitors, **mast cell stabilizers** and **xanthine agents** are older therapies that may be introduced. Cromolyn is a mast cell stabilizer that is inhaled. It blocks mast cell activity. Mast cells contribute to the overreactive inflammatory process in asthma.

Xanthine agents include theophylline and aminophylline. These oral agents are similar in chemical structure to caffeine. They are direct bronchodilators that can also be used to treat COPD. Currently, these agents tend not to be used, in part due to their side effects, which include anxiety, headache, insomnia, dizziness, tremors, heart palpitations, and increased urination. Blood levels may be checked periodically to monitor xanthine therapy. Certain drugs (e.g., erythromycin) may elevate xanthine blood concentrations.

Another asthma agent that is used in specialized cases is omalizumab. **Omalizumab** is a recombinant DNA-derived humanized monoclonal antibody that binds selectively to human immunoglobulin E (IgE). This medication is used to treat patients older than age 12 whose asthma symptoms are not controlled with inhaled corticosteroids.

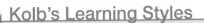

Kolb's Learning Styles

If you like having time to think things through, as Assimilators do, you might enjoy making a list or chart of all of the inhaler medications for asthma and COPD. See if you can find a picture of each inhaler online (manufacturers' websites are often good sources) and place them on a chart. Then, for each inhaler, list the generic name, brand name, drug class, use (such as *asthma rescue inhaler* or *COPD long-term therapy*, and so on), and the method of delivery (for example, *MDI* or *DPI*). Simply making this chart can be a learning experience, and you will have produced a useful reference for memorizing the inhalers.

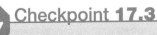

Checkpoint 17.3

Take a moment to review what you have learned so far and answer these questions.

1. What are the main types of medications used to treat asthma?

2. What are the common side effects of short-acting beta agonists?

3. What are the various ways asthma medications can be administered?

COPD

Chronic obstructive pulmonary disease (COPD) refers to a group of chronic lung diseases that impede airflow and cause breathing difficulty. COPD is the fourth leading cause of chronic disease and death in the United States. In fact, the World Health Organization predicts that this disorder will be the third leading cause of death worldwide by 2030.

COPD is a long-term, progressive condition in which airflow is limited by an abnormal inflammatory response. COPD is not reversible, which means lung function does not significantly improve with administration of bronchodilators. In fact, COPD is a disease that progressively worsens, even with treatment.

On the positive side, COPD is largely preventable. Although some patients are genetically predisposed to developing COPD, studies show that 85% of people with COPD are smokers. Most patients with COPD have a history of smoking or exposure to pollution or occupational hazards. Repeated respiratory infections can also contribute to COPD.

COPD has several subtypes, including chronic bronchitis and emphysema (see Figure 17.5). **Chronic bronchitis** is defined as a persistent cough that produces sputum lasting at least three months out of the year for at least two consecutive years. It is caused by an overgrowth of mucous glands and airway narrowing in the lungs.

Emphysema occurs when alveolar walls are damaged or destroyed, causing enlargement of the air spaces deep within the lungs. Having fewer alveoli walls reduces the surface area available within the lungs for gas exchange. Patients can have a mixture of chronic bronchitis and emphysema symptoms, depending on their condition.

FIGURE 17.5 | Chronic Bronchitis and Emphysema

Chronic bronchitis and emphysema are the two main types of COPD.

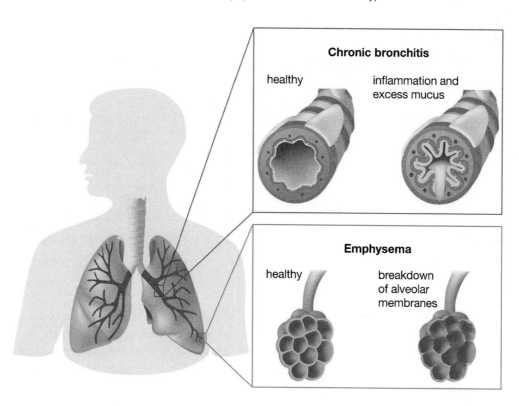

Drug Regimens and Treatments

For patients with COPD who smoke, tobacco cessation is the cornerstone of therapy. Drug therapy for COPD does not prevent progression of the disease; it simply relieves symptoms. COPD treatment can improve quality of life and allow patients to exercise or be physically active without getting out of breath. Most agents used to treat COPD act on the bronchoconstriction that occurs as the condition gets worse. In the most severe states, patients may need oxygen to help them breathe. Some patients with COPD carry portable oxygen packs or pull oxygen tanks on wheels. A tube called a **nasal cannula** delivers the gas into the nostrils. Healthcare professionals recommend that patients with COPD get a flu shot every year because patients with COPD are at an increased risk of serious flu-related complications.

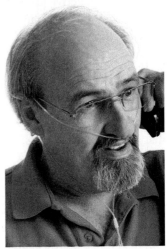

A nasal cannula delivers oxygen to an individual who has COPD.

Anticholinergics

Used as a first-line treatment for bronchoconstriction related to COPD, **anticholinergic agents** (see Table 17.8) work by inhibiting acetylcholine, a neurotransmitter that stimulates smooth muscle in the lungs to constrict. Anticholinergics are used when long-term bronchodilation is needed. The purpose of these agents is to prevent frequent COPD exacerbations, not to treat acute breathing problems after they begin. These agents improve the quality of life for patients with COPD and can reduce the need for hospitalization.

TABLE 17.8 Common Anticholinergic Agents

Generic (Brand)	Dosage Form	Route of Administration	Common Dosage
Aclidinium (Tudorza Pressair)	Powder for inhalation	Inhalation	400 mcg twice a day
Ipratropium (Atrovent)	Aerosol (MDI), nasal spray, nebulizer solution	Inhalation, intranasal	MDI: 2 puffs 4 times a day Nasal spray: 2 sprays per nostril 3–5 times a day Nebulizer: 500 mcg 3–4 times a day
Ipratropium/albuterol (Combivent, DuoNeb)	Aerosol (MDI), nebulizer solution, oral inhalation solution	Inhalation	MDI: 2 puffs 4 times a day Nebulizer: 3 mL treatment 4 times a day Oral solution: 1 inhalation 4 times a day
Tiotropium (Spiriva)	Powder for inhalation	Inhalation	Inhale contents of 1 capsule a day
Umeclidinium/vilanterol (Anoro Ellipta)	Powder for inhalation	Inhalation	1 inhalation once a day

Side Effects The most common side effects of anticholinergics are dry mouth, nervousness, dizziness, headache, cough, nausea, bitter taste, nasal dryness, upper respiratory tract infection, and nosebleeds. Patients who have glaucoma or urination problems, such as prostate enlargement, should not use anticholinergics because they can worsen these conditions.

Contraindications Aclidinium does not have any contraindications. Ipratropium is contraindicated in patients with a hypersensitivity to atropine. The Combivent brand of ipratropium/albuterol should not be used by patients with a hypersensitivity to soy or peanuts. Tiotropium should not be used by patients with lactose sensitivity. Umeclidinium is contraindicated in patients with a hypersensitivity to milk proteins.

Cautions and Considerations Ipratropium inhalers require priming before first use, whereas aclidinium and tiotropium inhalers do not need to be primed. Priming the inhaler involves holding the inhaler away from the body and pushing the canister against the mouthpiece so the medication sprays into the air. When starting use of a new canister, priming may take up to seven sprays. In cases where the inhaler has not been used for more than 24 hours, patients should prime the inhaler twice.

Tiotropium capsules are used only with an inhaler device; they should not be swallowed. Patients should take care to follow instructions for puncturing the capsule and inhaling the powder using the inhaler device. Counseling patients on the correct administration of tiotropium is an important responsibility for allied health personnel.

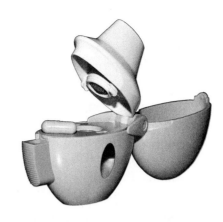

Tiotropium therapy requires the use of an inhaler. The capsules containing the powdered medication are punctured, and the powder is placed in the inhaler. Warn patients that tiotropium capsules are not to be swallowed.

Long-Acting Beta Agonists

Used for both COPD and asthma, **long-acting beta agonists** work in a way that is similar to the action of short-acting beta agonists (discussed earlier in this chapter); they simply do not have to be administered as frequently. Although they are used more frequently for COPD, the long-acting agents can also be used for severe asthma when bronchodilator therapy is needed multiple times a day on a regular basis. For a list of common long-acting beta agonists, see Table 17.9.

Quick Study

It can be difficult to remember which medication is an anticholinergic and which medication is a long-acting beta agonist. Remember that the anticholinergic agents that target the respiratory system end in *–ium*. The long-acting beta agonists that are used for respiratory disorders end in *–erol*.

TABLE 17.9 Common Long-Acting Beta Agonists

Generic (Brand)	Dosage Form	Route of Administration	Common Dosage
Arformoterol (Brovana)	Nebulizer solution	Inhalation	15 mcg twice a day
Formoterol (Foradil, Perforomist)	Nebulizer solution, powder capsule for inhalation	Inhalation	12 mcg every 12 hr
Indacaterol (Arcapta Neohaler)	Powder capsule for inhalation	Inhalation	75–300 mcg a day
Salmeterol (Serevent Discus)	Powder for inhalation	Inhalation	1 inhalation twice a day

Side Effects As is true for short-acting beta agonists, common side effects for long-acting beta agonists include dizziness, heartburn, nausea, and tremors. Long-acting beta agonists can cause cardiac effects including increased blood pressure and tachycardia. Patients with high blood pressure or heart problems should discuss the side effects of these beta agonists with their physicians before using them.

Contraindications Arformoterol is contraindicated in patients with a hypersensitivity to formoterol. The Foradil brand of formoterol should not be used in acute episodes of asthma or exacerbations of COPD.

Long-acting beta agonists should not be used as monotherapy for patients with asthma. Patients with asthma should always take an inhaled corticosteroid, such as fluticasone, concurrently with the long-acting beta agonist.

Cautions and Considerations Warnings and drug interactions for long-acting beta agonists are similar to those for short-acting beta agonists. Patients should not take these agents with beta blockers. In addition, MDIs need to be shaken before each use to distribute the drug evenly and to ensure proper, equal doses.

 Checkpoint 17.4

Take a moment to review what you have learned so far and answer these questions.

1. What are the main types of medications used to treat COPD?

2. What are the generic drug names of the anticholinergics and long-acting beta agonists used to treat respiratory disorders? Provide a minimum of two generics for each drug class.

Pneumonia

Pneumonia is a lower respiratory tract infection caused by bacterial, viral, or fungal pathogens. Pneumonia can be acquired from the general community or from exposure to pathogens during hospitalization. Patients who get pneumonia from exposure outside of an inpatient facility have **community-acquired pneumonia (CAP)**. Pneumonia that is acquired while an individual is hospitalized or living in a long-term care facility is called **nosocomial pneumonia**. Nosocomial pneumonia is severe and difficult to treat because it is usually caused by pathogens that are more virulent than those that cause CAP. Patients in the hospital setting encounter such pathogens because they are in proximity to other sick patients who have these infections.

Drug Regimens and Treatments

Drug therapy for pneumonia will not be covered here in detail because most agents that treat this respiratory disorder are addressed in the "Infectious Diseases" section of Chapter 23. Before appropriate drug therapy can begin, however, prescribers must determine if a patient has CAP or nosocomial pneumonia. This process takes time; therefore, a two-step treatment process is typically undertaken.

Initially, the patient is treated according to **empirical therapy**, or a therapy based on common knowledge of the pathogens typically causing certain types of pneumonia. Empirical therapy is prescribed according to the patient's symptoms, general medical history, and the suspected location of exposure. These factors provide clues to the likely pathogen and, therefore, drug therapy can be started immediately. An antibiotic that covers a broad range of pathogens will be chosen first to increase the chances that the appropriate pathogen is being targeted.

While the first therapy is in process, a second process, called **narrowing treatment**, begins. Specimens are obtained for laboratory tests and cultures to determine exactly what pathogens are present in the lungs. The patient and healthcare practitioners must then wait, typically for a few days, to receive the test results. Allied health personnel may be asked to retrieve these results when they become available. Drug therapy is modified, if necessary, to target any pathogen identified. Patients who have labored breathing may also be administered bronchodilators and corticosteroids to assist breathing.

Tuberculosis

Tuberculosis (TB) is an infectious disease caused by a mycobacterium that infects the lungs and causes tubercles (nodular lesions) to form. Formerly called *consumption*, this disease claimed the lives of millions of individuals and is still difficult to cure. Drug therapy for TB became available in the twentieth century; however, TB has not been completely eradicated. In fact, TB is on the rise now that drug-resistant strains have emerged and immunocompromised conditions are more prevalent. According to the Centers for Disease Control and Prevention (CDC), tuberculosis is the second leading cause of adult mortality worldwide among infectious diseases.

Healthcare professionals who work in inpatient or long-term care settings are usually required to get annual skin tests using **purified protein derivative (PPD)** to check for exposure to TB. In a PPD skin test, an injection of tuberculin is placed just under the skin and then checked again 48 to 72 hours later for **induration** (i.e., inflammation and swelling). On testing positive for TB exposure, an individual receives a chest X-ray and other tests to see if drug therapy is needed. Not everyone who is exposed will develop the full disease with active organisms. Symptoms of active disease include night sweats, weight loss, coughing blood, chest pain, and fatigue.

In the inpatient setting, patients with TB should be placed in airborne infection isolation rooms. These isolation rooms should employ negative pressure to prevent the escape of potentially infectious droplets from the room. Healthcare personnel and visitors entering the room of a patient having TB must take special precautions to protect against transmission. Some precautions include special masks with filters, gloves, and protective clothing. Signs are posted on the door and in areas outside these hospital rooms warning individuals to wear appropriate personal protective clothing and to use universal precautions when entering the rooms of infected patients.

Work Wise

Allied health professionals may hear other healthcare personnel use the acronym TST to refer to the tuberculin skin test. The TST and PPD are the same test. *PPD* is the acronym for *purified protein derivative*, which is the intradermal injection administered into the skin of the inner forearm during a TST.

Drug Regimens and Treatments

Because drugs for TB are often specialized, they are covered only briefly here (see Table 17.10). Allied health personnel working in settings where TB is seen regularly, such as hospitals and long-term care facilities, should refer to additional resources for further information. Bacille Calmette-Guerin (BCG) vaccine is available and is used in countries with a high prevalence of TB to prevent childhood tuberculous meningitis and miliary TB. The BCG vaccine is not usually recommended in the United States for several reasons: the low risk of infection with *Mycobacterium tuberculosis*, the vaccine's variable effectiveness in the prevention of adult pulmonary TB, and the vaccine's interference with the PPD skin test (may cause a false-positive result). For the latter reason, a chest X-ray is recommended.

One reason for the reemergence of TB is the high rate of nonadherence to drug therapy for the disease. The course of therapy for most infections is 5 to 14 days, but the course of therapy for TB is 6 months or longer. For many patients, adhering to therapy for that long is challenging, and many do not complete the entire course. Instead, they stop taking the TB medications once they begin to feel better. However, stopping therapy too soon allows the bacteria to regain a foothold and grow even stronger. Incomplete therapy only promotes the emergence of **drug-resistant TB**—in other words, some strains of TB that current drugs cannot eradicate.

Another reason patients find it hard to complete TB therapy is the side effects. For example, isoniazid can cause liver toxicity. Kanamycin and streptomycin are aminoglycosides, so they can cause kidney damage and hearing loss. Rifampin causes flulike symptoms such as fever, chills, and a general feeling of illness. Ethambutol can cause changes in vision, which should be reported to the physician.

In addition to these side effects, most of these drugs must be taken on an empty stomach to ensure proper absorption. Patients do not always follow this requirement and may take the doses inconsistently. Consequently, each of these agents can be difficult to take for the entire course of therapy. Patients can lose motivation before therapy is complete.

Work Wise

Allied health professionals have the opportunity to educate, motivate, and encourage patients to complete their TB therapy. Acknowledging the challenges to therapy completion and offering suggestions to ease side effects may be helpful.

TABLE 17.10 Common TB Drugs

Generic (Brand)	Dosage Form	Length of Therapy	Common Dosage
Cycloserine (Seromycin)	Capsule	18–24 months	500 mg–1 g a day
Ethambutol (Myambutol)	Tablet	6–9 months	15 mg/kg/day
Isoniazid (INH)	Injection, syrup, tablet	6–24 months	5 mg/kg/day or 15 mg/kg/day 2–3 times a week
Pyrazinamide	Tablet	6–9 months	15–30 mg/kg/day
Rifampin (Rifadin)	Capsule, injection	6–9 months	10 mg/kg/day
Streptomycin	IM injection only	Up to 12 months	15 mg/kg/day or 1–2 g daily

Kolb's Learning Styles

If you like to learn with others, as Divergers and Accommodators do, try this exercise to put a "face" on TB. Collaborate with other students and use the library and Internet to identify some historical figures (authors, politicians, world leaders, and others) who died of "consumption." Also, think about how TB is depicted in movies and theater productions. Then get together with a few other students to discuss your findings. Which historical figures were victims of TB? What findings surprised you? Why?

Cystic Fibrosis

Cystic fibrosis (CF) is a genetic disease that affects exocrine glands and their ability to transport chloride across cell membranes. This abnormal chloride transport results in production of thick, sticky mucus in the lungs, pancreas, liver, intestines, and reproductive tract. It also leads to increased salt content in sweat gland secretions. However, most hospitalizations and deaths from CF occur because of pulmonary problems. The mucus accumulating in the lungs clogs airways, and infections easily take hold. In the gastrointestinal (GI) system, mucous accumulation causes intestinal obstructions and affects nutrient absorption. General pancreatic function is also reduced. Therefore, treatment of CF must address nutritional needs and include pancreatic enzyme supplementation in addition to addressing respiratory complications. CF is a fatal disease from which some patients die before early to middle adulthood.

Drug Regimens and Treatments

Because drugs for CF are specialized and not dispensed regularly in all settings, they are covered only briefly here. Respiratory therapy for CF includes percussion (nondrug treatment), antibiotics, and mucolytics.

Percussion is a tapping, pounding movement performed on the back and chest to break up and help expectorate mucus from the lungs. Nebulizer therapy with bronchodilators, hypertonic saline, acetylcysteine, and other specialized medications is often used in conjunction with percussion to help clear airways.

Several antibiotics are used to combat the pathogens that take root in the respiratory mucous secretions. These antibiotics are selected based on isolated organisms and include cefazolin, nafcillin, vancomycin, linezolid, piperacillin/tazobactam, ceftazidime, cefepime, imipenem/cilastin, meropenem, ciprofloxacin, tobramycin, amikacin, colistin, and aztreonam.

Theophylline, which may cause bronchodilation, can also be used in CF. Of note, patients with CF have pharmacokinetic profiles that are vastly different from those of healthy patients. Special dosing and monitoring is needed.

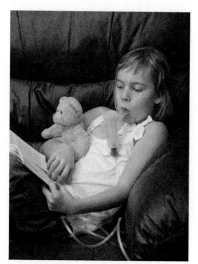

Lastly, **mucolytics** are administered to liquefy and promote expulsion of thick mucus from the lungs. Dornase alfa and inhaled hypertonic saline are the most commonly used mucolytics. Both medications are inhaled by nebulizer once or twice a day. The most common side effects include chest pain, fever, rash, pharyngitis, rhinitis, dyspnea, and voice alteration. Dornase alfa is contraindicated in patients with a hypersensitivity to Chinese hamster ovary cells, which are often used in recombinant protein production.

This patient is receiving inhaled antibiotics for cystic fibrosis.

Because the GI system and pancreas are also affected, physicians often prescribe special vitamins and **pancreatic enzyme supplements** for patients with CF. These supplements help prevent ductal obstructions and **steatorrhea** (fatty, foul-smelling diarrhea caused by fatty foods not being absorbed). They improve growth and life expectancy for children with CF. The number of pancreatic enzyme supplements is large, so it is not possible to cover them all here. However, they all contain varying amounts of **lipase**, **protease**, and **amylase**. Pancreatic dysfunction also contributes to

malabsorption, especially for fat-soluble vitamins. Therefore, you will see many patients with CF on supplements containing vitamins A, D, E, and K. You may be more likely to encounter these oral agents in pediatric specialty centers and outpatient settings.

Smoking and the Respiratory System

According to the CDC, smoking causes nearly a half million deaths each year in the United States and increases the risk of death from all causes. Its impact on the respiratory system is especially destructive, resulting in damaged airways and alveoli. In fact, cigarette smoking causes the most cases of lung cancer in the United States and is responsible for nearly 80% of all deaths from COPD. Asthma can also be caused or exacerbated by smoking or by exposure to cigarette smoke. In addition, smoking harms other organs in the body, increasing the risk for heart disease and stroke, cancer, Type 2 diabetes mellitus, rheumatoid arthritis, reproductive disturbances, and decreased bone health.

Because nicotine in cigarettes is addictive, smoking can be a difficult habit to quit. However, there are compelling reasons for **smoking cessation**, including a reduction in morbidity and mortality. For example, within one year after smoking cessation, an individual's risk for a heart attack drops sharply. Within two to five years after smoking cessation, a person's risk for a stroke falls to that of a nonsmoker and his or her risk of cancer of the mouth, throat, esophagus, and bladder drops by half. After 10 years of smoking cessation, an individual's risk for lung cancer drops by half.

Nicotine Dependence

Nicotine dependence is an addiction to tobacco products that contain nicotine. Nicotine is a chemical in tobacco that produces temporary, pleasing, physical and mood-altering effects. These pleasing effects make an individual want to continue using tobacco products. Nicotine dependence also involves behavioral factors, such as actions or cues that can be associated with smoking. Symptoms of nicotine dependence include the following:

- an inability to stop smoking
- withdrawal symptoms when attempting cessation
- the forfeiture of social or recreational activities in order to smoke

Nicotine Withdrawal

Abrupt discontinuation of nicotine-containing products can lead to **nicotine withdrawal**. Symptoms of nicotine withdrawal include the following:

- anxiety
- decreased blood pressure and heart rate
- depression
- drowsiness
- headache
- increased appetite and weight gain
- insomnia
- irritability, frustration, and restlessness

Nicotine withdrawal symptoms can make quitting smoking difficult. However, tobacco cessation can be achieved via behavioral counseling, pharmacologic treatments, and alternative therapies (acupuncture, aversive therapy, financial incentives, and hypnosis). Because the exploration of behavioral and alternative therapies is beyond the scope of this book, the following discussion focuses only on pharmacologic treatments for smoking cessation.

Drug Regimens and Treatments for Smoking Cessation

Prescription and over-the-counter (OTC) medications can reduce nicotine withdrawal symptoms for patients trying to quit smoking (see Table 17.11). In combination with smoking-cessation programs and social support, these medications can help patients quit smoking successfully. Drug therapy for smoking cessation includes nicotine supplements, an antidepressant, and a nicotine blocker.

TABLE 17.11 Common Smoking-Cessation Products

Generic (Brand)	Dosage Form	Route of Administration	Common Dosage
Bupropion (Wellbutrin, Zyban)	Tablet	Oral	150 mg twice a day
Nicotine (Commit, NicoDerm, Nicorette, Nicotrol)	Gum, inhaler, patch, spray	Buccal, inhalation, nasal, transdermal	Varies, depending on product and patient
Varenicline (Chantix)	Tablet	Oral	1 mg twice a day

Nicotine Supplements

Nicotine supplements are used to reduce absorbed nicotine slowly over time, thereby reducing many withdrawal symptoms. They are available in several OTC dosage forms, including gum, inhaler, patch, and spray.

Nicotine gum works best for users of smokeless tobacco products. These forms are chewed briefly and then "parked" in the cheek until the craving for nicotine returns. Inhaled forms mimic the use and effects of smoking while eliminating the harmful toxins from inhaling smoke. In the patch form, nicotine is absorbed transdermally and provides the most continuous nicotine delivery. However, this form does not allow the smoker to adjust nicotine exposure throughout the day. Nicotine nasal spray is administered intranasally and results in more rapid absorption compared to oral dosage forms. Its use is limited due to side effects such as rhinitis, sneezing, tearing, and nose and throat irritation. The dose of nicotine supplements usually depends on the number of cigarettes smoked daily. Doses should be tapered gradually as nicotine withdrawal symptoms subside.

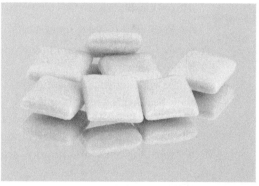

Nicotine gum must be carefully chewed. If the gum is chewed too vigorously, too much nicotine can be released, causing unpleasant side effects.

Side Effects Side effects of nicotine supplements mimic those of excess nicotine. These effects include abdominal pain, confusion, diarrhea, dizziness, headache, hearing loss, hypersalivation, nausea, sweating, vision changes, vomiting, and weakness. Removing or discontinuing the medication will alleviate or eliminate these effects. Inhaled dosage forms can cause mouth irritation, coughing, runny nose, headache, and indigestion. If side effects are bothersome, patients should switch to another dosage form.

Contraindications Nicotine supplements are contraindicated in patients who smoke after a recent heart attack and in patients who have life-threatening arrhythmias or worsening chest pain. These supplements should be avoided by pregnant patients as well. Nicotine gum should not be used by patients with active temporomandibular joint disease.

Cautions and Considerations Nicotine can increase heart rate and blood pressure. Risk/benefit analysis should occur for patients who require nicotine replacement and who have concurrent heart disease, hypertension, or arrhythmias. Dental problems may worsen with the gum form of nicotine. Airway irritation may result from the inhaled form of nicotine, and caution must be used in patients with airway disease. Nicotine patches should be used cautiously in patients who are allergic to adhesive tape or in those individuals who have skin problems. Nicotine nasal spray is not recommended for use in patients with chronic nasal disorders such as allergy, rhinitis, nasal polyps, and sinusitis.

Bupropion

Bupropion, an antidepressant, is used to combat the mood changes and emotional instability associated with smoking cessation. It can also reduce cravings for nicotine. Bupropion is available only by prescription.

Side Effects Side effects of bupropion include drowsiness, dizziness, blurred vision, and insomnia. To reduce these effects, patients should avoid drinking alcohol while taking this medication and take the medication in the morning.

Contraindications Contraindications to bupropion include seizure disorder, history of anorexia or bulimia, abrupt discontinuation of ethanol or sedatives, use of MAOIs, and use of linezolid or methylene blue.

Cautions and Considerations When discontinuing bupropion therapy, doses must be tapered to avoid a rebound of depressive symptoms. Patients should not stop taking bupropion abruptly.

As with starting any antidepressant therapy, patients using bupropion should talk with their healthcare prescribers if they notice symptoms of depression or suicidal ideation. The US Food and Drug Administration (FDA)–approved labeling for bupropion includes a black box warning that alerts users of serious mental health events. Patients should be observed for agitation, hostility, depression, and changes in behavior.

Varenicline

Varenicline stimulates the nicotinic acetylcholine receptors in the brain, thus reducing the craving for and the withdrawal symptoms of nicotine use. This agent also blocks these nicotine receptors if an individual resumes smoking, which makes smoking less desirable. Varenicline must be started one week prior to the desired quit date. The medication is taken for 12 weeks and is used in conjunction with a formal smoking-cessation program for best results. It is available only by prescription and has the added benefit of reducing weight gain. In fact, potential weight gain is a common reason why smokers do not want to participate in smoking-cessation programs.

Name Exchange

Varenicline is the generic name of the smoking-cessation medication widely known by the brand name Chantix.

Side Effects Side effects of varenicline include nausea and unusual dreams. Patients should take varenicline with food and a full glass of water to decrease nausea. In rare cases, patients using this medication have experienced serious mental status changes and neuropsychiatric events (see the "Cautions and Considerations" section for more details).

Contraindications Varenicline does not have any contraindications.

Cautions and Considerations The FDA-approved labeling for varenicline includes a black box warning that alerts users to serious neuropsychiatric events. Patients should be observed for agitation, hostility, depression, and changes in behavior. Patients with suicidal ideation should stop taking varenicline immediately and talk with their healthcare prescribers.

 Checkpoint 17.5

Take a moment to review what you have learned so far and answer these questions.

1. When treating pneumonia, what is meant by empirical therapy?
2. What are three common smoking-cessation drugs?

Herbal and Alternative Therapies

Echinacea, **zinc**, and **vitamin C** are herbal and supplement products that patients often take to boost immune function and fight off cold and flu virus infections that can progress to pneumonia. With varying success, these products have been found to reduce the severity and length of symptoms of the common cold or flu. Although some success with these products has been seen, standardized regimens have not been proven in the scientific literature. Little is known about their true clinical effects on lower respiratory tract infections such as pneumonia. If echinacea or zinc is used, it must be started at the first sign of infection to have any significant effects on the severity or length of symptoms. Vitamin C is best taken as a preventive agent during cold and flu season.

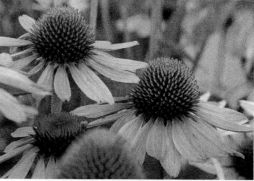

Extract from the roots of *Echinacea purpurea*, commonly known as the purple coneflower, is used in the herbal supplement echinacea. This OTC product is used by patients with the aim of boosting immune function.

Chapter Review

Chapter Summary

Respiratory diseases and conditions are common in the healthcare setting. Symptoms such as runny nose (rhinitis), sinus congestion, and cough frequently accompany upper respiratory tract infections. Antihistamines, decongestants, cough suppressants, and expectorants are used to combat symptoms of colds and respiratory tract infections, but they do not cure the infections. Many drugs used to treat symptoms of the upper respiratory system are taken orally; however, some treatments are delivered intranasally and topically.

Diseases and conditions of the lower respiratory tract—such as asthma, COPD, and pneumonia—are commonly encountered in healthcare settings. To help patients manage these disorders, allied health professionals can provide support through patient teaching and follow-up.

Patients depend on drug therapy to breathe effectively. Inhaled therapies are delivered via MDIs, dry powder inhalers, and nebulizer machines. Short-acting beta agonists dilate and open airways when immediate relief is needed, whereas inhaled corticosteroids reduce inflammation and improve breathing in asthma over the long term. Although COPD gets progressively worse, drug therapy can help improve symptoms and quality of life. Unfortunately, too many patients still misunderstand how to use inhalers to better control their condition. Proper education is important for patient adherence to the drug regimen.

Pneumonia and TB are infectious diseases that require drug treatment. TB agents must be taken for more than six months to be successful.

Smoking cessation is something most people must attempt multiple times before succeeding. Drug therapies that aid smoking cessation include nicotine supplements, an antidepressant, and a nicotine blocker.

Chapter Checkup

The Navigator+ learning management system that accompanies this textbook offers many opportunities to help you master chapter content, including end-of-chapter exercises, a glossary of key terms, flash cards, and additional interactive activities.

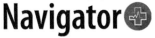

 Career Exploration

If you enjoyed learning about the respiratory system in this chapter, you may want to explore the following career options:

- athletic trainer
- cardiopulmonary rehabilitation specialist
- computed tomography (CT) technician
- emergency medical technician (EMT)/paramedic
- exercise physiologist
- magnetic resonance imaging (MRI) technician
- medical assistant
- pharmacy technician
- respiratory therapist

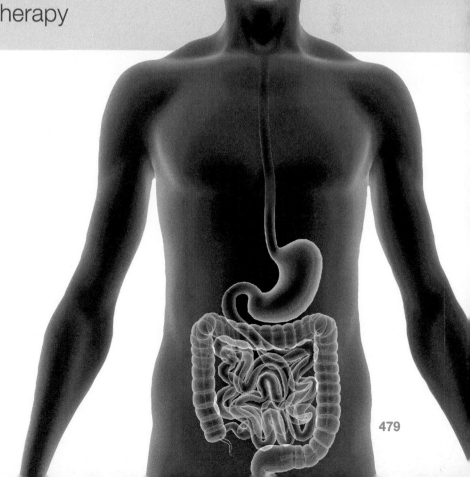

Pharmacotherapy for the Gastrointestinal and Endocrine Systems

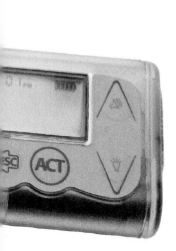

18

The Gastrointestinal System and Drug Therapy

Pharm Facts

- Despite its name, the small intestine is the largest of your internal organs. It is about four times as long as an individual's height. The tight loops of this organ allow it to fit inside the abdominal cavity.

- The liver is the heaviest internal organ (weighing 3.5 pounds) and performs more than 500 different functions, including producing bile and detoxifying the blood.

- Stomach cells have one of the shortest life cycles in the body (three to four days) due to their constant contact with hydrochloric acid, a substance so strong that it can dissolve razor blades.

- The colon is home to at least 400 types of bacteria.

- The sensation of "butterflies in the stomach" is part of the body's "fight-or-flight" response to stress. During that response, bloodflow is diverted from the stomach to the muscles and lungs, causing a nauseous or "fluttery" sensation.

"I got into nuclear medicine by accident. Originally, I was going to tour a hospital's ultrasound department and listen to a presentation, but the tour was canceled at the last minute. I ended up going to a presentation on nuclear medicine and was immediately hooked. I signed up right then and there to go through the program.

Nuclear medicine is different from other types of radiology. Because the average scan takes 30 to 60 minutes and many of our patients must have periodic scans, I have the opportunity to build relationships with my patients. That patient interaction has been the driving force of my longevity as a nuclear tech."

—**Paul Backstrom**, BS, NMTCB, ARRT(N)
Nuclear Medicine Technologist

Nausea, vomiting, diarrhea, constipation, and heartburn are common gastrointestinal (GI) complaints that all individuals encounter at some point in their lives. In fact, every day, patients visit pharmacies, clinics, and hospitals for treatment of chronic and acute GI disorders. Regardless of work setting, all healthcare professionals have a role in helping patients manage GI problems, many of which are treated with drug therapy.

This chapter describes the GI system and the prescription medications, nonprescription medications, and alternative therapies used to treat the most common problems affecting the GI system. Treatment of diarrhea, constipation, gastroesophageal reflux disease, peptic ulcer disease, and nausea and vomiting is discussed. Both over-the-counter (OTC) and prescription medications are used to treat these conditions. Also discussed are two less common conditions: irritable bowel syndrome and ulcerative colitis. Probiotic products, a growing segment of the nutraceutical market used to combat irregularity (constipation and diarrhea), are explained as well.

Anatomy and Physiology of the GI System

The **gastrointestinal (GI) system** is the system of organs that processes food and liquids. This action includes **digestion** (breakdown of large food molecules to smaller ones) and **absorption** (uptake of essential nutrients into the bloodstream). The GI system is composed of the **GI tract** (also known as the **alimentary tract**) and a number of supportive organs. Specifically, the GI tract includes the **mouth, esophagus, stomach, small intestine, colon,** and **rectum** (see Figure 18.1).

Digestive Process in the Upper GI System

When food is swallowed, smooth muscle along the walls of the esophagus propels it into the stomach. This process of coordinated muscle contraction, called **peristalsis**, keeps food particles moving through the GI tract.

FIGURE 18.1 Diagram of the GI Tract

The mouth, esophagus, and stomach are part of the upper GI system, and the intestines, colon, and rectum are part of the lower GI system.

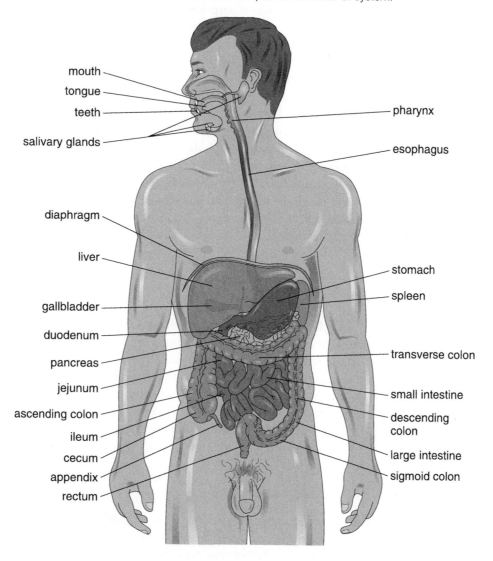

Once food reaches the stomach, acid and enzyme secretions digest large particles and proteins in ingested food. **Gastrin**, a hormone that stimulates acid secretion, is released when the walls of the stomach stretch in response to food. **Parietal cells**, which line the walls of the stomach, are responsible for producing acid from specialized structures known as **proton pumps**. Gastrin stimulates **histamine** release, which increases the number of active proton pumps.

Acidity in the GI system is measured by **pH**, a scale that indicates the degree of acidity present. Normally, the pH of the stomach is approximately 1 to 2 (very acidic). Most body tissues would not tolerate these acidic conditions, but the cells lining the stomach walls are protected by a layer of mucus. In addition to helping to digest food particles, the low pH of the stomach is protective because it kills a majority of the bacteria that are ingested. Furthermore, a low pH is critical for absorption of certain drugs that dissociate poorly in a neutral or basic environment.

Digestive Process in the Lower GI System

When food particles leave the stomach, they enter the small intestine. The **small intestine** is the site where most digestion and nutrient absorption occur. This organ has an enormous surface area, which allows for maximal nutrient absorption. In fact, a large percentage of drugs administered orally are absorbed in the small intestine. Movement of food through the intestines is referred to as **GI motility**. The parasympathetic nervous system controls GI motility (see Chapter 12). Increased GI motility can result in diarrhea, whereas decreased GI motility can result in constipation.

Once food moves through the small intestine, the remaining food particles proceed to the **large intestine**. The large intestine has four distinct segments: **ascending colon**, **transverse colon**, **descending colon**, and **sigmoid colon**. Normally, the GI tract is very efficient, absorbing all carbohydrates, fats, and proteins that are consumed. Only nonabsorbable substances, such as fiber and bacteria, remain as waste material. This waste material, or **stool**, exits the body through the rectum and **anus** via **defecation** (bowel movement). Because carbohydrates, fats, and proteins have already been absorbed through the small intestine, the large intestine absorbs additional salt and water, bringing the stool to the proper consistency for elimination.

Sphincters and the Digestive Process

To regulate the speed at which food particles move through the GI tract, the body uses sphincters. These **sphincters**, or muscle rings wrapped around the GI tract, are important because they prevent food and other digested substances from moving in the wrong direction. For example, a very important sphincter called the **lower esophageal sphincter** is located between the esophagus and stomach. This sphincter relaxes to allow chewed-up food to pass into the stomach; it then closes to prevent the acidic contents of the stomach from traveling back up into the esophagus. Without a properly functioning lower esophageal sphincter, acid travels up into the esophagus, causing pain and tissue damage.

Auxiliary Organs of the GI System

Other components of the GI system include the **salivary glands, gallbladder, pancreas,** and **liver** (see Figure 18.2). These organs release secretions that aid in the digestion of food and the absorption of nutrients. **Saliva** provides lubrication for food, making swallowing easier, and contains enzymes that begin the process of digesting sugars. The gallbladder is a holding area where bile is stored. **Bile**, an alkaline fluid, is produced by the liver and assists in the digestion and absorption of fat and cholesterol from the small intestine. The pancreas produces many enzymes that help digest carbohydrates, fats, and proteins. The pancreas is also important because it releases secretions that neutralize the acid from the stomach.

In addition to making bile, the liver is the major organ for drug metabolism. After being absorbed from the small intestine, molecules travel in the blood via the portal vein directly to the liver. The liver removes harmful substances before they reach the general circulation. Before orally administered drugs enter the circulation, they must pass through the liver. The liver metabolizes drugs before they reach their target in the body; this is called the **first-pass effect** (see Figure 18.3).

FIGURE 18.2 Auxiliary Organs of the GI System

Without neutralization by pancreatic secretions, acid from the stomach would damage the small intestine.

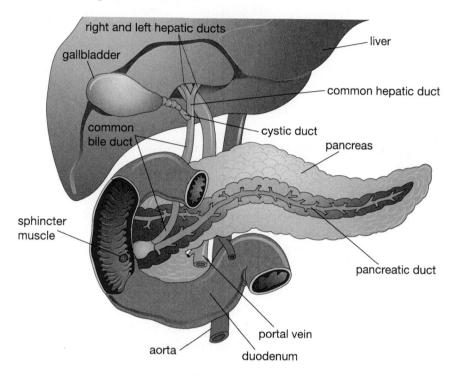

FIGURE 18.3 Liver Function and First-Pass Effect

Alternatives to oral administration are necessary for drugs that will lose their efficacy if they undergo the first-pass effect.

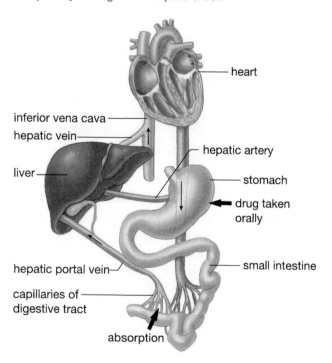

Checkpoint 18.1

Take a moment to review what you have learned so far and answer these questions.

1. How does food move through the GI tract? Trace the movement of food as it is ingested, digested, and eliminated from the body, as well as the organs involved in the transmission.

2. What is the first-pass effect?

Common GI System Disorders

Work Wise

Because GI disorders are the most common disorders for which patients self-medicate with OTC medications, it is very important that allied health professionals carefully screen for these kinds of medications when taking patients' complete medication histories.

Diarrhea, constipation, heartburn, and hemorrhoids are common GI disorders and are most often treated with OTC medications. Nausea, vomiting, gastroesophageal reflux disease, and peptic ulcer disease are also common conditions but may require prescription medications for successful treatment.

Diarrhea

Diarrhea is defined as excessive, soft, or watery stools. Excessive stool can mean large stool volume (greater than 250 g of stool a day) or a larger number of bowel movements than normal. In diarrhea, increased GI motility leads to frequent bowel movements. Acute diarrhea is a common condition that can be caused by infections such as **traveler's diarrhea** and **food poisoning**, as well as certain drugs (see Table 18.1). Common infectious causes of diarrhea include *Salmonella*, *Escherichia coli (E. coli)*, *Giardia*, and *Norovirus*. Drugs used to treat infections are discussed in Chapter 23. Chronic diarrhea is less common but can be caused by irritable bowel syndrome, ulcerative colitis, or Crohn disease.

TABLE 18.1 Drugs That Can Cause Diarrhea

Angiotensin-converting enzyme (ACE) inhibitors	H2 receptor antagonists
Antibiotics	Magnesium-containing laxatives or antacids
Chemotherapy drugs (specifically, fluoropyrimidines and irinotecan)	Nonsteroidal anti-inflammatory drugs (NSAIDs)
Digoxin	Proton pump inhibitors (PPIs)

Drug Regimens and Treatments

Antidiarrheal medications slow the transit of food through the GI tract or decrease secretions into it, which reduces stool volume and makes stool less watery. Diarrhea is a symptom of a disease, not a disease itself. Therefore, antidiarrheal medications do not treat the underlying cause of the diarrhea but only help reduce diarrhea symptoms. Some types of diarrhea are caused by an infection. If this is the case, the patient may receive an antibiotic in addition to an antidiarrheal medication. Antibiotics used to treat infectious diarrhea are discussed in Chapter 23. Patients with diarrhea lose a large amount of water, so fluid or electrolyte replacement may be needed along with antidiarrheal medications (see Chapter 26).

Opiate Derivatives

Acute diarrhea can be treated on a short-term basis with medications derived from opiates. These medications are similar to narcotic analgesics in that they too are derivatives of opium (see Chapter 25). Unlike the powerful pain medications, however, these **opiate derivatives** are poorly absorbed and do not reach the brain in high concentrations. Instead of affecting the central nervous system (CNS), they work by inhibiting peristalsis and slowing the progression of food through the GI tract. They also reduce the liquid content of stool. They are taken only when needed for short-term relief of diarrhea. **Loperamide** is available over the counter, and **diphenoxylate/ atropine** is a controlled substance (Schedule V). Table 18.2 lists opiate derivatives and other commonly used antidiarrheal drugs. Although these agents can potentially be used in children, they are usually avoided in that patient population. Parents or caregivers seeking an opiate derivative for an infant or a child younger than two years old should first talk with their pharmacists or healthcare practitioners. These medications take about six to eight hours to work.

Quick Study

Because hydration is key to treating diarrhea, familiarize yourself with hydration products in a local pharmacy. Oral re-hydration products come in a variety of brands and dosage forms:

- liquid products (Ora-lyte, Pedialyte, and Resol)
- powdered products for reconstitution (CeraORS, Pedia-Care, and Pedialyte)
- child-friendly freeze pops (Oralyte and Pedialyte)

TABLE 18.2 | **Commonly Used Antidiarrheal Drugs**

Generic (Brand)	Dosage Form	Route of Administration	Common Dosage
Opiate Derivatives			
Diphenoxylate/atropine (Lomotil, Lonox)	Oral solution, tablet	Oral	5 mg 4 times a day (maximum 20 mg a day)
Loperamide (Imodium)	Capsule, oral solution, tablet	Oral	4 mg, then 2 mg after each loose stool (maximum 16 mg a day)
Bismuth Subsalicylate			
Bismuth subsalicylate (Kaopectate, Pepto-Bismol)	Chewable tablet, oral suspension	Oral	534 mg every 0.5–1 hr (maximum 8 doses or 4,272 mg a day)

Side Effects Loperamide can cause dizziness and constipation, even when used correctly. Diphenoxylate/atropine has very few side effects, but some patients may experience dizziness and drowsiness. However, blurred vision, dry mouth, and difficulty urinating are potential side effects of atropine. Patients can minimize these effects by not exceeding the recommended daily dose. If high doses are taken, respiratory depression is possible. Children are more likely than adults are to experience adverse events.

Drug Alert

Diphenoxylate/atropine (Lomotil) is a controlled substance (Schedule V). Although it is usually dispensed upon prescription order, Lomotil can be purchased without a prescription in many states. This medication is kept behind the counter in pharmacies so that the pharmacist can assess whether it is appropriate for a patient to use. If Lomotil is dispensed without a prescription, special documentation is required.

Contraindications Diphenoxylate/atropine is contraindicated in children younger than two years of age. This drug is also contraindicated in patients with obstructive jaundice and diarrhea associated with pseudomembranous enterocolitis or enterotoxin-producing bacteria. Loperamide should be avoided in children younger than two years of age and in patients who have abdominal pain without diarrhea.

 Note: *Allied health professionals should be aware that an allergy to a particular drug contraindicates its use. This warning applies to all Contraindications sections in this chapter.*

Cautions and Considerations Diphenoxylate can cross the blood-brain barrier and cause euphoria, giving this drug the potential for abuse. Atropine is added to diphenoxylate to discourage misuse because it has undesirable side effects including blurred vision, urinary retention, and dry mouth. Still, pharmacies must follow state laws regarding controlled substance dispensing. In some states, special restrictions apply to the purchase of these products, and all sales are documented in a logbook. Opiate derivatives are not appropriate for treating all types of diarrhea. If fever or bloody stool is present, the patient should consult a physician. In addition, if diarrhea continues for 48 hours after use of an opiate derivative, the patient needs further evaluation by a medical professional.

Because opiate derivatives may cause dizziness and drowsiness, patients should be reminded that activities such as driving might not be safe while taking these medications. Caution patients to take careful note of the effects of these drugs before attempting such activities.

Drug Alert

Lomotil sounds similar to Lamictal, an anticonvulsant, and Lamisil, an antifungal medication. Be careful not to get these medications mixed up.

Bismuth Subsalicylate

Acute diarrhea can be treated with **bismuth subsalicylate**. Bismuth subsalicylate has both antibacterial and **antisecretory** action. In addition, it has anti-inflammatory effects, making it beneficial in treating ***Helicobacter pylori (H. pylori)*** infection and traveler's diarrhea. This product may be used in small children, but specialized doses may be required. Bismuth subsalicylate is available over the counter.

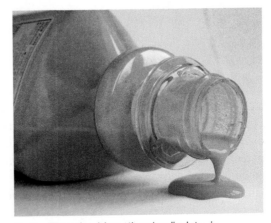

Pepto-Bismol, a bismuth subsalicylate, is frequently taken to treat acute diarrhea.

Side Effects Bismuth subsalicylate may cause constipation, nausea, vomiting, and darkening of the tongue and/or stools. Taking bismuth subsalicylate with food and plenty of water may relieve nausea symptoms. Although rare, neurotoxic symptoms such as tinnitus (ringing in the ears), confusion, and weakness are also potential side effects. To avoid these more serious side effects, patients should not take excessive doses of bismuth subsalicylate.

Contraindications Bismuth subsalicylate should not be used in patients with a history of severe GI bleeding or coagulation problems. In addition, patients with aspirin hypersensitivity should avoid products containing bismuth subsalicylate because such products may trigger an allergic-like reaction.

Cautions and Considerations Patients should be warned that their tongue and stools might darken while taking this medication. These changes are harmless and temporary. Patients should also be told to stop taking bismuth subsalicylate if they experience confusion, dizziness, or vision changes and to report these problems to their healthcare practitioners.

Bismuth subsalicylate may decrease the effectiveness of tetracycline antibiotics, so patients should not take the two medications concurrently. In addition, these products may enhance the anticoagulant effects of warfarin, thereby increasing a patient's risk of bleeding. Patients should tell their physicians and pharmacists about all prescription and nonprescription products they are taking to avoid or limit these potential drug interactions. Patients with renal failure or gout should consult their healthcare practitioners before using bismuth subsalicylate.

Patients should consult their pharmacists or physicians before giving this product to children. Children and adolescents are at risk of a condition known as **Reye syndrome**, a potentially life-threatening disorder caused by salicylate use for viral infections.

Oral suspensions must be shaken well before ingestion to ensure adequate mixing and proper dosing.

Constipation

Constipation is the opposite of diarrhea. It is characterized by infrequent bowel movements, small stool size, hard stools, or the feeling of incomplete bowel evacuation. Most people pass at least three stools a week, so fewer stools could constitute constipation. However, diagnosis depends on the individual patient. Many episodes of constipation are related to a diet low in fiber or fluid intake. Constipation can also be caused by certain foods or drugs (see Table 18.3). Although many drugs have the potential to cause diarrhea or constipation, the ones most associated with constipation include pain medications such as opiates and antacids. Stress may also exacerbate constipation, whereas light exercise promotes GI motility.

TABLE 18.3	Drugs That Can Cause Constipation	
Antiemetics		Diuretics
Antihistamines		Iron
Calcium- and aluminum-containing laxatives or antacids		Nonsteroidal anti-inflammatory drugs (NSAIDs)
		Opiates (hydrocodone, morphine, oxycodone, etc.)
Calcium-channel blockers		Tricyclic antidepressants (TCAs)

Drug Regimens and Treatments

Dietary modification and lifestyle changes should accompany pharmacologic treatment of constipation. Adequate dietary intake of fiber (including fruits, vegetables, and cereals) and regular exercise (even light walking) regulates GI motility. Patients with repeat bouts of constipation should drink plenty of fluids, eat adequate fiber, and exercise regularly.

Drugs that relieve constipation are known as **laxatives**. Typically, laxatives are used only as needed on a short-term basis. Electrolyte abnormalities may occur if laxatives are used too frequently. If patients are using laxatives on a regular basis, they should consult their physicians for a full evaluation.

In addition to oral dosage forms, many laxatives are available as **suppositories** or **enemas**. These dosage forms are used for rapid treatment of moderate-to-severe constipation. Rectal suppositories take 15 to 60 minutes to work. They are useful for hospitalized patients who are unable to swallow oral laxatives. Before inserting a rectal suppository, the patient should squat or lie on his or her side with one leg straight and the other bent. The patient should then remove the foil wrapping from the suppository and insert it—pointed end first—into the rectum (see Figure 18.4). The suppository needs to be inserted far enough into the rectum so that it does not slip out. Afterward, the patient should wash his or her hands.

An enema is a liquid solution that is delivered directly into the rectum. Enemas are used to rapidly empty the bowels prior to surgery or diagnostic procedures such as a colonoscopy or barium enema. They also can remove excessive fecal matter that is blocking the GI tract. To use an enema, the patient should lie down and insert the enema tip into the rectum. He or she should allow the liquid to drain into the rectum via gravity or by squeezing the bottle. After holding the enema liquid in the rectum for a specific period (2 to 60 minutes, depending on the product), the patient should then defecate normally.

FIGURE 18.4 Suppository Insertion

A suppository must be inserted past the rectal sphincter so that it does not slip out.

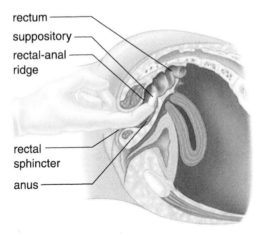

Bulk-Forming Laxatives

Mild constipation can be treated with **bulk-forming laxatives**. As with dietary fiber, bulk-forming agents are poorly absorbed and remain in the GI tract, drawing water and other electrolytes into the GI system. Increased volume in the GI tract triggers peristalsis and facilitates bowel movements. In general, these agents take between one and three days to work. Bulk-forming laxatives work best for preventing constipation rather than as acute treatment. Patients with repeated problems with constipation may consider using a bulk-forming laxative on a daily basis to remain regular. These laxatives may also have beneficial effects in patients who have diabetes or high cholesterol because these

TABLE 18.4 Commonly Used Laxatives

Generic (Brand)	Dosage Form	Route of Administration	Common Dosage
Bulk-Forming Laxatives			
Methylcellulose (Citrucel, Maltsupex, Unifiber)	Powder for oral solution, tablet	Oral	See individual product; used 3–4 times a day
Polycarbophil (Equalactin, FiberCon, Fiber-Lax, Konsyl Fiber)	Chewable tablet, tablet	Oral	2 tablets 1–4 times a day
Psyllium (many brand names, including Fiberall, Genfiber, Konsyl, and Metamucil)	Capsule, powder for oral solution, wafer	Oral	See individual product
Wheat dextrin (Benefiber)	Caplet, chewable tablet, powder for oral solution	Oral	3 g up to 3 times a day
Stool Softeners			
Calcium, docusate sodium, and potassium (many brands, including Colace)	Capsule, enema, oral solution, syrup, tablet	Oral, rectal	PO (adult): 5–500 mg a day divided in 1–4 doses PO (pediatric): 5–150 mg a day Rectal (adult and pediatric): Add 50–100 mg of docusate liquid to enema fluid
Stimulant Laxatives			
Bisacodyl (many brands)	Enema, suppository, tablet	Oral, rectal	Adult or Pediatric (12 years or older): 5–15 mg PO once a day or one suppository or one enema once a day Pediatric (6–12 years): 5 mg PO once a day
Senna (many brands, including Ex-Lax, Fletcher's)	Chewable tablet, oral solution, syrup, tablet	Oral	Adult: 15 mg once a day Pediatric: 3.75–8.6 mg once a day

medications absorb fat and reduce glucose. Bulk-forming laxatives are available over the counter. Table 18.4 contains information on commonly used laxatives.

Side Effects Although rare, obstruction of the esophagus or bowels is possible with bulk-forming laxatives. To avoid obstruction, patients should take bulk-forming laxatives with a full glass of liquid (at least eight ounces).

Contraindications Bulk-forming laxatives are contraindicated in patients with impaired intestinal motility and in patients with intestinal stenosis.

Cautions and Considerations Bulk-forming laxatives should be used with caution in patients with esophageal strictures, ulcers, intestinal adhesions, or difficulty swallowing. Products should be taken with at least eight ounces of water to prevent choking or obstruction.

Because they increase GI motility, bulk-forming laxatives can affect drug absorption. Patients should separate doses of these laxatives from other medications by at least two hours to ensure that other drugs are absorbed properly.

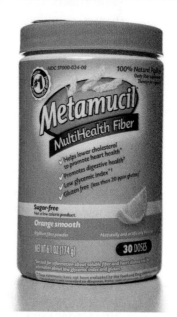

Patients dissolve powdered dosage forms of bulk-forming laxatives, such as Metamucil, in water or juice and then drink the solution.

Stool Softeners

For patients who are at risk of becoming constipated, **emollient laxatives** (another term for **stool softeners**) are used. They are not as effective for treatment of acute constipation as they are for helping reduce or prevent constipation when it is likely to occur. Stool softeners are typically taken on a regular or daily basis. They work by increasing water and electrolyte secretions in the GI tract, which makes stools softer and easier to pass.

Side Effects Although well tolerated, side effects of stool softeners can include throat irritation, abdominal pain, diarrhea, and intestinal obstruction. Drinking plenty of fluids each day can reduce these effects.

Contraindications Docusate is contraindicated for patients with intestinal obstruction, acute abdominal pain, nausea, or vomiting. This drug should not be used concomitantly with mineral oil.

Cautions and Considerations The syrup dosage form has a bitter taste. Taking these products with eight ounces of milk or juice can mask the bad taste. Drinking plenty of fluids while taking stool softeners enhances their effect. As with many laxatives, excessive or long-term use may lead to electrolyte imbalance. Patients should inform their health-care practitioners if constipation continues or abdominal pain occurs while taking a stool softener.

Stimulant Laxatives

Acute constipation can be treated with **stimulant laxatives**. These medications work by stimulating parasympathetic neurons that control bowel muscles, thereby enhancing peristalsis and GI motility. To avoid electrolyte imbalances, stimulant laxatives are taken only when needed on a short-term basis. These drugs are commonly used to treat opiate-induced constipation.

Side Effects Common side effects of stimulant laxatives include mild abdominal pain, nausea, vomiting, and rectal burning. Patients should take these agents at bedtime to avoid these side effects. Serious electrolyte abnormalities are very rare but can occur with chronic use. For this reason, long-term use is not recommended.

Contraindications Bisacodyl is contraindicated in patients with abdominal pain or obstruction, nausea, or vomiting. Senna should be avoided in patients with intestinal obstruction, acute intestinal inflammation, colitis, ulcerative colitis, appendicitis, and abdominal pain of unknown origin.

Cautions and Considerations Patients should take bisacodyl with a full glass of water on an empty stomach to achieve the best effect. Dairy products and antacids can decrease the effects of bisacodyl, so patients should not ingest these substances simultaneously. Senna should not be taken if a patient has intestinal obstruction, Crohn disease, or abdominal pain.

Bowel Preparation Laxatives

Evacuating the bowels prior to surgery or a diagnostic procedure requires quick-acting, powerful laxatives. Bowel evacuation may also be necessary for clearing poisons or parasitic worms from the GI tract and for treating bowel impaction from severe constipation. **Bowel preparation ("prep") laxatives** work by drawing water and electrolytes into the GI tract. They prepare the bowel for examination by completely cleaning it out.

Magnesium citrate and sodium phosphate are available over the counter in oral and rectal dosage forms. Polyethylene glycol is available over the counter (MiraLAX) and by prescription (GlycoLax, GoLYTELY) as a powder for an oral solution. MiraLAX can be used for occasional constipation in smaller doses taken daily, whereas GlycoLax is usually used the day before a bowel procedure. These agents take only a few hours to work if taken orally, or less than an hour if used rectally. Therefore, patients should use these products at home, where a toilet is readily accessible.

Side Effects Common side effects of bowel prep laxatives include abdominal pain, diarrhea, and electrolyte loss or imbalance. Polyethylene glycol electrolyte solution has higher rates of side effects than other fast-acting laxatives and can cause anal irritation, bloating, nausea, and vomiting. Although bothersome, these effects are brief and abate within a few hours of using the product.

Contraindications Sodium phosphate has contraindications based on its route of administration. Sodium phosphate enemas are contraindicated in ascites, kidney impairment, heart failure, imperforate anus, known or suspected GI obstruction, and congenital or acquired megacolon. The intravenous (IV) form of sodium phosphate is contraindicated in diseases accompanied by hyperphosphatemia, hypocalcemia, or hypernatremia. Oral sodium phosphate should be avoided in acute phosphate nephropathy, bowel obstruction, bowel perforation, gastric bypass or stapling surgery, toxic colitis, and toxic megacolon. Polyethylene glycol and magnesium citrate do not have contraindications.

Cautions and Considerations Products containing magnesium or sodium should be used with caution in patients with congestive heart failure, given the potential accumulation of these ions. These products should also be used with caution in patients with kidney problems and in children younger than two years old. To avoid significant electrolyte loss, these laxatives should only be used occasionally. If a patient is using one of these products on a regular basis, he or she should consult a healthcare practitioner for a full evaluation.

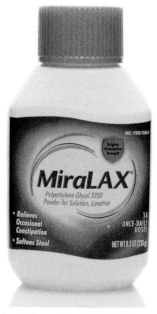

Polyethylene glycol (MiraLAX) softens stool and relieves occasional constipation.

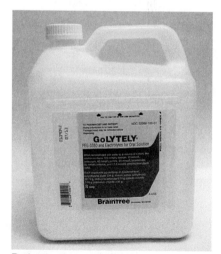

Patients who are taking bowel prep laxatives should fill the 4-liter container with water and drink an 8-ounce glass of the laxative solution every 10 minutes until the entire container is empty.

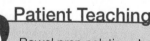 **Patient Teaching**

Bowel prep solutions have an unpleasant taste. Tell patients that refrigerating bowel prep solutions prior to drinking them can make them more palatable for consumption.

Miscellaneous Laxatives

A few other laxative agents bear mentioning because healthcare professionals will see them used in select cases. **Milk of magnesia** is used frequently over the counter and in the long-term care setting for mild constipation. It is available as a liquid and as chewable tablets. **Glycerin suppositories** are used in children with occasional constipation. **Lactulose** is an oral solution used for patients with ammonia toxicity and delirium in end-stage liver failure. It pulls ammonia from the bloodstream into the GI tract, where diarrhea is stimulated to eliminate the ammonia rapidly. Healthcare professionals working in the inpatient setting may be more likely to see lactulose used because of the additional benefit of helping patients with delirium in end-stage liver failure.

Kolb's Learning Styles

Learners who like fieldwork and authentic laboratory exercises, as Accommodators and Convergers do, may find a trip to a pharmacy useful. Check out the laxatives available over the counter. Can you find the OTC bowel prep products? What brand names of bisacodyl and senna can you find?

Checkpoint 18.2

Take a moment to review what you have learned so far and answer these questions.

1. What are the common causes of diarrhea and constipation?
2. What drugs are used to treat diarrhea and how do they work?
3. What drugs are used to treat constipation and how do they work?

Heartburn and Ulcers

Gastroesophageal reflux disease (GERD), the medical term for **heartburn**, is a common complaint for which patients seek medication. It is estimated that 10% of people in the United States get heartburn every week. Heartburn is characterized by a burning or sensation of warmth starting in the gut or chest that may radiate to the neck. In GERD, the lower esophageal sphincter allows stomach contents to move up into the esophagus, where acidic juices can cause tissue damage and pain. GERD is most likely caused by a faulty lower esophageal sphincter that does not close properly (see Figure 18.5). Spicy or fatty foods, caffeine, smoking, and drinking alcohol decrease the closing pressure of this lower esophageal sphincter (see Table 18.5). Large meals and obesity increase pressure in the stomach and force its contents up to the esophagus. Weight loss, elevating the head of the bed at night, not eating before bedtime, remaining upright after a meal, reducing meal size, and decreasing alcohol and tobacco use can relieve GERD symptoms.

GERD not only produces bothersome symptoms for patients, but also, over time, causes permanent changes in the tissue lining of the esophagus. When chronically exposed to acid, the cells of the esophageal lining change. These changes have been linked to narrowing of the esophagus (esophageal stricture) and esophageal cancers. Repeated bouts of GERD indicate a condition the patient should not ignore. Long-term treatment involves reducing the acidity of the stomach contents to limit damage to the esophagus.

FIGURE 18.5 Lower Esophageal Sphincter Function

GERD is common during pregnancy, because as the growing fetus requires more room, the uterus expands and pushes upward on the stomach.

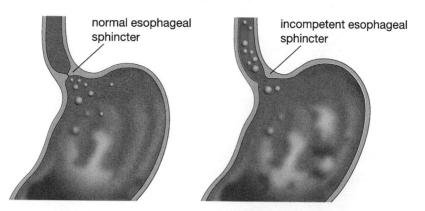

normal esophageal sphincter

incompetent esophageal sphincter

TABLE 18.5 Foods and Medications That May Worsen GERD

Foods	Medications
Alcohol	Alendronate
Caffeine	Anticholinergics
Chocolate	Aspirin
Coffee or soft drinks	Barbiturates
Fatty foods	Dopamine
Garlic	Iron
Onions	Nicotine
Orange juice	Nitrates
Peppermint and spearmint	Nonsteroidal anti-inflammatory drugs (NSAIDs)
Spicy foods	Tetracycline

Ulcers occur when the protective lining of the GI tract is worn away and bleeding occurs. Ulcers are sores or patches of dead tissue along the walls of the GI tract. A bacterial parasite, *H. pylori*, is the most common culprit that causes **peptic ulcer disease (PUD)**, or ulcers in the stomach. *H. pylori* is a spiral-shaped, gram-negative organism that attaches to the lining of the stomach. It releases chemicals that cause inflammation and damage the stomach lining, leading to ulcer formation. In addition, *H. pylori* elicits an immune response whereby activated immune cells damage neighboring cells in the stomach and small intestine in the process of killing bacteria. **Duodenal ulcers** occur in the portion of the small intestine just below the stomach. These ulcers are caused by hyperacidity, not usually by *H. pylori* (see Figure 18.6).

Stress ulcers occur in critically ill patients who are bedridden. The exact mechanism by which they form is not well understood, but it is thought that serious illness, stress, and trauma lead to a decrease in the protective mucous layer of the stomach and an increase in acid secretion in the stomach. Patients in intensive care settings are routinely given medications that reduce stomach acid to prevent stress ulcers.

Nonsteroidal anti-inflammatory drugs (NSAIDs), such as **ibuprofen** and **aspirin**, can cause ulcers. These acidic drugs irritate and erode GI tissue. More importantly, they inhibit production of prostaglandins. Prostaglandins produce inflammation and pain

FIGURE 18.6 Peptic Ulcers

Peptic ulcers are erosions of the mucosal lining of the GI tract. Proton pump inhibitors are commonly used to treat these ulcers.

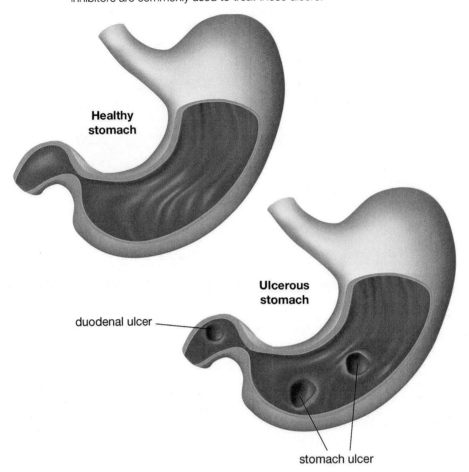

Healthy stomach

Ulcerous stomach

duodenal ulcer

stomach ulcer

throughout most of the body, but in the stomach, they protect the lining from acid secretion. Prolonged use of NSAIDs removes the protective effects of prostaglandins in the stomach and can result in GI ulceration. When ulceration erodes into a blood vessel, a **GI bleed** can occur. GI bleeds may be asymptomatic for many patients and are particularly dangerous for elderly patients or patients who are critically ill. Patients taking long-term NSAIDs, aspirin, and anti-coagulation therapy are at high risk for ulcers and life-threatening bleeding.

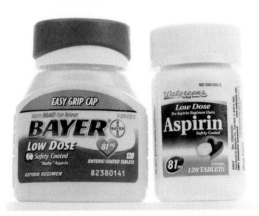

Patients who are on long-term NSAID therapy, such as low-dose aspirin for anticoagulation, are at a higher risk for stress ulcer formation.

Drug Regimens and Treatments

Although the underlying problems of GERD and GI ulcers relate to damage in the GI tract from stomach acid, most treatments for these conditions do not directly fix this problem. Antacids, proton pump inhibitors (PPIs), and H2 blockers relieve symptoms of GERD by decreasing acid production in the stomach. This means that stomach contents may still regurgitate into the esophagus or reach an ulcer in the stomach or intestines, but less damage will occur because the gastric juices are less acidic.

Antacids

Mild-to-moderate GERD can be treated with antacids. **Antacids** contain special ions that react with hydrogen ions in the stomach and neutralize acid. They are effective for only a few hours, so it may be necessary to take these medications after every meal. Antacids are available over the counter. See Table 18.6 for information on antacids.

TABLE 18.6 Commonly Used Antacids

Generic (Brand)	Dosage Form	Route of Administration	Common Dosage
Aluminum hydroxide (ALternaGEL, Gaviscon)	Chewable tablet, suspension	Oral	Doses vary depending on product, dosage form, and indication for use. Refer to product packaging for proper dosing instructions.
Aluminum hydroxide/magnesium hydroxide (Maalox, Mylanta)	Suspension	Oral	
Calcium carbonate (Maalox, Tums)	Chewable tablet	Oral	
Calcium carbonate/magnesium hydroxide (Mylanta, Rolaids)	Gelcap, suspension, tablet	Oral	

Side Effects Common side effects of antacids include constipation, diarrhea, stomach pain, nausea, and vomiting. These effects are generally mild. Calcium- and aluminum-containing antacids tend to cause constipation, whereas magnesium-containing antacids tend to cause diarrhea.

Contraindications There are no contraindications to antacids.

Cautions and Considerations Antacids provide short-term relief for patients with heartburn. Patients requiring repeated or constant use of antacids should see their prescribers and discuss other treatment options. Continuous use of calcium-containing antacids can cause acid hypersecretion, particularly when the medication is discontinued, so long-term use of calcium products should be discouraged.

Antacids bind to several other oral drugs, decreasing their absorption. Antibiotics such as tetracyclines, quinolones, and isoniazid should not be given at the same time as antacids for this reason. Other interacting medications include iron supplements containing ferrous sulfate and the sulfonylureas (treatment for diabetes). Antacids should be taken more than two hours before or after the other medication.

Antacids must be used with caution in patients with renal failure because aluminum and magnesium can accumulate in the blood. Patients should let their pharmacists or physicians know if they have kidney failure.

Antacid suspensions need to be shaken well before use to ensure adequate mixing of contents and proper dosing.

Name Exchange

OTC antacids are commonly used products. Allied health professionals may find it helpful to learn the generic and brand names of antacids, as patients often refer to these products by their brand names. Calcium carbonate is commonly known by the brand names Tums or Maalox; calcium carbonate/magnesium hydroxide is sold under the brand names Mylanta and Rolaids.

Proton Pump Inhibitors

GERD, PUD, and *H. pylori* infection can all be treated with **proton pump inhibitors (PPIs)**, which work by binding to proton pumps in the stomach lining, rendering them inactive. When fewer proton pumps are functioning in the stomach, less acid is produced. PPIs are long-acting agents, with effects lasting approximately 24 hours. Patients with chronic GERD problems take PPIs on a daily basis to continually suppress stomach acid production. Because PPIs are most effective when taken on an empty stomach, patients should take them one hour before the first meal of the day. Esomeprazole, lansoprazole, and omeprazole are available over the counter, whereas other PPIs are available only by prescription.

Infants can have GERD in the first weeks or months of life and are prescribed liquid forms of PPIs. These specially compounded products can be made in the pharmacy for such pediatric patients.

Some PPI medications are available for IV use, and these drugs may be given to patients who are critically ill in the hospital and at risk for stress ulcers.

Patients with gastric tubes are also prescribed PPIs. Although medications are often crushed and given through the gastric tube into the stomach, many PPI products are delayed-release or produced as capsules that cannot be crushed. Liquid dosage forms can be given via gastric tube, but tablet and capsule forms cannot. Table 18.7 has more information on common PPIs.

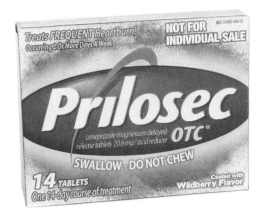

Prilosec is available as both a prescription medication and an OTC drug and is used to treat heartburn, stomach ulcers, and GERD.

TABLE 18.7 Commonly Used PPIs

Generic (Brand)	Dosage Form	Route of Administration	Common Dosage	Dispensing Status
Dexlansoprazole (Dexilant)	Capsule	Oral	Adult: 30–60 mg once a day	Rx
Esomeprazole (Nexium)	Capsule, granules for oral suspension, powder for reconstitution for IV injection	IV, oral	Adult: 20–40 mg once a day Pediatric: 10–20 mg once a day	OTC, Rx
Lansoprazole (Prevacid)	Capsule, oral dispersible tablet, oral suspension (premixed)	Oral	Adult: 15–30 mg once a day Pediatric: 15–30 mg once a day	OTC, Rx
Omeprazole (Prilosec)	Capsule, granules for suspension, tablet	Oral	Adult: 20–40 mg once a day Pediatric: 5–20 mg once a day	OTC, Rx
Pantoprazole (Protonix)	Granules for suspension, powder for reconstitution, tablet	IV, oral	Adult: 40 mg once a day Pediatric (≥ 5 years old): 20–40 mg once a day	Rx
Rabeprazole (AcipHex)	Capsule sprinkle, tablet	Oral	Adult: 20–60 mg once a day Pediatric: 5–20 mg once a day	Rx

Side Effects PPIs are very well tolerated. Rarely, patients may experience headache, nausea, vomiting, and diarrhea. If these side effects become bothersome, patients should consult their healthcare practitioners. PPIs have been associated with an increased risk for developing certain infections, such as respiratory tract infections. The significance of this association is not clear.

Contraindications Hypersensitivity to one PPI contraindicates use of all other PPIs.

Cautions and Considerations It is important that patients know that delayed-release capsules or tablets cannot be crushed or chewed. Lansoprazole is available as oral dispersible tablets that are placed on the tongue and allowed to dissolve. The dissolved particles must be swallowed without chewing.

Quick Study

PPIs are sold under various brand names. One way to easily identify a PPI is to look at the generic name. They all have the suffix *–prazole*.

PPIs may decrease the absorption of drugs that need an acidic environment to dissolve. Ketoconazole (an antifungal drug) is an acid-soluble drug that may not work if used simultaneously with PPIs. Because PPIs have long-lasting effects on stomach acidity, alternatives to PPIs should be sought for patients taking ketoconazole.

In addition to decreasing the absorption of some drugs, PPIs seem to decrease the effectiveness of clopidogrel (Plavix) by an unknown mechanism. Clopidogrel is an antiplatelet drug (see Chapter 16) that is used following cardiac surgery to help prevent heart attack and stroke. The importance of this interaction is currently unclear and is still being studied.

OTC omeprazole should be used for only 14 days. If symptoms have not resolved after two weeks, patients should consult their healthcare practitioners.

H2 Blockers

Similar to PPIs, **H2 blockers** treat GERD and PUD. They work by blocking type 2 histamine receptors in the stomach, which decreases proton pump activity and limits acid secretion. Their effects last approximately eight hours, and they can be taken daily or on an as-needed basis (see Table 18.8). They all have OTC versions available, in addition to prescription dosing. In the inpatient setting, IV dosage forms may be useful for critically ill patients at risk for stress ulcers (see Figure 18.7).

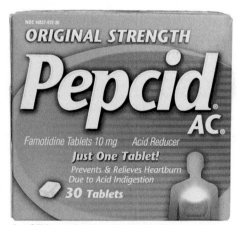

An OTC medication, Pepcid AC is an H2 blocker used to treat occasional heartburn.

Side Effects H2 blockers are well-tolerated medications. However, patients may experience headache, diarrhea, and dizziness occasionally. Rarely, these agents may cause temporary confusion. If this occurs, patients should discontinue treatment and contact their healthcare practitioners or pharmacists. H2 blockers have been associated with an increased risk for developing certain infections, such as respiratory tract infections. The significance of this association is not clear.

Contraindications Patients with hepatitis should not take ranitidine. Although rare, reports of liver failure and death have occurred in patients with hepatitis who are taking ranitidine.

TABLE 18.8 Commonly Used H2 Blockers

Generic (Brand)	Dosage Form	Route of Administration	Common Dosage	Dispensing Status
Cimetidine (Tagamet)	Oral solution, solution for injection, tablet	IV, oral	Adult: 400–1,200 mg a day IV or PO (divided 2–4 times a day) Pediatric: weight-based	OTC, Rx
Famotidine (Pepcid)	Gelcap, premixed infusion, solution for injection, tablet	IV, oral	Adult: 20 mg twice a day IV or PO Pediatric: weight-based	OTC, Rx
Nizatidine (Axid)	Capsule, oral solution, tablet	Oral	Adult: 150 mg twice a day Pediatric: weight-based	OTC, Rx
Ranitidine (Zantac)	Capsule, premixed infusion, solution for injection, syrup, tablet	IV, oral	Adult: 50 mg every 6–8 hours IV or 150 mg twice a day PO Pediatric: weight-based	OTC, Rx

Cautions and Considerations Cimetidine interacts with several other drug therapies. For example, it increases the levels of theophylline, warfarin, phenytoin, nifedipine, and propranolol in the bloodstream. Therefore, patients taking these other medications should talk with their pharmacists or prescribers before taking cimetidine. Other H2 blockers do not interact with these medications, so patients can be switched to one of them if drug interactions are a concern. Allied health professionals can help avoid these drug-drug interactions by taking a complete medication history, including all prescription, OTC, and herbal/dietary supplements.

H2 blockers decrease the absorption of drugs that require an acidic environment to dissolve. Ketoconazole (an antifungal) is an acid-soluble drug that may not be effective if used simultaneously with H2 blockers. Because H2 blockers have long-lasting effects on stomach acidity, alternatives should be sought for patients taking ketoconazole.

FIGURE 18.7 Medication Label for IV Famotidine

The H2 blocker famotidine is available in oral dosage forms and intravenously (as shown here).

Sucralfate

Sucralfate coats the walls of the stomach and small intestine, forming a protective barrier against stomach acid. It must be taken four times a day. For best results, sucralfate should be taken on an empty stomach one hour before or two hours after a meal.

Side Effects Because sucralfate is not absorbed systemically, it causes very few side effects. Constipation, diarrhea, headache, GI discomfort, and indigestion are possible.

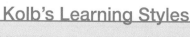

Kolb's Learning Styles

If you like to learn in a hands-on way, as Accommodators do, look through your medicine cabinet at home, and gather all medications for treating heartburn. What are the active ingredients in each product? Think about when and why you choose to use them. What is the difference in dose between OTC and prescription GERD medications? Talk with your family about the proper use of these products. Seeing, handling, and talking about these medications will give them relevance and cement their names and uses in your memory.

Contraindications Sucralfate has no contraindications.

Cautions and Considerations Sucralfate interacts with many other medications because it coats the lining of the stomach and forms a barrier, thereby preventing absorption. Patients should avoid taking sucralfate simultaneously with other medications, particularly quinolone antibiotics, antifungals, phosphate supplements, and levothyroxine. Sucralfate suspensions must be shaken well before use to ensure adequate mixing of contents.

Misoprostol

Misoprostol is approved by the US Food and Drug Administration for prevention of NSAID-induced ulcers. Misoprostol is a prostaglandin analog and replaces prostaglandins reduced or inhibited by NSAIDs. It is generally taken four times a day with food and is available as a tablet. Misoprostol must be taken during the duration of NSAID therapy to be effective. Other uses of misoprostol include cervical ripening, labor induction, and termination of pregnancy.

Side Effects Diarrhea and abdominal pain are common side effects with misoprostol use. Taking doses with or right after meals may decrease the incidence of these conditions. Other side effects include flatulence, dyspepsia, and uterine contractions.

Contraindications Hypersensitivity to prostaglandins contraindicates misoprostol use. When used to treat NSAID-induced ulcers, pregnancy contraindicates the use of this medication.

Cautions and Considerations Misoprostol should be used only to treat patients who have a high risk for gastric ulcers. This medication has abortifacient properties; therefore, it should not be given to women of childbearing age unless they are able to comply with effective contraceptive measures. When used in pregnancy, misoprostol may cause abortion, birth defects, or premature birth. Because of these risks, patients should be instructed not to share their medication with others.

Regimens for *H. pylori*

If a patient with PUD is *H. pylori* positive (+), a multidrug regimen is prescribed (see Table 18.9). These drug combinations treat the ulcer, reduce symptoms, and kill *H. pylori* in the GI tract at the same time. All regimens consist of a PPI to heal the ulcer and antibiotics to destroy the bacteria. Combination products are also available.

TABLE 18.9 Commonly Used Regimens for *H. pylori* Eradication

PPI	Plus Antibiotic	Plus Antibiotic	
Esomeprazole (Nexium) Lansoprazole (Prevacid) Omeprazole (Prilosec) Pantoprazole (Protonix) Rabeprazole (AcipHex)	Clarithromycin 500 mg twice a day	Amoxicillin 1 g twice a day or metronidazole 500 mg twice a day	

Brand name of combination product: Prevpac

PPI	Plus Antibiotic	Plus Antibiotic	Plus Antacid
PPI listed above or Cimetidine (Tagamet) Famotidine (Pepcid) Nizatidine (Axid) Ranitidine (Zantac)	Metronidazole 250–500 mg 4 times a day	Tetracycline 500 mg 4 times a day, or amoxicillin 500 mg 4 times a day, or clarithromycin 250–500 mg 4 times a day, or doxycycline 100 mg twice a day	Bismuth subsalicylate (Pepto-Bismol) 524 mg 4 times a day

Brand names of combination products: Helidac and Pylera

 Checkpoint 18.3

Take a moment to review what you have learned so far and answer these questions.

1. How do the causes of peptic ulcers and stress ulcers differ?

2. What classes of drugs are used to treat ulcers?

Nausea and Vomiting

Nausea is the feeling of the need to vomit. **Vomiting** is the expulsion of stomach contents out of the mouth. It involves coordinated muscle contractions along the upper GI tract (**reverse peristalsis**). Vomiting is a defense mechanism to protect the body from harmful substances that have been consumed.

The impulse to vomit or the feeling of nausea begins in the brain (see Figure 18.8). The **chemoreceptor trigger zone (CTZ)** and **vomiting center** in the medulla receive input from the cerebral cortex, hypothalamus, GI tract, and blood-borne stimuli (e.g., bacteria) to cause nausea and vomiting. For instance, when a harmful or foreign substance is detected in the stomach or normal balance is thrown off in the inner ear, the vomiting center signals the nausea sensation and stimulates vomiting.

Nausea and vomiting are related symptoms and are caused by a variety of diseases and conditions. Intestinal infections such as traveler's diarrhea are a common cause of nausea and vomiting. **Morning sickness** is nausea and vomiting in the first weeks of pregnancy. It is related to hormonal changes. **Motion sickness** is nausea and vomiting following movement (e.g., on a roller coaster or boat ride). It is related to vestibular responses in the inner ear that affect the sense of balance. Anesthesia used during surgery is also associated with nausea and vomiting.

Nausea and vomiting can also be induced by drugs. All drugs are foreign substances to the body and have the potential to trigger stomach irritation, nausea, and vomiting. However, medications most commonly associated with nausea and vomiting are chemotherapy agents. Radiation treatments, such as those for cancer, can also cause nausea and vomiting (see Table 18.10).

FIGURE 18.8 Chemoreceptor Trigger Zone (CTZ) and Vomiting Center

Blocking the receptors for serotonin, dopamine, histamine, and substance P in the CTZ can relieve symptoms of nausea and vomiting.

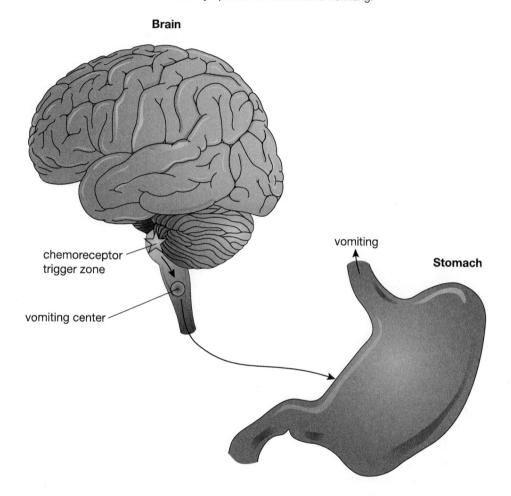

Brain

chemoreceptor trigger zone

vomiting center

vomiting

Stomach

TABLE 18.10 Treatments That Can Cause Nausea and Vomiting

Antibiotics	Digoxin
Antiseizure medications (carbamazepine, levetirace-tam, phenytoin, etc.)	Opiates (hydrocodone, morphine, oxycodone, etc.)
	Radiation therapy
Chemotherapy agents	Theophylline

Drug Regimens and Treatments

The act of vomiting is also known as **emesis**. Therefore, drugs used to prevent vomiting are called **antiemetics**. Treatment depends on the cause and severity of the nausea and vomiting. For nausea and vomiting due to heartburn, antacids and H2 blockers can be used. For mild nausea and vomiting related to motion sickness, OTC anticholinergic agents can be used. For moderate-to-severe nausea and vomiting, more potent antiemetics are needed. These medications are prescribed in clinics and hospitals for nausea and vomiting associated with severe dehydration, chemotherapy, and anesthesia following surgical procedures. Sometimes, these potent agents are used in combination with oral corticosteroids (see Chapter 24).

Anticholinergic Antiemetics

In general, **anticholinergic antiemetics** are similar in chemical structure to antihistamines. They are used as antiemetics for mild motion sickness. They work by blocking histamine and acetylcholine, two neurotransmitters in the CTZ and vomiting center. One combination product, doxylamine/pyridoxine (Diclegis), is used for pregnancy-associated nausea and vomiting. (See Table 18.11 for more information.)

TABLE 18.11 Commonly Used Anticholinergic Antiemetic Agents

Generic (Brand)	Dosage Form	Route of Administration	Common Dosage
Dimenhydrinate (Dramamine)	Liquid injection, tablet	IM, IV, oral	Varies by age and use; usually taken 1 hr prior to when motion sickness is expected and once a day thereafter (when needed)
Doxylamine/pyridoxine (Diclegis)	Delayed-release tablet	Oral	2 tablets at bedtime (doxylamine 20 mg and pyridoxine 20 mg)
Hydroxyzine (Atarax, Vistaril)	Capsule, injection, suspension, syrup, tablet	IM, oral	Varies by age and use; usually taken 1–2 hr prior to when motion sickness is expected and once a day thereafter (when needed)
Meclizine (Bonine)	Capsule, tablet	Oral	Varies by age and use; usually taken 1 hr prior to when motion sickness is expected and once a day thereafter (when needed)
Scopolamine (Scopace, Transderm Scop)	Tablet, transdermal patch	Oral, transdermal	PO: 0.4–1 mg, usually taken 1 hr prior to when motion sickness is expected; Transdermal: 1 patch every 72 hr applied 1 hr prior to when motion sickness is expected

Side Effects Common side effects of anticholinergic antiemetics are drowsiness, dry mouth, and urinary retention. Patients who take other medications that also cause drowsiness should be careful because sedation could be excessive. Patients should avoid drinking alcohol and take care when driving until they know how the medication affects them. Patients who have prostate enlargement may want to avoid anticholinergic antiemetics because they can make urination even more difficult.

In some children, anticholinergic antiemetics have a paradoxical effect, where excitation occurs rather than drowsiness. Parents should be aware of the potential for this side effect.

Contraindications Anticholinergic antiemetics should not be given to infants or mothers who are breast-feeding. In addition, patients with glaucoma or those individuals using monoamine oxidase inhibitors (MAOIs) should not take these agents. Dimenhydrinate injection should not be used in neonates, as it contains benzyl alcohol. Hydroxyzine should not be used in early pregnancy, and it should not be injected via subcutaneous, intra-arterial, or IV routes. Contraindications to scopolamine include hypersensitivity to belladonna alkaloids and narrow-angle glaucoma. Meclizine does not have contraindications.

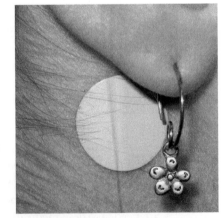

Many people use the scopolamine patch to prevent motion sickness while traveling on boats or airplanes.

Cautions and Considerations Patients who have high blood pressure or heart problems should talk with their prescribers before taking anticholinergic antiemetics.

General Antiemetics

A handful of agents make up the majority of prescription orders for antiemetics, especially in the inpatient setting. **Metoclopramide** works by increasing GI motility, which allows food to pass quickly through the stomach, thereby preventing vomiting. **Promethazine** blocks histamine (H1) receptors.

Phenothiazines are potent antiemetic drugs that work by blocking dopamine. They are first-generation antipsychotics when used in higher doses. Healthcare professionals working in an inpatient setting will likely dispense phenothiazines daily because they are frequently ordered in that setting.

These medications are available in many different dosage forms (see Table 18.12), an important feature because patients with nausea and vomiting may not be able to swallow a pill or oral solution. Patients can receive an intramuscular (IM) or an IV injection, or a rectal suppository to relieve symptoms.

TABLE 18.12 Commonly Used General Antiemetics

Generic (Brand)	Dosage Form	Route of Administration	Common Dosage
Metoclopramide (Reglan)	Solution for injection, syrup, tablet	IM, IV, oral	10–20 mg 3–4 times a day
Promethazine (Phenergan, others)	Liquid, solution for injection, suppository, tablet	IM, IV, oral, rectal	12.5–25 mg 4–6 times a day
Phenothiazines			
Chlorpromazine (Thorazine)	Liquid, solution for injection, tablet	IM, IV, oral	IM/IV: 25–50 mg every 4–6 hr PO: 10–25 mg every 4–6 hr
Prochlorperazine (Compazine)	Liquid, solution for injection, suppository, tablet	IM, IV, oral, rectal	IM/IV: 2.5–10 mg 3–4 times a day PO: 5–10 mg 3–4 times a day Rectal: 25 mg twice a day

Side Effects Common side effects of general antiemetics include drowsiness and sedation. Movement disorders such as tardive dyskinesia and dystonia (called **extrapyramidal symptoms [EPS]** or **EPS side effects**) are also possible with phenothiazines, particularly at high doses. EPS effects include uncontrollable movements of the eyes, face, and limbs that may become permanent. Patients, especially the elderly, have to be closely monitored for the appearance of EPS. If any symptoms of EPS appear, patients should stop taking the antiemetic. Diphenhydramine may be used to treat dystonia.

Contraindications Metoclopramide is contraindicated in GI obstruction, perforation, or hemorrhage; pheochromocytoma; history of seizures; and concomitant use of other agents likely to increase extrapyramidal reactions. Promethazine is contraindicated for patients who are in a coma or experiencing lower respiratory tract symptoms. Promethazine is also contraindicated in children younger than two years of age, and for intra-arterial or subcutaneous administration. Chlorpromazine and prochlorperazine should not be used in patients with severe CNS depression or coma. In addition, prochlorperazine is contraindicated in pediatric surgery and in children younger than two years or weighing less than 9 kg.

Cautions and Considerations The sedative effects of these medications may make it difficult for patients to drive or accomplish other activities. Alcohol may make the sedation worse.

Patients with liver problems cannot eliminate these agents from the bloodstream properly, increasing the risk for EPS. Patients should inform their prescribers if they have liver problems so that this risk can be assessed and other therapy chosen if necessary.

Serotonin Type 3 (5-HT3) Receptor Antagonists

These agents are potent antiemetics used to prevent and treat severe nausea and vomiting associated with chemotherapeutic medications, radiation treatment, or anesthesia. **Serotonin type 3 receptor antagonists** work by blocking serotonin type 3 (5-HT3) receptors in the brain and GI tract. Blocking these receptors stops nausea signals traveling from the brain to the stomach. These powerful antiemetics are prescription-only products (see Table 18.13) that healthcare professionals in the inpatient and oncology specialty clinics will encounter.

Quick Study

An easy way to identify a 5-HT3 receptor antagonist is to look at the generic name. The generic names all end in –*setron*.

TABLE 18.13 | **Commonly Used 5-HT3 Receptor Antagonists**

Generic (Brand)	Dosage Form	Route of Administration	Common Dosage
Dolasetron (Anzemet)	Solution for injection, tablet	IV, oral	IV: 12.5 mg PO: 100 mg
Granisetron (Granisol, Kytril, Sancuso)	Solution for injection, tablet, transdermal patch	IV, oral, transdermal	IV: 1 mg or 10 mcg/kg PO: 2 mg Transdermal: 1 patch at least 24 hr prior to chemotherapy (may be worn for up to 7 days)
Ondansetron (Zofran)	Oral disintegrating tablet, pre-mixed infusion bag, solution for injection, tablet	IM, IV, oral	IM/IV: 4–12 mg PO: 8–24 mg
Palonosetron (Aloxi)	Solution for injection	IV	0.075–0.25 mg

Side Effects Common side effects of 5-HT3 receptor antagonists include headache, fatigue, constipation, drowsiness, and muscle weakness. Although extremely rare, serious side effects such as anaphylaxis, hypotension, or swelling of the throat or tongue have been reported. Because these potentially life-threatening reactions are possible, it is recommended that patients not be alone when they take their first dose of a 5-HT3 receptor antagonist.

Work Wise

A few of the 5-HT3 receptor antagonist medications are expensive. For a patient's insurance plan to cover these drugs, the prescriber may need to complete a prior authorization request. As an allied health professional, you may be asked to prepare the documentation needed for such a request.

Contraindications Dolasetron is contraindicated via the IV route when used for the prevention of chemotherapy-associated nausea and vomiting. Granisetron, ondansetron (see Figure 18.9), and palonosetron do not have contraindications.

Cautions and Considerations Because 5-HT3 receptor antagonists may cause dizziness and drowsiness, patients should be reminded that activities such as driving may not be safe while taking these medications.

FIGURE 18.9 Medication Label for IM or IV Ondansetron

There are times when patients experiencing nausea and vomiting are unable to tolerate oral antiemetics. In these cases, IM, IV, or transdermal administration is used. This label shows the injectable form of the 5-HT3 receptor antagonist, ondansetron.

Dronabinol

Dronabinol is the active substance in *Cannabis sativa* (marijuana). As an orally active cannabinoid, dronabinol has effects on the sympathetic nervous system, which influence appetite. The principal uses of dronabinol are to treat nausea and vomiting associated with chemotherapy and appetite stimulation in patients with acquired immunodeficiency syndrome (AIDS). Dronabinol is given in doses of 2.5–20 mg, three to four times a day for the prevention of vomiting. The dosing for appetite stimulation is lower, with a maximum of 20 mg a day. Because of the potential for abuse, dronabinol is a Schedule III controlled substance.

Side Effects As an active cannabinoid substance, dronabinol can have psychoactive effects such as easy laughing, elation or euphoria, heightened awareness, anxiety, hallucination, confusion, and paranoia. It can also cause dizziness, sleepiness, heart palpitations, and flushing. Patients taking dronabinol should not drive or engage in hazardous activity until they know how it affects them. Discontinuing dronabinol after prolonged use can produce withdrawal effects such as irritability, insomnia, restlessness, hot flashes, sweating, runny nose, loose stools, and hiccups. Use and appropriate dosing of this medication should be monitored closely to reduce unwanted side effects.

Contraindications Dronabinol is contraindicated in patients with a hypersensitivity to cannabinoids, sesame oil, or marijuana.

Cautions and Considerations Patients with depression, mania, or schizophrenia should talk with their healthcare practitioners before taking dronabinol. Careful psychiatric monitoring would be needed in such patients so as not to make their conditions worse. Dronabinol should be used with caution in patients with a history of substance abuse or dependence. The potential for abuse of dronabinol is higher in such patients.

Neurokinin-1 Receptor Antagonists

Emend, the brand name for aprepitant and its injectable form fosaprepitant, belongs to the class of drugs called **neurokinin-1 receptor antagonists** (also known as *neurokinin-1 inhibitors*). Aprepitant and fosaprepitant are used to prevent nausea and vomiting induced by chemotherapy drugs or anesthesia. They work by blocking NK1 receptors, thereby preventing **substance P**—a neuropeptide involved in mediating responses such as pain, pleasure, thirst, and hunger—from stimulating nausea. Blocking NK1 receptors stops the nausea signal as it travels from the brain to the GI tract. Fosaprepitant is given as an IV infusion 20 to 30 minutes prior to chemotherapy.

Side Effects Common side effects of aprepitant and fosaprepitant include fatigue, muscle weakness, and constipation. Hypotension, slow heart rate, diarrhea, GI pain, kidney and liver dysfunction, and blood abnormalities are rare but significant side effects. If a patient experiences severe side effects while taking aprepitant or fosaprepitant, he or she should call for medical help immediately.

Contraindications Aprepitant and fosaprepitant are contraindicated in patients using cisapride or pimozide. Fosaprepitant is also contraindicated in patients with a hypersensitivity to polysorbate 80, which is an emulsifier used in food products and cosmetics that has been associated with contact dermatitis.

Cautions and Considerations Fosaprepitant inhibits the metabolism of corticosteroids and chemotherapy medications. Consequently, patients taking fosaprepitant may require lower doses of corticosteroids and chemotherapy medications. Patients taking warfarin should be monitored closely after initiating fosaprepitant therapy because the drug can speed up the metabolism of warfarin.

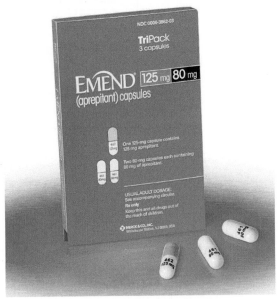

The oral form of aprepitant, sold under the brand name Emend, is used to prevent chemotherapy-induced nausea and vomiting.

Hemorrhoids

The anus contains two sphincters that control defecation. The **hemorrhoidal cushion** protects the anal sphincters from becoming damaged over time. However, in response to straining during defecation and passing hard stools, blood vessels from the hemorrhoidal cushion can be forced into the anal cavity, where they are at risk of rupturing. These displaced blood vessels, or **hemorrhoids**, are similar to varicose veins, except they occur near the anus rather than in the legs. **Hemorrhoid disease** is bleeding and irritation when a blood vessel of the hemorrhoidal cushion ruptures.

Drug Regimens and Treatments

For mild hemorrhoids, increasing dietary **fiber** or taking a fiber product such as a bulk-forming laxative may make passing stools easier and resolve symptoms. Patients with hemorrhoids should increase water intake, avoid straining when defecating, take sitz baths, and treat constipation promptly. Serious hemorrhoids may require topical corticosteroids or surgery. **Topical hemorrhoid agents** such as hydrocortisone ointment are used to decrease symptoms of itching and pain caused by hemorrhoids. **Witch hazel** is an astringent that may also help stop bleeding. **Pramoxine** is a local anesthetic. Most available hemorrhoidal products are over the counter (see Table 18.14). Medications for hemorrhoids decrease symptoms, but they do not reduce bleeding or cure the underlying problem.

TABLE 18.14 Commonly Used Treatments for Hemorrhoids

Generic (Brand)	Dosage Form	Route of Administration	Common Dosage
Hydrocortisone (Preparation H Hydrocortisone)	Cream, enema, ointment, suppository	Rectal, topical	Enema: once a day Suppository: 1 suppository twice a day Topical: 3–4 times a day
Pramoxine (Anusol, others)	Cream, gel, medicated cloth, ointment, solution, topical foam	Topical	Apply 3–4 times a day as needed
Pramoxine/hydrocortisone (ProctoFoam-HC)	Cream, gel, ointment, solution, topical foam	Topical	Apply 3–4 times a day as needed
Witch hazel (Tucks, others)	Medicated pads	Topical	Apply 3–4 times a day as needed

Side Effects Any side effects associated with use of these products should be mild and short-lived. Both witch hazel and pramoxine products can cause mild itching or burning when used to treat hemorrhoids. Rarely, pramoxine can cause swelling of the tongue (angioedema). If this occurs, the patient should seek medical care immediately.

Contraindications Hydrocortisone rectal enemas are contraindicated in systemic fungal infections and ileocolostomy. Pramoxine, pramoxine/hydrocortisone, and witch hazel do not have contraindications.

Cautions and Considerations None of these products should be used for long periods. If hemorrhoid symptoms do not resolve, the patient should consult a healthcare practitioner. Topical foams need to be shaken well before use to ensure adequate mixing and proper dosing.

Other GI System Disorders

Other GI conditions include irritable bowel syndrome (IBS), ulcerative colitis, and Crohn disease. These disorders are chronic conditions that are often managed with drug therapy.

Irritable Bowel Syndrome

Irritable bowel syndrome (IBS) is a chronic disease that features frequent and painful constipation or diarrhea without any structural or dietary problems. There are three types of IBS: constipation-predominant (IBS-C), diarrhea-predominant (IBS-D), and mixed IBS. The exact cause of IBS is still unknown, but it is thought to be due to muscle dysfunction in the intestines, leading to altered GI motility. For reasons that are not well understood, IBS is more common in women than in men.

Drug Regimens and Treatments

Drug therapy options for IBS are tried only after other dietary treatments have failed. For IBS-C, increased fiber (i.e., psyllium) and polyethylene glycol (PEG) can be used. Because it is an OTC medication and widely available, PEG is often given first. The dose can be adjusted as needed. If psyllium and PEG do not work, linaclotide or lubiprostone can be used. Linaclotide works on the inner lining of the intestines to stimulate production of intestinal fluid. This action accelerates GI transit and reduces abdominal pain.

The capsules should be swallowed whole, not chewed or crushed, at least 30 minutes prior to the first meal of the day. Lubiprostone works by activating chloride channels in the lining of the intestines, which stimulates production of intestinal fluid and increases passage of stools.

In addition to loperamide (discussed previously in this chapter), drug therapy options for IBS-D include bile acid sequestrants, alosetron (a 5HT-3 receptor antagonist), and antispasmodic agents such as dicyclomine and hyoscyamine (see Table 18.15). All of these agents slow peristalsis and reduce the amount of stool present in the GI tract. Bile acid sequestrants work for patients with IBS-D because up to half of these patients have malabsorption of bile acids needed to stimulate colon motility. These agents are also occasionally used to treat high cholesterol. Alosetron works by blocking 5-HT3 receptors. These receptors close channels in the intestinal lining, which allows fluid to enter the GI tract. Alosetron is used only in women who have had severe IBS-D for more than six months and who have had unsuccessful alternate drug therapies. The antispasmodic agents are anticholinergic drugs that affect the autonomic nervous system regulation of the GI tract.

Side Effects The most common side effect associated with agents used to treat IBS-C and even some IBS-D agents is diarrhea. If this occurs, patients should alert their healthcare practitioners. In some cases, the dose can be adjusted downward to reduce this unwanted side effect.

Antispasmodics are anticholinergic drugs and thus can cause dry mouth or eyes, blurred vision, reduced urination, and constipation. These effects should be monitored in patients taking dicyclomine or hyoscyamine, and the doses of these medications should be adjusted accordingly. Anticholinergic drugs can also alter mental status. Patients taking these medications who experience confusion, memory loss, hallucinations, anxiety, insomnia, and agitation should seek medical care right away.

TABLE 18.15 Drug Treatments for IBS

Generic (Brand)	Dosage Form	Route of Administration	Common Dosage
Agents for IBS-C			
Linaclotide (Linzess)	Capsule	Oral	290 mcg a day
Lubiprostone (Amitiza)	Capsule	Oral	8–24 mcg twice a day
Polyethylene glycol 3350, PEG (Dulcolax Balance, GlycoLax, MiraLAX)	Powder for oral solution	Oral	17 g (1 heaping tablespoon or 1 capful) dissolved in 8 oz of water or juice a day
Agents for IBS-D			
Alosetron (Lotronex)	Tablet	Oral	0.5–1 mg twice a day
Bile acid sequestrants: Cholestyramine (Prevalite, Questran) Colesevelam (Welchol) Colestipol (Colestid)	Granules, powder packet	Oral	1–2 packets or scoopfuls 1–6 times a day
Antispasmodics			
Dicyclomine (Bentyl)	Capsule, oral solution, tablet	Oral	20 mg 4 times a day
Hyoscyamine (Anaspaz, Levbid, Levsin, Oscimin, others)	Tablets (dispersible, oral, and sublingual)	Oral, sublingual	0.125–0.25 mg 3–4 times a day as needed

Contraindications All agents for IBS are contraindicated in patients with a history of bowel obstruction or in those individuals who are suspected of having this condition. Antispasmodics are contraindicated in patients with glaucoma, ulcerative colitis, and myasthenia gravis. Linaclotide is contraindicated in patients younger than six years old. Cholestyramine is contraindicated in complete biliary obstruction. Colesevelam should not be used in patients with hypertriglyceridemia-induced pancreatitis or in patients whose serum triglycerides levels are greater than 500 mg/dL. Colestipol and polyethylene glycol 3350 do not have contraindications.

In addition to bowel obstruction and ulcerative colitis, alosetron is contraindicated in patients with a history of severe or chronic constipation, ischemic colitis, intestinal stricture, toxic megacolon, GI perforation, adhesions, diverticulitis, Crohn disease, severe liver impairment, impaired intestinal circulation, thrombophlebitis, or hypercoagulable state. Alosetron should not be initiated in patients who are constipated and should not be administered concomitantly with fluvoxamine.

Besides bowel obstruction, ulcerative colitis, and glaucoma, dicyclomine is contraindicated in patients with reflux esophagitis, unstable cardiovascular status in acute hemorrhage, obstructive uropathy, and myasthenia gravis. In addition, dicyclomine should not be used in patients who are breast-feeding and in infants younger than six months of age.

Contraindications to hyoscyamine, besides those listed above, include patients with a hypersensitivity to belladonna alkaloids, obstructive uropathy, myasthenia gravis, paralytic ileus, toxic megacolon, unstable cardiac status, and myocardial ischemia. Hyoscyamine also should be avoided in elderly or debilitated patients who have intestinal atony.

Cautions and Considerations Antispasmodics should be used with caution in patients with heart disease or an enlarged prostate.

Alosetron can completely shut down the GI tract and cause severe complications requiring hospitalization, blood transfusion, and surgery. To ensure patient safety, distribution is restricted to pharmacies that participate in a specialized program called the Prescribing Program for Lotronex (see Drug Alert feature box).

Drug Alert

Alosetron (Lotronex) may cause serious GI side effects, including ischemic colitis and severe constipation. These side effects may lead to hospitalization and, in rare cases, death. Due to the serious side effects, only certain registered prescribers are able to write prescriptions for alosetron. Patients who are considering therapy with alosetron must receive an information sheet, called a Medication Guide, before beginning treatment and with each prescription refill. The Medication Guide includes important information such as side effects, appropriate use, contraindications, precautions, and administration instructions.

Ulcerative Colitis and Crohn Disease

Ulcerative colitis and Crohn disease are two conditions that cause chronic diarrhea. **Ulcerative colitis** involves excessive inflammation of the GI tract, causing ulcers. This damage causes abdominal pain and weight loss as well as diarrhea. The damage tends to be limited to specific portions of the colon or large intestine, and some patients can be cured surgically by removing the affected portion.

Crohn disease is similar to ulcerative colitis in that it involves inflammation of the GI tract and causes chronic diarrhea. It also has manifestations outside the GI tract. However, it is different in that it is an autoimmune disease in which the immune system malfunctions and attacks tissue lining of the entire GI tract. Although surgery is sometimes performed, it cannot cure Crohn disease. Despite these differences, ulcerative colitis and Crohn disease share similar symptoms and many of the same treatments.

Drug Regimens and Treatments

The first-line therapies for ulcerative colitis and Crohn disease are immunosuppressants and anti-inflammatory medications. Corticosteroids such as prednisone, methylprednisolone, hydrocortisone, and budesonide (a nonsystemic glucocorticoid) are used most often. Other options for therapy include azathioprine and cyclosporine, which are also immunosuppressants. (For a detailed discussion of corticosteroids and immunosuppressants, see Chapter 24.) Sometimes, aminosalicylates are used with some success. These medications, including sulfasalazine and mesalamine, work through anti-inflammatory action (see Table 18.16).

TABLE 18.16 Commonly Used Drugs for Ulcerative Colitis and Crohn Disease

Generic (Brand)	Dosage Form	Route of Administration	Common Dosage
Aminosalicylates			
Mesalamine (Apriso, Asacol, Canasa, Delzicol, Lialda, Pentasa)	Capsule, enema, pellet, suppository, tablet	Oral, rectal	PO: dose varies depending on dosage form and indication Rectal: administered once a day
Sulfasalazine (Azulfidine, Sulfazine)	Tablet	Oral	2–4 g a day, divided
Corticosteroids			
Budesonide (Entocort EC)	Capsule	Oral	2 mg twice a day
Hydrocortisone (A-Hydrocort, Cortef, Solu-Cortef)	Enema, foam, solution for injection, suppository, tablet	IM, IV, oral, rectal	IM, IV, PO: 100–500 mg a day Rectal: apply twice a day
Methylprednisolone (A-MethaPred, Depo-Medrol, Medrol, Solu-Medrol)	Solution for injection, tablet	IM, IV, oral	4–48 mg a day
Prednisone (Sterapred)	Oral solution, tablet	Oral	5–60 mg a day
Immunosuppressants			
Azathioprine (Imuran)	Tablet	Oral	2–3 mg/kg a day
Cyclosporine (Gengraf, Neoral, Sandimmune)	Capsule, oral solution	Oral	Dose varies depending on dosage form and indication

Aminosalicylates

Aminosalicylates are used for both induction and maintenance of remission in patients with Crohn disease and ulcerative colitis. Although their exact mechanism is unknown, it is thought that aminosalicylates modulate chemical mediators of the inflammatory response. Aminosalicylates can be administered orally or rectally, depending on the product.

Side Effects Common side effects of aminosalicylates include upset stomach, headache, arthralgia, and pharyngitis. Ulcerative colitis may worsen in patients, particularly children, using aminosalicylates.

Contraindications Hypersensitivity to one aminosalicylate contraindicates the use of all others. Sulfasalazine should be avoided in patients with sulfa hypersensitivity.

Cautions and Considerations There are reports of cardiac hypersensitivity in patients using aminosalicylates; therefore, these drugs should be used cautiously in patients predisposed to heart conditions. Hepatic failure has been reported. Patients with hepatic or renal impairment should be monitored closely when using aminosalicylates.

Corticosteroids

Corticosteroids are used for their anti-inflammatory and immunosuppressant properties. Patients with ulcerative colitis and Crohn disease typically use corticosteroids orally or intravenously. (Refer to Chapter 24 for additional information concerning corticosteroids.)

Side Effects Common side effects of corticosteroids include headache, dizziness, insomnia, and hunger. Taking oral corticosteroids first thing in the morning will lessen the effects of insomnia. Long-term use can affect metabolism in the body and cause facial swelling (typically referred to as "moon facies" or "moon face"), significant weight gain, fluid retention, and fat redistribution to the back and shoulders ("buffalo hump"). Other side effects include high blood pressure, loss of bone mass, electrolyte imbalance, cataracts and glaucoma, and insulin resistance (diabetes). Patients taking corticosteroids for an extended period will need to work with their healthcare practitioners to monitor these effects. If possible, corticosteroid therapy should be used on a short-term basis and only when needed. For those patients taking corticosteroids for extended periods, the medication regimen must be tapered because adrenal suppression may ensue if these drugs are abruptly withdrawn.

Contraindications Prednisone and methylprednisolone are contraindicated in systemic fungal infections. Administration of live or live-attenuated vaccines should be avoided when immunosuppressive doses of prednisone are used. Hydrocortisone use is contraindicated in systemic fungal infection, serious infections, and tubercular skin lesions. Contraindications to budesonide include primary treatment of status asthmaticus, acute episodes of asthma, and acute bronchospasm.

Cautions and Considerations Because corticosteroids suppress the immune system, patients taking them are at an increased risk of infection. With prolonged use, corticosteroids have been found to stunt growth in children. Patients who are taking budesonide should be instructed to swallow the capsule whole rather than crush or chew it.

Immunosuppressants

Medications that suppress the immune system are called immunosuppressants. These medications may induce response and remission in patients with Crohn disease or ulcerative colitis. (Refer to Chapter 24 for additional information concerning immunosuppressants.)

Side Effects Common side effects of immunosuppressants include sore throat, cough, dizziness, nausea, muscle aches, fever, chills, itching, and headache. These effects are usually mild to moderate. Taking acetaminophen can alleviate some of these effects if they are bothersome.

Rare but serious effects include changes in heart rhythm or blood pressure, chest pain, unusual bleeding, bruising, anemia, and hyperlipidemia. Therefore, patients taking these agents need close monitoring for cardiac function and periodic blood tests. Some evidence in studies shows that long-term immunosuppressant use may increase the risk of cancer.

Contraindications Azathioprine is contraindicated in pregnancy and in patients with rheumatoid arthritis and a history of treatment with alkylating agents. Cyclosporine is contraindicated in patients with a hypersensitivity to polyoxyethylated castor oil.

Cautions and Considerations Because these agents suppress the immune system, patients taking them are at an increased risk of infection. Patients are often instructed to take special precautions to minimize exposure to infection. They may be directed to wear face masks and stay out of crowded public areas. Of course, frequent hand washing to prevent disease is recommended.

Checkpoint 18.4

Take a moment to review what you have learned so far and answer these questions.

1. What classes of drugs are used to treat nausea and vomiting?

2. What drugs are used to treat IBS?

3. What is the difference between Crohn disease and ulcerative colitis?

Herbal and Alternative Therapies

Ginger can be used to reduce nausea associated with surgery, vertigo, and motion sickness. This supplement has shown some benefit in pregnant women with morning sickness but has not undergone rigorous safety testing in this patient population. The exact mechanism of action of ginger is unknown, but it may exert its effects by inhibition of serotonin receptors (5-HT3) in a manner similar to that of other antiemetics. The standard dose for preventing nausea and vomiting is 500–1,000 mg. Ginger may cause heartburn, gas, bloating, mouth and throat irritation, and diarrhea. Because ginger has antiplatelet effects, its use should be avoided in patients taking aspirin, warfarin, or other anticoagulants (see Chapter 16).

Probiotics are products that contain live cultures of yeast or bacteria. They are not herbal products or dietary supplements. Probiotics are used as nonpharmacologic adjunctive treatment for diarrhea, constipation, *H. pylori* infection, and antibiotic-induced diarrhea. They may even be used to treat diarrhea associated with rotavirus, Crohn disease, ulcerative colitis, and IBS. Probiotic organisms are not pathogenic and are commonly available in capsules, powders, beverages, or yogurts, some of which need to be refrigerated to keep the microorganisms alive. These products are used to colonize the GI tract with beneficial organisms for digestion and regular GI motility.

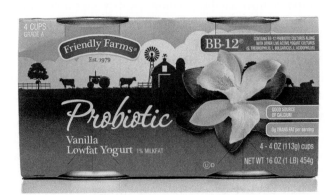

Probiotic yogurt contains beneficial microorganisms to help individuals digest food and maintain regular GI motility.

These bacteria compete with harmful bacteria, hopefully replacing or displacing them. They may enhance the immune response to pathogenic organisms and break down toxins. Patients with poor immune system function should not use probiotic products. Doses vary based on the product and indication.

Lactobacilli are gram-positive bacteria that are normal flora of the human GI tract. Common lactobacilli products contain *Lactobacillus acidophilus*, *Lactobacillus helveticus*, *Lactobacillus bulgaricus*, and *Lactobacillus rhamnosus*. Lactobacilli products are taken each day, divided into three or four doses. They are usually well tolerated with few side effects, the most common of which are gas and bloating.

Saccharomyces boulardii (S. boulardii) is a yeast organism that lives in the human GI tract. This organism can be found in Florastor, a brand-name product that is used for the prevention of antibiotic-associated diarrhea. Typically, 250–500 mg of Florastor is taken two to four times a day. *S. boulardii* can cause gas, bloating, and constipation.

Bifidobacteria agents are not as well studied as lactobacilli and *S. boulardii* products. However, they might be effective for diarrhea associated with a variety of causes. Doses vary based on specific products and indications. As with other probiotics, bifidobacteria are well tolerated in general but have the potential to cause gas and bloating.

Chapter Review

Chapter Summary

Diarrhea, constipation, and hemorrhoids are common complaints from patients seeking self-treatment in the pharmacy. These disorders can be caused by many factors, including infection, food poisoning, medication, and chronic conditions. Diarrhea can be treated with OTC medications such as loperamide, diphenoxylate/atropine, and bismuth subsalicylate. Drugs that relieve constipation are known as laxatives and come in many varieties. Some take a few days to work, whereas others produce a bowel movement in less than an hour. Hemorrhoids are treated with topical agents.

GERD and PUD are caused by irritation and damage to the esophagus, stomach, or small intestine from stomach acid. GERD produces heartburn and is usually caused by eating large meals, fatty or spicy foods, or certain medications. PUD is usually caused by a bacterial organism called *H. pylori*, or drugs such as NSAIDs. PPIs and H2 blockers treat both GERD and PUD by increasing the pH of the stomach. If a patient has PUD secondary to *H. pylori* infection, he or she needs antibiotics in addition to a PPI or H2 blocker. Antacids are commonly used for GERD to relieve heartburn associated with meals.

Nausea and vomiting are common problems associated with motion sickness, food poisoning, and anesthesia for surgery. In addition, they are common side effects of medications, most notably chemotherapy agents. Anticholinergic antiemetics are used to treat mild nausea and vomiting. General antiemetics such as promethazine are given to hospital patients who become nauseated. Patients taking chemotherapy are given powerful antiemetics known as 5-HT3 receptor antagonists.

Other problems of the GI tract include IBS, Crohn disease, and ulcerative colitis. IBS is a chronic disease that results in frequent and painful constipation or diarrhea. Dietary treatment should be tried before initiating drug therapy. Drug treatment includes psyllium, PEG, linaclotide, lubiprostone, loperamide, alosetron, bile acid sequestrants, and antispasmodic agents. Crohn disease and ulcerative colitis involve inflammation of the GI tract and cause chronic diarrhea. Drug treatment includes corticosteroids, immunosuppressants, and aminosalicylates.

Herbal and alternative products that may supplement GI functioning include ginger, probiotics, and products containing lactobacilli, *S. boulardii*, and bifidobacteria agents.

Chapter Checkup

The Navigator+ learning management system that accompanies this textbook offers many opportunities to help you master chapter content, including end-of-chapter exercises, a glossary of key terms, flash cards, and additional interactive activities.

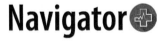

Career Exploration

If you enjoyed learning about the gastrointestinal system in this chapter, you may want to explore the following career options:

- certified clinical nutritionist
- computed tomography (CT) technician
- diagnostic sonographer
- endoscopy technician
- magnetic resonance imaging (MRI) technician
- medical assistant
- nuclear medicine technologist
- pharmacy technician
- registered dietitian

Nutrition and Drugs for Metabolism

Pharm Facts

- In addition to relieving stress, crying has other beneficial effects. Tears contain a high concentration of manganese, a trace element involved in metabolic and enzymatic reactions in the body. Elevated levels of manganese can cause nervousness, anxiety, and irritability. Crying lowers these levels, thus improving a person's mood.

- Originally, vitamins were named alphabetically. However, after moving through the beginning of the alphabet, scientists then discovered that vitamin B was not a single substance but rather a complex of various substances. Consequently, vitamin B was assigned numbers: *vitamin B_1, vitamin B_2,* etc. The numbering of B vitamins is also out of numeric order because some substances initially identified as members of the B complex were not accurate and, thus, were removed.

- The human body can produce only three vitamins from sources other than diet: vitamin B_7, vitamin D, and vitamin K.

"More than ever before, individuals are taking charge of their own health and using the wealth of information and technology available to individualize their nutritional approach. Much of this information, however, contains conflicting messages about the foods they need to eat—thus leading to confusion. Registered dietitians who understand and can communicate the science of nutrition and metabolism can resolve this confusion and help individuals achieve optimal health."

—**Lindsey Schnell**, MS, RD
Registered Dietitian

Learning Objectives

1 Describe the basic physiology of nutrition and weight management, including the intake of essential vitamins and minerals.

2 Explain the therapeutic effects of vitamins and minerals.

3 Identify recommended adequate intakes and common doses of vitamin and mineral products.

4 Describe the disorders associated with overnutrition and undernutrition.

5 Explain the therapeutic effects of prescription medications and nonprescription medications used to treat obesity.

6 Identify the generic names, brand names, indications, dosage ranges, side effects, contraindications, and cautions and considerations associated with the drugs that are commonly used to treat obesity.

7 Describe parenteral and enteral nutrition therapies.

8 Identify common herbal and alternative therapies that are related to the treatment of obesity.

P roper nutrition is important to an individual's overall health and well-being. Although some allied health professionals specialize in nutrition or dietetics, the majority of allied health personnel will likely need a working knowledge of nutrition, including its associated disorders and drug therapies. Whether taking a patient's health history; gathering height and weight measurements to calculate body mass index (BMI); handling prescription drugs or over-the-counter (OTC) nutrition-related drugs or supplements; or answering patients' questions about dietary supplements, allied health workers will likely be addressing patients' nutritional concerns.

Dietary supplements, in particular, are garnering quite a bit of patient interest. According to a 2013 Government Accountability Office report, dietary supplements are taken by more than 50% of US adults. Consequently, allied health professionals must have access to useful, up-to-date, and reliable nutritional information to help patients navigate a variety of nutrition-associated products and services.

This chapter describes the roles of essential vitamins and minerals; discusses the contributing factors and physiologic processes that affect nutritional status; addresses nutritional disorders such as obesity and malnutrition and their common pharmacologic therapies; and explains the use of alternative feeding methods to achieve optimal nutrition.

Nutritional Needs of the Body

Micronutrients are materials that are essential to human health, development, and growth. In most cases, micronutrients cannot be synthesized by the body and must be supplied through an individual's diet. They play a crucial role in prevention and treatment of disease, as well as the optimization of physical and mental functioning.

Micronutrients

Micronutrients are substances such as vitamins and minerals that are essential for the growth of a living organism. They play a key role in many metabolic processes, such as supporting coenzyme and cofactor production. For a given micronutrient, there is a range of intakes between inadequate, which can lead to clinical deficiency, and excess, which can lead to toxicity. Between these extremes is a level of adequate micronutrient intake that sufficiently supports normal health.

To help provide information on sufficient micronutrient intake, the US Department of Agriculture (USDA) and the Institute of Medicine publish **dietary reference intakes (DRIs)** of macronutrients (proteins, carbohydrates, and fats) and micronutrients (vitamins and minerals). The purpose of the DRIs is to serve as a practical guide for healthcare professionals to assess and plan for the nutrient needs of individuals. DRIs include reference values for nutrition and comprise four different categories: **estimated average requirements**, **recommended dietary allowances (RDAs)**, **adequate intakes (AIs)**, and **tolerable upper intake levels**.

Recommended values of micronutrients are often reported by mass, frequently in the metric system as milligrams (mg) or micrograms (mcg). Package labels for micronutrients may list measurements by mass or by using **international units (IUs)**. IUs are units of measurement developed for each substance based on its biologic effect. For example, vitamin E exists in a number of different forms, with each form having different biologic activity. Rather than specifying the precise type and mass of vitamin E in a preparation, the biologic activity is presented in IUs. It is important to read labels and dosing information carefully to get the appropriate amounts of micronutrients. There are cases when individual needs of micronutrients are higher or lower than those recommended by the USDA. For instance, when a patient has a deficiency of a particular vitamin or mineral, intake may need to be higher to replenish lost stores.

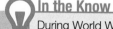

In the Know

During World War II, the National Academy of Sciences was tasked with providing recommendations on nutrient intake. At the time, food was in short supply, and the US government needed guidance on the amounts of nutrients needed for its citizens. The recommendations provided by the National Academy of Sciences were called the *recommended dietary allowances* or *RDAs*. The RDAs have received numerous updates since World War II, and they recently were replaced with the dietary reference intakes (DRIs). The DRIs provide a more complete set of nutritional information and include, among other things, information provided previously by the RDAs.

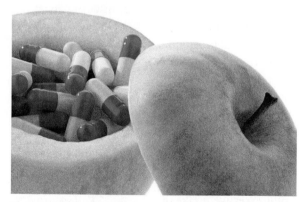

The body better absorbs nutrients from fresh fruits and vegetables—most of which provide a multitude of vitamins and minerals—than from supplements.

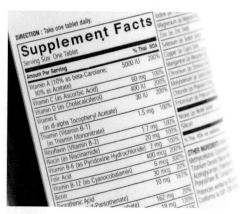

Vitamin supplement labels show measurements by mass (mg or mcg) or by IUs.

Vitamins

A **vitamin** is an organic substance that is required in the diet in small amounts for the maintenance of normal metabolic integrity. Deficiency of a particular vitamin causes disease that can be cured only by restoring adequate physiologic levels of that vitamin. Vitamin deficiency can be diagnosed based on clinical signs and symptoms and by interpretation of specially ordered laboratory test results. Vitamins generally do not have contraindications, except in the case of hypersensitivity and evidence of vitamin toxicity.

Fat-Soluble Vitamins

Fat-soluble vitamins are absorbed with dietary fats and are maintained in stores in the body. Deficiency usually develops only after several months of restricted intake. It is possible to ingest too much of a fat-soluble vitamin, which leads to excessive levels and toxicity. Fat-soluble vitamins include vitamins A, D, E, and K; their DRI values are shown in Table 19.1.

TABLE 19.1 DRI Values for Fat-Soluble Vitamins

Vitamin	DRIs for Men	DRIs for Women
A (as retinol activity equivalents)	900 mcg	700 mcg
D (as cholecalciferol)	15 mcg	15 mcg
E (as alpha-tocopherol)	15 mg	15 mg
K (as phytonadione)	120 mcg*	90 mcg*

Red type indicates that the value is an RDA; an asterisk indicates that the value is an AI.

Source: USDA's National Agricultural Library

Vitamin A

Vitamin A is actually a family of compounds referred to as **retinoic acids**. Vitamin A can be found in two forms: provitamin A carotenoids such as beta-carotene and preformed vitamin A such as retinol, retinal, retinoic acid, and retinyl esters. Vitamin A is needed for vision, growth, bone formation, reproduction, immune system function, and skin health.

Provitamin A carotenoids must be metabolized into active vitamin A via a highly regulated process. Provitamin A carotenoids can be found in green, leafy vegetables; sweet potatoes; and carrots. Because the conversion to active vitamin A is regulated on an as-needed basis by the body, excessive intake of provitamin A is unlikely to cause toxicity.

In the Know

IUs are often used to describe vitamins A, D, and E on supplement and food labels. There are different guidelines for converting milligrams (mg) to IU for each vitamin's specific form. For example, the conversion of 3,000 IU of vitamin A supplied as retinol would be 900 mcg; the conversion of 3,000 IU of vitamin A supplied as beta-carotene would be 1.8 mg.

Preformed vitamin A is more active and is found mostly in animal sources and supplements. Liver, kidney, egg yolk, and butter are common food sources of preformed vitamin A. Absorption and storage of preformed vitamin A are efficient, and toxicity can occur if excessive quantities are ingested.

Carrots and sweet potatoes are great sources of beta-carotene. In fact, the compound beta-carotene gives these vegetables their orange color.

Indications for Vitamin A Supplementation

Vitamin A supplements are used primarily to treat deficiency. Deficiency is rarely seen in the United States but is the third most common nutritional deficiency in the world. Vitamin A deficiency may result in **keratomalacia**, a softening and ulceration of the cornea of the eye. Signs and symptoms of keratomalacia include corneal degeneration, night blindness, and dry eyes. Other manifestations of vitamin A deficiency include poor bone growth, dermatologic problems, and impairment of the immune system.

Vitamin A is also used in the treatment of cataracts and for reducing complications of human immunodeficiency virus (HIV), measles, and malaria.

Vitamin A Toxicity Excessive intake of vitamin A, usually from ingestion of preformed vitamin A, may cause toxicity. Signs and symptoms of vitamin A toxicity include nausea, vomiting, vertigo, blurry vision, hair loss, headache, irritability, skin peeling, and bone and liver problems.

Vitamin A can be highly teratogenic, especially in the first trimester of pregnancy, and can lead to spontaneous abortions and fetal malformations. The USDA suggests an RDA of 750 mcg (as retinol activity equivalents) of vitamin A during pregnancy. Doses in excess of this dietary allowance are contraindicated in pregnant women.

Name Exchange

Topical vitamin A, also known as *tretinoin*, is sold by prescription under the names Avita, Renova, Retin-A, and Tretin-X. This medication is used for a variety of dermatologic issues including acne, fine wrinkles, hyperpigmentation, and skin roughness.

Vitamin D

Vitamin D, or **calciferol**, was first identified in the early twentieth century as a vitamin and is now recognized also as a hormone. Vitamin D and its metabolites play an important role in maintaining calcium and phosphate levels in the body. There is evidence to suggest that vitamin D plays a role in insulin resistance, obesity, metabolic syndrome, and various cancers.

Vitamin D has two major forms: ergocalciferol (vitamin D_2) and cholecalciferol (vitamin D_3). **Ergocalciferol** is largely human-made and added to foods. **Cholecalciferol** is synthesized in the skin in response to sunlight and can be consumed in the diet through the intake of animal-based foods. Sunlight usually provides 80%–90% of the body's vitamin D stores. Both forms of vitamin D are made commercially and can be found in dietary supplements or fortified foods.

There are few naturally occurring food sources of vitamin D. These sources include fatty fish, fish liver oil, and egg yolks.

Indications for Vitamin D Supplementation Vitamin D is used to treat **rickets**, a childhood disease in which a lack of vitamin D results in bone softening and muscle weakness. A hallmark of rickets is bowlegs. Vitamin D can also be used to treat **osteomalacia**, a disorder of bone that is manifested by bone pain, muscle weakness, difficult walking, and fracture.

Vitamin D Toxicity Excessive intake of vitamin D can lead to toxicity. Signs and symptoms of vitamin D toxicity include high blood calcium levels, kidney stones, nausea, vomiting, thirst, increased urination, muscle weakness, and bone pain.

Vitamin E

The physiologic role of **Vitamin E**, or **tocopherol**, is still being defined; it is thought to work as an antioxidant. Vitamin E is found in a variety of food products including oils; meat; eggs; and green, leafy vegetables. The form that is best known for its role in human health, alpha-tocopherol, is abundant in olive oil and sunflower oil. Gamma-tocopherol can be found in soybean oil and corn oil.

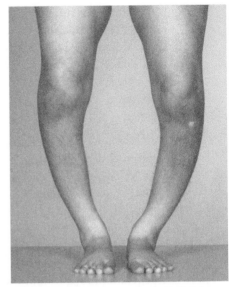

Rickets is caused by a vitamin D deficiency. This deficiency softens the bones, causing the legs to bow outward from the weight of the body.

Indications for Vitamin E Supplementation Vitamin E deficiency rarely occurs, except in cases of specific genetic or malabsorption disorders. Vitamin E deficiency can cause neuromuscular disorders, fragile red blood cells (RBCs), and hemolysis, and it may be treated with supplementation.

Laboratory studies support the use of vitamin E in the treatment of macular degeneration and Alzheimer's disease. Vitamin E also has been shown to reduce the risk of some cancers and dementia and to improve immune system function. Other indications for the use of vitamin E include diabetic retinopathy and cardiovascular disease. Topical use of vitamin E can improve skin health, healing, and hydration.

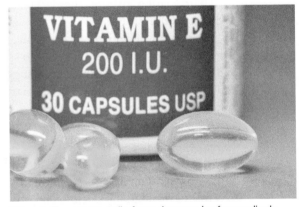

Vitamin E protects cells from damage by free radicals and boosts the body's immune system.

Vitamin E Toxicity Very high doses of vitamin E may result in bleeding or stroke.

Vitamin K

Vitamin K functions as a coenzyme for the hepatic production of blood-clotting factors and for bone metabolism. Dietary forms of vitamin K (phylloquinone and phytonadione) are found in green, leafy vegetables such as spinach, broccoli, and Brussels sprouts, and in fats such as plant oils and margarine.

Indications for Vitamin K Supplementation Vitamin K deficiency is rare in otherwise healthy adults. Signs and symptoms of vitamin K deficiency usually are associated with impaired coagulation (such as easy bruising, mucosal bleeding, melena, and hematuria).

Therefore, vitamin K is administered in situations where blood clotting is desired. One of these situations is the reversal of warfarin, a common anticoagulant.

Another indication for the administration of vitamin K is in cases of deficiency caused by drug therapy (for example, salicylates, sulfonamides, quinine, quinidine, and broad-spectrum antibiotics). Vitamin K injection may also be administered to neonates.

Vitamin K Toxicity Vitamin K toxicity is rare. Signs of toxicity include anemia and jaundice.

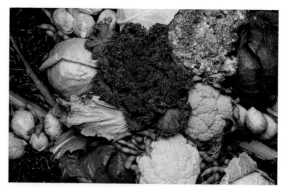

Vitamin K can be found naturally in many commonly consumed vegetables, including broccoli, cauliflower, and cabbage.

Patient Teaching

Allied health professionals should instruct their patients who are taking warfarin, a common anticoagulant, to monitor their intake of foods rich in vitamin K. These foods include green, leafy vegetables (broccoli, spinach, cabbage, turnip greens, parsley, lettuce, kale, and endive) as well as blueberries, blackberries, and avocados. Most patients can consume these foods as long as they keep their intake consistent.

Water-Soluble Vitamins

Water-soluble vitamins are easily excreted from the body in the urine; consequently, other than occasional incidents of stomach upset or diarrhea, toxic levels of these vitamins are difficult to achieve. Examples of water-soluble vitamins include the B vitamins: B_1 (thiamine), B_2 (riboflavin), B_3 (niacin), B_5 (pantothenic acid), B_6 (pyridoxine), B_7 (biotin), B_9 (folate or folic acid), and B_{12} (cyanocobalamin). Vitamin C (ascorbic acid) is also considered a water-soluble vitamin. The DRI values of water-soluble vitamins are shown in Table 19.2.

TABLE 19.2 DRI Values of Water-Soluble Vitamins

Vitamin	DRIs for Men	DRIs for Women
B_1 (thiamine)	1.2 mg	1.1 mg
B_2 (riboflavin)	1.3 mg	1.1 mg
B_3 (niacin)	16 mg	14 mg
B_5 (pantothenic acid)	5 mg*	5 mg*
B_6 (pyridoxine)	1.3 mg	1.3 mg
B_7 (biotin)	30 mcg*	30 mcg*
B_9 (folate or folic acid)	400 mcg	400 mcg
B_{12} (cyanocobalamin)	2.4 mcg	2.4 mcg
C (ascorbic acid)	90 mg	75 mg

Red type indicates that the value is an RDA; an asterisk indicates that the value is an AI.

Source: USDA's National Agricultural Library

Vitamin B$_1$

Vitamin B$_1$, or **thiamine**, is an important coenzyme involved in carbohydrate metabolism. It also plays a role in nerve impulse propagation. Thiamine is found in food products such as yeast, legumes, pork, rice, and cereals. Thiamine, however, is denatured at high temperatures, and cooking, baking, canning, and pasteurization can destroy it.

Indications for Vitamin B$_1$ Supplementation Thiamine supplements are used to treat vitamin B$_1$ deficiency. Signs and symptoms of vitamin B$_1$ deficiency include impaired memory, lactic acidosis, visual disturbances, and mental status changes. Thiamine deficiency is most common during pregnancy and in **Wernicke-Korsakoff syndrome**, which can occur in patients who abuse alcohol. Patients with known alcohol abuse may be given thiamine supplements when hospitalized to combat symptoms of alcohol withdrawal. In addition, thiamine supplements are used to treat patients who have **beriberi**, a disease that results from a diet low in vitamin B$_1$. Beriberi presents with numbness and tingling, edema, and heart failure.

Vitamin B$_2$

Vitamin B$_2$, or **riboflavin**, is a coenzyme involved in tissue respiration and normal cell metabolism. Riboflavin is found in many foods such as cereal, green vegetables, milk, and some meats. It is also made in the intestines by bacteria.

Indications for Vitamin B$_2$ Supplementation Riboflavin is usually used to treat vitamin B$_2$ deficiency, but it can also be used in doses of 400 mg a day to decrease migraine headaches. Signs of vitamin B$_2$ deficiency include mucositis, skin rash, cracked lips, photophobia, tearing, poor vision, poor wound healing, and anemia.

Vitamin B$_3$

Vitamin B$_3$, or **niacin**, is essential for reactions in the body that produce **adenosine triphosphate (ATP)**, a critical molecule in cellular energy production. The two most common forms of niacin are nicotinic acid and nicotinamide. Niacin also helps regulate production and activity of cholesterol molecules in the blood. Vitamin B$_3$ is found in yeast, peanuts, peas, beans, whole grains, potatoes, and lean meats.

Indications for Vitamin B$_3$ Supplementation Niacin is most frequently used to treat patients with **dyslipidemia**, a condition signified by elevated total or low-density lipoprotein (LDL) cholesterol levels or low levels of high-density lipoprotein (HDL) cholesterol. It lowers triglycerides and LDL levels and raises HDL levels. The dose required for these effects is at least 1,200–1,500 mg a day.

In addition, niacin supplements are used to treat vitamin B$_3$ deficiency. This deficiency may result from the use of certain medications such as isoniazid, 5-fluorouracil, pyrazinamide, 6-mercaptopurine, hydantoin, ethionamide, phenobarbital, azathioprine, and chloramphenicol.

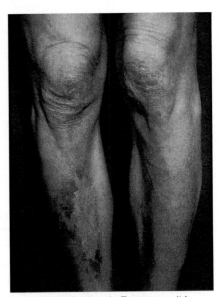

A deficiency in vitamin B$_3$ can result in pellagra. Signs of this disorder include cracked, inflamed areas on exposed skin.

In the Know

Some individuals theorize that the myth of vampires stems from a deficiency of niacin that results in pellagra. Although rare today, pellagra was common years ago before complete nutrition sources were readily available. Its symptoms—including sensitivity to sunlight, swollen mouth, and dementia—are thought to mimic those associated with vampires.

A deficiency in vitamin B_3 may result in **pellagra**, a disease that presents with hyper-pigmented rash in areas of exposed skin, red tongue, swelling of the mouth and tongue, diarrhea, sensitivity to light, and neurologic symptoms such as insomnia, anxiety, and disorientation. Pellagra often develops in patients who have certain gastrointestinal (GI) diseases or alcoholism.

Patient Teaching

Niacin products commonly cause flushing, hot flashes, and a sensation of prickly skin. Some prescription formulations slow the release and absorption of niacin, thereby reducing this effect. However, these side effects are still quite common and can be the reason patients stop taking niacin. To avoid these effects, remind patients to take the supplement with food or, with prescriber approval, to swallow an aspirin 30 minutes prior to taking niacin. In addition, recommend that patients take niacin at bedtime so that if flushing occurs, the patient is less likely to be bothered by it while sleeping.

Vitamin B_5

Vitamin B_5, or **pantothenic acid**, is a precursor to coenzyme A. Coenzyme A has an important role in the synthesis of many molecules such as vitamins A and D, cholesterol, steroids, heme, fatty acids, amino acids, and proteins. Vitamin B_5 is found in walnuts, whole grains, potatoes, chicken, beef, egg yolk, liver, kidney, broccoli, and milk. Pantothenic acid can also be produced by bacteria in the colon.

Indications for Vitamin B_5 Supplementation Pantothenic acid supplements are usually used to treat vitamin B_5 deficiency. Signs of deficiency include paresthesia, dysesthesia, fatigue, malaise, headache, insomnia, vomiting, and abdominal cramps.

Vitamin B_6

Vitamin B_6, or **pyridoxine**, is converted in the body to the coenzymes responsible for amino acid metabolism. Common forms include pyridoxine, pyridoxal, and pyridoxamine. Pyridoxine and pyridoxamine are predominantly found in plant-based foods such as vegetables, whole grains, and nuts. Pyridoxal is most commonly derived from animal foods. Cooking, processing, and storage can reduce vitamin B_6 levels by up to 50%.

Indications for Vitamin B_6 Supplementation
Pyridoxine is used to treat vitamin B_6 deficiency. Signs of deficiency include skin rash, nerve pain, loss of reflexes, convulsions, and anemia. Other indications for vitamin B_6 supplements include certain types of anemia and seizure disorders. Pyridoxine is also given to alcoholic patients with nerve damage and to patients who take isoniazid for tuberculosis because isoniazid depletes vitamin B_6.

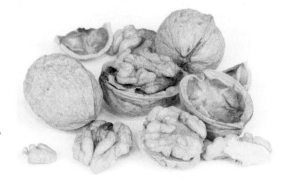

Walnuts are a good source of pantothenic acid.

Vitamin B$_7$

Vitamin B$_7$, or **biotin**, a coenzyme involved in metabolism, plays an essential role in many processes including cell replication. Biotin can be found in a variety of plants (particularly peanuts and green, leafy vegetables), liver, egg yolk, soybeans, and yeast.

Indications for Vitamin B$_7$ Supplementation Biotin supplements are taken for vitamin B$_7$ deficiency. Signs of deficiency include skin rash, hair loss, change in hair color, depression, tiredness, hallucinations, and numbness and tingling. Biotin deficiency is typically associated with altered absorption, such as short-bowel syndrome. Consumption of large quantities of raw egg whites can also lead to biotin deficiency.

Vitamin B$_9$

Vitamin B$_9$, also known as **folic acid** or **folate**, plays a major role in intracellular metabolism and the breakdown of **homocysteine**, an amino acid associated with cardiovascular disease. It is also involved in the production of the neurotransmitter serotonin. Folic acid is frequently added to foods but is naturally found in green, leafy vegetables; fruits; cereals; grains; and red meat.

Indications for Vitamin B$_9$ Supplementation
Folic acid supplements are used to treat vitamin B$_9$ deficiency. Signs of deficiency include anemia, diarrhea, and a swollen or painful tongue. A lack of vitamin B$_9$ also has a deleterious effect on the cardiovascular system and is associated with a higher risk of coronary heart disease, stroke, and peripheral vascular disease.

Deficiencies in folic acid cause anemia and neural tube defects in a developing fetus; consequently, folic acid supplements are highly recommended for all women who are pregnant or planning to get pregnant. Taking folic acid can greatly reduce the incidence of some birth defects.

To reduce homocysteine levels, vitamin B$_9$ supplements are also used to treat patients with end-stage kidney disease. Other uses include treatment for chronic fatigue syndrome, depression, and vitiligo.

The Centers for Disease Control and Prevention (CDC) recommends that women take folic acid at least one month prior to conception, and that they continue the supplement throughout pregnancy. Folic acid has been shown to prevent neurologic birth defects.

Vitamin B$_{12}$

Vitamin B$_{12}$, or **cyanocobalamin**, is a coenzyme necessary for cell reproduction, normal growth, and RBC production. It is found in fish, milk, bread, and meats. Intestinal absorption of vitamin B$_{12}$ requires intrinsic factor, which is produced in the stomach. Patients who have undergone a gastrectomy will need to take lifelong vitamin B$_{12}$ injections due to their lack of intrinsic factor production.

Indications for Vitamin B$_{12}$ Supplementation Cyanocobalamin deficiency takes a long time to develop and is easily treated with supplements. It is most common in older adults and strict vegetarians. Signs of B$_{12}$ deficiency include anemia, swollen or painful tongue, and nerve pain and degeneration.

Other indications for cyanocobalamin supplements are pernicious anemia and end-stage renal disease.

Vitamin C

Vitamin C, or **ascorbic acid**, is best known for its role in immune system function and as an antioxidant. **Antioxidants** are substances that can prevent cell damage caused by free radicals and are thought to be protective. Vitamin C is found in citrus fruits, tomatoes, potatoes, Brussels sprouts, cauliflower, broccoli, strawberries, blueberries, cabbage, and spinach.

Indications for Vitamin C Supplementation Small doses (100–250 mg a day) of vitamin C supplements are used to treat deficiency. Signs of deficiency include poor wound healing, fatigue, and depression. Vitamin C is most effective for treating a severe deficiency known as **scurvy**, a disease rarely seen in the United States. Scurvy presents with fatigue, anemia, hemorrhages, nosebleeds, spongy gums, and enlargement of hair follicles. Other indications for vitamin C supplements are macular degeneration, seasonal allergies, improved iron absorption, and protein metabolism in premature infants.

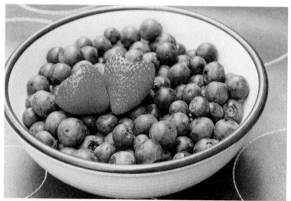

Many individuals also take large doses of vitamin C supplements (1–3 g a day) to prevent illness, such as the common cold, with some individuals taking the vitamin as part of their drug regimen for prevention of cancer, atherosclerosis, and sunburn. However, they should be aware that high doses of supplemental vitamin C may increase their risk for kidney stones.

Strawberries and blueberries are high in antioxidants, substances that have been proven to prevent cardiovascular disease and keep individuals "heart healthy."

Checkpoint 19.1

Take a moment to review what you have learned so far and answer these questions.

1. What are the fat-soluble vitamins and their DRI values?

2. What are the water-soluble vitamins and their DRI values?

3. What are the dietary sources of vitamin K?

Trace Minerals

A **trace mineral** is a metallic substance found in minimal amounts in the human body. Trace minerals play a significant role in cellular structure and are required for physiologic function. These minerals are present in food as well as produced naturally in the body. Because trace minerals are integral to basic metabolic processes, deficiencies or excesses can cause significant morbidity. Mineral deficiencies can be measured with specially ordered laboratory tests. A diagnosis of deficiency usually starts with clinical presentation of signs and symptoms. Trace minerals generally do not have contraindications, except in the case of a hypersensitivity and evidence of toxicity. Most side effects of trace element supplements result from excess intake and mimic conditions of toxicity.

TABLE 19.3 DRI Values of Trace Minerals

Trace Mineral	DRI for Men	DRI for Women
Chromium	35 mcg*	25 mcg*
Copper	900 mcg	900 mcg
Iodine	150 mcg	150 mcg
Iron	8 mg	18 mg
Manganese	2.3 mg*	1.8 mg*
Selenium	55 mcg	55 mcg
Zinc	11 mg	8 mg

Red type indicates that the value is an RDA; an asterisk indicates that the value is an AI.

Source: USDA's National Agricultural Library

The recommended daily intake of trace minerals is relatively low and typically easy to obtain through normal food consumption (see Table 19.3). Supplements are used primarily as additives to enteral and parenteral nutrition formulas (see the section titled "Enteral and Parenteral Nutrition" for more information).

Chromium

Chromium is part of a complex of molecules called **glucose tolerance factor**, which helps regulate glucose tolerance and insulin levels. It is found in grains, cereals, fruits, vegetables, and processed meats.

Indications for Chromium Supplementation True deficiency in chromium usually occurs only in patients with malnutrition. Other patients at risk for chromium deficiency include those with short-bowel syndrome, burns, traumatic injuries, or those receiving parenteral nutrition without trace mineral supplementation. Signs of deficiency include glucose intolerance, peripheral neuropathy, weight loss, elevated LDL cholesterol levels, and glucose in the urine. (For more information on parenteral nutrition, see the section titled "Enteral and Parenteral Nutrition.")

Chromium levels are low in many patients with diabetes, but its role in diabetes is not fully understood. Chromium picolinate is taken in doses of 200–400 mcg a day to improve glucose tolerance and control in Type 1 and Type 2 diabetes. However, unless the patient is extremely deficient (which is rare), the clinical effect may not be noticeable. Glucose tolerance improves during chromium supplementation, but patients do not find that they can eliminate drug or insulin therapy for diabetes. Chromium has not been found to be useful in prediabetes to prevent the onset of this condition.

Chromium Toxicity Excessive intake of chromium may result in skin or nasal lesions, skin rash, or lung cancer.

Copper

Copper is a catalyst and coenzyme in a wide variety of chemical reactions in the body. Without it, RBC and white blood cell counts decline, causing anemia, leukopenia, and neutropenia. More than half of dietary copper in Western diets comes from food products such as vegetables, grains, and seeds. Smaller amounts come from meat, fish, and poultry.

Indications for Copper Supplementation Copper supplementation is used almost exclusively for cases of deficiency. Copper deficiency is rare and usually encountered only in patients who are receiving long-term parenteral nutrition without trace mineral supplementation. Signs of copper deficiency include neutropenia, leukopenia, anemia, osteoporosis, hair or skin depigmentation, anorexia, diarrhea, mental status changes, and high cholesterol. Acquired copper deficiency can occur in patients with gastrectomy or gastric bypass surgery, chronic diarrhea or other malabsorptive condition, chronic dialysis, and excessive zinc ingestion.

Copper Toxicity Signs of copper toxicity include diarrhea, vomiting, a metallic taste in the mouth, and cirrhosis.

Iodine

Iodine is used in the body to make thyroid hormones, which regulate metabolic rates. Iodine is found in highest concentrations in seafood and seaweed and is added to salt in developed countries.

Indications for Iodine Supplementation Iodine supplements are used to treat deficiency, a condition that is more commonly seen in underdeveloped countries. This deficiency may cause **goiter**, or thyroid gland enlargement. Other signs of deficiency include hypothyroidism, neuromuscular problems, deafness, decreased mental function, and bone softening/slowed growth. Iodine is also used to treat some thyroid conditions and for radiation emergencies in which radioactive iodides have been used.

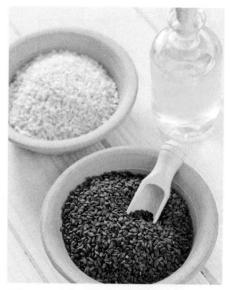

Although both white and black sesame seeds are good sources of copper, unhulled black sesame seeds are also rich in calcium. Black sesame seeds have a nuttier taste and are a staple of Asian and Middle Eastern cuisines.

> **In the Know**
>
> Did you know that iodine might have made the United States smarter? In the early twentieth century, goiter was prevalent in the Pacific Northwest and regions near the Great Lakes. The Swiss practice of adding iodine to table and cooking salt was adopted in the United States, and iodized salt was commercially available across the country. A report later published in a paper for the National Bureau of Economic Research associated introduction of iodinated salt with a national average IQ increase of 3.5 points.

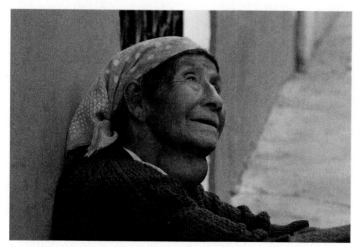

A swollen thyroid gland may indicate a diet that is deficient in iodine.

Iodine Toxicity Signs of iodine toxicity include a metallic taste in the mouth, sore teeth and gums, irritation of the mouth and throat, toxic thyroid, upset stomach, diarrhea, weight loss, tachycardia (rapid heartbeat), muscle weakness, fever, and infertility.

Iron

Iron is found in hemoglobin inside RBCs and myoglobin in muscles. It is a cofactor for neurotransmitter production and is a part of the functional groups of many important enzymes. Without iron, the production of RBCs is diminished, and the oxygen-carrying capacity of RBCs is reduced. Most people first think of red meat, poultry, and fish as sources of iron. Other sources of iron include whole-grain cereals, spinach, walnuts, and green peas.

Indications for Iron Supplementation Iron is used to treat **anemia of chronic disease** and **iron-deficiency anemia**. Two common signs of anemia are weakness and fatigue. Other signs include pallor, weakness, a swollen or painful tongue, headache, difficulty swallowing, fingernail changes, and numbness or tingling. Iron supplements may cause significant constipation. Therefore, some formulations contain a stool softener to lessen this unwanted side effect.

Iron Toxicity Too much iron may cause a liver condition called **hemochromatosis**. Other signs of iron toxicity are cirrhosis, heart problems, pancreatic damage, and changes in skin pigmentation.

Manganese

Manganese is a cofactor in many metabolic and enzymatic reactions in the body. Some believe it is involved in the development of osteoporosis. Manganese is found in nuts; legumes; seeds; tea; whole grains; and green, leafy vegetables.

Indications for Manganese Supplementation Manganese supplements are used to treat deficiency. Signs of deficiency include nausea, vomiting, skin rash, hair color changes, low cholesterol, growth retardation, and problems with carbohydrate or protein metabolism.

Manganese Toxicity Manganese toxicity can occur in workers who are exposed to manganese aerosols or dust (such as welders) and in individuals who have consumed well water with high manganese concentrations. Signs of manganese toxicity include changes in gait when walking, loss of balance, irritability, hallucinations, and changes in libido.

Selenium

Selenium is a metallic trace element that is incorporated into amino acids; it plays a role in multiple biologic functions. Selenium reduces oxidative stress in the body. Seafood, kidney, liver, and other animal protein are often good sources of selenium. Although grains and seeds may contain selenium, the amount varies based on the selenium content of the soil in which they were grown.

Indications for Selenium Supplementation Selenium deficiency is associated with skeletal muscle dysfunction, enlarged heart, and mood disorders. Historically, trace element mixtures added to parenteral nutrition did not include selenium; consequently, patients who were administered long-term parenteral nutrition therapy developed selenium deficiency.

Selenium Toxicity Signs of selenium toxicity include nausea, vomiting, hair and nail loss, tooth decay, skin lesions, irritability, fatigue, and peripheral neuropathy.

Zinc

Zinc is a cofactor in many physiologic processes, including the synthesis of DNA and protein. It plays an important role in immune function, wound healing, blood clotting, reproduction, and appropriate growth. Zinc is found in nuts, legumes, meat, seafood, dairy products, and whole grains.

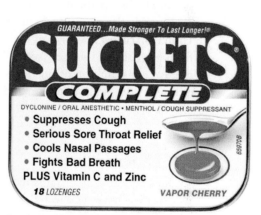

Indications for Zinc Supplementation Zinc supplements are used to treat deficiency, boost immune function, aid wound healing, and treat Wilson's disease. Zinc lozenges are used to reduce the symptom severity and length of the common cold. Zinc is also used topically to heal burn and skin wounds. Zinc supplements may cause nausea, vomiting, diarrhea, and a metallic taste in the mouth.

Studies have shown that zinc lozenges may slightly reduce the duration of the common cold if they are taken when symptoms first arise. This effect may be due to zinc's inhibition of rhinovirus replication.

Zinc Toxicity Signs of zinc toxicity are upset stomach, nausea, dizziness, and decreased HDL cholesterol levels.

Kolb's Learning Styles

For those of you who enjoy outside-of-the-box learning activities and entertainment, as Divergers do, develop a news story (either written or videotaped) on the claims made about the use of supplements to cure disease. Although scientific literature does not always support these claims, the media and the Internet heighten awareness with anecdotal stories about miraculous cures. You can see how easy it is for patients to become enamored of such products. Be sure to report both sides of the issue. Present your findings in class and invite feedback from students regarding your information.

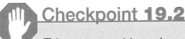

Checkpoint 19.2

Take a moment to review what you have learned so far and answer these questions.

1. What are the signs of copper toxicity?

2. What are the manifestations of iodine deficiency?

Nutritional Status

Maintenance of adequate nutrition involves both external and internal physiologic processes, and it is typically assessed by a variety of factors including an individual's height and weight. Comparing an individual's actual body weight (ABW) with his or her ideal body weight (IBW) is one method (see discussion on ABW and IBW below). The best indicator of nutritional status in children is appropriate growth (including height and weight by age). **Growth charts** with population averages are used to determine whether a child is growing appropriately for his or her age, gender, and development. The 50th percentile for a particular age on a growth chart is considered ideal.

Outside the range of adequate nutrition are undernutrition and overnutrition. **Undernutrition** is a form of malnutrition resulting from a reduced supply of food or from an inability to digest, assimilate, and use necessary nutrients. **Overnutrition** is the overconsumption of nutrients and food to the point at which health is adversely affected. Both undernutrition and overnutrition are associated with deleterious health effects.

ABW and IBW

Evaluating nutritional status requires comparing what is considered "normal" body weight for a patient's age and development with the patient's **actual body weight (ABW)**. An individual within the normal range generally shows no signs of nutritional deficiency and maintains an appropriate body weight and makeup for his or her age and frame size.

Ideal body weight (IBW) is the weight for a given height that is associated with maximum longevity and health. IBW is calculated in adults as follows:

Men: IBW (kg) = 50 + (2.3 × height in inches over 5 feet)

Women: IBW (kg) = 45.5 + (2.3 × height in inches over 5 feet)

TABLE 19.4 Evaluating ABW

Undernutrition	ABW < 70% IBW	Severe malnutrition
	ABW 70% to 80% IBW	Moderate malnutrition
	ABW 80% to 90% IBW	Mild malnutrition
Normal	ABW 90% to 120% IBW	Normal
Overnutrition	ABW 120% to 150% IBW	Overweight
	ABW 150% to 200% IBW	Obese
	ABW ≥ 200% IBW	Morbidly obese

As mentioned previously, comparing a patient's ABW with the IBW is a basic method for assessing nutritional status (see Table 19.4). ABW is typically used to calculate weight-based doses unless patients are overweight and, in some cases, underweight.

BMI

Another way to assess appropriate weight for height is to calculate **body mass index (BMI)**. BMI is used to identify both undernutrition and overnutrition. Table 19.5 shows the general interpretations of BMI that have been accepted by most healthcare practitioners. Due to increased muscle mass, certain individuals (such as bodybuilders and athletes) may not be considered overweight until their BMI reaches higher levels. In children and adolescents, the BMI calculation is slightly different and takes into account age and gender differences. In these age-groups, BMI must be compared to averages in growth in order to be interpreted correctly.

$$\text{BMI (adults)} = \frac{\text{weight (kg)}}{[\text{height (m)}]^2}$$

Caloric Needs

Good nutritional status is maintained through appropriate energy intake and expenditure. Typically, energy intake is measured in **calories** (kcal/kg). Maintaining caloric balance over time is important to maintaining a healthy weight. Appropriate daily caloric needs depend on age, gender, weight, and activity level, and various formulas exist to approximate goals. In general, an intake of 25 kcal/kg of body weight a day is usually adequate to

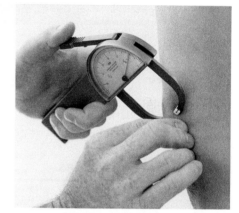

BMI is an indicator of an individual's body fat. Other assessments to determine body fat may include skinfold thickness measurements obtained with calipers.

TABLE 19.5 Evaluating BMI

Age-Group	BMI (kg/m²)	Interpretation
Adults	< 16.00	Severe thinness
	16.00–16.99	Moderate thinness
	17.00–18.49	Mild thinness
	18.50–24.99	Normal range
	25.00–29.99	Pre-obese or overweight
	30.00–34.99	Obese class I
	35.00–39.99	Obese class II
	≥ 40.00	Obese class III
Children and Adolescents	BMI for age < 5th percentile	Underweight
	BMI for age 5th to 85th percentile	Healthy
	BMI for age 85th to 95th percentile	Overweight
	BMI for age 95th percentile or higher	Obese

Source: World Health Organization's Global Database on Body Mass Index

maintain the basal metabolic rate in adults. Malnourished and critically ill patients need more calories.

Macronutrients

In addition to calories, the body needs appropriate amounts of macronutrients. **Macronutrients** are substances consumed in larger quantities than micronutrients; they provide bulk energy. The main macronutrients are carbohydrates, proteins, and fats. The USDA suggests that total caloric intake should be broken down by percentage of macronutrient intake (see Table 19.6).

TABLE 19.6 USDA Macronutrient Recommendations*

Macronutrients	Recommended Percentage of Total Daily Calories
Carbohydrates	45%–65%
Proteins	10%–35%
Fats	20%–35%

* The USDA macronutrient guidelines are currently under review. Check with your instructor regarding any updates to the information in this table.

Source: US Department of Agriculture and US Department of Health and Human Services. 2010. *Dietary Guidelines for Americans.*

Carbohydrates

Carbohydrates are often referred to as sugars or starches. Their primary role is to provide energy to cells in the body, notably the cells of the brain. Due to a lack of information, the USDA does not recommend a specific daily allowance of carbohydrates. Carbohydrates are often rated based on their **glycemic index**, or the food's effect on an individual's blood glucose level. It has been suggested that one way of achieving a healthy diet is to replace high-glycemic-index carbohy-

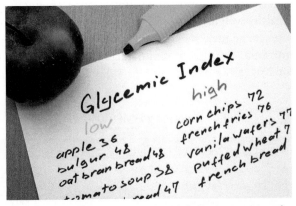

To maintain a healthy diet, an individual may want to refer to a list of low- and high-glycemic-index foods.

drates with low-glycemic-index ones. Examples of high-glycemic-index carbohydrates include white bread, pancakes, baked white potatoes, candy, and white rice. Examples of low-glycemic-index carbohydrates include fruits and vegetables.

Proteins

Proteins are a necessary component of all cells in the body. Proteins are made up of amino acids that contain nitrogen in their chemical structure. The RDA of proteins suggested by the USDA for healthy adult men and women is 0.8 g/kg. However, protein needs vary depending on age, disease state, and clinical condition. For instance, older adults need relatively more protein to compensate for the lean muscle mass lost with advancing age. In patients with wounds or severe burns, healing and tissue growth is a high priority, and adequate protein is needed to form the building blocks for tissue regeneration. On the other hand, protein intake may be restricted in patients with kidney or liver failure because nitrogen cannot exit the body normally. Albumin, prealbumin, and transferrin are proteins in the blood; these can be measured with the use of laboratory tests to assess a patient's protein and nutritional status. Lower than normal amounts of any of these substances in the blood usually indicate malnutrition.

Fats

Fats are an energy source for the body, and they aid in absorption of vitamins A, D, E, and K as well as carotenoids. Due to insufficient data, the USDA does not recommend a specific RDA of fats. However, an acceptable range of 20%–35% of daily calories is suggested. The type of fat consumed is important to health status. **Trans fats** and **saturated fats** appear to have deleterious health effects with no known health benefits and have been associated with cardiovascular disease. Conversely, there is some evidence to support health benefits of **omega-3 fatty acids** (such as those found in oily fish), for example, in the reduction of cardiovascular disease.

Checkpoint 19.3

Take a moment to review what you have learned so far and answer these questions.

1. What BMI is considered normal for adults?
2. What is the equation for IBW for men?
3. What is the equation for IBW for women?

Nutritional Disorders

Nutrition is an important component of health and wellness. When an individual receives too much or too little of the daily caloric, protein, or micronutrient needs for his or her age and size, overnutrition (obesity) or undernutrition (malnutrition) can result. Both obesity and malnutrition can have negative health impacts and result in higher morbidity and mortality. According to the World Health Organization, global obesity has more than doubled since 1980, and more than 1.9 billion adults were overweight in 2014. Once a problem associated with high-income countries, obesity is now on the rise in low- and middle-income countries. In fact, most of the world's population lives in countries where being overweight kills more people than being underweight. Malnutrition, however, is still a major concern. It is estimated that malnutrition contributes to more than one-third of child deaths worldwide.

Obesity

Obesity is a condition characterized by the excessive accumulation and storage of fat in the body. Obesity is a major healthcare concern. The CDC estimates that in 2010 nearly 70% of adults and 32% of children in the United States were overweight. The CDC also reports that more than one-third of the population in the United States is obese. This statistic has climbed over the past few decades. Obesity in adults is most commonly defined using BMI (see Table 19.5). If a patient's BMI is 30 or higher, the patient is considered *obese*.

Environmental factors that contribute to obesity include leading a sedentary lifestyle, having a readily available food supply, and consuming increased amounts of fats and refined sugars and decreased amounts of fruits and vegetables. In the United States, these environmental factors are readily apparent: Food portion sizes are large in comparison with those in other industrialized countries, and the lifestyle of many individuals has become sedentary, as technology has taken over many manual labor tasks.

Genetic correlation is a major factor in obesity and the distribution of body fat. For instance, obesity among first-degree relatives (parents and siblings) is a strong predictor of obesity in adulthood.

Physiologic factors affect appetite control. Peptides such as leptin and incretins as well as neurotransmitters such as serotonin, norepinephrine, and dopamine are involved in **satiety**, the sensation of feeling full and satisfied. As weight and adipose (fat) tissue accumulate, it is thought that normal release and sensitivity to these hormones and neurotransmitters are affected. Other physiologic contributors include medical conditions such as hypothyroidism and Cushing's syndrome. Certain drugs, such as corticosteroids, also cause fat redistribution and appetite changes that foster weight gain.

Obesity is associated with serious health risks and mortality (see Table 19.7). **Centrally distributed fat** is adipose tissue that accumulates in the abdominal area, rather than in the hips, thighs, or buttocks. This kind of fat distribution is linked to heart disease and diabetes. Obese people also have greater rates of depression and psychological disturbances. Consequently, preventing and treating obesity is an important effort within health care. Reducing body weight has been shown to reduce morbidity and mortality in overweight and obese patients.

Drug Regimens and Treatments

The preferred treatment for obesity is lifestyle intervention, a combination of diet and exercise, and behavior modification. Initial treatment should create a caloric deficit by reducing caloric intake and/or increasing caloric expenditure. Patients who restrict caloric intake and also perform physical activity will lose weight. Some individuals find these interventions difficult. Changes must be permanent to keep off lost weight. Consequently, providing products and services for weight loss and physical fitness is a billion-dollar industry.

FIGURE 19.1 | Prevalence of Self-Reported Obesity among US Adults by State and Territory, 2013

Prevalence estimates reflect BRFSS methodological changes started in 2011. These estimates should not be compared to prevalence estimates before 2011.

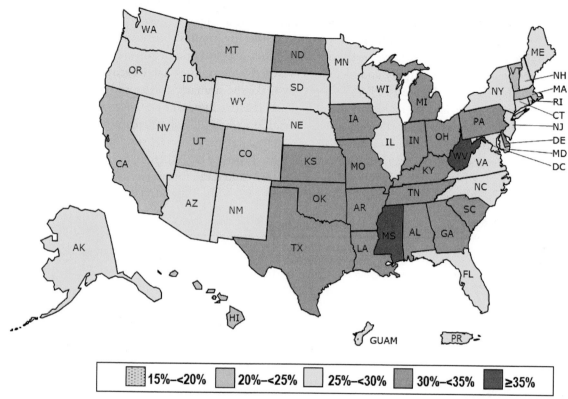

| | 15%–<20% | | 20%–<25% | | 25%–<30% | | 30%–<35% | | ≥35% |

Source: Behavioral Risk Factor Surveillance Systems (BRFSS), CDC.

TABLE 19.7 | Comorbid Conditions of Obesity

Breast and colon cancer	Hypertension
Congestive heart failure	Inflammatory disorders
Coronary artery disease	Obstructive airway disease
Degenerative bone and joint disease	Osteoarthritis
Depression	Polycystic ovarian syndrome
Eating disorders	Pulmonary hypertension
Gallbladder inflammation	Skin tags, stretch marks, and other dermatologic problems
Gastroesophageal reflux disorder	Sleep apnea
Hiatal hernia	Stroke
High cholesterol	Type 2 diabetes

Special diets tend to restrict specific components of nutrition to achieve weight loss. Popular weight-loss programs include those that restrict the intake of carbohydrates and/or fats. These programs are not often sustainable because they do not represent a balanced way to eat that ensures adequate nutrition in the long term. The most successful and healthy diets are those that restrict caloric intake while maintaining a proper balance of nutrients.

Some patients are candidates for more aggressive therapy options. Medications and/or surgical intervention can achieve significant weight loss. Surgical options are collectively referred to as **bariatric surgery** and include (1) restrictive procedures (**laparoscopic or gastric banding** [see Figure 19.2]) that effectively make the stomach smaller and prevent excess food intake, and (2) malabsorptive techniques (**gastric bypass**) that bypass parts of the intestine, thus preventing nutrients from foods from being fully absorbed. Whether surgical or drug therapy is chosen for weight loss, patients must first meet specific criteria. Usually, surgical methods are limited to patients with a BMI of 40 or higher. Some patients with a BMI of 30 or higher will be considered candidates for surgery if they have comorbid health conditions.

| **FIGURE 19.2** | Laparoscopic or Gastric Banding |

One type of bariatric surgery involves the placement of a gastric band around the stomach. This band restricts the size of the stomach, thereby promoting weight loss in morbidly obese patients.

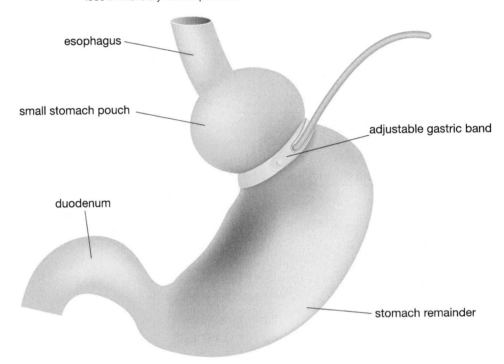

Lipase Inhibitors

Medications that are commonly used to treat obesity are lipase inhibitors. As the name suggests, **lipase inhibitors** work by binding to gastric and pancreatic lipase enzymes in the intestines, thereby preventing the enzymes from breaking down fats into a form that can be absorbed. Fat then passes through the intestines and out of the rectum, where it is excreted in stool. Orlistat, a commercially available lipase inhibitor, is available over the counter and by prescription. It is taken three times a day with each meal that contains fat (see Table 19.8).

TABLE 19.8 Lipase Inhibitors

Generic (Brand)	Dosage Form	Route of Administration	Common Dosage	Dispensing Status
Orlistat (Alli)	Capsule	Oral	60 mg with each meal	OTC
Orlistat (Xenical)	Capsule	Oral	120 mg with each meal	Rx

Side Effects Common side effects of orlistat include fatty or oily stools, fecal incontinence or urgency, gas, and diarrhea. These effects may decrease over time. Patients can reduce or avoid these effects by limiting fat intake to less than 30% of total calories. If not, they may find the side effects become intolerable.

Contraindications Orlistat is contraindicated in chronic malabsorption syndrome, cholestasis, and pregnancy.

➕ *Note: Allied health professionals should be aware that an allergy to a particular drug contraindicates its use. This warning applies to all Contraindications sections in this chapter.*

Cautions and Considerations Because orlistat interferes with the absorption of fat, it can also prevent absorption of fat-soluble vitamins. Patients should take multivitamin supplements to combat potential vitamin deficiency.

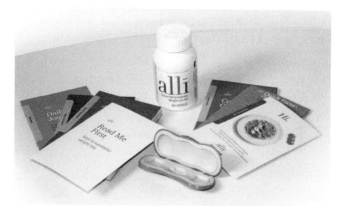

Orlistat is sold over the counter under the brand name Alli.

Sympathomimetic Drugs

One class of drugs used to treat obesity, **sympathomimetics**, stimulates the central nervous system (CNS) as much as amphetamines do. These medications are used in conjunction with exercise, behavior modification, and reduced caloric intake to produce weight loss in patients with a BMI of 30 or higher (or over 27 with the presence of other risk factors, such as high blood pressure, diabetes, or high cholesterol). The sympathomimetics stimulate dopamine and norepinephrine and prevent reuptake of serotonin. Increased neurotransmitter levels signal a sense of satiety. In effect, patients do not feel as hungry. Fast-acting dosage forms are taken 30 minutes to 1 hour prior to eating, and long-acting forms are taken once a day (see Table 19.9).

Side Effects Common side effects of sympathomimetics are headache, stomachache, insomnia, nervousness, tachycardia, and irritability. Taking these medications in the morning may help reduce insomnia, but other effects can be limiting if they are bothersome. Sympathomimetics can also cause dry mouth, difficulty urinating, and constipation. Patients with urinary problems should not take these medications, and drinking plenty of water can help with these effects. In men, sympathomimetics can cause impotence. Patients should discuss the risks versus benefits of sympathomimetics with their healthcare practitioners.

A possible serious side effect of sympathomimetics is **serotonin syndrome**, a condition causing a dangerous rise in blood pressure and heart rate. In fact, deaths have occurred

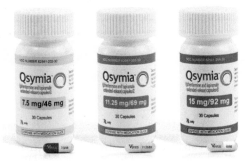

Qsymia, a sympathomimetic drug, was formerly known by the brand name Qnexa. The Food and Drug Administration (FDA) asked the manufacturer to change the brand name to avoid potential mix-ups with other, similar-sounding drug names.

TABLE 19.9 Common Sympathomimetic Drugs

Generic (Brand)	Dosage Form	Route of Administration	Common Dosage
Benzphetamine (Didrex, Regimex)	Tablet	Oral	25–50 mg 1–3 times a day
Diethylpropion	Tablet	Oral	25 mg 3 times a day (1 hour prior to meals)
Phendimetrazine (Bontril)	Capsule, tablet	Oral	35 mg 2–3 times a day (1 hour prior to meals)
Phentermine (Adipex-P, Suprenza)	Capsule, tablet	Oral	15–37.5 mg once a day (2 hours prior to breakfast)
Combination Product			
Phentermine/topiramate (Qsymia)	Capsule	Oral	Phentermine 7.5 mg/topiramate 46 mg once a day

from this syndrome when it is linked to the use of appetite suppressants. These medications should not be taken with other drugs that also increase serotonin (for example, antidepressants). Cardiac function must be closely monitored. Some patients with cardiovascular problems may not be good candidates for this class of medications.

Contraindications The sympathomimetics are contraindicated in patients with coronary heart disease, high blood pressure, hyperthyroidism, and in patients with a history of drug abuse.

Cautions and Considerations All CNS stimulants are controlled substances (Schedules II–IV) and have addiction and abuse potential. For Schedule II stimulants, no refills are allowed, and limited amounts can be dispensed at one time. Patients must be informed that a new prescription is needed each time they need a refill.

Serotonin Agonists

Serotonin is a neurotransmitter that can affect mood, social behavior, sleep, memory, sexual desire, and appetite and digestion. It is manufactured in the brain and intestines and generally reduces food intake in animals and human beings. **Serotonin agonists** activate serotonin receptors and therefore reduce appetite and food intake. Lorcaserin, the serotonin agonist available in the United States, may be used in addition to a reduced-calorie diet and exercise regimen in patients with a BMI of 30 or higher (or 27 or higher with the presence of other risk factors, such as high blood pressure, diabetes, or high cholesterol). Lorcaserin is taken twice a day, with or without food (see Table 19.10).

Side Effects Common side effects of serotonin agonists include headache, upper respiratory infection, back pain, dizziness, and nausea.

Contraindications Lorcaserin is contraindicated in pregnancy and in patients with renal dysfunction.

Cautions and Considerations Lorcaserin-induced weight loss may pose risks in patients who are taking oral medications to treat Type 2 diabetes. In these patients, weight loss may increase the risk for hypoglycemia; therefore, dose reduction of diabetes medications may be warranted. Lorcaserin should not be continued if it is not efficacious, meaning it should be discontinued in patients who do not lose 5% of body weight after 12 weeks of drug therapy.

Serotonin syndrome is a risk with serotonin agonist use. Lorcaserin should not be used in combination with medications that increase serotonin activity. For example, many types of antidepressants—such as selective serotonin reuptake inhibitors (SSRIs), serotonin-norepinephrine reuptake inhibitors (SNRIs), bupropion, tricyclic antidepressants (TCAs), and monoamine oxidase inhibitors (MAOIs)—should not be taken concurrently with lorcaserin.

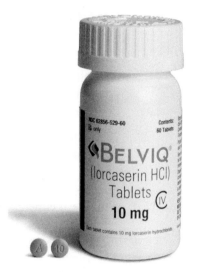

Belviq is a Schedule IV prescription weight-loss medication used to treat obesity. Patients who take this drug must continue this therapy for life; once discontinued, appetite and food consumption return to their high levels.

TABLE 19.10 Serotonin Agonist

Generic (Brand)	Dosage Form	Route of Administration	Common Dosage
Lorcaserin (Belviq)	Tablet	Oral	10 mg twice a day

Glucagon-Like Peptide Receptor Agonists

Glucagon-like peptide is a gastric hormone that stimulates glucose-dependent insulin secretion and inhibits glucagon release and gastric emptying. It acts as a regulator of appetite and caloric intake. **Glucagon-like peptide receptor agonists** act similarly to endogenous glucagon-like peptide, and there is evidence to suggest these medications decrease body weight through decreased caloric intake. Liraglutide, a glucagon-like peptide receptor agonist, is indicated as an adjunct to a reduced-calorie diet and increased physical activity for long-term weight management in adults with a BMI of 30 or higher (or 27 or higher with the presence of other risk factors, such as high blood pressure, diabetes, or high cholesterol). Liraglutide is approved by the FDA and is available as a solution for subcutaneous injection (see Table 19.11).

TABLE 19.11 Glucagon-Like Peptide Receptor Agonist

Generic (Brand)	Dosage Form	Route of Administration	Common Dosage
Liraglutide (Saxenda)	Solution for injection	Sub-Q	3 mg a day

Side Effects Liraglutide may cause nausea, hypoglycemia, diarrhea, constipation, vomiting, headache, decreased appetite, dyspepsia, fatigue, dizziness, abdominal pain, and increased lipase.

Contraindications Liraglutide is contraindicated in patients with a personal or family history of medullary thyroid carcinoma or multiple endocrine neoplasia type 2. Liraglutide should not be used by pregnant patients.

Cautions and Considerations Because liraglutide can cause insulin secretion, it should be used cautiously with other secretagogues. There may be an increased risk of thyroid tumors with use, and patients should be counseled about their symptoms. Liraglutide has been associated with acute pancreatitis and gallbladder disease. Patients should discontinue use if either of these conditions is suspected or confirmed.

Checkpoint 19.4

Take a moment to review what you have learned so far and answer these questions.

1. What drug classes are used to treat obesity?

2. Which drug used to treat obesity is available without a prescription?

Malnutrition

Malnutrition is a lack of adequate nutrient intake to supply basic metabolic needs. It can be related to an overall lack of calorie or protein consumption, or it may be associated with a deficiency in a specific micronutrient (for example, a vitamin or mineral). Malnutrition is most prevalent in underdeveloped countries. Children living in these poorer nations are especially vulnerable to malnutrition. They often develop **marasmus**, a chronic condition caused by inadequate caloric and protein intake over a prolonged period. Muscle and fat tissue wasting is observed, a condition known as **cachexia**. Individuals in these underdeveloped countries are also at risk for **kwashiorkor**, a condition in which caloric intake is adequate but protein intake is deficient. These patients, paradoxically, usually appear well nourished because heightened metabolic rates break down protein stores but leave adipose tissue intact. However, patients may acquire fluid accumulation in the abdomen, hands, face, and feet.

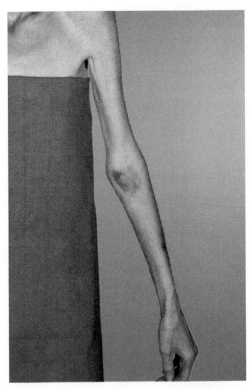

Often patients with malnutrition appear to be wasting away, a condition called *cachexia*.

In the United States, malnutrition is most often encountered in the inpatient setting, where it is associated with disease states, acute illness, and even drug therapy. Some causes for malnutrition include the following:

- anorexia
- food allergies/intolerance
- chronic infection or inflammatory conditions
- cancer
- endocrine disorders
- pulmonary disease
- cirrhosis of the liver
- renal failure
- nausea, vomiting, or diarrhea
- trauma, burns, or sepsis
- inflammatory bowel disease, Crohn disease, or short-bowel syndrome
- inadequate parenteral or enteral nutrition
- psychiatric or psychological conditions

Signs of malnutrition include weight loss, skin changes (too dry, shiny, or scaly), hair loss, fatigue, poor wound healing, pallor (pale skin), sunken eyes, dry mouth and eyes, visible loss of muscle mass, and fluid accumulation in the abdomen or around the ankles and tailbone.

Drug Regimens and Treatments

Vitamins and minerals are used to either treat or prevent malnutrition. Because caloric and protein requirements increase in critically ill patients, treatment must focus on meeting patients' heightened nutritional needs. Individuals with long-term chronic conditions, fever, or sepsis must have their caloric needs increased from 25 kcal/kg a day to 30–40 kcal/kg a day. Patients who are recovering from major surgery, trauma, or burns also must have an increase in their daily caloric needs. For these patients who have wounds, healthcare personnel must pay particular attention to their protein and amino acid intake because wound healing requires proteins, the building blocks of new tissue.

An individual cannot go longer than 7 to 10 days without food or nutrition; malnutrition will ensue and negatively affect health outcomes. When a patient cannot be fed normally, alternative methods of supplying nutrition must be employed. Enteral nutrition and parenteral nutrition are artificial ways to feed patients that do not involve swallowing.

Enteral Nutrition

Enteral nutrition is a method of feeding a patient liquid nutrients through a tube inserted into the GI tract. The tube can be inserted manually or surgically. A nasogastric (NG) tube is manually inserted. A gastrostomy (G) tube and a jejunostomy (J) tube are placed surgically in the stomach and jejunum, respectively (see Figure 19.3). A liquid nutrient formula is put through the tube, either in bolus doses to mimic eating a meal or continuously with an enteral pump.

FIGURE 19.3 | **Enteral Feeding Tube Sites**

NG tubes are uncomfortable for patients, so such tubes are suitable for only short-term use. If enteral feeding is necessary for more than a few days, a G tube or J tube will be placed surgically.

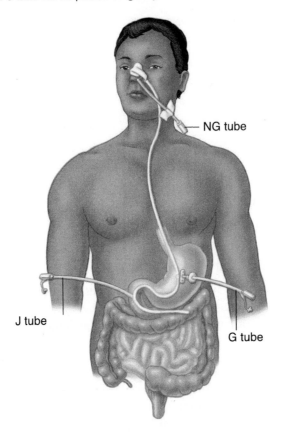

Indications for enteral feeding include bowel obstruction, short-bowel syndrome, and Crohn disease. Patients in long-term care who are unable to swallow foods voluntarily because of a severe stroke or prolonged coma may have an enteral feeding tube placed to supply them with adequate nutrition. In addition to an enteral feeding formula, water can also be given via an enteral tube to maintain a patient's hydration status.

Specialized enteral feeding products are available for specific conditions, so patients must be matched with appropriate formulas. Healthcare personnel should never administer enteral nutrition through an intravenous (IV) line. These preparations are neither sterile nor formulated for that use. Enteral feeding is preferred to parenteral feeding because it keeps the GI tract functional and prevents abdominal infections.

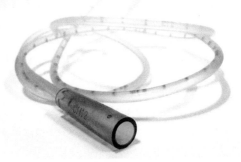

An NG tube, also known as a Levin tube, is made from lightweight polyurethane material and is inserted manually through a nostril and threaded down the esophagus and into the stomach. This tube delivers liquid nutrients to a patient.

Parenteral Nutrition

Parenteral nutrition (often referred to as **total parenteral nutrition [TPN]**) is provided by feeding a patient through an IV line. TPN is used when the digestive tract cannot be used at all. Indications for TPN include severe burns, intolerance to enteral feeding, anorexia nervosa (refusal to eat), pancreatitis, severe gallbladder disease, inflammatory bowel disease, and severe diarrhea. TPN may also be necessary in pregnancy, acquired immunodeficiency syndrome (AIDS), and cancer.

TPN carries risks for complications. TPN is complex in that it supplies all the fluids, electrolytes, nutrients (carbohydrates, proteins, and fats), vitamins, and minerals that a patient needs through a vein. If an essential nutrient or trace element is not included, a patient can easily become nutritionally deficient or imbalanced. Regular laboratory monitoring is necessary to guide TPN therapy and protect against infection. Special care must be taken when adding trace minerals to a TPN formula because of the heightened risk of underdosing or overdosing these elements.

Mixing of a TPN Formula Parenteral nutrition can be supplied commercially or it can be compounded, usually by a pharmacist or a specially trained pharmacy technician. Careful calculations and mixing techniques must be used to ensure that the end product is both safe and appropriate for an individual patient.

When preparing a TPN formula, the order of mixing is important. Some electrolytes and trace minerals must be added separately to reduce the chance of precipitating out of solution. When minerals precipitate out of solution, they bind together and form visible clumps or specks of material. These specks could block capillary blood flow and endanger the patient if introduced through an IV line. Vitamins are usually added to the solution last, just before administration.

Proper agitation and mixing of each TPN bag is also important to ensure even concentrations throughout. TPN bags are large, so this mixing requires special effort. TPN solutions can be infused temporarily through a peripherally inserted central catheter (PICC) line, but they are most often administered through a surgically placed central line because they are **hypertonic** (they have a higher concentration and osmolality than blood plasma).

TPN solutions can be mixed in two ways: two-in-one and three-in-one mixtures. **Two-in-one TPN mixtures** contain only proteins (amino acids) and carbohydrates (dextrose); **three-in-one TPN mixtures** contain proteins and carbohydrates plus lipids (fats). Patients receiving TPN will need all

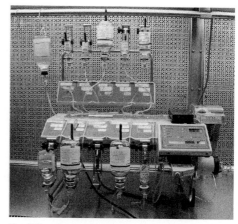

Facilities that prepare large numbers of TPN solutions each day use a special automated device called a *micronutrient compounder*. This device automatically injects vitamins, minerals, and electrolytes into the TPN solution.

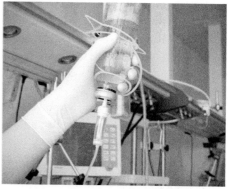

Physicians and pharmacists work closely with registered dietitians and nurses to monitor the patient for appropriate TPN therapy.

Quick Study

To remember the difference between parenteral and enteral nutrition, just break down the words. The suffix *-enteral* means "relating to or affecting the intestines." Therefore, enteral nutrition goes through the intestines. The prefix *para-* means "around or outside." Therefore, parenteral nutrition goes around or takes place outside of the intestines.

three nutrient components (carbohydrates, proteins, and lipids), but adding the lipids into the same bag poses complications. In particular, lipids are cloudy and hide the appearance of precipitates, and TPN solutions with lipids are less stable and do not last as long as those with only proteins and carbohydrates.

Checkpoint 19.5

Take a moment to review what you have learned so far and answer these questions.

1. What are the causes of malnutrition?

2. What are the key differences between enteral nutrition and parenteral nutrition?

Herbal and Alternative Therapies

Fiber is a natural substance in fruits and vegetables. It can also be found in psyllium husk, beans, oat bran, legumes, and flaxseeds. Fiber creates a sense of fullness and speeds GI motility, thus limiting fat and calorie absorption. Alone, it may not produce significant weight loss, but fiber can contribute to an overall diet program that results in weight loss. Patients can increase the fiber content of their diet by eating more fruits and vegetables (and reducing meat and carbohydrates). Fiber can also be ingested via supplements. In addition, fiber has been found to produce laxative effects, lower cholesterol, and promote colon health.

Ephedra (also known as *ma huang*) is currently banned from sale in the United States because serious effects and deaths have occurred following the use of ephedra. This natural supplement is a CNS stimulant with anorexiant effects.

Drug Alert

Ephedra was connected with the death of a young baseball pitcher for the Baltimore Orioles in 2003. This news story prompted efforts to remove ephedra from the market. The FDA banned the sale of ephedra supplements in 2004.

Chapter Review

Chapter Summary

Proper nutrition is important for health and wellness and includes the adequate intake of micronutrients (such as vitamins and trace minerals) and macronutrients (carbohydrates, proteins, and fats). Failure to ingest adequate amounts of either substance can lead to deficiency and physiologic consequences. Vitamins are either fat-soluble or water-soluble. A lack of vitamins can cause illness, whereas an excess of vitamins tends to occur only with fat-soluble vitamins, which accumulate in fatty tissue and may cause illness as well. Trace minerals are needed in small quantities only but play a significant role in wellness. The USDA publishes DRIs for many micronutrients. Macronutrients are required in larger quantities, and the USDA suggests percentages of total calories that each should comprise.

Nutritional status is often assessed by BMI or comparison of ABW to estimated IBW. Overnutrition (obesity) and undernutrition (malnutrition) are serious health conditions and can lead to significant morbidity and mortality. Obesity occurs when excess nutrition results in a body composition that has too much fat tissue. Treatment for obesity usually begins with diet and lifestyle changes but may progress to drug therapy if the obesity is severe. Medications for obesity include lipase inhibitors, sympathomimetics, serotonin agonists, and glucagon-like peptide agonists. Lipase inhibitors are available as prescription and OTC products. They are easy to use but do come with undesirable side effects if the patient does not follow a low-fat diet. Sympathomimetics are CNS stimulants and are controlled substances because they can be addictive. They also can have significant cardiovascular side effects, so they are used only for patients with a BMI of 30 and higher (or over 27 with the presence of other risk factors, such as high blood pressure, diabetes, or high cholesterol). Serotonin agonists may increase feelings of fullness but may also increase the risk for serotonin syndrome. Glucagon-like peptide agonists may decrease caloric intake and increase feelings of fullness.

Malnutrition (or undernutrition) results from a lack of appropriate intake or from disease states that affect absorption or digestion. When malnutrition is a problem, enteral and parenteral nutrition may be needed. Enteral nutrition is feeding patients through a tube placed in the digestive tract. Parenteral nutrition is feeding patients through an IV. Special considerations and preparations are involved in both products.

Finally, fiber is a natural diet supplement that can promote weight loss. Allied health professionals can help educate patients about nutrition and drugs for obesity so that patients can make informed decisions about their health care.

Chapter Checkup

The Navigator+ learning management system that accompanies this textbook offers many opportunities to help you master chapter content, including end-of-chapter exercises, a glossary of key terms, flash cards, and additional interactive activities.

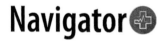

Navigator

Career Exploration

If you enjoyed learning about nutrition and its associated disorders in this chapter, you may want to explore the following career options:

- certified clinical nutritionist
- clinical dietitian specialist
- medical assistant
- pharmacy technician

- registered dietetic technician
- registered dietitian
- weight consultant

The Endocrine System and Drug Therapy

Pharm Facts

- Two of the major stress hormones in the body, cortisol and adrenaline, may adversely affect the immune system. However, the levels of both hormones decline with laughter.

- The term *hormone* comes from the ancient Greek root word *hormon*, which means "to set in motion."

- The adrenal glands shrink as a human ages. For a fetus in the seventh month of development, the glands are similar in size to the kidneys. In an elderly individual, the glands are almost imperceptible.

- Although the majority of the body's hormones are secreted by endocrine glands, other organs and tissues secrete additional hormones. Ghrelin, a hormone released by the stomach, is an appetite stimulant that signals the brain that you are hungry. Leptin, a hormone secreted by fat cells, is an appetite suppressant. Both of these "hunger hormones" play a role in energy balance, appetite, and weight gain.

"Diabetes is a complicated, labor-intensive, chronic illness, and individuals diagnosed with diabetes provide 99% of their own care. When they arrive for my diabetes education class, they are overwhelmed by their diagnosis. Management of diabetes requires them to change their eating habits, increase their physical activity, monitor their blood glucose, take their medications as ordered, go to the eye doctor, check their feet daily, keep a detailed diary, problem solve, and manage their stress. My job is to customize a diabetes self-care plan that fits into their lives. My joy comes from empowering them to live long, healthy lives with diabetes."

—**Kathy Warwick**, RD, CDE

Registered Dietitian and
Certified Diabetes Educator

Learning Objectives

1 Understand the basic anatomy and physiology of the endocrine system.

2 Describe the common conditions that affect the endocrine system.

3 Explain the therapeutic and adverse effects of prescription medications and nonprescription medications commonly used to treat diseases of the endocrine system.

4 Identify the generic names, brand names, indications, dosage ranges, side effects, contraindications, and cautions and considerations associated with the drugs commonly used to treat the endocrine system.

5 Identify common herbal and alternative therapies that are related to the endocrine system.

The endocrine system regulates many different body functions and includes several different glands. This chapter focuses on the normal structure and function of the endocrine system as well as the common disorders that affect this body system. These disorders include diabetes, thyroid disorders, and adrenal gland disorders. Pharmacologic options for treating diabetes are expanding, so these drug classes are covered in depth. Glucose monitoring systems are also mentioned because they are the key tools used by patients to manage their disease. Thyroid disorders are common and easily treated with drug therapy. Adrenal and pituitary gland disorders affect hormone production. Treatment with drug therapy is useful for normalizing hormone levels and alleviating unwanted effects of these disorders.

Anatomy and Physiology of the Endocrine System

Work Wise

An endocrinologist is a physician who specializes in hormone-related disorders. Because hormones affect several body systems, these internists work as members of a multidisciplinary team in the healthcare setting. For example, endocrinologists work in tandem with dietitians, diabetes educators, ophthalmologists, and podiatrists to treat a patient with diabetes.

The **endocrine system** is a collection of glands located in various parts of the body that produce hormones that regulate physiologic functions (see Figure 20.1). **Hormones** are secreted substances that regulate metabolism, maintain fluid balance, control the life cycle, stimulate growth, and generate responses to stressful stimuli. Hormone release is regulated by a **negative feedback system**. As more hormones are released into the bloodstream, receptors detect the rise in hormone concentration and signal the associated gland to slow further production. Often, this feedback loop includes a series of hormones, each one controlling the release of the next hormone. For instance, the hypothalamus produces hormones that regulate the pituitary gland, which in turn releases several different hormones.

Figure 20.1 Endocrine System

Endocrine glands release hormones directly into the bloodstream, where they travel throughout the body to trigger responses in specific target tissues.

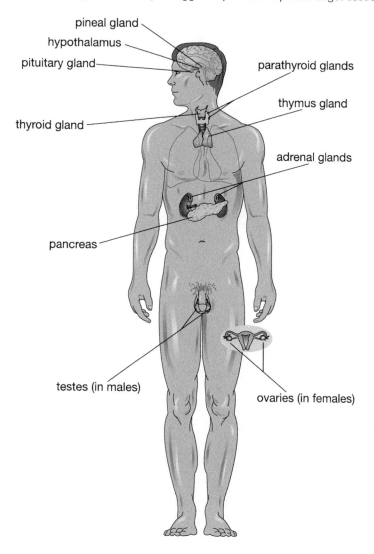

pineal gland
hypothalamus
pituitary gland
parathyroid glands
thymus gland
thyroid gland
adrenal glands
pancreas
testes (in males)
ovaries (in females)

Pituitary Gland and the Hypothalamus

The **pituitary gland** plays an important role in controlling several other endocrine glands and body functions. The hormones produced by this gland vary widely in the target tissues they affect (see Figure 20.2). The pituitary gland is an integral part of the **hypothalamic-pituitary-adrenal (HPA) axis**, a core feedback mechanism that controls endocrine and adrenal function. The **hypothalamus** is an area of the brain that works in concert with the pituitary gland to regulate the production of hormones that affect body temperature, hunger, thirst, sleep, and mood.

FIGURE 20.2 | Pituitary Gland

The pituitary gland plays a key role in growth, onset of puberty, and reproductive cycles.

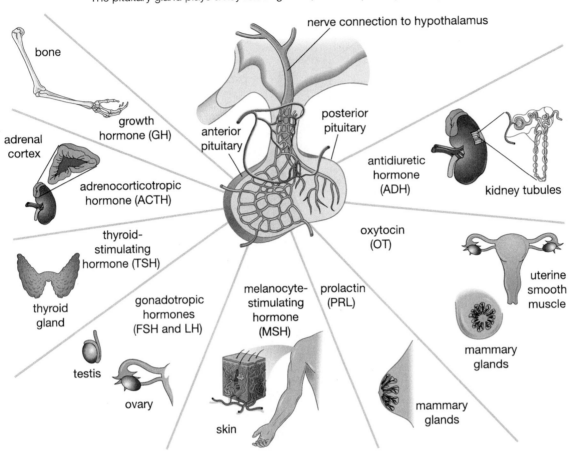

Thyroid and Parathyroid Glands

The **thyroid gland** is found in the neck surrounding the trachea (see Figure 20.3). This gland releases **tri-iodothyronine (T_3)** and **thyroxine (T_4)** in response to **thyroid-stimulating hormone (TSH)**, which is released from the pituitary gland. Iodine is necessary for formation of thyroid hormones. Whereas T_3 is more physiologically active, both T_3 and T_4 regulate basal metabolic rate and affect the metabolism of carbohydrates, fats, and proteins. Thyroid hormones increase the conversion of food to energy and thereby raise body temperature. A third hormone released from the thyroid gland is **calcitonin.** This hormone lowers blood concentrations of calcium and causes calcium to be stored in bone.

The **parathyroid glands** exist as two paired small structures that are embedded in the posterior thyroid gland. These glands release **parathyroid hormone**, which raises blood concentrations of calcium and, therefore, has the opposite action of calcitonin. Together, this antagonistic pair of hormones (calcitonin and parathyroid hormone) regulates calcium and phosphorus balance within the body. Maintaining normal blood concentrations of calcium is important for nerve and muscle function and also in blood clotting.

In the Know

A carbonated beverage contains phosphorus. If this beverage is consumed in large quantities, it can affect the balance of phosphorus and calcium in the blood. When the phosphorus level increases in the blood, the calcium level decreases, thereby putting bone health at risk.

FIGURE 20.3 Thyroid and Parathyroid Glands

The thyroid and parathyroid glands not only work together, but they are also located next to each other.

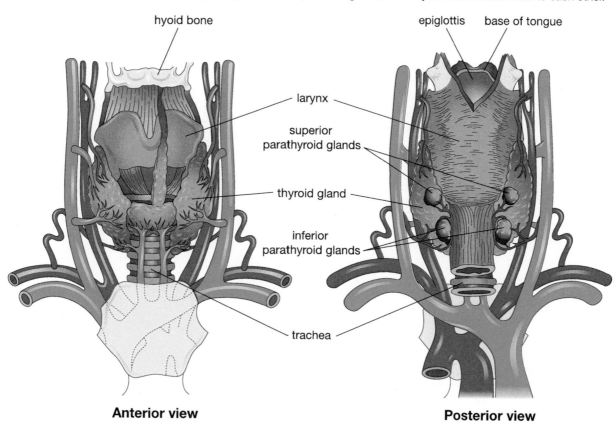

Anterior view   **Posterior view**

Adrenal Glands

The **adrenal glands** are located on the tops of the kidneys. The inner layer of these glands, called the **adrenal medulla**, produces **adrenaline (epinephrine)**. Heavy physical activity, stress, and low blood glucose trigger the adrenal medulla to produce adrenaline. Adrenaline, also called epinephrine, elevates blood pressure and diverts blood from body organs to muscles (see Figure 20.4). In addition, adrenaline prompts the release of stored glucose and fats into the blood. These actions prepare the body's **"fight-or-flight" response** in stressful situations.

The outer layer of the adrenal glands, called the **adrenal cortex**, releases **corticosteroids**, including mineralocorticoids and glucocorticoids. **Mineralocorticoids** regulate fluid and electrolyte balance; **glucocorticoids** affect day/night cycles and metabolism. The hypothalamus produces corticotropin-releasing factor, which stimulates the pituitary gland to make **adrenocorticotropic hormone (ACTH)**. ACTH travels through the blood to the adrenal glands, where it stimulates release of **cortisol**, the primary glucocorticoid, according to a **circadian rhythm**. This rhythm cycles every 24 hours, with cortisol levels peaking in the morning and decreasing at night (see Figure 20.5). Cortisol affects glucose metabolism, fat deposition, water retention, and the anti-inflammatory action of the immune system. Although the ovaries and testes produce most of the sex hormones, aromatase (an enzyme made by the adrenal glands) converts estrogen and testosterone to active forms in other parts of the body.

FIGURE 20.4 **Adrenal Glands**

Adrenaline can provide an individual with tremendous strength or speed when a frightful circumstance is encountered.

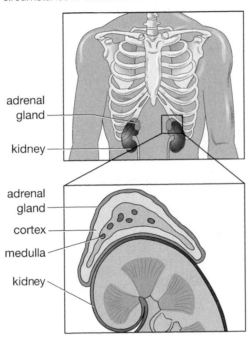

FIGURE 20.5 **Circadian Rhythm of Cortisol**

Cortisol ramps up metabolism in the morning, in advance of daily activity and meals, and slows down metabolism for rest and sleep at night.

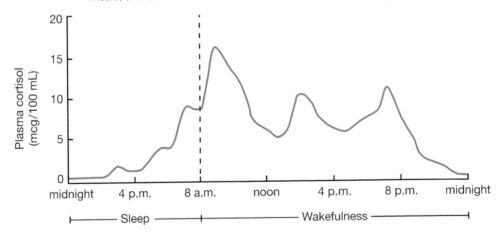

Pancreas

The **pancreas** is a large gland located in the abdomen, just behind the stomach. In addition to producing digestive enzymes and releasing them into the duodenum (a section of the small intestine), the pancreas produces **glucagon** and **insulin**. **Alpha islet cells** produce glucagon, and **beta islet cells** produce insulin. Insulin is released in response to a rise in blood glucose, such as what happens after eating a meal, especially if that meal is high in **carbohydrates** (see Figure 20.6). Insulin connects with receptors on the surfaces of cells to activate channels in the membrane. In effect, insulin is the key that opens the door, allowing glucose to enter cells. Glucose provides the energy all cells need to live.

FIGURE 20.6 Pancreas and Normal Glucose Metabolism

The pancreas releases insulin to lower blood glucose after you eat, and it releases glucagon to maintain adequate blood glucose when you are fasting.

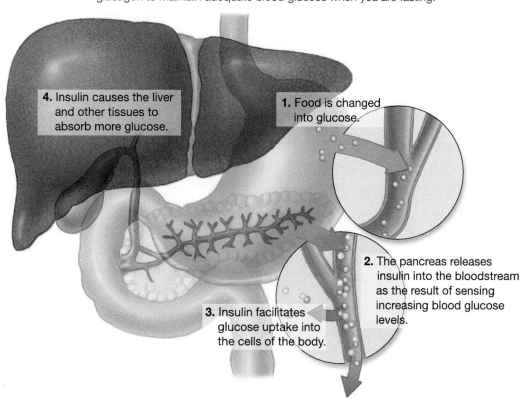

4. Insulin causes the liver and other tissues to absorb more glucose.

1. Food is changed into glucose.

2. The pancreas releases insulin into the bloodstream as the result of sensing increasing blood glucose levels.

3. Insulin facilitates glucose uptake into the cells of the body.

Glucagon, on the other hand, raises blood glucose levels. It activates liver cells to break down stored glycogen molecules into glucose and release it into the blood. Glucagon is released in response to low blood glucose, such as in between meals and overnight (see Figure 20.7). Glucagon also facilitates the breakdown of fats and proteins as alternative sources of energy. Although this process is useful in the short term to maintain life, **ketones** (by-products of this alternative energy source) are produced. Ketones have toxic effects when they accumulate in the blood.

 Checkpoint **20.1**

Take a moment to review what you have learned so far and answer these questions.

1. What are the glands and structures within the endocrine system?

2. What hormones are released by each of the glands within the endocrine system?

Disorders of the Endocrine System

Disorders of the endocrine system are on the rise. As obesity rates climb in the United States, the incidence of Type 2 diabetes is increasing dramatically. In fact, diabetes has been compared to an epidemic in scale because of its effect on the healthcare system.

FIGURE 20.7 Maintaining Blood Glucose Levels

Hormones produced by the pancreas, adrenal glands, and pituitary gland participate in maintaining appropriate blood glucose levels after eating and in between meals.

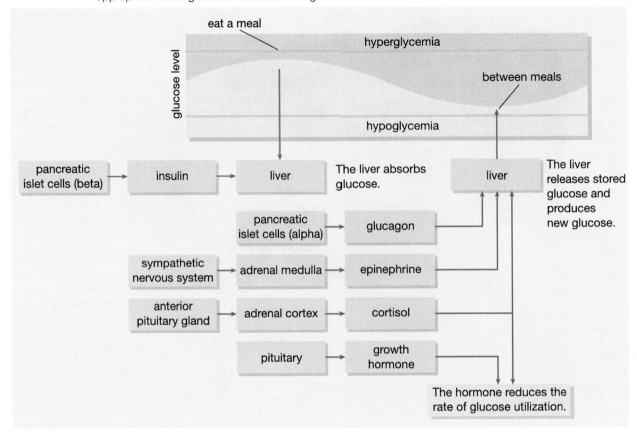

The Centers for Disease Control and Prevention (CDC) estimates that the direct medical costs attributed to diabetes in 2012 was $176 billion. The CDC also notes that people diagnosed with diabetes have medical expenditures approximately 2.3 times higher than people without diabetes.

Other disorders of the endocrine system affect the thyroid, pituitary, and adrenal glands. Thyroid disease affects up to 10% of adults and is more common among women. Conditions related to the pituitary and adrenal glands include Cushing's syndrome and Addison's disease. Myriad drug therapies treat these conditions, but none completely cure them. Therefore, healthcare professionals must work with patients to ensure that they are taking their medications as prescribed.

Diabetes

In simple terms, **diabetes mellitus** (commonly known as diabetes) refers to elevated blood glucose that results in damage to small blood vessels and nerve tissue. This damage has significant and life-threatening effects. Diabetes has multiple causes and is categorized into Type 1, Type 2, and gestational diabetes. **Type 1 diabetes** (sometimes called juvenile diabetes) is the least common, affecting only about 5% of patients with diabetes. It is an autoimmune process that destroys the islet cells within the pancreas, thereby impairing and eliminating its ability to make insulin (see Figure 20.8). Patients with Type 1 diabetes must be given insulin to stay alive. If insulin is not present, glucose remains in the blood

FIGURE 20.8 Type 1 Diabetes

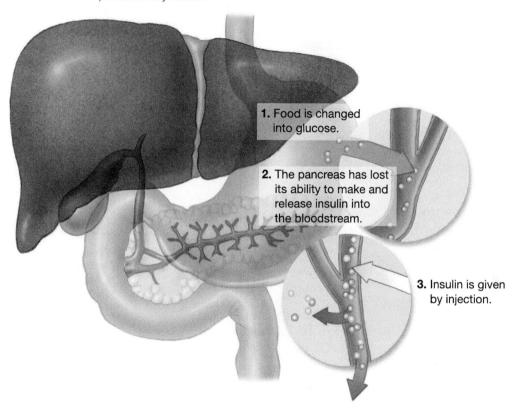

Insulin is given to patients with Type 1 diabetes because their pancreas no longer produces any insulin.

1. Food is changed into glucose.

2. The pancreas has lost its ability to make and release insulin into the bloodstream.

3. Insulin is given by injection.

and climbs to dangerous levels. The body also begins using alternative energy sources, thereby producing ketones. **Ketoacidosis** is a life-threatening emergency in which ketones accumulate to toxic levels in the blood.

Type 2 diabetes is a multifactorial disorder that causes high blood glucose (see Figure 20.9). It accounts for approximately 95% of patients with diabetes. Usually, Type 2 diabetes starts with accumulation of abdominal fat (**central obesity**), which is highly resistant to the effects of insulin. The pancreas still makes insulin, but the insulin does not work as well as it should. In fact, insulin receptors around the body become less sensitive to its effects. This **insulin resistance** triggers a cascade of other abnormal metabolic processes, one of which is overproduction of glucagon from the pancreas. Glucagon further increases blood glucose by promoting release of unneeded glucose from the liver into the blood. At first, the beta islet cells compensate for the additional glucose by producing excess insulin, but eventually they cannot keep up and their ability to make insulin diminishes. Thus, Type 2 diabetes is characterized first by insulin insensitivity and then by **relative insulin insufficiency**. Type 2 diabetes is a progressive disease that worsens over time, necessitating changes in treatment every few years.

Many people with Type 2 diabetes have **metabolic syndrome**. This condition refers to a triad of problems: high blood pressure, high cholesterol and triglyceride levels, and high blood glucose. Patients do not have to be diagnosed with diabetes to have metabolic syndrome. Patients may not have high blood glucose all of the time. They may have **impaired fasting glucose** (elevated blood glucose on waking) or **impaired glucose tolerance** (elevated blood glucose after eating) along with hypertension and high triglycerides. Patients with metabolic syndrome are at a high risk for cardiovascular disease.

FIGURE 20.9 Type 2 Diabetes

Type 2 diabetes is a multifactorial disorder including insulin insensitivity, impaired insulin production, and altered glucagon release.

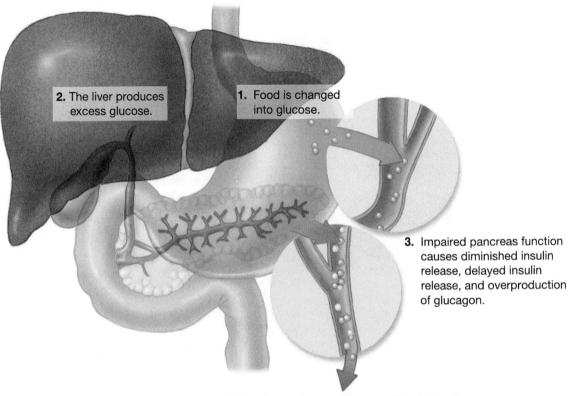

2. The liver produces excess glucose.

1. Food is changed into glucose.

3. Impaired pancreas function causes diminished insulin release, delayed insulin release, and overproduction of glucagon.

4. The tissues become less sensitive to insulin.

Gestational diabetes results from insulin resistance caused by hormones that are produced in excess during pregnancy. Pregnancy hormones, especially progesterone and human chorionic somatomammotropin, cause insulin resistance in the mother to preserve glucose availability for the developing fetus. Therefore, gestational diabetes mimics Type 2 diabetes and often precedes it.

Patients should be aware of risk factors for developing diabetes. Risk factors for Type 2 diabetes include the following:

- age over 45 years
- family history of diabetes (parents or siblings)
- overweight (body mass index higher than 25 kg/m²)
- habitual physical inactivity
- race/ethnicity (African American, Asian, or Latino)
- impaired fasting glucose or impaired glucose tolerance
- hypertension (blood pressure higher than 140/90 mm Hg)
- cholesterol abnormalities (low high-density lipoproteins and high triglycerides)
- history of gestational diabetes or birth of baby weighing more than nine pounds
- polycystic ovary syndrome

Prominent symptoms of diabetes, no matter the cause, include increased urination (**polyuria**), excessive urination at night (**nocturia**), glucose in the urine (**glycosuria**), excessive thirst (**polydipsia**), excessive hunger (**polyphagia**), blurred vision, and fatigue. Other symptoms of diabetes include frequent infections, slow wound healing, weight gain or loss, and numbness and tingling in fingers and toes. Onset of these symptoms is sudden in Type 1 diabetes but is slow to appear in Type 2 diabetes. Unfortunately, many patients do not realize they have Type 2 diabetes until they have had it for years.

When glucose cannot enter cells, it remains in the bloodstream and causes damage to tiny blood vessels and capillaries leading to the kidneys, eyes, and nerves. These **microvascular complications** are leading causes of dialysis and kidney transplants, blindness, and lower leg amputations (see Table 20.1). **Macrovascular complications** of Type 2 diabetes include heart disease, heart attack, and stroke. Someone with diabetes is half as likely to survive a heart attack as someone without it. Consequently, the ultimate concern about diabetes is preventing long-term complications.

TABLE 20.1 Microvascular Complications of Untreated Diabetes

Nephropathy	Damage to kidneys, affecting their ability to filter the blood. If left untreated, it can lead to kidney failure. In fact, the leading cause of dialysis and kidney transplant is diabetic nephropathy.
Neuropathy	Damage to tiny nerves in the extremities. In the feet, loss of sensation can lead to ulcers, infection, and, ultimately, amputation. The leading cause of lower leg amputations is diabetic neuropathy.
Retinopathy	Damage to retinal tissue in the eyes. If left untreated, it can progress to blindness. The leading cause of blindness (other than congenital causes) is diabetic retinopathy.

 Patient Teaching

You can help patients with diabetes take good care of themselves by reminding them to get eye examinations, cholesterol tests, and foot examinations annually. It is also recommended that people with diabetes get annual flu shots because high blood glucose impairs the immune system and thus the ability to fight off infection.

If a patient is taking insulin or other medication for diabetes, **hypoglycemia** (low blood glucose or low blood sugar reaction) is possible. In individuals with diabetes, hypoglycemia commonly results from injecting too much insulin or skipping meals when taking medication for diabetes.

Symptoms of hypoglycemia include the following:

- shakiness
- dizziness
- sweating
- headache
- irritability
- confusion
- vision changes
- hunger

Patients who are experiencing these symptoms should test their blood glucose, if possible, and immediately ingest a food or beverage that contains sugar. To treat hypoglycemia, patients should ingest 15–30 g of carbohydrate in the form of simple sugar. Fruit juice, nondiet soda, hard candy, and glucose tablets are good sources of such carbohydrates. Although foods such as pasta, bread, and rice are carbohydrates, they consist of complex carbohydrates that take time for the body to break down. The glucose in foods or beverages with simple sugar will reach the bloodstream more quickly. Patients should understand that ingesting large amounts of food is not necessary and will raise blood glucose levels too much.

Diabetes is detected by measuring **blood glucose** (sugar) concentrations in the blood. Concentrations can be determined with the use of laboratory blood tests or **glucose meters** at home (see Patient Teaching feature box below). The normal range for blood glucose is 70–120 mg/dL. Any random blood glucose result of 200 mg/dL or greater or a fasting result (at least eight hours since eating) of 126 mg/dL or greater is diagnostic of diabetes. Blood glucose measurements, taken both randomly and after fasting, are easy to administer, and results are often available quickly. If a patient's random or fasting blood glucose level is elevated but not diagnostic of diabetes or is elevated due to a clinical condition such as pregnancy, a glucose tolerance test may be appropriate. Glucose tolerance tests are also used to diagnose diabetes: Patients drink a solution that contains concentrated glucose and then have their blood glucose levels measured over the next three hours. The purpose of measuring blood glucose is to determine trends in its concentration throughout the day so that treatment can be selected and adjusted appropriately.

The test used to assess overall blood glucose control is the **hemoglobin A1c** test. The normal range for hemoglobin A1c (or glycolated hemoglobin) is 4%–6%, but patients with untreated diabetes can have an A1c result of 10% or greater; a result of 6.5% or greater is diagnostic of diabetes. This test can be run via a blood draw in the laboratory or a finger stick in a clinic or pharmacy. The hemoglobin A1c test measures the percentage of red blood cells (RBCs) with glucose attached to the hemoglobin molecules contained inside. Glucose irreversibly binds to hemoglobin and remains there for the life span of the

Patient Teaching

Many glucose meters are available for home use to allow patients to monitor their blood glucose levels. Immediate feedback about blood glucose levels at any time of day can help patients determine trends of high and low glucose concentrations. These results guide drug therapy as well as help patients to make changes in diet and exercise. The goal is to maintain blood glucose concentrations within the normal range.

Some factors that patients should consider when choosing a glucose meter are cost (or third-party coverage for the meter and/or strips); ease of use; patient dexterity and eyesight (some strips are small and thus difficult to handle); and patient preference for size, portability, and speed (time it takes for the machine to produce a result). Most meters can test blood from multiple body sites including fingers, palms, and arms.

To help patients control their diabetes, many meter manufacturers offer software programs that allow patients to download glucose results to a computer for analysis. Research the programs that you could use as a teaching tool when working with this patient population.

RBC. Because RBCs live for about three months in the body, this test provides an overall average of glucose concentration in the blood over the previous three months.

Drug Regimens and Treatments

As the incidence of diabetes increases, drug therapy options available to treat it expand. Unfortunately, none of these options cure the disorder. However, the variety of medication choices can be customized to achieve good outcomes for individuals. Patients must often be reminded that although high blood glucose does not necessarily make them feel ill, it does cause long-term damage to vital organs. The leading causes of death in patients with diabetes are heart disease and stroke. Fortunately, treating diabetes dramatically reduces the risk of developing long-term complications.

Type 1 diabetes requires treatment with insulin because patients with this disorder cannot make their own insulin. Treatment for Type 2 diabetes begins with **lifestyle modifications**: changes in diet to reduce carbohydrate, fat, and calorie intake; regular exercise for 30 minutes most days of the week; smoking cessation; and weight loss. Drug therapy begins with metformin, progresses to combination therapy, and often requires insulin eventually to achieve goals for blood glucose levels and hemoglobin A1c.

Metformin

Initial drug therapy for Type 2 diabetes is **metformin**. This drug can be used alone or in combination with other agents and works by inhibiting excess hepatic glucose production, a process that normally occurs at a slow rate overnight. Metformin also increases insulin sensitivity in muscle and other body tissues. Metformin is typically taken two to three times a day with food or meals. When treatment begins, a low dose is prescribed so as to avoid upset stomach, abdominal cramps, and diarrhea. Slowly, the dose is increased. Metformin can take as long as three weeks to reach full effect. It usually does not cause hypoglycemia unless it is taken in combination with other agents for diabetes. In addition, metformin can promote mild weight loss (five to six pounds) and improve cholesterol profiles. The best time to test blood glucose when taking metformin is in the morning, just after waking. See Table 20.2 for metformin products. Metformin is paired with other antidiabetic agents into several combination products, which are not discussed in this text. You should be aware that these products exist and be ready to look them up when needed.

TABLE 20.2 Metformin Products

Generic (Brand)	Dosage Form	Route of Administration	Common Dosage
Metformin (Glucophage)	Oral solution, tablet	Oral	500–1,000 mg twice a day
Combination Products			
Glipizide/metformin (Metaglip)	Tablet	Oral	2.5 mg/250 mg to 5 mg/500 mg twice a day
Glyburide/metformin (Glucovance)	Tablet	Oral	1.25 mg/250 mg to 5 mg/500 mg twice a day
Pioglitazone/metformin (ACTOplus Met)	Tablet	Oral	15 mg/500 mg to 15 mg/850 mg once or twice a day
Repaglinide/metformin (PrandiMet)	Tablet	Oral	1 mg/500 mg to 2 mg/500 mg two or three times a day
Rosiglitazone/metformin (Avandamet)	Tablet	Oral	2 mg/500 mg to 4 mg/1,000 mg a day
Sitagliptin/metformin (Janumet)	Tablet	Oral	50 mg/500 mg to 50 mg/1,000 mg once or twice a day

Side Effects Common side effects of metformin include upset stomach, abdominal cramps, nausea, diarrhea, flatulence, and a metallic taste. These effects can be diminished or avoided by taking the medication with food and increasing the dose slowly. Over time, these side effects will decrease.

Serious but rare side effects include **lactic acidosis**, a potentially fatal condition that requires medical care and hospitalization. This side effect can usually be avoided if patients stop taking metformin when they are severely ill or hospitalized. The risk for lactic acidosis increases under the following circumstances:

- severe dehydration or altered fluid balance
- excessive alcohol consumption
- liver or kidney impairment (or taking other drugs that contribute to impairment)
- sepsis (a serious, acute infection in the bloodstream that requires intravenous [IV] antibiotics)
- unstable or acute heart failure

Contraindications Metformin is contraindicated for patients who have kidney dysfunction, liver problems, or heart failure because these conditions raise the risk for lactic acidosis. Metformin should also be avoided in the presence of shock, sepsis, or metabolic acidosis. This medication should also not be used in patients 80 years old or greater unless they have normal kidney function. The dose generally should not be increased to the maximum dose in older adults (over 80 years old).

➕ *Note: Allied health professionals should be aware that an allergy to a particular drug contraindicates its use. This warning applies to all Contraindications sections in this chapter.*

Cautions and Considerations Patients who are taking metformin should temporarily discontinue the medication when undergoing procedures in which contrast dye or iodine substances are used. Such patients are usually instructed to stop taking metformin the day before the procedure and resume the medication 48 hours after the procedure. Drug interactions between these substances and metformin can precipitate kidney failure and lactic acidosis.

Patient Teaching

Be sure to remind patients who are scheduled for imaging procedures to stop taking their metformin the day before their procedure and to hold off taking it until 48 hours after their procedure. Drug interactions between metformin and the contrast dye or iodine substance can lead to lactic acidosis and kidney failure.

Insulin Secretagogues

Agents that stimulate insulin production from the pancreas to directly lower blood glucose levels are known as **insulin secretagogues**. Two common classes of insulin secretagogues are **sulfonylureas** and **meglitinides**. Sulfonylureas and meglitinides differ in their onset and duration of action. Sulfonylureas can take 30 minutes or more to start working and can last for 8 hours or longer. Meglitinides act within 10 minutes and last for around 2 hours.

Sulfonylureas are used alone or in combination with other agents to treat Type 2 diabetes. They are taken before breakfast each day and sometimes again before dinner. Meglitinides are used in combination with other agents to treat Type 2 diabetes. They

TABLE 20.3 Common Insulin Secretagogues

Generic (Brand)	Dosage Form	Route of Administration	Common Dosage
Sulfonylureas			
Glimepiride (Amaryl)	Tablet	Oral	2–4 mg a day
Glipizide (Glucotrol)	Tablet	Oral	5–10 mg a day
Glipizide ER (Glucotrol XL)	Tablet	Oral	5–10 mg a day
Glyburide (DiaBeta, Glynase, Micronase)	Tablet	Oral	5–10 mg a day
Meglitinides			
Nateglinide (Starlix)	Tablet	Oral	60–120 mg prior to meals
Repaglinide (Prandin)	Tablet	Oral	0.5–2 mg prior to meals

are taken just before eating and provide an extra boost of insulin for a specific meal. Table 20.3 provides information on common insulin secretagogues.

Side Effects Low blood glucose reactions (hypoglycemia) are the most common side effect of these medications. Symptoms of hypoglycemia include shakiness, headache, blurred vision, dizziness, confusion, irritability, hunger, and tiredness. Hypoglycemia tends to occur when a patient takes the medication but then skips a meal or does more physical activity than usual. Patients can avoid this effect by not skipping meals or omitting a dose when they anticipate eating significantly less than usual on a particular day. Other side effects include nausea, diarrhea, and constipation.

Contraindications All sulfonylureas and meglitinides are contraindicated in the presence of diabetic ketoacidosis. Glipizide, glyburide, nateglinide, and repaglinide should not be used in Type 1 diabetes mellitus. In addition, glyburide use is contraindicated with bosentan use, and repaglinide should not be used with gemfibrozil.

Cautions and Considerations Because sulfonylureas and meglitinides increase the risk of hypoglycemia, patients should be informed of the symptoms of low blood glucose and know how to treat it. Patients should monitor their blood glucose level at home regularly and whenever they feel their level may be low. The best times to check blood glucose when taking sulfonylureas are first thing in the morning before eating (fasting) and then occasionally before other meals during the day. The best time to check blood glucose when taking meglitinides is one to two hours after meals. Patients with liver or kidney disease may not be able to take sulfonylureas depending on the agent chosen. Patients with these conditions should talk with their prescribers before taking one of these agents.

Kolb's Learning Styles

If you are a visual learner or like to learn in small groups (as Convergers and Accommodators do), try using pictures to learn the drugs for Type 2 diabetes. Draw a diagram of the organs and abnormal functions involved in diabetes; then write the drug names that address each abnormal process next to the organ involved. Explain your diagram to a classmate and ask him or her to do the same for you. Teaching someone else is one of the best ways to solidify concepts in your own mind.

TZDs

Agents known as **thiazolidinediones (TZDs)**—or **glitazones**—are used in combination with metformin or sulfonylureas to treat Type 2 diabetes (see Table 20.4). They work by directly increasing insulin sensitivity in cells of the body. TZDs connect with intracellular receptors to stimulate production of more insulin receptors. This process can take weeks to months to occur, and thus onset of effect is not immediate. The best time to check blood glucose levels when using TZDs is first thing in the morning before eating (fasting), and occasionally after meals during the day.

Quick Study

TZDs are often referred to as *glitazones* due to their similar generic-drug endings.

TABLE 20.4 TZDs

Generic (Brand)	Dosage Form	Route of Administration	Common Dosage
Pioglitazone (Actos)	Tablet	Oral	15–30 mg a day
Rosiglitazone (Avandia)	Tablet	Oral	4–8 mg once or twice a day

Side Effects Common side effects of TZDs include fluid accumulation (edema) and weight gain. If patients notice rapid weight gain or swelling, especially with shortness of breath, they should talk with their prescribers right away.

Rare but serious effects include liver toxicity and macular edema (swelling of the eye, resulting in distorted vision). If patients experience unexplained nausea, vomiting, abdominal pain, fatigue, or dark urine, they should report these symptoms to their healthcare prescribers. Regular blood tests are conducted to monitor liver function.

Patients with diabetes should see an eye doctor annually for an eye examination in which their pupils are dilated and their retinas are examined.

Contraindications Because TZDs can cause fluid retention and edema, pioglitazone and rosiglitazone therapies should not be initiated in patients with New York Heart Association (NYHA) Class III or Class IV heart failure.

Cautions and Considerations Because TZDs can cause fluid retention and edema, they can worsen heart failure. Patients with heart failure should not take TZDs. Patients with edema or other heart problems may not be good candidates for TZD therapy.

In some women with fertility problems, TZDs have increased ovulation and increased pregnancy rates. Patients who are sexually active but do not want to become pregnant should use birth control to avoid the possibility of pregnancy.

Incretin Therapies

Incretin drugs either mimic endogenous incretin hormones or change their metabolism to increase their activity. **Glucagon-like peptide-1 (GLP-1)** and **glucose-dependent insulinotropic polypeptide** are **endogenous incretin hormones**, which are produced in response to glucose arriving from the intestines. They have multiple physiologic effects. First, incretins facilitate proper timing and function of phase I and phase II insulin response. **Phase I insulin response** refers to the immediate burst of insulin that occurs with, or even slightly before, the first bite of food. **Phase II insulin response** refers to the continued but somewhat slower release of insulin in the hours after eating. In Type 2 diabetes, both phase I and phase II insulin responses are blunted. Second, incretins inhibit glucagon production from the pancreas that otherwise promotes an undesirable increase in blood glucose. Third, incretins have some effect on appetite by producing **satiety**, a sensation of fullness and satisfaction. Many patients experience significant and sustained weight loss on incretin mimetics. (Other medications to treat diabetes—such as sulfonyl-ureas, TZDs, and insulin—are associated with weight gain.) Incretin drug therapies are used most often in combination with other medications used to treat Type 2 diabetes. Common incretin drugs are listed in Table 20.5.

TABLE 20.5 Incretin Therapies

Generic (Brand)	Dosage Form	Route of Administration	Common Dosage
GLP-1 Agonists			
Exenatide (Byetta)	Injection	sub-Q	5–10 mcg twice a day
Exenatide ER (Bydureon)	Injection	sub-Q	2 mg once a week
Liraglutide (Victoza)	Injection	sub-Q	1.2–1.8 mg once a day
Pramlintide (Symlin)	Injection	sub-Q	15–120 mcg per dose
DPP-4 Inhibitors			
Saxagliptin (Onglyza)	Tablet	Oral	2.5–5 mg a day
Sitagliptin (Januvia)	Tablet	Oral	100 mg a day

Exenatide and liraglutide are injectable products that mimic the action of GLP-1. Because GLP-1 is released only when glucose is introduced to the bloodstream, hypoglycemia between meals does not occur. Like GLP-1, then, exenatide and liraglutide do not carry a risk of causing low blood glucose levels.

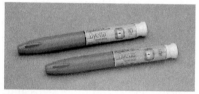

Exenatide is available in a self-injector pen device that patients can easily learn to use.

Pramlintide mimics **amylin**, a hormone copro-duced with insulin that reduces glucagon produc-tion, slows gastric emptying, and produces satiety. This incretin mimetic can be used by patients with Type 1 diabetes to supplement insulin. The addition of pramlintide to an insulin regimen can dramatically reduce the amount of insulin a patient has to take. Pramlintide is injected 30 minutes prior to each meal or snack containing at least 30 g of carbohydrate.

Saxagliptin and sitagliptin are oral **dipeptidyl peptidase-4 (DPP-4) inhibitors** that slow inactivation of incretin hormones, thereby allowing them to persist longer and produce beneficial effects. Satiety does not seem to be as pronounced with these agents, and thus weight loss is not usually an added benefit. They are taken daily without regard to food.

Patient Teaching

Injectable incretin therapies tend to be expensive, so insurance plans may require prior authorization by the prescriber. Insurance coverage may not pay for one of these products until other, less expensive medications have been tried. You can reduce frustration by helping patients understand this process.

Side Effects Common side effects of GLP-1 drugs include nausea, vomiting, diarrhea, diz-ziness, fatigue, and headache. Nausea is common at the beginning of therapy but dimin-ishes over time. Side effects can be minimized by beginning treatment at a low dose and increasing the dose slowly. Timing injections immediately before eating can reduce nausea, vomiting, and upset stomach. Over a period of several weeks, the patient can move the time of injection further ahead of eating until reaching 30 to 60 minutes prior to a meal.

Common side effects of DPP-4 inhibitors include headache, nasopharyngitis (runny nose and sore throat), and upper respiratory tract infection. The reason for these unusual side effects is not fully understood.

Contraindications Contraindications for exenatide ER and liraglutide include a patient or family history of medullar thyroid carcinoma and multiple endocrine neoplasia type 2. Pramlintide use is contraindicated in patients with gastroparesis and hypoglycemia unawareness.

DPP-4 inhibitors should not be used for patients with pancreatitis.

Drug Alert

Although GLP-1 agonists can be associated with significant weight loss, they are not approved as weight-loss drugs. Therefore, insurance companies will not pay for these agents if used solely for weight loss. Patients should be aware of this third-party rejection, especially because these agents can be expensive.

Cautions and Considerations Exenatide use has been associated with pancreatitis (inflammation of the pancreas). Patients should stop taking exenatide immediately and seek medical attention if they experience persistent or serious abdominal pain, especially if it is accompanied by vomiting.

If pramlintide is given with insulin, the patient can be at serious risk for low blood glucose levels, and those signs and symptoms can appear within three hours of taking the medications. Blood glucose levels should be checked before and after the injection. In addition, patients should be instructed on how to treat low blood glucose when it occurs.

Doses of DPP-4 inhibitors are cleared by the kidneys, so they must be adjusted for patients with kidney disease. Patients with kidney problems should alert their prescribers so that proper dosing is ordered.

Injectable incretin products must be stored in the refrigerator until dispensed. Once these products reach room temperature, they begin to degrade. Injectable incretin products are good at room temperature for only 30 days. Therefore, patients should keep these products in the refrigerator until they begin using them. Once opened, they can be kept at room temperature. Patients should protect these products from temperature extremes.

Checkpoint 20.2

Take a moment to review what you have learned so far and answer these questions.

1. What drug classes are used to treat Type 2 diabetes?

2. What are the generic names of the oral medications used to treat Type 2 diabetes?

3. Although all drugs for diabetes can, when used in combination, increase the risk of hypoglycemia, which oral therapies have the greatest risk of causing low blood glucose levels?

Insulin

Insulin is normally produced in a combination of basal and bolus rates to maintain steady glucose concentrations in the blood (see Figure 20.10). **Basal insulin** is slowly released throughout the day and night to allow energy for basic cellular function. In contrast, **bolus insulin** is released at mealtimes to react with glucose entering the body from food intake. When insulin is given by injection, the goal is to mimic this natural physiologic insulin production. For patients with Type 1 diabetes, multiple injections each day of combination basal and bolus insulins are necessary to achieve physiologic insulin dosing. Patients with Type 2 diabetes may be given insulin using a similar physiologic dosing schedule or as one injection at bedtime of long-acting insulin added to oral medications.

FIGURE 20.10 | **Normal Glucose Production**

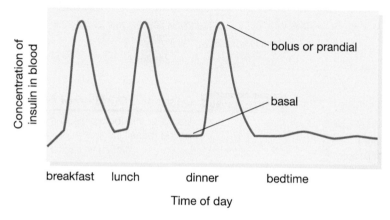

The timing of bolus insulin released with meals is called *prandial*, which means "with meals."

Insulin is essential for survival in an individual with Type 1 diabetes. In Type 2 diabetes, insulin is used later in the course of treatment as an adjunct to other therapies. **Rapid-acting insulin** begins to work in 10 minutes and, for practical purposes, lasts as long as 2 hours. It is given just before meals to reduce **prandial** (mealtime) elevations in blood glucose. **Short-acting insulin** begins to work in around 30 minutes and lasts up to 4 hours in most cases. It is also taken prior to meals. **Intermediate-acting insulin** begins to be effective in 30 to 60 minutes and lasts 6 to 8 hours in most cases. It is used either once or twice a day. **Long-acting insulin** works for approximately 24 hours and is injected once a day (see Table 20.6 and Figure 20.11).

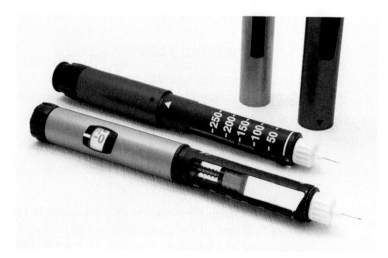

Some patients find using an insulin pen, such as the ones pictured above, more convenient than using an insulin vial and syringe.

TABLE 20.6 Commonly Used Insulins

Generic (Brand)	Onset of Action	Maximum Peak and Duration	Appearance and Dispensing Status
Rapid-Acting			
Insulin aspart (NovoLog)	10–15 min	1–2 hr; 4 hr	Clear; Rx only
Insulin glulisine (Apidra)	Few minutes	1 hr; 2 hr	Clear; Rx only
Insulin lispro (Humalog)	10–15 min	1–2 hr; 4 hr	Clear; Rx only
Short-Acting			
Regular insulin (Humulin R, Novolin R)	30 min	4 hr; 8 hr	Clear; OTC
Intermediate-Acting			
NPH insulin (Humulin N, Novolin N)	1 hr	6–8 hr; 24 hr	Cloudy; OTC
Long-Acting			
Insulin detemir (Levemir)	1 hr	Peak is possible with Levemir but absent with Lantus; 24–36 hr	Clear; Rx only
Insulin glargine (Lantus)	1 hr	None; 24–36 hr	Clear; Rx only

Name Exchange

You may hear other healthcare practitioners refer to insulin glargine more frequently by the brand name Lantus.

FIGURE 20.11 Onset and Duration of Action for Insulin

Rapid-acting (bolus) insulins are used most often with long-acting (basal) insulins to mimic normal pancreatic function.

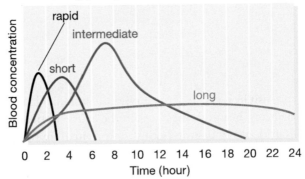

Kolb's Learning Styles

If you like working with abstract concepts (as Divergers do), re-create Figure 20.11 by drawing on a piece of paper and label each curved line representing insulin with its corresponding generic and brand-name insulin products. For each type of insulin, identify the time of day and frequency patients should check their blood glucose to see if the medication is working.

Insulin is available by injection only because it is a protein. If taken orally, the protein structure is denatured and deactivated by stomach acid before it reaches the bloodstream. Therefore, patients who need insulin must learn to self-inject into the subcutaneous (sub-Q) tissue. Figure 20.12 shows sites where sub-Q injections of insulin are given. The abdomen is the preferred **insulin injection site** because the rate of insulin absorption into the blood is most consistent at this location. Physical activity increases bloodflow to large leg muscles, thereby dramatically increasing insulin absorption. Patients using this site should inject immediately before bedtime, when they will be inactive for a few hours.

FIGURE 20.12 | Insulin Injection Sites

Patients should rotate injection sites to different areas of the body, keeping injections at least one to two inches away from previous injections on the skin.

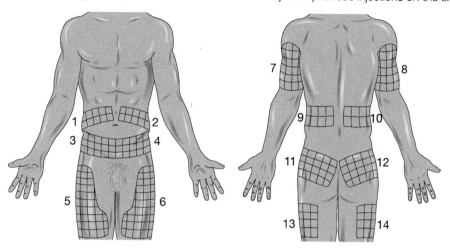

Insulin is available in **vials** for use with **syringes** as well as in **self-injector pens. Insulin pumps** are also available; these deliver insulin through a tiny tube inserted just under the skin. These pumps can be programmed to deliver just the right amount of insulin each hour of the day for an individual patient. The tube must be reinserted every three days. Pumps eliminate the need for multiple injections a day but must be well understood and properly maintained to work effectively. Inhaled insulin was available for a short period but was taken off the market due to limited market performance. Other inhaled insulins are currently in clinical trials and are expected to reach the market soon.

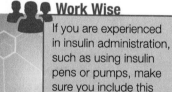

Work Wise

If you are experienced in insulin administration, such as using insulin pens or pumps, make sure you include this skill on your résumé. Potential employers may be impressed with this competency.

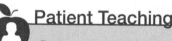

Patient Teaching

Patients must be instructed on how to use a self-injector pen or a syringe to self-administer insulin. They should also follow basic medication safety and hygiene standards associated with insulin injection:

- Remind patients to choose an appropriate injection site and to rotate the sites.
- Instruct patients to cleanse the injection site with an alcohol swab before the injection and to use a new needle for each injection.
- Dispose of the used needle in an approved sharps container to avoid the risk of injury or infection from inadvertent contact with the needle.

Side Effects The most common "side effect" of insulin is hypoglycemia. Although often listed as a side effect, hypoglycemia is, in fact, the intended effect of insulin. However, someone using insulin is at an increased risk of developing serious hypoglycemia when doses are too high or meals are skipped. If blood glucose concentrations are lower than 40 mg/dL, loss of consciousness and brain damage can occur. Diabetic coma is life-threatening if not treated immediately. Symptoms of hypoglycemia include shakiness, headache, blurred vision, dizziness, confusion, irritability, hunger, and tiredness.

Patient Teaching

Patients taking insulin or other drugs that have the potential to quickly lower blood glucose (i.e., secretagogues) must be educated about the signs and symptoms of hypoglycemia and know how to treat it if symptoms occur. They should test their blood glucose levels and immediately ingest a food or beverage containing sugar. Good sources of sugar include ½ glass of fruit juice, ½ can of nondiet soft drink, hard candy, or glucose tablets.

Other side effects are rare but can include lipodystrophy (fat accumulation or depletion at injection site). This effect can be largely avoided by rotating injection sites.

Contraindications Insulin glulisine, insulin lispro, and regular insulin are contraindicated during episodes of hypoglycemia.

Cautions and Considerations Because most hospitalizations and emergency room visits for patients with Type 1 diabetes result from hypoglycemic events, the risk of hypoglycemia cannot be overemphasized. Patients must be instructed to recognize and treat low blood glucose when it occurs. Family members of an individual who uses insulin should be taught how to administer glucagon. This medication is given when the patient is unconscious because of hypoglycemia and cannot self-treat by ingesting a food or beverage containing sugar.

All insulin products must be stored in the refrigerator until dispensed or used by the patient. Once insulin warms to room temperature, the protein begins to degrade. Therefore, patients should keep insulin vials or pens in the refrigerator until they use them. Once opened, insulin vials will expire in 28 to 30 days. Most insulin pens are also good for 1 month after opening, but a few expire in 14 days. If exposed to extreme heat or cold, insulin can become damaged. Patients should protect insulin from heat (e.g., do not keep it in a car during the summer) or freezing temperatures. For patients who are traveling by plane, recommend that they keep insulin with them in a carry-on bag because air cargo areas on planes are not climate-controlled. Finally, patients should discard any insulin package that contains clumps or appears frosty.

Drug Alert

Insulin is involved in up to 11% of all hospital medication errors. These life-threatening errors occur for a couple of reasons. First, it is easy to confuse insulins that have different onsets of action because the boxes of insulin look the same and are similar in size. Second, the timing of insulin doses with food is difficult to achieve in the inpatient setting and is critical to the effectiveness of the drug. With that in mind, healthcare personnel must double-check insulin labels prior to the drug's administration and should be vigilant in adhering to proper insulin dosage guidelines.

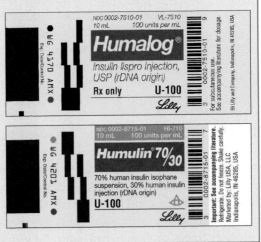

SGLT-2 Inhibitors

Sodium-glucose linked transporter-2 (SGLT-2) inhibitors, such as canagliflozin and dapagliflozin, are a class of new medications used for Type 2 diabetes (see Table 20.7). SGLT-2 inhibitors are taken once a day, often in combination with other oral agents such as metformin. They work by blocking the reabsorption of glucose that the kidney filters out of the bloodstream, thus increasing the excretion of glucose in the urine.

Side Effects Patients taking SGLT-2 inhibitors can experience urinary tract infections and genital fungal infections such as yeast infections. Patients who have a history of these types of infections prior to taking these medications should talk with their healthcare prescribers before taking SGLT-2 inhibitors. Some patients have experienced low blood pressure and high potassium blood levels from taking these drugs.

TABLE 20.7 SGLT-2 Inhibitors

Generic (Brand)	Dosage Form	Route of Administration	Common Dosage
Canagliflozin (Invokana)	Tablet	Oral	100–300 mg once a day
Dapagliflozin (Farxiga)	Tablet	Oral	5–10 mg once a day

Contraindications The use of canagliflozin and dapagliflozin is contraindicated for patients with severe kidney impairment and end-stage kidney disease, as well as for patients who are on dialysis.

Cautions and Considerations Patients over 80 years old and those who take diuretics or blood pressure medications should work closely with their healthcare prescribers as they start therapy with SGLT-2 inhibitors.

 Checkpoint **20.3**

Take a moment to review what you have learned so far and answer these questions.

1. How does insulin work?
2. What is the peak action time of each insulin product currently available?
3. What are the symptoms of hypoglycemia and how should it be treated?

Hypothyroidism

Hypothyroidism is a disorder in which too little thyroid hormone is produced by the thyroid gland. Causes of hypothyroidism, other than general dysfunction, include autoimmune destruction of thyroid tissue (known as **Hashimoto's disease**), radioactive iodine therapy, surgical removal of the thyroid, and pituitary or hypothalamus dysfunction. Symptoms of hypothyroidism include constipation; bradycardia; depression; fatigue; dry skin, nails, and scalp; tremors; reduced mental acuity; memory loss; intolerance to cold; lower voice pitch; and weight gain.

Thyroid disorders are diagnosed by combining symptom history with interpretation of laboratory tests. The primary laboratory test used to detect and monitor thyroid disorders is a blood test that measures the concentration of thyroid-stimulating hormone (TSH). TSH is released from the pituitary gland to stimulate the thyroid to make T_3 and T_4 (see

Figure 20.13). If the patient's TSH level is high, the pituitary gland is sensing low T$_3$ and T$_4$ levels in the blood (via the feedback loop) and producing extra TSH to stimulate the thyroid.

FIGURE 20.13 The Feedback Loop between the Thyroid Gland and the Pituitary Gland for Thyroid Hormones

A high TSH test result means that T$_3$ and T$_4$ levels are low (hypothyroidism).

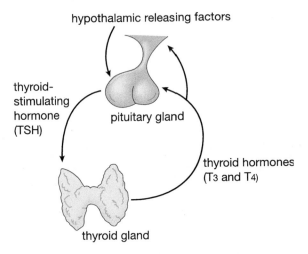

Drug Regimens and Treatments

In hypothyroidism, thyroid hormone supplementation is needed and accomplished by taking oral medications. Even though the US Food and Drug Administration (FDA) has approved generic substitution for thyroid hormone products, variability among products is still possible. Therefore, patients are instructed to choose one brand or generic version of thyroid hormone and continue with it consistently. Switching between brands and generic forms of thyroid hormone can result in variability in drug delivery and corresponding hormone levels measured in the laboratory. Because doses are adjusted and maintained according to results obtained from one product, the patient should avoid switching thyroid hormone products if at all possible.

Thyroid Hormone Products

Hypothyroidism is treated with thyroid hormone supplementation (see Table 20.8) to maintain appropriate blood levels of T$_3$ and T$_4$. Doses are individualized to each patient using blood tests to measure hormone levels. Once an appropriate dose is found for a patient, it is taken once a day.

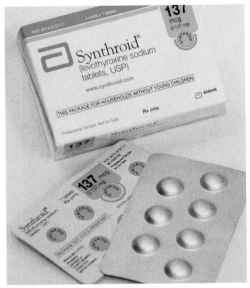

Levothyroxine is available as a generic drug or as the brand-name product Synthroid.

TABLE 20.8 Common Thyroid Hormone Products

Generic (Brand)	Dosage Form	Route of Administration
Levothyroxine (Synthroid, Tirosint)	Capsule, tablet	Oral
Liothyronine (Cytomel)	Tablet	Oral
Liothyronine (Triostat)	Solution for injection, tablet	Injection, oral
Liotrix (Thyrolar)	Tablet	Oral
Thyroid extract (Armour Thyroid)	Tablet	Oral

Side Effects Common side effects of thyroid hormone are usually related to therapeutic overdose, a situation in which a patient exhibits hyperthyroid symptoms due to excess thyroid hormone. Such symptoms include heart palpitations, rapid heart rate, elevated blood pressure, fever, tremors, headache, nervousness, insomnia, anxiety, hyperactivity, irritability, diarrhea, vomiting, abdominal cramps, skin flushing, sweating, heat intolerance, and weight loss. Patients should notify their prescribers if any of these effects begin to occur. Long-term overdosage can also cause loss of bone density and impair fertility. If gross overdosing continues, cardiac arrest can occur.

Contraindications Levothyroxine and liothyronine use is contraindicated in the presence of an acute heart attack, untreated thyrotoxicosis, and uncorrected adrenal insufficiency. Armour Thyroid, which contains beef and pork products, should not be used in patients with a hypersensitivity to beef or pork.

Contraindications exist for various forms of common thyroid hormone products. The capsule form of levothyroxine should not be used in individuals who cannot swallow capsules. The injection form of liothyronine should not be used in patients who are undergoing artificial rewarming.

Cautions and Considerations Thyroid medications can produce weight loss, but it is not an effective weight-loss therapy and can be toxic. Serious and potentially life-threatening toxic effects can occur with higher doses, especially in patients with normal levels of thyroid hormones.

Patients should be reminded to get regular blood tests to check thyroid hormone levels. Various brands of thyroid hormone may contain slightly different amounts, enough for changes in therapy to be experienced by individual patients. Once one brand of thyroid hormone is chosen, the patient should continue receiving that brand at each refill.

Hyperthyroidism

Hyperthyroidism is a disorder in which too much thyroid hormone is produced. This condition is less common than hypothyroidism. Causes of hyperthyroidism include **Graves' disease**, thyroid nodules or tumors, and pituitary nodules or tumors. Symptoms of hyperthyroidism include diarrhea, skin flushing, nervousness, hyperactivity, insomnia, heat intolerance, perspiration, tachycardia, decreased menses, and weight loss. One visible sign of hyperthyroidism is **exophthalmos**, a condition in which fat collects behind the eyeball, causing protrusion of the eye and an inability of the eyelids to fully close. In addition to natural causes of hyperthyroidism, taking too much thyroid hormone can cause an individual to experience these symptoms.

Patient Teaching

Thyroid pills are color-coded, so patients may refer to their dose by the color of the pill. You might consider keeping a handy reference card listing the color for each dose available near your workstation, so you can be sure you are documenting the correct dose in the patient's record.

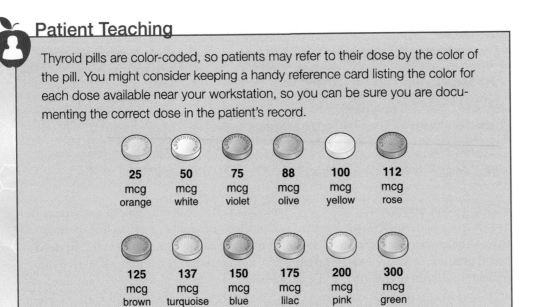

25 mcg orange	50 mcg white	75 mcg violet	88 mcg olive	100 mcg yellow	112 mcg rose
125 mcg brown	137 mcg turquoise	150 mcg blue	175 mcg lilac	200 mcg pink	300 mcg green

Drug Regimens and Treatments

Treatment for hyperthyroidism usually involves surgery, which removes or reduces the malfunctioning gland, or **ablation**, which destroys the thyroid gland via radioactive iodine. Propylthiouracil and methimazole are sometimes used for short-term suppression of thyroid hormones. Afterward, **oral thyroid supplementation** is given to artificially provide adequate hormone levels.

Addison's Disease

Addison's disease is a deficiency, or underproduction, of glucocorticoids and mineralocorticoids from the adrenal glands. Symptoms include fatigue, weakness, hyperkalemia (high potassium levels), hyperpigmentation of skin, low blood sodium, low blood glucose, low blood pressure, and weight loss. This condition can be serious and must be treated with oral corticosteroids.

Drug Regimens and Treatments

Acute adrenal deficiency can be life-threatening and is treated with IV fluids and **dexamethasone**. Chronic adrenal deficiency is treated with corticosteroids given in a schedule that mimics the normal circadian rhythm. When using **hydrocortisone**, a short-acting steroid, a larger dose (10 mg) is taken in the morning, followed by a smaller dose (5 mg) in the afternoon. When using oral dexamethasone, a longer-acting steroid, the dose is taken once a day in the morning. Individual response needs to be monitored and the dose adjusted to relieve symptoms.

Side Effects Common side effects of corticosteroids include headache, dizziness, insomnia, and hunger. Taking corticosteroids in the morning may lessen these effects, especially insomnia. Long-term or excessive use can affect normal metabolism in the body and cause symptoms of steroid overproduction (see Cushing's syndrome). Severe effects include high blood pressure, loss of bone mass (osteoporosis), electrolyte imbalance, cataracts or glaucoma, and insulin resistance (diabetes). Patients taking corticosteroids long term need special monitoring to avoid or treat these effects.

Contraindications There are no contraindications for propylthiouracil and methimazole. Dexamethasone use is contraindicated in systemic fungal infections and cerebral malaria. Contraindications to hydrocortisone include serious infections (except septic shock or tuberculous meningitis) and skin lesions of viral, fungal, or tubercular origin. Injectable hydrocortisone should not be administered intramuscularly in patients with idiopathic thrombocytopenic purpura or via the intrathecal route.

Cautions and Considerations Patients should not stop taking corticosteroids abruptly. Untoward and life-threatening effects can occur if a patient who has been taking chronic corticosteroids discontinues them suddenly. Because these medications can suppress the immune system if taken in large doses, patients taking them may be at an increased risk for infection. Growth and development must be monitored closely in children taking corticosteroids long term because these drugs have the potential to stunt growth.

Cushing's Syndrome

Whereas Addison's disease is caused by an underproduction of corticosteroid hormones, **Cushing's syndrome** is an overproduction or overdose of corticosteroid hormones. Normal sleep and wake cycles may also be affected as the circadian rhythm is disrupted. Cushing's syndrome is often caused by tumors of some kind in the adrenal glands, but elevated steroid hormone levels can also be caused by overmedication with corticosteroids. Symptoms include a round, puffy face (called moon face); abdominal weight gain; osteoporosis; mood changes and psychosis; hypertension; cataracts; peptic ulcer disease; and fat accumulation over the shoulder blades (called buffalo hump).

Drug Regimens and Treatments

Surgery is used most often to remove tumors causing Cushing's syndrome. Sometimes cytotoxic or chemotherapy drugs are used to treat the tumor and suppress corticosteroid production. (See Chapter 27 for more information on chemotherapeutic agents.)

 Checkpoint 20.4

Take a moment to review what you have learned so far and answer these questions.

1. What are the symptoms of hypothyroidism?
2. What are the brand names of the thyroid hormone products commonly used to treat hypothyroidism?
3. What is the difference between Addison's disease and Cushing's syndrome?

Herbal and Alternative Therapies

Chromium is an essential trace element that has been used for diabetes prevention and treatment. Its effectiveness is somewhat controversial, in that patients should not expect dramatic reductions in blood glucose levels from taking it. Patients with diabetes have been found to be deficient in chromium, but little definitive evidence is available to verify that correcting chromium deficiency is beneficial for improving blood glucose levels. Typical doses range from 200–1,000 mg a day. Side effects are rare but may include headache, insomnia, diarrhea, and hemorrhage. Patients with kidney or liver disease should not take chromium.

Cinnamon is often taken for Type 2 diabetes. One initial study showed potential benefits, but all subsequent trials have shown that cinnamon has little effect on blood glucose levels. Although manufacturers of cinnamon products claim benefits, patients should know that taking cinnamon may not produce any noticeable effect on their blood glucose or hemoglobin A1c results. Patients with liver disease probably should not take cinnamon because it has the potential to exacerbate hepatic conditions.

Chapter Review

Chapter Summary

The endocrine system regulates various body functions via hormone production. This system of glands regulates metabolism, growth, and fluid balance in a variety of ways.

The pancreas produces insulin and glucagon, which regulate blood glucose levels. Without glucose, cells in the body die from lack of energy. Type 1 diabetes is an autoimmune disorder that destroys beta cells in the pancreas, thereby eliminating their ability to produce insulin. Type 2 diabetes begins with central obesity that causes insulin insensitivity. Eventually, insulin and glucagon production are altered, and blood glucose rises. Type 1 diabetes is treated with insulin and products that supplement insulin. Agents for Type 2 diabetes include metformin, insulin secretagogues, TZDs, incretins, insulin, and SGLT-2 inhibitors. Because Type 2 diabetes is prevalent in the US population, the medications prescribed to treat this condition are among the top 100 drugs dispensed in pharmacies.

The thyroid gland controls the metabolic rate, which has effects on weight, heart rate, and digestion. Hypothyroidism is the underproduction of thyroid hormone and is treated with oral thyroid hormone supplementation. Hyperthyroidism is the overproduction of thyroid hormone and is usually treated by removing or destroying the thyroid gland. This procedure is typically followed by providing the patient with oral thyroid hormone supplementation.

The adrenal glands produce steroid hormones that affect metabolism, appetite, daily wake/sleep cycles, and fat deposition in the body. Addison's disease is a deficiency of steroid hormones, whereas Cushing's syndrome is an excess of these hormones.

Chapter Checkup

The Navigator+ learning management system that accompanies this textbook offers many opportunities to help you master chapter content, including end-of-chapter exercises, a glossary of key terms, flash cards, and additional interactive activities.

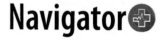

Career Exploration

If you enjoyed learning about the endocrine system in this chapter, you may want to explore the following career options:

- certified clinical nutritionist
- diabetes educator
- medical assistant
- nuclear medicine technologist
- pharmacy technician
- registered dietitian

UNIT 7

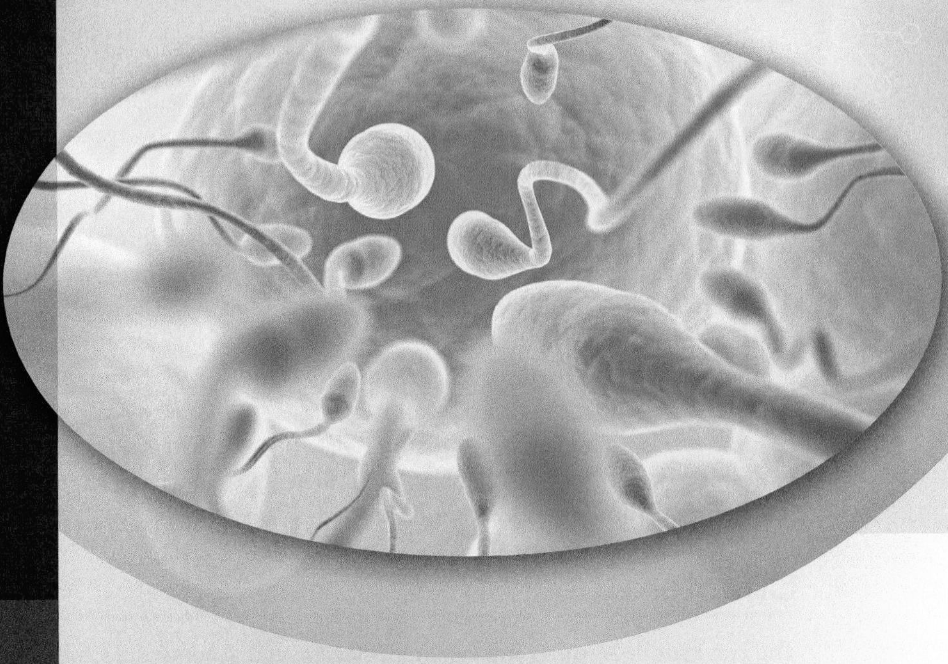

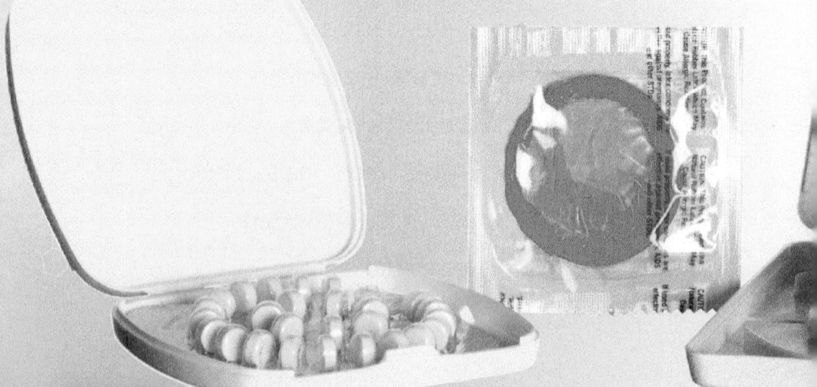

Navigator

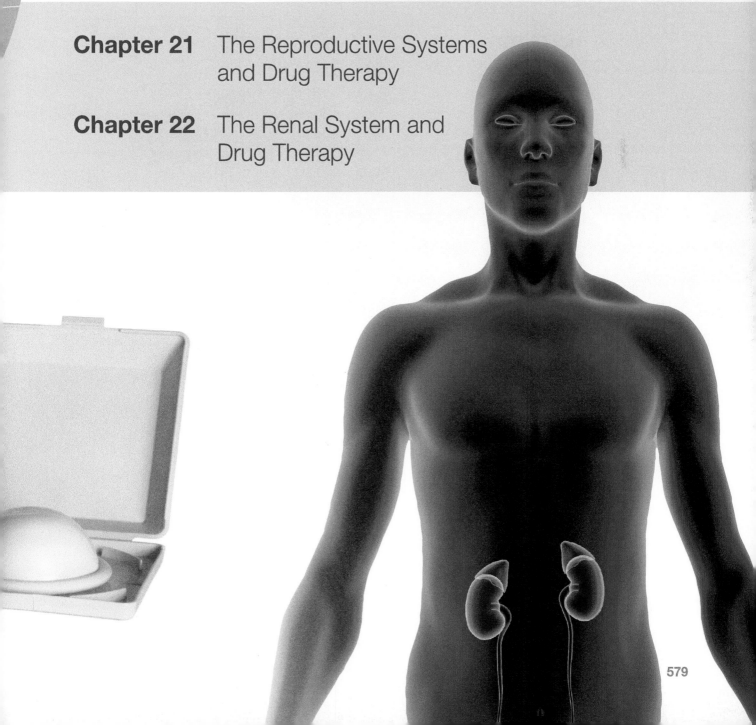

Pharmacotherapy for the Genitourinary System

The Reproductive Systems and Drug Therapy

Pharm Facts

- All humans begin the first hour of life as a single cell.

- The largest cell in the female body is the ovum, which is visible to the human eye. In the male body, a sperm is the smallest cell, consisting of little more than a nucleus.

- A female is born with approximately one to two million ovarian follicles, each containing an oocyte. Half of these are lost by puberty, and about 400 to 500 primary follicles will ripen into mature follicles during her reproductive life.

- A male produces about 1,000 sperm cells per second.

- The placenta is unusual in that it is the only temporary organ in the human body. It only grows when there is a developing embryo and fetus and is expelled from the mother with the birth of the baby.

- At around the 28th week of pregnancy, a fetus can smell the same things as his or her mother can smell.

"I am constantly impressed by the role that ultrasound sonography plays in medicine. My work as a diagnostic medical sonographer has helped both parents and healthcare practitioners make informed decisions about maternal and fetal health. In addition, some of my most joyous moments have come from introducing parents to their baby for the first time and informing them of their baby's gender. After 18 years in the sonography field, I can truly say that my decision to be a sonographer was one of the best choices that I have ever made."

—**Wendy Fuller**, BBA, RDMS
Diagnostic Medical Sonographer

Learning Objectives

1   Understand the basic anatomy and physiology of the male and female reproductive systems.

2   Describe the common conditions that affect the male and female reproductive systems.

3   Explain the therapeutic effects of prescription medications and non-prescription medications commonly used to treat the male and female reproductive systems.

4   Identify the generic names, brand names, indications, dosage ranges, side effects, contraindications, and cautions and considerations associated with the drugs commonly used to treat the male and female reproductive systems.

5   Identify common herbal and alternative therapies that are related to the male and female reproductive systems.

Navigator

Oral contraceptives, estrogen replacement therapies, drugs for erectile dysfunction, and antibiotics for sexually transmitted infections are commonly prescribed medications in healthcare settings. In fact, oral contraceptives and estrogen replacement therapies are among the top 200 most commonly dispensed medications in the United States. Due to the sensitive nature of the conditions that they treat, these products generate many questions from patients that require confidentiality. Armed with information, allied health professionals should feel confident in helping to dispel myths and assist patients with their reproductive healthcare needs.

To that end, this chapter begins with an overview of the anatomy and physiology of the male and female reproductive systems, followed by descriptions of common disorders affecting these systems. Because the reproductive systems are regulated by hormones, many of the drugs used to treat their disorders contain these chemical messengers. This chapter distinguishes the uses, similarities, and differences in hormone therapies. For certain abnormal conditions—such as infertility, erectile dysfunction, and sexually transmitted infections—prescription medications are used. Other conditions related to a woman's life cycle may also require drug therapy, including contraceptives for the prevention of pregnancy and hormone replacement therapy for relief of menopausal symptoms.

Sex Hormone Production and Reproduction

The **reproductive system** is responsible for procreation and fetal development. Males and females have **gonads** (specialized reproductive organs) that make **gametes**, or cells containing single strands of deoxyribonucleic acid, or DNA (the code for life and cell function). These cells are generated specifically so that when they combine—one from the male and one from the female—they produce a **zygote** (a normal cell containing double-stranded DNA). Females produce **ova** (the plural of *ovum*) from the **ovaries**, and males produce **sperm** from the **testes** (the plural of *testis*). The ovum and sperm combine during **fertilization** to form a zygote, which becomes an **embryo** as it develops. If properly supported inside the female uterus, an embryo grows into a fetus and is born. Both male and female reproductive systems are regulated by the **hypothalamic-pituitary-gonadal (HPG) axis**, as seen in Figure 21.1. In response to a negative feedback loop, the pituitary gland releases **follicle-stimulating hormone (FSH)** and **luteinizing hormone (LH)**, which stimulate sex hormone production from the ovaries and testes. The sex hormones include estrogen, progesterone, and testosterone. Testosterone is made by both males and females. However, testosterone is more prominent in males, and estrogen is more prominent in females. Although sex hormones are produced primarily from the ovaries and testes, approximately 5% of them come from a process called **aromatization**. This process occurs peripherally, in tissues other than the ovaries and testes.

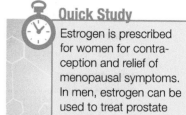

Quick Study

Estrogen is prescribed for women for contraception and relief of menopausal symptoms. In men, estrogen can be used to treat prostate cancer.

FIGURE 21.1 HPG Axis

The HPG axis controls sexual maturation and reproduction in humans.

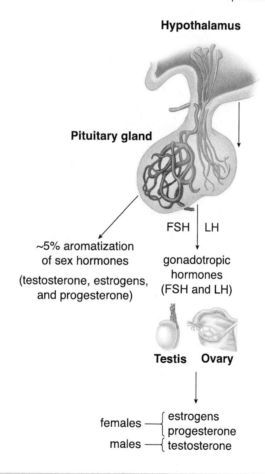

Hypothalamus

Pituitary gland

FSH | LH

~5% aromatization
of sex hormones

(testosterone, estrogens,
and progesterone)

gonadotropic
hormones
(FSH and LH)

Testis   Ovary

females —{ estrogens
         { progesterone
males —{ testosterone

Anatomy and Physiology of the Male Reproductive System

The male reproductive system includes the testes, epididymis, ductus deferens (also called *vas deferens*), seminal vesicles, prostate gland, urethra, and penis (see Figure 21.2). The purpose of the male reproductive system is to facilitate sexual reproduction and to eliminate urine from the body. During a male's lifetime, trillions of sperm cells originate in the testes, or testicles, which are located in the **scrotum**. After maturing in a part of the scrotum known as the **epididymis**, sperm move through the **ductus deferens**. During sexual stimulation, sperm combine with **semen**, the fluid produced by the **seminal vesicles** and **prostate gland**. The semen then travels through the **urethra** and is ejaculated from the **penis**. The purpose of ejaculation is to deliver sperm into a woman's vagina near the cervix, thus enabling the sperm to travel to the fallopian tubes to fertilize an ovum.

FIGURE 21.2	Anatomy of the Male Reproductive System

The prostate gland and seminal vesicles contribute to the nourishment and energy of sperm. The prostate gland produces a fluid that keeps sperm viable; the seminal vesicles produce a fluid that contains fructose (sugar), which gives sperm energy to move.

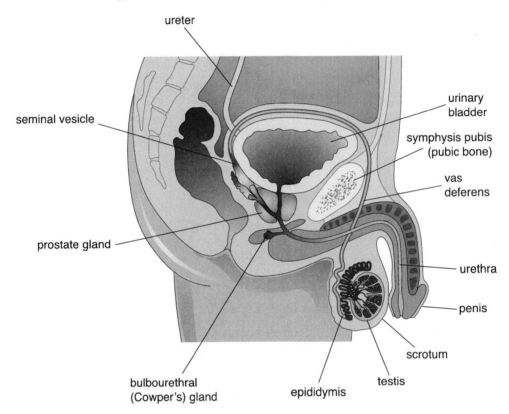

Male Sex Hormones

Both female and male sex hormones are produced in response to FSH and LH from the pituitary gland. However, in males this process is continuous and does not cycle every 28 days. FSH and LH stimulate androgen production from **Leydig cells** in the testes.

Testosterone

Testosterone, the primary **androgen** in males, is responsible for sperm production and maturation of male genitalia. Testosterone is also associated with secondary sexual characteristics, which develop during puberty in males, including pubic hair growth, increased libido (sex drive), fat distribution away from hips and thighs to the abdomen, and development of greater bone and muscle mass than in females. Testosterone is also responsible for male-pattern hair growth (such as on the chest) and baldness. Testosterone levels decline with age but do not typically cause the dramatic symptoms in men that menopause causes in women. Changes men may experience with reduced testosterone associated with age include decreased testicular size, muscle weakness, reduced bone density, and decreased energy, mood, and libido.

Anatomy and Physiology of the Female Reproductive System

The female reproductive system includes the ovaries, fallopian tubes, uterus, cervix, and vagina (see Figure 21.3). These organs develop and present mature ova for fertilization and then support the growth of the embryo and fetus when fertilization occurs.

FIGURE 21.3 Anatomy of the Female Reproductive System

When a woman is not pregnant, the uterus measures a mere three inches long and two inches wide. However, because the uterus has some of the strongest muscles in the female body, this organ can expand to accommodate a growing fetus.

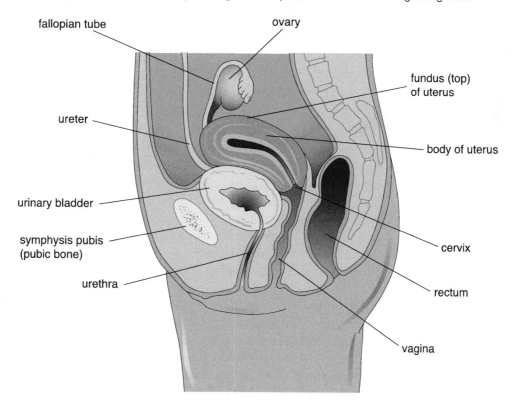

The ovaries produce ova in response to FSH from the pituitary gland. After release from the ovary, the ovum travels through the **fallopian tube** to the **uterus**. If sperm is present, fertilization typically happens within the fallopian tube. If the ovum is fertilized, a zygote is formed and begins dividing into a clump of cells that gradually develops into an embryo. As this cell division occurs, the zygote, now referred to as a *blastocyst*, travels to the uterus and implants in the endometrial lining (see Figure 21.4). If the ovum is not fertilized, the egg passes through the uterus and out through the **cervix** to the **vagina**. The uterine lining then sloughs off, and the whole process starts over. This sloughing of the endometrial tissue is called **menstruation** (commonly referred to as a woman's *period* or *monthly cycle*).

FIGURE 21.4 Fertilization and Implantation

Fertilization typically occurs in the fallopian tube within a day or two of ovulation if sperm are present. When fertilization does not occur, the ovum travels through the fallopian tube and uterus and leaves the body through the vagina.

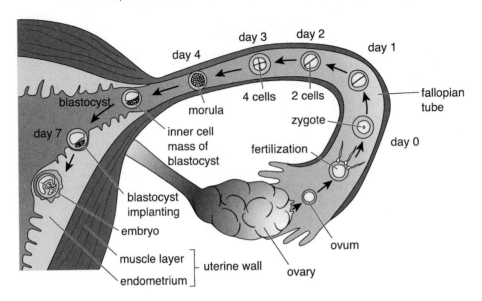

Menstrual Cycle

The **menstrual cycle** is regulated by FSH, LH, estrogen, and progesterone. It restarts about every 28 days, unless pregnancy occurs (see Figure 21.5). The cycle begins with FSH production from the pituitary gland. FSH stimulates follicles in the ovaries to grow and produce estrogen. Even though a handful of follicles begin to grow with each cycle, generally only one will release an ovum. As the ova inside the follicles reach maturity, the pituitary gland senses a rise in estrogen in the bloodstream and releases LH. The surge in LH causes the most mature follicle to burst and release an ovum. Ovulation occurs approximately every 28 days from puberty to menopause resulting in as many as 450 to 650 released ova over a lifetime. However, decreased ovum reserve and poor quality of aging **oocytes** begin to affect a woman's fertility in her late 30s and 40s. LH also stimulates the leftover follicle tissue (corpus luteum) to begin releasing progesterone, which facilitates endometrial lining growth and supports implantation. If implantation occurs, the placenta begins to develop and release **human chorionic gonadotropin (hCG)**, the pregnancy hormone. In the presence of hCG, progesterone and estrogen levels continue to rise. Without fertilization and the presence of hCG, progesterone levels drop and menstruation ensues.

Female Sex Hormones

Sex hormone production varies throughout a woman's life cycle. Production begins significantly at puberty. Hormone production begins to taper off and affect fertility during the fifth decade (ages 40 to 49) of a woman's life. During the sixth decade (ages 50 to 59), hormone production dramatically decreases during menopause.

FIGURE 21.5 | Female Menstrual Cycle

In pregnancy, the estrogen and progesterone levels continue to rise (instead of fall at the end of the luteal phase) to support embryo implantation and uterine/placental growth.

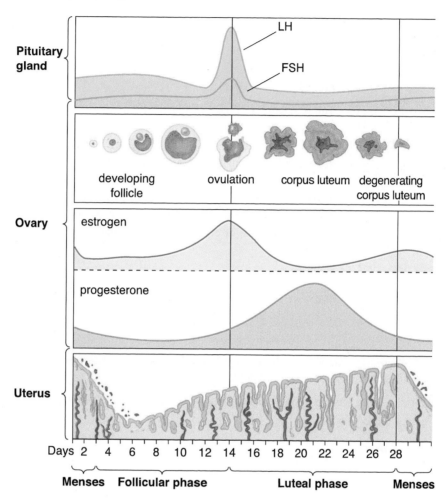

Estrogen

Estrogen is considered the primary female sex hormone because it is responsible for female sex characteristics, such as breast enlargement. It is also responsible for endometrial growth, production of cervical mucus, vaginal mucosa maintenance, bone health, and cessation of growth in height for females.

Estrogen has effects on sodium retention, the skin's blood vessels, cholesterol levels, blood coagulation, calcium utilization, and carbohydrate metabolism. A rise in estrogen levels coincides with bloating, weight gain, cravings, headaches, and mood swings during the days leading up to menstruation. When estrogen levels decline with age, menopausal symptoms (described later in this chapter) begin.

Progesterone

Progesterone, also referred to as progestin when produced in the body, is the hormone necessary for zygote implantation and the maintenance of pregnancy. Progesterone suppresses LH production, thickens cervical mucus, and alters the endometrial lining to support implantation. It has effects on insulin levels, glucose tolerance, fat deposition, and body temperature, all changes that prepare a woman's body for pregnancy. Progesterone levels rise in pregnancy and decline in menopause. Exogenous progesterone is prescribed for women for contraception, infertility, and menopausal symptoms.

hCG

The hormone hCG is considered the pregnancy hormone because its presence indicates that a zygote is implanted in the uterus and a placenta has started to form. The steep rise in this hormone level signals pregnancy to the body, which starts the physiologic changes that prepare for and maintain pregnancy. Thus, hCG is the hormone measured by home pregnancy tests. When it is present in measurable concentrations in the blood or urine, a diagnosis of pregnancy can be made.

Checkpoint 21.1

Take a moment to review what you have learned so far and answer these questions.

1. What are the anatomic parts of the male reproductive system with which sperm comes into contact as it is produced and as it exits the body?

2. What are the anatomic parts of the female reproductive system with which an ovum comes into contact as it is produced and as it exits the body?

3. What are the effects of the following hormones in and female body?

   - estrogen

   - progesterone

   - FSH

   - LH

Conditions and Disorders of the Male Reproductive System

Common conditions of the male reproductive system include low testosterone (also called *hypogonadism*), erectile dysfunction, and infertility. Another related condition, benign prostatic hyperplasia (BPH), is covered in Chapter 22. Sexually transmitted infections (STIs) that affect the male reproductive organs and methods of contraception affecting the male reproductive system are covered later in this chapter.

Hypogonadism

Hypogonadism, sometimes called *low testosterone*, is the underproduction of testosterone in men. Insufficient testosterone production can contribute to infertility in men. **Andropause** is the decline in androgen (testosterone) production that occurs with age. Symptoms include fatigue, low sexual desire, weakness, erectile dysfunction, poor sleep, depression, irritability, and memory loss. Many men attribute these symptoms simply to getting older. Recent research shows that low testosterone is associated with obesity and Type 2 diabetes. Hypogonadism can also be caused by previous radiation or chemotherapy, excessive consumption of alcohol, and long-term use of ketoconazole or opiates.

Drug Regimens and Treatments

Treatment of low testosterone can significantly improve quality of life and can improve fertility. Supplementation with the hormone that is missing or low is the aim of therapy. Removal of drugs that contribute to low testosterone should be attempted if possible before starting testosterone therapy.

Exogenous Testosterone

Exogenous testosterone is prescribed most commonly for testosterone deficiency (hypogonadism) in men. Dosing is adjusted individually and guided by laboratory tests and relief of symptoms. Exogenous testosterone is a controlled substance (Schedule III) because it can be used as a physical performance enhancement drug. Athletes, as reported in the media, use such agents to produce larger muscle mass and improve strength and speed. In general, exogenous testosterone and related compounds are referred to as **anabolic steroids**.

 Patient Teaching

> Exogenous testosterone is available as a topical gel. During its application, the gel can rub off onto another person, which can cause unwanted side effects in the other individual. To reduce the transfer of medication, advise the patient to wash his or her hands after application of the gel, avoid skin contact in the application area until the gel has dried, and avoid getting the application site wet for five hours after application.

Side Effects Topical exogenous testosterone products can cause local skin irritation. Other forms of this drug can have systemic effects. For example, exogenous testosterone can cause or exacerbate an enlarged prostate. Regular examinations with a healthcare practitioner can monitor for this effect. In addition, this medication can suppress LH release and thus affect sperm production. Consequently, patients who are taking exogenous testosterone on a long-term basis can experience problems with fertility. Finally, when taken in large amounts, exogenous testosterone can cause irritability, rage, and psychosis.

Contraindications Patients with prostate or breast cancer (men or women) and those with high prostate-specific antigen (PSA) laboratory test results should not take exogenous testosterone.

✚ *Note: Allied health professionals should be aware that an allergy to a particular drug contraindicates its use. This warning applies to all Contraindications sections in this chapter.*

Cautions and Considerations Unfortunately, many serious risks are associated with exogenous testosterone when it is not medically needed and is improperly used. Healthcare professionals should be aware of federal and state laws regarding dispensing exogenous testosterone products. Besides special storage, labeling, and handling issues related to controlled-substance laws, some states also require that prescriptions written for exogenous testosterone state the patient's medical diagnosis on the face of the document. Without this wording, a prescription is not considered legal and cannot be filled.

Patients with sleep apnea should be careful about taking exogenous testosterone because the medication can worsen this condition.

Erectile Dysfunction

Erectile dysfunction (ED) is the failure to initiate or maintain an erection until ejaculation. This condition is also referred to as **male impotence**. Causes include testosterone deficiency, high blood pressure, heart disease, alcoholism, cigarette smoking, diabetes with microvascular (blood vessel) problems, psychological factors, and medication. Cardiovascular disease is probably the condition most closely associated with ED. Some studies show that 40%–50% of patients with heart disease have some form of ED.

Certain medications can cause or contribute to ED (see Table 21.1). Many blood pressure medications, in particular, have been studied for their effects on sexual function. Not all these drugs cause problems with sexual function, but some researchers believe that drugs, such as beta blockers, can contribute to the problem.

TABLE 21.1 Drugs Associated with ED

Alcohol
Antidepressants, especially selective serotonin reuptake inhibitors (SSRIs)
Cimetidine
Clonidine
Ketoconazole
Methyldopa
Nicotine
Spironolactone
Thiazide diuretics

Drug Regimens and Treatments

Navigator

Table 21.2 lists common ED medications. By far the drugs most frequently used to treat ED are the **phosphodiesterase-5 (PDE-5) inhibitors**. In fact, PDE-5 inhibitors are usually listed in the top 50 drugs dispensed in pharmacies today. Even though much of the media attention is paid to these drugs, there are other treatment options for patients to consider. However, the routes of administration for these products are not as convenient as the oral route of PDE-5 inhibitors. One of these alternative treatment options is alprostadil. Considered a second-line choice of therapy for ED, **alprostadil** is a prostaglandin that works by relaxing smooth muscle in the vasculature of the penis. Alprostadil is injected into the base of the penis or inserted as a pellet into the urethra.

TABLE 21.2 | Common ED Medications

Generic (Brand)	Dosage Form	Route of Administration	Duration of Action	Common Dosage
PDE-5 Inhibitors				
Avanafil (Stendra)	Tablet	Oral	5 hours	100–200 mg taken 30 minutes prior to sexual activity
Sildenafil (Viagra)	Tablet	Oral	4 hours	50–100 mg taken 1–4 hours prior to sexual activity
Tadalafil (Cialis)	Tablet	Oral	36 hours	40 mg taken 1–36 hours prior to sexual activity
Vardenafil (Levitra)	Tablet	Oral	4 hours	10 mg taken 1 hour prior to sexual activity
Other				
Yohimbine (Aphrodyne, Yocon)	Tablet	Oral	Unknown	1 tablet (5.4 mg) 3 times a day

PDE-5 Inhibitors

PDE-5 inhibitors work by relaxing smooth muscle in the corpus cavernosum of the penis, which eases bloodflow into the area, facilitating erection. This effect, however, occurs only with excitatory or sexual stimulation. PDE-5 inhibitors do not cause erection directly or immediately. Instead, they create conditions whereby erection is allowed to occur more easily if sexual stimulation is applied. These medications are taken at least 30 to 60 minutes or more prior to sexual activity, depending on the agent. The duration of action varies among products, so planning for sexual activity must occur.

Side Effects Common side effects of PDE-5 inhibitors include headache, heartburn, nausea, and flushing. If an erection lasts longer than four hours or is painful (a condition called **priapism**), the patient should seek medical attention so that permanent tissue damage does not occur.

Contraindications PDE-5 inhibitors are contraindicated in patients who take nitrates or alpha blockers. The combination of PDE-5 inhibitors and these other medications can cause a dangerous drop in blood pressure. Alprostadil is an alternative when PDE-5 inhibitors are contraindicated. Patients must be appropriately instructed in the preparation and administration of alprostadil.

Cautions and Considerations Patients taking other medications for blood pressure should first discuss the use of PDE-5 inhibitors with their prescribers. Drinking alcohol while taking a PDE-5 inhibitor can worsen blood pressure effects. Patients may also experience increased heart rate, dizziness, and headache. PDE-5 inhibitors interact with several other medications. The patient should be sure that his pharmacist and prescriber know all the medications and

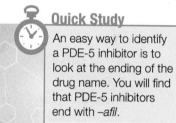

Quick Study

An easy way to identify a PDE-5 inhibitor is to look at the ending of the drug name. You will find that PDE-5 inhibitors end with *-afil*.

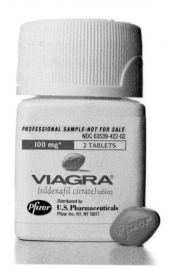

Viagra, a PDE-5 inhibitor, was initially used in clinical trials to treat angina and hypertension. Although the drug was unsuccessful for these indications, it did have an unexpected side effect in men: increased erections.

over-the-counter (OTC) dietary supplements he takes to avoid any dangerous interactions. You can help by obtaining thorough medication histories for patients who bring in prescriptions for PDE-5 inhibitors.

Yohimbine

Another drug therapy choice, **yohimbine,** works by blocking alpha-2 receptors and enhancing parasympathetic nervous system effects. This drug is taken three times a day continuously to promote conditions conducive to erection on sexual stimulation. It does not cause erection directly or immediately.

Side Effects Common side effects of yohimbine include changes in blood pressure, nervousness, irritability, tremor, dizziness, nausea, headache, and skin flushing.

Contraindications Yohimbine should not be used in the elderly or in patients with renal disease or a peptic or duodenal ulcer. In addition, patients with hypertension should not take yohimbine.

Cautions and Considerations This medication can interact with several antidepressant medications; therefore, patients taking antidepressants (other than monoamine oxidase inhibitors [MAOIs]) should avoid taking yohimbine or only do so if recommended by their prescribers.

Infertility

Infertility is the inability to achieve pregnancy after one year of regular, unprotected sexual intercourse. Infertility can be associated with problems in the male or female reproductive system, or both. It is estimated that up to 10% of the US population faces fertility issues at some point.

Common causes of infertility in men include infectious diseases, anatomic abnormalities, immunologic factors, and anything that hinders sperm production or prevents semen (and sperm) from exiting through the urethra. **Hyperprolactinemia** (overproduction of prolactin) and hypogonadism (low testosterone) are other causes of low sperm production and infertility. Lifestyle factors—such as excessive alcohol or caffeine consumption, tight-fitting underclothes, the use of hot tubs (which increase temperature of the testes), and the use of street drugs such as cocaine or marijuana—can also affect the growth and maturation of sperm.

Drug Regimens and Treatments

Making lifestyle changes such as smoking cessation, reduced alcohol consumption, and avoidance of street drugs can help enhance male fertility. Men with low sperm counts should wear loose-fitting underclothes (i.e., boxer shorts) to decrease the internal temperature in the testes. Hot tubs, saunas, and other activities that can raise body temperature should be avoided when trying to conceive if male fertility is a concern. Often an artificial method such as in vitro fertilization (IVF) may be necessary if the man is the major contributor to a couple's infertility. (For more information on IVF, see the section titled "Assistive Reproductive Technology" later in this chapter.)

For patients with hypogonadism, **gonadotropin therapy** may improve fertility. Such therapies include human chorionic gonadotropin, or hCG (Novarel, Ovidrel,

Pregnyl); human menopausal gonadotropin, or hMG (Menopur, Repronex); gonadotropin-releasing hormone, or GnRH (Nafarelin); and follicle-stimulating hormone, or FSH (follitropin alpha and beta). Mildly low testosterone levels can be treated with clomiphene (Clomid).

Checkpoint 21.2

Take a moment to review what you have learned so far and answer these questions.

1. What is hypogonadism and how is exogenous testosterone used to treat it?

2. What drugs are used to treat ED?

3. What are some nondrug methods of treatment for male infertility?

Conditions and Disorders of the Female Reproductive System

Common conditions of the female reproductive system covered in this chapter include pregnancy, infertility, and menopause. Most of these conditions are not necessarily abnormal conditions but are encountered almost daily by healthcare professionals. Many of these conditions involve drug therapy treatment. Your likelihood of working with patients who have these conditions is high. Sexually transmitted infections that affect the female reproductive organs and methods of contraception affecting the female reproductive system are covered later in this chapter.

Pregnancy

Pregnancy is the normal physiologic process that a woman's body goes through as a fetus develops within her uterus. Pregnancy rarely requires pharmacologic intervention. In fact, drug therapy is avoided during pregnancy whenever possible because many medications can affect the developing fetus in the womb. Still, a few drugs bear mentioning because they are used to treat the side effects and complications of pregnancy.

Nausea and vomiting are common side effects during the first trimester of pregnancy. Typically, these effects can be treated with the following measures. Patients should eat a snack before rising in the morning; consume small, frequent meals throughout the day; and drink small sips of water through a straw. However, sometimes nausea and vomiting are so severe that they interfere with daily living and can cause dehydration requiring hospitalization. This condition is called **hyperemesis gravidarum**.

Another complication, which occurs especially in the later stages of pregnancy, is **preeclampsia,** or the development of high blood pressure and proteinuria (protein in the urine). Symptoms include severe headache, blurred vision, stomach pain, nausea, vomiting, chest pain, and altered mental status. If left untreated, preeclampsia can progress to **eclampsia,** in which life-threatening seizures and coma can occur.

Testing for pregnancy at home allows a woman to make informed decisions about lifestyle and health care early in a pregnancy. Because vital organs begin to develop in the embryo in the first weeks of gestation, a woman's diet, alcohol consumption, caffeine intake, and medication use can affect this critical development. Early confirmation of pregnancy allows a woman to make choices that will improve her prenatal care. Several home pregnancy test kits are available on the market for patients to use. Although each one is slightly different in the technique and wait time, most patients get reliable results with these products.

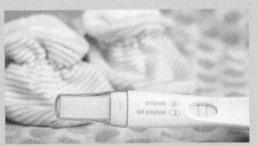

Home pregnancy test kits have an absorbent tip on the test stick that tests the urine for the presence of hCG. The test stick window displays the results.

Home pregnancy tests measure the presence of hCG in the urine. The hormone hCG is produced by the placenta once implantation has occurred. It can be detected as soon as six to eight days after conception, so home pregnancy tests can be used on day one of a missed period. Some test products claim to detect pregnancy hormone as soon as three or four days prior to a missed menstrual cycle. However, home pregnancy tests are most accurate on the first day of a missed period and after. Patients should realize that testing too soon may not detect a pregnancy and thus produce a false-negative result. It is best to test again in a couple of days after a negative result if the menstrual cycle has not begun. For patients to get the most accurate result from a home pregnancy test, healthcare professionals should advise them to use the first morning urine, as it will contain the highest concentration of hCG, if present. Patients should dip the test stick into the urine stream midway through urinating and then read the test stick results according to the manufacturer's guidelines.

Drugs Regimens and Treatments

Initial treatment of nausea and vomiting during pregnancy involves nonpharmacologic interventions. Drinking peppermint tea, sucking on peppermint candy, avoidance of foods and odors that trigger nausea, acupuncture or acupressure, and even hypnosis can be helpful. Ginger used in powder, tea, or candy form can also help alleviate nausea and vomiting. Vitamin B_6, antihistamines (diphenhydramine, meclizine, and dimenhydrinate), metoclopramide, and rectal promethazine have also been used with some success. Diclegis is a new prescription drug indicated for nausea and vomiting in pregnancy. This medication combines the antihistamine doxylamine with vitamin B_6.

Preeclampsia is treated with antihypertensive medications. Hydralazine and labetalol are often used to bring blood pressure down quickly during pregnancy. Anticonvulsants are used to treat or prevent seizures. Intravenous magnesium sulfate is typically used first, followed by phenytoin or diazepam.

Pregnancy Termination

Uterine evacuation procedures are undertaken for both elective **pregnancy termination** as well as for the management of spontaneous abortion, intrauterine fetal demise, and other medical conditions. The majority of pregnancy terminations occur surgically. However, pregnancy termination within the first trimester can be achieved with the assistance of drug therapy.

Patient Teaching

Healthcare professionals should help patients understand that drug therapy for pregnancy termination is not the same thing as emergency contraception. Medication-assisted pregnancy termination ends a pregnancy after blastocyst implantation in the uterine lining, whereas emergency contraception prevents ovulation or implantation from occurring in the first place.

Drug Regimens and Treatments

Drug therapy for pregnancy termination is only supplied to physician offices (not pharmacies) that agree to abide by strict monitoring and therapy guidelines. One of those guidelines requires three visits to a prescribing physician in a clinic, medical office, or hospital to determine the gestational age of the embryo. Two medications are approved for first-trimester pregnancy termination: mifepristone and misoprostol.

Mifepristone and Misoprostol

Mifepristone (Korlym, Mifeprex) and **misoprostol** (Cytotec) are taken to terminate a uterine pregnancy during the first 49 days of pregnancy. After taking one of these agents, the patient will experience cramps, spotting, and bleeding. This is an expected effect of taking these medications and is related to termination of the pregnancy.

Side Effects Common side effects include headache, diarrhea, nausea, and abdominal pain. These effects subside over time. Rarely, cardiovascular changes such as arrhythmia, high blood pressure, and chest pain can occur. The patient should seek medical attention if any of these rare side effects occur.

Name Exchange

Mifepristone may be referred to by the brand names Korlym or Mifeprex. You may also hear mifepristone referred to as RU-486, the name that was used during drug development.

Contraindications Patients who have a suspected **ectopic pregnancy** (embryo implanted outside of the uterus) or an intrauterine device in place should not take mifepristone. Patients who are taking long-term corticosteroids, concurrent anticoagulants, or immunosuppressive therapy should not take mifepristone. In addition, the presence of anemia, hemorrhagic disorders, or inherited porphyrias contraindicates mifepristone use. Patients with an allergy to prostaglandins should not take misoprostol.

Cautions and Considerations Patients must return for a follow-up visit after taking one of these agents. Prolonged and heavy vaginal bleeding will occur as a result of these medications, but patients should return for care to verify that pregnancy termination has occurred.

After pregnancy termination, patients are at an increased risk for bacterial infection. Patients should report fever, abdominal pain, or pelvic tenderness to their healthcare practitioners right away. Adrenal insufficiency, hypokalemia (low potassium), and alterations in cardiac rhythm can occur. Patients should adhere to instructions about follow-up so that their practitioners can monitor for these effects.

Infertility

As mentioned earlier in this chapter, infertility is the inability to achieve pregnancy after one year of regular, unprotected sexual intercourse. For women 35 years of age and older, infertility may be diagnosed sooner, after only six months, because egg production and quality decline quickly after that age. Infertility can be associated with problems in the female or male reproductive system, or both. It is estimated that up to 10% of the US population faces fertility issues at some point.

Common causes of infertility in women include pelvic inflammatory disease, hormonal imbalance, anatomic abnormalities, fibroids, and polycystic ovary syndrome (PCOS). **Endometriosis** is another common cause of infertility in women and has a negative effect on general health and well-being. This condition is the presence of endometrial tissue outside of the uterus. It can be in the fallopian tubes, ovaries, or pelvic abdominal cavity. Why this tissue grows outside of the uterus in some women is not fully understood, but such growth can cause pelvic or abdominal pain, heavy menstrual flow, severe cramping, and painful intercourse. Women with endometriosis tend to have more problems with irritable bowel symptoms and infections of the urinary tract and vagina. Endometriosis can also be silent—a woman may not realize she has it until she encounters problems when trying to become pregnant.

Patient Teaching

Allied health professionals who are caring for female patients who want to become pregnant may be involved in a discussion about home ovulation test kits. Remind these patients that if intercourse is timed to take place during the ideal period of ovulation, the likelihood of sperm and egg meeting in the fallopian tube is increased and the chances of pregnancy improved. Explain to them that one method for predicting ovulation is based on body temperature: Immediately before ovulation, a slight decrease in body temperature occurs, followed by a slight rise after the egg is released. Tell patients that by measuring basal body temperature daily and charting the results over time, they can detect trends and predict when ovulation is most likely to occur.

Inform patients that several types of home test kits exist for ovulation prediction. These tests tend to be more sensitive and are used more often than temperature charting. One type is a home ovulation kit that measures hormonal fluctuation, which predicts when ovulation is about to occur. Another type is a urine test kit that detects the LH surge that occurs just prior to ovulation. Tell patients that urine tests are easy to use, but the instructions should be followed closely. Most kits include five to seven tests, so it is important to test appropriately—on those days when ovulation is expected. A meter with test strips is available but is not usually covered by insurance. Patients should determine how often they plan to use ovulation tests to be sure that purchasing a meter is cost-effective.

Drug Regimens and Treatments

Assistive reproductive technology may be performed to achieve fertilization of an ovum. These treatments are often done in tandem with drug therapy.

Assistive Reproductive Technology

A complicated and specialized practice, **assistive reproductive technology (ART)** matches drug therapy and other modes of treatment to the specific cause of infertility. For example, the process of **ovulation induction** uses hormones (such as FSH and LH) to stimulate the ovaries to produce and release multiple ova. In **artificial insemination**, semen that contains sperm is collected from a man and introduced into a woman's uterus during peak ovulation. These two methods are often used together to bring more ova and sperm into potential contact and thus improve the chances of fertilization. **In vitro fertilization (IVF)** is a procedure whereby multiple eggs are retrieved from a woman (after ovulation induction) and artificially fertilized with sperm (from a designated man) in a laboratory (see Figure 21.6). The embryos are then placed into the woman's uterus for implantation. Additional drug therapy is often given after fertilization to improve the chances of implantation and to help maintain a pregnancy once initiated.

Therapies used for ovulation induction and IVF include GnRH (Nafarelin), FSH (follitropin alpha and beta), hCG (Novarel, Ovidrel, Pregnyl), and hMG (Menopur, Repronex).

FIGURE 21.6 | In Vitro Fertilization

According to the American Society of Reproductive Medicine, the average cost of a single IVF procedure (shown here) is $12,400.

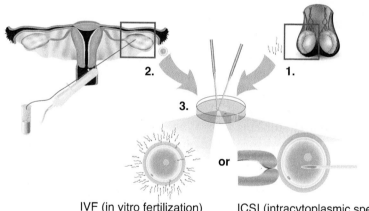

1. The sperm is collected.
2. The eggs are removed from the ovary.
3. The eggs are fertilized with sperm in a laboratory.
4. The fertilized eggs are growing.
5. The embryos are transferred to the uterus.

IVF (in vitro fertilization)   ICSI (intracytoplasmic sperm injection)

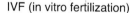

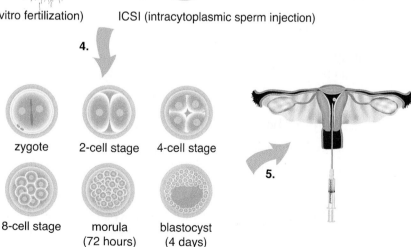

zygote   2-cell stage   4-cell stage

8-cell stage   morula (72 hours)   blastocyst (4 days)

Side Effects Infants conceived through ART may have a higher risk of low birth weight, preterm birth, and perinatal death. Research in this area is ongoing.

Contraindications ART therapies are contraindicated in patients with abnormal uterine bleeding, liver disease, ovarian cysts, and thyroid or pituitary tumors.

Cautions and Considerations Although a few medications in ART are taken orally, many ART agents are costly injectables that require precise dosing and close monitoring. Insurance plans generally do not cover ART or the medications involved, so patients pay their own costs. In fact, just one cycle of drug therapy alone for ovulation induction can cost the patient more than $5,000. Due to their high cost and specialized use, ART agents are usually dispensed by specialty pharmacies. Healthcare professionals who have the opportunity to work with these patients and fertility medications should be mindful of the emotional and financial toll that ART takes on patients.

The use of ART therapies increases the possibility of multiple births. Patients should understand and be prepared for this potential result. Pregnancy and delivery of multiple births have complications for both the mother and babies involved. If multiple births are not desired, ovulation induction should be halted and barrier methods of contraception used to prevent pregnancy.

Clomiphene Therapy

Clomiphene (Clomid) is often the first drug therapy used for ovulation induction, especially in women who have irregular menstrual cycles and inconsistent ovulation. The advantage is that it is inexpensive and does not necessarily require complex monitoring with ultrasound and laboratory tests. In women with PCOS, metformin can be used in addition to clomiphene to increase the chance of ovulation.

Side Effects Common side effects of clomiphene include visual disturbances, nausea, vomiting, hot flashes, headache, and breast tenderness. Ovarian hyperstimulation syndrome (OHSS) is also a potential side effect of clomiphene for which all patients will be closely monitored. Symptoms of OHSS include ovarian enlargement, abdominal pain, bloating, nausea, vomiting, diarrhea, weight gain, difficulty breathing, and frequent urination. If not treated, OHSS can cause severe low blood pressure, electrolyte imbalance, pulmonary distress, blood clots, and liver problems. OHSS can develop rapidly and may require hospitalization, so patients should seek medical attention if any of these symptoms occur during clomiphene therapy.

Contraindications Clomiphene is contraindicated in liver disease, abnormal uterine bleeding, enlargement or development of ovarian cyst, uncontrolled thyroid or adrenal dysfunction, and pregnancy.

Cautions and Considerations Clomiphene may increase the risk of ovarian cancer. Caution should be exercised in patients with PCOS, as lower doses may be necessary. Uterine fibroids may enlarge with clomiphene use.

Gonadotropin Therapy

Depending on the cause of infertility, **gonadotropin therapy** may be used. This therapy is used to produce multiple ova in advance of IVF or to control development and release of an ovum to accurately time artificial insemination (see Table 21.3). Gonadotropin therapy involves receiving daily injections of FSH in the early part of the menstrual cycle and monitoring ovum development with laboratory and ultrasound tests. Once a mature ovum is present, the ovum can be collected for IVF or stimulated for release by using hCG. Often, a progestin will be given in the latter half of the menstrual cycle to support uterine lining growth and thus improve the chances of implantation and survival of a viable embryo.

TABLE 21.3 Gonadotropin Therapy Agents

Hormone	Function	Medication
Ovulation Stimulants		
FSH	Stimulates ovum development	Follitropins: Bravelle, Follistim, Gonal-f Menotropins: Menopur, Repronex
hCG and r-hCG	Mimic LH surge to trigger ovulation	hCG: Novarel, Pregnyl Recombinant hCG: Ovidrel
Implantation Supporters		
Progestins	Promote uterine lining growth to support implantation and viability of a fertilized embryo	Hydroxyprogesterone, medroxyprogesterone, megestrol, norethindrone, progesterone

Side Effects Common side effects of gonadotropin therapy include headache, nausea, vomiting, irritability, and mood swings. These effects can be bothersome but are usually manageable. OHSS is also a potential side effect for gonadotropin therapy. Refer to the side effects of clomiphene for more information about the symptoms of OHSS. Patients should seek medical attention if any of the symptoms occur during gonadotropin therapy.

Contraindications Gonadotropins are contraindicated in pregnancy. FSH is contraindicated in patients with high FSH levels; sex hormone–dependent tumors of the reproductive tract and accessory organs; intracranial lesions; uncontrolled thyroid, pituitary, or adrenal dysfunction; abnormal uterine bleeding; and ovarian cysts or enlargement not due to PCOS. The Repronex form of menotropins is contraindicated with infertility due to any cause other than anovulation, or failure to release ova over a period of three months.

The hormone hCG is contraindicated in precocious puberty and prostatic carcinoma. Additional contraindications associated with r-hCG include primary ovarian failure, uncontrolled thyroid or adrenal dysfunction, uncontrolled intracranial lesion, abnormal uterine bleeding, ovarian cyst or enlargement, and sex hormone–dependent tumors.

Progestins are contraindicated in patients with current thrombosis or a history of thrombosis or thromboembolic disorders; liver impairment; liver tumors or cholestatic jaundice of pregnancy; carcinoma of the breast or other hormone-sensitive cancers; undiagnosed vaginal bleeding unrelated to pregnancy; and uncontrolled hypertension.

Cautions and Considerations The risk of spontaneous abortion, ectopic pregnancy, and ovarian enlargement is increased with the use of gonadotropin therapy. Serious pulmonary effects and thromboembolic events have been reported with gonadotropin use.

Menopause

The life change of **menopause**, or cessation of sex hormone production in women, is not an abnormal physiologic process. Rather, it is part of the normal life cycle and typically occurs during the fifth or sixth decade of a woman's life. This process begins with perimenopause—a period of three to five years during which menstrual cycles become erratic, hormone levels fluctuate, and fertility declines. Menopause is permanent cessation of menstruation, defined by the absence of menses for at least 12 months. During menopause, ovarian follicle activity stops; estrogen levels drop 40%–60%; and progesterone levels fall dramatically. The release of FSH and LH, in fact, increases due to the negative feedback loop, but the ovaries lose sensitivity to these hormones.

Menopause has a significant impact on quality of life. Lack of estrogen causes vasomotor spasms (hot flashes), irregular menstrual bleeding, vaginal dryness and atrophy (tissue shrinkage), weight gain, insomnia, fatigue, loss of libido, depression, mood swings, and memory impairment. To mitigate the impact of these effects, many women take estrogen supplements—hormone replacement therapy (HRT).

Menopause is associated with several adverse outcomes, such as **osteoporosis** (bone thinning) and increased risk for heart disease and stroke. Because estrogen has beneficial effects on bone resorption, cholesterol metabolism, and blood coagulation, lack of estrogen after menopause causes bone thinning; elevations in blood cholesterol that contribute to atherosclerosis and heart disease; and increased potential for blood clot formation, resulting in stroke. Prior to menopause, estrogen provides protection against these conditions. Incidences of osteoporosis, heart disease, and stroke increase dramatically after menopause.

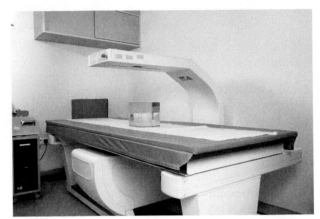

A bone densitometry machine measures bone density by estimating the amount of bone in a patient's hip, spine, or other bones. A menopausal woman over age 50 with a family history of osteoporosis is a likely candidate for such a procedure.

Drug Regimens and Treatments

For many years, hormones such as estrogen and progesterone were prescribed to provide relief from menopausal symptoms as well as to protect against life-threatening conditions, such as heart disease, stroke, and osteoporosis. However, research has shown that this therapy also carries risks. For example, increased rates of breast cancer are observed in women who take estrogen after menopause. Recent well-designed studies now report that the potential benefits and protections against heart disease and stroke originally thought to be associated with hormone replacement are not accurate. Therefore, the risks and benefits of HRT must be weighed for each patient individually.

Paroxetine (Paxil), an SSRI, is approved for use of vasomotor symptoms of menopause. Please see Chapter 13 for more information on SSRIs.

Hormone Replacement Therapy

Hormone replacement therapy (HRT) may be used in postmenopausal women with moderate-to-severe symptoms. However, doses should be kept as low as possible, and length of therapy should be as short as possible to minimize adverse effects. In addition, replacing multiple hormones in proportions that more closely mimic physiologic levels may produce better results than simply replacing lost estrogen and/or progesterone alone.

Although most people think of estrogen when referring to HRT, the hormones progesterone and estrogen are both prescribed for relief of menopausal symptoms. The current standard of practice is to use the lowest dose necessary for the shortest time possible. Women who have had a hysterectomy (removal of the uterus) can take estrogen alone. For most women (those retaining the uterus), estrogen and progesterone are taken in combination to reduce endometrial cancer risk, which is increased when estrogen is taken alone. Dosing is individualized to each patient (see Table 21.4).

Estrogen products usually include **ethinyl estradiol,** either from natural or equine (horse) sources. Conjugated estrogens are sodium salt forms of estrogen collected from pregnant mare urine. Progesterone preparations include synthetic agents such as medroxyprogesterone acetate or natural progesterone. Synthetic hormone products are available commercially and are taken orally or applied transdermally. Natural-source estrogen and progesterone products are specially compounded in pharmacies and are often used topically (on the skin). Some controversy exists about whether HRT compounded in a pharmacy has the same risks that synthetic products carry; most likely, they pose the same long-term risks. Natural HRT is an attractive choice for some women because it may produce fewer short-term side effects.

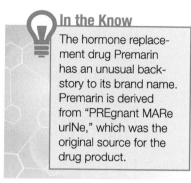

In the Know

The hormone replacement drug Premarin has an unusual backstory to its brand name. Premarin is derived from "PREgnant MARe urINe," which was the original source for the drug product.

TABLE 21.4 **Commercially Available Female Hormone Replacement Products**

Generic (Brand)	Dosage Form	Route of Administration
Conjugated estrogen (Premarin)	Cream, tablet	Oral, vaginal
Esterified estrogen (Menest)	Tablet	Oral
Estradiol (Estrace, Femtrace)	Tablet	Oral
Estradiol cypionate (Depo-Estradiol)	Oil	IM
Estradiol valerate (Delestrogen)	Oil	IM
Estropipate (Ortho-Est)	Tablet	Oral
Progesterone (Prometrium)	Capsule	Oral
Combination Products		
Conjugated estrogen/medroxyprogesterone (Premphase, Prempro)	Tablet	Oral
Estradiol/levonorgestrel (Climara Pro)	Patch	Transdermal
Ethinyl estradiol/norethindrone (Activella, Femhrt)	Tablet	Oral
Ethinyl estradiol/norethindrone (CombiPatch)	Patch	Transdermal

Side Effects Common side effects of HRT agents include dizziness, abdominal pain or bloating, diarrhea, nausea, headache, breast tenderness, vaginal discharge, fluid retention, hair loss, and depression. These side effects may subside with continued therapy. Sometimes, HRT can cause dark skin patches on the face, called *melasma*. Patients should inform their prescribers about these effects so that necessary dose changes can be made. Some women find that specialty and extemporaneous compounded forms of estrogen and progesterone produce fewer such effects.

Contraindications Because of the increased risks for breast, endometrial, and ovarian cancers associated with HRT use, patients with a history of these conditions should not begin this type of therapy. Patients with no personal history but with a significant family history of cancer should discuss the risks and benefits of HRT with their prescribers.

Patients with cardiovascular disorders, such as a previous heart attack, deep-vein thrombosis (DVT), or pulmonary embolism (PE), probably should not begin HRT. Patients with a family history of these conditions should discuss the risks and benefits with their prescribers.

Cautions and Considerations Patients with a history of stroke should discuss the risks and benefits of HRT with their healthcare practitioners before taking it. In some cases, HRT has been associated with an increased risk of stroke and heart attack.

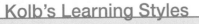

Kolb's Learning Styles

If you like to learn by discussing topics in a small group, as Divergers and Accommodators do, get together with at least two other individuals and discuss the pros and cons of HRT. What are some reasons that women choose or refuse to take HRT?

Sexual Dysfunction

Sexual dysfunction is reported by 40% of women worldwide. The hallmarks of this condition include low sexual desire, inability to reach orgasm, and pain during intercourse. These symptoms should be evaluated and diagnosed by a healthcare practitioner to determine the most likely cause and to provide appropriate treatment.

In premenopausal women, low sexual desire that causes distress or interpersonal difficulty is called **acquired, generalized hypoactive sexual desire disorder (HSDD)**. This disorder develops in a patient who has had no previous issues with sexual desire. In many cases, the causes of HSDD are not known.

Drug Regimens and Treatments

Premenopausal women with HSDD may be prescribed flibanserin, the first drug approved by the US Food and Drug Administration (FDA) to treat this disorder (see Table 21.5).

Flibanserin

Flibanserin (Addyi) is a mixed serotonin inhibitor, but its exact mechanism of action is unknown. This medication is taken once daily at bedtime to minimize the potential for low blood pressure and fainting. If no improvement in sexual desire is seen after taking flibanserin for eight weeks, the patient should discontinue taking it.

Flibanserin has been approved with a risk evaluation and mitigation strategy (REMS), a plan that manages the safe use of a medication with a known or potential serious risk. The REMS requires that prescribers must complete training to learn about flibanserin's interaction with alcohol and subsequently become certified to counsel patients when prescribing this medication. Only REMS-certified pharmacies and pharmacists may dispense flibanserin, and pharmacists must provide counseling to patients. This drug also must have a black box warning on the package insert that alerts prescribers and pharmacists to the risk of severe hypotension and syncope in patients who consume alcohol while taking flibanserin.

Side Effects Flibanserin can cause severe low blood pressure and fainting.

Contraindications Flibanserin should not be used in conjunction with alcohol consumption. Severe low blood pressure and fainting can occur. Patients must avoid drinking alcohol and using products that contain alcohol.

Patients with liver disease cannot take flibanserin. Patients with liver disease such as hepatitis should talk with their healthcare practitioners before taking flibanserin.

Cautions and Considerations There are many drugs that cannot be taken with flibanserin. Of note, patients should not take flibanserin with any OTC products, natural or herbal products (such as St. John's wort), or medications used to treat hepatitis or human immunodeficiency virus (HIV). Antibiotics, carbamazepine, phenobarbital, phenytoin, rifabutin, and rifampin also should not be taken with flibanserin. Because of the many drug interactions, flibanserin is distributed through the REMS program.

TABLE 21.5 Flibanserin

Generic (Brand)	Dosage Form	Route of Administration	Common Dose
Flibanserin (Addyi)	Tablet	Oral	100 mg a day at bedtime

Checkpoint 21.3

Take a moment to review what you have learned so far and answer these questions.

1. What drugs are used to treat infertility in women?

2. What is menopause and how is estrogen used to treat it?

3. When would a woman use a home pregnancy test kit versus a home ovulation test kit?

Contraception

Contraception is any practice that serves to prevent pregnancy during sexual activity. These practices can be either nonpharmacologic or pharmacologic. Contraceptive methods that are nonpharmacologic include **abstinence** and **temporary abstinence**. Contraceptive methods that are pharmacologic include oral contraceptives; various barrier products, such as male and female condoms; transdermal and vaginal contraceptives; and various injections, implants, and intrauterine devices. Because of the pharmacology foundation of this textbook, the pharmacologic methods of contraception are discussed in depth in this section.

Rates of Effectiveness

Choosing a method of contraception is a personal decision, and individuals must consider several factors including rates of effectiveness, ease of use, and adherence requirements. Patients should understand that rates of effectiveness for preventing pregnancy reported in product labeling refer to "perfect use." These rates are only achieved when the patient follows instructions exactly and uses the product every time he or she engages in sexual intercourse. If a product is difficult to use or undesirable for a particular patient, adherence will not be ideal. Perfect use is not representative of actual use in many cases, and all products have some failures, even if such failures are rare.

Contraceptive Products for the Male Reproductive System

Birth control products on the market that work for the male reproductive system generally use physical barriers that prevent sperm and ova from coming into contact. Drug therapy that alters sperm production and thus affects male fertility has been researched, but no effective products have been brought to market.

Barrier Products

Barrier birth control products are used when intercourse is anticipated. These products form a physical barrier that prevents sperm from entering the uterus through the cervix. To be effective, the products are put in place prior to intercourse, left there for a specific amount of time, and then removed.

Contraceptive Device

The only contraceptive device for men is the male condom.

Male Condom

The **male condom** is placed over the erect penis before penetration into the vagina. Condoms collect the ejaculate (semen and sperm) and prevent it from coming into contact with the vagina or cervix. Ejaculate material is removed along with the condom. Condoms are the only birth control method other than abstinence that also prevents or lowers the risk of transmission of sexually transmitted infections (STIs), also referred to as sexually transmitted diseases (STDs). Latex and polyurethane condoms provide the best protection because they are impermeable.

Condoms are available in a variety of options and may contain spermicides. Although **spermicides** may help reduce the likelihood of pregnancy when used with condoms, they are not considered highly effective when used alone.

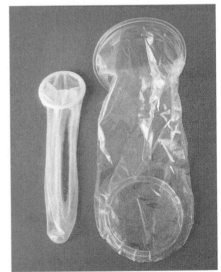

Side Effects Other than latex allergy and skin irritation, no apparent side effects are typically associated with condom use. In condoms with spermicide, side effects also include irritation, burning, or itching of mucous membranes.

Contraindications Latex allergy is a contraindication to latex condom use. Men and women who have a latex allergy should use polyurethane condoms. Condoms with spermicide include nonoxynol 9. Patients with a hypersensitivity to nonoxynol 9 should avoid condoms with spermicide.

Cautions and Considerations Getting the proper fit, keeping the condom on during the entire sexual activity, and maintaining an erection while wearing a condom have been reported as problems that decrease the ease of use and effectiveness of condoms.

The male condom (left) and female condom (right) are barrier methods of contraception. Both devices are OTC products that prevent sperm from entering the vagina.

Water-based lubricants such as K-Y Jelly and Astroglide can be used with latex condoms. However, oil-based lubricants can facilitate condom breakage and are not recommended for use with condoms. Some other vaginal products and medications can contain oil-based ingredients such as butoconazole and mineral oil. Therefore, patients using these therapies should abstain from intercourse or use polyurethane condoms until this therapy is completed. Finally, concurrent use of male and female condoms is not recommended because friction between the condoms can cause them to break.

Contraceptive Products for the Female Reproductive System

Birth control products on the market today that affect the female reproductive system generally apply one or more of the following contraception approaches:

- physical or pharmacologic barriers that prevent sperm and ova from coming into contact

- drug therapy that prevents ovulation from occurring

- drug therapy that prevents implantation of a fertilized ovum in the uterus

As mentioned earlier in the chapter, patients should understand that rates of effectiveness for contraception methods are only achieved when the patient follows instructions exactly and uses the product every time he or she engages in sexual intercourse. However, there are circumstances that may hinder the effectiveness of certain types of birth control, despite perfect adherence by the patient. For example, specific drugs and conditions may adversely affect the efficacy of the oral contraceptive pill.

Barrier Products

As mentioned earlier, barrier birth control products are used when intercourse is anticipated. These products form a physical barrier that prevents sperm from entering the uterus through the cervix. To be effective, the products are put in place prior to intercourse, left there for a specific period, and then removed. Barrier products do not alter normal ovulation, cervical mucus, or endometrial lining formation.

Contraceptive Devices

Contraceptive devices for women include barrier products such as the female condom, diaphragm, and cervical cap.

Female Condom

The **female condom** is worn by a woman and forms a physical barrier between the penis and the vagina. The female condom is made of nitrile material instead of latex, and it is inserted up to eight hours before sexual activity. When used properly, the condom holding the ejaculate material is removed after intercourse. As mentioned earlier, condoms also prevent or lower the risk of STI transmission.

Side Effects Few if any side effects are typically associated with the use of female condoms.

Contraindications The female condom is not contraindicated in any specific patient population. This type of condom can be used as an alternative barrier method of birth control when one of the partners has a latex allergy.

Cautions and Considerations To ensure effectiveness of this contraceptive, partners must be sure that the penis does not slip between the vagina and the outer surface of the condom or that the outer ring does not get pushed inside of the vagina. Although the female condom can be removed at any time after intercourse, it is most effective when removed before the woman stands up, to avoid spilling semen. To remove the condom, the outer ring is twisted to seal it and then pulled out.

Patients should also be aware that concurrent use of male and female condoms is not recommended, as friction between the condoms can cause them to break. Finally, patients should understand that the female condom is more expensive than the male condom and has a slightly lower rate of effectiveness at preventing pregnancy.

Diaphragm and Cervical Cap

The **diaphragm** and the **cervical cap** are made of rubber, latex, or silicone and are bordered by a rounded ring that fits over the cervix inside the vagina. They form a barrier that covers the cervical opening and prevents sperm from entering the uterus and traveling to the fallopian tubes. A diaphragm is larger than a cervical cap and covers a larger area over the cervix. These products work best when used with a spermicide that kills sperm cells on contact. Diaphragms and cervical caps are prescription items that must be fitted or sized to a woman's internal anatomy by her prescriber. They are self-inserted prior to sexual intercourse and left in place for at least six hours.

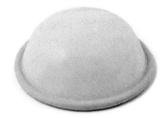

A diaphragm should be used concurrently with a spermicide for maximum effectiveness. This device should be replaced every one to two years.

Side Effects Some women can experience more frequent urinary tract infections when using diaphragms or cervical caps. This effect is thought to be related to changes in the normal vaginal flora from exposure to the spermicide that is used along with these devices. Use of a diaphragm without a spermicide, however, will diminish its effectiveness at preventing pregnancy. Therefore, to reduce the incidence of urinary tract infections, it is recommended that women urinate before insertion of these devices and right after intercourse. Diaphragms and cervical caps are often used with spermicide; if irritation, burning, or rash occurs with spermicide use, an alternative form of birth control should be used.

Contraindications Diaphragms and cervical caps should not be used by women with an allergy to spermicide. The diaphragm should not be used by women who have an allergy to latex or who have frequent urinary tract infections or a history of toxic shock syndrome. Some anatomic differences (such as uterine prolapse) can make it difficult to get a proper fit for a diaphragm and will preclude some patients from being able to use one.

Cautions and Considerations Diaphragms and cervical caps do not protect against transmission of STIs. These contraceptives are meant to be reused, but they must be thoroughly cleaned with mild soap and water and properly stored after each use. In addition, women should be refitted for a diaphragm or cervical cap after pregnancy, miscarriage, abortion, pelvic surgery, or significant weight loss or gain because the shape of the uterus and vagina changes.

Oral Contraceptives

Pharmacologic contraception involves manipulating hormones to prevent ovulation and change the texture of cervical mucus. These drugs contain ethinyl estradiol, a synthetic estrogen, and one of several synthetic progesterones. **Oral contraceptives** that contain synthetic estrogens work by suppressing production of LH, the hormone that triggers ovulation. Oral contraceptives that contain progesterones suppress LH production and thicken cervical mucus, making travel difficult for sperm.

Drug Regimens and Treatments

Oral contraceptives are taken daily at the same time to maintain a steady and elevated hormone level. Depending on the product chosen, patients begin therapy on the first day of their menstrual flow, the first Sunday after their menstrual flow, or whenever desired. In any case, backup birth control, such as a barrier method, must be used to prevent pregnancy for at least the first seven days of therapy, if not for the entire first cycle.

There are several oral contraceptive products on the market. Some options include placebo pills. **Placebo pills** do not include any active drug but rather are used to help reinforce the user's daily habit of taking a pill. Some placebo pills include an iron supplement, as iron needs are thought to increase during menstruation.

No matter the brand, all oral contraceptive products have special packaging and dispensing regulations. These regulations state that all patients, upon receipt of their prescriptions, must receive a patient-information leaflet that has been approved by the FDA.

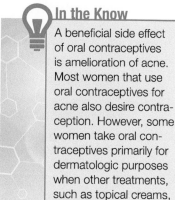

In the Know

A beneficial side effect of oral contraceptives is amelioration of acne. Most women that use oral contraceptives for acne also desire contraception. However, some women take oral contraceptives primarily for dermatologic purposes when other treatments, such as topical creams, have failed.

Ethinyl Estradiol Combinations and Other Products

Oral contraceptives contain either a combination of estrogen and **progestin** or progestins only (see Table 21.6). Combination oral contraceptives come in monophasic, biphasic, and triphasic dosing regimens. Monophasic regimens contain the same dose throughout the cycle, whereas biphasic and triphasic regimens increase the dosage once or twice during a menstrual cycle. The color of the tablet usually changes as the dose changes.

New approaches to oral contraception have brought about extended oral regimens. Such products (Seasonale and Seasonique) involve taking a steady dose for 84 days before allowing a hormone-free week during which menstruation occurs. In effect, patients experience bleeding only once every three or four months. Although concern about endometrial thickening exists, such a regimen works well for patients who have menstrual cycle–related migraines, severe premenstrual symptoms (premenstrual syndrome [PMS]), endometriosis, or PCOS. Prescribers occasionally order a similar extended regimen of monophasic oral contraceptives. The patient skips use of the placebo pills in the dose pack until the end of the extended regimen.

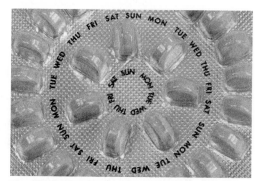

The first oral contraceptive was approved by the FDA in 1960. Today, "the Pill" is the most common form of temporary birth control, appearing on the list of the most popular prescribed drugs in the United States.

Side Effects Common side effects of oral contraceptives include weight gain, nausea, vomiting, bloating, increased appetite, tiredness, fatigue, breast tenderness or enlargement, headache, and edema (fluid retention). These effects tend to subside with continued use but can be a reason to stop or change therapy if bothersome. Patients should discuss these effects with their prescribers. Breakthrough bleeding (bloodflow in the middle of a menstrual cycle) can occur, especially at the start of therapy. If it continues, the patient should talk with her prescriber. An increase in blood pressure can occur in the first few months of oral contraceptive therapy. Patients with high blood pressure should be encouraged to use other methods of contraception, if possible.

TABLE 21.6 Common Oral Contraceptive Products

Generic Names	Brand Names
Estrogen and Progestin Combination Products	
Ethinyl estradiol/desogestrel	Apri, Azurette, Caziant, Cesia, Cyclessa, Desogen, Kariva, Mircette, Velivet, Viorele
Ethinyl estradiol/drospirenone	Ocella, Yasmin, Yaz
Ethinyl estradiol/ethynodiol diacetate	Kelnor, Zovia
Ethinyl estradiol/levonorgestrel	Alesse, Amethia, Aviane, Camrese Lo, Daysee, Lessina, Levlite, Lutera, Seasonale, Seasonique, Tri-Levlen, Triphasil
Ethinyl estradiol/norethindrone	Brevicon, Estrostep, Femhrt, Lo Minastrin Fe, Loestrin, Necon, Norinyl, Nortrel, Ortho-Novum, Ovcon, Tri-Norinyl
Ethinyl estradiol/norgestimate	MonoNessa, Ortho-Cyclen, Ortho Tri-Cyclen, Ortho Tri-Cyclen Lo, Previfem, Sprintec, TriNessa
Ethinyl estradiol/norgestrel	Cryselle 28, Lo/Ovral, Norgestrel, Ogestrel, Ovral
Progestin-Only Product	
Norethindrone	Camila, Errin, Jolivette, Lyza, Nor-QD, Ortho Micronor

Drug Alert

Many oral contraceptives contain *Ortho* in the name (e.g., Ortho-Novum, Ortho-Cyclen, and Ortho Tri-Cyclen). Be careful that you have the correct drug name on all orders and prescriptions.

Contraindications Patients with clotting disorders should not take oral contraceptives because these agents can increase the formation of blood clots. Patients with heart or cerebral vascular disease should not take oral contraceptives. Blood clots, depending on their location and severity, may be fatal.

Patients who have disorders that affect potassium levels, such as kidney disease, liver dysfunction, or adrenal insufficiency, should not take ethinyl estradiol/drospirenone products. These products contain drospirenone, which has actions similar to a diuretic and can adversely affect potassium levels.

Cautions and Considerations Patients with a history of breast, endometrial, ovarian, or cervical cancer should discuss the risks and benefits of oral contraceptives with their healthcare practitioners. Some controversy exists about whether oral contraceptives increase a woman's risk of cancer in these organs, so patients should make informed decisions about their own care.

The advantage of products containing only progestin is that the lower hormone dose reduces side effects, such as headaches and elevated blood pressure. With appropriate risk assessments, these products may be used in patients for whom oral contraceptives are typically not appropriate (i.e., women who have high blood pressure or heart disease, women older than 35 years old, and women with blood-clotting disorders, especially those who smoke). Smoking in conjunction with hormone therapy increases the risk of heart attack, blood clots, and stroke.

The disadvantage of products containing only progestin is that missed doses affect failure rate more quickly than contraceptives containing estrogen. If a dose of a progestin-only pill is missed by more than three hours, the patient should take it as soon as she remembers and use a backup birth control method, such as condoms, for at least 48 hours.

Allied health professionals should remind patients that oral contraceptives do not prevent transmission of STIs. To avoid transmission, patients must use a barrier method (such as a condom) along with an oral contraceptive.

Finally, other medications, herbal preparations, and supplements can interact with oral contraceptives and reduce their effectiveness. These drugs and supplements include the following:

- antibiotics (especially penicillins and tetracyclines)

- barbiturates

- carbamazepine

- lamotrigine

- phenytoin

- protease inhibitors

- St. John's wort

Patients should use additional or alternative methods of birth control to prevent pregnancy while taking these interacting medications.

Kolb's Learning Styles

If you are particularly musical or kinesthetic (as are some Divergers when they learn), you may find that putting the brand and generic drug names for oral contraceptives to a rhyme, tune, or dance will help you recall them better.

Emergency Contraceptives

Emergency contraceptives work primarily by preventing ovulation (if it has not occurred). They may also alter tubal transport of sperm and ovum or inhibit implantation. These contraceptives are not effective if implantation of a fertilized egg has already begun, and they will not affect a pregnancy if it has already started. Emergency contraceptives are not intended to be used as a primary method of birth control.

Drug Regimens and Treatments

There are different options for emergency contraception. Products containing levonorgestrel, ulipristal, and estradiol plus levonorgestrel are used. Levonorgestrel products include Plan B, Plan B One-Step, Next Choice, Next Choice One Dose, and Take Action.

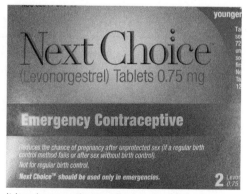

It has been estimated that up to 10% of women of childbearing age may need an emergency contraceptive, such as Next Choice, at some time during their lives.

One-pill products including Plan B One-Step, Next Choice One Dose, and Take Action are OTC products with no age restrictions for purchase. Ulipristal, branded as ella, is available by prescription only. Two-pill products such as Plan B and Next Choice are available by prescription. Estradiol plus levonorgestrel is not sold in a form specific to emergency contraception. This method uses commercially available oral contraceptives at increased doses.

Levonorgestrel and Ulipristal

Levonorgestrel products should be started within 72 hours of unprotected sexual intercourse or the failure of another form of birth control. Ulipristal can be started within 120 hours after intercourse. The cost of emergency contraceptives varies depending on where the products are obtained.

Side Effects Nausea and vomiting are the most common side effects of emergency contraceptives. Antiemetic medication (meclizine or metoclopramide) can be given prior to the emergency contraceptive to reduce these side effects. If a patient vomits within three hours of taking emergency contraception, the medication should be taken again along with an antiemetic medication to reach its full effectiveness. Headache, dizziness, and abdominal pain are also possible.

Contraindications Levonorgestrel and ulipristal list pregnancy as a contraindication to their use. There are no other contraindications. Even conditions that would typically make long-term oral contraception use dangerous (clotting disorders and cardiovascular or liver disease) are not contraindicated in the short-term use of emergency contraception.

Cautions and Considerations Some medications that affect liver function can alter the effectiveness of emergency contraception. These medications may include antiseizure and antiretroviral (HIV) agents.

Transdermal and Vaginal Contraceptives

Transdermal and vaginal contraceptives deliver active drug systemically through the skin or locally in the vagina to produce effectiveness. They provide alternatives for patients who do not want or cannot remember to take a daily oral medication. Patients who experience unwanted side effects of oral contraceptives often find these alternatives an attractive choice.

Medication-Dispensing Devices

Transdermal and vaginal contraceptives include the transdermal patch, the vaginal ring, and the sponge. These devices dispense hormone medications that prevent pregnancy.

Transdermal Contraceptives

Transdermal contraceptives use a stick-on patch to deliver a combination of estrogen and progesterone in a steady supply through the skin (see Table 21.7). As is true for oral contraceptives, the hormones that are delivered alter the menstrual cycle and prevent follicle maturation and ovulation. They also thicken cervical mucus, making it difficult for sperm to pass through the cervix. One patch is applied each week for three weeks and then left off for one week while menstruation occurs. The patch should be removed and replaced the same day of the week. It is placed on a clean, dry, intact area of the skin on the buttock, abdomen, upper-outer arm, or upper torso (not the breasts). The area of patch application should be rotated.

TABLE 21.7 Transdermal and Vaginal Hormonal Contraceptives

Brand Name	Active Ingredient	Dosage Form	Route of Administration
NuvaRing	Etonogestrel and ethinyl estradiol	Ring	Intravaginal
Ortho Evra	Norelgestromin and ethinyl estradiol	Patch	Transdermal
Today	Nonoxynol 9	Sponge	Intravaginal

Side Effects Common side effects of transdermal contraceptives are similar to those of oral contraceptives and include breast tenderness, headache, irritation at the application site, nausea, menstrual cramps, and abdominal pain. These effects tend to subside with continued use. If these effects remain bothersome, an alternative contraceptive agent should be tried.

Contraindications As with all estrogen and progesterone hormone products, risks and benefits of therapy must be weighed. Hormone therapy can increase the risk of cardio-vascular events, stroke, and blood clots. Risk of blood clots is especially high for patients 35 years and older who smoke. These hormones can exacerbate depression and migraine headaches. Patients with these conditions should discuss use of hormone contraception with their healthcare practitioners.

Cautions and Considerations If the patch detaches (fully or partially) from the skin, it should be reapplied if possible. If detachment lasts for less than a day, no backup birth control is needed. If detachment lasts longer than a day, then nonhormonal methods of birth control such as a barrier method should be used for seven days. If the patch cannot be reapplied, a new patch should be used and backup birth control used for seven days. A new cycle then begins, and the day to change the patch must be altered.

Vaginal Ring

The **vaginal ring** is a combination birth control that contains synthetic estrogen and progesterone. The ring is inserted into the vagina where the hormones are absorbed through the vaginal mucosa. This device is left in place for three weeks and then removed for a week while menstruation occurs.

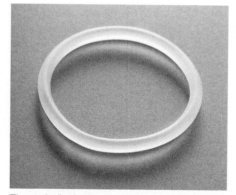

The soft, flexible vaginal ring is compressed and inserted into the vagina to prevent ovulation.

Side Effects Common side effects of the vaginal ring include headache, nausea, vaginal secretion, vaginitis, bloating, cramps, and weight gain. Use of the vaginal ring appears to be associated with fewer side effects than experienced with oral contraceptives, presumably because the ring delivers a lower hormonal dose to a localized area. These effects may subside with continued use. If these effects continue to be bothersome, patients should discontinue therapy and talk with their prescribers.

Contraindications Vaginal rings, such as the NuvaRing, should not be used in patients with breast cancer or other estrogen- or progestin-dependent tumors, liver tumors or disease, pregnancy, or undiagnosed uterine bleeding. Women at high risk for arterial or venous thrombosis (for example, those individuals with cerebrovascular disease, coronary artery disease, diabetes mellitus with vascular disease, DVT or PE, migraine, uncontrolled

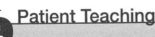
hypertension, or inherited coagulopathies) should not use vaginal rings. In addition, women over the age of 35 who smoke should also not use these devices due to their high risk of thrombosis.

Cautions and Considerations When stored in a pharmacy, vaginal rings must be kept in the refrigerator to maintain their potency until patients pick up their prescribed products. Patients should be directed to keep their vaginal rings in the refrigerator until they plan to use them.

Vaginal Sponge

The **vaginal sponge** is an OTC contraceptive that is made of a porous, polyurethane material. The polyurethane is infused with a spermicide that kills sperm on contact. Although the sponge forms a partial barrier over the cervix, the true mechanism of action comes from the spermicidal foam that is released on insertion of the device into the vagina. The sponge should be inserted prior to sexual intercourse (12 to 24 hours in advance) and left in place for 6 hours after intercourse.

Prior to insertion, the vaginal sponge must be moistened with two tablespoons of water to activate the spermicide. The sponge is then rolled (dimple side in) and inserted into the vagina.

Side Effects A common side effect of the sponge is vaginal irritation. If this effect is bothersome, an alternative choice of contraception is recommended.

Contraindications Patients who are allergic to polyurethane should not use the sponge because it is made of polyurethane. The sponge also should not be used if the male partner is allergic to polyurethane.

Cautions and Considerations If the sponge is left in the vagina longer than 24 hours, the risk of infection and toxic shock syndrome increases. The sponge should be left in place for six hours after sexual intercourse to avoid pregnancy, but it should be removed as soon as possible to avoid bacterial growth and infection.

Injections, Implants, and Intrauterine Devices

Injections, implants, and intrauterine devices (IUDs) are contraception methods used to prevent pregnancy for long periods of time (i.e., months to years). All of these methods use hormonal therapy in some way. The advantage is that the patient does not have to remember to take or use the product regularly to prevent pregnancy. Once administered, these methods continue working for a period of time during which the patient is protected without having to think about it.

Drug Regimens and Medication-Dispensing Devices

Long-term contraceptives include medroxyprogesterone injections, etonogestrel implants, and IUDs. All of these contraceptive methods require intervention by healthcare practitioners.

Medroxyprogesterone

Medroxyprogesterone (Depo-Provera) is an intramuscular injection given in the deltoid or gluteus maximus every 12 weeks. It is administered by a healthcare practitioner and works by inhibiting ovulation, thickening the cervical mucus, and changing the endometrium to inhibit implantation (see Figure 21.7).

Side Effects Common side effects of medroxyprogesterone injection include menstrual irregularity, abdominal pain, weight changes, dizziness, headache, weakness, fatigue, and nervousness. Also possible are decreased libido, inability to achieve orgasm, pelvic pain, backache, breast pain, leg cramps, hair loss, depression, bloating, nausea, rash, insomnia, edema, hot flashes, acne, sore joints, and vaginitis. Patients should understand the risks of these potential side effects along with the benefits when choosing this long-term contraception option. Because the drug is long-acting, these effects are unavoidable once they occur and will probably continue for three months.

Contraindications Patients with clotting disorders should not take medroxyprogesterone because it can increase the formation of blood clots. In addition, patients with heart or cerebrovascular disease should not take systemic contraceptive medications. A clot in either a coronary artery or cerebral artery could be fatal.

Cautions and Considerations Medroxyprogesterone should not be used if conception has already occurred. For this reason, the patient may be required to take a pregnancy test before administration. It can take weeks for a normal menstrual cycle to resume after the patient has used medroxyprogesterone. Patients desiring greater control over fertility in the near weeks to months should use an alternative method of birth control.

FIGURE 21.7 Depo-Provera Contraceptive Injection

Women who use Depo-Provera, the birth-control shot, are less likely to have uterine cancer or pelvic inflammatory disease than women who use other forms of birth control.

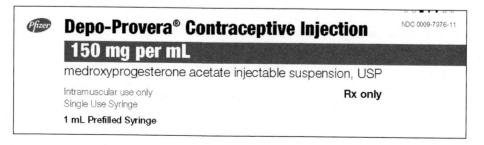

Etonogestrel

Etonogestrel (Implanon) is an implant placed just under the skin on the upper-inner arm every three years to prevent pregnancy. This product must be inserted by a healthcare practitioner. It works by inhibiting ovulation, thickening the cervical mucus, and changing the endometrium to inhibit implantation.

Side Effects Common side effects of etonogestrel include changes in menstrual bleeding, weight gain, and mood swings. Other potential side effects include upper respiratory tract infection, vaginitis, breast pain, acne, and abdominal pain. These effects, if particularly bothersome, can be sufficient reason to have the implant removed.

Contraindications Etonogestrel should not be used if conception has already occurred. For this reason, the patient may be required to take a pregnancy test before insertion of the implant. Patients with clotting disorders should not take etonogestrel because it can increase the formation of blood clots. In addition, patients with heart or cerebrovascular disease should not take systemic contraceptive medications. A clot in either a coronary artery or cerebral artery could be fatal.

Cautions and Considerations Because this product is a long-term option for contraception, patients should understand the risks and potential complications of using this drug. It can take three to four weeks for ovulation to resume after removing this implant.

Intrauterine Device

An **intrauterine device (IUD)** is a small device placed into the uterus by a healthcare practitioner every five years. There are several types of IUDs on the market. Some IUDs contain **levonorgestrel,** a hormone that alters the endometrium to prevent implantation. Some IUDs contain copper, and some IUDs that are available in foreign countries do not contain any active ingredient at all. These IUDs may be reasonable options for long-term contraception for patients who cannot take hormones such as women with recent breast cancer.

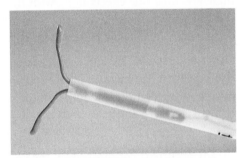

The presence of the IUD within the uterus changes the endometrium itself, and the drug that leaches from the device affects ovulation.

Although the exact mechanism of action is not well understood, IUDs primarily prevent pregnancy by impeding fertilization. The presence of the IUD device in the uterus causes an inflammatory response that is toxic to sperm and ova and impairs implantation.

Side Effects Common side effects of IUDs can include spontaneous abortion, septicemia, pelvic infection, perforation of the uterus, vaginitis, abnormal menstrual bleeding, anemia, pain, cramping, backaches, and tubal damage. These effects can be serious and should be fully discussed and understood before patients choose this contraception method.

Contraindications Women with an abnormal or distorted uterine shape, active pelvic inflammatory disease (PID), endometriosis, Wilson's disease, allergy to copper, or unexplained uterine bleeding should not use IUDs. Pregnancy or suspected pregnancy contraindicates IUD use. For this reason, a patient may be required to take a pregnancy test before insertion of the device. Women with breast cancer should not use an IUD that contains an active hormone (levonorgestrel).

Cautions and Considerations An IUD is a long-term but reversible option for contraception. Patients should understand the risks and potential complications of using an IUD before choosing one.

Checkpoint 21.4

Take a moment to review what you have learned so far and answer these questions.

1. What are the barrier methods of contraception useful in both men and women?
2. How is the vaginal ring used?
3. How do oral contraceptives work?

Gender Reassignment

Transsexualism is a condition wherein an individual identifies with a gender different from his or her own. Consequently, an individual may decide to switch his or her gender through anatomic, psychological, and hormonal changes. The goal of **gender reassignment** is to transition to the opposite gender through hormonal and surgical treatment. Transitioning to the opposite gender begins with counseling to ensure proper diagnosis and to discuss the risks and benefits of gender reassignment therapy. The patient must be supported psychosocially as he or she begins living with a new gender identity and learns to manage expectations for what can be achieved during the transitional phase.

Hormonal Therapy

Hormonal therapy, which suppresses characteristics of the **natal sex** and enhances characteristics of the desired gender, is often the next step. This therapy allows the patient to transition in appearance to the new gender and provides time for the patient to experience life as a member of the opposite sex. The last step is to undergo surgical intervention to remove sexual organs of the natal sex and to create anatomic features of the new gender.

Drug Regimens and Treatments

Male-to-female hormone therapy involves suppression of androgen secretion and administration of estrogen. Drugs used to block androgen production include spironolactone, cyproterone acetate, medroxyprogesterone, gonadotropin-releasing hormone (GnRH) agonists (goserelin), and finasteride. A variety of estrogen products are used to enhance female characteristics. Although estrogen alone can achieve some androgen inhibition, most individuals find taking androgen suppression therapy in addition to estrogen preferable. Many characteristics of women such as reduced facial and body hair growth, increased libido, some growth of breast tissue, and fat redistribution can be achieved through hormone therapy. Patients must understand that results are not always complete. Facial hair growth may be difficult to fully eliminate, and a deep voice cannot be altered.

Female-to-male hormone therapy involves primarily administration of testosterone. Many testosterone preparations and products are available. These medications can help individuals achieve hair growth in the male pubertal pattern (including male-pattern baldness), a deepening voice, changes in body mass, a decrease in breast tissue, increased libido, and clitoral enlargement. Many patients also experience an increase in acne.

STIs

Sexually transmitted infections (STIs) are infections that are transmitted through sexual contact and affect the male and female reproductive systems. Although abstinence from sexual activity is the only sure way to prevent transmission, some barrier methods (such as the male or female condom) have shown some effectiveness in preventing transmission of some STIs. Causes of STIs include bacteria and viruses. Bacterial infections can be cured with antibiotics, but viral STIs can only be treated symptomatically. Once someone contracts a viral STI, the goals of treatment change from curing the infection to reducing the severity of symptoms and risk of transmission.

Table 21.8 provides an overview of the most commonly used drugs for the STIs discussed in this chapter. Refer to Chapter 23 for additional discussion of the antibiotics, antivirals, and vaginal candidiasis agents listed in Table 21.8. Drugs for HIV are also discussed in Chapter 23.

TABLE 21.8 Common Drug Therapy for STIs

STI	Drugs of Choice
Acquired immunodeficiency syndrome (AIDS)	Enfuvirtide, non-nucleoside reverse transcriptase inhibitors (NNRTIs), nucleoside reverse transcriptase inhibitors (NRTIs), and protease inhibitors (PIs)
Chlamydia	Azithromycin, doxycycline, or erythromycin
Genital herpes	Acyclovir, famciclovir, or valacyclovir
Gonorrhea	Ceftriaxone or a fluoroquinolone
Human papillomavirus (HPV)	Imiquimod or podofilox
Syphilis	Doxycycline, penicillin, or tetracycline
Vaginosis (bacterial)	Clindamycin, metronidazole
Vaginosis (yeast)	OTC or prescription vaginal candidiasis products

Bacterial STIs

As mentioned earlier, antibiotics are prescribed to treat bacterial STIs. These infections include chlamydia, gonorrhea, syphilis, and vaginosis.

Chlamydia

Chlamydia trachomatis is the bacterium that causes **chlamydia**, which is the most common STI in the United States. This disease can also infect the eyes and pharyngeal (throat) tissue. The eyes of infants born to women with chlamydia or gonorrhea can become infected during a vaginal delivery. Cesarean birth can reduce transmission, but most newborns receive either erythromycin or silver nitrate treatment in their eyes to prevent infection and blindness. In males, common symptoms of chlamydia include painful urination, urinary frequency, and urethral discharge. These symptoms occur 7 to 21 days after exposure. Women are often asymptomatic and do not realize they have the disease. The infection can progress to involve the entire pelvic region (i.e., PID). Women with PID have abdominal pain and can become infertile as inflammation scars and blocks fallopian tubes. Chlamydia frequently accompanies gonorrhea, so testing for both diseases when either one is suspected is standard procedure.

Gonorrhea

Gonorrhea is a gram-negative bacterial infection caused by *Neisseria gonorrhoeae* that attaches to mucosal tissue in the male and female reproductive systems, rectum, eyes, and pharyngeal (throat) area. Symptoms are most pronounced in men, who have painful urination and pus-like discharge from the urethra (i.e., urethritis). These symptoms usually develop within two to eight days of exposure, prompting most men to seek treatment and avoid further complications. Women are usually asymptomatic but can

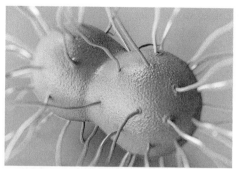

Neisseria gonorrhoeae, the bacterium that causes gonorrhea, is commonly treated with a dual therapy: ceftriaxone (a cephalosporin) and either azithromycin or doxycycline.

have vaginal discharge and abdominal pain that develop within 7 to 14 days of exposure. If left untreated, the bacterial infection can progress to PID in women and can affect the heart, brain, eyes, pharynx, and joints.

Syphilis

Syphilis is a bacterial infection caused by *Treponema pallidum*. It is transmitted through contact with reproductive mucous membranes and/or genital skin lesions. If left untreated, syphilis can slowly progress to affect the central nervous and cardiovascular systems. Primary syphilis develops first, within 10 to 90 days after exposure. At this stage, a painless lesion or chancre appears as a round or oval red lump or blister in the genital area, ulcerates, and then heals on its own within one to eight weeks.

If not treated during the primary phase, syphilis continues to the secondary phase, two to eight weeks after the first phase is over. In this phase, multiple lesions appear on the skin, often on the palms of the hands or soles of the feet. Swelling, fever, headache, sore throat, loss of appetite, and joint pain usually accompany these skin lesions. Most patients seek treatment before or at this secondary phase of the disease.

However, when treatment is not sought, the patient enters the latent phase, during which no symptoms are present; the disease can remain latent for years. Patients are contagious to others through the early part of this latent phase.

Tertiary syphilis is the final stage of disease, in which a generalized inflammatory response occurs throughout the body. In this stage, patients can develop blindness, deafness, dementia, aortic aneurysm, and destructive skin lesions. Because antibiotic treatment is easy, inexpensive, and highly successful, few patients reach the tertiary stage of syphilis.

Vaginosis

Inflammation and infection of the vaginal mucosa is known as **vaginosis**. It can be caused by bacteria, such as *Gardnerella vaginalis* and *Trichomonas vaginalis*, or by yeast-like fungi, such as *Candida albicans*. Symptoms of bacterial vaginosis include frothy or discolored vaginal discharge, fishy odor, and vaginal itching and pain. Symptoms of vaginal yeast infection (also considered a fungal-type infection) include white discharge (often described as looking like cottage cheese) in addition to vaginal odor, itching, and irritation. All vaginosis infections can be transmitted sexually, and yeast infections can develop even without sexual activity. Poor exposure to air, such as from wearing tight underwear and/or wet clothing, can create a damp atmosphere that is conducive to yeast growth.

Taking antibiotics can also kill normal vaginal flora, allowing yeast and other bacteria to grow and cause infection. Vaginal yeast infections can be treated with OTC or prescription antifungal products; bacterial infections usually require prescription antibiotic treatment.

Viral STIs

Some STIs are caused by viruses. Unlike bacterial STIs, these infections are not curable and, unfortunately, become chronic conditions that the patient must treat for life. Vaccines are not available to prevent most of these viral infections. Viral STIs include genital herpes, human papillomavirus, and HIV.

Genital Herpes

Genital herpes is a viral infection caused by the herpes simplex virus. Herpes simplex virus type 1 (HSV-1) is associated with canker sores in and around the mouth, whereas herpes simplex virus type 2 (HSV-2) is associated with genital herpes. HSV-2 appears as painful blister-like lesions on the skin, typically in the pubic region, within 2 to 14 days of exposure. Vesicles (or blisters) containing infectious material form and then heal in about two weeks. Fever, headache, and body aches can also occur in this phase. Once healed, the lesions become latent but can reappear at any time. Recurrent outbreaks are less severe but tend to occur in response to stress, menstruation, or during illness. Up to half of patients are asymptomatic, however. Genital herpes is not curable and usually recurs. Although patients are most contagious during an outbreak, they can pass the virus to someone else through sexual contact at any time. Antiviral drug therapy can reduce frequency and severity of outbreaks but does not completely eliminate the possibility of transmission.

HPV

The most common viral STI in the United States is **human papillomavirus (HPV)**. Symptoms of HPV include wart-like lesions that appear in the genital region—although not all patients have them. The warts are not usually painful but are unsightly and difficult to remove. The virus is closely linked to development of cervical cancer in women, and no cure is available. A vaccine for preventing HPV is now available for females and males ages 9 to 26. The vaccine helps reduce the transmission of certain strains of HPV and thus significantly reduces the risk of cervical cancer. (For more information about the HPV vaccine, see Chapter 24.)

Work Wise

Because of the highly sensitive nature of personal information regarding HIV infection, it is even more imperative that the allied health professional remember his or her ethical and legal obligation to maintain patient confidentiality. Additional information regarding the Health Insurance Portability and Accountability Act (HIPAA) rules for protecting personal patient information is discussed in Chapter 4 and in Chapter 8.

HIV

Human immunodeficiency virus (HIV) is a viral infection that is transmitted through exchange of body fluids, such as during sexual activity. It can also be passed via blood transfusion and from an infected mother to her developing fetus, if not treated. HIV is a retrovirus that attacks the DNA of T cells, destroying their ability to attack foreign cells and fight infection. Thus, HIV not only destroys the body's ability to rid itself of the virus but also damages the immune response to all infections. Although drug therapy is possible to subdue the virus to almost immeasurable levels, there is no cure for this condition.

HIV is deadly for infected individuals because the immune system cannot fight infection, and patients eventually die from opportunistic infections. Patients who are infected with HIV and have experienced opportunistic infections because of that infection are diagnosed with acquired immunodeficiency syndrome (AIDS), the illness caused by HIV. See Chapter 23 for more information on HIV/AIDS.

Herbal and Alternative Therapies

Soy, also known as isoflavone or **phytoestrogen**, is a plant source of protein used to treat several conditions. In the United States, it is used most frequently for hot flashes associated with menopause. Soy is a source of fiber and protein found most commonly in milk and dairy substitutes. It can be obtained from dietary sources alone or from a combination of food and oral supplements. It has estrogenic effects that can be beneficial for menopausal symptoms, diabetes, high cholesterol, osteoporosis, kidney disease, and, possibly, breast cancer prevention. Soy is usually well tolerated but can cause upset stomach upset, diarrhea, constipation, bloating, nausea, and even insomnia in some cases. It can also worsen migraine headaches, especially for women whose headaches are related to hormonal fluctuations of the menstrual cycle.

Black cohosh is a plant product with estrogenic effects used for menopausal symptoms such as hot flashes. It is sometimes used in combination with St. John's wort for psychological symptoms that may be associated with menopause such as depression and mood swings. Studies have not produced standard dosing, so success varies. Side effects of black cohosh include upset stomach, rash, headache, dizziness, weight gain, cramping, breast tenderness, and vaginal spotting (bleeding). Some concern exists about black cohosh and liver disease because some women have experienced hepatitis-type symptoms after taking black cohosh. Women with liver disease, or who are pregnant or breast-feeding, should probably avoid black cohosh.

Evening primrose oil is sometimes used to reduce symptoms of menopause or PMS. However, studies have found mixed results and do not currently support its effectiveness for these conditions. Evidence for the use of evening primrose oil for osteoporosis is also mixed. It is considered safe to take and few side effects have been reported.

Wild yam, also called Mexican yam, is a phytoestrogen similar to soy with mild estrogenic effects. It is applied topically or ingested orally as a tincture. Some use it for menopausal symptoms such as hot flashes. Published research does not recommend a formulation or dose that is consistently effective. Ingestion of large amounts can cause vomiting. More research is needed to determine the clinical usefulness of wild yam.

 Checkpoint **21.5**

Take a moment to review what you have learned so far and answer these questions.

1. What are the steps for gender reassignment and how are drugs used in this process?

2. What are the bacterial (curable) and viral (incurable) STIs?

3. What drugs are used to treat genital herpes, chlamydia, and vaginosis?

Chapter Review

Chapter Summary

The male and female reproductive systems are complex sets of organs regulated by hormones, such as estrogen, testosterone, progesterone, FSH, and LH. Female ovaries produce ova, and male testes produce sperm. Conditions affecting the male reproductive system are hypogonadism, erectile dysfunction, infertility, and STIs. Conditions affecting the female reproductive system are pregnancy, pregnancy termination, infertility, menopause, and STIs.

Drug therapies used for the reproductive system include a variety of contraceptive products, hormones (primarily estrogen, progesterone, and testosterone), and PDE-5 inhibitors. Oral contraceptives and their transdermal, vaginal, and subcutaneous counterparts are among the most commonly dispensed medications. Understanding the hormones used in contraception is not an easy task. Familiarity with the normal female reproductive cycle provides a good start for understanding how estrogen or progesterone can prevent ovulation. Familiarity with these agents is useful because they are a source of many patient questions. In addition, drug therapies for these conditions are associated with considerable risks. Hormone therapy is also used for patients undergoing gender reassignment.

Chapter Checkup

The Navigator+ learning management system that accompanies this textbook offers many opportunities to help you master chapter content, including end-of-chapter exercises, a glossary of key terms, flash cards, and additional interactive activities.

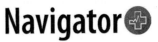

Career Exploration

If you enjoyed learning about the reproductive systems in this chapter, you may want to explore the following career options:

- cytogenetics technologist
- diagnostic medical scientist
- diagnostic medical sonographer
- genetic counselor
- HIV/AIDS counselor
- lactation consultant
- medical assistant
- obstetric (OB) technician
- pharmacy technician

The Renal System and Drug Therapy

Pharm Facts

- Every 24 hours, a human's kidneys filter about 50 gallons of blood through approximately 140 miles of tubules, or passages.

- Indigenous people of Mexico and Central America believed that nephrite, a form of jade, had healing powers for kidney problems. Nephrite, from the Greek word *nephros*, meaning "kidney," was placed over the kidneys as a form of crystal therapy.

- Each kidney has close to 1 million filtering units called *nephrons*.

- The appearance and smell of urine provide insights into a person's health. Pink-tinged urine may indicate bleeding in the urinary tract, a sign of kidney disease or a bladder infection. Brownish urine may indicate liver disease, and foamy urine may be a sign of a kidney problem or excess dietary protein. Urine that smells sweet may be a sign of diabetes. In fact, physicians in the eighteenth century would not only smell a patient's urine if they suspected diabetes but also taste it for sugar.

"As a hemodialysis technician, I work directly with patients who have chronic kidney disease, a terminal condition if left untreated. I am responsible for administering their dialysis treatment, monitoring their vital signs, and encouraging them to adopt healthy habits for optimal clinical outcomes. I have built caring, professional relationships with my regular dialysis patients, and they have taught me patience, empathy, and sincerity. I would highly recommend a position in the renal dialysis field."

—**Jordan Struthers**, AA, CCHT
Hemodialysis Technician

Learning Objectives

1 Understand the basic anatomy and physiology of the renal system.

2 Describe the common conditions that affect the renal system.

3 Explain the therapeutic effects of prescription medications and non-prescription medications commonly used to treat diseases of the renal system.

4 Identify the generic names, brand names, indications, dosage ranges, side effects, contraindications, and cautions and considerations associated with the drugs commonly used to treat diseases of the renal system.

5 Identify common herbal and alternative therapies related to the renal system.

Understanding the renal system is important when studying pharmacology because most drugs and their metabolites eventually exit the body through the kidneys and into the urine. This elimination process is affected by several factors. One of these factors is the patient's kidney function. Any diminished function leaves the patient vulnerable to drug accumulation and toxicity. Therefore, a prescriber must make adjustments in a patient's dosage regimen to compensate for kidney dysfunction. Another factor that prescribers must consider is the properties of the drug itself. Medications vary as to their rate and amount of renal clearance. In fact, some drugs directly damage the kidneys and need to be closely monitored (see the section titled "Nephrotoxicity and Renal Dosing" later in this chapter). All of these factors need to be considered when prescribing drug therapy.

Renal and urinary tract problems account for several frequently dispensed medications. Conditions such as urinary tract infections, spastic bladder, and prostate enlargement all have common drug treatments. Diuretics are used to treat high blood pressure and heart failure, but their site of action is in the kidneys and on the regulatory systems that affect renal function. This chapter begins with a description of the anatomy and physiology of the renal system, including the importance of the kidney's functional unit called the nephron. Common disorders of the renal system and kidney function are covered along with the drug treatments for them. Drug classes such as antimuscarinics and diuretics are described, including the treatments for benign prostatic hyperplasia.

Anatomy and Physiology of the Renal System

The **renal system**, also called the *urinary system*, is responsible for clearing waste products from the blood while maintaining proper fluid and electrolyte balance. The kidneys are the primary filters for this process, which is known as **elimination**. Blood flows through the kidneys, which clear it of metabolic by-products and waste substances. These compounds build up and become toxic if not eliminated from the body. In addition, the kidneys are responsible for the following functions:

- balancing fluids and electrolytes, such as sodium, potassium, and calcium

- regulating the blood pH and blood pressure

- producing hormones that regulate systemic and kidney hemodynamics (renin, angiotensin II, and prostaglandins); red blood cell production (**erythropoietin**); and mineral metabolism

The kidneys perform the filtering function, and then the ureters transport the waste products and excess fluid to the urinary bladder, where these substances are held until **voiding** (see Figure 22.1). Urine exits the body through the urethra. The female urethra is short, and the male urethra is long and passes through the center of the prostate gland before exiting the body.

FIGURE 22.1 Anatomy of the Renal System

The proximity of the kidneys to the abdominal aorta, the largest artery in the body, makes these delicate organs highly susceptible to changes in blood pressure. High blood pressure damages the filtering ability of the kidneys, and low blood pressure can cause acute renal failure.

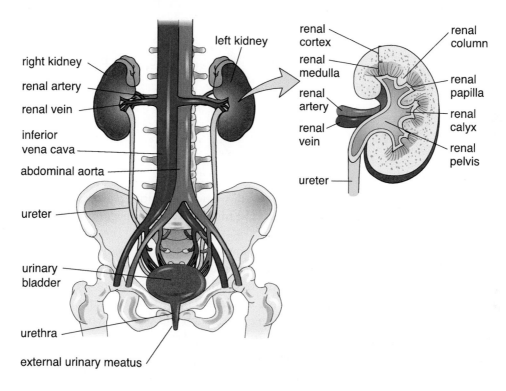

Kidneys

The **kidneys** are bean-shaped organs located in the rear upper torso. The upper part of the kidneys are anterior to the ribs. The lower part of the kidneys are inferior to the ribs. Although they are in the abdominal region, they are not inside the peritoneal cavity, where the stomach, pancreas, and intestines are located. The adrenal glands (discussed in detail in Chapter 20) are located on top of the kidneys, almost like two little caps, and produce hormones. The **renal artery** branches off the abdominal aorta and brings blood into the kidneys. Blood that has been filtered in the kidneys returns to the bloodstream via the **renal vein** (see Figure 22.2).

The **renal cortex** is the outer layer of the kidneys and is responsible for filtration. The **renal medulla**, in the body of each kidney, also performs filtration. The renal cortex and renal medulla are made up of thousands of microscopic-sized **nephrons**, the

FIGURE 22.2 Anatomy of the Kidney

Erythropoietin, which is released from the renal cortex, is the hormone that stimulates red blood cell production.

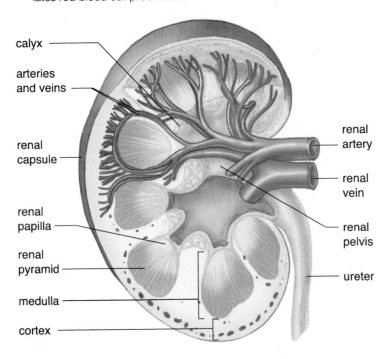

- calyx
- arteries and veins
- renal capsule
- renal papilla
- renal pyramid
- medulla
- cortex
- renal artery
- renal vein
- renal pelvis
- ureter

functional filtering units of the kidney. Urine formation, a multistep process including glomerular filtration, tubular reabsorption, and tubular secretion, begins in the nephron (see Figure 22.3).

Blood containing fluid and waste products enters the nephron through the **afferent arteriole** into the **Bowman's capsule**. Here, the capillary is tightly folded, forming the **glomerulus**. The tight folding in the glomerulus and the small amount of space inside the capsule create the high pressure that forces fluid and other substances from the blood. **Glomerular filtration** is the first step in urine production and the maintenance of fluid balance. Large molecules, such as proteins, are not filtered out in the glomerulus, but most fluids and other smaller substances are. Blood leaves the Bowman's capsule via the **efferent arteriole**. **Filtrate**, the fluids and by-products filtered from the blood in the glomerulus, continues through the nephron.

As filtrate passes through the tubules and **loop of Henle**, molecules selectively reenter the bloodstream through several mechanisms. Some substances are reabsorbed through simple diffusion. Others are exchanged between blood and urine by secretion, an active transport process. Still others move across the membranes due to force of pressure, which is another way to describe **filtration**. Those substances that are filtered out or secreted into the urine (but that do not reenter the blood) are then eliminated from the body.

Proper urine production and maintenance of fluid balance rely on the tubular **reabsorption** and **secretion** processes. In fact, reabsorption of water and sodium is essential for main-

Quick Study

To remember the difference between the afferent and efferent arterioles, just break down the words. The suffix *–ferent*, means "carrying." The prefix *af–* means "toward." Therefore, the *afferent* arteriole is carrying fluid and waste toward the nephron into the Bowman's capsule. The prefix *ef–* means "out of" or "from." So the *efferent* arteriole is carrying fluid and waste out of or from the Bowman's capsule.

FIGURE 22.3 The Nephron and Urine Formation

Each part of the microscopic-sized nephron performs specific functions: filtration, reabsorption, and secretion of select electrolytes, fluids, and other substances.

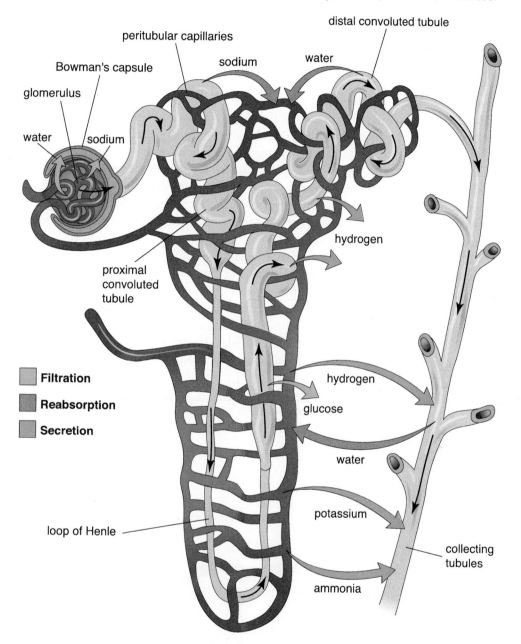

taining good hydration. If kidney failure occurs, the proper balance of excretion and reabsorption is not maintained. Inability to produce urine is called **anuria**. It signals kidney failure, which results in toxins building up in the blood and poisoning the body.

Hormones such as **aldosterone** and **antidiuretic hormone (ADH)** regulate the rate and volume of urine production. These hormones are released in response to changes in fluid status, blood pressure, and the concentrations of various substances in the blood. They can stimulate or inhibit urine production in the nephron to maintain overall body fluid status.

Ureters

The **ureters** are paired muscular ducts that extend from the renal pelvis to the bladder. The main function of the ureters is to move urine from the kidney to the bladder. Movement is facilitated by smooth-muscle contraction in the ureter wall.

Urinary Bladder

The **urinary bladder** is located in the pelvic region. It collects and holds urine until the fluid exits the body during urination. The bladder is made of elastic epithelial and smooth-muscle cells, which allow it to expand and hold up to 1 L of fluid. However, the functional capacity of the bladder (the volume held before voluntary voiding) is much smaller—around 300–400 mL in adults. The **internal urinary sphincter** is an involuntary smooth muscle located at the junction of the inferior aspect of the bladder and the proximal urethra. It functions to contain urine within the urinary bladder. In contrast, the **external urinary sphincter** is a voluntary muscle that holds urine in the bladder before it exits the body.

When the bladder is full and distended, stretch receptors sense the pressure and cause the **detrusor muscles** in the bladder to contract and the external urinary sphincter to relax. Urine is pushed out, and the bladder empties (see Figure 22.4). This urination process is called **micturition**. **Urinary retention** occurs when the kidneys produce urine, but the micturition process does not function properly. Consequently, urine accumulates in the bladder. This problem is a malfunction of the bladder. The inability to control the external urinary sphincter, thus allowing urine to leak out of the bladder, is called **incontinence**.

FIGURE 22.4 | Anatomy of the Bladder

Although the bladder can hold up to 1 L of urine, stretch receptors typically trigger the urge to urinate when only 30%–40% of that volume has accumulated.

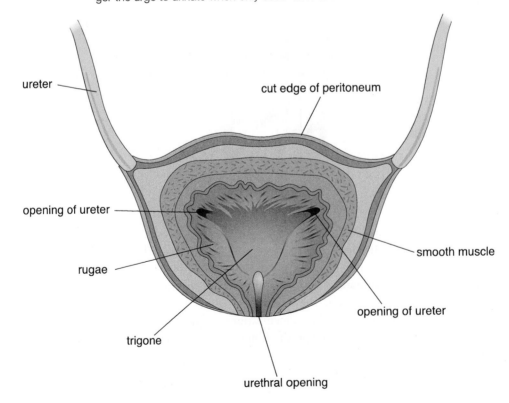

Assessment of Kidney Function

Laboratory blood tests are used to diagnose and monitor kidney function. The most common tests are **blood urea nitrogen (BUN)** and **serum creatinine (SCr)**. When kidney function is impaired, the elimination of urea, nitrogen, and creatinine (a by-product of muscle metabolism) is also impaired, and the concentrations of these substances increase in the blood. Although results of these tests vary according to age, weight, and gender, as well as other factors such as exercise, these tests are good markers for kidney function.

Typically, the normal range for SCr is 0.5–1.5 mg/dL. SCr can be used to calculate **creatinine clearance** (CrCl), which estimates **glomerular filtration rate** (GFR). A low CrCl (<60 mL/min) is a sign of impaired kidney function. CrCl and GFR estimate the level of kidney function while taking into account such factors as age, ideal body weight (IBW), and gender. The most common formula used to estimate CrCl is the **Cockcroft and Gault equation**:

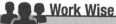

Work Wise

For allied health professionals, learning healthcare jargon is an important communication skill. Abbreviations used to describe kidney function are pronounced in different ways. For example, the abbreviations *BUN* and *GFR* are generally pronounced by saying the letters individually. The abbreviation *CrCl* is generally spoken by saying "creatinine clearance."

$$\text{Men:} \qquad \text{CrCl in mL/min} \approx \frac{(140 - \text{age}) \times \text{IBW in kilograms (kg)}}{\text{SCr in mg/dL} \times 72}$$

$$\text{Women:} \qquad \text{CrCl in mL/min} \approx \frac{(140 - \text{age}) \times \text{IBW in kilograms (kg)} \times 0.85}{\text{SCr in mg/dL} \times 72}$$

Allied health professionals in the inpatient setting may find themselves calculating GFR estimates many times a day when monitoring patients' drug therapy. Although other formulas for estimating kidney function exist, the Cockcroft and Gault equation is used most often when adjusting drug dosing for impaired renal function. For instance, the dose is decreased or the interval between doses is increased for many drugs when CrCl drops below 30 mL/min or 60 mL/min.

 Checkpoint 22.1

Take a moment to review what you have learned so far and answer these questions.

1. What are the main functions of the kidneys?

2. Which hormones help regulate the rate and volume of urine production?

Nephrotoxicity and Renal Dosing

Because of the importance of the kidneys to the pharmacokinetic process, healthcare practitioners need to be especially mindful of lowering medication doses for patients with impaired renal function. Dose adjustment often depends on the degree of renal dysfunction present. Some drugs need dose adjustment only in the case of severe renal failure, whereas others cannot be used (are contraindicated) even in mild kidney impairment.

Drug accumulation in a patient's blood can lead to serious side effects and toxicities. Certain drugs can also cause **nephrotoxicity** or direct damage to kidney tissue. Nephrotoxicity is usually reversible; however, if it is not addressed quickly, this condition can cause kidney failure. For that reason, a patient who is taking a drug that is considered nephrotoxic or potentially nephrotoxic under certain conditions (such as dehydration) must be closely monitored. Examples of nephrotoxic or potentially nephrotoxic drugs include nonsteroidal anti-inflammatory drugs (NSAIDs), amphotericin B, contrast media (dye for imaging procedures), aminoglycosides, and cisplatin and carboplatin.

NSAIDs

NSAID-induced nephrotoxicity affects up to 2 million individuals in the United States each year. Low urine volume and low urine sodium content are common presentations of NSAID-induced nephrotoxicity. Increases in weight, edema, BUN levels, SCr levels, and potassium levels may also be seen. Sulindac, a potent NSAID, may have a lower propensity for nephrotoxicity. Alternative therapies, such as acetaminophen, may be substituted for NSAIDs as another preventive measure. If nephrotoxicity is suspected, NSAIDs should be discontinued and supportive care should be initiated.

Amphotericin B

The risk of amphotericin-related nephrotoxicity increases with higher doses. It generally presents with potassium, sodium, and magnesium wasting. SCr levels increase and GFR decreases. Amphotericin-related nephrotoxicity may be prevented by avoiding other nephrotoxic drugs and by using intravenous (IV) hydration prior to each dose.

Contrast Media

Contrast media is one of the leading causes of acute kidney injury. Nephrotoxicity caused by contrast media presents initially with transient diuresis and proteinuria. SCr levels rise, and approximately 50% of patients develop **oliguria**, or low urine output. Hydration with IV fluids 6 to 12 hours before administration of contrast media may prevent nephrotoxicity. Some prescribers choose to use medications such as acetylcysteine, ascorbic acid, or theophylline in addition to hydration as a preventive measure.

Aminoglycosides

Aminoglycoside-induced nephrotoxicity occurs in 2%–50% of patients. It presents with an increase in SCr levels and a decrease in GFR. Wasting of electrolytes, commonly potassium and magnesium, may also be seen. To prevent aminoglycoside-induced nephrotoxicity, healthcare prescribers should monitor patients for adequate hydration, lower the total daily dose of aminoglycosides, ensure that patients avoid other nephrotoxic drugs, and prescribe extended-interval dosing. Aminoglycosides should be avoided in patients who are at high risk for nephrotoxicity, including individuals with a history of chronic kidney disease and older adults (defined as older than 65 years).

Cisplatin and Carboplatin

Cisplatin and **carboplatin** are chemotherapy agents that are associated with nephrotoxicity. Toxicity presents with an increase in SCr levels that peaks around 10 days after therapy initiation. SCr levels may continue to rise with subsequent chemotherapy cycles and administration. Decreased magnesium, potassium, and calcium may also present. Preventive measures for cisplatin- and carboplatin-induced nephrotoxicity include avoidance of other nephrotoxic drugs, administration of the smallest possible dose of the chemotherapeutic agent, and adequate patient hydration. Amifostine, a preventive chelating agent, may be used in patients at risk for nephrotoxicity that require cisplatin or carboplatin.

Disorders of the Renal System

Disorders of the renal system vary widely in prevalence, symptoms, and treatment. Some are treatable conditions, such as urinary tract infections, urinary incontinence, and benign prostatic hyperplasia. However, acute kidney injury and chronic kidney disease are serious disorders. In fact, kidney disease affects one in three individuals (many of whom are unaware that they have this condition) and is the ninth leading cause of death in the United States.

Urinary Tract Infections

Urinary tract infections (UTIs) usually occur in the bladder but can affect any part of the renal system. **Cystitis** is a lower UTI that involves the bladder, and **pyelonephritis** is an upper UTI that affects the kidneys. Symptoms of UTIs include pain or burning during urination, a frequent urge to void, abdominal pain, fever, chills, and cloudy urine. Symptoms of pyelonephritis may also include back pain (just inferior to the ribs), nausea, and vomiting.

UTIs commonly occur in sexually active women because the opening of the urethra is in proximity to the vagina and anus, where bacteria are commonly found. The urethra is short in women, so bacterial access to the bladder is relatively easy (see Figure 22.5). Most UTIs in women are considered uncomplicated in that they do not involve structural or neurologic problems. Bladder infections in men are rare, however, and considered complicated infections to treat. Complicated UTIs involve structural, obstructive, or other problems that contribute to their development.

Drug Regimens and Treatments

Treatment of UTIs usually involves prescription antibiotics, such as penicillins, nitrofurantoin, sulfamethoxazole/trimethoprim, and fluoroquinolones (see Chapter 23 for a discussion of these antibiotics). Whereas antibiotics are prescription drugs, one drug—phenazopyridine—is an over-the-counter (OTC) agent that has anesthetic effects.

Phenazopyridine

Phenazopyridine is specifically used for the pain, burning, itching, and urinary urgency associated with UTIs.

FIGURE 22.5 Anatomy of the Female Urinary System

The urethra in females is approximately 1.5 inches in length. Consequently, bacteria from the vagina or anus can easily access the bladder and cause a UTI.

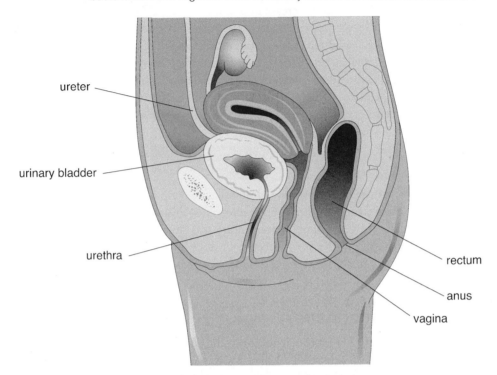

ureter

urinary bladder

urethra

rectum

anus

vagina

Side Effects Phenazopyridine can turn the urine orange, which can be alarming to patients. The colored urine may also stain clothing. Headache and stomach cramps are also common side effects.

Contraindications Phenazopyridine is contraindicated in patients with kidney or liver disease.

➕ ***Note:*** *Allied health professionals should be aware that an allergy to a particular drug contraindicates its use. This warning applies to all Contraindications sections in this chapter.*

Cautions and Considerations Phenazopyridine should be limited in length of use to two to three days only. It acts as an analgesic and does not treat a UTI.

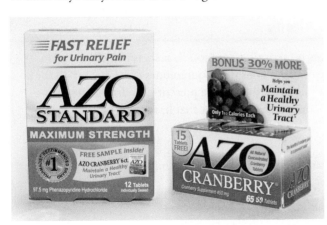

Patients suffering from the discomfort of UTIs can find several OTC phenazopyridine products to relieve the pain, burning, and urinary urgency.

Urinary Incontinence

Urinary incontinence is the complaint of involuntary loss of urine. Common types of urinary incontinence include urge incontinence—often referred to as *overactive bladder*—and overflow incontinence. The prevalence of urinary incontinence is correlated with age. In addition to involuntary loss of urine, patients may feel pain and the urge to urinate often.

Drug Regimens and Treatments

Urinary incontinence can be treated with drugs. Drug treatment often depends on the specific type of urinary incontinence experienced. **Urge incontinence** or **overactive bladder** is generally treated with **antimuscarinic agents**, also known as *anticholinergic agents*. A **beta-3 adrenoreceptor agonist** (mirabegron) is also used to treat overactive bladder (see Table 22.1). **Overflow incontinence** is often treated with alpha-adrenergic antagonists (alpha blockers) and 5-alpha-reductase inhibitors. Alpha-adrenergic antagonists and 5-alpha-reductase inhibitors are discussed in more detail in the section titled "Benign Prostatic Hyperplasia."

TABLE 22.1 Commonly Used Agents for Overactive Bladder

Generic (Brand)	Dosage Form	Route of Administration	Common Dosage
Antimuscarinics			
Darifenacin (Enablex)	Tablet	Oral	7.5 mg a day
Fesoterodine (Toviaz)	Tablet	Oral	4–8 mg a day
Flavoxate	Tablet	Oral	100 mg 3–4 times a day
Oxybutynin (Ditropan)	Patch, syrup, tablet	Oral, transdermal	PO: 5 mg 2–3 times a day Transdermal: 3.9 mg patch applied every 3–4 days
Solifenacin (VESIcare)	Tablet	Oral	5 mg a day
Tolterodine (Detrol)	Capsule, tablet	Oral	2–4 mg a day
Trospium (Sanctura)	Capsule, tablet	Oral	20 mg twice a day or 60 mg extended-release form once a day
Beta-3 Adrenoreceptor Agonist			
Mirabegron (Myrbetriq)	Tablet	Oral	25–50 mg a day

Antimuscarinics

Urinary antimuscarinics work by inhibiting acetylcholine in the autonomic nerves that control involuntary bladder contraction and emptying. In effect, they relax the smooth detrusor muscles and enhance muscle waves in the ureters.

Side Effects Common side effects of antimuscarinics include dry mouth, constipation, blurred vision, and urine retention. These effects can subside over time but may not completely disappear. Drinking plenty of water or sucking on hard candy can help alleviate dry mouth. Staying hydrated and taking a stool softener may help with constipation. Other side effects can include hallucinations, drowsiness, and upset stomach. If

Work Wise

As an allied health professional, you will likely encounter patients with overactive bladder or incontinence. Many of these patients will feel embarrassed and uncomfortable about their condition. With that in mind, show these patients empathy and avoid judgment when addressing their health-care concerns.

abdominal pain, eye pain, or difficulty with urination occurs, the patient should consult his or her prescriber. Allergic reactions are rare but can happen. Patients should inform their prescribers if they experience a skin rash while taking one of these medications.

Contraindications Antimuscarinics are contraindicated in patients with gastric retention and narrow-angle glaucoma.

Cautions and Considerations Antimuscarinics should be used with caution in older adults. This patient population may be particularly susceptible to adverse effects such as hallucinations, dry mouth, blurred vision, and constipation.

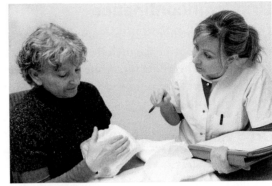

An allied health professional should discuss incontinence measures, such as the use of an incontinence pad, in a private setting.

Beta-3 Adrenoreceptor Agonists

Beta-3 adrenoreceptor agonists work by promoting relaxation of the detrusor smooth muscle during urine storage. In effect, this action increases bladder capacity.

Side Effects Common side effects of beta-3 adrenoreceptor agonists, such as mirabegron, include hypertension, tachycardia, headache, dizziness, constipation, dry mouth, diarrhea, UTI, back pain, nasopharyngitis, and flulike symptoms.

Contraindications There are no contraindications to mirabegron.

Cautions and Considerations Mirabegron should not be used in patients with uncontrolled hypertension due to reported dose-related increases in blood pressure. It should be used cautiously in patients with controlled hypertension, as exacerbations of hypertension have been reported. The risk of urinary retention may be increased, so mirabegron should be used carefully in patients with bladder obstruction. Doses of mirabegron should be decreased in patients with hepatic and renal impairment. Mirabegron use is not recommended in patients with severe hepatic impairment or end-stage renal disease.

Benign Prostatic Hyperplasia

Benign prostatic hyperplasia (BPH) is a chronic male condition that occurs as the prostate gland enlarges with age. Although prostate enlargement happens in all men, this condition is especially common among men ages 60 to 85. Prostate enlargement is not harmful in and of itself; however, the enlarged gland can impinge on the urethra and obstruct urine flow (see Figure 22.6).

The incidence of symptoms varies, but symptoms may include a weak or slow urine stream, a delayed start of urination, and straining to void. Because urine flow is obstructed, the bladder cannot be fully emptied. This incomplete or partial emptying can cause frequent urges to urinate. Men with this condition feel the need to urinate often, but they void only small amounts each time. The condition is diagnosed by a review of symptoms and a digital rectal examination, in which a gloved finger is inserted into the rectum to palpate the prostate gland directly.

Prostate-specific antigen (PSA) is a laboratory test that can screen for BPH and more serious prostate gland problems. When properly interpreted, elevations in PSA can indicate whether the prostate tissue growth is benign or potentially malignant (prostate

FIGURE 22.6 Anatomy of the Male Urinary System

Unvoided urine can promote infection. Most males will not have UTIs, but men with BPH may find they have bladder infections frequently.

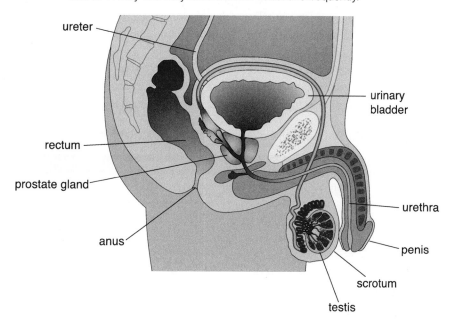

cancer). In fact, one in six men receive a diagnosis of prostate cancer in their lifetime, making prostate cancer the second most common type of cancer among men. Fortunately, prostate cancer is highly treatable, especially when caught early. Symptoms of prostate cancer are similar to those of BPH and include difficulty starting or stopping urination, frequent voiding, painful urination, and blood in the urine.

Drug Regimens and Treatments

Close monitoring of the patient's symptoms precedes the initiation of drug therapy for BPH. When symptoms become bothersome, alpha-adrenergic antagonists (alpha blockers) or 5-alpha-reductase inhibitors are prescribed. If symptoms become severe or cause complications, more invasive action may be needed. Procedures to remove part of the prostate gland and open an obstructed urethral lumen include transurethral resection of the prostate and transurethral needle ablation, among others.

Healthcare practitioners should also be aware that some drug therapies cause urinary retention (see Table 22.2). These agents can exacerbate urination problems and should not be used by patients with BPH.

TABLE 22.2 Drugs to Avoid in BPH and Possible Substitutions

Drugs to Avoid	Possible Drug Substitutions
Anticholinergics	Antacid, H2 blockers, sucralfate
Calcium-channel blockers	Alpha-adrenergic antagonists
Disopyramide	Quinidine
Oral bronchodilators	Inhaled bronchodilators
Tricyclic antidepressants (TCAs)	Selective serotonin reuptake inhibitors (SSRIs)

Alpha-Adrenergic Antagonists

Alpha-adrenergic antagonists, or *alpha blockers*, are used to treat patients with BPH, especially those individuals who also have high blood pressure. These two conditions are a common combination in older men. These medications work by inhibiting the alpha-1 receptors that contract smooth muscle in the prostate gland and bladder (as well as relax blood vessels in the rest of the body).

Commonly used alpha-adrenergic antagonists for BPH appear in Table 22.3. In the urinary system, alpha-adrenergic antagonists reduce urinary resistance and improve urine flow. They are sometimes used to help pass kidney stones that have become lodged in the ureters.

TABLE 22.3 Commonly Used Alpha-Adrenergic Antagonists for BPH

Generic (Brand)	Dosage Form	Route of Administration	Common Dosage
Alfuzosin (Uroxatral)	Tablet	Oral	10 mg a day
Doxazosin (Cardura)	Tablet	Oral	4–8 mg a day
Tamsulosin (Flomax)	Capsule	Oral	0.4–0.8 mg a day
Terazosin (Hytrin)	Capsule	Oral	10 mg a day

Side Effects Common side effects of alpha-adrenergic antagonists include dizziness, drowsiness, fatigue, headache, fainting, and **orthostatic hypotension**, which is a drop in blood pressure that causes dizziness on sitting or standing up. Rising slowly from a seated or lying position can alleviate this effect.

Alpha-adrenergic antagonists also have sexual side effects that are very rare but serious. One such effect is **priapism**, a prolonged and painful erection. If this condition occurs, patients should seek medical attention immediately to avoid permanent damage and impotence.

Contraindications Alfuzosin is contraindicated in moderate-to-severe liver insufficiency and with medications—such as itraconazole, ketoconazole, and ritonavir—that may increase the levels of alfuzosin in the blood. Doxazosin should be avoided in patients with a hypersensitivity to quinazolines. Tamsulosin and terazosin do not have any contraindications.

Cautions and Considerations Alpha-adrenergic antagonists can have a first-dose effect whereby blood pressure drops dramatically and causes dizziness or fainting. Patients are often observed closely during the first dose to monitor for this effect. Repeated blood pressure measurements may be required for four to six hours after taking the first dose. Consequently, patients should be careful about driving or operating machinery until they know how the medication affects them.

These agents must be used with caution in patients with gastrointestinal (GI) disorders, liver disease, or kidney impairment. Alpha-adrenergic antagonists can exacerbate GI motility disorders. Patients should inform their prescribers if they have any of these conditions before taking an alpha-adrenergic antagonist.

Quick Study

Allied health personnel should note that many of the generic names for alpha-adrenergic antagonists end in *-osin*.

In addition, alpha-adrenergic antagonists interact with several other prescription medications. Patients should inform their prescribers and pharmacists of all medications they take so that interactions can be identified and evaluated appropriately.

Healthcare practitioners should tell patients to take alpha-adrenergic antagonists before bedtime and to avoid crushing or chewing alfuzosin, doxazosin, and tamsulosin. These medications should be swallowed whole.

5-Alpha-Reductase Inhibitors

The drug class known as **5-alpha-reductase inhibitors** is used to treat BPH, but these medications can also be used to treat male-pattern hair loss (see Table 22.4). The 5-alpha-reductase inhibitors work by inhibiting the conversion of testosterone into its active form dihydrotestosterone (DHT) in the prostate gland, hair follicles, and other androgen-sensitive tissues. Impeding this process reduces the size of the prostate because prostate tissue growth is testosterone dependent. Although blocking testosterone altogether would reduce prostate size, the side effects of reduced androgen production in the body are undesirable for most patients. With this class of drugs, only DHT is blocked, which thereby reduces prostate size while allowing adequate levels of testosterone to remain in the bloodstream.

TABLE 22.4 Common 5-Alpha-Reductase Inhibitors for BPH

Generic (Brand)	Dosage Form	Route of Administration	Common Dosage
Dutasteride (Avodart)	Capsule	Oral	0.5 mg a day
Finasteride (Propecia, Proscar)	Tablet	Oral	5 mg a day

Side Effects Common side effects of 5-alpha-reductase inhibitors include decreased libido, erectile dysfunction, and ejaculation disorders. These medications can also cause **gynecomastia** (breast enlargement in men or boys). If these effects are bothersome, patients should speak with their prescribers to determine if drug therapy should be discontinued.

Contraindications Dutasteride and finasteride are contraindicated in women of child-bearing age.

Cautions and Considerations Because these agents block an active form of testosterone production, they could be harmful to a developing fetus in utero. Women of childbearing age must not handle these agents with bare skin. They should wear gloves to prevent measurable absorption of 5-alpha-reductase inhibitors, especially if handling broken tablets or opened capsules. They should also avoid contact with semen from a male partner exposed to 5-alpha-reductase inhibitors.

 Checkpoint 22.2

Take a moment to review what you have learned so far and answer these questions.

1. Which drugs are nephrotoxic or potentially nephrotoxic?
2. What are the side effects of antimuscarinic drugs?

 Kolb's Learning Styles

Accommodators and Divergers may enjoy this particular learning activity to help them remember the drugs used to treat urinary bladder problems. Antimuscarinic agents and 5-alpha-reductase inhibitors (drugs for BPH) are frequently advertised on television and in magazines. Take some time to locate a few such advertisements and make note of the brand names mentioned. Think of the generic name for each drug and then describe how each drug works.

Acute Kidney Injury and Chronic Kidney Disease

Kidney disease can be acute or chronic. **Acute kidney injury** is a decrease in kidney function or GFR that occurs over hours, days, or even weeks. If supportive care is provided and the cause for failure resolved, kidney function may return to normal. If the insult is sufficiently severe, acute kidney injury can be life-threatening and might result in some level of permanent damage.

Chronic kidney disease (CKD), on the other hand, involves progressive damage to the kidney tissue, resulting in the death of this tissue over time. Common causes of CKD include diabetes and untreated hypertension. CKD is more common than acute kidney injury and cannot be reversed. As it worsens, it can be categorized into stages that guide the approach and degree of urgency for treatment (see Table 22.5). Drug therapies, such as diuretics and other renal-protective medications, can help slow the progression of the disease in early stages, but in later stages, these agents are of no use. Eventually, in end-stage kidney failure, dialysis and kidney transplantation are the only means of treatment.

TABLE 22.5 Stages of CKD

Stage	GFR (mL/min/1.73 m²)	Description
I	≥ 90	Normal kidney function but urine findings, structural abnormalities, or a genetic trait point to kidney disease
II	60–89	Mildly reduced kidney function but urine findings, structural abnormalities, or a genetic trait point to kidney disease
IIIa	45–59	Moderately reduced kidney function
IIIb	30–44	Moderately reduced kidney function
IV	15–29	Severely reduced kidney function
V	< 15	End-stage kidney failure (sometimes called *established renal failure*)

Drug Regimens and Treatments

Acute kidney injury typically improves or reverses as its cause is resolved. Therefore, drug treatment for acute kidney injury is limited and short term.

CKD is more frequently treated with medication. Hypertension management is a key strategy used in patients with CKD. In order to decrease hypertension, angiotensin-converting enzyme (ACE) inhibitors and angiotensin receptor blockers (ARBs) are given initially, followed by diuretics.

In addition to these medications, hematopoietic therapy and iron supplements are used to treat anemia that results from decreased erythropoietin production. Various drugs are also used to supplement imbalances of sodium, potassium, calcium, phosphorus, aluminum, and vitamin D.

Finally, treatment for advanced stages of CKD often includes dialysis. This procedure, as well as the drug regimens mentioned previously, is discussed later in this chapter.

ACE Inhibitors and ARBs

An **angiotensin-converting enzyme (ACE) inhibitor** or an **angiotensin receptor blocker (ARB)** is usually used to treat patients with CKD (see Table 22.6). ACE inhibitors and ARBs are used for a variety of conditions, including kidney protection and blood pressure management. For a more detailed discussion of ACE inhibitors and ARBs, see Chapter 15.

TABLE 22.6 Common ACE Inhibitors and ARBs

Generic (Brand)	Dosage Form	Route of Administration	Common Dosage
ACE Inhibitors			
Benazepril (Lotensin)	Tablet	Oral	5–40 mg a day
Captopril (Capoten)	Tablet	Oral	25–100 mg a day
Enalapril (Epaned, Vasotec)	Injectable solution, tablet	IV, oral	IV: 1.25 mg every 6 hr infused over 5 min PO: 5–20 mg a day
Fosinopril	Tablet	Oral	10–40 mg a day
Lisinopril (Prinivil, Zestril)	Tablet	Oral	5–40 mg a day
Moexipril (Univasc)	Tablet	Oral	7.5–30 mg a day
Perindopril (Aceon)	Tablet	Oral	4–16 mg a day
Quinapril (Accupril)	Tablet	Oral	10–80 mg a day
Ramipril (Altace)	Capsule	Oral	2.5–20 mg a day
Trandolapril (Mavik)	Tablet	Oral	1–4 mg a day
ARBs			
Azilsartan (Edarbi)	Tablet	Oral	40–80 mg a day
Candesartan (Atacand)	Tablet	Oral	8–32 mg once or twice a day
Eprosartan (Teveten)	Tablet	Oral	400–800 mg a day
Irbesartan (Avapro)	Tablet	Oral	150 mg a day
Losartan (Cozaar)	Tablet	Oral	25–100 mg a day
Olmesartan (Benicar)	Tablet	Oral	20–40 mg a day
Telmisartan (Micardis)	Tablet	Oral	20–80 mg a day
Valsartan (Diovan)	Tablet	Oral	80–320 mg a day

Side Effects Common side effects of ACE inhibitors include headache, dizziness, fatigue, mild diarrhea, and a dry hacking cough. A cough is a frequent but odd side effect that patients often do not associate with their blood pressure medication. **Angioedema** is a rare but serious side effect of ACE inhibitors.

Common side effects of ARBs include headache, dizziness, fatigue, and mild diarrhea. Dizziness occurs most frequently in patients who also have heart failure. Patients taking ARBs may also have more respiratory tract infections, but the reason for this side effect is unknown.

Contraindications ACE inhibitors should not be used in patients who experienced angioedema with previous ACE inhibitor use or in patients who are pregnant, because of the risk of severe birth defects. Other contraindications for ACE inhibitor use include idiopathic or hereditary angioedema and bilateral renal artery stenosis. ACE inhibitors and ARBs are contraindicated with concomitant use of aliskiren in patients with diabetes mellitus.

Cautions and Considerations In rare instances, **hypotension**, or low blood pressure, can occur with ACE inhibitor or ARB use. ACE inhibitors may cause elevated potassium levels (hyperkalemia); consequently, periodic blood tests for potassium levels should be conducted. Patients who take diuretics along with an ACE inhibitor should be warned against taking potassium supplements. Patients with other types of kidney problems can still take ACE inhibitors, but doses are adjusted downward. Patients with kidney or liver impairment may need special dosing and monitoring if they are to take ARBs.

Diuretics

Diuretics are most often used as adjunct therapy to improve urine output in patients with kidney disease or to reduce blood volume in patients with high blood pressure. (Figure 22.7 shows the sites of action for the commonly used diuretics.) Thiazide diuretics and potassium-sparing diuretics tend to be used more often for treating hypertension, whereas loop diuretics are used more for treating kidney failure or reducing edema. Carbonic anhydrase inhibitors are usually used in patients with edema that have acid-base balance concerns. Combinations of these diuretic classes may be used in certain kidney failure situations to maximize urine output. Table 22.7 lists diuretics commonly used in the treatment of CKD; two of these medications, furosemide and spironolactone, are shown in Figure 22.8.

FIGURE 22.7 | **Diuretic Sites of Action**

Thiazide diuretics work in the distal convoluted tubule, and loop diuretics work in the loop of Henle.

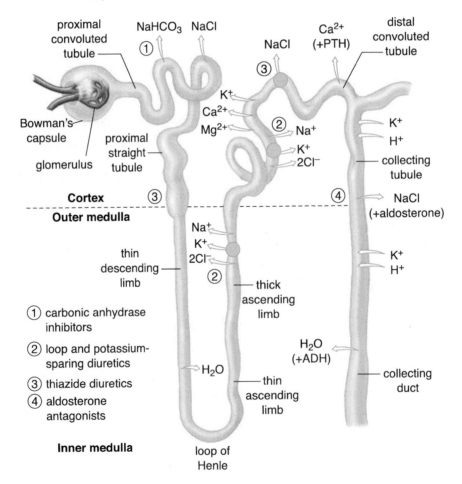

Patient Teaching

As an allied health professional, you are in an excellent position to educate patients on appropriate timing of diuretics. Patients taking diuretics almost always experience increased urinary frequency and volume. For this reason, most patients prefer to take diuretics in the morning. Bedtime dosing can lead to night-time awakenings, incontinence, and—in older adults—falls.

TABLE 22.7 Commonly Used Diuretics

Generic (Brand)	Dosage Form	Route of Administration	Common Dosage
Carbonic Anhydrase Inhibitor			
Acetazolamide (Diamox)	Capsule, injection, tablet	IV, oral	250–375 mg a day or every other day
Loop Diuretics			
Bumetanide	Injection, tablet	IM, IV, oral	Individualized to patient
Ethacrynate (Edecrin)	Injection, tablet	IV, oral	Individualized to patient
Furosemide (Lasix)	Injection, oral solution, tablet	IV, oral	Individualized to patient
Torsemide (Demadex)	Tablet	Oral	Individualized to patient
Potassium-Sparing Diuretics			
Amiloride	Tablet	Oral	5–20 mg a day
Spironolactone (Aldactone)	Tablet	Oral	25–200 mg a day
Triamterene (Dyrenium)	Capsule	Oral	200–300 mg a day
Thiazide Diuretics			
Chlorothiazide (Diuril)	Injection, suspension, tablet	IV, oral	Varies by age
Chlorthalidone	Tablet	Oral	30–120 mg a day
Hydrochlorothiazide (Microzide)	Capsule, tablet	Oral	12.5–50 mg a day
Indapamide	Tablet	Oral	1.25–2.5 mg a day
Methyclothiazide (Enduron)	Tablet	Oral	2.5–10 mg a day
Metolazone (Zaroxolyn)	Tablet	Oral	2.5–20 mg a day
Combination Products			
Spironolactone/hydrochlorothiazide (Aldactazide)	Tablet	Oral	25–100 mg/25–100 mg a day
Triamterene/hydrochlorothiazide (Dyazide, Maxzide)	Capsule, tablet	Oral	37.5–75 mg/25–100 mg a day

FIGURE 22.8 Diuretic Labels

These medication labels show widely used diuretics for the treatment of CKD.

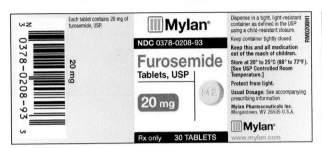
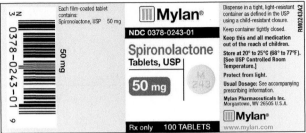

Carbonic Anhydrase Inhibitors

Carbonic anhydrase inhibitors work in the nephrons by increasing excretion of bicarbonate ions, which carry sodium, potassium, and water into the urine. They are similar to sulfonamides in their chemical structure. These medications are used more frequently for open-angle glaucoma but are occasionally used for diuresis (urine production) in congestive heart failure.

Side Effects Common side effects of carbonic anhydrase inhibitors include **tinnitus** (ringing in the ears), tingling, nausea, vomiting, diarrhea, drowsiness, and changes in taste.

Contraindications Acetazolamide should not be used in patients with a hypersensitivity to sulfonamides, liver disease or insufficiency, decreased sodium or potassium levels, adrenocortical insufficiency, cirrhosis, hyperchloremic acidosis, and severe kidney disease or dysfunction. Long-term use in narrow-angle glaucoma is contraindicated. It should also be avoided with concurrent aspirin use.

Cautions and Considerations Carbonic anhydrase inhibitors can cause sulfa allergy and Stevens-Johnson syndrome. If patients experience a skin rash while taking one of these agents, they should notify their prescribers immediately.

Loop Diuretics

Loop diuretics work by inhibiting reabsorption of sodium, chloride, and water in the ascending loop of Henle. This unique site of action produces fast and profound diuresis. Sodium, chloride, magnesium, calcium, and potassium are all excreted quickly and efficiently with the use of a loop diuretic. For this reason, loop diuretics are used to pull fluid out of the body rapidly. Typically, these agents are used to treat swelling and fluid accumulation due to heart or kidney failure.

Name Exchange

Even though the loop diuretic furosemide is widely available as a generic drug, it is often referred to in practice by its brand name, Lasix.

Side Effects Side effects for loop diuretics are similar to those for thiazide diuretics and include hypotension, dizziness, headache, skin rash, hair loss (alopecia), upset stomach, diarrhea, and constipation. Patients should be reminded to rise slowly from seated or lying positions to help with dizziness and decreases in blood pressure.

Contraindications Loop diuretics are contraindicated in patients with anuria. Bumetanide should not be used in patients with hepatic coma or severe electrolyte depletion. Ethacrynate should not be used in patients with a history of severe watery diarrhea upon use and should not be used in infants.

Cautions and Considerations Loop diuretics deplete potassium levels in the body. Taking potassium supplements is often necessary with these diuretics to maintain proper electrolyte balance (see the section titled "Potassium Supplements").

Potassium-Sparing Diuretics

Potassium-sparing diuretics work by blocking the exchange of potassium for sodium that takes place in the distal tubule. Therefore, more sodium is excreted while potassium is preserved in the body. Water follows sodium, so water is excreted along with sodium ions without depleting the body of potassium, as may happen with thiazide and loop diuretics. These drugs are used primarily to treat hypertension.

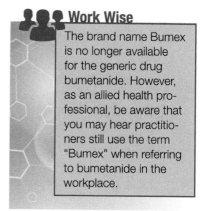

Work Wise

The brand name Bumex is no longer available for the generic drug bumetanide. However, as an allied health professional, be aware that you may hear practitioners still use the term "Bumex" when referring to bumetanide in the workplace.

Aldosterone antagonists can be considered potassium sparing, but these agents work by inhibiting a hormone that promotes fluid retention. Spironolactone, an older medication with this activity, works by inhibiting aldosterone, which promotes sodium and water reabsorption in the distal tubule and collecting duct of the nephron. Spironolactone is used primarily for hypertension and heart failure and sometimes may be used in **hyperaldosteronism** (a condition in which the body produces too much aldosterone).

Side Effects Side effects of potassium-sparing diuretics can include gynecomastia. If bothersome, this effect may limit therapy because there is no treatment for it, other than to stop taking the drug. Other, less common side effects include upset stomach, headache, confusion, and drowsiness.

Contraindications Potassium-sparing diuretics should not be used in the presence of elevated serum potassium, kidney insufficiency or impairment, and anuria. Amiloride should not be used if a patient is using other potassium-conserving agents or supplements or if that patient has diabetic nephropathy. Spironolactone is contraindicated in Addison's disease or other conditions associated with elevated potassium levels and with concomitant eplerenone use. Contraindications to triamterene include severe liver disease and coadministration with other potassium-sparing agents.

Cautions and Considerations Potassium-sparing agents can cause hyperkalemia (high potassium levels) because they promote potassium retention. Periodic laboratory tests are needed to monitor for this effect.

Thiazide Diuretics

Thiazide diuretics work by inhibiting reabsorption of sodium and chloride ions in the distal tubule of the nephron. Because water follows sodium, water is excreted along with the sodium. In effect, water is pulled into the urine and eliminated from the body, thereby reducing blood volume. The loss of both water and sodium contributes to the decline in blood pressure. Because of a sodium-potassium exchange mechanism in the distal tubule, most diuretics (like thiazides) cause both potassium and sodium to be lost.

Side Effects Possible side effects include hypotension, dizziness, headache, skin rash, hair loss (alopecia), upset stomach, diarrhea, and constipation. Patients should be reminded to rise slowly from seated or lying positions to help with dizziness and decreases in blood pressure.

Contraindications Thiazide diuretics are related to sulfonamide-derived drugs and therefore are contraindicated in patients with a hypersensitivity to sulfonamides. Thiazide diuretics are also contraindicated in anuria. Metolazone has the additional contraindication of hepatic coma or precoma.

Cautions and Considerations Thiazide diuretics deplete potassium levels in the body. Taking potassium supplements is often necessary with these diuretics to maintain proper electrolyte balance (see the subsequent section titled "Potassium Supplements"). Patients should understand that taking these supplements is important because potassium is essential for effective cardiac function.

Thiazide diuretics can interact with alcohol to contribute to drops in blood pressure. Patients should use caution when drinking alcohol while taking these medications. Thiazides also interact with drugs used to treat diabetes because they can raise blood glucose levels. However, this interaction is not a concern if a low-dose drug regimen is followed. In addition, thiazide diuretics interact with corticosteroids and lithium, so they are not usually used in conjunction with them.

Potassium Supplements

Prescription potassium supplements are used to replenish a potassium deficiency caused by thiazide and loop diuretics. These supplements are taken daily in tablet, capsule, oral liquid, or oral packet form. Most potassium tablets are quite large and can be difficult to swallow. Brand names include K-Dur, K-Lor, Klor-Con, K-Lyte, K-Tab, Kaon-CL, and Micro-K.

Side Effects Common side effects of potassium supplements include nausea, vomiting, diarrhea, gas, and upset stomach. These effects are usually mild and can be reduced by taking the supplement with food or a full glass of water.

Contraindications Because most salt-substitute products contain potassium rather than sodium, patients who take potassium supplements should not use salt substitutes. If they do, they can ingest too much potassium, which is harmful to cardiac function. In addition, patients with digestive problems that affect the motility of stomach or intestinal contents should not take potassium supplements. If the potassium tablet becomes stagnant, the lining of the GI tract can become irritated and damaged.

Cautions and Considerations Most potassium tablets are quite large and can be difficult to swallow. Many of these supplements are extended-release formulations, so they should be swallowed whole, not chewed or crushed. Effervescent tablets should be dissolved in three to eight ounces of water and then drunk slowly.

Drug Alert

Although potassium supplements may seem benign, they can be harmful if not used appropriately. Patients with kidney disease, diabetes, heart disease, Addison's disease, stomach ulcers, or potassium-altering conditions or disorders should not take potassium supplements without talking to a healthcare practitioner first. Potassium supplements cause hyperkalemia, or high levels of potassium in the blood. This condition may result in cardiac dysfunction and even death. Acute hyperkalemia may be treated with Kayexalate, or sodium polystyrene sulfonate.

Dialysis

Dialysis is an artificial method of filtering blood and correcting the electrolyte imbalances caused by kidney failure. When indicated, dialysis is accomplished by one of two common methods: hemodialysis or peritoneal dialysis. **Hemodialysis** is accomplished by diverting bloodflow through a machine that mechanically filters the blood and returns the blood to the body (see Figure 22.9). **Peritoneal dialysis** is accomplished by putting **dialysate** (a special fluid that draws toxins from the body into itself) into the abdominal cavity and leaving it there for a certain period—typically, a few days (see Figure 22.10).

FIGURE 22.9 | Hemodialysis

In hemodialysis, a patient is connected to a machine in a dialysis center and must remain at the center for several hours.

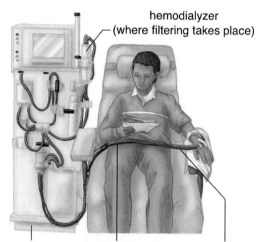

hemodialyzer
(where filtering takes place)

hemodialysis
machine

unfiltered blood
flows to hemodialyzer

filtered blood flows
back to body

FIGURE 22.10 | Peritoneal Dialysis

In peritoneal dialysis, a patient has the freedom to receive treatment at home, at work, or while traveling.

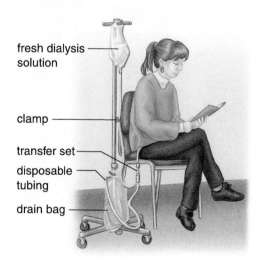

fresh dialysis
solution

clamp

transfer set

disposable
tubing

drain bag

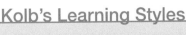
During this time, toxins and electrolytes diffuse into the dialysate fluid from the many capillaries in the abdominal cavity. With proper instruction, the dialysate fluid can be drained and changed at home. The risk of infection and other complications is greater with peritoneal dialysis.

Kidney Transplantation

Kidney transplantation is the treatment of choice for Stage V, or *end-stage*, kidney disease. The process involves a kidney from a living or deceased donor being surgically implanted into a recipient. Kidney transplantation is one of the most common transplant operations in the United States.

Potential kidney recipients undergo evaluation for transplant. If determined to be an eligible candidate for the procedure, patients are placed on a **national waiting list**. Waiting list priority depends on key factors such as type of kidney problem, disease severity, and likelihood of transplant success. Kidney transplant surgery takes approximately three hours. After the procedure, patients can expect to stay in the hospital for several days. Procedure recovery time varies but is, on average, six months. Almost all patients who undergo kidney transplantation will require maintenance immunosuppression to help prevent organ rejection. Close follow-up care with a healthcare practitioner is necessary for many years after the procedure.

In the Know

According to the National Kidney Foundation, there were more than 100,000 patients awaiting kidney transplants in 2014. In addition, approximately 3,000 patients are added to the national kidney waiting list each month. Donor organs are matched to patient recipients through the National Organ Procurement and Transplantation Network. To become an organ donor, an individual can visit the Donate Life America website via http://PharmEssAH.emcp.net/DonateLife and select his or her state of residence to learn about donation options.

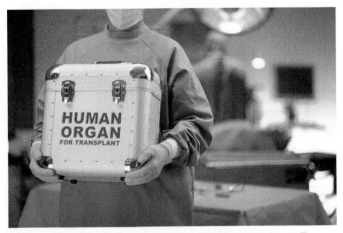

A donated kidney may be from a living or deceased donor. To transport the kidney to a hospital, the organ is placed in a cool saline solution to preserve its viability for up to 48 hours.

Take a moment to review what you have learned so far and answer these questions.

1. What drugs are commonly used to treat CKD?

2. What are the main types of diuretics discussed in this chapter?

3. What are the key differences between hemodialysis and peritoneal dialysis?

Herbal and Alternative Therapies

Saw palmetto is used to treat BPH symptoms, such as frequent or painful urination, as well as urinary hesitancy and urgency. Clinical studies have shown that this herbal treatment may have efficacy similar to that of finasteride in reducing these symptoms. Saw palmetto does not shrink overall prostate gland size; it works by reducing the thickness of the inner layer. It inhibits 5-alpha-reductase, which prevents conversion of testosterone to DHT. It has some anti-inflammatory effects but

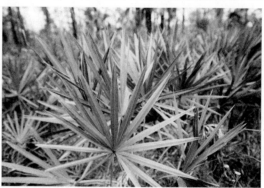

Saw palmetto supplements come from the saw palmetto plant and may be used to treat BPH.

does not reduce PSA levels. Side effects are mild and include dizziness, headache, nausea and/or vomiting, constipation, and diarrhea. Drug interactions with anticoagulants and some hormone therapies are possible. Patients should inform their physicians and pharmacists if they take saw palmetto. Typical doses are 160 mg twice a day or 320 mg once a day. Saw palmetto teas do not generally provide a high-enough dose to be effective.

Cranberry juice is used for prevention of recurrent UTIs. When consumed on a daily basis, it has been shown in clinical trials to be effective in preventing UTIs in elderly women, pregnant women, and inpatients. Oral capsules are not as effective. Although initially thought to acidify urine, cranberry juice is now thought to work by adhering to bacterial cells and preventing them from attaching to the inner walls of the bladder. Cranberry juice does not release bacteria that have already adhered to the bladder wall, so it does not treat an active UTI. Although side effects are few, cranberry juice, when consumed in large quantities, can cause upset stomach and diarrhea. Cranberry juice can interact with warfarin, so patients drinking it on a regular basis or in large amounts should let their healthcare practitioners know.

Chapter Summary

Concepts regarding renal function are particularly important to know when studying pharmacology because so many drugs rely on kidney function for their elimination from the body. Kidneys are the primary organs that filter the blood and remove toxins, metabolic by-products, and drugs. The nephron is the part of the kidney responsible for filtration. The blood concentration of SCr is used as a laboratory marker for kidney function. It is used to calculate GFR, a guide to estimating renal function and dosing drug therapy. Kidney damage can be acute or chronic. Acute kidney injury is often reversible, whereas CKD is irreversible and progressive. Stages of CKD have been established to guide treatment.

Other problems with the urinary system include UTIs, urinary incontinence, and prostate gland enlargement. Antimuscarinics and a beta 3-adrenoreceptor agonist (mirabegron) are used to treat overactive bladder. Alpha-adrenergic antagonists, 5-alpha-reductase inhibitors, and saw palmetto (a natural plant product) are used to treat BPH. ACE inhibitors and ARBs are used to lower blood pressure and protect the kidneys. Diuretics are used to improve kidney function and urine production. At low doses, they are used most often to treat hypertension, but at high doses they can treat early stages of renal failure. Thiazide, loop, and potassium-sparing diuretics work in different parts of the nephron and are used in different situations. Thiazide diuretics and potassium-sparing diuretics are commonly used to treat hypertension. Loop diuretics are used when large amounts of fluid need to be removed from patients with heart or kidney failure.

Dialysis is an artificial method of filtering blood and correcting the electrolyte imbalance caused by kidney failure. This procedure is accomplished by one of two common methods: hemodialysis or peritoneal dialysis. End-stage kidney disease typically requires kidney transplantation.

Chapter Checkup

The Navigator+ learning management system that accompanies this textbook offers many opportunities to help you master chapter content, including end-of-chapter exercises, a glossary of key terms, flash cards, and additional interactive activities.

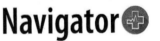

Career Exploration

If you enjoyed learning about the renal system in this chapter, you may want to explore the following allied health career options:

- diagnostic medical sonographist
- medical assistant
- pharmacy technician
- renal dialysis technician
- renal registered dietitian
- renal social worker
- urinalysis technician

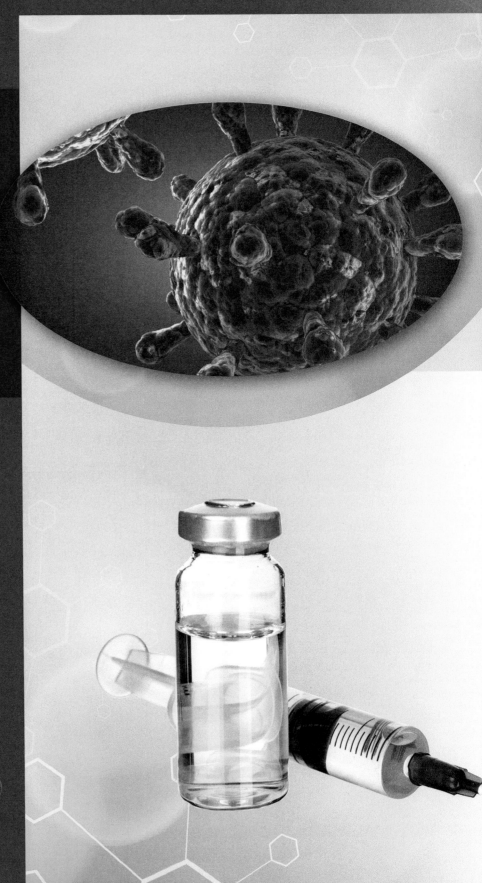

UNIT

8

Navigator

Pharmacotherapy for the Immune System

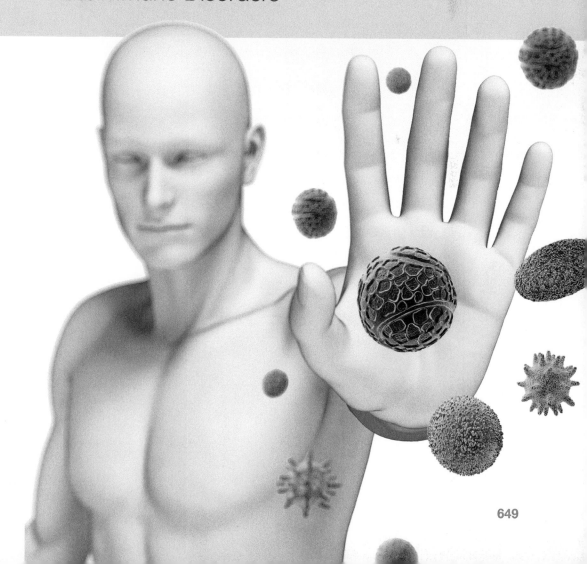

23 The Immune System and Infectious Disease Therapy

Pharm Facts

- Bacterial cells outnumber human cells in the body 10 to 1! There are 10 trillion human cells but *100* trillion bacterial cells.

- Severe combined immunodeficiency (SCID), a hereditary disorder, affects 1 in 100,000 infants. In this disorder, individuals have a malfunctioning immune system that leaves them vulnerable to potentially deadly infections. SCID is commonly known as "bubble boy disease," a moniker that stemmed from a boy diagnosed with the disorder who lived inside a plastic bubble for 12 years.

- Research conducted by Dr. Steven Cole, a professor at UCLA, has shown that happiness can alter immune-cell structure. Having a sense of well-being and a purpose in life can increase levels of the antiviral response in immune cells and decrease the body's inflammatory response.

- According to 2013 statistics from the World Health Organization, 35 million individuals worldwide have HIV, with more than 70% of those affected living in sub-Saharan Africa.

"As a community health educator, you learn firsthand the needs of the community, the barriers to accessing health care, and the factors that prevent individuals from achieving behavioral change. Community health educators build independent and collaborative relationships with community members to tailor their healthcare services and improve their quality of life. These relationships have made a great impact on addressing the health, social, and psychological concerns of patients living with HIV/AIDS. For example, I have seen an increase in consistent HIV testing and in accessible, quality health care and a decrease in STI/HIV transmission and new HIV and AIDS diagnoses within the community. For me, these positive changes have made my work fulfilling."

—**T. Jibri Douglas**, BSHP
Community Health Educator

The immune system is a complex network of barriers, organs, and molecules that has evolved over millions of years to work in concert to defend the body against invading pathogens. Before the twentieth century, infection was the most common cause of death in the United States. Since then, the development of antibiotics and vaccines has helped treat and prevent infection.

The purpose of this chapter is to describe the immune system and explain the use of antimicrobial agents in treating infections that commonly affect the immune system as well as other body systems. The most frequently encountered pathogens (bacteria, viruses, and fungi) are described along with the typical infections they cause. The number of antimicrobial drugs is large, making this a long chapter. However, knowing these drugs will be useful because allied health professionals work with such medications on a daily basis in patient care settings. Other related immune system topics, such as acquired immunity and autoimmune disorders, are discussed in Chapter 24.

Anatomy and Physiology of the Immune System

The **immune system** is the body's built-in defense mechanism against invading **pathogens**, the foreign organisms that cause infection. The immune system works on two levels: a local level, at the site of a cut or wound, and a systemic level, throughout the body. The immune system comprises specialized cells, tissues, and organs located throughout the body.

Cells of the Immune System

The cells of the immune system are known as **leukocytes**, or white blood cells. Leukocytes are categorized as **agranulocytes** (those that do not contain granules in the cytoplasm) and **granulocytes** (those that do contain granules in the cytoplasm). Agranulocytes include monocytes, macrophages, and lymphocytes. Granulocytes include neutrophils, eosinophils, and basophils. **Neutrophils** and **monocytes** circulate throughout the body in the blood and move into tissue when an infection is present. Once there, monocytes mature into **macrophages**. Both neutrophils and macrophages ingest foreign invaders. The two main types of **lymphocytes** are B cells and T cells, and they detect specific pathogens and support an organism's immunity in different ways. **B cells** secrete antibodies into the blood when a foreign substance is detected, whereas **T cells** attack infected cells. **Eosinophils** are proinflammatory leukocytes that destroy invading organisms and are utilized in inflammatory processes, particularly allergic disorders, and in many parasitic infections. **Basophils** are involved with inflammation and allergic response. (For clarification on the types of leukocytes, see Figure 23.1.)

FIGURE 23.1 Types of Leukocytes

Human blood contains 4,000 to 11,000 leukocytes per microliter (mcL) of blood. The blood differential test determines the percentage of leukocytes that are in the blood. Neutrophils make up the largest percentage (40%–60%) of leukocytes.

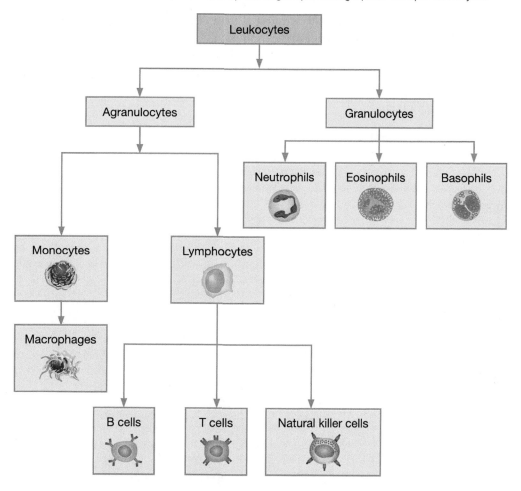

Tissues and Organs of the Immune System

The major tissues and organs of the immune system can be classified as primary or secondary. Primary lymphoid tissues and organs are the sites where lymphocytes develop. Secondary lymphoid tissues and organs are the sites where mature lymphocytes activate and perform their functions.

The major components of the primary lymphoid tissues and organs are the bone marrow and thymus. **Bone marrow** is a flexible tissue found in the interior of bones and is an important lymphoid tissue. Bone marrow is the primary source of **erythrocytes** (red blood cells), leukocytes (white blood cells), and **thrombocytes** (platelets). The **thymus** is the major primary lymphoid organ, the main function of which is the production of T cells. T cells are lymphocytes that assist in acquired or innate immunity (see the section titled "Types of Immunity").

The major secondary lymphoid organs include the spleen, tonsils, and lymph nodes. The **spleen** is an organ located in the abdomen that acts as a filter of the blood. The spleen removes defective or old erythrocytes, stores and removes thrombocytes, and stores various immune cells. The **tonsils** are located in the oral cavity and activate the immune system when pathogens are detected. The **lymph nodes** are small organs found primarily between the groin and neck. These organs contain and filter immune cells, trap pathogens, and activate antibody production.

Lymph nodes are part of the lymphatic system, a component of the immune system. The **lymphatic system** is a network of organs, nodes, ducts, and vessels that produce and transport lymph throughout the body (see Figure 23.2).

Lymph is a clear or white fluid comprising leukocytes (especially lymphocytes) and **chyle**, which is intestinal fluid containing fat and protein. The lymphatic system includes the lymph nodes, spleen, tonsils, and thymus.

FIGURE 23.2 **Lymphatic System**

Lymph nodes are typically clustered in different regions of the body. Three major regions include the neck (cervical) area, the armpit (axillary) area, and the groin (inguinal) area.

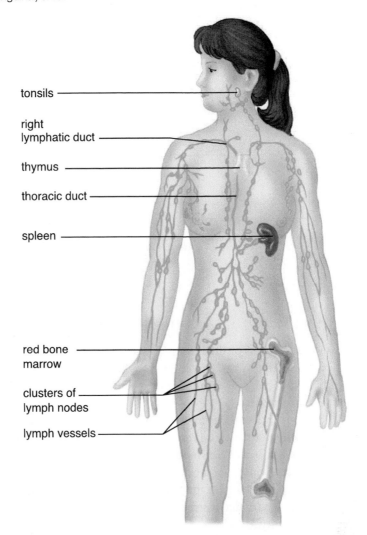

tonsils

right lymphatic duct

thymus

thoracic duct

spleen

red bone marrow

clusters of lymph nodes

lymph vessels

Types of Immunity

The localized immune process can be referred to as innate immunity or nonspecific immunity. **Innate immunity**, although limited, is present from birth and is usually the first line of defense against pathogens (see Figure 23.3). Innate immunity consists of cells, enzymes, and proteins that are readily available and work quickly to mobilize and fight pathogens. A simple form of innate immunity includes the physical defense provided by the integumentary and gastrointestinal (GI) systems. These systems provide a barrier between the body's interior and potentially damaging pathogens. Defenses that are more complex involve **phagocytic leukocytes**, which break down pathogens. Phagocytic leukocytes include eosinophils, macrophages, and neutrophils. Other innate immune responses involve the **complement system** (a component of the innate immune system that consists of enzymes and proteins) and mediator chemicals—for example, histamine, leukotrienes, and prostaglandins.

When an invading pathogen infiltrates the body, a systemic immune response ensues. This process, called **acquired immunity** or **adaptive immunity**, destroys invading pathogens. Adaptive immunity can differentiate between host cells and foreign cells and has memory. The adaptive immune response is carried out by specific leukocytes called **lymphocytes**. As previously discussed, the two main types of lymphocytes are B cells and T cells, and these cells detect specific pathogens. T cells are lymphocytes responsible for **cellular immunity**, the process of detecting cells that are

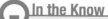

In the Know

Laboratory tests can detect exposure to certain viruses. Two options are available for patients who would prefer to test for human immunodeficiency virus (HIV) at home. The OraQuick In-Home HIV Test allows a person to use an oral fluid sample and a tube of solution to test for the presence of the virus. The result is available in 20 minutes.

Another home collection kit, called the Home Access HIV-1 Test System, requires the user to obtain a blood sample using the kit and to send the sample to a licensed laboratory. Results are quick and confidential.

It is recommended that any positive test result be followed up with a confirmation test provided by a healthcare practitioner.

FIGURE 23.3 Innate Immunity and the Inflammatory Response

Increased numbers of leukocytes or white blood cells (WBCs), improved bloodflow, and fluid accumulation from increased vascular permeability combine at the site of an infection to cause redness and swelling.

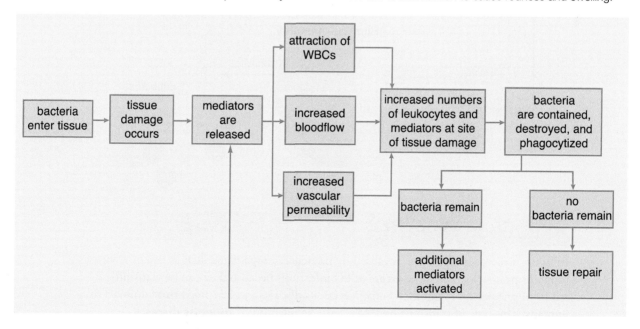

infected with viruses and initiating the immune response. **Killer T cells** attack cells of the body that have already been infected with a virus, and **helper T cells** release lymphokines that stimulate B cells into action. B cells provide **humoral immunity**, which is the process of making antibodies to prevent further infection. B cells mature into plasma cells that release antibodies, which fight off viruses before the viruses infect cells. **Antibodies** help the body remember specific pathogens in the event they are encountered again. They allow the body to detect an infection early and respond before the infection causes symptoms or illness (see Figure 23.4).

Laboratory tests to detect antibodies for specific viruses, such as the hepatitis B virus, can be used to check for exposure. If antibodies to a particular virus are found in a blood sample, that individual has been exposed either through natural contact or through a vaccine. Depending on the type and amount of antibodies measured, one can determine whether someone has been infected through exposure or is immune due to vaccination.

FIGURE 23.4 Adaptive Immunity

Killer T cells directly attack cells infected with viruses, whereas helper T cells release substances that stimulate B cells to produce antibodies.

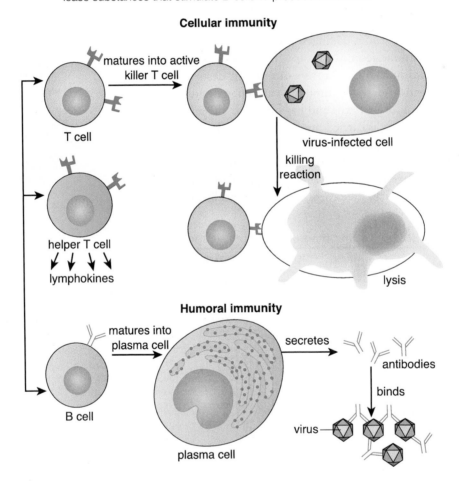

Infectious Diseases

Infectious diseases are disorders caused by pathogenic organisms such as bacteria, viruses, fungi, or protozoa. These diseases are called infectious because they can be transmitted from one person to another. Some infectious diseases can be spread from animals to humans. This type of transmission leads to the acquisition of **zoonotic diseases**.

Infectious disease is an important health topic worldwide. In fact, infectious diseases kill more people globally than any other single cause. In the United States, a 2010 report issued by the Centers for Disease Control and Prevention (CDC) states that 23.6 million physician office visits were attributable to infectious and parasitic diseases. Infections can cause significant morbidity and mortality, especially for older adults, infants, and children.

Infectious Disease Prevention

Infectious diseases can be prevented using various methods. Two methods of prevention, hand washing and blood-borne pathogen precautions, are discussed in this chapter. A third method, vaccination, is discussed in Chapter 24.

Hand Washing and Hand Hygiene

According to the CDC, simple hand washing and hand hygiene are the two most important practices for minimizing touch contamination and reducing the transmission of infectious agents. **Hand washing** involves using soap and water to clean the hands, whereas **hand hygiene** is defined as cleaning the hands using special alcohol-based rinses, gels, or foams that do not require water. Both hand washing and hand hygiene require friction to be effective. All allied health professionals should know the correct procedures for keeping their hands clean (see Table 23.1).

TABLE 23.1 Hand-Washing and Hand-Hygiene Guidelines
The hand-washing and hand-hygiene guidelines described herein are appropriate for infection-control procedures in a hospital setting. These procedures are followed by healthcare personnel in several departments, including pharmacy and nursing. *However, it should be noted that special, aseptic hand washing must be performed by personnel preparing sterile products.*   • When washing hands with soap and water, wet hands first with water, apply an amount of product recommended by the manufacturer to hands, and rub hands together vigorously for at least 20 (preferably 30) seconds, covering all surfaces of the hands and fingers. Rinse hands with water and dry thoroughly with a disposable towel. Use the towel to turn off the faucet. Avoid using hot water; repeated exposure to hot water may increase the risk of skin irritation.   • Liquid, bar, or powdered forms of plain soap are acceptable when washing hands with a non-antimicrobial soap and water. When bar soap is used, a soap rack facilitating drainage should be available.   • Dry hands with single-use towels, or air-dry. Multiple-use cloth towels of the hanging or roll type are not recommended for use in healthcare settings because they can transfer infectious agents.   • When disinfecting hands with an alcohol-based hand rub, apply product to the palm of one hand and rub hands together, covering all surfaces of hands and fingers, until hands are dry. Follow the manufacturer's recommendations regarding the volume of product to use.

Source: The Centers for Disease Control and Prevention

Blood-Borne Pathogen Precautions

Blood-borne pathogens are disease-causing microorganisms that can be transmitted through blood and other bodily fluids. Healthcare personnel may be exposed to blood-borne pathogens as part of their job responsibilities. The Occupational Safety and Health Administration (OSHA) enforces workplace controls concerning blood-borne pathogens. Following workplace safety rules is especially important when needles are used to draw blood or to give injections.

Universal precautions are established personal safety standards designed to protect against accidental exposure to pathogens. These standards must be adhered to by all healthcare professionals without exception. Another important safety standard (noted previously) is proper hand washing before and after a procedure. Hand washing is the most effective means of preventing the spread of disease.

Each medical facility must ensure that the proper equipment is used whenever a procedure poses a risk of exposure to bodily fluids. This equipment may include **personal protective equipment** (gloves, gowns, eye protection, and facemasks), disposable syringes and needles with retractable safety caps, and puncture-resistant (sharps) containers for disposal of contaminated waste. Medical facilities must also ensure that such procedures are performed in complete compliance with OSHA standards. OSHA enforces its safety and health standards through a system of on-site inspections and by levying fines against the employer. Serious violations may result in a mandatory $7,000 fine per citation. When violations are willful and serious, employers may be fined up to $70,000 per citation.

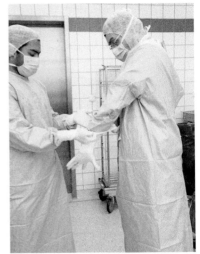

Healthcare personnel must don personal protective equipment to safeguard themselves against exposure to infectious bodily fluids.

Checkpoint 23.1

Take a moment to review what you have learned so far and answer these questions.

1. What is the role of bone marrow?

2. What are the benefits of hand washing and hand hygiene?

Infectious Disease Treatment

Many, but not all, infectious diseases can be treated. Infectious diseases are treated based on their suspected or confirmed underlying cause. For example, bacterial infections are treated with antibiotics, and viral infections are treated with antivirals.

Bacterial Infections

Bacteria are single-celled microorganisms that live practically everywhere. For example, many bacteria can be found on the skin and in the bowel at all times. These skin and bowel organisms may be beneficial but may cause disease when they grow out of control or gain entry to the blood. Other bacteria are harmful whenever they invade. This type of bacteria, known as **pathogenic bacteria**, may produce toxins that cause many of the signs and symptoms experienced when infection is present.

Bacteria are either **aerobic**, which means they need oxygen to live, or **anaerobic**, meaning they can survive in an environment void of oxygen. Bacteria are classified by their shape and arrangement of growth (see Figure 23.5). If bacterial cells grow in chains or lines, their name begins with *strep–*. If they grow in clusters, their name begins with *staph–*. If they grow in pairs, their name begins with *diplo–*. For instance, *Staphylococcus aureus*, a common bacterium found on the skin, is round and grows in clusters like grapes.

Work Wise

Often the names of bacteria are abbreviated in workplace communications. For example, you may hear *Streptococcus pneumoniae* called "Strep. pneumo." *Clostridium difficile* may be called "C. diff," and *Escherichia coli* is often referred to as "E. coli."

FIGURE 23.5 Characteristic Bacteria Shapes

Spherical bacteria (a) are called *cocci*. Rod-shaped bacteria (b) are called *bacilli*. Spiral-shaped bacteria (c) are called *spirochetes*. *Streptococcus pyogenes*, the bacterium that causes strep throat, is spherical and grows in chains.

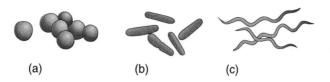

(a)   (b)   (c)

Finally, bacteria are said to be either *gram positive* or *gram negative*. This classification originates from a staining technique named after its developer, Hans Christian Joachim Gram. In this technique, a purple stain called crystal violet is applied to the bacteria, and then they are viewed under a microscope. **Gram-positive bacteria** have a thick cell wall that absorbs this stain and appears purple. **Gram-negative bacteria** have a thin cell wall that does not absorb this stain. (See Tables 23.2 and 23.3 for more information on the classification of common and miscellaneous types of bacteria.)

Drug Regimens and Treatments

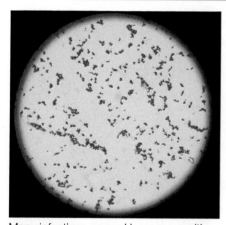

Many infections caused by gram-positive bacteria (shown here) have become resistant to drug therapies. These "superbugs" have created worldwide concern as scientists scramble to develop new medications to combat these dangerous strains.

Antibiotics are used to treat bacterial infections. They are not effective against viral infections. Antibiotics are either *bacteriostatic* or *bactericidal*. **Bacteriostatic** means the drug does not necessarily kill the pathogen but hinders its growth and progression, allowing the body's immune system to fight off the bacterial invasion. **Bactericidal** means that the drug kills the pathogen. Bactericidal drugs are used on the most difficult infections to treat, especially for patients whose immune systems are not functioning well.

Antibiotics are chosen based on the type of pathogen that is suspected of causing the infection, the antibiotic's spectrum of activity on that particular pathogen, and the location of the pathogen. An antibiotic's **spectrum of activity** is the range of bacteria against which it is effective. For example, penicillin is effective for infections caused by gram-positive, aerobic bacteria, such as *Streptococcus pyogenes* (a pathogen that can cause strep throat). To identify the bacteria and facilitate the choice of drug treatment, a sample or swab of the bacteria is obtained from the patient and grown in culture in the laboratory. Then, various antibiotics are tested on the culture to determine which drug has the best effect on the pathogen. This laboratory test is called a **culture and sensitivity (C&S) test**. The amount of drug needed to inhibit growth of the bacteria is called the **minimum inhibitory concentration (MIC)**, a result often reported along with the C&S results.

When choosing appropriate drug therapy, the prescriber must also take into account **antibiotic resistance**. Bacteria have the ability to develop defense mechanisms that resist or

 In the Know

The overuse of antibiotics has led to some grim statistics in the United States. At least 2 million individuals every year acquire serious bacterial infections that are resistant to antibiotic therapies, and more than 23,000 patients die from their infections. Gram-negative bacteria, in particular, are resistant to nearly all drugs commonly used to treat the pathogens.

TABLE 23.2 | Common Bacteria and Associated Infections

Gram Stain	Shape	Bacteria	Associated Infection(s)
Aerobic			
Positive	Cocci	*Streptococcus pneumoniae* *Streptococcus pyogenes* (Group A)	Respiratory tract infection (RTI) and/or pneumonia Strep throat
Positive	Cocci	*Staphylococcus aureus* and other *Staphylococcus* spp.	Skin infection Endocarditis
Positive	Cocci	*Enterococcus faecalis, Enterococcus faecium*	Intestinal infection, urinary tract infection (UTI)
Positive	Bacilli	*Bacillus anthracis*	Anthrax
Positive	Bacilli	*Gardnerella vaginalis* *Lactobacillus* spp.	Vaginal infections
Positive	Bacilli	*Listeria monocytogenes*	Meningitis
Positive	Bacilli	*Clostridium tetani* *Clostridium perfringens* *Clostridium botulinum* *Clostridium difficile*	Tetanus Gangrene Botulism Intestinal infection
Positive	Bacilli	*Corynebacteria diphtheriae*	Diphtheria
Negative	Cocci	*Neisseria meningitidis* *Neisseria gonorrhea*	Meningitis Gonorrhea
Negative	Bacilli	*Escherichia coli* *Klebsiella* spp. *Proteus* spp. *Enterobacter* spp. *Shigella* spp.	Intestinal infection, UTI
Negative	Bacilli	*Salmonella typhi*	Typhoid fever
Negative	Bacilli	*Yersinia pestis*	Plague
Negative	Bacilli	*Pseudomonas aeruginosa*	Various difficult-to-treat infections
Negative	Bacilli	*Haemophilus influenzae*	RTI
Negative	Bacilli	*Vibrio cholerae*	Cholera
Negative	Coccobacilli	*Bordetella pertussis*	Pertussis
Negative	Coccobacilli	*Helicobacter pylori*	Stomach ulcers
Anaerobic			
Positive	Cocci	*Peptococcus, Peptostreptococcus*	Dental infection
Negative	Bacilli	*Bacteroides fragilis*	Abdominal infection, sepsis

TABLE 23.3 | Miscellaneous Bacteria and Associated Infections

Bacteria	Associated Infection(s)
Treponema pallidum *Borrelia burgdorferi*	Syphilis Lyme disease
Mycoplasma pneumonia *Legionella* spp.	RTI and/or pneumonia
Mycobacterium tuberculosis	Tuberculosis
Chlamydia trachomatis	Chlamydia and pelvic inflammatory disease

FIGURE 23.6 Antibiotic Prescribing Rates in the United States (2012–2013)

According to the Centers for Disease Control and Prevention, the overuse of antibiotics is the leading cause of antibiotic resistance worldwide.

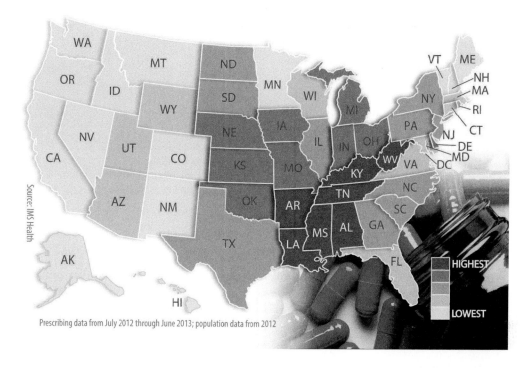

Source: IMS Health

Prescribing data from July 2012 through June 2013; population data from 2012

inactivate the antibiotics used on them. For instance, many bacteria that cause common respiratory tract infections (RTIs) are now resistant to the most frequently used drugs, like amoxicillin. Antibiotic resistance is a growing problem as more of these common drugs are prescribed. If a patient were to develop an infection that was resistant to the most powerful antibiotics, no therapy would exist to treat the infection, a grim situation that could result in death. To help prevent antibiotic resistance, prescribers must be mindful of using appropriate antibiotics only when necessary. Figure 23.6 shows the antibiotic prescribing rates in the United States in 2012 and 2013.

One type of infection that is often drug-resistant and difficult to treat is a **nosocomial infection**, also known as a **healthcare-associated infection (HAI)**. An HAI is acquired while a patient is in a hospital or nursing home. For this type of infection, the common first choice of therapy cannot be used because the bacteria are already known to be resistant. Because an HAI can be serious and even life-threatening, aggressive antibiotic therapy may be warranted. This therapy would start empirically with powerful drugs and then modified based on C&S results.

The route of administration chosen for antibiotic therapy depends on the site and severity of the infection as well as the bacteria suspected to be causing it. In most cases, antibiotics are best given at even intervals throughout the day. In children, antibiotics are often dosed for an entire day, based on the child's weight, but are given in divided doses. Dosages provided in this text are presented as general guides for recognizing when a prescribed dosage is out of the ordinary. Healthcare practitioners should always refer to the package insert or other reliable sources to verify proper dosing and to double-check dose calculations for children.

Work Wise

In addition to penicillins, other antibiotics such as cephalosporins, monobactams, and carbapenems also contain a beta-lactam ring. Therefore, you may hear healthcare practitioners refer to these antibiotics as "beta-lactams."

Penicillins

Penicillins were one of the first group of antibiotics used in the treatment of bacterial infections. There are many different types of penicillins, and they mainly treat infections caused by gram-positive bacteria (see Table 23.4). These antibiotics kill bacteria by inhibiting the formation of their cell wall, without which the cell cannot survive. Some bacteria, however, are resistant to penicillins because the pathogens produce an enzyme called **beta-lactamase**, which destroys the beta-lactam ring present in the molecular structure of all penicillins. This action renders the drug inactive. For this reason, some penicillin products are available as a combination of penicillin with a **beta-lactamase inhibitor**.

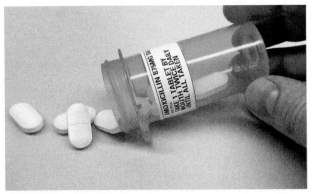

Amoxicillin is a widely prescribed antibiotic for bacterial infections. Patients must complete the full therapy regimen to avoid the risk of creating a strain of antibiotic-resistant bacteria.

Side Effects Common side effects of penicillins include upset stomach and diarrhea. Taking them with food can help with these side effects. Other rare but more severe side effects include mental disturbances, seizures, kidney damage, and bleeding abnormalities. These particular side effects tend to occur more often at higher doses and when the doses are administered by intravenous (IV) infusion.

Drug Alert

Up to 10% of patients in the United States report penicillin allergies. Although true penicillin allergies are serious and can be life-threatening, many self-reported allergies are in fact adverse drug reactions and not an allergic reaction. If you are taking a patient history, specifically ask what his or her reaction is to the offending agent. If a patient reports mild upset stomach or diarrhea, common side effects of penicillins, you may want to investigate the allergy claim.

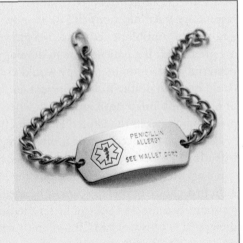

Contraindications Most penicillin contraindications are associated with hypersensitivity. If a person has a true hypersensitivity to one type of penicillin, use of the others is contraindicated. Amoxicillin/clavulanate is contraindicated in patients with liver dysfunction and severe renal impairment.

➕ *Note: Allied health professionals should be aware that an allergy to a particular drug contraindicates its use. This warning applies to all Contraindications sections in this chapter.*

Cautions and Considerations Approximately 10% of patients who are allergic to penicillin are also allergic to cephalosporins, another class of antibiotics that inhibits cell wall

TABLE 23.4 Common Penicillins

Generic (Brand)	Dosage Form	Route of Administration	Common Dosage
Aminopenicillins			
Amoxicillin (Moxatag)	Capsule, chewable tablet, oral suspension, tablet	Oral	Adult: 250–875 mg taken 2–3 times a day Pediatric: 20–90 mg/kg/day in divided doses
Ampicillin	Capsule, injection, oral suspension	IM, IV, oral	IM/IV: varies by age of patient; typical doses range in hundreds of milligrams a day in divided doses PO: 250–500 mg four times a day
Natural Penicillins			
Penicillin G	Injection, powder for injection	IM, IV	Varies by age of patient; typical doses range from thousands to millions of units a day in divided doses
Penicillin V (Pen VK)	Solution, tablet	Oral	Adult: 250–500 mg every 6 hr (and variations) Pediatric: 25–50 mg/kg/day in divided doses
Antistaphylococcal Penicillins			
Dicloxacillin	Capsule	Oral	Adult: 125–250 mg every 6 hr Pediatric: 12.5 mg/kg/day in divided doses
Nafcillin (Nallpen)	Injection	IV	1,000–2,000 mg every 4 hr
Oxacillin	Injection	IV	Varies by age of patient; typical doses range in hundreds of milligrams a day Adult: 500–2,000 mg every 4–6 hr Pediatric: 50–100 mg/kg/day in divided doses
Extended-Spectrum Penicillins			
Piperacillin	Injection	IM, IV	Varies depending on route and type of infection treated; usually given multiple times a day
Ticarcillin	Injection	IM, IV	Varies depending on route, patient age, and type of infection treated; usually given multiple times a day
Combination Penicillins			
Amoxicillin/clavulanate (Augmentin)	Chewable tablet, oral suspension, tablet	Oral	Adult: 250–500 mg every 8–12 hr Pediatric: 20–45 mg/kg/day in divided doses
Ampicillin/sulbactam (Unasyn)	Injection	IM, IV	Adult: 1.5–3 g every 6 hr Pediatric: 300 mg/kg/day in divided doses
Piperacillin/tazobactam (Zosyn)	Injection	IV	Adult: 3.375 g every 6 hr Pediatric: varies by age and weight of patient; usually given multiple times a day
Ticarcillin/clavulanate (Timentin)	Injection	IV	Varies by age of patient; typical doses range in hundreds of milligrams a day in divided doses

formation. Therefore, allied health professionals should always inquire about all drug allergies when taking a patient's medication history or when preparing to administer penicillins or cephalosporins.

Oral penicillins work best when taken on an empty stomach, but if upset stomach occurs, they can be taken with food. These medications should not be taken with acidic beverages such as fruit juice or carbonated drinks such as cola products because the acid in these beverages can deactivate the drug. Oral suspensions should be shaken well before every dose. Most of these suspensions must also be refrigerated. Suspensions prepared with water are good for only 14 days from the mixing date. Any medication left over after treatment should be disposed of properly.

Although IV preparations are often used in conjunction with other antibiotics (such as aminoglycosides, for difficult infections), they should not be mixed in the same IV bag.

Some bacteria have become resistant to methicillin, an older penicillin used for difficult staphylococcal infections. The antistaphylococcal penicillins (also called penicillinase-resistant) have largely replaced it in practice. **Methicillin-resistant *Staphylococcus aureus* (MRSA)** infections are resistant to all antistaphylococcal penicillins and, consequently, few drugs can treat them. Special precautions are used to protect against the spread of this bacteria to other patients. For instance, access to the affected patient's hospital room is restricted, and anyone who enters must don protective gear such as a gown, facemask, and gloves.

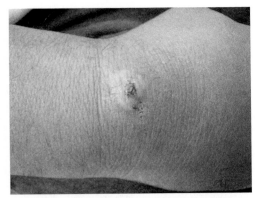

According to the CDC, most MRSA infections present as skin abscesses at sites of trauma (such as abrasions or cuts) or in areas covered by body hair. These lesions are red, painful, and often filled with pus.

Cephalosporins

Like penicillins, **cephalosporins** are drugs that kill bacteria by inhibiting the formation of their cell walls. Cephalosporins are divided into four groups, called **generations**. In general, first-generation cephalosporins work best on gram-positive bacteria. Activity against gram-negative bacteria increases through the subsequent generations (see Table 23.5).

Overall, cephalosporins are used to treat upper and lower RTIs, skin infections, and some urinary tract infections (UTIs). These medications are also used for infection prophylaxis during surgical procedures. The second-generation cephalosporins are used for respiratory infections caused by *Haemophilus influenzae* and for otitis media (ear infections). The third-generation cephalosporins are used for severe gram-negative infections. The fourth-generation cephalosporin, cefepime, is used for *Pseudomonas* infections that are difficult to treat. Ceftaroline has been called a fifth-generation cephalosporin and may be used for MRSA.

Side Effects Common side effects of cephalosporins include nausea, vomiting, diarrhea, headache, and dizziness. Most of the time, these effects are tolerable. Other rare but more severe side effects include mental disturbances, seizures, heart palpitations, and bleeding abnormalities. These particular side effects tend to occur more frequently at higher doses and when the medication is administered using the IV route. Some of the more serious side effects can be worsened by alcohol intake, so patients should avoid alcohol while taking a cephalosporin.

Contraindications The cephalosporins are contraindicated in patients with a hypersensitivity to other cephalosporins. Ceftriaxone should not be used in neonates with elevated bilirubin levels or in neonates who are receiving IV calcium-containing products. Cefditoren is contraindicated in patients with milk-protein hypersensitivity or carnitine deficiency. Cefepime is contraindicated in patients with penicillin or beta-lactam hypersensitivity.

Cautions and Considerations Allergic reactions to cephalosporins are common. Approximately 10% of patients who are allergic to penicillins are also allergic to cephalosporins. Therefore, you should always inquire about all drug allergies when taking a patient's medication history or when preparing to administer either cephalosporins or penicillins.

Some cephalosporins should be taken with food, and others should be taken on an empty stomach. For example, cefditoren should be taken with food but not with antacids. Refer to the package insert for proper dosing instructions.

TABLE 23.5 Common Cephalosporins

Generic (Brand)	Dosage Form	Route of Administration	Common Dosage
First Generation			
Cefazolin (Ancef)	Injection	IM, IV	250–1,000 mg taken every 6, 8, or 12 hr (depends on type of infection being treated); also given before or during surgical procedures
Cephalexin (Keflex)	Capsule, oral suspension, tablet	Oral	Adult: 250–750 mg every 6 hr Pediatric: 25–50 mg/kg/day in divided doses
Second Generation			
Cefaclor (Ceclor)	Capsule, chewable tablet, oral suspension, tablet	Oral	Adult: 250 mg every 8 hr or 375–500 mg every 12 hr Pediatric: 20–40 mg/kg/day divided every 8–12 hr
Cefotetan	Injection	IM, IV	500–3,000 mg every 12 hr
Cefoxitin (Mefoxin)	Injection	IV	1–2 g every 6–8 hr; also given before or during surgical procedures
Cefuroxime (Zinacef)	Injection, oral suspension, tablet	IM, IV, oral	IM/IV: 750–1,500 mg every 8 hr; also given before or during surgical procedures PO: 250–1,000 mg twice a day (adult); 20–30 mg/kg/day divided twice a day (pediatric)
Third Generation			
Cefdinir	Capsule, oral suspension	Oral	Adult: 300–600 mg every 12–24 hr Pediatric: 7 mg/kg every 12 hr or 14 mg/kg every 24 hr
Cefditoren (Spectracef)	Tablet	Oral	200–400 mg twice a day
Cefixime (Suprax)	Oral suspension	Oral	Adult: 400 mg a day Pediatric: 8 mg/kg/day
Cefotaxime (Claforan)	Injection	IM, IV	IM/IV: 1–2 g every 4–12 hr depending on severity of infection
Ceftazidime (Fortaz, Tazicef)	Injection	IM, IV	Adult: 1–2 g every 8–12 hr Pediatric: 30–50 mg/kg every 8–12 hr
Ceftibuten (Cedax)	Capsule, oral suspension	Oral	400 mg once a day
Ceftriaxone (Rocephin)	Injection	IM, IV	Adult: 1–2 g once or twice a day Pediatric: 50–100 mg/kg once or twice a day
Fourth Generation			
Cefepime (Maxipime)	Injection	IV	1–2 g every 8–12 hr
Fifth Generation			
Ceftaroline (Teflaro)	Injection	IV	600 mg every 12 hr

Most oral liquid dosage forms are suspensions and should be shaken well before every dose. Most of these suspensions must also be refrigerated. Cefixime (Suprax) is one of the few suspensions that does not have to be refrigerated after reconstitution. When a suspension is prepared with water, it is good for only 14 days from mixing. Any medication left over after treatment should be disposed of properly. Some suspension products, such as cefdinir, are high in sugar content, so patients with diabetes should be aware of this information.

Name Exchange

Cefdinir is available exclusively as a generic product. However, you may hear some healthcare practitioners continue to refer to this drug by its brand name, Omnicef.

Some of the products in this class can be taken twice a day instead of three times a day. This feature is good for parents with children in daycare or school, when it may be difficult to administer medications in the middle of the day.

Carbapenems and Monobactams

The drug classes carbapenems and monobactams are grouped together here because they differ only slightly in their molecular structure from penicillins and cephalosporins. These drug classes kill bacteria by inhibiting the formation of the cell wall. **Carbapenems** are used for mixed infections that have both gram-positive and gram-negative bacteria; **monobactams** are used only for gram-negative bacterial infections. Both drug classes are used in special situations for serious HAIs. Carbapenems include ertapenem, imipenem, and meropenem. Aztreonam is a monobactam.

Side Effects Side effects of carbapenems include skin rash, headache, anemia, and pain. Aztreonam inhalation can cause sore throat, cough, nasal congestion, wheezing, fever, and chest discomfort. The IV form of aztreonam may cause neutropenia, increased liver enzymes, and skin rash.

Contraindications Hypersensitivity to one carbapenem contraindicates use of other agents in the class. Intramuscular use of ertapenem is contraindicated in patients with a hypersensitivity to amide-type anesthetics. Aztreonam does not have contraindications.

Cautions and Considerations Seizures have been reported during treatment with carbapenems. These reactions occurred most commonly in patients with central nervous system (CNS) disorders such as a history of seizures and in patients with renal impairment. Carbapenems require dosage adjustment in patients with kidney dysfunction. Aztreonam has rare cross-allergenicity to penicillins, cephalosporins, or carbapenems and should be used with caution in patients with a history of beta-lactam hypersensitivity. Aztreonam requires dosage adjustment in patients with renal impairment.

Vancomycin

A single drug in a class by itself is **vancomycin**. Its mechanism is not fully understood, but it probably works by inhibiting cell wall formation. Vancomycin has activity against gram-positive bacteria and is used primarily to treat MRSA infections; in fact, it is the drug of choice. Unfortunately, some enterococci are resistant to vancomycin; these are called **vancomycin-resistant** *Enterococcus* (**VRE**).

Vancomycin is most frequently administered intravenously because the oral form is poorly absorbed into the bloodstream. The oral dosage form is used, therefore, only for infections that are localized within the intestines. Dosages range from 500–2,000 mg a day in divided doses.

Work Wise

Vancomycin, a commonly used antibiotic in the hospital setting, is often referred to as *vanco* (pronounced "van-ko").

Side Effects Vancomycin may cause **nephrotoxicity** (kidney damage) and **ototoxicity** (hearing loss). With proper monitoring of blood levels and laboratory tests, these effects can be avoided or minimized. However, these side effects limit vancomycin's use to the treatment of difficult infections.

Contraindications Vancomycin does not have contraindications.

Cautions and Considerations Vancomycin must be administered slowly (usually over 60 minutes) to avoid an effect called **red man syndrome**. This syndrome involves hypotension, redness in the neck and face, and skin rash.

Lincosamides and Macrolides

Lincosamides and **macrolides** work by blocking bacteria's ability to produce needed proteins for survival. At low doses, they are bacteriostatic, but at high doses, they can be bactericidal.

Clindamycin is the most commonly prescribed lincosamide and is used to treat infections caused by various organisms including anaerobes, *Staphylococcus aureus*, *Streptococcus pneumoniae*, and *Streptococcus pyogenes*. Clindamycin is used for bone and joint infections, gynecologic infections, intra-abdominal infections, sepsis, and skin and soft-tissue infections.

Macrolides have a broad spectrum of activity in that they work against some gram-positive and gram-negative bacteria. Macrolides are used mainly to treat respiratory infections and pneumonia. They are also used with other drugs to treat infections caused by *Helicobacter pylori*, the bacteria found in association with stomach ulcers. The duration of therapy for one macrolide, azithromycin, is unusually short but convenient (typically 3 to 5 days) relative to other antibiotics (usually 7 to 14 days). See Table 23.6 for additional dosing information.

TABLE 23.6 | Common Lincosamides and Macrolides

Generic (Brand)	Dosage Form	Route of Administration	Common Dosage
Lincosamide			
Clindamycin (Cleocin)	Cream, foam, gel, injection, lotion, oral solution, suppository, tablet, topical solution	IM, IV, oral, topical	IM/IV: 600–2,700 mg a day in divided doses PO: 150–300 mg every 6 hr (adult); 8–20 mg/kg/day in 3–4 divided doses (pediatric) Topical: varies depending on product; usually given 1–2 times a day
Macrolides			
Azithromycin (Zithromax)	Injection, oral suspension, tablet	IV, oral	IV: 500 mg daily for 2–10 days depending on type of infection PO: 250–500 mg daily for 3–5 days or 2 g one time only (adult); varies by age and weight of patient as well as type of infection (pediatric)
Clarithromycin (Biaxin)	Oral suspension, tablet	Oral	Adult: 250–500 mg every 12 hr Pediatric: 15 mg/kg/day divided every 12 hr
Erythromycin (EES, Eryc, EryPed, Ery-Tab, Erythrocin, Pediazole)	Capsule, gel, injection, oral suspension, pledget, solution, tablet	IM, IV, oral, topical	Varies depending on age of patient and type of infection; usually given 3–4 times a day

Side Effects Common side effects of lincosamides and macrolides include upset stomach, nausea, vomiting, heartburn, abdominal pain, and diarrhea. To reduce these effects, patients should take lincosamides and macrolides with food. If abdominal pain or diarrhea is severe, patients should seek medical attention immediately because such pain could indicate a serious problem.

Liver toxicity has also occurred with the use of erythromycin. Patients with prior liver problems should not take this medication. If jaundice (yellowing of skin and eyes) occurs with erythromycin use, medical attention should be sought immediately.

Contraindications Clindamycin is contraindicated in patients with a hypersensitivity to lincomycin.

Macrolides are contraindicated in patients with a hypersensitivity to other macrolides. Azithromycin and clarithromycin are contraindicated in patients with liver dysfunction associated with prior use. Other contraindications to clarithromycin include a history of QT prolongation or ventricular cardiac arrhythmia; concomitant use with cisapride, pimozide, ergotamine, dihydroergotamine, simvastatin, lovastatin, astemizole, or terfenadine; and concomitant use with colchicine in patients with liver or kidney impairment. Erythromycin is contraindicated with patients who are taking pimozide, cisapride, ergotamine or dihydroergotamine, terfenadine, astemizole, lovastatin, or simvastatin.

Cautions and Considerations Macrolides, especially erythromycin and clarithromycin, have many drug interactions. Some of the effects caused by these interactions can be severe.

Oral suspension products should be shaken well before every dose. Most of these suspensions must also be refrigerated. Any of these suspensions prepared with water are good for only 14 days from mixing. Any medication left over after treatment should be disposed of properly.

Clindamycin has a black box warning because it can cause severe and possibly fatal colitis. Its use should be reserved for treatment of serious infections for which use of other antimicrobials is inappropriate.

Aminoglycosides

A class of drugs called **aminoglycosides** kills bacteria by blocking their ability to make essential proteins for survival. These powerful bactericidal medications are used to treat peritonitis, severe infection of the gums, and life-threatening infections such as sepsis. Aminoglycosides are often used in conjunction with other antibiotics (e.g., penicillins, cephalosporins, and vancomycin). Aminoglycosides work synergistically with these other drug classes. **Synergistic drug therapy** is when two or more drugs are used together because they employ different mechanisms of action (in this case, the inhibition of protein synthesis [aminoglycosides] and cell wall lysis [penicillins, cephalosporins, vancomycin]) that work better together than either drug works alone. The aminoglycosides gentamicin and tobramycin are used to treat eye infections in patients with immunodeficiency.

Many healthcare institutions have instituted **pulse dosing**, whereby aminoglycosides are given once a day instead of multiple times a day. Because the side effects of aminoglycosides can be serious, less exposure to the drug during the day seems to help reduce its toxic effects. Special nomograms (dosing charts) are used for dosing in these situations. Table 23.7 includes common aminoglycosides and their routes of administration.

TABLE 23.7 Common Aminoglycosides

Generic (Brand)	Dosage Form	Route of Administration
Amikacin	Injection	IM, IV
Gentamicin (Garamycin, Gentak)	Injection, ophthalmic ointment, ophthalmic solution	IM, IV, ophthalmic
Tobramycin (TOBI, Tobrex)	Injection, ophthalmic ointment, ophthalmic solution, solution for nebulizer inhalation	IM, inhalation, IV, ophthalmic

Side Effects Side effects of aminoglycosides can include nephrotoxicity (kidney damage) and ototoxicity (tinnitus, hearing loss, and balance problems). With proper monitoring of blood levels and laboratory tests, these effects can be avoided or minimized. However, these side effects limit the use of aminoglycosides to the treatment of difficult infections.

Contraindications Cross-sensitivity may exist among aminoglycosides; therefore, hyper-sensitivity to one aminoglycoside contraindicates the use of others.

Cautions and Considerations Aminoglycosides have been known to cause neuromuscular blockade in some cases. If a patient complains of muscle weakness, difficulty breathing, numbness, tingling, twitching, or seizures, the drug should be discontinued. Patients with muscular disorders, such as myasthenia gravis or Parkinson's disease, should not be given aminoglycosides. Caution must be used if aminoglycosides are given after surgery because they may interact with neuromuscular blockers, a class of drugs used in many surgical procedures.

Although aminoglycosides are often used in conjunction with other antibiotics such as cephalosporins or penicillins, they should not be mixed in the same IV infusion bag. Ophthalmic preparations should be kept as sterile as possible. Patients should be instructed not to touch the tip of the applicator to the eye or other surfaces during medication administration.

> **Quick Study**
>
> It is easy to recognize aminoglycosides by looking at their name. The aminoglycosides end in the suffix –*cin*.

Tetracyclines

Another class of drugs for bacterial infections is **tetracyclines**, which are bacteriostatic drugs that inhibit protein synthesis within bacterial cells. Consequently, they require a functioning immune system to cure an infection.

Tetracycline itself is probably used most often for acne treatment. Tetracyclines as a class are also drugs of choice for Lyme disease and Rocky Mountain spotted fever. Doxycycline is used frequently to treat sexually transmitted infections such as gonorrhea and chlamydia. Occasionally, tetracyclines are used to treat RTIs and some abdominal infections. Table 23.8 contains dosage information for tetracyclines.

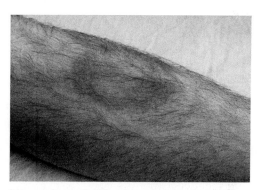

Tetracycline is first-line therapy for Lyme disease. A hallmark of Lyme disease is erythema migrans, or a "bull's eye" rash that appears, on average, seven days after the tick bite and can reach a diameter of 12 inches across.

TABLE 23.8 Common Tetracyclines

Generic (Brand)	Dosage Form	Route of Administration	Common Dosage
Doxycycline (Doryx, Vibramycin)	Capsule, injection, oral suspension, syrup, tablet	IV, oral	100–200 mg twice a day
Minocycline (Minocin)	Capsule, injection, oral suspension, tablet	IV, oral	100 mg every 12 hr
Tetracycline	Capsule	Oral	250–500 mg 2–4 times a day

Side Effects Common side effects of tetracyclines include upset stomach, nausea, and vomiting. They can be taken with food (but not dairy products or antacids) to reduce these effects. Tetracyclines also cause photosensitivity. Patients should be informed that their skin will burn faster when exposed to the sun and a skin rash may develop. When taking a tetracycline, patients should apply sunscreen and wear sun-protective clothing when spending time outside.

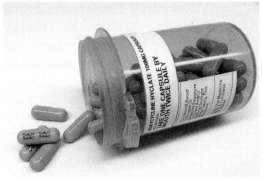

Doxycycline, an antibiotic prescribed for bacterial infections of the skin, must have an auxiliary warning label affixed to the drug container. This label alerts the patient to the risk of photosensitivity while taking this medication.

Contraindications Hypersensitivity to one tetracycline contraindicates the use of other tetracyclines.

Cautions and Considerations Tetracyclines bind with metals and ions, such as calcium, aluminum, and magnesium. When this occurs, the tetracyclines cannot be absorbed into the bloodstream. Therefore, patients should avoid food, drink, and other products that contain these substances (such as cheese, milk, antacids, or laxatives).

Tetracyclines also accumulate in teeth and bones and can cause permanent discoloration and enamel hypoplasia. Consequently, children younger than eight years of age and pregnant or lactating women cannot use tetracyclines because of possible permanent damage to teeth.

Tetracyclines break down over time to become toxic. Therefore, expired tetracyclines should be discarded properly and never saved for future use.

Fluoroquinolones

The class of drugs known as **fluoroquinolones** (also called **quinolones**) kills bacteria by inhibiting the enzyme that helps deoxyribonucleic acid (DNA) to coil. If DNA cannot coil, it is rendered useless and the cell dies because it cannot function. Quinolones have strong activity against gram-negative bacteria. They are often used to treat bone and joint infections, eye infections, and serious RTIs and UTIs. Ciprofloxacin and levofloxacin may be used to treat infections caused by *Pseudomonas aeruginosa*. Quinolones also have a special use as treatment for anthrax, a potential bioterrorism agent.

Due to overprescribing, resistance to quinolones has developed. Therefore, their use is discouraged in ordinary and frequently seen infections. Quinolones should be reserved for more serious and difficult-to-treat gram-negative bacterial infections. Table 23.9 gives dosing information for common quinolones.

TABLE 23.9 | Common Quinolones

Generic (Brand)	Dosage Form	Route of Administration	Common Dosage
Ciprofloxacin (Cipro)	Injection, oral suspension, tablet	IV, oral	IV: 200–400 mg every 12 hr PO: 250–750 mg every 12 hr (adult); 6–20 mg/kg every 8–12 hr (pediatric)
Levofloxacin (Levaquin)	Injection, oral solution, tablet	IV, oral	250–750 mg a day
Moxifloxacin (Avelox, Vigamox)	Injection, ophthalmic solution, tablet	IV, ophthalmic, oral	IV and PO: 400 mg a day Ophthalmic: 1 drop 2–3 times a day

Side Effects Common side effects of quinolones include nausea, vomiting, dizziness, diarrhea, and a bitter or unpleasant taste in the mouth. If the patient cannot tolerate these effects, different antibiotics will need to be chosen. Taking quinolones with food does not necessarily reduce these effects. These drugs also cause photosensitivity, so patients should wear sunscreen when outside.

Less common but serious side effects include liver toxicity and alterations in glucose metabolism. Elongation of the QT interval on electrocardiography has occurred with quinolone use. Consequently, these drugs may not be the best choice for patients with heart problems. Quinolones may also cause tendon ruptures, especially in younger patients.

Changes in mental function and seizures have been reported with quinolones, especially ciprofloxacin. If a patient is exhibiting confusion, agitation, dizziness, hallucinations, insomnia, nightmares, or paranoia, use of the drug should be stopped and the patient should seek medical attention immediately.

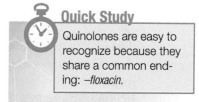

Stockpiles of Cipro (ciprofloxacin) have been accumulated in key locations around the country in anticipation of bioterrorist attacks, such as anthrax. Pharmacies are sometimes asked to report their inventory of ciprofloxacin to assess readiness for homeland security.

Contraindications Ciprofloxacin is contraindicated with concurrent administration of tizanidine. Levofloxacin and moxifloxacin do not have contraindications.

Quick Study

Quinolones are easy to recognize because they share a common ending: –*floxacin*.

Cautions and Considerations Allied health professionals should be aware that many drugs interact with quinolones. For example, quinolones may inhibit clearance of caffeine and theophylline, leading to increased blood levels. Quinolones may prolong QT intervals and may enhance QT-prolonging effects of other drugs. Quinolones should not be taken with antacids, calcium-fortified juices, or dairy products because the absorption of the quinolones will be reduced.

Sulfonamides and Nitrofurantoin

Another common class of drugs is **sulfonamides**, or **sulfa drugs**, which are bacteriostatic and work by blocking bacteria from making folic acid, an essential substance for survival. Although humans can absorb folic acid from food, bacteria cannot, and thus must make folic acid. Sulfa drugs are used most often to treat UTIs. The most common sulfa drug is a combination containing trimethoprim. This combination is especially good for UTIs caused by *Escherichia coli*. Sulfa drugs are also used to treat community-acquired MRSA skin infections and as prophylaxis against *Pneumocystis carinii* pneumonia, a common deadly lung infection in patients who have end-stage acquired immunodeficiency syndrome (AIDS).

Like sulfa drugs, **nitrofurantoin** is used to treat UTIs (see Figure 23.7). Its mechanism of action is not well understood, but its spectrum of activity is similar to that of sulfonamides. It works best if taken with food and plenty of fluids. Table 23.10 lists dosing information for common sulfonamides and nitrofurantoin.

TABLE 23.10 Common Sulfonamides and Nitrofurantoin

Generic (Brand)	Dosage Form	Route of Administration	Common Dosage
Nitrofurantoin (Macrobid, Macrodantin)	Capsule, oral suspension	Oral	Adult: 5–100 mg 1–4 times a day Pediatric: 5–6 mg/kg/day in divided doses
Trimethoprim/sulfamethoxazole (Bactrim, Septra)	Injection, oral suspension, tablet	IV, oral	Varies depending on age and infection treated

FIGURE 23.7 Medication Label for Macrobid

Nitrofurantoin is sold under several brand names, one of them being Macrobid.

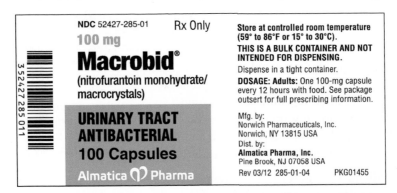

NDC 52427-285-01   Rx Only

100 mg

Macrobid®
(nitrofurantoin monohydrate/macrocrystals)

URINARY TRACT ANTIBACTERIAL
100 Capsules

Almatica ♡ Pharma

Store at controlled room temperature (59° to 86°F or 15° to 30°C).
THIS IS A BULK CONTAINER AND NOT INTENDED FOR DISPENSING.
Dispense in a tight container.
DOSAGE: Adults: One 100-mg capsule every 12 hours with food. See package outsert for full prescribing information.

Mfg. by:
Norwich Pharmaceuticals, Inc.
Norwich, NY 13815 USA
Dist. by:
Almatica Pharma, Inc.
Pine Brook, NJ 07058 USA
Rev 03/12 285-01-04   PKG01455

Side Effects Common side effects of sulfa drugs are nausea, vomiting, fever, and photosensitivity. Rarely, jaundice and Stevens-Johnson syndrome, a severe and possibly fatal skin rash condition, have occurred. Patients should know that if they have yellowing of their skin or eyes, or any kind of skin rash, they should stop taking the sulfa drug and notify their prescribers right away. Kidney damage has also occurred with sulfa drugs, so patients should be sure to drink six to eight glasses of water a day when taking these medications.

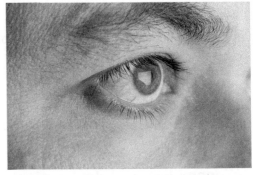

Jaundice is a rare side effect of sulfa drugs and can present as scleral icterus, or the yellowing of the sclera of the eye.

Contraindications Trimethoprim/sulfamethoxazole is contraindicated in patients with a history of drug-induced immune thrombocytopenia; in megaloblastic anemia due to folate deficiency; in infants younger than two months of age; and in marked liver or kidney dysfunction.

Contraindications to nitrofurantoin include anuria, oliguria, or significant impairment to kidney function; previous history of jaundice or hepatic dysfunction associated with prior nitrofurantoin use; pregnant patients at term, during labor and delivery, or when the onset of labor is imminent; and in neonates younger than one month of age.

Cautions and Considerations Taking sulfa drugs with food can help alleviate the common side effects of nausea and vomiting. Sulfa allergy is common, so allied health professionals should always inquire about drug allergies when dispensing a sulfa drug.

Nitrofurantoin turns urine brown. Patients should be alerted to this harmless but sometimes alarming effect.

Metronidazole

The drug metronidazole is chemically structured like an antifungal drug but works like an antibiotic. It also has activity on some protozoa. The agent is used to treat common infections including *Giardia* infection, amoebic dysentery, bacterial vaginosis, trichomoniasis, rosacea, and *Helicobacter pylori* ulcers. Metronidazole (Flagyl, MetroGel, Vandazole) comes in tablet, lotion, cream, vaginal gel, and injectable dosage forms.

Side Effects The most common side effects of metronidazole are headache, anorexia, vomiting, diarrhea, and abdominal cramps. Taking metronidazole with food can help alleviate these effects.

Contraindications Metronidazole is contraindicated in patients with a hypersensitivity to nitroimidazole derivatives. This medication is also contraindicated in the first trimester of pregnancy, use of disulfiram within the past two weeks, and use of alcohol during therapy or within three days of therapy discontinuation.

Cautions and Considerations One of the most important things to remember about metronidazole is that it interacts with alcohol to cause a severe reaction. Patients can become quite ill with nausea, vomiting, flushing, sweating, and headache if they ingest any alcohol while taking metronidazole and for three days after stopping the medication. Some cough medications and other over-the-counter (OTC) products have alcohol in them. Patients should be warned not to consume these products (in addition to alcoholic beverages) when taking metronidazole.

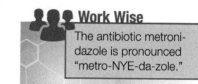

Work Wise

The antibiotic metronidazole is pronounced "metro-NYE-da-zole."

Kolb's Learning Styles

If you enjoy active learning, as Convergers do, or practical application, as Accommodators do, seek out someone who works in infectious diseases (such as a physician, nurse, or pharmacist). Which antibiotics do they most often prescribe or use? Based on what you know about these drugs, try to guess which types of infections these practitioners are treating most often.

Checkpoint 23.2

Take a moment to review what you have learned so far and answer these questions.

1. What are the main classes of antibiotics?

2. Which antibiotics should not be taken with alcohol products or beverages?

Viral Infections

Viruses are not whole-cell organisms like bacteria. They are segments of nuclear material (DNA or ribonucleic acid [RNA]) surrounded by a capsid, or protein coating. They attach to human cells and inject their nucleic material into the cell, which then alters that cell's function so that it begins replicating viruses. The cell's normal function is halted and it dies, releasing newly formed viruses that invade other cells. This process continues as the infection spreads.

There is rich diversity in the virus world. Viruses can vary in structure, gene expression, replication method, transmission, and physiologic effects. Signs and symptoms of a viral infection depend on the type of cells destroyed by the virus. For example, a cold virus attacks cells in the respiratory mucosa, causing runny nose, sinus congestion, and coughing.

Common viral infections include influenza and **herpes**, a family of viruses causing chicken pox (herpes varicella), shingles (herpes zoster), cold sores (herpes labialis), and sexually transmitted infections (herpes simplex). Other viral infections include hepatitis (A, B, and C), measles, mumps, rubella, West Nile, rabies, respiratory syncytial virus (RSV), and rotavirus.

Drug Regimens and Treatments for Nonretroviral Infections

The number of antiviral agents is growing but does not rival the number of antibiotics available. Because viruses use a living cell to replicate, most drug therapy used to kill the virus also kills the cell. Antiviral drugs either prevent viruses from entering cells or alter their ability to replicate (see Figure 23.8). In most cases, it is preferable to prevent viral infections before they occur, using vaccines when possible.

FIGURE 23.8 | Mechanisms of Action for Antiviral Agents

Antiviral drugs stop a virus from attaching to a cell, block its replication within the cell, or prevent its assembly into intact viruses for release.

Three methods to block viral infection or progression using medication:

1. block attachment of virion to cell surface

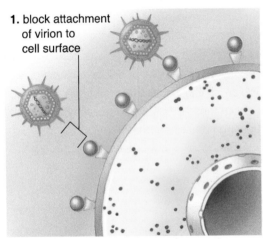

2. block virion replication and/or insertion into cell DNA (multiple methods, such as blocking enzymes that uncoil and splice DNA, are possible)

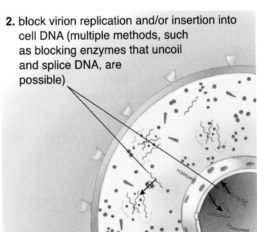

3. prevent release by disrupting viral assembly

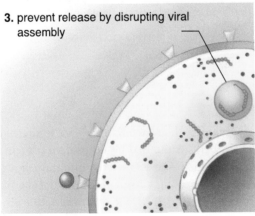

Common Antiviral Agents

For common viral infections such as influenza, cold sores, and shingles, drug therapy must be started as soon as the first symptoms begin. These agents do not eradicate the virus; they simply limit viral replication, which lessens the severity of symptoms and shortens the length of illness. Agents used to treat common viral infections are taken only when symptoms indicate an infection has started and therapy is needed. Agents used to treat hepatitis and genital herpes are taken on a long-term basis to suppress the virus and prevent or lessen outbreaks. Table 23.11 lists some common antivirals and their dosages. Please refer to other resources for details on antiviral treatment specifically used to treat hepatitis B.

TABLE 23.11 Antiviral Drugs for Common Infections

Generic (Brand)	Dosage Form	Route of Administration	Indication and Common Dosage
Antiherpes Agents			
Acyclovir (Zovirax)	Capsule, injection, ointment, oral suspension, tablet	IV, oral, topical	Chicken pox (pediatric): 　PO: Children ≥ 2 years and ≤ 40 kg: 20 mg/kg 4 times a day; children > 40 kg: 800 mg 4 times a day 　Topical: Varies by age, product, and indication Genital herpes (acute): 　IV: 5 mg/kg/dose 3 times a day for 5–7 days, followed with oral therapy for a minimum of 10 days total treatment 　PO: 200 mg 5 times a day or 400 mg 3 times a day for 7–10 days Genital herpes (chronic suppression): 　PO: 400 mg twice a day for 1 year Herpes zoster (shingles) and chicken pox (adult): 　IV: 10 mg/kg/dose 3 times a day for 7–10 days 　PO: 800 mg 5 times a day for 7–10 days
Famciclovir (Famvir)	Tablet	Oral	Genital herpes (acute): 1,000 mg twice a day for 1 day Genital herpes (chronic suppression): 250 mg twice a day for 1 year Herpes labialis (cold sores): 1,500 mg single dose Herpes zoster (shingles): 500 mg every 8 hr
Valacyclovir (Valtrex)	Tablet	Oral	Genital herpes (acute): 1,000 mg twice a day for 10 days Genital herpes (chronic suppression): 1,000 mg a day Herpes labialis (cold sores): 2,000 mg every 12 hr for 1 day Herpes zoster (shingles): 1,000 mg 3 times a day for 7 days
Anti-influenza Agents			
Amantadine (Symmetrel)	Capsule, syrup, tablet	Oral	Adult: 100–200 mg a day Pediatric: varies by age and weight of patient
Oseltamivir (Tamiflu)	Capsule, oral suspension	Oral	Adult: 75 mg twice a day for 5 days Pediatric: varies by age and weight of patient
Rimantadine (Flumadine)	Tablet	Oral	Adult: 100 mg twice a day Pediatric: 5 mg/kg/day
Zanamivir (Relenza)	Powder for inhalation	Inhalation	2 inhalations twice a day
Other Antiviral Agents			
Ribavirin (Virazole, various)	Capsule, oral solution, powder for inhalation, tablet	Inhalation, oral	RSV: 20 mg/mL inhaled for 12–18 hr a day

Side Effects Common side effects of antivirals include headache, malaise, fatigue, nausea, vomiting, diarrhea, cough, and skin rash. Usually, these effects are tolerable or indistinguishable from the viral infection being treated.

Contraindications Acyclovir is contraindicated in patients with a hypersensitivity to valacyclovir. Famciclovir is contraindicated in patients with a hypersensitivity to penciclovir. Valacyclovir should not be used in patients with a hypersensitivity to acyclovir.

Rimantadine is contraindicated in patients with a hypersensitivity to drugs of the adamantine class. Zanamivir is contraindicated in patients with a hypersensitivity to milk protein. Amantadine and oseltamivir do not have contraindications.

Contraindications to ribavirin include pregnancy; use in male patients whose female partners are pregnant; patients with hemoglobinopathies; patients with autoimmune hepatitis; and concomitant use with didanosine.

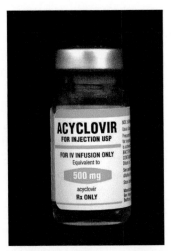
Acyclovir injection is used to treat herpes simplex infections.

Cautions and Considerations Famciclovir and zanamivir both contain milk products and should be used prudently by patients with milk-product sensitivities.

Amantadine and rimantadine may have CNS side effects such as dizziness, headache, and weakness. Older adults are at higher risk for such side effects and should use caution when taking these drugs. Acyclovir and valacyclovir may have CNS side effects such as confusion, hallucinations, and seizures. Use of these agents in older adults should be done with caution due to the aforementioned CNS side effects.

Ribavirin has a serious side effect of hemolytic anemia and may worsen underlying cardiac disease and lead to fatal and nonfatal heart attacks. Patients with heart disease should avoid using ribavirin.

Drug Regimens and Treatments for Retroviral Infections

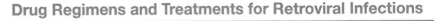

Work Wise

When a person is exposed to HIV, prophylactic therapy can be initiated to prevent infection. The sooner postexposure prophylaxis is started—ideally within two hours—the more effective it is. Healthcare workers must report any such exposure immediately to their supervisors so that proper testing and preventive therapy can begin. If warranted, postexposure prophylaxis therapy will include a combination of agents for three to six months.

A **retrovirus** is a virus that uses RNA as its genetic material. Retroviruses use an enzyme called **reverse transcriptase** to become part of the host's DNA, which allows replication of the virus.

Human immunodeficiency virus (HIV) is a retrovirus that attaches to receptors on the surface of T cells and injects its contents. Once inside, an intracellular enzyme, reverse transcriptase, uses this material to make pro-DNA fragments. The pro-DNA fragments insert themselves into the host cell's DNA, which then alters the cell's function to produce parts of the virus. Another enzyme, **protease**, then promotes assembly of the viral parts into intact HIVs, which are then released for further invasion. Patients with advanced and severe forms of HIV are said to have AIDS. In AIDS, even simple infections that typically would not cause any problems can become deadly.

The drugs used against HIV and AIDS save lives, but these agents have numerous severe side effects and drug interactions, making them difficult medications to tolerate. These drugs can be combined into therapy, called a **cocktail**, to take advantage of the effects of synergistic drug therapy. By attacking the viral replication process in multiple stages, more viruses can be destroyed. Although these medications can reduce the number of viruses in the body to almost undetectable levels, patients must continue to take the drugs throughout their lives to prevent progression of the illness and death and must follow medication instructions carefully to receive optimal effect.

Different classes of drugs are used to treat HIV, including nucleoside reverse transcriptase inhibitors (NRTIs), nucleotide reverse transcriptase inhibitors (NtRTIs), nonnucleoside reverse transcriptase inhibitors (NNRTIs), protease inhibitors (PIs), and integrase inhibitors.

A patient with HIV generally takes a combination of three or more antiviral drugs from the different classes, such as one NNRTI plus two NRTIs or a PI combined with ritonavir and two NRTIs. Some of these cocktails are available packaged in a single tablet (e.g., Atripla, Stribild, and Truvada). Patients who are new to treatment may start with one of those combination pills. Over time, the virus develops resistance to the different antiviral agents, so patients will change drug treatments periodically throughout the course of the disease. Table 23.12 identifies common HIV treatment combinations.

The same drugs used to treat HIV can also be used to help prevent virus transmission. **Pre-exposure prophylaxis** (or **PrEP**) is used to prevent HIV transmission to an HIV-negative individual when taken prior to HIV exposure. **Postexposure prophylaxis** may be used to prevent transmission of HIV from an HIV-positive patient to an HIV-negative individual after viral exposure.

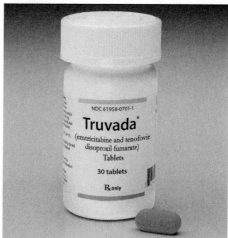

One HIV cocktail is Truvada, a combination of emtricitabine and tenofovir. Truvada is used to suppress HIV in patients who have the virus but is also used as a pre-exposure prophylaxis to prevent HIV transmission.

TABLE 23.12 Combination Treatments for HIV

Generic (Brand)	Common Dosage
Abacavir/lamivudine (Epzicom)	1 tablet a day
Efavirenz/emtricitabine/tenofovir (Atripla)	1 tablet a day
Elvitegravir/cobicistat/emtricitabine/tenofovir (Stribild)	1 tablet a day
Emtricitabine/tenofovir (Truvada)	1 tablet a day
Lamivudine/zidovudine (Combivir)	1 tablet twice a day

NRTIs and NtRTIs

Nucleoside reverse transcriptase inhibitors (NRTIs) and **nucleotide reverse transcriptase inhibitors (NtRTIs)** are HIV agents that work by inhibiting reverse transcriptase, which forms pro-DNA molecules inside of T cells. Table 23.13 covers common dosing information for these drug classes.

Side Effects Common side effects of NRTIs and NtRTIs are nausea and vomiting, which can be severe. Rarely, some of these agents can also cause lactic acidosis with liver enlargement, a life-threatening condition. These drugs can also cause pancreatitis, a painful

TABLE 23.13 Common NRTIs and NtRTIs

Generic (Brand)	Dosage Form	Route of Administration	Common Dosage
Abacavir/lamivudine (Epzicom)	Tablet	Oral	600 mg/300 mg a day
Abacavir/lamivudine/ zidovudine (Trizivir)	Tablet	Oral	300 mg/150 mg/300 mg a day
Didanosine (Videx)	Capsule, powder for oral solution	Oral	Capsule: 125–200 mg twice a day or 250–400 mg once a day Oral solution: 167–250 mg twice a day
Efavirenz/emtricitabine/ tenofovir (Atripla)	Tablet	Oral	600 mg/200 mg/300 mg a day
Emtricitabine (Emtriva)	Capsule, oral solution	Oral	Capsule: 200 mg a day Oral solution: 240 mg a day
Emtricitabine/tenofovir (Truvada)	Tablet	Oral	200 mg/300 mg a day
Lamivudine (Epivir)	Oral solution, tablet	Oral	100 mg a day
Lamivudine/zidovudine (Combivir)	Tablet	Oral	150 mg/300 mg twice a day
Stavudine (Zerit)	Capsule, powder for oral solution	Oral	30–40 mg every 12 hr
Tenofovir (Viread)	Oral powder, tablet	Oral	300 mg a day
Zidovudine (Retrovir)	Capsule, injection, oral solution, syrup, tablet	IV, oral	IV: 1 mg/kg/dose infused over 1 hr, given 5–6 times a day PO: 600 mg a day in divided doses

inflammation of the pancreas, and peripheral neuropathy, a painful nerve condition in the legs and hands. Alcohol increases the incidence and severity of these toxicities. Avoiding alcohol is especially important when taking didanosine.

Contraindications Patients with moderate-to-severe liver impairment should not use products containing abacavir. Didanosine is contraindicated in patients currently using allopurinol or ribavirin. Products containing emtricitabine, lamivudine, stavudine, tenofovir, or zidovudine do not have contraindications.

Cautions and Considerations NRTIs have black box warnings for the risk of lactic acidosis. NRTIs and NtRTIs are metabolized in the liver, where many other drugs are also metabolized. Consequently, these agents can interact with other drugs and should only be prescribed by experienced healthcare practitioners. Didanosine cannot be taken with members of its own class (stavudine). Abacavir has a unique boxed warning for the risk of hypersensitivity reactions. These reactions can be extremely harmful and even fatal. Patients should undergo special testing prior to abacavir therapy to help determine the likelihood of an allergic reaction.

Patients must follow specific instructions regarding which drugs should be taken with or without food. For example, didanosine must be taken on an empty stomach to work properly.

NNRTIs

Non-nucleoside reverse transcriptase inhibitors (NNRTIs) are agents used exclusively for the treatment of HIV infection. NNRTIs inhibit reverse transcriptase, which forms

TABLE 23.14 Common NNRTIs

Generic (Brand)	Dosage Form	Route of Administration	Common Dosage	Side Effects
Delavirdine (Rescriptor)	Tablet	Oral	400 mg 3 times a day	Central obesity/weight gain, Stevens-Johnson syndrome
Efavirenz (Sustiva)	Capsule, tablet	Oral	600 mg a day	Dizziness; insomnia; drowsiness; abnormal dreams; hallucinations; CNS effects such as depression, suicidal tendencies, paranoia, mania
Etravirine (Intelence)	Tablet	Oral	200 mg twice a day	Skin rash, nausea, hypersensitivity, fat redistribution
Nevirapine (Viramune)	Oral suspension, tablet	Oral	200 mg 1–2 times a day	Liver problems, severe allergic reaction, Stevens-Johnson syndrome
Rilpivirine (Edurant)	Tablet	Oral	25 mg daily	Skin rash, depression, insomnia, headache

pro-DNA molecules. Table 23.14 describes common dosages of these drugs, as well as their side effects.

Side Effects The side effects of NNRTIs vary and can be found in Table 23.14.

Contraindications Contraindications to delavirdine include concurrent use of alprazolam, astemizole, cisapride, ergot alkaloids, midazolam, pimozide, rifampin, terfenadine, or triazolam. Nevirapine is contraindicated in patients with moderate-to-severe liver impairment and should not be used for postexposure prophylaxis. Rilpivirine contraindications include coadministration with anticonvulsants, antimycobacterials, proton-pump inhibitors, systemic dexamethasone, and St. John's wort. Efavirenz contraindications include concurrent use of bepridil, cisapride, midazolam, pimozide, triazolam, St. John's wort, and ergot alkaloids. Etravirine does not have contraindications.

Cautions and Considerations Nevirapine has a black box warning for fatal and nonfatal hepatitis and skin rashes, including Stevens-Johnson syndrome. Delavirdine cannot be taken with antacids or it will not be absorbed properly. Efavirenz should not be taken with a high-fat meal and should be avoided in the first trimester of pregnancy due to teratogenicity. Etravirine should be taken with food. Due to lack of data, rilpivirine should be used with caution in patients with a viral load greater than 100,000 copies/mL. A **viral load** is a measurement taken from a blood sample that determines the level of HIV activity and the effectiveness of antiretroviral therapy.

PIs

Protease inhibitors (PIs), another class of drugs, work by blocking the enzyme that affects the assembly of proteins into working HIVs. In effect, the infection cycle is halted because nonfunctional and noninfectious viruses are produced. Table 23.15 covers common dosing for PIs.

Side Effects Many PIs can cause severe diarrhea, which usually decreases with use. Loperamide, an OTC antidiarrheal product, can be used to control this side effect. Other side effects include

Work Wise

Many ineffective herbal products and remedies are promoted and sold to patients with HIV and AIDS. These products do not cure this disease, but patients with this terminal illness often look for "miracle cures." Encourage patients to talk with their healthcare practitioners about herbal products they want to take.

TABLE 23.15 Common PIs

Generic (Brand)	Dosage Form	Common Dosage
Atazanavir (Reyataz)	Capsule	300 mg once a day with food (must be taken with ritonavir)
Darunavir (Prezista)	Oral suspension, tablet	600 mg twice a day with food (must be taken with ritonavir)
Fosamprenavir (Lexiva)	Oral suspension, tablet	700–1,400 mg twice a day (must be taken with ritonavir)
Indinavir (Crixivan)	Capsule	800 mg every 8 hr
Lopinavir/ritonavir (Kaletra)	Oral solution, tablet	400 mg/100 mg twice a day
Nelfinavir (Viracept)	Tablet	1,250 mg 2 times a day with food
Ritonavir (Norvir)	Capsule, oral solution	Up to 600 mg twice a day
Saquinavir (Invirase)	Capsule, tablet	1,000 mg twice a day (must be taken with ritonavir)
Tipranavir (Aptivus)	Capsule, oral solution	500 mg twice a day (must be taken with ritonavir)

headache, fatigue, dizziness, nausea, vomiting, bleeding problems, pancreatitis, depression, and Stevens-Johnson syndrome. Many patients also develop allergic reactions.

All of these agents cause fat redistribution, where fat and weight gain in the abdominal area is significant. In this process, normal fat and sugar metabolism is altered, causing many patients to get diabetes. Therefore, many patients who have HIV and are taking PIs will also need treatment for diabetes.

Contraindications Many contraindications to PIs are connected with drug interactions. Contraindications to atazanavir, darunavir, and lopinavir/ritonavir include concurrent therapy with alfuzosin, cisapride, ergot derivatives, indinavir, irinotecan, lovastatin, midazolam, nevirapine, pimozide, rifampin, sildenafil, simvastatin, St. John's wort, or triazolam; and coadministration with drugs that strongly induce cytochrome P450 (CYP450) 3A4 and may lead to lower atazanavir exposure and loss of efficacy.

Contraindications to fosamprenavir and indinavir include concurrent therapy with alfuzosin, cisapride, ergot derivatives, irinotecan, lovastatin, midazolam, nevirapine, pimozide, rifampin, sildenafil, simvastatin, St. John's wort, or triazolam.

Nelfinavir should not be used concurrently with alfuzosin, amiodarone, cisapride, ergot derivatives, lovastatin, midazolam, pimozide, quinidine, rifampin, sildenafil, simvastatin, St. John's wort, or triazolam.

Ritonavir is contraindicated with concurrent use of alfuzosin, amiodarone, cisapride, ergot derivatives, flecainide, lovastatin, midazolam, pimozide, propafenone, quinidine, sildenafil, simvastatin, St. John's wort, triazolam, or voriconazole.

Contraindications to saquinavir include congenital or acquired QT prolongation, refractory hypokalemia or hypomagnesemia, concomitant use of medications that both increase saquinavir plasma concentrations and prolong QT interval, complete atrioventricular block, and severe liver impairment. Saquinavir combined with ritonavir is contraindicated with concurrent use of alfuzosin, amiodarone, bepridil, cisapride, dofetilide, ergot derivative, flecainide, lidocaine, lovastatin, midazolam, pimozide, propafenone, quinidine, rifampin, sildenafil, simvastatin, trazodone, or triazolam.

Tipranavir is contraindicated in moderate-to-severe liver impairment. Tipranavir in combination with ritonavir should not be used with alfuzosin, amiodarone, bepridil, cisapride, ergot derivatives, flecainide, lovastatin, midazolam, pimozide, propafenone, quinidine, rifampin, sildenafil, simvastatin, St. John's wort, or triazolam.

Cautions and Considerations All of the PIs have numerous drug interactions, many of which are severe. For example, commonly used OTC antihistamines may have a serious interaction with PIs. Allied health professionals should be mindful of potential drug interactions between PIs and both prescription and nonprescription agents when taking patients' medication histories.

Most of these drugs cause liver and kidney problems. At times, these effects can be severe and life-threatening. Patients with such conditions should work closely with their prescribers when using PIs.

Darunavir must be coadministered with ritonavir.

Patients taking indinavir should drink six to eight glasses of water a day to prevent kidney stones. This drug cannot be taken with food or grapefruit juice.

Tipranavir capsules contain dehydrated ethanol and should be avoided in patients with cautions, contraindications, and a hypersensitivity to ethanol. The oral solution formula contains vitamin E. Those individuals using the oral solution should avoid vitamin E use.

Miscellaneous Therapies

HIV-1 integrase is essential for viral replication. **Chemokine coreceptor (CCR5) inhibitors** exert their antiviral activity by binding to the CCR5 receptor and preventing fusion on HIV entry into the host cell. Maraviroc (Selzentry) is the only CCR5 inhibitor available. It works only for certain strains of HIV, so special testing is performed to select appropriate patients for this therapy.

Fusion inhibitors work by blocking HIV from attaching to cellular membranes. Enfuvirtide (Fuzeon) is a fusion inhibitor available for patients.

Integrase inhibitors work by inhibiting strand transfer of viral DNA to host cells. Raltegravir and elvitegravir are two of the integrase inhibitors currently available; they are used in combination with cobicistat, tenofovir, and emtricitabine. Another integrase inhibitor, dolutegravir, is used in combination with either abacavir/lamivudine or tenofovir/emtricitabine.

Table 23.16 lists the common dosage forms and dosages of these miscellaneous therapies.

Side Effects The side effects of the miscellaneous antiretroviral agents vary and can be found in Table 23.16.

Contraindications Maraviroc is contraindicated in patients with severe kidney impairment. Enfuvirtide and raltegravir do not have contraindications. Dolutegravir should not be used with dofetilide. Elvitegravir does not have contraindications. The elvitegravir combination product is contraindicated with concurrent use of alfuzosin, cisapride, ergot derivatives, lovastatin, midazolam, pimozide, rifampin, sildenafil, simvastatin, St. John's wort, or triazolam.

Cautions and Considerations Maraviroc may induce liver toxicity, so baseline liver function tests should be taken. Dolutegravir may cause fat redistribution and hypersensitivity reaction. Enfuvirtide may cause hypersensitivity reactions and pneumonia. Elvitegravir may contribute to lactic acidosis. It should be avoided in patients with severe liver impairment. Elvitegravir does not have contraindications. The elvitegravir combination product

TABLE 23.16 Miscellaneous HIV Therapies

Generic (Brand)	Dosage Form	Common Dosage	Side Effects
CCR5 Inhibitor			
Maraviroc (Selzentry)	Tablet	300 mg twice a day	Abdominal pain, cough, dizziness, and fever
Fusion Inhibitor			
Enfuvirtide (Fuzeon)	Solution for sub-Q injection	90 mg twice a day	Diarrhea, nausea, fatigue, and injection site irritation
Integrase Inhibitors			
Dolutegravir (Tivicay)	Tablet	50 mg a day	Elevated serum lipase, insomnia, elevated liver enzymes, hyperglycemia
Elvitegravir (Vitekta)	Tablet	85–150 mg a day	Kidney toxicity, nausea, diarrhea, proteinuria
Raltegravir (Isentress)	Chewable tablet, film-coated tablet, oral suspension	400 mg twice a day	Nausea, headache, diarrhea, pyrexia, creatine kinase elevation

may decrease bone mineral density and cause fat redistribution. It may also contribute to lactic acidosis. It should be avoided in patients with severe liver impairment. Raltegravir has multiple drug interactions, so caution should be exercised when used in combination with other drugs.

Patient Teaching

Treatment adherence is extremely important with HIV therapy. Make sure patients know that adherence affects how well HIV medications decrease viral load and prevent drug resistance. To help patients adhere to their therapy regimens, provide them with written copies of their treatment plans, including all medications and dosages; learn the possible side effects of their therapies; and understand why adherence is important to their treatment outcomes.

Kolb's Learning Styles

If you like to study on your own, as Assimilators do, research the Internet to look for new combination antiviral products that will be part of the HIV drug arsenal if approved by the US Food and Drug Administration. Make note of at least two of these combination products (brand name, generic name, and directions for use) and think about how they could improve patient adherence to therapy.

Checkpoint 23.3

Take a moment to review what you have learned so far and answer these questions.

1. What classes of antivirals are used to treat HIV?

2. Which class of antivirals used to treat HIV has the side effect of fat redistribution?

Fungal Infections

Fungi (or *funguses*) include **yeasts** and molds that are one-celled organisms. These organisms do not have chlorophyll, the substance that gives plants their green color. They do have a plant-like cell wall, the target for most antifungal medications. Usually, fungal infections are topical and mild. **Dermatophytes**, fungi of the skin, cause some of the most frequent and ordinary infections, such as athlete's foot and ringworm. **Candidiasis** is a fungal infection caused by **Candida**, a genus of yeast. Common examples include vaginal yeast infections and thrush. However, when a fungus gains entry to the bloodstream or cannot be destroyed due to immunodeficiency, it can cause serious systemic infections. Table 23.17 lists common fungi and related infections.

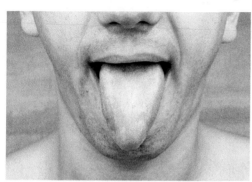

Oral thrush, also known as *oral candidiasis*, is caused by the fungus *Candida albicans*. This fungal infection is characterized by white, painful lesions or patches in the mouth.

TABLE 23.17 Fungal Organisms and Common Infections

Organism	Associated Infection
Aspergillus spp.	Lung infection and other difficult-to-treat infections
Candida spp.	Meningitis, oral or vaginal thrush (yeast infection), pneumonia, sepsis
Cryptococcus spp.	Meningitis and other difficult-to-treat infections
Histoplasma spp.	Lung infection
Tinea spp.	Skin infections (athlete's foot and ringworm), toenail and fingernail infections

Drug Regimens and Treatments

Antifungals are drugs used to treat fungal infections (see Table 23.18). Most fungal infections of the skin and nails, mucocutaneous tissue (such as the tissue lining the mouth and vagina), and the entire body system require treatment with antifungals.

Antifungal Drugs

Many antifungal drugs damage **ergosterol**, a substance in the cell wall of fungi. Without this molecule, the cell wall cannot form properly and the fungal cell dies. Many fungal infections and their treatments are topical. Oral or IV drug therapy is needed to treat systemic fungal infections. However, most antifungal agents can be toxic to the liver when used systemically. Sometimes pulse dosing, in which the drug is given one week a month, is used to reduce the amount of time the drug comes into contact with the liver, which decreases the toxic effects. Laboratory tests are used periodically to check liver function in patients who take antifungal drugs systemically.

TABLE 23.18 Common Antifungal Drugs

Generic (Brand)	Dosage Form	Common Dosage	Dispensing Status
Oral Thrush Agents			
Clotrimazole (Mycelex)	Lozenge	Dissolve in mouth 5 times a day	Rx
Nystatin (Mycostatin)	Oral suspension, powder, tablet	500,000–1 million units 3 times a day	Rx
Posaconazole (Noxafil)	Oral suspension	100–400 mg twice a day	Rx
Skin and Nail Agents			
Butenafine (Lotrimin Ultra, Mentax)	Topical cream	Once a day for 2 weeks	OTC, Rx
Ciclopirox (Loprox, Penlac)	Cream, gel, lotion, nail lacquer, shampoo, topical suspension	Depends on dosage form and site of infection but can take up to 12 weeks for cure	Rx
Clotrimazole (Desenex, Lotrimin AF)	Cream, lotion, topical solution	Twice a day for 2–4 weeks	OTC
Clotrimazole/betamethasone (Lotrisone)	Cream, lotion	Twice a day for 4 weeks	Rx
Griseofulvin (Grifulvin V, Gris-PEG)	Oral suspension, tablet	Varies depending on age and weight of patient (4 weeks for athlete's foot, 4–6 months for nail infections)	Rx
Ketoconazole (Nizoral)	Cream, foam, gel, shampoo	200–400 mg a day for 2–4 weeks	Rx
Miconazole (Micatin, Neosporin AF)	Gel, ointment, solution, spray, topical cream	Twice a day for 2 weeks	OTC
Nystatin (Nyamyc, Nystop)	Cream, ointment, powder	Twice a day until lesions heal	Rx
Terbinafine (Lamisil AT)	Cream, gel, spray	Once a day for 1–2 weeks	OTC
Systemic Agents			
Amphotericin B	Powder for injection	Varies by patient and disease being treated	Rx
Caspofungin (Cancidas)	Powder for injection	70 mg as initial dose followed by 50 mg a day	Rx
Flucytosine (Ancobon)	Capsule	50–150 mg/kg/day in divided intervals every 6 hr	Rx
Itraconazole (Sporanox)	Capsule, oral solution	200–400 mg a day	Rx
Ketoconazole (Nizoral)	Tablet	200–400 mg a day	Rx
Liposomal amphotericin B (Abelcet, Amphotec, AmBisome)	Oral suspension for injection	Varies by patient and disease being treated	Rx
Micafungin (Mycamine)	Powder for injection	Active treatment: 150 mg/day Preventive therapy: 50 mg/day	Rx
Voriconazole (Vfend)	Oral suspension, powder for injection, tablet	IV: 4–6 mg/kg every 12 hr PO: 200 mg every 12 hr	Rx
Vaginal Agents			
Butoconazole (Gynazole-1)	Vaginal cream	Once a day for 1–3 days	OTC, Rx
Clotrimazole (Gyne-Lotrimin)	Vaginal cream and suppository	Once a day for 3–7 days	OTC
Fluconazole (Diflucan)	Oral suspension, oral tablet, solution for injection	IV: varies depending on infection being treated PO: 150 mg in 1 dose	Rx
Miconazole (Monistat)	Vaginal cream	1,200 mg at bedtime for 1 day 200 mg a day for 3 days 100 mg a day for 7 days	OTC
Tioconazole (Vagistat-1)	Vaginal ointment	1 applicator at bedtime for 1 day	OTC

Side Effects Generally, antifungal drugs that are administered systemically (either orally or by injection) have more bothersome side effects compared with antifungals administered topically.

Amphotericin B is an antifungal drug that is particularly toxic to the liver and kidneys. Thus, its use is reserved for the most serious and life-threatening fungal infections. This drug should be infused slowly or fever, chills, nausea, vomiting, and headache can occur. Amphotericin B is also available in an IV **liposome** dosage form (see Figure 23.9), which surrounds the drug molecules with a fat/oil layer. This protective layer decreases the drug's ability to come into direct contact with body tissues and thus reduces its toxic effects.

Antifungals ending in the suffix *–azole* are in the **azole** family and are generally well tolerated. When ingested orally, nausea, vomiting, abdominal pain, and diarrhea are most frequently reported. Itraconazole and ketoconazole are particularly likely to cause stomach symptoms. Voriconazole is associated with transient vision changes (such as seeing flashes of light or having sensitivity to light), visual hallucinations, alopecia, nail changes or loss, and skin rash. Topically applied azoles are associated with application site reactions such as burning, discomfort, edema, and pain.

The generic names of the **echinocandin** class of antifungals end in the suffix *–fungin*. The echinocandins are injectables and may result in infusion and hypersensitivity reactions including skin rash, redness, hypotension, and—in some cases—angioedema. Injection site pain is another potential side effect.

Other antifungals are related to certain side effects. Flucytosine is associated with leukopenia; thrombocytopenia; GI symptoms such as nausea, diarrhea, and vomiting; and hepatic side effects. Nystatin is associated with diarrhea, nausea, stomach pain, and vomiting. Ciclopirox, which is applied topically, is associated with acne, alopecia, contact dermatitis, dry skin, skin burning, eye pain, and headache. Side effects of griseofulvin include dizziness, fatigue, skin rash, photosensitivity, and diarrhea. Terbinafine may cause headache, skin rash, diarrhea, dyspepsia, and nasopharyngitis.

FIGURE 23.9 Liposome Dosage Form

Liposomal amphotericin B is available as a suspension for injection, depending on the brand chosen. Be sure to remind patients to follow preparation instructions closely, for mistakes can be costly.

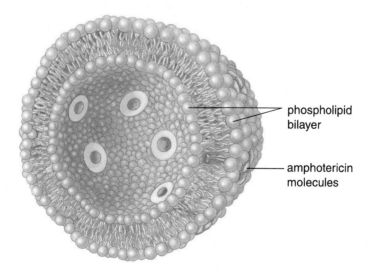

phospholipid bilayer

amphotericin molecules

Contraindications Azole antifungals are associated with multiple drug-drug interactions. They should not be used with quinidine; benzodiazepines such as alprazolam, chlordiazepoxide, clonazepam, diazepam, estazolam, flurazepam, halazepam, quazepam, and triazolam; dofetilide; pimozide; and statins such as lovastatin, simvastatin, and atorvastatin.

Griseofulvin is contraindicated in patients who are pregnant or have liver failure or porphyria. Miconazole is contraindicated in patients with milk-protein allergy.

Amphotericin B, butenafine, ciclopirox, flucytosine, nystatin, and terbinafine do not have contraindications. In addition, there are no contraindications for the echinocandins.

Cautions and Considerations Systemic antifungals are associated with liver function abnormalities. Liver function is usually assessed in patients using these medications.

Antifungals are involved in many serious drug-drug interactions. Patients using antifungals should make sure their prescribers and pharmacists are aware of all medications and alternative therapies being used concomitantly.

Reports of anaphylaxis are associated with amphotericin B use, and infusions should be supervised. If patients exhibit signs of anaphylaxis, administration should be discontinued immediately.

Fluconazole may cause QT prolongation, and caution should be exercised when used with other medications that can cause arrhythmia.

Name Exchange

Diflucan is the brand name of fluconazole, a commonly used antifungal.

Flucytosine carries a black box warning to use extreme caution in patients with renal dysfunction. The agent should be used only in combination with other antifungals due to development of resistance. Patients with bone marrow depression, hematologic disease, or those undergoing therapy that suppresses the bone marrow should use flucytosine with caution.

Griseofulvin should be discontinued if granulocytopenia occurs. There is a potential cross-reaction between penicillin hypersensitivity and griseofulvin hypersensitivity. Severe skin reactions have been reported with griseofulvin use; it is recommended that patients discontinue therapy and seek emergency medical care if severe skin reactions occur.

Depression has been reported with terbinafine use. Patients should contact their healthcare practitioners immediately if they experience any signs and symptoms of depression.

Parasitic and Protozoan Infections

Parasites are organisms that live off a host. Most parasites do not kill their host, but they can create great discomfort and severe symptoms. Some examples of parasites include pinworms, hookworms, roundworms, and tapeworms. **Protozoa** are single-celled organisms that usually cause infection through the oral–fecal route. These parasites are transmitted when hands, food, or water are contaminated with feces from an infected human or animal. **Giardiasis** is an intestinal infection caused by protozoa that live in soil, water, and food. Individuals who ingest or are exposed to these parasites have symptoms such as diarrhea and bloating. Malaria, caused by a sporozoan species, affects millions of people who live in tropical areas where mosquitoes thrive. Table 23.19 covers common parasitic and protozoan infections.

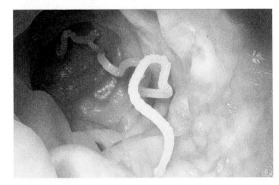

Approximately 50 million people worldwide are infected with tapeworms. This type of parasite, shown here in the human intestines, can grow up to 30 inches long.

TABLE 23.19 Common Parasitic and Protozoan Organisms and Infections

Parasite or Protozoa	Associated Infection
Giardia lamblia	Intestinal infection
Plasmodium vivax	Malaria
Pneumocystis carinii or *Pneumocystis jiroveci*	Lung infection
Toxoplasma gondii	Toxoplasmosis
Trichomonas vaginalis	Vaginal infection

Drug Regimens and Treatments

Most of the drugs used for parasitic and protozoan infections have already been covered in this chapter. For example, metronidazole is used to treat several common intestinal infections caused by protozoa such as *Giardia*. Malaria, however, is treated using several other drugs. Therapy often combines two or three drugs, including quinine, chloroquine, primaquine, doxycycline, tetracycline, clindamycin, atovaquone, proguanil, and mefloquine. Because malaria is not a common disease in the United States, allied health professionals are not often in contact with patients who are undergoing treatment. Such prescriptions will be filled only when a patient is traveling to or from a country where malaria is common. For these reasons, greater detail on these agents is not provided in this text.

 Checkpoint 23.4

Take a moment to review what you have learned so far and answer these questions.

1. What antifungals are used to treat oral thrush?

2. Which drug classes are associated with the suffixes *–azole* and *–fungin*?

Herbal and Alternative Therapies

Echinacea (*Echinacea purpurea*) is an herb some patients use to treat the common cold, RTIs, and even vaginal yeast infections. It has been found to reduce the severity and length of symptoms. Echinacea does not cure infections, but it may be used to augment drug therapy. Echinacea causes macrophage activation and the release of interleukins. It also has antioxidant activity. Echinacea products contain various concentrations of this herbal remedy. A standard dose has not been established. However, for echinacea to be effective, patients must use it multiple times a day and initiate its use at the very first signs of infection. Dosing is heaviest during the first 5 days of infection and continues for up to 10 days.

Garlic (*Allium sativum*) is a plant whose aromatic bulb may be used for immune system stimulation and prevention of infections (such as the common cold). It is also used topically for dermatophyte infections. The exact antimicrobial mechanism is unknown, but garlic has been shown to exert activity against various bacterial strains. When used topically, garlic gel has been shown to be **fungistatic** (able to inhibit fungal growth) and **fungicidal** (able to kill fungus). Topical garlic may also cause dermatitis or burns. Common side effects of oral garlic include malodorous breath, body odor, nausea, and vomiting. Garlic has antiplatelet activity and should be used with caution by patients who are using anticoagulants.

American **ginseng** (*Panax quinquefolius*) is a perennial plant whose root may be used for various health concerns including prevention of infections. Ginseng has been found to decrease the duration of colds and reduce the risk of recurring colds. Ginseng is thought to work by activating monocytes and cytokines and stimulating T-cell activity and

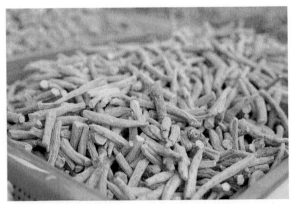

Dried American ginseng root is often coarsely ground to release its active components (ginsenosides) and placed in a tea infuser to brew a cup of tea.

B-cell proliferation. Headaches are the most common adverse effects associated with ginseng ingestion. Ginseng may decrease the efficacy of the anticoagulant warfarin and, therefore, should not be used by patients who are taking warfarin.

Zinc is a required component in many biologic processes in the body, including protein synthesis. It also boosts immune function. Like echinacea, zinc can be used to treat infections, including the common cold, flu, and RTIs. Zinc is available as a pill or lozenge. Dosages range from 24–200 mg multiple times a day. Zinc should not be taken with caffeine because caffeine reduces its absorption by up to 50%. Zinc also interacts with several other prescription medications, so patients should check with their pharmacists and healthcare practitioners about taking zinc along with other medications.

Vitamin C, or ascorbic acid, is a substance that boosts immune function and has antioxidant effects. This vitamin can be taken in high doses, but these higher amounts can cause diarrhea, upset stomach, and kidney stones. Vitamin C is best taken during cold and flu season, when the likelihood of encountering infection is greatest. Doses for fighting infection are in the range of 1–3 g a day.

Chapter Review

Chapter Summary

Infections are caused by pathogenic organisms or normal floras that grow uncontrolled. Organisms that cause disease are bacteria, viruses, fungi, and protozoa. Most infections can be treated with medication. Unfortunately, some pathogens develop resistance to the drugs typically used. When this happens, more expensive therapies must be tried, and, in some cases, effective drug therapy is not available.

Common classes of antibiotics used to treat bacterial infections are penicillins, cephalosporins, vancomycin, aminoglycosides, macrolides and lincosamides, tetracyclines, sulfonamides, quinolones, and metronidazole. These agents are chosen based on the type, site, and severity of infection.

Viral diseases such as influenza and herpes are treated with antiviral agents. These drugs do not eradicate the infection but can lessen the symptoms and duration of illness. Several antiviral drugs, including NRTIs, NtRTIs, NNRTIs, and PIs, are available to treat HIV infection and AIDS. These drugs are usually taken as a cocktail, in combinations of two or three, and can be difficult to take because of side effects and toxicities.

Antifungal drugs are used to treat simple fungal infections, such as athlete's foot, as well as life-threatening systemic infections.

These drugs come in a wide variety of dosage forms. Allied health professionals are likely to be in contact with patients who are undergoing treatment for infectious diseases. Becoming familiar with this large set of medications can be challenging but important in the practice setting.

Chapter Checkup

The Navigator+ learning management system that accompanies this textbook offers many opportunities to help you master chapter content, including end-of-chapter exercises, a glossary of key terms, flash cards, and additional interactive activities.

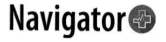

Career Exploration

If you enjoyed learning about the immune system and infectious diseases in this chapter, you may want to explore the following career options:

- clinical immunology technologist
- community health worker
- cytotechnologist
- environmental health officer/public health inspector
- histotechnologist
- HIV/AIDS counselor
- hospital occupational health and safety officer
- medical assistant
- occupational health and safety technician
- pharmacy technician
- sterile processing technician

24 Acquired Immunity and Autoimmune Disorders

Pharm Facts

- In the sixteenth century, Asian healthcare practitioners deliberately infected individuals with smallpox by blowing dried, pulverized smallpox scabs into their noses. The individuals would then contract a mild form of smallpox but would recover and have lifelong immunity from the disease.

- A 2012 study in the journal *SLEEP* revealed that vaccines are more effective in patients who get a full night's sleep than in those who sleep less than six hours. Sleep deprivation weakens the body's immune system response to germs.

- Researchers have identified more than 80 different autoimmune disorders, many of which have a genetic relationship.

- In 1938, US citizens were asked to mail a dime to the White House to combat polio, a disease that afflicted the current US president, Franklin D. Roosevelt. Within the first three days, the White House received 230,000 dimes. This campaign, dubbed the March of Dimes, led to the establishment of an organization that continues to advocate for the vaccinations of children to provide resistance to infectious diseases.

"Laboratory test findings provide a better understanding of a patient's pathology and aid in the early diagnosis of disorders. As a medical technologist, I conduct a variety of laboratory tests, including blood banking, clinical chemistry, hematology, serology, microbiology, and immunology. For example, I perform immunologic tests that are used to gauge the body's ability to resist infections as well as to determine the production of immune cells and antibodies. These tests guide the treatments of patients with immunodeficiency and autoimmune diseases. As better diagnostic technologies emerge, medical technology will continue to play a vital role in shaping individualized, quality patient care."

—Pamela Campbell, BSMT, ASCP
Medical Technologist

Learning Objectives

1 Understand the basic physiology of acquired immunity and the types of immunity.

2 Identify the generic names, brand names, routes of administration, prophylactic use, side effects, contraindications, and cautions and considerations for common vaccines.

3 Understand the CDC Immunization Schedule for Adults and know the locations of other immunization schedules for children and healthcare personnel.

4 Become familiar with the Vaccine Adverse Event Reporting System and its role in vaccination safety.

5 Describe common autoimmune disorders and their impact on various body systems.

6 Identify the generic names, brand names, indications, dosage ranges, and routes of administration for immunologic medications commonly used to prevent and treat autoimmune disorders.

7 Explain the indications and regimens for antitoxins and antivenoms.

Whereas Chapter 23 covered the anatomy and physiology of the immune system and the conventional treatment of infectious diseases, this chapter describes the drug therapies that prevent infection and provide immunosuppression. Preventive strategies are preferred for difficult-to-treat infectious diseases. The administration of vaccines provides **prophylaxis** (or prevention) for diseases that are associated with high risks of mortality or that result in significant illness. Vaccination, or immunization, is a way to boost the immune system in advance of exposure to disease-causing pathogens that impact public health and productivity.

Immunosuppressants are used to boost the immune systems of patients who have been diagnosed with autoimmune disorders such as multiple sclerosis, systemic lupus erythematosus, autoimmune hepatitis, and cancer. For patients who have undergone organ transplantation, immunosuppressants are used to prevent organ rejection, a process in which the organ recipient's immune system recognizes transplanted tissue as foreign and mounts an attack. These medications suppress the immune system's reaction.

Learning about immunizations is important to all allied health professionals. Some allied health personnel are permitted to administer vaccines in their state of practice. All healthcare workers—including student externs—who work in hospitals or other facilities accredited by The Joint Commission are mandated by law to have certain vaccinations or proven immunity to a variety of illnesses that can be transmitted to patients. In fact, a healthcare facility may require more than what is mandated by law.

Becoming familiar with immunosuppressants is important to allied health professionals as well. Pharmacy technicians with advanced education and training may be involved in the preparation and handling of these medications. Other allied health personnel most certainly will be involved in patient documentation and adherence to the prescribed immunosuppressant therapy regimen.

Physiology of Acquired Immunity

The immune response is a complex system that protects and fights against infectious disease. Acquired immunity discriminates between the body's own cells (*self cells*) and foreign cells (*pathogens*). In an **acquired immune response**, pathogens are carried to the lymph nodes where lymphocytes (T cells and B cells) detect and destroy them.

T Cells

As shown in Figure 24.1, **helper T cells** detect specific antigens (molecules on foreign pathogens) and stimulate killer T cells and B cells to become active. **Killer T cells** start killing any cells of the body infected with the foreign antigens. These cells can also help rid the body of cancerous cells in a similar manner. In organ transplantation, this part of the body's immune system must be suppressed to keep it from attacking new tissue.

FIGURE 24.1 | **Acquired Immune Response**

T cells and B cells can distinguish the body's own cells from foreign pathogens. These foreign cells quickly become targets for killer T cells.

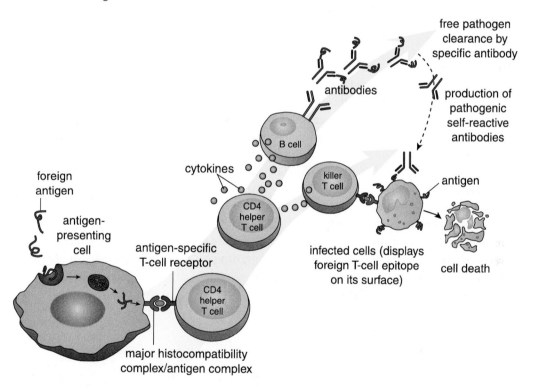

B Cells

B cells produce antibodies, which are also called *immunoglobulins*. There are five types of immunoglobulins, and each **immunoglobulin (Ig)** plays a role in the immune system (see Table 24.1). Immunoglobulins fight infection by binding pathogens and preventing them from infecting healthy cells. Sometimes, the immune system can malfunction and begin producing antibodies against normal, healthy cells. Autoimmune disorders are defined by such activity and include diseases such as systemic lupus erythematosus, rheumatoid arthritis, and multiple sclerosis.

TABLE 24.1 Immunoglobulins

Type	Location(s)	Function(s)
IgA	• Mucous membranes of the gastrointestinal system and respiratory tract • Tears, sweat, and saliva • Breast milk, from which immunity is transferred to child during breast-feeding	• Defends mucous membranes against exposure to external pathogens
IgD	• Plasma • Surfaces of lymphocytes	• May be involved in B-cell maturation
IgE	• Skin, lungs, and mucous membranes	• Mounts allergic response and fights parasites
IgG	• Blood • Lymph	• Activates other immune system cells to destroy foreign bodies • Provides passive immunity (mother to fetus) via the placenta
IgM	• Surfaces of red blood cells	• Provides a natural defense against bacteria • Activates the complement system • Is responsible for ABO blood typing

Hypersensitivity Reactions

The immune system also mediates **allergic reactions**, which are cases of **hypersensitivity**. Hypersensitivity is categorized into four types. **Type I hypersensitivity** reactions are anaphylactic reactions that can be life threatening. **Anaphylaxis** is a process mediated by antibodies, basophils, and mast cells that—if not treated quickly—causes swelling of the airways, blood vessel dilation, and shock. Some drugs can cause anaphylaxis. **Type II hypersensitivity** reactions stimulate the complement system, another component of the immune system. Antibodies attach to foreign cells and attract complement molecules, which poke holes in the foreign cells and kill them. This kind of reaction can occur when blood of the wrong type is given to a patient. Individuals having a Type II hypersensitivity reaction will often experience hemolytic anemia, thrombocytopenia, or neutropenia. Reactions of this type usually occur five to eight days after causative exposure. **Type III hypersensitivity** reactions involve toxins and antibodies. Normally, this process occurs in the spleen but, if

sufficiently severe, can cause inflammation of blood vessels. A **Type IV hypersensitivity** reaction is the immune response mediated by killer T cells. Type IV hypersensitivity reactions are called *delayed responses* because they take 12 to 72 hours to occur. A tuberculin skin test for tuberculosis is an example of a Type IV hypersensitivity reaction. When drugs cause this type of allergy, patients will have hives or an itchy rash. This hypersensitivity is not harmful if the drug is stopped but can progress to anaphylaxis if the drug continues to be administered.

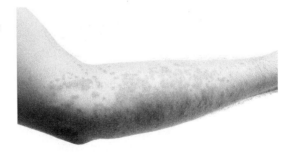

Urticaria, more commonly known as *hives*, is a type of rash notable for red, itchy welts that appear in clusters on the skin. These welts are a Type IV hypersensitivity reaction and occur in approximately 20% of the population during their lifetime.

Types of Immunity

You may recall from Chapter 23 that immune responses can be either innate (localized and nonspecific) or adaptive (antigen-specific). Once an antigen has been recognized, the adaptive immune system creates antibodies designed to attack that particular antigen. Adaptive immunity also includes a "memory" that makes future responses against a specific antigen more efficient.

Immunization is the process whereby a person acquires adaptive immunity or resistance to an infectious disease. There are two general ways people acquire immunity: passively and actively. Passive immunity occurs when preformed antibodies are transferred to an individual; active immunity occurs when an individual is exposed to a certain pathogen and makes his or her own antibodies. Both passive and active immunity can be acquired naturally or artificially. See Figure 24.2 for a graphic representation of the types of immunity.

FIGURE 24.2 Types of Immunity

Immunity is gained innately or adaptively. Adaptive immunity can be acquired naturally or artificially.

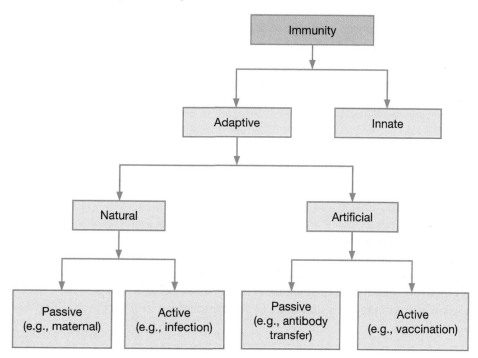

Passive Immunity

Passive immunity is a type of immunity gained by the transfer of antibodies from one individual to another. The antibodies received are ready-made, meaning the recipient does not create them. Passive immunity provides immediate protection, but the body does not develop memory. Without memory, the recipient of passive immunity may be susceptible to infection from the same pathogen in the future. Passive immunity occurs either naturally (from mother to fetus during pregnancy) or artificially (through the injection of immunoglobulin agents).

Natural Immunity

Newborns, with characteristically weak immune responses, benefit from naturally acquired passive immunity. While in utero, fetuses receive antibodies from their mothers (via the placenta) that provide immune protection for a short duration. Nursing babies may also receive protective antibodies naturally transmitted via breast milk.

Artificial Immunity

Although natural immunity has occurred for thousands of years, artificial acquisition of passive immunity is a more recent phenomenon. **Artificial passive immunity** occurs when ready-made exogenous antibodies are transferred to an individual. Exogenous antibodies may come in a variety of forms: via human or animal immunoglobulins or in the form of **monoclonal antibodies**, or antibodies cloned in a laboratory.

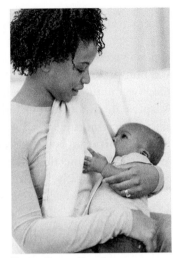

Protective antibodies are naturally transmitted to nursing babies via breast milk.

    Immunoglobulins are administered when rapid immunity is needed for a specific disease for a defined period. For instance, a patient recently exposed to a disease for which immunity status is uncertain may be given an immunoglobulin product. The onset of immunity is quick and usually lasts only a few months. Immunoglobulin use is approved by the US Food and Drug Administration (FDA) for the following conditions: immune thrombocytopenia, primary immunodeficiency states, secondary immunodeficiency in chronic lymphocyte leukemia, pediatric human immunodeficiency virus (HIV) infection, Kawasaki syndrome, and prevention of graft-versus-host disease (discussed in detail later in this chapter). Immunoglobulins may be used for other disorders that may not have FDA indications such as chronic neuropathy and hypogammaglobulinemia.

Active Immunity

In contrast to passive immunity, where ready-made antibodies are transferred to an individual, **active immunity** is the process of a person making their own antibodies to a pathogen. Active immunity, like passive immunity, can be obtained naturally or artificially. Active immunity acquired naturally occurs when a person is exposed to certain pathogens; active immunity acquired artificially typically results from the administration of vaccinations.

In the Know

In the fourteenth century, it was discovered that patients that recovered from the bubonic plague would never become reinfected. In other words, patients acquired immunity to the plague through exposure—an example of naturally acquired active immunization.

Natural Immunization

Naturally acquired active immunization occurs when an individual is exposed to foreign antigens in daily life, and his or her body produces antibodies against them. Consequently, the next time the individual encounters that disease, the body recognizes the pathogens and quickly builds a defense to provide immunity. This type of immunity is called *natural immunization* because the pathogen exposure was not deliberate. The strength and duration of natural immunity varies according to the type and amount of antigen encountered, genetics, and disorders of the immune system (such as immunodeficiency and immunosuppression).

Artificial Immunization

Artificially acquired active immunization is the process by which a person gains immunity or resistance to a disease through deliberate exposure to an antigen. The most common method of artificial immunization is **vaccination**. Vaccination is a proven tool for the prevention and elimination of infectious diseases. In fact, it is estimated that vaccination averts 2–3 million deaths worldwide annually.

Vaccination may reduce and prevent serious diseases when used universally. For example, vaccination practices have effectively eliminated smallpox worldwide. Vaccination also reduces many other diseases that cause great sickness and disability, especially among children. For instance, **vaccines** have reduced the impact of measles, polio, and influenza.

Various types of vaccines are available. **Live attenuated vaccines** use live but weakened pathogens to produce an immune response. **Inactivated vaccines** use pathogens that have been killed with chemicals, heat, or radiation.

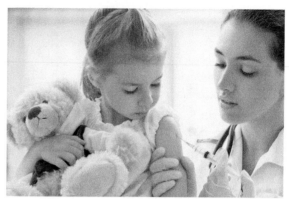

An allied health professional administers a vaccine to a young girl.

Immunization Schedule

Several vaccines require multiple doses to produce an adequate immune response and confer full immunity to a disease. The **Centers for Disease Control and Prevention (CDC)** publishes a schedule for childhood and adult vaccines. Certain immunizations are recommended for children, whereas others are more appropriate for adults (see Figure 24.3). In most cases, specific vaccines are required for children to enter public school. When the vaccine regimen is complete, most childhood vaccinations lead to lifetime immunity. Others, such as the tetanus and pertussis vaccines, must be readministered periodically as booster shots to continue immunity protection.

Allied health professionals should be informed of immunization schedules and be certain they are personally up-to-date on their immunizations. Working in the healthcare field without being properly vaccinated increases an individual's risk of exposure to diseases and promotes disease transmission. Certain vaccines are recommended for healthcare personnel. These immunizations include hepatitis B vaccination and an annual influenza shot. Many healthcare employers require their employees to get these vaccinations and keep all others current as part of employment. Furthermore, allied health professionals who manage health records may be responsible for maintaining immunization records as part of their job responsibilities.

In the Know

Community immunity, or *herd immunity*, describes a situation in which a sufficient proportion of a population has immunity to an infectious disease (usually through vaccination or prior exposure). Community immunity, in theory, makes it less likely for disease to spread from person to person; in other words, protection is extended to those individuals within the community who do not have immunity.

FIGURE 24.3 CDC Immunization Schedule for Adults (2015)

The first adult immunization schedule was published by the CDC in 2002 and is updated annually. The CDC also publishes an adult immunization schedule based on medical and other indications that is designed for use by healthcare professionals. To view these immunization schedules, go to http://PharmEssAH.emcp.net/ImmunizationSchedule.

VACCINE ▼ AGE GROUP ▶	19-21 years	22-26 years	27-49 years	50-59 years	60-64 years	≥ 65 years
Influenza*	1 dose annually					
Tetanus, diphtheria, pertussis (Td/Tdap)*	Substitute 1-time dose of Tdap for Td booster; then boost with Td every 10 yrs					
Varicella*	2 doses					
Human papillomavirus (HPV) Female*	3 doses	3 doses				
Human papillomavirus (HPV) Male*	3 doses	3 doses				
Zoster					1 dose	1 dose
Measles, mumps, rubella (MMR)*	1 or 2 doses					
Pneumococcal 13-valent conjugate (PCV13)*					1-time dose	
Pneumococcal polysaccharide (PPSV23)	1 or 2 doses					1 dose
Meningococcal*	1 or more doses					
Hepatitis A*	2 doses					
Hepatitis B*	3 doses					
Haemophilus influenzae type b (Hib)*	1 or 3 doses					

*Covered by the Vaccine Injury Compensation Program

For all persons in this category who meet the age requirements and who lack documentation of vaccination or have no evidence of previous infection; zoster vaccine recommended regardless of prior episode of zoster

Recommended if some other risk factor is present (e.g., on the basis of medical, occupational, lifestyle, or other indication)

No recommendation

Common Vaccines

Many vaccines are administered in physicians' offices, clinics, or inpatient settings. Greater numbers of vaccines are administered in community pharmacies every day. For example, many patients now receive their annual **influenza vaccine** at their local pharmacies. To learn more about common vaccines, their routes of administration, and their reason for use, see Table 24.2.

Numerous clinics and pharmacies operate **travel immunization clinics**. These clinics can help prepare people for travel and provide immunizations and advice about what vaccines are recommended or necessary for global travel. Examples of travel vaccines include those for hepatitis and cholera. These diseases are not common enough to warrant mass vaccination in the United States but are found in other parts of the world. When traveling from an area of low rates

Work Wise

Yellow fever is a vaccine recommended by the CDC for individuals traveling to or living in high-risk areas of South America and Africa. If one of your patients is traveling to these areas, you have an opportunity to educate him or her on vaccination best practices. You should also tell your patient that some countries do not allow foreigners to enter without documentation of yellow fever immunization.

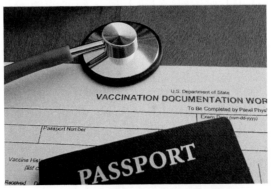

The CDC offers a travelers' health website (http://PharmEssAH.emcp.net/CDCtravel) that provides guidance on vaccines needed to travel to certain countries.

TABLE 24.2 Common Vaccines

Generic (Brand)	Route of Administration	Prophylaxis
Bacille Calmette-Guerin (BCG)	Injection	• Recommended for patients at high risk of exposure to tuberculosis • Recommended for healthcare workers in high-risk settings only (refer to Chapter 17 for an explanation of these settings)
Diphtheria, pertussis, and tetanus (various combinations available)	Injection	• Diphtheria, pertussis (whooping cough), and tetanus in children and adults
Haemophilus influenzae type B or Hib (ActHIB, PedvaxHIB)	Injection	• *Haemophilus influenzae* type B in children
Hepatitis A or HAV (Havrix, Vaqta)	Injection	• Recommended for patients at high risk of exposure to hepatitis A
Hepatitis B or Hep B (Engerix-B, Recombivax HB)	Injection	• Hepatitis B in children • Recommended for adults at high risk of exposure to hepatitis B • Recommended for healthcare workers
Hib + Hep B (Comvax)	Injection	• *Haemophilus influenzae* type B and hepatitis B in children
Human papillomavirus or HPV (Cervarix, Gardasil, Gardasil 9)	Injection	• Recommended for girls and women 9–26 years old to prevent cervical cancer and genital warts due to HPV • Recommended for boys and men 9–26 years old to prevent anal cancer and genital warts
Influenza (Afluria, Fluarix, Flu-Laval, Fluvirin, Fluzone)	Injection	• Influenza in children and adults • Recommended for healthcare workers
Influenza (FluMist)	Intranasal	• Influenza in patients 2–50 years old • Recommended for healthcare workers
Japanese encephalitis (JE-VAX)	Injection	• Recommended for patients at high risk of exposure to Japanese encephalitis
Measles, mumps, rubella (MMR II, ProQuad)	Injection	• Measles, mumps, and rubella in adults and children
Meningococcal (Menactra, Menomune)	Injection	• Recommended for patients at high risk of exposure to *Neisseria meningitidis*
Pneumococcal, conjugate (Prevnar)	Injection	• Pneumonia and otitis media (ear infections) in children
Pneumococcal, polyvalent (Pneumovax 23)	Injection	• Pneumonia in patients under 2 years old or over 50 years old
Polio, inactivated or IPV (IPOL)	Injection	• Poliovirus in children
Rotavirus (Rotarix, RotaTeq)	Oral	• Rotavirus in infants and children
Typhoid (Typhim Vi)	Injection	• Recommended for patients at high risk of exposure to typhoid fever
Typhoid (Vivotif Berna)	Oral	• *Salmonella typhi* in adults and children
Varicella (Varivax)	Injection	• Chickenpox in children
Yellow fever (YF-Vax)	Injection	• Recommended for patients at high risk of exposure to yellow fever
Zoster (Zostavax)	Injection	• Herpes zoster (shingles) in patients 60 years old and older

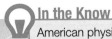
of infection to areas with high rates of infection, travel vaccines are recommended or required. **Travel vaccines** must be given well in advance of travel to allow the immune system enough time to mount the appropriate response and confer full immunity. Time to level of immunity differs among vaccines. Many immunizations should be given two or more weeks before travel.

Side Effects Common side effects of vaccines include fever, headache, upset stomach, local injection-site irritation, mild skin rash, and irritability. These symptoms are related to the humoral, or systemic, immune response (see Chapter 23), which makes a person feel generally tired and achy. It can feel like the onset of the flu, which is why many patients mistakenly believe that the influenza shot gave them the flu. Such symptoms can also occur after injection of other vaccines. All guidelines state specifically that taking acetaminophen for 24 to 48 hours after immunization usually alleviates these symptoms.

Patient Teaching

As an allied health professional, you will most likely encounter parents who have chosen not to vaccinate their children and have based their decision on a study that links autism with the preservatives contained in the measles, mumps, and rubella (MMR) vaccine. This situation presents you with the opportunity to have a teachable moment with parents. Explain to 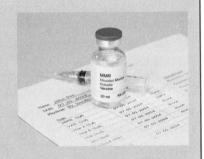 these parents and/or caregivers that this study has since been retracted and that subsequent studies in Europe and the United States have found no association between the MMR vaccine and autism. In addition, explain that organizations such as the Institute of Medicine and the American Academy of Pediatrics established panels of independent scientists to study a potential link. All panels concluded that there is no association between the MMR vaccine and autism. Finally, inform these parents that although subsequent studies have not found a connection between the preservatives and autism, vaccine manufacturers have eliminated the use of these preservatives in vaccines.

Contraindications The Bacille Calmette-Guerin (BCG) vaccine should not be administered to pregnant women or to patients who are **immunocompromised**, a state in which patients have impaired or weakened immune systems due to drug therapy (such as immunosuppressants or corticosteroids) or autoimmune disorders.

The diphtheria, pertussis, and tetanus vaccine is contraindicated in patients with encephalopathy not attributable to another identifiable cause within seven days of administration of a previous dose of that vaccine, and in patients with progressive or unstable neurologic disorder. Certain formulations include latex and those should not be administered to patients with a latex allergy.

The *Haemophilus influenzae* type B (Hib) vaccine is contraindicated in patients younger than six weeks of age.

The hepatitis A vaccine should not be given to patients with a history of a severe reaction to a prior dose of the hepatitis A vaccine or to patients who have a serious sensitivity to vaccine additives. The hepatitis B vaccine is contraindicated in individuals with a history of a hypersensitivity to yeast.

The vaccine for human papillomavirus (HPV) is contraindicated in patients with a yeast hypersensitivity.

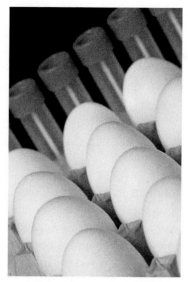

The influenza vaccine comes in both inactivated and live formulas. The inactivated influenza vaccine is grown in chicken eggs and is contraindicated in patients with egg or chicken allergies. This vaccine should be withheld in children with moderate-to-severe acute febrile illness and administered only after symptoms resolve. However, minor illness with or without fever is not a contraindication. Some inactivated influenza vaccine formulations contain thimerosal or gelatin; patients with allergies to either of these substances should avoid those formulations.

The inactivated form of the influenza vaccine is grown in chicken eggs and should not be administered to patients with egg or chicken allergies.

Contraindications to the live influenza vaccine include the following: age younger than 2 years; history of an anaphylactic reaction to gelatin or arginine; long-term aspirin or salicylate therapy; history of Guillain-Barré syndrome; asthma in children younger than 5 years; recurrent wheezing in children ages 2 to 4 years; chronic pulmonary, cardiovascular, renal, hepatic, neurologic, hematologic, or metabolic disorders; pregnancy; known or suspected immunodeficiency; or receipt of other live virus vaccines within the previous four weeks.

The Japanese encephalitis vaccine contains protamine sulfate; therefore, its use should be avoided in patients with a protamine hypersensitivity.

Contraindications to the MMR vaccine include an anaphylactic reaction to neomycin, pregnancy, and known altered immunodeficiency states. The MMR vaccine is a live vaccine and use should be withheld in severe febrile illness until the acute illness has subsided.

The rotavirus vaccine is contraindicated in patients with a history of intussusception (a gastrointestinal [GI] disorder) and severe combined immunodeficiency disease.

The oral typhoid vaccine is contraindicated in patients who are immunocompromised or in those patients who have acute febrile illness.

Contraindications to the varicella vaccine include patients who are immunocompromised, as this vaccine contains a live virus.

The yellow fever vaccine should not be given to patients who have a hypersensitivity to egg or chicken protein; children younger than six months of age; patients who are immunosuppressed (from disorders or use of medications that induce immunosuppression); patients with thymus disorder associated with abnormal immune function; and patients who have undergone organ transplantation.

Contraindications to the zoster vaccine include a history of anaphylactic reaction to gelatin or neomycin; immunosuppression; primary and acquired immunodeficiency states; acquired immunodeficiency syndrome (AIDS) or clinical manifestations of HIV; immunosuppressive therapy; or pregnancy.

The meningococcal, pneumococcal, polio (inactivated), and injectable typhoid vaccines do not have contraindications.

Note: Allied health professionals should be aware that an allergy to a particular drug contraindicates its use. This warning applies to all Contraindications sections in this chapter.

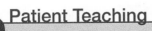
The typhoid vaccine is available in an oral dosage form. The oral vaccine is given as three capsules, one capsule every other day. Oral typhoid capsules must be refrigerated and should be taken with cold or lukewarm water about one hour prior to eating a meal. Antibiotics and some malaria medications can decrease the vaccine's effectiveness; consequently, concurrent use should be avoided.

Cautions and Considerations Like any drug therapy, immunization is not without risk. Patients must receive written information about risks before getting a vaccination. A **vaccine information sheet (VIS)** is available from the CDC for all vaccines on the market. Allied health professionals can find samples of these sheets at the CDC website (http://PharmEssAH.emcp.net/VaccineInfo). Prior to vaccination, patients must sign a consent form stating that they are making an informed decision to receive a vaccine and verifying they have received a VIS for the appropriate vaccine. Quite often, obtaining these signatures and maintaining documentation records are the

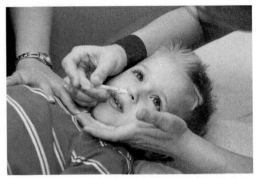

FluMist is a nasal spray option for those who want to get the influenza (flu) vaccine without an injection. This dosage form is only for patients 2 to 50 years of age and contains a live attenuated virus, rather than a deactivated virus. Patients should be aware of the extra precautions and limitations for use of FluMist.

responsibilities of allied health professionals. These responsibilities should not be taken lightly because the patient consent form is required by law.

Healthcare personnel giving immunizations must be trained in administering cardiopulmonary resuscitation and other necessary treatments in the event of an anaphylactic reaction.

Work Wise

If you are trained or certified in vaccine administration, note this skill on your résumé and, if appropriate, during a job interview. Vaccine administration is a special skill in which potential employers may be interested.

Most vaccines require storage in either the refrigerator or freezer. The recommended storage temperature range can differ from vaccine to vaccine and must be strictly followed. Most vaccine products cannot be used if frozen. If allowed to warm to room temperature, most vaccines must be used right away (not refrigerated again). Daily temperature measurement of refrigerators and freezers is required to ensure that stored vaccines are kept at the appropriate temperature and do not spoil. Vaccines that are supplied as powder for injection usually must be used within minutes to hours after reconstitution. Advance mixing and preparation of multiple doses are not recommended.

Vaccine Adverse Event Reporting System

A separate reporting system, called the **Vaccine Adverse Event Reporting System (VAERS)**, is a postmarketing national safety surveillance system operated by the FDA and the CDC to collect and analyze information about adverse events that occur after a vaccination. Since 1990, VAERS has received over 123,000 reports, most of which describe mild side effects such as fever. As with medications, hundreds of thousands of vaccine administrations may be required to detect a potential problem. In fact, it may take more than a million doses of a vaccine for a few adverse effects to occur and be investigated.

The FDA and the CDC use VAERS information to ensure the safest strategies of vaccine use and to further reduce the rare risks associated with vaccines. Healthcare personnel are mandated by the National Childhood Vaccine Injury Act of 1986 to report serious adverse reactions from vaccines. In addition, patients can report any problems with a vaccine. A VAERS report can be made online or by mail or fax using a form downloaded from the VAERS website (http://PharmEssAH.emcp.net/VAERS).

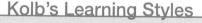

Kolb's Learning Styles

No matter what learning style(s) you prefer, you can learn from applying vaccination concepts to your own health history. Look up your vaccination records and determine your immunization status for hepatitis A and B. Depending on your age, you may have been vaccinated against these diseases as a child, as is recommended currently. Did you get all three doses of the hepatitis B series? Did you get boosters of the hepatitis A vaccine? This practical application exercise is useful for remembering vaccinations and completes a task that is necessary for anyone hoping to be employed in the healthcare field.

Checkpoint 24.1

Take a moment to review what you have learned so far and answer these questions.

1. How many doses of the HPV vaccine should female patients receive?

2. What are common side effects of vaccines?

Autoimmune Disorders

Autoimmune disorders occur when the body's immune system attacks and destroys healthy organs, tissues, and cells. When an individual has an autoimmune disorder, his or her body does not accurately distinguish between self and foreign bodies, meaning the body produces antibodies to attack its own cells. This reaction may have a negative effect on blood vessels, tissue, endocrine glands, joints, muscles, red blood cells, or skin.

Each autoimmune disorder affects different parts of the body, depending on the types of antibodies produced and the cells that are attacked. There are more than 80 distinct autoimmune disorders, and the National Institutes of Health estimates that up to 22 million Americans are afflicted with one or more. Common autoimmune disorders include the following: Crohn disease (see Chapter 18), multiple sclerosis, myasthenia gravis, psoriasis (see Chapter 9), rheumatoid arthritis (see Chapter 10), systemic lupus erythematosus, thyroid disorders (see Chapter 20), and Type 1 diabetes (see Chapter 20).

MS

Multiple sclerosis (MS) is an autoimmune disorder in which antibodies destroy the myelin sheath surrounding many nerve cells. Damaged myelin tissue forms scars (sclerosis) that interfere with coordinated signal conduction along these nerves. Symptoms usually start with visual disturbances or numbness in the limbs. Eventually, this tissue destruction leads to loss of nerve axons and white matter in the brain, causing more severe symptoms such as vision loss and paralysis. Disease progression and symptoms are variable among individual patients and can be difficult to predict.

Of the four main types of MS, **relapsing-remitting MS (RRMS)** is the most frequently diagnosed. The National Multiple Sclerosis Society estimates that up to 85% of patients with MS have RRMS. In RRMS, severe symptoms flare up, but these exacerbations are followed by periods of partial or complete remission. Most people with RRMS eventually transition to secondary-progressive MS. Secondary-progressive MS is characterized by the disappearance of remissions and steadily worsening symptoms.

Drug Regimens and Treatments

Acute relapses of MS are generally treated with corticosteroids. Patients commonly receive intravenous methylprednisolone or oral prednisone. More information about corticosteroids can be found later in this chapter in the discussion concerning autoimmune hepatitis.

Disease-modifying therapies are also used for patients who have MS. Although they do not cure the disorder, these therapies may decrease relapse rate and slow disease progression. Interferon betas, glatiramer, natalizumab, fingolimod, and teriflunomide are all commonly used therapies in MS treatment. A summary of the disease-modifying therapies can be found in Table 24.3.

Interferon Betas

Interferon betas are used for a variety of conditions affecting the immune system, including MS. Interferon betas closely resemble interferons (cytokines) naturally produced by the body. The exact way that interferon betas help in the treatment of MS is not fully understood. However, they can prevent central nervous system inflammation and demyelination. Interferon therapy is costly (tens of thousands of dollars a year) and often dispensed only in specialty pharmacies or hospitals.

Side Effects Interferon betas have many side effects, which are described in Table 24.3. Injection-site reactions are common and can include skin necrosis.

Contraindications Interferon betas are contraindicated in patients with a hypersensitivity to human albumin.

Cautions and Considerations Hypersensitivity reactions are a concern with interferon betas. Anaphylaxis is associated with interferon use and may occur immediately after initiation of therapy or after prolonged use.

Interferon betas are associated with asymptomatic liver dysfunction. Caution should be exercised in patients using other potentially hepatotoxic drugs.

Hematologic abnormalities including leukemia and anemia have been reported with use of interferon betas. Routine monitoring of blood cell counts is recommended.

TABLE 24.3 | Disease-Modifying Therapies for the Treatment of MS

Generic (Brand)	Route of Administration	Common Dosage	Side Effects
Interferon Betas			
Interferon beta-1a (Avonex)	IM	30 mcg once a week	Flulike symptoms, anemia, injection-site reactions
Interferon beta-1a (Rebif)	Sub-Q	22–44 mcg 3 times a week	Flulike symptoms, injection-site reactions, leukopenia, increased liver enzymes
Interferon beta-1b (Betaseron)	Sub-Q	0.25 mg every other day	Flulike symptoms, injection-site reactions, asthenia, menstrual disorders
Other Disease-Modifying Therapies (Non-Interferon)			
Dimethyl fumarate (Tecfidera)	Oral	240 mg twice a day	Flushing, abdominal pain, diarrhea
Fingolimod (Gilenya)	Oral	0.5 mg once a day	Increased liver enzymes, infections, diarrhea
Glatiramer (Copaxone)	Sub-Q	20 mg once a day	Injection-site reactions, chest pain, flushing, dyspnea
Mitoxantrone	IV	12 mg/m^2 every 3 months up to a lifetime dose of 140 mg/m^2	Nausea, alopecia, menstrual disorders
Natalizumab (Tysabri)	IV	300 mg every 4 weeks	Headache, fatigue, arthralgia
Teriflunomide (Aubagio)	Oral	7–14 mg once a day	Diarrhea, nausea, hair thinning

In the Know

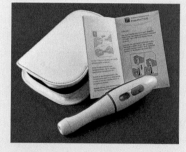

As health care shifts from a clinical setting to a home setting, medical-equipment manufacturers are using cutting-edge technology to produce devices, such as monitoring test kits and drug delivery devices, that allow patients to perform self-care. Patients with chronic disorders such as diabetes, asthma, and hypertension have benefitted from the use of these technologies. Now, patients who have MS may also be assisted in their self-care through the use of a new drug delivery device that administers interferon beta-1b.

The ExtaviPro 30G auto-injector allows patients to hold the ergonomic device securely with one hand—despite the presence of tremors—and safely inject interferon beta-1b subcutaneously. In addition to the ergonomic design, the auto-injector has additional safety features including a hidden, ultrathin needle and a syringe safety cap that can remain in place during the loading of the medication. Developed through the collaborative efforts of Novartis (a pharmaceutical company), Cambridge Consultants (a product-design and development firm), healthcare professionals, and patients with MS, the ExtaviPro 30G was recently launched in Europe and is currently under review by the FDA in the United States.

Patient Teaching

Injection-site reactions are most common with interferon betas that are administered subcutaneously. To help prevent reactions, provide patients with the following self-administration tips:

- Bring the drug to room temperature before injection.
- Apply ice to the injection site.
- Alternate injection sites.

Other Disease-Modifying Therapies

There are several disease-modifying therapies for MS in addition to the interferon betas (see Table 24.3). Unlike interferon betas, which are injectable products, these medications are available in various dosage forms.

Side Effects Side effects of disease-modifying therapies for MS are detailed in Table 24.3.

Contraindications Fingolimod is contraindicated in heart disease, stroke, heart failure, atrioventricular block or sick sinus syndrome, or with concurrent use of a class Ia antiarrhythmic (disopyramide, procainamide, quinidine) or class III antiarrhythmic. Contraindication to glatiramer includes a mannitol hypersensitivity. Natalizumab should not be used by patients with a history of progressive multifocal leukoencephalopathy. Teriflunomide is contraindicated in patients with severe liver impairment, women of childbearing age who do not use contraception reliably, and pregnancy. Dimethyl fumarate and mitoxantrone do not have contraindications.

Cautions and Considerations Dimethyl fumarate may decrease lymphocyte counts; consequently, these counts should be monitored while patients are undergoing therapy. Fingolimod is associated with the risk of varicella-zoster virus infections and tumor development. Mitoxantrone therapy may lead to bone marrow suppression and typically should not be used in patients with neutropenia. Myocardial toxicity may occur with mitoxantrone use, and the risk increases with cumulative dosing. Severe local tissue damage can occur with mitoxantrone extravasation. Natalizumab may increase the risk of developing fatal or disabling progressive multifocal leukoencephalopathy. Routine monitoring of signs and symptoms of this condition is required. Teriflunomide use is associated with a risk of liver toxicity; therefore, caution should be taken in patients with known liver disease. This agent is not recommended in pregnancy, and caution should be taken in women of childbearing age.

Kolb's Learning Styles

If you are a Converger and enjoy hands-on learning, consider making arrangements to shadow a healthcare professional such as a nurse, pharmacist, or physician at an MS clinic. What drugs do you see used most frequently? Compare and contrast the side effects of these commonly used drugs. Use the Internet or drug information references to estimate the monthly cost of therapy.

Systemic Lupus Erythematosus

Systemic lupus erythematosus (SLE), also known as *lupus*, is a chronic autoimmune disease that can affect the skin, joints, kidneys, lungs, nervous system, mucous membranes, and other organs. Like MS, SLE is characterized by periods of acute relapses and of remission. Common symptoms of SLE include fatigue, fever, and weight gain. Symptoms that patients may experience depend on the areas that are affected. Some of these symptoms include arthritis, skin lesions, Raynaud phenomenon (a disorder characterized by cold-induced color changes of the hands and feet), kidney dysfunction, GI problems (such as gastritis), pulmonary dysfunction, cardiovascular dysfunction, neurologic complications, ophthalmic issues, and hematologic dysfunction (such as thromboembolism).

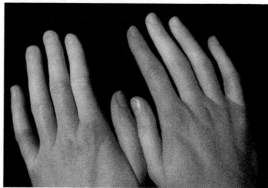

One symptom of SLE is Raynaud phenomenon, a disorder characterized by reduced bloodflow to the fingers and toes. This disorder creates a blanching of the extremities, as shown in this photo.

Drug Regimens and Treatments

Treatment of SLE is based on a myriad of factors, including patient preference, disease activity, and comorbidities. Most patients with SLE see a specialized physician called a rheumatologist. A **rheumatologist** is a physician who has completed additional training and experience in the diagnosis and treatment of musculoskeletal and immune system disorders.

Most patients with SLE are treated with hydroxychloroquine or chloroquine, which are drugs traditionally used for malaria. Oral corticosteroids (such as prednisone) or injectable corticosteroids (such as methylprednisolone) may also be used. Corticosteroids are covered more thoroughly later in this chapter. Immunosuppressants such as azathioprine or methotrexate may also be used. (Methotrexate is discussed in the graft-versus-host disease section later in this chapter.) Typical dosages of SLE medications are included in Table 24.4.

TABLE 24.4 Common Treatments for SLE

Generic (Brand)	Dosage Form	Route of Administration	Common Dosage	Side Effects
Antimalarials				
Chloroquine (Aralen)	Tablet	Oral	250 mg a day	Upset stomach, skin discoloration, agitation, anxiety
Hydroxychloroquine (Plaquenil)	Tablet	Oral	200–400 mg a day	Upset stomach, alopecia, skin discoloration
Immunosuppressants				
Azathioprine (Imuran)	Tablet	Oral	2 mg/kg a day	Malaise, nausea, vomiting, leukopenia, neoplasia, thrombocytopenia, liver toxicity, increased susceptibility to infection, myalgia, fever
Methotrexate (Otrexup, Rasuvo, Rheumatrex)	Solution for injection, tablet	IM, IV, oral, sub-Q	7.5–20 mg a week	Mouth sores, nausea, vomiting, abdominal distress, anemia and blood disorders, liver and kidney damage, Stevens-Johnson syndrome, eye irritation, heart problems

Antimalarials

Antimalarials are a class of medications traditionally used to treat malaria. However, these agents can improve SLE by decreasing autoantibody production, protecting the skin, and improving skin lesions. Hydroxychloroquine and chloroquine are the most frequently used antimalarials for the treatment of SLE.

Side Effects Side effects of antimalarials are detailed in Table 24.4.

Contraindications Contraindications to hydroxychloroquine and chloroquine include previous retinal and visual field changes. Hydroxychloroquine should not be used on a long-term basis in children.

Cautions and Considerations Chloroquine and hydroxychloroquine have been associated with cardiovascular effects, including QT prolongation. Use should be avoided in patients with QT prolongation. Ophthalmic effects (such as macular degeneration and irreversible retinal damage) have occurred with use of both chloroquine and hydroxychloroquine. Monitoring for ophthalmic effects should occur, and treatment should be discontinued immediately if signs or symptoms of visual changes occur.

Autoimmune Hepatitis

Hepatitis literally means inflammation of the liver. Viral disease (which causes hepatitis A, B, and C), alcohol use, medications, poisons, or autoimmune diseases all can cause hepatitis. **Autoimmune hepatitis** is a chronic disease in which the body's immune system attacks the liver, resulting in inflammation and liver damage. Autoimmune hepatitis may even result in liver cirrhosis (scarring) or failure.

Symptoms of autoimmune hepatitis may include fatigue, joint pain, nausea, loss of appetite, pain or discomfort in the abdominal area, skin rashes, dark yellow urine, light-colored stools, and jaundice. Symptoms can vary from mild to severe and are patient specific.

Drug Regimens and Treatments

Treatment for autoimmune hepatitis relieves symptoms but does not cure the disease. Autoimmune hepatitis is typically treated with corticosteroid therapy. The immunosuppressant azathioprine may also be used.

Corticosteroids

Systemic corticosteroids are used for their anti-inflammatory and immunosuppressant properties. They work by modifying the immune response. Systemic corticosteroids slow leukocyte function and decrease fever, redness, and swelling.

Systemic corticosteroids have many functions and are used to treat a variety of disorders. They are frequent choices for treating autoimmune disorders and hypersensitivity and allergic reactions. They also help reduce inflammation and improve breathing during asthma exacerbations and protect against organ transplant rejection. Table 24.5 includes commonly used systemic corticosteroids. (Other corticosteroids, such as topical corticosteroids and nasal/inhaled corticosteroids, are discussed in Chapter 9 and Chapter 17, respectively.)

Side Effects Common side effects of corticosteroids include headache, dizziness, insomnia, and hunger. Using corticosteroids first thing in the morning will mimic the

TABLE 24.5 Commonly Used Systemic Corticosteroids

Generic (Brand)	Dosage Form	Route of Administration	Common Dosage
Betamethasone (Celestone)	Oral solution, solution for injection	IM, intrabursal, intradermal, oral	Varies depending on preparation and indication
Budesonide (Entocort EC)	Tablet	Oral	9 mg a day
Cortisone	Tablet	Oral	25–300 mg a day
Dexamethasone (Baycadron, Dexamethasone, DexPak)	Elixir, oral solution, tablet	Oral	0.75–9 mg a day
Hydrocortisone (A-Hydrocort, Cortef, Solu-Cortef)	Oral solution, solution for injection, tablet	IM, IV, oral	IM/IV: 100–500 mg a day PO: 20–240 mg a day
Methylprednisolone (A-MethaPred, Depo-Medrol, Medrol, Solu-Medrol)	Solution for injection, tablet	IM, IV, oral	Varies depending on preparation and indication
Prednisolone (Flo-Pred, Orapred, Pediapred, Prelone)	Oral solution, suspension, syrup, tablet	Oral	Varies depending on preparation and indication
Prednisone (Prednisone Intensol, Rayos)	Oral solution, tablet	Oral	5–60 mg a day

typical daily cycle of cortisol in the bloodstream, which may lessen these effects, especially insomnia. Long-term therapy can affect normal metabolism and may result in facial swelling ("moon face"), significant weight gain, fluid retention, and fat redistribution to the back and shoulders ("buffalo hump"). For these reasons, systemic corticosteroid agents are taken on a short-term basis whenever possible. Severe effects include high blood pressure, loss of bone mass (osteoporosis), electrolyte imbalance, cataracts or glaucoma, and insulin resistance (diabetes). In some cases, long-term use of high-dose corticosteroids may cause steroid-induced psychosis. Patients taking corticosteroids long term will need special monitoring and treatment for these effects.

Contraindications Intramuscular betamethasone is contraindicated in idiopathic thrombocytopenic purpura.

Budesonide should not be used for acute bronchospasm.

Contraindications to cortisone include serious infections and administration of live virus vaccines. Dexamethasone should not be used in patients with a hypersensitivity to sulfites in the presence of systemic fungal infections or cerebral malaria.

Hydrocortisone is contraindicated in systemic fungal infections; serious infections, except septic shock or meningitis; and viral, fungal, or tubercular skin lesions. Intrathecal hydrocortisone administration is contraindicated.

Methylprednisolone should not be used in systemic fungal infections and administration of live virus vaccines.

Prednisolone and prednisone are contraindicated in acute superficial herpes simplex keratitis, live or attenuated virus vaccines, systemic fungal infections, and varicella.

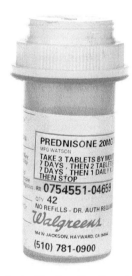

As indicated by the directions for use on this medication label, prednisone therapy must be tapered. Stopping any corticosteroid abruptly can lead to adverse or life-threatening effects for the patient.

Cautions and Considerations Patients taking corticosteroids longer than a couple of weeks should slowly decrease the dose over time when discontinuing therapy. Abruptly changing corticosteroid levels can cause untoward and even life-threatening effects.

Because corticosteroids suppress the immune system, patients taking these medications are at an increased risk of infection. Patients may have to follow precautions similar to those for other immunosuppressants.

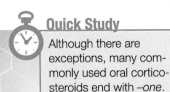

Quick Study

Although there are exceptions, many commonly used oral corticosteroids end with *-one*.

Corticosteroids can increase blood glucose levels. Use with caution in patients with diabetes.

Budesonide should be swallowed whole, not crushed or chewed.

With prolonged use, corticosteroids have been found to stunt growth in children. Again, therapy should be as brief as possible but is often necessary to properly treat conditions such as asthma.

Graft-Versus-Host Disease

Organ transplantation is indicated when an existing organ no longer functions properly or effectively. Organs that are routinely transplanted include the heart, intestines, kidney, liver, lung, and pancreas. In 2013, nearly 30,000 organs were transplanted in the United States.

When an individual receives an organ or a stem cell transplant, host T cells may detect and attack the foreign tissue, and host B cells make antibodies against it. Unless **immunosuppressive therapy** is begun, the body will reject an implanted organ. Before transplant surgery, tissue typing is performed to find a good match for organ donation, which helps reduce the chance of **organ rejection**. However, tissue typing never completely eliminates this risk. If nothing is done to prevent a body's natural immune response to foreign tissue, the new organ will be destroyed. In addition, T cells remaining in the transplanted organ can mount an attack against the recipient's body after transplantation, a reaction called **graft-versus-host disease**.

Acute graft-versus-host disease presents within six months of transplantation. Symptoms of acute disease include abdominal pain, nausea, vomiting, jaundice, and skin rash or itching. Chronic graft-versus-host disease usually begins three or more months after transplantation but can last indefinitely. Chronic disease can present with dry eyes or vision changes, dry mouth, fatigue, joint pain, shortness of breath, or weight loss.

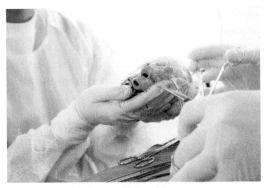

The heart is a commonly transplanted organ. According to the Mayo Clinic, the US survival rate for patients who have heart transplants is approximately 88% after one year and about 75% after five years.

Drug Regimens and Treatments

Drug therapy for graft-versus-host disease depends on the individual patient. Factors such as particular organ involvement, symptom severity, and the use of other prescribed medications all determine treatment. Corticosteroids (discussed previously in this chapter) are a mainstay of therapy. Methylprednisolone, in particular, is frequently used. Immunosuppressants, also used for prevention of graft-versus-host disease, may also be used in its treatment.

Immunosuppressants

Medications that suppress immune system activity are used perioperatively to prevent organ rejection. Although some agents mentioned in Table 24.6 are used on a short-term basis, other immunosuppressants are taken by transplant recipients to prevent organ rejection for the remainder of their lives.

Side Effects Common side effects of immunosuppressants include sore throat, cough, dizziness, nausea, muscle aches, fever, chills, itching, and headache. Most of the time, these effects are mild to moderate. Taking acetaminophen can alleviate some of these effects if they are bothersome.

Rare but serious effects include changes in heart rhythm or blood pressure, chest pain, unusual bleeding, bruising, anemia, and hyperlipidemia. Therefore, patients taking these agents need close monitoring for cardiac function and periodic blood tests. Some evidence in studies also shows that long-term immunosuppressant use may increase a patient's risk of cancer.

Drug Alert

Methotrexate may cause kidney damage leading to acute kidney failure. For that reason, patients should be instructed to drink plenty of fluids while taking this medication.

TABLE 24.6 Commonly Used Immunosuppressants for Graft-Versus-Host Disease

Generic (Brand)	Dosage Form	Route of Administration	Other Common Uses	Common Dosage for Graft-Versus-Host Disease
Cyclosporine (Gengraf, Neoral, Sandimmune)	Capsule, oral solution, solution for injection	IV, oral	Organ transplantation, psoriasis, rheumatoid arthritis	3–5 mg/kg a day
Etanercept (Enbrel)	Solution for injection	Sub-Q	Psoriasis, rheumatoid arthritis	0.4 mg/kg twice a week
Infliximab (Remicade)	Solution for injection	IV	Crohn disease, psoriasis, rheumatoid arthritis, ulcerative colitis	Varies depending on regimen
Methotrexate (Rheumatrex)	Solution for injection, tablet	IM, IV, oral, sub-Q	Acute lymphoblastic leukemia, breast cancer, Crohn disease, psoriasis, rheumatoid arthritis	10–15 mg/m²/dose; frequency varies
Mycophenolate (CellCept, Myfortic)	Capsule, solution for injection, tablet	IV, oral	Organ transplantation, SLE	Varies depending on dosage form
Sirolimus (Rapamune)	Oral solution, tablet	Oral	Organ transplantation	2 mg a day
Tacrolimus (Prograf)	Capsule, solution for injection	IV, oral	Organ transplantation, rheumatoid arthritis	Varies depending on dosage form

Contraindications Cyclosporine is contraindicated in patients with a hypersensitivity to polyoxyethylated castor oil. When used for rheumatoid arthritis or psoriasis, cyclosporine is contraindicated with abnormal kidney function, uncontrolled high blood pressure, and malignancies. Additional contraindications for prescribing cyclosporine to treat psoriasis include concomitant use of methotrexate, other immunosuppressive agents, coal tar, or radiation therapy.

Etanercept is contraindicated in sepsis.

Infliximab should not be used in patients with a hypersensitivity to murine proteins and in doses higher than 5 mg/kg for patients with moderate-to-severe heart failure.

Methotrexate is contraindicated in women who are breast-feeding.

CellCept, a brand-name drug for mycophenolate, should not be used in patients with a hypersensitivity to polysorbate 80.

Sirolimus and tacrolimus do not have contraindications.

Drug Alert

CellCept and Myfortic are both brand names for mycophenolate. CellCept is the mofetil form of mycophenolate; Myfortic is mycophenolic acid. Although the forms are similar, these drugs are not the same and should never be used interchangeably.

Cautions and Considerations Because these agents suppress the immune system, patients taking immunosuppressants are at an increased risk of infection. Patients are often instructed to take special precautions to minimize exposure to infection, such as wearing facemasks and avoiding crowded public areas. Frequent hand washing to prevent disease is always recommended.

Special administration instructions apply to each of these agents. For instance, oral tacrolimus cannot be taken with antacids. Sirolimus can be taken with or without food, but once one method is chosen, the patient should continue using that method throughout treatment. Allied health professionals should ensure patients follow administration directions carefully.

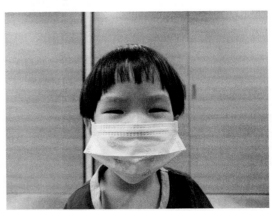

A patient who is immunocompromised should wear a facemask to reduce the risk of acquiring an infection.

Checkpoint 24.2

Take a moment to review what you have learned so far and answer these questions.

1. What interferons are available for treating MS?

2. What are common side effects of corticosteroids?

Antitoxins and Antivenoms

Antitoxins and **antivenoms** are injected antibodies used to reduce the effects of toxins and venoms in the bloodstream. The antibodies in these agents combine with the toxin or venom and neutralize it. For instance, Rh factor immunoglobulin is used to bind up antigens in the bloodstream of an Rh-negative pregnant woman who may be carrying a fetus who is Rh-positive. This immunoglobulin inactivates the antibodies the mother makes to the foreign antigens of the Rh-positive baby. Otherwise, these antibodies would build up and harm the developing fetus.

Antivenoms (also called *antivenins*) are used to treat spider bites and snakebites. If you work in an inpatient setting, you may encounter antivenoms for black widow spiders and snakes, including rattlesnakes, copperheads, and North American coral snakes. To be effective, most antivenoms must be administered intravenously within four hours of the bite. Therefore, these antivenoms are kept for use in the emergency room (ER). Orders for these products must be prepared immediately and rushed to the ER for administration.

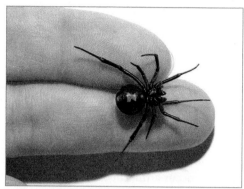

An antivenom may be administered to a patient who has been bitten by a black widow spider.

Chapter Review

Chapter Summary

The immune response is complex and can fight and protect against infectious disease. Immunization can occur naturally such as in transmission from mother to fetus and through infection exposure. It can also occur artificially, through administration of antibodies or through vaccination. The administration of vaccines is the most common form of artificial immunization and is estimated to prevent millions of deaths each year. Vaccination recommendations and schedules are released by the Centers for Disease Control and Prevention (CDC).

Autoimmune disorders occur when the immune system malfunctions and attacks healthy organs, tissues, and cells. Multiple sclerosis (MS) is such a disorder and results in central nervous system damage. MS is often treated with corticosteroids and disease-modifying therapies, including interferon betas. Systemic lupus erythematosus (SLE), or lupus, is a chronic autoimmune disorder that can affect various parts of the body. Treatment of SLE is based on patient-specific factors but often includes the use of antimalarials, hydroxychloroquine, and chloroquine. Oral corticosteroids may also be used. Autoimmune hepatitis is a condition that results in liver damage. Drug regimens for autoimmune hepatitis usually include systemic corticosteroids.

Thousands of organs, such as the heart, intestines, kidney, liver, lung, and pancreas are transplanted each year. Transplantation can result in organ rejection and graft-versus-host disease. Graft-versus-host disease is treated with corticosteroids and immunosuppressants.

Finally, antitoxins and antivenoms provide antibodies to reduce the effects of toxins and venoms. These medications usually need to be used within hours of toxin or venom exposure.

Chapter Checkup

The Navigator+ learning management system that accompanies this textbook offers many opportunities to help you master chapter content, including end-of-chapter exercises, a glossary of key terms, flash cards, and additional interactive activities.

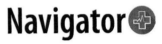 Navigator

 Career Exploration

If you enjoyed learning about acquired immunity and autoimmune disorders in this chapter, you may want to explore the following career options:

- allergy technician
- clinical immunology technologist
- clinical laboratory scientist/technologist
- diagnostic medical scientist
- histotechnologist
- medical assistant
- medical laboratory technician
- medical laboratory technologist
- pharmacy technician

UNIT

9

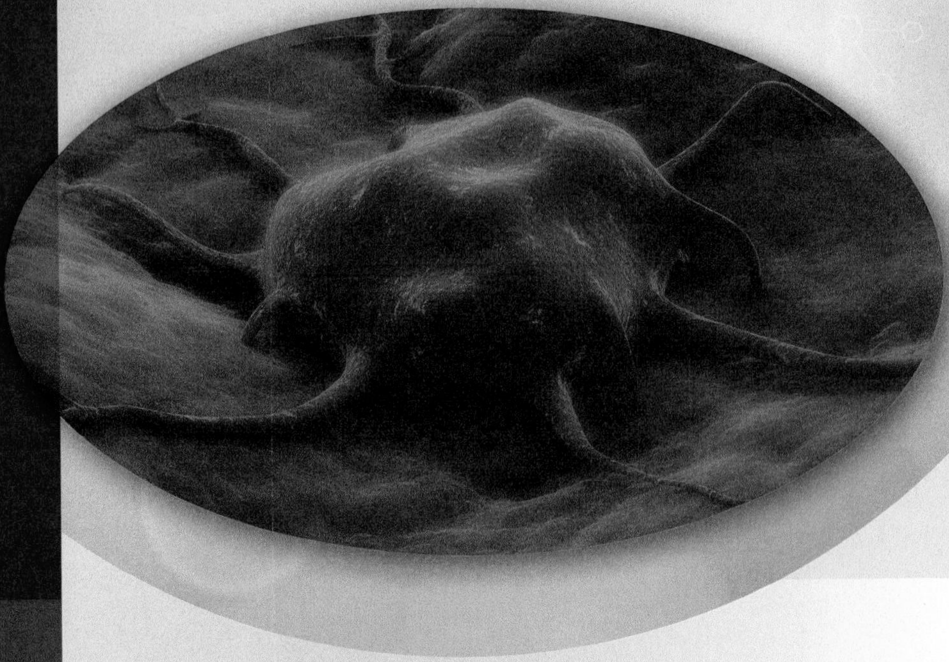

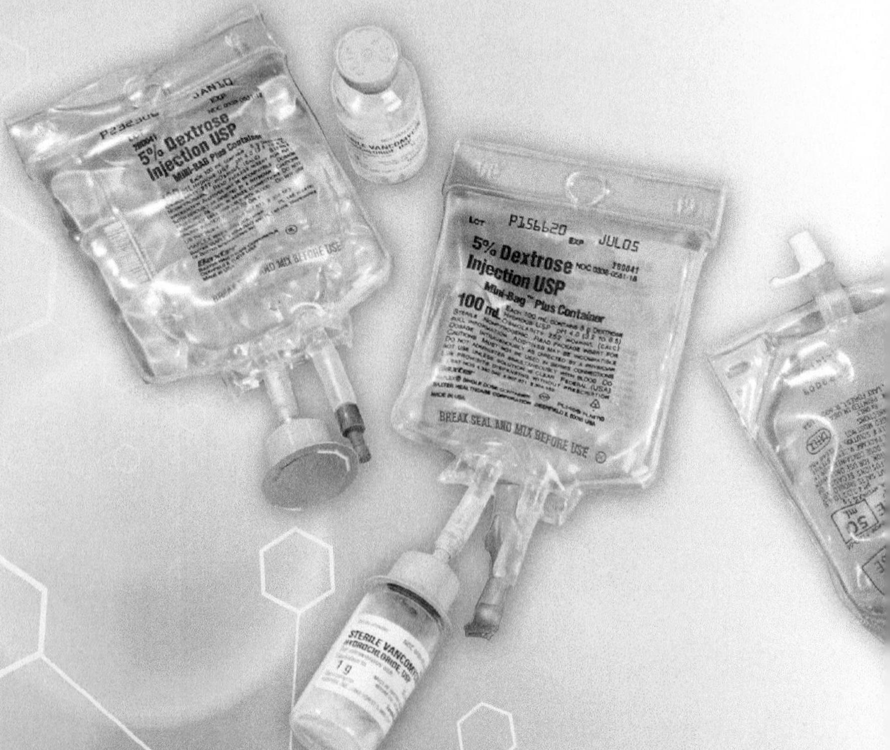

Navigator

Pharmacotherapy for Multisystems

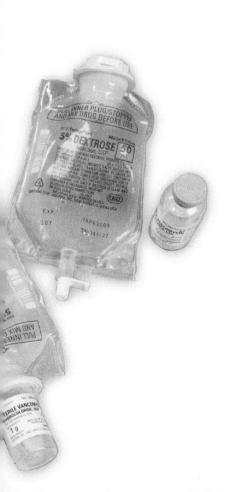

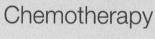

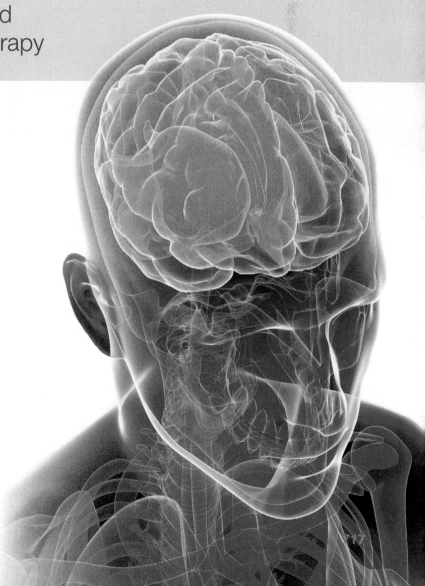

Pharm Facts

- Although the brain is the organ in which pain sensation is perceived, the brain itself does not "feel" pain. In fact, the brain lacks pain receptors. Neurosurgeons can probe brain tissue to assess muscle movement and speech while a patient is awake and feeling no pain whatsoever.

- According to the US Drug Enforcement Administration, approximately 100,000 Americans died from overdoses of painkillers in the past decade.

- A study published in *Anesthesiology*, a journal for the profession, provides evidence that a genetic mutation in natural redheads may result in an increased sensitivity to pain in this patient population.

- More than 45 million Americans suffer from chronic, recurring headaches, and 28 million of those individuals experience migraines.

- In 2013, almost 207 million opioid prescriptions were written in the United States.

"As a certified anesthesia technician, I am passionate about making a difference in the health and well-being of my patients. I work in the operating room alongside other members of the anesthesia team, including certified registered nurse anesthetists and anesthesiologists. We work in tandem to deliver outstanding care to our patients by preparing them for surgery, easing their pain, and helping them to awaken from anesthesia after a procedure. Knowing that I have helped patients on their journey to stabilization or recovery is very satisfying. Every day brings new challenges and learning experiences, and I welcome them."

—**Susan Kwiatek**, AS, Cer AT
Anesthesia Technology, Program Chair

Learning Objectives

1 Describe the basic anatomy and physiology of the nervous system as it relates to pain and sensation.

2 Describe how pain is categorized by duration, origin, or location and is assessed using different pain scales.

3 Explain the therapeutic effects of the prescription and nonprescription medications used to treat mild-to-moderate and moderate-to-severe pain disorders and to induce anesthesia.

4 Identify the generic names, brand names, indications, dosage ranges, side effects, contraindications, and cautions and considerations associated with the drugs commonly used for pain and anesthesia.

5 Identify herbal and alternative therapies that are commonly used for pain and anesthesia.

Pain is a physiologic process regulated by the nervous system. Peripheral nerves sense painful stimuli, and the central nervous system (CNS) perceives and responds. Pain is so pervasive in health care that it is considered the "fifth vital sign," something that should be assessed in all patients. Whereas acute pain is often the reason patients seek care, chronic pain usually coexists with other conditions. Treating pain is challenging because it is subjective and sometimes involves drug therapy that can promote dependence and addiction. The goal is to gain adequate pain relief without undue misuse, abuse, and addiction.

This chapter explains the physiologic process of pain perception. It also discusses analgesic options for drug therapy, including nonopioid and opioid medications. Allied health professionals should be aware of the desired and undesired effects of pain medications in order to work as a member of the healthcare team. In addition, allied health personnel must also be familiar with the legal and ethical ramifications of dispensing controlled substances, which constitute a large part of the pain-relief drug arsenal.

Finally, this chapter covers anesthesia. Anesthetic drugs work on the sensory nervous system, but they do more than treat pain. Local anesthetic drugs temporarily block or reduce pain, and general anesthetics produce a loss of the conscious sensation of pain. Anesthetic agents produce a total lack of sensation so that procedures including surgery can be performed without discomfort.

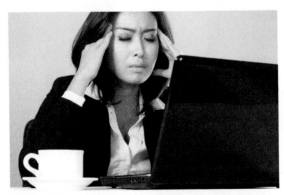

Stress, fatigue, anger, and anxiety are catalysts for a tension headache. Symptoms of a tension headache include soreness or pain at the temples and a band-like sensation encircling the head.

Anatomy and Physiology of Pain and Sensation

Pain is an unpleasant sensation and an emotional response with an important biologic function. It is a normal physiologic response to stimuli and is usually associated with tissue damage of some kind. The **peripheral nervous system** is responsible for detecting temperature, pressure, and touch as well as pain. **Sensation** starts with heat, cold, pressure, or chemical stimulus to sensory receptors and nerve endings in the peripheral nervous system. These signals travel up the spinal cord to the cerebral cortex, where sensation is perceived (see Figure 25.1). When **pain receptors** are stimulated, and the signal is sufficient, the sensation is perceived as pain. Pain alerts the body to injury or inflammation.

Inflammation causes a cascade of events starting with the release of **arachidonic acid**, which is acted on by the enzyme **cyclooxygenase** to form prostaglandins. **Prostaglandins** are chemical triggers for pain and cause local redness and swelling. They are also **pyrogens** (substances that produce fever). Some pain medications, including aspirin and other nonsteroidal anti-inflammatory drugs (NSAIDs), treat pain and fever by inhibiting prostaglandin production. Agents that treat fever are referred to as **antipyretics**.

FIGURE 25.1 | The Perception of Pain

Pain is experienced when the peripheral nervous system sensory receptors detect stimulus. This detection results in an impulse that travels to the spinal cord and ultimately the cerebral cortex, where sensation is perceived.

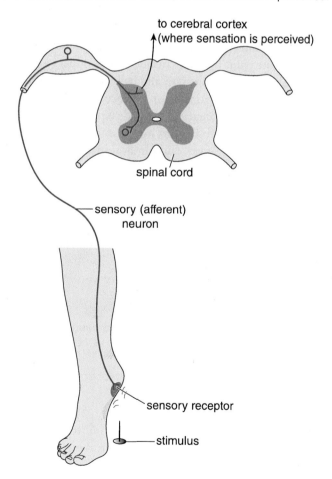

Types of Pain

Pain has a significant impact on a patient's overall health and quality of life. In addition to causing physical symptoms, it affects the patient's social, emotional, and psychological well-being. Misconceptions, however, can create barriers to detecting and adequately treating pain. In fact, pain is often undertreated. Fear of medication addictions and the subjective nature of pain make it a challenging condition to treat. Adequate pain treatment involves a good assessment of the quality, intensity, and location of the pain, along with realistic and appropriate expectations for treatment.

There are different ways to categorize pain. Pain can be described by duration, origin, or location. It is important to understand the types of pain because treatment is often designed for different categories.

Acute Pain

Acute pain describes pain that lasts less than six months and can range from mild to severe. Acute pain may be a result of injuries that heal quickly (such as mild sunburn or a sprained ankle) or relatively quickly (broken wrist). The body's response to acute pain involves the sympathetic nervous system: increases in pulse, blood pressure, and breathing rate; tensing of muscles; and dilation of pupils. Other **physiologic responses** include altered functions of the gastrointestinal (GI), urinary, and lymphatic systems.

Chronic Pain

Chronic pain lasts longer than six months and may not be associated with sympathetic manifestations such as acute pain. Instead, chronic pain produces a **compensatory response** that commonly involves depression and behavioral adaptation over time. When an individual first experiences acute pain, he or she focuses on it, talks about it, cries, moans, rubs the painful area, and grimaces. Someone with chronic pain may suffer from more subtle changes—for example, feelings of hopelessness, sleep disturbances, lack of facial expression, isolation, fatigue, anger, and physical inactivity.

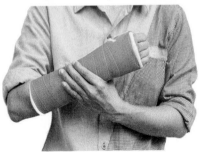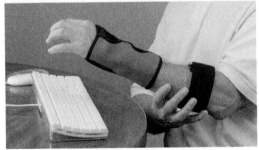

Acute pain (left) may result from a sudden injury such as a fractured wrist. Chronic pain (right) may result from a repetitive stress injury such as the compression of the median nerve in carpal tunnel syndrome.

Somatic Pain

Pain is also categorized according to where it is generated. **Somatic pain** comes from injury to body tissue. Usually somatic pain is localized, but it may vary in intensity and description. Examples of somatic pain include postsurgical incision pain and bone pain from metastases in patients with cancer.

Visceral Pain

Visceral pain comes from problems with internal organs, such as the kidneys or intestines. Because typical sensory nerves do not receive innervation from these internal organs, pain from these areas is experienced differently. Symptoms of visceral pain include nausea, vomiting, and sweating. Patients may also describe the pain as originating somewhere else in the body (referred pain). A well-known example of referred pain is the pain experienced in the left shoulder and arm that accompanies a heart attack.

Neuropathic Pain

Neuropathic pain comes from damage to nerve tissue itself. Symptoms include a tingling, burning, or stabbing pain in the area of injury. This type of pain is frequently radiating, meaning that it spreads throughout the area of the body supplied by the injured nerve. For example, nerve compression from an injured disc in the cervical spine may be experienced as pain down the arm of the affected side.

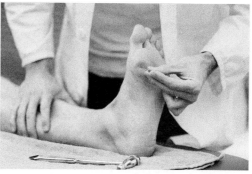

A healthcare practitioner must regularly assess the feet of a patient with diabetes to check for diabetic neuropathy, or peroneal nerve damage that results from high blood glucose levels. This condition is often treated with neuropathic pain agents.

Peripheral nerves commonly associated with neuropathic pain are the sciatic nerve in the legs, the trigeminal nerve in the face, and the peroneal nerves in the feet. This kind of pain does not always respond to typical analgesics, so alternative agents (such as antidepressants or anticonvulsants) that alter nerve signal transmission are used. Stress and painful stimuli can trigger damaged nerve tissue to begin firing in a cyclic manner. Patients may be able to reduce the occurrence or severity of these **pain cycles** through nonpharmacologic treatment, such as practicing relaxation techniques, avoiding known triggers, getting good sleep and rest, and pursuing alternative therapies such as acupuncture.

Sympathetic-Mediated Pain

Sympathetic-mediated pain is associated with nerve overactivity. In this kind of pain, the patient feels pain when there is no obvious stimulus for it. An example of sympathetic pain is phantom limb pain, which is a difficult problem to treat. **Phantom limb pain** is a condition in which a patient feels pain in a limb that is no longer there, such as an amputated leg. Nerve-blocking agents are sometimes useful for sympathetic-mediated pain.

Pain Assessment Scales

Pain intensity is subjective and requires communication from the patient to his or her healthcare practitioner. Pain measurement instruments were created to facilitate this communication. Commonly used instruments include a visual analog scale, a numeric rating scale, and a face scale.

Visual Analog Scale

A **visual analog scale** utilizes a straight line with labels at each end describing extremes. For example, one end of the visual analog scale could say *no pain*, and the other end could say *worst pain* or *pain as bad as it could be*. Patients are asked to indicate where between the two extremes their pain lies (see Figure 25.2).

FIGURE 25.2	Visual Analog Scale

A visual analog scale is one method that healthcare personnel can use to assess a patient's level of pain.

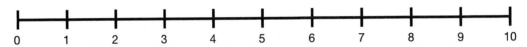

no pain ——————————————————————— pain as bad as it could be

Numeric Rating Scale

A **numeric rating scale** can be either verbal or visual and uses the numbers 0 (indicating no pain) through 10 (indicating the worst possible pain). Patients are asked to rate their pain using the scale. Numeric rating scales tend to be used more commonly by healthcare practitioners (see Figure 25.3).

FIGURE 25.3	Numeric Rating Scale

A numeric rating scale is a pain assessment tool that is commonly used by healthcare practitioners.

0 1 2 3 4 5 6 7 8 9 10

Face Scale

A **face scale** is a graphic pain assessment tool that is particularly useful in two patient populations: children and patients who have difficulty communicating. Patients are asked to point to the face that best expresses their level of pain (see Figure 25.4).

FIGURE 25.4	Face Scale

A face scale provides a visual representation of pain level. Some face scales, such as the one shown here, also provide a corresponding numeric scale and an explanation of the pain level category.

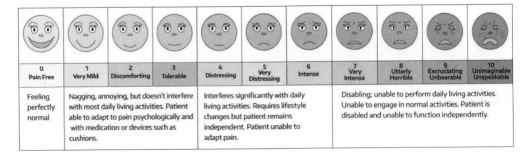

0 Pain Free	1 Very Mild	2 Discomforting	3 Tolerable	4 Distressing	5 Very Distressing	6 Intense	7 Very Intense	8 Utterly Horrible	9 Excruciating Unbearable	10 Unimaginable Unspeakable
Feeling perfectly normal	Nagging, annoying, but doesn't interfere with most daily living activities. Patient able to adapt to pain psychologically and with medication or devices such as cushions.			Interferes significantly with daily living activities. Requires lifestyle changes but patient remains independent. Patient unable to adapt pain.			Disabling; unable to perform daily living activities. Unable to engage in normal activities. Patient is disabled and unable to function independently.			

Mild-to-Moderate Pain Disorders

Assessing pain level is useful for determining treatment regimens. Pain can be grouped into mild, moderate, or severe intensity. In general, **mild pain** is described as 1 to 4 on a numeric rating scale. **Moderate pain** is a 5 to 6 on this scale.

Mild-to-moderate pain can be experienced due to a variety of disorders. As mentioned earlier, it is important to remember that pain is subjective. Whereas headache is frequently thought to cause mild-to-moderate pain, some patients experience higher pain categories. For example, cluster-type headaches are frequently described by patients as severe (7 to 10 on a numeric rating scale).

Drugs for Pain

Mild pain can be managed with over-the-counter (OTC) **analgesics**, or drugs that treat pain. Moderate pain can also be treated with the same analgesics, as well as prescription analgesics. Prescription NSAIDs and cyclooxygenase-2 (COX-2) inhibitors are used to treat moderate pain.

Nonopioid Analgesics

Analgesics can be thought of as *nonopioid* or *opioid*. A **nonopioid analgesic** (or *non-narcotic analgesic*) is a pain reliever that works independently of opioid receptors. Opioid analgesics and opioid receptors are discussed later in this chapter.

Acetaminophen

Mild pain and fever can be relieved with **acetaminophen**. This medication works by inhibiting prostaglandin production in the CNS. Acetaminophen is especially effective for pain associated with headache and for children experiencing pain or fever. It is also used in combination with opioids for moderate-to-severe pain. Combining this nonopioid analgesic with opioid drugs achieves pain relief through **synergistic drug therapy**. In this type of therapy, smaller doses are needed and fewer side effects occur than by using either agent alone (see Table 25.1). Note that acetaminophen, unlike NSAIDs, does not have a noticeable anti-inflammatory effect.

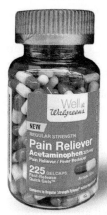

Acetaminophen is an ingredient in a variety of pain-relief products.

TABLE 25.1 Acetaminophen and Aspirin Analgesics

Generic (Brand)	Common Abbreviation	Dosage Form	Route of Administration	Common Dosage
Acetaminophen (Ofirmev, Tylenol, others)	APAP	Chewable tablet, liquid, oral disintegrating tablet, rectal suppository, solution for injection, tablet	IV, oral, rectal	IV: 650–1,000 mg every 6 hr (max 4 g a day) PO/rectal: 325–650 mg every 4–6 hr (max 4 g a day)
Aspirin (Bayer, Ecotrin, others)	ASA	Effervescent tablet, suppository, tablet	Oral, rectal	PO: 325–650 mg every 4–6 hr (max 4 g a day) Rectal: 300–600 mg every 4–5 hr (max 4 g a day)

Side Effects Acetaminophen is usually well tolerated, but common side effects may include an upset stomach or vomiting.

Contraindications Acetaminophen is contraindicated in patients with severe liver impairment or severe active liver disease.

✚ *Note: Allied health professionals should be aware that an allergy to a particular drug contraindicates its use. This warning applies to all Contraindications sections in this chapter.*

Cautions and Considerations When taken in high doses (more than 4 g a day) or used chronically at daily maximum dose levels, acetaminophen can cause liver toxicity. Intentional overdose can cause permanent liver damage or death. Patients who drink alcohol regularly should limit the total daily dose of acetaminophen to 2 g because serious liver impairment can occur. To avoid liver damage and toxicity, acetaminophen should be taken in the lowest doses possible for short-term use.

Work Wise

The pain reliever acetaminophen is used by itself and in combination with other products. Either way, you may see acetaminophen referred to by its common abbreviation: *APAP*. *APAP* stands for acetaminophen's chemical name, *N-acetyl-p-aminophenol*. Healthcare practitioners often pronounce the abbreviation "ay-pap."

Aspirin

Mild-to-moderate pain and fever in patients 16 years of age and older can be relieved with aspirin. **Aspirin** (an NSAID) works by inhibiting cyclooxygenase, the enzyme that converts arachidonic acid to prostaglandins. It is useful for pain associated with inflammation, such as menstrual cramps. It is also used in low doses for stroke and heart attack prevention based on its ability to make platelet cells less adherent to one another during blood clot formation (thrombogenesis). Aspirin is sometimes used in combination with opioids for treating moderate-to-severe pain. Combining this nonopioid analgesic with opioid drugs relieves pain through synergistic drug therapy. Other NSAIDs, such as COX-1 and COX-2 inhibitors, are described in detail in Chapter 10.

Side Effects Common side effects of aspirin can include upset stomach, GI irritation and erosion, bleeding, headache, dizziness, and skin rash. Taking aspirin with food can help avoid upset stomach and irritation. Signs of bleeding include blood in the urine or stool; black, tarry stools; bleeding in the mouth or gums; unusual or unexplained bruising; vomiting blood (which can look like coffee grounds to some people); and nosebleeds. If such effects occur, the patient should see his or her healthcare practitioner. Aspirin should not be used in patients who are already at risk for bleeding, such as during surgical procedures. Patients will usually be instructed to stop taking aspirin prior to a procedure and until well after it. Aspirin can also cause or exacerbate gout. Patients with a history of gout should use other medications for pain or fever relief.

Signs of aspirin toxicity include ringing in the ears (tinnitus), dizziness, and confusion. Patients taking aspirin who experience these effects should stop taking it and contact their healthcare practitioners.

Contraindications Aspirin is contraindicated in patients who are pregnant. Aspirin is also contraindicated in patients with a hypersensitivity to salicylates or other NSAIDs; asthma; rhinitis; nasal polyps; inherited or acquired bleeding disorders; and in children younger than 16 years of age recovering from viral infections due to a potential association with Reye syndrome. Symptoms of Reye syndrome include lethargy, confusion, disorientation, agitation, amnesia, seizures, coma, and respiratory failure. Permanent brain damage can occur. Most pediatric aspirin products have been removed from the market.

Cautions and Considerations Some patients are allergic to aspirin. For that reason, allied health professionals should take a thorough drug allergy history when conducting a

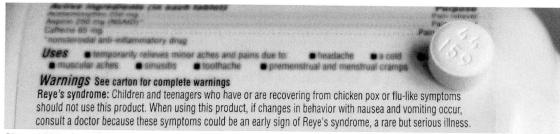

Since 1985, the US Food and Drug Administration has required that all aspirin products be labeled with a warning regarding Reye syndrome (also known as Reye's syndrome).

prescription intake with patients. They should inform patients that aspirin is contained in many OTC products—a fact that many patients do not realize.

Aspirin should not be used by patients with bleeding disorders or a history of ulcers because the risk of severe hemorrhage is high. For this same reason, patients should not take other NSAIDs along with aspirin. Other NSAIDs not only affect platelet activity and increase bleeding risk, but they also compete for activity with aspirin and decrease its effectiveness.

Drug Alert

Many patients are prescribed low-dose aspirin (typically 81 mg) to prevent blood clots and, therefore, reduce the risk of a stroke or a heart attack. Low-dose aspirin is sometimes marketed or sold as "baby aspirin" because it is a smaller dose. Unfortunately, the name "baby aspirin" can cause confusion and be mistaken for something that is safe for babies or children. Aspirin should not be used in pediatric patients to treat fever or pain, due to its association with Reye syndrome.

Checkpoint 25.1

Take a moment to review what you have learned so far and answer these questions.

1. Which analgesics can be used to treat mild-to-moderate pain?
2. What is a caution associated with acetaminophen use?

Moderate-to-Severe Pain Disorders

Moderate-to-severe pain can be caused by various disorders or injuries. Pain perception is subjective but can be assessed using a numeric rating scale. Moderate pain, as mentioned earlier, is a 5 to 6 on this scale. **Severe pain** is described as a 7 or above. Some causes of moderate-to-severe pain include fibromyalgia, shingles, and nerve damage. Some headaches, such as migraine or cluster headaches, can also cause moderate-to-severe pain. Additional information on migraines can be found in Chapter 12.

Drugs for Pain

Moderate-to-severe pain often requires prescription medications, many of which are opioids. Other treatments include neuropathic pain agents and combination products.

Opioid Analgesics

Relief for moderate-to-severe pain may require **opioid analgesics** or **opioids** (sometimes referred to as *narcotic analgesics*), alone or in combination with other analgesics (see Table 25.2). Opioid analgesics work by binding to CNS opioid receptors, specifically mu-opioid and kappa-opioid pain receptors. Natural endorphins work at these receptors to produce analgesia and a sense of well-being. When these drugs connect with opioid receptors, pain perception and processing decrease. Additional effects include cough suppression and generalized **CNS depression**.

Opioid analgesics can produce **euphoric effects** that mimic the natural endorphins that the body makes. **Endorphins** are produced in response to pain and stress in order to help the body deal with pain. Opioids, including natural endorphins, may reduce anxiety and feelings of restlessness and create feelings of well-being. Due to these effects, opioid analgesics can promote dependence, which can lead to addiction. For this reason, opioids are controlled substances with regulations for handling and storage in the pharmacy. (For more information about controlled substances, see Chapter 8.)

Name Exchange

In the workplace setting, you will often hear patients and healthcare practitioners refer to opioid analgesics by their brand names. For example, products that contain hydrocodone and acetaminophen are referred to as "Vicodin," and oxycodone and acetaminophen products are referred to as "Percocet."

Addiction is a compulsive behavioral disorder in which a patient becomes preoccupied with habit-forming substances (such as opioids or alcohol). The patient displays decreased general function and ability to participate in normal life activities and begins altering normal behavior to obtain more of the substance of addiction. Patients who are addicted may see multiple prescribers and visit many pharmacies to satisfy their need for more of the drug. They will likely need counseling in addition to medical treatment. Patients are usually more successful at overcoming addiction if withdrawal symptoms are treated appropriately. For example, drugs such as benzodiazepines can help with alcohol withdrawal. Methadone, an opioid analgesic with less of a euphoric effect than other opioids, can be substituted for other opioids (including heroin) when addiction is present.

Fear of addiction is a major barrier to adequate pain control. When pain is not controlled adequately, patient behavior can appear to be drug seeking and inappropriate when instead it is simply an attempt to get adequate pain relief. Allied health professionals can help patients to understand the nature of the tolerance and dependence effects inherent in opioid drug use. Many times, patients believe that tolerance and dependence are conditions that indicate addiction, so they resist appropriate therapy. (For more information about drug dependence and drug-seeking behavior, see Chapter 2.)

Codeine and Morphine

Codeine and morphine are known as natural opiates. As the name suggests, **natural opiates** are derived from sources found in nature. Codeine and morphine are alkaloids of the poppy plant, *Papaver somniferum*, and are difficult to synthesize.

Codeine can be used to treat moderate pain or cough. For analgesia, codeine is available by itself or in combination with nonopioid analgesics. Morphine is commonly used to treat moderate-to-severe pain. Morphine is available in oral, rectal, and injectable dosage forms.

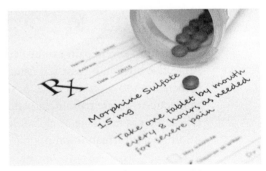

Morphine, an opiate compound, was discovered in the early 1800s by Friedrich Wilhelm Serturner, a pharmacist's assistant. Because of the compound's sleep-inducing properties, he named it *morphine*, after the Greek god of dreams, Morpheus.

TABLE 25.2 Commonly Used Opioid Analgesics

Generic (Brand)	Dosage Form	Route of Administration	Common Dosage	Drug Classification
Natural Opioids				
Acetaminophen/codeine (Tylenol No. 3 and No. 4)	Oral solution, suspension, tablet	Oral	Every 3–4 hr to every 4–6 hr	Schedule III and Schedule V
Morphine (Duramorph, MS Contin, others)	Capsule, oral solution, solution for injection, suppository, tablet	IM, IT, IV, oral, rectal	Varies depending on dosage form	Schedule II
Semisynthetic Opioids				
Hydrocodone/acetaminophen (Lortab, Vicodin)	Capsule, elixir, oral solution, tablet	Oral	PO (capsule and tablet forms): 1–2 capsules or tablets every 4–6 hr (do not exceed 4 g of acetaminophen a day) PO (elixir and oral solution): 2.5–10 mg of the hydrocodone component every 4–6 hr (max dose may be limited by the acetaminophen component)	Schedule II
Hydrocodone/ibuprofen (Vicoprofen)	Tablet	Oral	1–2 tablets every 4–6 hr	Schedule II
Hydromorphone (Dilaudid, Dilaudid-HP, Exalgo)	Liquid, solution for injection, suppository, tablet	IV, oral, rectal	IV: 0.2–1 mg every 2–3 hr PO: 1–4 mg every 4–6 hr Rectal: 3 mg every 6–8 hr	Schedule II
Oxycodone (OxyContin)	Capsule, liquid, oral solution, tablet	Oral	Acute pain: 5 mg every 6 hr Chronic pain: 10–160 mg every 12 hr	Schedule II
Oxycodone/acetaminophen (Endocet, Percocet, others)	Capsule, oral solution, tablet	Oral	PO (capsule and tablet forms): 1–2 capsules or tablets every 4–6 hr (do not exceed 4 g of acetaminophen a day) PO (solution): 5–10 mg of the oxycodone component every 4–6 hr (do not exceed 4 g of acetaminophen a day)	Schedule II
Oxycodone/aspirin (Endodan, Percodan)	Tablet	Oral	1–2 tablets every 4–6 hr	Schedule II
Synthetic Opioids				
Fentanyl (Abstral, Duragesic, Fentora, Lazanda, Onsolis, Subsys)	Film for buccal application, liquid spray, lozenge, patch, solution for injection, sublingual tablet, tablet	Buccal, IM, IV, nasal, oral, sublingual, transdermal	Varies depending on dosage form	Schedule II
Methadone (Dolophine)	Liquid concentrate, oral solution, solution for injection, tablet	IM, IV, oral, sub-Q	Varies depending on dosage form and use	Schedule II
Tramadol (Ultram)	Tablet	Oral	50–100 mg every 4–6 hr (400 mg a day max)	Rx only
Tramadol/acetaminophen (Ultracet)	Tablet	Oral	2 tablets every 4–6 hr (8 tablets a day max)	Rx only

Side Effects Side effects of codeine and morphine include drowsiness, fever, xerostomia (dry mouth), bradycardia, anxiety, euphoria, fatigue, hallucination, skin rash, and hypersensitivity reaction.

Contraindications Codeine and morphine are contraindicated in patients with **respiratory depression** (a decreased breathing rate), acute or severe bronchial asthma, and paralytic ileus. Codeine should not be used for postoperative pain management in children who have undergone tonsillectomy and/or adenoidectomy.

Specific morphine dosage forms have contraindications. Epidural or intrathecal morphine should not be used in the presence of upper airway obstruction. Extended-release morphine should not be used in patients with GI obstruction. Injectable forms are contraindicated in heart failure due to chronic lung disease, cardiac arrhythmias, increased intracranial pressure, head injuries, brain tumors, acute alcoholism, delirium tremens, seizure disorders, and during labor when a premature birth is anticipated. Morphine rectal suppositories should not be used in the presence of severe CNS depression, cardiac arrhythmias, heart failure due to chronic lung disease, increased intracranial or cerebrospinal pressure, head injuries, brain tumor, acute alcoholism, delirium tremens, seizure disorders, biliary tract surgery, suspected acute abdomen, surgical anastomosis, and concurrent use of monoamine oxidase inhibitors (MAOIs) or use of these medications within the past two weeks.

Cautions and Considerations Respiratory depression is a concern with all opioid products. In fact, the extended-release formulation of morphine has a black box warning for serious, life-threatening, or fatal respiratory depression. Patients using the extended-release formulations should be advised to swallow the capsule or tablet whole as expedited absorption (from crushing, chewing, or dissolving) can increase the risk of respiratory depression. All forms of morphine also carry a black box warning for abuse potential and addiction.

Opioids carry the risk of CNS depression that may impair physical or mental abilities. Patients must be warned not to complete tasks that require alertness (such as driving).

Constipation is common with opioids, particularly with chronic use. Bowel obstruction may occur in patients with underlying GI disorders.

Opioids may also cause hypotension, and patients at risk for hypotension or falls should use caution when taking opioids.

Hydrocodone, Hydromorphone, and Oxycodone

Semisynthetic opioids are made by chemically modifying natural opioids. Commonly used semisynthetic opioids include hydrocodone, hydromorphone, and oxycodone, which are used to treat moderate-to-severe pain. More information about semisynthetic opioids can be found in Table 25.2.

Side Effects Side effects of semisynthetic opioid analgesics are similar to those of other opioids. They include sedation, dizziness, upset stomach, fatigue, headache, and constipation. Taking these medications with food may alleviate upset stomach. Patients on high doses or taking an opioid for longer than a few days may need to take a stool softener to help with constipation. Patients should drink plenty of fluids and maintain good fiber intake to counteract constipation. Less common side effects include changes in blood pressure and heart rate.

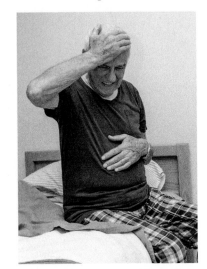

Constipation is a common side effect of opioid pain relievers, especially in older adults. A healthcare practitioner often prescribes a stool softener for a patient who is taking an opioid for more than a few days.

Contraindications Contraindications to hydrocodone/acetaminophen include CNS depression and severe respiratory depression. Hydrocodone/ibuprofen should not be used in patients who have a history of asthma or urticarial or allergic reactions to aspirin or other NSAIDs. This medication should also be avoided to treat perioperative pain in the setting of coronary artery bypass graft.

Hydromorphone has general contraindications and ones that are specific to particular dosage forms. Generally, hydromorphone is contraindicated in acute or severe asthma and severe respiratory depression. Liquid and tablet forms should not be used in the setting of obstetric analgesia. Dilaudid injections should not be used in opioid-nontolerant patients. Dilaudid-HP should not be used in patients who are at risk for developing GI obstruction. The Exalgo product should not be used in opioid-nontolerant patients, or in settings of paralytic ileus, preexisting GI surgery resulting in narrowing of the GI tract, loops in the GI tract, or GI obstruction. Hydromorphone suppositories are contraindicated in intracranial lesions associated with increased intracranial pressure and respiratory depression.

Contraindications to oxycodone include significant respiratory depression, hypercarbia (a condition of abnormally high carbon dioxide levels), acute or severe bronchial asthma, paralytic ileus, and GI obstruction.

Cautions and Considerations Hydrocodone, hydromorphone, and oxycodone products carry a black box warning for abuse potential and addiction as well as for respiratory depression.

Opioids may interact with alcohol, and combined use may result in potentiation of dangerous side effects, including respiratory depression. Concomitant use is not advised. Opioids may also cause hypotension, and patients at risk for hypotension or falls should use caution when taking these medications.

Semisynthetic opioids are associated with constipation, and preventive constipation measures should be considered.

Fentanyl, Methadone, and Tramadol

Synthetic opioids are opioid analgesics that are not naturally occurring. Instead, they are manufactured in laboratories and have a chemical structure similar to that of natural opioids. Commonly used synthetic opioids for moderate-to-severe pain include fentanyl, methadone, and tramadol. Dosing information about the synthetic opioids can be found in Table 25.2.

Fentanyl is a synthetic opioid that can be used for pain or as an adjunct to anesthesia. Fentanyl comes in various dosage forms and can be administered via the oral, intramuscular (IM), intravenous (IV), sublingual, transdermal, buccal, and nasal routes. The injectable form of fentanyl can be used for acute severe pain. Other forms, such as the lozenge, buccal film, liquid spray, and transdermal patch, should be used only for chronic pain in patients who are **opioid tolerant** (describing a patient who is already using opioids on a long-term basis).

Methadone is used for severe pain relief as well as for drug abuse treatment. Methadone has opioid analgesic effects with fewer euphoric effects. Consequently, it is useful for heroin addiction. Heroin can be a difficult drug to stop using due to severe withdrawal effects and dependence. Patients are switched to methadone, and then doses are slowly tapered. Methadone allows patients to get assistance for their addiction and dependence.

Tramadol is an opioid analgesic used for short-term treatment (five days or fewer) of moderate-to-severe pain. It is an alternative to other opioids when strong pain control is needed but the side effects of other opioids are intolerable or addiction potential is high. Tramadol works by modulating serotonin and norepinephrine in addition to blocking mu-opioid receptors, so its effects differ slightly from those of other opioid analgesics. Although tolerance and dependence can occur, tramadol is not typically habit-forming, nor is it a controlled substance in every state.

Side Effects Side effects of synthetic opioids include feelings of nervousness, restlessness, and anxiety. Some patients experience insomnia, whereas others may experience drowsiness. Other side effects include flushing, dizziness, and muscle weakness.

Contraindications Fentanyl has contraindications based on different formulations. Transdermal fentanyl patches should not be used in severe respiratory disease or depression, paralytic ileus, or in patients who require short-term therapy or are nontolerant to opioids. Buccally administered fentanyl lozenges, sublingual tablets, and liquid spray are contraindicated in the management of acute or postoperative pain and in patients who are nontolerant to opioids.

Contraindications to methadone include significant respiratory depression, acute or severe bronchial asthma, or concurrent use of selegiline. Methadone should not be used on an as-needed basis.

Tramadol is contraindicated in acute intoxication with alcohol, hypnotics, centrally acting analgesics, opioids, or psychotropic drugs; severe/acute bronchial asthma; or respiratory depression.

Cautions and Considerations Methadone has two black box warnings. One is for QT prolongation and cardiac arrhythmias. Patients using methadone should be closely monitored for changes in cardiac rhythm. The other black box warning is for serious, life-threatening, or fatal respiratory depression. Fentanyl also carries the black box warning for respiratory depression.

Methadone's pharmacokinetic properties are complex, and there is a risk of drug accumulation. For those reasons, only experienced clinicians should prescribe methadone, and use of the drug requires close patient monitoring.

Because opioids are CNS depressants, they should not be used with alcohol because excessive sedation and respiratory depression can occur.

Tramadol can lower the **seizure threshold** (the level at which your brain will have a seizure), so patients with seizure disorders should discuss therapy with their healthcare practitioners before taking this medication.

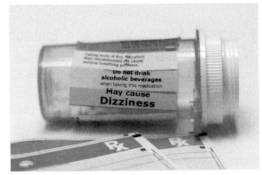

Opioid medication containers must have auxiliary warning labels that alert patients to the dangers of taking these drugs.

Drug Alert

A patient using one opioid may need to be switched to another opioid for various reasons. This situation calls for dose conversion of one opioid to another. Many opioid conversion charts and calculators exist on the Internet, and their use often results in doses that are inappropriate. Caution must be used when converting one opioid to another, and any questions about the conversion should be directed to a pharmacist or a prescriber.

Checkpoint 25.2

Take a moment to review what you have learned so far and answer these questions.

1. Consider the medications discussed in this chapter. Can you identify an example of a natural opiate, a semisynthetic opiate, and a synthetic opiate?

2. What are common side effects of opioids?

Neuropathic Pain Agents

As mentioned previously, neuropathic pain does not always respond to conventional analgesics. Anticonvulsants, the serotonin/norepinephrine reuptake inhibitor duloxetine, and tricyclic antidepressants (TCAs) are frequently used to treat this type of pain. These agents are usually taken on a long-term basis for conditions such as spinal cord injury, sciatica, trigeminal neuralgia, and diabetic peripheral neuropathy. Table 25.3 shows agents that are commonly used to treat neuropathic pain.

Work Wise

Chronic pain can be both physically and psychologically taxing for patients. As an allied health professional, it is important for you to show empathy and respect for patients. You can do this by actively listening and displaying sensitivity.

Gabapentin and Pregabalin

Gabapentin and pregabalin are indicated for the treatment of neuropathic pain. Both drugs have similar mechanisms of action. These drugs are often referred to as anticonvulsants or antiepileptics because they can be effective in seizure prevention.

Side Effects See Table 25.3 for the side effects of anticonvulsants used to treat neuropathic pain.

Contraindications Gabapentin and pregabalin do not have contraindications.

Cautions and Considerations Gabapentin and pregabalin are associated with CNS side effects such as dizziness and drowsiness. Patients should be cautioned against performing tasks that require mental alertness, such as driving.

Peripheral edema may occur in patients with heart failure, so caution should be exercised in this patient population.

TABLE 25.3 | Commonly Used Agents to Treat Neuropathic Pain

Generic (Brand)	Dosage Form	Route of Administration	Side Effects
Anticonvulsants			
Gabapentin (Gralise, Neurontin)	Capsule, oral solution, tablet	Oral	Blurred vision, drowsiness, dry mouth, headache, peripheral edema, tremors, weight gain
Pregabalin (Lyrica)	Capsule, oral solution	Oral	
Serotonin/Norepinephrine Reuptake Inhibitor			
Duloxetine (Cymbalta)	Capsule	Oral	Drowsiness, dry mouth, fatigue, headache, nausea, weight loss
TCAs			
Amitriptyline (Elavil)	Solution for injection, tablet	IM, oral	Blurred vision, constipation, drowsiness, dry mouth, urinary retention
Nortriptyline (Aventyl, Pamelor)	Capsule, oral solution	Oral	

Duloxetine

Duloxetine is classified as a serotonin/norepinephrine reuptake inhibitor (SNRI) and an antidepressant. More information on the antidepressant properties of duloxetine can be found in Chapter 13.

Side Effects See Table 25.3 for the side effects of duloxetine.

Contraindications Contraindications to duloxetine include use of MAOIs within 14 days. Initiation of duloxetine is contraindicated in patients receiving linezolid or IV methylene blue.

Cautions and Considerations Duloxetine has a black box warning about increased risk of suicidal thinking and behavior in children, adolescents, and young adults with major depression and other psychiatric disorders.

TCAs

Like duloxetine, TCAs have properties of SNRIs. More information on the antidepressant properties of TCAs can be found in Chapter 13.

Side Effects Please see Table 25.3 for the side effects of TCAs for neuropathic pain.

Contraindications TCAs should not be used concurrently with MAOIs. Amitriptyline should not be used with cisapride or in the phase or time period directly after a heart attack.

Cautions and Considerations TCAs are associated with a risk of suicidal thoughts and behaviors. For this reason, patients using TCAs should be monitored for behavior changes that may indicate suicidal thoughts.

TCAs can cause cardiotoxicity and heart arrhythmias. Patients with preexisting heart conditions or those who have recently had a heart attack should not take TCAs. These drugs can also cause orthostatic hypotension (a drop in blood pressure on sitting or standing up). Patients should take care to change positions slowly.

TCAs can lower the seizure threshold, so most patients with seizure disorders should not take these drugs. Because these agents can also cause liver toxicity, patients with liver problems should not take TCAs. Periodic blood tests are required to monitor liver function.

TCAs should not be taken with MAOIs because serotonin syndrome could develop.

Selective Serotonin Receptor Agonists (Triptans)

The class of drugs known as **triptans** is the mainstay of abortive therapy for migraine pain and may be used to treat cluster headaches. Triptans work by stimulating serotonin receptors to cause vasoconstriction. Constricting cerebral blood vessels counteracts the vasodilation that causes throbbing headache pain.

Migraine headaches are characterized by a throbbing pain on one side of the head that affects daily activities. A migraine is not fully understood but is thought to be a vascular phenomenon that occurs when cerebral surface blood vessels constrict and then rapidly dilate. Serotonin, a potent vasoconstrictor and neurotransmitter, is possibly involved. Unlike typical headaches, migraines often are accompanied by nausea, vomiting, and/or sensitivity to light. Increased sensitivity to sound is also common.

Migraines are categorized as occurring with or without *aura*. **Aura** is defined as symptoms that precede a migraine and are usually sensory disturbances. Examples of aura include visual disturbances (including seeing halos, flashing lights, floating spots, or areas of darkness or blurriness) and tingling of the face or hands. Aura is associated with the initial blood vessel constriction of a migraine and is part of the **prodrome** (or early) phase of this disorder. Aura is a warning for patients to seek immediate treatment.

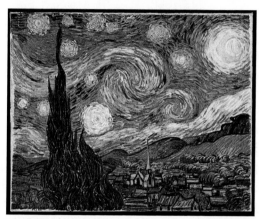

In 1889, Vincent van Gogh was being treated for "migraine personality" (which at the time was classified as *mild insanity*) at the St. Remy Asylum in France. While there, van Gogh painted *The Starry Night*, which many researchers believe depicts the aura associated with migraine headaches.

Treating migraines involves using acute pain medication (such as NSAIDs) and abortive therapies (such as triptans) that stop a headache. Preventing migraines requires that the patient avoid known triggers including certain foods, stress, sleep deprivation, medications, and environmental irritants. The hormone fluctuations associated with menstrual cycles also trigger migraines; therefore, hormonal regulation and careful timing of preventive drug therapies are employed.

For best results, triptans must be used at the first sign that a headache is starting. They begin to work in as little as 15 minutes and last anywhere from 2 hours to several hours. Once severe throbbing pain has started, these agents are not as effective. Each of the triptans has limits on the total number of doses or total dosage that patients can take every 24 hours. Injectable forms are used less frequently because fast-acting oral forms have become available (see Table 25.4).

Patient Teaching

A migraine headache can be accompanied by nausea and vomiting. For this reason, oral tablets for abortive migraine therapy are not always the best option. If you have a patient who experiences nausea and vomiting with a migraine, you may suggest that he or she explore options such as oral disintegrating tablets, nasal sprays, and injections.

TABLE 25.4 Commonly Used Triptans

Generic (Brand)	Dosage Form	Route of Administration	Common Dosage
Almotriptan (Axert)	Tablet	Oral	6.25–12 mg, may repeat in 2 hr (12–24 mg max a day)
Eletriptan (Relpax)	Tablet	Oral	20–40 mg, may repeat in 2 hr (80 mg max a day)
Frovatriptan (Frova)	Tablet	Oral	2.5 mg, may repeat in 2 hr (7.5 mg max a day)
Naratriptan (Amerge)	Tablet	Oral	1–2.5 mg, may repeat in 4 hr (5 mg max a day)
Rizatriptan (Maxalt)	Oral disintegrating tablet, tablet	Oral	5–10 mg, may repeat in 2 hr (30 mg max a day)
Sumatriptan (Imitrex)	Nasal spray, oral disintegrating tablet, solution for injection, tablet	Nasal, oral, sub-Q	Nasal: 1 spray, may repeat in 2 hr (40 mg max a day) PO: 25 mg, may repeat in 2 hr (100 mg max a day) Sub-Q: 6 mg, may repeat in 1 hr (12 mg max a day)
Zolmitriptan (Zomig)	Nasal spray, oral disintegrating tablet, tablet	Nasal, oral	Nasal: 2.5 mg, may repeat in 2 hr (5 mg max a day) PO: 2.5 mg, may repeat in 2 hr (10 mg max a day)

Side Effects Common side effects of triptans include dizziness, hot flashes, tingling, chest tightness, muscle aches, weakness, increased blood pressure, and sweating. When administered by injection, bruising sometimes occurs at the injection site. These effects are normal; if they are bothersome, alternative therapy will be required.

Contraindications Triptans are contraindicated in patients with recent use of another serotonin agonist or ergotamine-containing product. These medications are also contraindicated in patients with ischemic heart disease, arrhythmias, stroke or transient ischemic attacks, uncontrolled hypertension, hemiplegic or basilar migraine, and peripheral vascular disease. Eletriptan is contraindicated in recent use of ketoconazole, itraconazole, nefazodone, troleandomycin, clarithromycin, ritonavir, or nelfinavir. Naratriptan should not be used in patients with severe kidney impairment. Rizatriptan, sumatriptan, and zolmitriptan should not be used concurrently or within two weeks of an MAOI. Sumatriptan should be avoided in patients with severe liver disease.

Quick Study

The generic names of selective serotonin receptor agonists end in –*triptan*. For this reason, the drug class is often referred to as "the triptans."

Cautions and Considerations Patients with high blood pressure, heart disease, or angina should not take triptans because these medications can worsen these conditions. Patients taking MAOIs should not use triptans because serotonin syndrome could occur. Patients on ergotamine drug therapy should not take triptans; ergotamine therapy is saved for when triptans do not work.

Checkpoint 25.3

Take a moment to review what you have learned so far and answer these questions.

1. What are ways to prevent a migraine headache?

2. For best results, when should triptans be administered?

Combination Agents

Combinations of nonopioid analgesics and caffeine are used to treat mild migraine headaches. Using analgesics from multiple classes attacks different mechanisms of pain, thereby producing an advantage due to the effects of synergistic drug therapy. Caffeine is sometimes combined with other analgesics (see Table 25.5) because it improves pain control by constricting blood vessels, but to a lesser extent than do triptans.

Barbiturate products are sometimes used for migraines, and only a few such products are used for acute headache pain. Butalbital is available in combinations with acetaminophen and caffeine or aspirin. It is used to treat tension and migraine headache pain. The combination of butalbital and caffeine with aspirin is a controlled substance (Schedule III), but the combination with acetaminophen is not controlled.

Butorphanol, a **mixed opioid receptor agonist-antagonist**, is useful for treating migraine headache pain and is available as a nasal spray and as a solution for IM and IV administration.

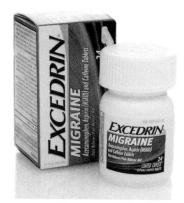

The combination product of acetaminophen, aspirin, and caffeine can be found in Excedrin Migraine.

Side Effects Common side effects of combination agents include drowsiness, dizziness, confusion, nervousness, skin rash, nausea, vomiting, heartburn, and constipation. If severe, these effects can limit therapy.

Common side effects of barbiturate-containing medications include drowsiness, dizziness, upset stomach, nasal congestion, and "hangover" feelings the day after administration. Therefore, these medications should be used with caution and on a limited basis when needed.

Butorphanol can cause drowsiness, dizziness, nausea, and vomiting. The nasal spray formulation of butorphanol can also cause insomnia.

TABLE 25.5 **Commonly Used Combination Products to Treat Headache Pain**

Generic (Brand)	Dosage Form	Route of Administration	Common Dosage	Drug Classification
Acetaminophen/aspirin/caffeine (Excedrin Migraine)	Caplet, tablet	Oral	Acetaminophen 500 mg Aspirin 500 mg Caffeine 130 mg	OTC
Isometheptene/dichloralphenazone/ acetaminophen (Midrin)	Capsule	Oral	Isometheptene 130 mg Dichloralphenazone 200 mg Acetaminophen 650 mg	Schedule IV
Barbiturates and Opiates				
Butalbital/acetaminophen/caffeine (Fioricet, others)	Capsule, liquid, tablet	Oral	Butalbital 50 mg Acetaminophen 325–650 mg Caffeine 40 mg	Rx
Butalbital/aspirin/caffeine (Fiorinal)	Capsule, tablet	Oral	Butalbital 50 mg Aspirin 325 mg Caffeine 40 mg	Schedule III
Butorphanol (Stadol)	Nasal spray, solution for injection	IM, IV, nasal	IM/IV: 1–4 mg every 3–4 hr Nasal: 1 spray in 1 nostril, may repeat in 60–90 minutes	Schedule IV

Contraindications Acetaminophen/aspirin/caffeine is contraindicated in pregnancy. Isometheptene/dichloralphenazone/acetaminophen should not be used in patients with heart or vascular insufficiency, severe kidney or liver disease, glaucoma, high blood pressure, or concomitant MAOI therapy. Butalbital products are contraindicated in porphyria. Butalbital/aspirin/caffeine is contraindicated in pregnancy. Butorphanol does not have contraindications.

Cautions and Considerations Patients should be warned about the drowsiness and dizziness effects of barbiturates and should be instructed to not drink alcohol while taking these medications because these effects could worsen.

Barbiturates produce tolerance and dependence, so they may be habit forming. The use of these medications should be limited to short term and only when needed.

Patients allergic to aspirin or other NSAIDs should not take combination products that contain aspirin.

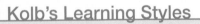

Kolb's Learning Styles

Although all learners may find this exercise useful, Assimilators and Accommodators may find it matches their learning styles best. Make a set of painkiller flash cards. Use a differently colored card for each drug classification type of product (e.g., OTC, prescription drug, and/or controlled substances). Assign each drug class (NSAIDs, opioids, nonopioids, triptans, and combination products) a different color of ink. Write the brand name on one side of the card, and the generic name on the other side of the card. Use your cards to quiz yourself and your classmates.

Anesthesia

Anesthesia inhibits sensation and pain during major procedures (such as heart transplants) and minor procedures (such as dental work). Anesthetics are also used during obstetric and diagnostic procedures. Depending on the type of procedure, general or local anesthesia will be used.

For short diagnostic procedures or to enhance relaxation, pain control, and amnesia associated with surgery, **preanesthetic medications** are sometimes used. Selected benzodiazepines (see Chapter 13) and opioid pain medications are frequently used in advance of general anesthesia. The most common preanesthetics are midazolam (Versed), diazepam (Valium), and lorazepam (Ativan), followed by fentanyl in various forms. These agents are administered systemically so they alter consciousness and cause amnesia. They reduce patient anxiety and resistance to therapy.

General Anesthesia

General anesthesia affects the entire body, and loss of consciousness occurs. Bodywide, skeletal muscle relaxes, and the patient has no memory of the event upon recovery. General anesthesia affects respiratory function and urination. Breathing slows, respiratory mucous production increases, and urination stops. Cardiac function slows, causing a decrease in blood pressure. Due to these effects, general anesthesia requires close monitoring of blood pressure, ventilation, pulse rate, oxygen level in the blood, and urinary output.

General Anesthetics

General anesthetics are used for surgery and other procedures for which overall muscle relaxation is necessary to keep the patient still during manipulation. With one exception (nitrous oxide), these agents cause loss of consciousness. Nitrous oxide is used during dental procedures to relax patients and provide analgesia.

General anesthetics are available in inhaled and injectable forms. Although these agents have varying lengths of effect, most act for only a few minutes. Therefore, an anesthesiologist or anesthetist administers and adjusts these medications throughout the procedure to individualize therapy and achieve proper sedation, relaxation, analgesia, and ventilation.

Inhaled Anesthetics

Inhaled anesthetics are stored in steel containers as compressed gas or liquid and then inhaled through a facemask. Most of these medications reduce blood pressure, so concomitant IV fluids must be administered to counteract this effect.

Side Effects Inhaled anesthetics, with the exception of nitrous oxide, are associated with decreases in blood pressure. Nitrous oxide is associated with no change or a slight increase in blood pressure. In addition, inhaled anesthetics are associated with an increase in respiratory rate.

After use of inhaled anesthetics, patients may experience shivering or trembling. Blurred vision, dizziness, nausea, and vomiting may also occur.

Contraindications Desflurane, enflurane, and isoflurane are contraindicated in patients with known or suspected genetic susceptibility to malignant hyperthermia. Desflurane is not for pediatric use. Enflurane is contraindicated in seizure disorder. Nitrous oxide should not be used without oxygen.

Cautions and Considerations General anesthetics can lower the seizure threshold, so anticonvulsants may be ordered along with these agents. For this reason, general anesthesia should be avoided when possible in patients with seizure disorders.

Malignant hyperthermia is a rare but life-threatening effect of certain general anesthetics. In this condition, body temperature increases suddenly and rapidly to dangerous levels; muscles become rigid; and patients may develop heart arrhythmias and have difficulty breathing. Hyperthermia is caused by a marked increase in intracellular calcium. Dantrolene, an intracellular calcium blocker, is used to treat malignant hyperthermia. One serious potential aspect of malignant hyperthermia is **rhabdomyolysis**. In this process, skeletal muscle is degraded, and the products of muscle breakdown can lead to acute renal failure.

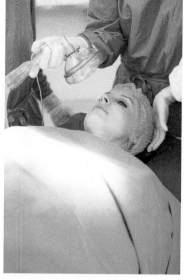

An inhaled anesthetic is administered via a facemask and renders the patient unconscious during a surgical procedure.

In the Know

The famous musician Michael Jackson died in 2009. His autopsy revealed his cause of death was acute propofol intoxication with concurrent benzodiazepine use.

In the Know

Nitrous oxide is used as a general anesthetic. There are several other uses for this agent. Nitrous oxide is used as a propellant in the food industry for items such as whipped cream. It can also be used alone or mixed with air in car engines, where it can enhance combustion and energy supply.

TABLE 25.6 Commonly Used General Anesthetics

Generic (Brand)	Dosage Form	Drug Classification
Inhaled Agents		
Desflurane (Suprane)	Gas	Rx
Enflurane (Ethrane)	Gas	Rx
Isoflurane	Gas	Rx
Nitrous oxide	Gas	Rx
Injectable Agents		
Etomidate (Amidate)	Solution for injection	Rx
Ketamine (Ketalar)	Solution for injection	Schedule III
Methohexital (Brevital)	Solution for injection	Schedule IV
Propofol (Diprivan)	Solution for injection	Rx
Remifentanil (Ultiva)	Solution for injection	Schedule II
Sufentanil (Sufenta)	Solution for injection	Schedule II

Injectable Anesthetics

Injectable anesthetics, like those that are inhaled, can be used for general anesthesia. They are administered via continuous infusion and used to induce or maintain anesthesia. Injectables are generally faster acting than their inhaled counterparts. The names and drug classifications of injectable anesthetics can be found in Table 25.6.

Side Effects Common side effects of injectable anesthetics are nausea, vomiting, decreased blood pressure, and reduced renal function. Antiemetic medications are often ordered along with the anesthetics to alleviate nausea. IV fluids are coadministered to counteract drops in blood pressure and reduced renal function.

Respiratory function is usually suppressed during general anesthesia. Because breathing slows and respiratory secretions increase, proper ventilation must be monitored throughout the procedure, and oxygen is sometimes administered.

Contraindications Ketamine is contraindicated in conditions in which an increase in blood pressure would be hazardous. Contraindications to methohexital are a hypersensitivity to barbiturates and porphyria. Propofol should not be used in patients with a hypersensitivity to eggs or soy. Remifentanil is not for intrathecal or epidural administration and should be avoided in patients with a fentanyl hypersensitivity. Sufentanil should not be used in patients with a hypersensitivity to opioids. Etomidate does not have contraindications.

Cautions and Considerations As discussed with inhaled anesthetics, general anesthesia can lower the seizure threshold, so anticonvulsants may be ordered along with these agents. For this reason, general anesthesia should be avoided when possible in patients with seizure disorders.

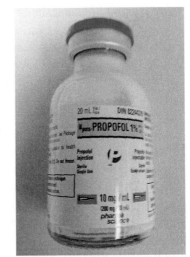

Propofol, a commonly used general anesthetic, appears cloudy or opaque. This appearance is due to its lipid- or fat-based formulation.

Like inhaled anesthetics, malignant hyperthermia is also a concern in injectable anesthetics.

Local Anesthesia

Local anesthesia affects only a designated part of the body, causing loss of pain, temperature, and tactile sensation. Skeletal muscle in the anesthetized area also relaxes. A person receiving local anesthesia may also lose the ability to recognize body position in that area. However, the patient does not lose consciousness and recalls everything that happened during the procedure.

Local Anesthetics

Local anesthetics are used when loss of sensation is desired in a defined area of the body. Procedures that may require local anesthetic action include dental work and placement of sutures. Local anesthetic agents come in a variety of dosage forms to accommodate the level of anesthesia needed in the location and size of the area being treated (see Table 25.7). For instance, they can be used topically for pain and burn relief, injected locally for dermatologic procedures, and injected as epidurals for obstetric procedures (i.e., cesarean delivery).

Local anesthetics work by depressing first the nerve activity of small axons, followed by that of larger myelinated nerve fibers. Onset of action typically occurs within a few minutes, but the duration of action depends on drug choice, drug concentration, and the size of the area to which the drug is administered.

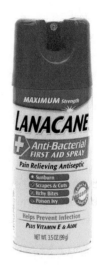

Lanacane is a spray product that contains benzocaine, a local anesthetic used as a topical pain reliever for sunburn.

TABLE 25.7 Commonly Used Local Anesthetics

Generic (Brand)	Dosage Form	Prescription Status
Esters		
Benzocaine (Anacaine, Anbesol, Cepacol, Lanacane, others)	Cream, eardrops, gel, lozenge, ointment, spray, topical liquid	OTC
Chloroprocaine (Nesacaine)	Solution for injection	Rx
Dyclonine (Sucrets)	Lozenge	OTC
Tetracaine (Pontocaine)	Solution for injection	Rx
Amides		
Bupivacaine (Marcaine)	Solution for injection	Rx
Lidocaine (AneCream, Topicaine, others)	Cream, gel, oral solution	OTC
Lidocaine (Xylocaine)	Solution for injection	Rx
Lidocaine/prilocaine (EMLA)	Cream	Rx
Mepivacaine (Carbocaine)	Solution for injection	Rx

Esters and Amides

Esters and amides are both local anesthetics. They are structurally similar but differ slightly in their chemical makeup. **Esters** are short-acting drug molecules metabolized by local tissue fluids, whereas **amides** are longer-acting drug molecules metabolized in the liver.

Side Effects Common side effects of local anesthetics include allergic reaction, skin rash, and swelling at the application site. These symptoms are usually mild. If an allergy to one chemical form (e.g., an ester) occurs, the alternate form (an amide) should be used instead.

Other side effects include **CNS excitation**. Symptoms include anxiety, nervousness, confusion, and, possibly, seizure. These effects can be treated with diazepam. Sometimes these symptoms are followed by CNS depression, including sedation, loss of consciousness, and respiratory or cardiac arrest. These effects are life threatening, and patients must receive medical treatment immediately.

Occasionally, local anesthetics are absorbed into the bloodstream and cause cardiac arrhythmias. For this reason, clinicians administer the lowest dose to the smallest area possible.

Contraindications Benzocaine is applied topically; it should not be used in the eyes or when there is a secondary bacterial infection. Chloroprocaine should not be used for subarachnoid administration (injection into the spine). Tetracaine should not be used when spinal anesthesia is contraindicated. Dyclonine does not have contraindications.

Bupivacaine should not be used for obstetric paracervical block anesthesia. Lidocaine products and mepivacaine are contraindicated in patients with a hypersensitivity to amide local anesthetics.

Cautions and Considerations When absorbed systemically, local anesthetics can lower the seizure threshold. Patients with seizure disorders should consult their healthcare practitioners before receiving any prescription-strength local anesthetics.

Analgesic and Anesthetic Antagonists

Naloxone (Evzio) is an opioid receptor antagonist that counteracts opioid pain and preanesthetic medications. It is used to reverse opioid effects in overdoses (both intentional and accidental). **Flumazenil** (Romazicon) is a benzodiazepine receptor antagonist used to reverse excessive sedation. It is used to speed recovery of consciousness in accidental or intentional overdose situations. Both agents are usually administered in the emergency or operating rooms.

In the Know

Naloxone, an antidote for an opioid overdose, is now available without a prescription in many states, including Arkansas, California, Massachusetts, Minnesota, Mississippi, Montana, New Jersey, North Dakota, Pennsylvania, Rhode Island, South Carolina, Tennessee, Utah, and Wisconsin. This decisive step was taken, in part, as a response to a recent government study that showed that the use of naloxone reversed approximately 27,000 drug overdoses between 1996 and 2014.

Having naloxone accessible to relatives and friends of drug users allows them to intervene quickly in a drug overdose situation, thus saving lives. Individuals can order the drug through a pharmacist in participating states and receive counseling about its use.

Checkpoint 25.4

Take a moment to review what you have learned so far and answer these questions.

1. How would you describe the actions of a general anesthetic and a local anesthetic? What are the indications for the administration of each type of agent?

2. What medication would you use to counteract the effects of opioids?

Herbal and Alternative Therapies

Caffeine is a CNS stimulant used in combination with other analgesics to treat headache. It is sometimes used in doses of 100–200 to treat fatigue and drowsiness. It should not be used more than every three to four hours. Caffeine is available in tablets, capsules, and lozenges. Side effects include rapid heartbeat, palpitations, insomnia, restlessness, ringing in the ears, tremors, light-headedness, nausea, vomiting, stomach pain, and an itchy skin rash. Taking caffeine with food can help with these effects, and typically doses should be decreased if such effects occur.

Capsaicin is a chemical derived from cayenne peppers that is used as a topical treatment for pain. It has been found to be effective in diabetic neuropathy, arthritis, and headache pain. It works by exhausting the supply of substance P, a substrate in pain nerve endings in the skin. At first, burning, itching, and tingling occur, and then analgesic effects take hold once substance P is depleted. It should not be taken orally, inhaled, or applied to the eye because severe burning can occur. Patients should wear gloves during application and wash their hands thoroughly afterward to avoid these effects.

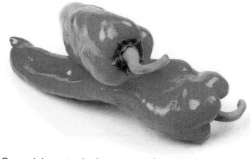

Capsaicin, a topical treatment for pain, is derived from cayenne peppers.

Feverfew is a plant product used orally for migraine pain. It is occasionally used to treat other pain conditions, including menstrual cramps and arthritis. It has been found to improve nausea, vomiting, and light sensitivity experienced during a migraine. Feverfew is generally well tolerated, but side effects include heartburn, nausea, diarrhea, constipation, abdominal pain, and gas. Chewing on feverfew leaves has caused mouth ulceration. Feverfew is taken 50–100 mg a day to prevent a migraine, rather than treating a migraine once it has already started.

Cannabis sativa, commonly known as *marijuana*, is a plant that is used for medical and recreational purposes. Synthetic and natural extracts may be used to provide relief of chronic or neuropathic pain. Medical marijuana can be administered via oral, sublingual, intramuscular, and inhalation routes, and its side effects include dizziness, weight gain, and heart disease. Inhaled marijuana may increase the risk of lung cancer.

Chapter Review

Chapter Summary

The peripheral nervous system is responsible for transmitting signals to the brain, some of which are interpreted as pain. Pain is a useful biologic response to harmful stimuli. It is categorized in multiple ways that help guide treatment. Acute pain is felt in response to injury to tissue and usually subsides as healing occurs. Chronic pain is a long-term condition that can cause changes in behavior (such as depression) in addition to the physical responses typically associated with pain. Pain is also categorized based on where it occurs and can be described as somatic, visceral, neuropathic, or sympathetic-mediated.

Mild-to-moderate pain can be managed with OTC and prescription analgesics. Nonopioid analgesics such as acetaminophen, NSAIDs, and COX-2 inhibitors are used to treat mild-to-moderate pain. Moderate-to-severe pain often requires prescription medications for treatment. Opioid analgesics are commonly used to treat moderate-to-severe pain. These medications have side effects including drowsiness and respiratory depression and have a tendency to promote toler-ance and dependence. Their euphoric effects make opioid analgesics a target for abuse and misuse. Natural and herbal products for pain include caffeine, capsaicin, and feverfew.

Neuropathic pain may not respond to typical pain therapies. Agents such as the anticonvulsants gabapentin and pregabalin, duloxetine, and TCAs can be used to treat neuropathic pain.

Migraine headaches are treated with acute pain medications and abortive therapies. Selective serotonin receptor agonists (triptans) are commonly used to abort migraine headaches. Combination agents of nonopioid analgesics and caffeine are also used to treat migraines.

Anesthesia is the loss of sensation to touch and pain, and it is used for procedures such as surgery or dental work. General anesthesia involves a loss of consciousness; local anesthesia results in a loss of sensation in a specific area of the body. General anesthetics are administered via the IV or inhalation route, whereas local anesthetics are given via the topical or injectable route.

Chapter Checkup

The Navigator+ learning management system that accompanies this textbook offers many opportunities to help you master chapter content, including end-of-chapter exercises, a glossary of key terms, flash cards, and additional interactive activities.

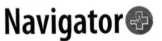

Career Exploration

If you enjoyed learning about pain and anesthesia therapies in this chapter, you may want to explore the following career options:

- anesthesia technician
- anesthesiologist assistant
- art therapist
- athletic trainer
- behavioral health technician
- dental assistant
- massage therapist
- medical assistant
- music therapist
- operating room technician
- physical therapist
- substance abuse counselor

26 Fluids and Electrolytes

Pharm Facts

- A human can survive about three weeks without food, but only three or four days without water.

- Approximately 20% of an individual's need for water is met through the ingestion of food. For example, an apple is approximately 84% water.

- In the United States, individuals drink up to 58 gallons of water a year.

- An individual in a high altitude (approximately 8,000 to 12,000 feet above sea level) requires an increased fluid intake. A high altitude causes a person to perspire more and breathe faster—two processes that result in fluid loss.

- The color of urine is a good indicator of a person's hydration status. Dark-colored urine indicates a greater concentration of waste products than water, which is a sign of dehydration.

"Choosing laboratory technology as a career was the best choice for my analytical mind. My job responsibilities involve producing quality results for physicians to interpret in order to provide a high standard of patient care. Many conditions, such as edema, acidosis, dehydration, and electrolyte imbalances, can be diagnosed and corrected with accurate lab results and proper medications. Knowing the work that I do in the lab saves patients' lives is extremely rewarding. As lab technology becomes more advanced and automated, I look forward to the challenge of learning new skills in this exciting field."

—**Jennifer Yates**, MLT, PBT (ASCP)
Medical Laboratory Technician

Learning Objectives

1 Describe the basic physiology of fluid and electrolyte balance.

2 Explain the therapeutic effects of fluids and electrolytes.

3 Describe the disorders associated with fluid imbalance, electrolyte imbalance, and acid-base imbalance.

4 Explain the indications and therapeutic effects of the products used to treat fluid and electrolyte imbalance.

5 Identify the products, dosage forms and strengths, and routes of administration of fluid and electrolyte products.

6 Identify alternative therapies related to fluid and electrolyte imbalance.

Maintaining fluid and electrolyte balance in the body is critical to the health and well-being of individuals. Daily needs for water and minerals are typically met through normal nutrition and fluid intake. When nutrition and fluid intake is altered or when disease processes affect normal fluid and electrolyte balance, supplementation is needed. Several types of intravenous (IV) fluids and electrolyte products are used to treat—as well as prevent—fluid imbalances. Some of these fluids, such as normal saline and dextrose in water, are also used as delivery vehicles for IV drug therapy.

Allied health professionals need to have an understanding and appreciation of the body's ability to maintain fluid and electrolyte balance despite conditions that challenge this state of equilibrium. They also need to be knowledgeable of the benefits and limitations of the products used to restore fluid and electrolyte balance in the body.

Physiology of Fluid and Electrolyte Balance

Body fluids and electrolytes are interdependent: A change in the level of one of these body components usually causes a change in the other component. Fluids and electrolytes move around the body in relation to each other. A loss of fluids in one area of the body prompts a shift in fluids from another area to replace what was lost. During this shift, electrolytes—or **solutes** dissolved in a **solvent** such as water or other body fluids—are exchanged in an effort to balance the concentration of electrolytes between fluid compartments of the body.

Body Fluids

Body fluids are compartmentalized into intracellular and extracellular spaces. Approximately two-thirds of body fluid is **intracellular fluid**, or fluid contained inside the cellular membrane. The remainder is **extracellular fluid**, or fluid located outside of the cells (see Figure 26.1).

Intracellular Fluid

The role of intracellular fluid is to assist in cell function and metabolism, including the transport of food and waste products. This fluid also helps maintain cell structure. Under normal conditions, the volume of intracellular fluid remains relatively constant.

Extracellular Fluid

Extracellular fluid plays a major role in maintaining overall fluid balance and hydration status. Three-quarters of extracellular fluid resides in the **interstitial spaces** between the cells in tissues. The remaining one-quarter of extracellular fluid is part of the **intravascular space**, a compartment particularly important to hydration. Extracellular fluid volume varies and contains the majority of substances that are active in maintaining proper solute concentrations.

FIGURE 26.1	Body Fluid Compartments

Extracellular fluid, the active fluid that maintains hydration status, consists of interstitial and intravascular fluid.

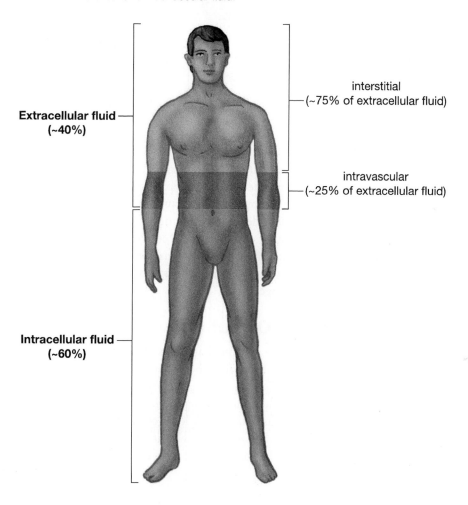

Extracellular fluid (~40%)

Intracellular fluid (~60%)

interstitial (~75% of extracellular fluid)

intravascular (~25% of extracellular fluid)

Water Content in Body Fluids

Most fluid in the body is water, with approximately two-thirds of water housed in the intracellular fluid and the other one-third of water found in extracellular fluid. In fact, one-half or more of an individual's body weight is water. Water content changes with gender, age, and body structure. As Figure 26.2 shows, 60% of body weight in men is water, whereas in women, this figure is 50%. The percentage of body weight that is water is lower than these stated figures in older adults and obese patients.

FIGURE 26.2 Body Water Content

In infants, water constitutes 70%–80% of body weight; in older adults, 45%–55% of body weight is water.

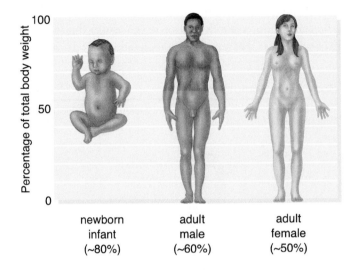

Water is a crucial medium for dissolving substances essential for life and transporting these important molecules throughout the body. Water passively moves across cellular membranes by **osmosis** to maintain the overall equilibrium in concentration of total molecules on both sides. If a solute is added to one side of the membrane, water moves to that side to keep concentration constant on both sides. More often than not, the concentration of intracellular and extracellular fluid remains constant. This fluid balance is one factor that allows the body to maintain a state of **homeostasis**, or the ability to maintain internal stability despite external changes.

Water Intake and Water Output

Homeostasis is maintained by multiple systems that regulate **water intake** and **water output** as well as distribute water into the various body compartments. Typically, water intake roughly matches water output (see Figure 26.3). Most adults take in approximately two liters of water a day by drinking fluids and eating food. A small amount of water is also produced during normal metabolism and breakdown of substances in the body. This water intake and production are necessary to replenish fluid lost through urination, feces production, and **insensible loss** (respiration and water lost through the skin).

Electrolytes

Electrolytes are molecular compounds that are present in both intracellular and extracellular fluid, though in differing concentrations, depending on the ion (see Table 26.1). Specific ion pumps (e.g., sodium/potassium ion pumps) and channels (e.g., chloride channels) in cellular membranes maintain these concentrations which are measured in **milliequivalents per liter (mEq/L)**.

Electrolytes form ions when dissolved in water. For example, sodium chloride (table salt) dissociates (or separates) into sodium (Na^+) and chloride (Cl^-) when dissolved in water. Because water forms the majority of body fluid, electrolytes exist throughout the body as positively or negatively charged ions. Positively charged ions are called **cations**, and negatively charged ions are called **anions**. Important cations in the body are sodium (Na^+), potassium (K^+), calcium (Ca^{2+}), and magnesium (Mg^{2+}). Important anions in the body include chloride (Cl^-), bicarbonate (HCO_3^-), and, at times, phosphate (PO_4^-).

Sodium

Sodium is the most abundant cation in the extracellular fluid. Sodium retains fluid in the body, helps generate and transmit nerve impulses, assists with acid-base balance, regulates enzyme activity, and serves as the primary active ion in maintaining fluid isotonicity. **Isotonicity** is a state of balanced electrolyte concentration across cell membranes.

FIGURE 26.3 | Daily Water Balance

Regulation mechanisms such as thirst and urine output help the body maintain proper water balance. The yellow box at the right provides an example of the average daily water intake and water output for an adult.

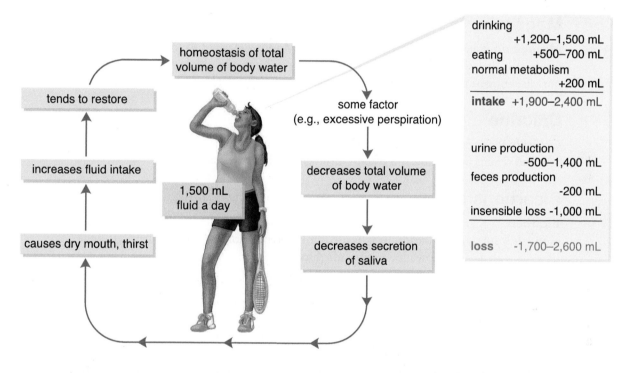

TABLE 26.1 | Normal Electrolyte Concentrations

Electrolyte	Extracellular Fluid		Intracellular Fluid (mEq/L)
	Plasma (mEq/L)	Interstitial Fluid (mEq/L)	
Sodium (Na^+)	136–145	146	15
Potassium (K^+)	3.5–5.5	5	150
Calcium (Ca^{2+})	4.3–5.3	3	2
Magnesium (Mg^{2+})	1.5–2.5	1	27
Chloride (Cl^-)	100–106	144	1
Bicarbonate (HCO_3^-)	27	30	10

Potassium

Potassium is the primary cation in intracellular fluid. Potassium is important in generating and transmitting nerve impulses and muscle contraction, such as in cardiac function and rhythm. Potassium also assists with acid-base balance, regulates enzyme activity, and is involved in carbohydrate metabolism.

Calcium

Calcium is most often associated with bone formation, and it is also essential for muscle contraction and the conduction of impulses. Proper blood coagulation depends on sufficient intake of this electrolyte. Calcium is a positively charged ion that is highly bound to **albumin**, a protein in plasma. Low albumin levels can therefore result in hypocalcemia (low calcium levels).

Magnesium

Magnesium is an abundant intracellular cation. Most magnesium in the body exists inside cells. It activates enzymes and facilitates normal nerve impulse production and muscle contraction. Magnesium is important in cardiac function.

Chloride

Chloride is an anion that transports carbon dioxide, forms hydrochloric acid in the stomach, and retains potassium. It is important in controlling acid-base balance.

Bicarbonate

Bicarbonate is an anion that helps to maintain pH balance in the blood. Its most common salt form, sodium bicarbonate, is used in IV preparations in the inpatient setting for patients with acidosis (low blood pH/acidic blood).

Phosphate

Phosphate is an anion that plays an important role in energy production within cells. Without sufficient phosphate, normal cell function is not possible. Phosphate commonly exists in counterbalance with calcium in the bloodstream. Excess intake of phosphate can deplete calcium levels and affect bone health.

 Checkpoint 26.1

Take a moment to review what you have learned so far and answer these questions.

1. How much total body water is distributed intracellularly versus extracellularly? What percentage of extracellular fluid is intravascular?

2. What is the most abundant cation in intracellular and extracellular fluid?

Disorders Associated with Fluid Imbalance

The human body constantly works to maintain fluid balance. The body loses fluid through urination, perspiration, and respiration. It is necessary for individuals to consume fluids to compensate for these losses.

When fluid intake is inadequate, dehydration may occur. In contrast, excess fluid can be a result of fluid overconsumption or underexcretion. Excess fluid may lead to edema, or swelling caused by an accumulation of excess fluid in the interstitial tissue space. Medical conditions may cause or promote fluid imbalance. For example, patients with diarrhea or vomiting may lose too much fluid. In contrast, patients with heart failure exacerbations often have excess fluid that collects in the blood vessels, body tissues, liver, and lungs.

Dehydration

Dehydration is the excess loss of body fluids, primarily water. This condition can result from vomiting, diarrhea, sweating from heat or fever, or excess urine output. Symptoms of dehydration include thirst, dry mucous membranes, weakness, dizziness, dry skin, **turgor** (reduced skin elasticity), hypotension, rapid heartbeat, and reduced or absent urine production.

Treatment of mild dehydration can be accomplished by drinking fluids. However, moderate-to-severe dehydration requires IV fluids and electrolytes. Simply drinking or administering water alone will not correct a moderate-to-severe fluid imbalance. In fact, water alone can be harmful. Fluids supplied for rehydration should be balanced with electrolytes so as not to cause further electrolyte imbalance while fluid status is being corrected.

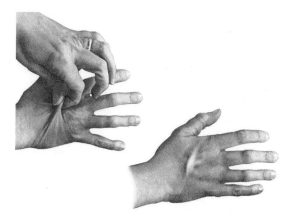

Reduced skin elasticity, or turgor, may be a sign of dehydration. Skin with decreased turgor may remain elevated after being pulled up and released.

Drug Regimens and Treatments

IV fluid products are used to replace lost fluids and electrolytes due to dehydration. In addition, they are used in total parenteral nutrition (TPN) solutions to supply essential trace minerals. (For more information on TPN solutions, refer to Chapter 19.) IV fluid products are also used as a liquid vehicle for administering IV drug therapy. IV fluids can be categorized by content (colloids versus crystalloids) or tonicity.

Drug Alert

Sterile water for injection is a commercially available IV fluid product. It is used for diluting other IV drugs or fluids and should *never* be administered by itself. Injecting or administering pure water through an IV line causes mass hemolysis as water rushes from plasma into red blood cells, quickly bursting them. Hemolysis destroys the blood and releases intracellular material in mass amounts, causing death.

Colloid solutions contain proteins and other large molecules (such as fats). Molecules in colloid products are so large that they do not quickly or easily move from the bloodstream to surrounding tissues. In that way, colloids act similarly to hypertonic solutions. They increase the osmolarity, or concentration of molecules, of blood plasma, which pulls fluid from interstitial spaces. Colloids are commonly referred to as *blood volume expanders*. Examples of colloids include albumin, dextran, and blood itself.

Crystalloid solutions contain small ions and molecules. They are used to replace lost fluid and treat dehydration. These solutions are used on a daily basis as a liquid vehicle for administering IV drugs. Both normal saline and dextrose in water are crystalloid solutions. Dextrose is desirable when a patient has need of caloric energy (such as with malnutrition) or when his or her glucose levels are low (such as with hypoglycemia). Table 26.2 contains examples of common crystalloid solutions along with their associated osmolarity.

Tonicity refers to the concentration of a solute (dissolved substance) in a solvent (fluid) and how that concentration affects movement of water across membranes. Figure 26.4 shows the effects of tonicity on cells in isotonic conditions (concentration

TABLE 26.2 Common Crystalloid Solutions

Tonicity	Solution	Osmolarity
Isotonic solutions	Dextrose 2.5% in 0.45% NaCl ($D_{2.5}W$ in ½ NS)	280 mOsm/L
	Dextrose 5% in sterile water (D_5W)	300 mOsm/L
	0.9% NaCl (normal saline [NS])	310 mOsm/L
	Lactated Ringer's solution (LR)	275 mOsm/L
Hypertonic solutions	Dextrose 5% in 0.45% NaCl (D_5W in ½ NS)	405 mOsm/L
	Dextrose 5% in 0.9% NaCl (D_5W in NS)	560 mOsm/L
	Dextrose 10% in sterile water ($D_{10}W$)	600 mOsm/L
	3%, 5%, 14.6%, and 23.4% NaCl concentrates	varies
Hypotonic (hydrating) solutions	0.45% NaCl (½ NS)	155 mOsm/L
	Dextrose 2.5% in sterile water ($D_{2.5}W$)	140 mOsm/L

FIGURE 26.4 Tonicity Effects on Cells in Solution

When a cell is in isotonic conditions, the amount of water entering and leaving the cell is the same. In hypotonic conditions, more water enters a cell and may result in cell rupture. In hypertonic conditions, more water leaves a cell and may result in cell shriveling.

IN HUMAN CELLS

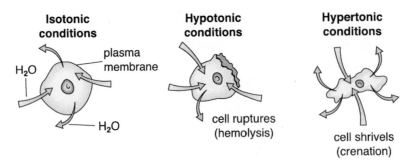

equal to blood plasma), hypotonic conditions (lower concentration of solute), and hypertonic conditions (higher concentration of solute).

The concept of tonicity refers only to molecules that do not move easily across membranes, such as ions and electrolytes. Fluid and electrolyte products have labeled concentrations in grams of solute per 100 mL of solvent, which is displayed as **percent concentration**.

Another related concept that affects tonicity is osmolarity. **Osmolarity** refers to the concentration of all molecules—both those that move across membranes and those that do not—in a set volume of fluid. Osmolarity is measured in **milliosmoles per liter (mOsm/L)**. The osmolarity of blood plasma, for example, is approximately 275–300 mOsm/L.

Isotonic Solutions

Isotonic solutions, also known as *maintenance solutions*, have a concentration similar to blood plasma. Isotonic fluid products replace daily fluid and electrolyte loss and prevent dehydration. When administered intravenously, normal balance between the vascular volume and interstitial spaces is maintained. The most common isotonic IV solution used is normal saline (0.9% NaCl).

Side Effects Solutions that contain albumin or **dextrans** (polysaccharides made of glucose molecules) may cause hypersensitivity reactions. Additionally, dextrans are associated with hypotension, chest tightness, and bleeding. Dextrose solutions may cause increased blood glucose levels. Lactated Ringer's solution contains potassium and its use is associated with hyperkalemia. Finally, normal saline products may cause hyperchloremic acidosis.

Contraindications Albumin-containing products are contraindicated in patients with severe anemia and cardiac failure.

Dextrans are contraindicated in patients with marked hemostatic defects, cardiac decompensation, and kidney disease that results in decreased urination.

Dextrose solutions are contraindicated in patients with a hypersensitivity to corn. These solutions should also be avoided in patients with diabetic coma from hyperglycemia;

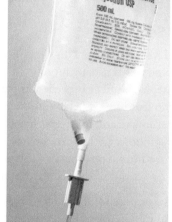
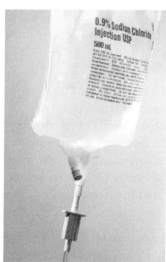

Isotonic solutions, such as 0.9% NaCl (normal saline) solution, rehydrate patients and distribute necessary electrolytes without disturbing the concentration within the bloodstream.

Drug Alert

Albumin should not be diluted with sterile water for injection, a hypotonic solution without electrolytes. A hypotonic solution may cause cell swelling and, possibly, cell rupture. In some cases, this effect can be fatal.

delirium tremens with dehydration; anuria; hepatic coma; or glucose-galactose malabsorption. Hypertonic dextrose solutions should not be used in patients with intracranial or intraspinal hemorrhage.

Lactated Ringer's solution should not be used in the treatment of lactic acidosis. Products containing normal saline are contraindicated in hypertonic uterus, hypernatremia, and fluid retention.

✚ *Note: Allied health professionals should be aware that an allergy to a particular drug contraindicates its use. This warning applies to all Contraindications sections in this chapter.*

Cautions and Considerations All IV fluid therapies may result in volume overload. They should be used with caution in patients at risk for volume overexpansion such as older adults and children.

Albumin may cause anaphylaxis and its use should be discontinued if allergic or anaphylactic reactions are suspected. Because albumin is a protein, it should be used cautiously in patients who have liver or kidney dysfunction. Albumin is a human plasma product and may contain infectious pathogens.

Dextrans may reduce hemoglobin concentrations. Patients who have heart failure and kidney impairment should use dextran products with caution.

Dextrose products with concentrations of 10% or higher are vesicants. Avoid extravasation and, in the event extravasation occurs, the dextrose solution should be discontinued immediately. Dextrose products without potassium may lead to hypokalemia.

Lactated Ringer's solution should not be infused simultaneously through the same IV line as calcium-containing products. Lactated Ringer's solution should also be used with caution in patients who have metabolic or respiratory alkalosis.

Normal saline should be used with caution in patients who have cirrhosis, edema, heart failure, hypertension, and kidney impairment.

Hypertonic Solutions

Hypertonic solutions contain a higher concentration of solute than body fluids. Osmolarity of these products is usually more than 350 mOsm/L. These products are used when urgent sodium replenishment is needed as part of hydration. They are indicated for severe sodium depletion from excess perspiration, vomiting, or diarrhea. They are also used to treat excess water intake and overuse of enemas or irrigating solutions (during surgery). In addition, these solutions are indicated when sodium-free fluids and electrolyte products have been used for fluid replacement. Cells placed in a hypertonic solution shrivel and shrink as water passes out of the cell membrane (see Figure 26.4).

Side Effects Hypertonic solutions have the same side effects as isotonic solutions. For this reason, see the "Side Effects" section in the discussion on isotonic solutions.

Contraindications Hypertonic solutions have the same contraindications as isotonic solutions. For this reason, see the "Contraindications" section in the discussion on isotonic solutions.

In addition, hypertonic solutions should not be used in patients with intracranial or intraspinal hemorrhage.

Cautions and Considerations Hypertonic solutions have the same cautions and considerations as isotonic solutions. For this reason, see the "Cautions and Considerations" section in the discussion on isotonic solutions.

In addition, hypertonic solutions can be quite irritating and corrosive to tissues and blood vessels. They must be administered via a central IV line (i.e., surgically inserted into a port in a central vein), not a peripheral IV line placed in the arm or hand.

Hypertonic solutions must also be administered slowly and monitored closely. If administered too quickly, the mass exodus of fluid from vital tissues can cause damage. Resulting fluid overload inside the blood vessels can cause heart failure.

Hypotonic Solutions

Hypotonic solutions contain a lower concentration of solute than solvent. Osmolarity of these products is usually less than 280 mOsm/L. These solutions treat dehydration by diluting the concentration within the bloodstream, which decreases osmolarity. Water leaves the blood and enters interstitial and intracellular spaces. Cells placed in a hypotonic solution swell and burst as water rushes into the cell. Hypotonic solutions are commonly referred to as *hydrating solutions* because they are used to correct dehydration.

Side Effects Hypotonic solutions have the same side effects as isotonic solutions. For this reason, see the "Side Effects" section in the discussion on isotonic solutions.

Contraindications Hypotonic solutions have the same contraindications as isotonic solutions. For this reason, see the "Contraindications" section in the discussion on isotonic solutions.

Cautions and Considerations Hypotonic solutions must be used with caution. If administered too quickly, fluid will shift into the cerebral compartment and cause increased intracranial pressure and brain damage.

Kolb's Learning Style

If you like hands-on experience, as Accommodators do, contact a hospital pharmacy employee. Ask if he or she can provide you with empty intravenous fluid containers. Determine the tonicity of each fluid container (isotonic, hypertonic, or hypotonic). Then explain to a friend the tonicity effects on cells in the body.

Edema

As mentioned earlier, **edema** is swelling caused by an accumulation of excess fluid in the interstitial tissue space. With edema, fluid most commonly accumulates in a patient's lower extremities and lungs, although the fluid can also accumulate in the brain (cerebral edema). Edema generally manifests as swelling in the ankles and legs or as difficulty breathing when it affects the lungs.

Edema can be caused by a number of factors. One of the most common causes is sodium and fluid retention in the extracellular space. Another cause of edema is renal failure. As kidney function weakens, fluid cannot exit the body and begins to collect in interstitial spaces. Still another cause of edema is reduced tissue perfusion, such as that which occurs in congestive heart failure. In this condition, the heart cannot efficiently pump blood

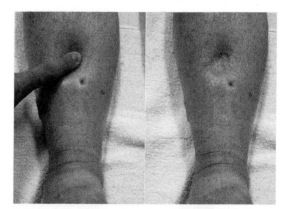

Edema generally manifests in several places, including the lower extremities. This photo shows an example of pitting edema, a condition that is visible when pressure applied with a finger leaves a temporary indentation, or pit, on the skin's surface.

through the vasculature; consequently, the blood pools in the capillaries. The resulting blood pressure buildup causes fluid to squeeze or leak into surrounding tissue.

Treating edema requires both removal of excess fluid as well as correction of electrolyte imbalances. **Diuretics** are the most common drug treatment for edema. These medications eliminate fluid from the body via the kidneys and urination. To review the side effects, contraindications, and cautions and considerations related to diuretics, refer to Chapters 15 and 22.

Disorders Associated with Electrolyte Imbalance

Electrolyte imbalances can be caused by depletion or excess production or intake of the electrolyte itself, or from a relative reduction or excess of fluid. Normal ranges for common electrolyte laboratory values in blood plasma are shown in Table 26.1. The electrolyte concentration in plasma is similar to extracellular levels. Intracellular levels cannot be directly measured, so laboratory values must be combined with clinical signs and symptoms to determine when deficits exist. It is useful to know the conditions in which fluid and electrolyte status should be monitored.

Electrolytes are most commonly prescribed for patients with an electrolyte deficiency, or in patients in which a deficiency is anticipated. Electrolytes are not administered in high doses to prevent disease, as is commonly the case with vitamins. Large quantities of electrolytes can be harmful.

Electrolytes in body fluids can be replaced in a variety of ways. When depletion is mild, electrolyte replacement can happen by changing the diet to include the absent mineral or taking an oral supplement. For instance, athletes consume sports drinks to replenish fluids and electrolytes lost from perspiration. Oral liquid electrolyte mixtures can also be consumed to treat mild dehydration caused by vomiting or diarrhea (see Table 26.3). These over-the-counter (OTC) products are generally safe to use because they contain only small amounts of electrolytes.

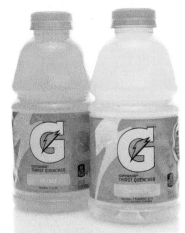

In mild cases of dehydration, sports drinks may be sufficient to replenish fluids and electrolytes. However, moderate-to-severe dehydration requires medical attention, especially in children.

When immediate correction is needed or severe deficiencies exist, IV electrolyte replacement products are used (see Table 26.4). Electrolytes are added to IV fluids, such as normal saline or dextrose in water. Laboratory results are used to guide therapy. Dosing must be individualized depending on the reason for the electrolyte imbalance and the fluid status of the patient.

TABLE 26.3 Common Oral Liquid Electrolyte Mixtures

Product	Electrolyte Content	Other content
Infalyte	Na, K, Cl	Rice syrup
Naturalyte	Na, K, Cl	Dextrose
Pedialyte	Na, K, Cl	Dextrose
Pedialyte Freezer Pops	Na, K, Cl	Dextrose
Rehydrate	Na, K, Cl	Dextrose

TABLE 26.4 Common Electrolyte Replacement Products

Generic (Brand)	Dosage Form and Strength	Route of Administration
Sodium		
Sodium chloride (Slo-Salt, Sustain)	Tablet: 600 mg, 650 mg, 1 g, 2.25 g (+ other combinations with potassium)	Oral
Sodium chloride	Injectable concentrate: 14.6%, 23.4% IV solution: 0.9% (NS), 0.45% (½ NS), 3%, 5% Solution for injection: 2.5 mEq/mL, 4 mEq/mL	IV infusion
Potassium		
Potassium acetate	IV additive: 10.2 mEq/g (diluted to 40–80 mEq/L)	IV infusion
Potassium chloride (K-Dur, K-Lor, K-Lyte, Klor-Con, Micro-K)	Capsule, effervescent powder, liquid, tablet: varying strengths, 8–25 mEq a dose	Oral
Potassium chloride	IV additive: 13.4 mEq/g (diluted to 40–80 mEq/L)	IV infusion
Calcium		
Calcium carbonate (Caltrate, Os Cal, Tums)	Suspension: 500 mg/5 mL, 1,250 mg/mL Tablet: 500 mg, 600 mg, 750 mg, 1,250 mg	Oral
Calcium chloride	Solution for injection: 1 g/10 mL	IV infusion
Calcium citrate (Cal-Citrate)	Tablet: 250 mg	Oral
Calcium gluconate	Tablet: 500 mg, 650 mg, 972 mg	Oral
Calcium lactate (Cal-Lac)	Tablet: 650 mg	Oral
Magnesium		
Magnesium chloride (Chloromag)	Solution for injection: 200 mg/mL	IV infusion
Magnesium gluconate (Mag-G, Magonate, Magtrate)	Liquid: 3.52 mg/mL, 1,000 mg/5 mL Tablet: 500 mg	Oral
Magnesium lactate (Mag-Tab)	Tablet: 84 mg	Oral
Magnesium oxide (Mag-Cap, Maox, Mag-Ox, Uro-Mag)	Capsule: 140 mg	Oral
Magnesium sulfate (Mag-200)	Capsule: 70 mg Solution for injection: 10 mg/mL, 20 mg/mL, 40 mg/mL, 80 mg/mL, 400 mg/mL, 500 mg/mL	Oral, IM, IV infusion
Phosphate		
Phosphorus (K-Phos, PHOS-NaK, Uro-KP)	Capsule and powder packets: 250 mg plus potassium and sodium	Oral

Hyponatremia and Hypernatremia

Hyponatremia is low sodium concentration relative to blood plasma's normal range. This condition is related to sodium loss or a relative excess of water in the extracellular space. Hyponatremia can be caused by excess water intake, overuse of salt-wasting diuretics, adrenal gland insufficiency, and kidney or liver failure. Low sodium concentrations can also occur with fluid loss caused by excess perspiration or vomiting.

Hypernatremia describes elevated sodium concentration relative to blood plasma's normal range. Hypernatremia can be caused by dehydration from lack of fluid intake, diarrhea, and/or a deficiency of antidiuretic hormone. Heart disease and kidney failure can also cause this condition.

Hyponatremia is usually treated with sodium-containing electrolyte supplements. These supplements are available as IV or oral products. Hypernatremia is treated with fluids as the condition is often due to fluid losses that have not been replaced.

Sodium-Containing Products

Sodium is available in various salt forms and can be administered orally or intravenously. Information regarding sodium-containing products can be found in Table 26.4.

Side Effects Common side effects of sodium-containing products include water retention and high blood pressure. Patients should talk with their prescribers if edema, swelling, or rapid weight gain occurs. These symptoms may indicate the need for a reduced dose or stoppage of the product.

Contraindications Contraindications to sodium-containing products include hypertonic uterus, hypernatremia, and fluid retention.

Cautions and Considerations Most electrolyte products, including sodium-containing products, cannot be used in patients who have kidney failure or impairment. If these products are used in this patient population, patients must be monitored closely. For this reason, patients with kidney problems should notify their healthcare practitioners before taking OTC electrolyte supplements or food products such as salt replacers and oral hydration fluids.

Hypokalemia and Hyperkalemia

Hypokalemia is a condition of lower-than-normal potassium concentration in blood plasma. Potassium can be lost through overuse of potassium-wasting diuretics, vomiting or gastric suctioning, or excess urine output. Signs of hypokalemia include reduced muscle tone (decreased reflexes), weakness, confusion, drowsiness, depression, low blood pressure, and cardiac arrhythmias.

Hyperkalemia results from an increase in potassium levels in blood plasma. High potassium is a dangerous condition because cardiac function and contractility are greatly affected. Cardiac arrest can occur when potassium levels are too high. Hyperkalemia can be caused by kidney failure, diarrhea, excess use of potassium-sparing diuretics, Cushing's syndrome, severe burns, and septic shock (severe systemic infection). Signs and symptoms of hyperkalemia include depressed breathing, diarrhea, nausea, vomiting, irritability, confusion, anxiety, upset stomach, and cardiac arrhythmias.

Drug Regimens and Treatments

Work Wise

Potassium supplementation is used for a variety of reasons. You may hear other healthcare practitioners refer to potassium supplements as *K* and potassium chloride supplements as *KCl*.

Hypokalemia is generally treated with potassium supplementation. Hyperkalemia can be treated using both rapid-acting products and slower-acting products. IV calcium, insulin with glucose (discussed in Chapter 20), beta blockers (discussed in Chapters 12 and 15), and sodium bicarbonate are quick-acting options to treat hyperkalemia.

Potassium-Containing Products

Oral potassium supplements are typically used to replace potassium lost from **diuresis**, or increased or excess production of urine. Some diuretics deplete potassium, so patients must take a potassium supplement while on those drug therapies. Doses are individualized to patients. More information on potassium-containing products can be found in Table 26.4.

Side Effects Common side effects of potassium-containing products include nausea, vomiting, diarrhea, and abdominal pain. In some cases, potassium supplements have been associated with gastrointestinal (GI) ulceration. At a minimum, they can be irritating to the GI tract. Patients should take oral potassium products with a full glass of water to reduce these effects. Effervescent powder products should also be mixed with plenty of water to avoid stomach and intestinal irritation. Taking potassium supplements with food may also decrease upset stomach.

Contraindications Potassium-containing products are contraindicated in patients with hyperkalemia. Potassium acetate should not be used in patients with severe renal impairment. Oral potassium chloride should not be used in patients with absorption or digestion delay or arrest.

Cautions and Considerations Before administration, an injectable potassium-containing product must be diluted, added to a large-volume IV solution, and mixed well so that the entire IV bag has a consistent concentration (see the following "Drug Alert"). Such infusions must also be administered slowly because these medications can be irritating to the veins and painful for the patient. Usually, 40 mEq of potassium is added to 1 L of IV fluid. The maximum safe concentration is 80 mEq/L. Administering too much potassium can be fatal because it can interfere with heart function and cause cardiac arrest.

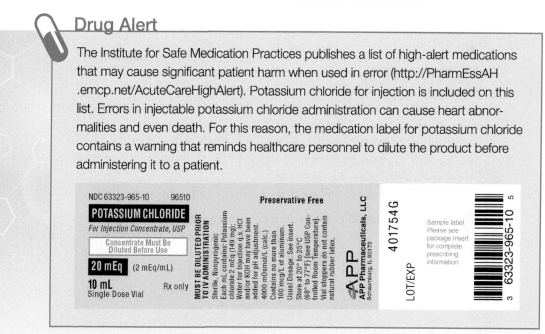

Drug Alert

The Institute for Safe Medication Practices publishes a list of high-alert medications that may cause significant patient harm when used in error (http://PharmEssAH .emcp.net/AcuteCareHighAlert). Potassium chloride for injection is included on this list. Errors in injectable potassium chloride administration can cause heart abnormalities and even death. For this reason, the medication label for potassium chloride contains a warning that reminds healthcare personnel to dilute the product before administering it to a patient.

Hypocalcemia and Hypercalcemia

Hypocalcemia is a depletion of calcium levels in blood plasma. Low calcium can be caused by insufficient calcium intake or parathyroid disease. Signs and symptoms of hypocalcemia include hyperexcitability of nerves and **tetany** (intermittent muscle spasms). As part of this condition, seizures and, possibly, death can occur.

Hypercalcemia is an excess of calcium in blood plasma. This condition can be caused by excess intake of calcium supplements and by some cancerous tumors. Patients with hypercalcemia may present without symptoms. Other patients may experience increased thirst, increased urination, dehydration, abdominal pain, anorexia, and muscle weakness.

Hypocalcemia is often treated with calcium supplements. Hypomagnesemia (discussed later in this chapter) often occurs concurrently with this condition; therefore, magnesium supplements may also be used during treatment. Hypercalcemia may be treated with fluids, calcitonin, or zoledronic acid. (For more information on calcitonin and zoledronic acid, see Chapter 10.)

Calcium-Containing Products

Oral calcium-containing products are used to prevent and treat bone loss from osteoporosis, rickets (which may be caused by calcium deficiency or vitamin D deficiency), and osteomalacia. These products are also used for tetany and for osteoporosis (see Chapter 10). Calcium-containing products are absorbed more efficiently when taken with vitamin D. For a listing of these products, see Table 26.4.

Side Effects Calcium-containing products can cause constipation. Taking these supplements with food and drinking plenty of water may decrease the likelihood of this condition. If hypercalcemia occurs from consuming these products, kidney stones can form. Patients should seek medical attention if they have back or flank pain and/or difficult or painful urination, especially if associated with nausea and vomiting. These signs can indicate kidney stone formation.

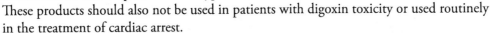

The formation of kidney stones is a possible side effect of consuming calcium-containing products.

Contraindications Calcium-containing products should not be used in patients with hypercalcemia. These products should also not be used in patients with digoxin toxicity or used routinely in the treatment of cardiac arrest.

Calcium gluconate is contraindicated in patients with ventricular fibrillation and in patients with hypercalcemia. In neonates, calcium gluconate should not be used with concomitant ceftriaxone administration.

Calcium lactate is contraindicated in patients with ventricular fibrillation.

Cautions and Considerations Calcium-containing products and phosphate salts can **chelate** (bond chemically to form an insoluble precipitate). The precipitate appears as small white specks or clumps of material within the IV bag. If infused through an IV line, the precipitate clogs a patient's capillaries and produces severe adverse effects. Therefore, mixing calcium-containing products and phosphate salts in the same IV bag should be avoided or done with caution.

Hypomagnesemia and Hypermagnesemia

Hypomagnesemia is a depletion of magnesium in blood plasma. Magnesium can be lost through alcohol abuse, preeclampsia, or drug therapy that causes increased magnesium excretion. Digoxin, estrogen, and diuretics can also deplete magnesium. Signs and symptoms of hypomagnesemia include muscle cramps, confusion, hypertension, tachycardia, arrhythmias, tremors, hyperactive reflexes, hallucinations, and seizures.

Hypermagnesemia is an excess of magnesium in blood plasma. This condition can be caused by renal failure, an overdose of IV magnesium infusion, or the use of enemas containing magnesium. Symptoms of hypermagnesemia may include nausea, drowsiness, diminished or absent tendon reflexes, bradycardia, low blood pressure, and hypocalcemia.

Drug Regimens and Treatments

Hypomagnesemia is treated with magnesium supplements. Hypermagnesemia often occurs in patients receiving magnesium products or in patients who have kidney disease. Discontinuation of magnesium-containing products can correct hypermagnesemia; however, in some cases, the administration of IV fluids containing diuretics or the use of dialysis may be necessary to treat this condition.

Magnesium-Containing Products

Oral or IV magnesium-containing products are typically used to treat hypomagnesemia. Magnesium supplementation may also be used to treat other disorders such as asthma. See Table 26.4 for more information on magnesium-containing products.

Side Effects Magnesium supplements can cause diarrhea. Taking these supplements with food can decrease this effect, although this effect usually improves over time.

Contraindications Magnesium chloride is contraindicated in kidney impairment and myocardial disease. Magnesium sulfate should not be used in heart block and myocardial damage. IV magnesium sulfate is contraindicated in the treatment of preeclampsia or eclampsia during the two hours prior to childbirth. Magnesium gluconate, magnesium lactate, and magnesium oxide do not have contraindications.

Cautions and Considerations Magnesium-containing products should be used cautiously in the presence of kidney impairment and neuromuscular disease (such as myasthenia gravis).

Hypophosphatemia and Hyperphosphatemia

Hypophosphatemia is a drop in phosphate level in blood plasma. This condition can be caused by anorexia or severe malnutrition. Low phosphate levels may also occur in patients who have kidney failure. Signs and symptoms of hypophosphatemia include weakness, respiratory failure, heart failure, hemolysis, and rhabdomyolysis (mass muscle tissue breakdown).

Hyperphosphatemia, or an abnormally high level of phosphate in blood plasma, can be caused by **tumor lysis syndrome** (a condition that can occur when receiving chemotherapy drugs for large cancer tumors), rhabdomyolysis, lactic acidosis, or diabetic ketoacidosis. Taking bisphosphonates or too much vitamin D, or overusing bowel preparation products containing phosphate, can also cause hyperphosphatemia. Symptoms of hyperphosphatemia are not always apparent to patients.

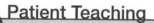 **Patient Teaching**

Many patients with hyperphosphatemia do not have symptoms. Individuals who are symptomatic may report hyperexcitability of nerves and tetany, which are manifestations of associated hypocalcemia. Other symptoms that patients might experience include fatigue, muscle pain, or shortness of breath. Because of the inconsistent presentation of symptoms, patients may not realize that they have hyperphosphatemia. To that end, allied health professionals can educate patients about this condition and encourage patients to have recommended blood tests to assess phosphate levels.

Hypophosphatemia is treated with phosphate supplementation. Hyperphosphatemia can be treated with phosphate binders, saline infusions, and dialysis.

Phosphorus-Containing Products

Phosphorus-containing products are used primarily in cases of malnourishment. Some patients are not able to take in sufficient phosphorus through their diet due to GI absorption abnormalities.

Side Effects Common side effects of phosphorus-containing products include upset stomach or diarrhea. Over time, these effects usually improve. Phosphorus supplements have also been associated with kidney stones. Patients should seek medical attention if they have back or flank pain and/or difficult or painful urination, especially if associated with nausea and vomiting. These signs could indicate kidney stone formation.

Contraindications Phosphorus-containing products are contraindicated in patients with hyperphosphatemia, hypocalcemia, and hypernatremia.

Cautions and Considerations As mentioned earlier, calcium-containing products and phosphate salts can chelate. The precipitate appears as small white specks or clumps of material within the IV bag. If infused through an IV line, the precipitate clogs a patient's capillaries and produces severe adverse effects. For this reason, mixing calcium-containing products and phosphate salts in the same IV bag should be avoided or done with caution.

Hypochloremia and Hyperchloremia

Hypochloremia is a depletion of chloride in blood plasma. This condition can be caused by a loss of fluid from excess production of urine or perspiration and from gastric suctioning. Some diuretics also deplete chloride.

Hyperchloremia is an excess of chloride in blood plasma. This condition can be caused by diarrhea, kidney disease, or diabetes.

Drug Regimens and Treatments

Hypochloremia and hyperchloremia rarely occur without the presence of other electrolyte or acid-base imbalances (see the following section titled "Disorders Associated with Acid-Base Imbalance"). Treatment is usually directed at fixing the underlying cause. Chloride itself is usually not supplemented and is given via supplementation with other electrolytes (such as potassium chloride or sodium chloride).

 Checkpoint 26.2

Take a moment to review what you have learned so far and answer these questions.

1. What do you call a solution that has a similar concentration to blood plasma?

2. What electrolyte abnormality may be caused by tumor lysis syndrome?

Disorders Associated with Acid-Base Imbalance

In addition to impacting fluid status, electrolytes affect the balance of **hydrogen ions (H⁺)** in the bloodstream. The concentration of hydrogen ions is reported on the **pH scale** and determines **acidity** or **alkalinity** of body fluids. A fluid with a low pH is **acidic**, whereas a fluid with a high pH is **basic**. The pH of blood is maintained between 7.35 and 7.45. The body uses an **acid-base pair buffer** system to keep the pH in this narrow range. **Carbonic acid** (acid) and **sodium bicarbonate** (base) are constantly produced through normal metabolism and respiration. This acid-base pair works together to mitigate, or buffer, large changes in the pH. If acid is added to the blood, sodium bicarbonate reacts and neutralizes it. Likewise, carbonic acid neutralizes bases.

Acid-base balance is also maintained by kidney function. Kidneys regulate the retention and excretion of electrolytes in the urine. For example, the retention of acidic electrolytes, such as phosphate and ammonium, lowers the blood pH.

Lung function can also help maintain the body's acid-base balance and can do so more quickly than kidney action can. During respiration, carbon dioxide combines with water in the blood to make carbonic anhydrase, an acid. Breathing faster or slower changes the rate at which carbon dioxide is exhaled and eliminated from the blood. The body then makes more or less carbonic acid, which changes the blood pH.

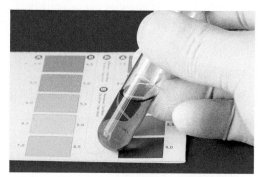

The pH scale determines the degree of acidity or alkalinity in a fluid. The fluid shown has basic properties, with a pH at the higher end of the scale.

Kolb's Learning Styles

If you like collaborative learning, as Convergers and Divergers do, find a classmate with whom to discuss acid-base balance. Explain to each other what happens if an acid or a base is added to the bloodstream. Talking through this process out loud is a way to solidify the concept. Teaching it to someone else helps you better understand the concept yourself.

Acid-base imbalance occurs when the body's pH deviates from the normal range. When a metabolic process is contributing to an acid-base imbalance, a respiratory process can make adjustments for it. By the same token, when a respiratory process is contributing to an acid-base imbalance, a metabolic process can make adjustments. Correction in the pH can occur quickly with respiratory changes, but metabolic correction takes time. In either case, if an imbalance is severe or urgent, drug therapy may be needed to address the imbalance.

Acidosis

Acidosis occurs when plasma contains excess hydrogen ions (commonly from an abundance of carbon dioxide), which causes the pH to drop below the normal range. **Metabolic acidosis** occurs when excess acid is produced; bicarbonate is lost (such as with diarrhea); or the kidneys do not excrete enough acid. **Respiratory acidosis** results from slow respiration and retention of carbon dioxide in the blood.

Drug Regimens and Treatments

Sometimes electrolyte products are used to correct acidosis rather than to correct electrolyte deficiencies. Basic (higher pH) products are also used to treat acidosis (see Table 26.5).

TABLE 26.5 Common Acidifying and Alkalinizing Products

Generic (Brand)	Dosage Form and Strength	Route of Administration
Acidifying Agent		
Ammonium chloride	Injection 5 mEq/mL (diluted and then infused)	IV infusion
Alkalinizing Agent		
Sodium bicarbonate	Injection 4.2%, 5%, 7.5%, 8.4%	IV infusion

Sodium Bicarbonate

Sodium bicarbonate is a basic substance used as an antacid for heartburn and acid indigestion, a systemic alkalinizer for treating metabolic acidosis, and a urinary alkalinizer for treating hemolytic emergencies and drug overdoses (e.g., salicylates and lithium). When using this product as an antacid, adult patients should take 1 to 2 tablets every 4 hours, up to a maximum of 24 tablets in 24 hours. Patients 60 years and older should not take more than 12 tablets in 24 hours. The oral powder is used by mixing ½ teaspoon in half (120 mL) of a glass of water and drinking as often as every 2 hours.

 Work Wise

Sodium bicarbonate is sometimes abbreviated in the workplace. You may hear your colleagues refer to it as *sodium bicarb.*

Much larger doses of sodium bicarbonate are needed when it is used as an oral systemic alkalinizer: 12 to 24 tablets (650 mg) are dissolved in 1–2 L of water and consumed during an hour. When using the IV form for systemic alkalization, 2–5 mEq/kg are administered over 4 to 8 hours, which allows the pH to be increased slowly. When using sodium bicarbonate as a urinary alkalinizer, the dose is 6 tablets (650 mg) initially, and then 2 to 4 tablets every 4 hours under the supervision of a physician.

Side Effects Sodium bicarbonate intake can result in sodium toxicity, which causes fluid overload. Renal function and cardiac function are impaired when sodium and water retention occurs. Tetany can also occur with sodium bicarbonate use.

Contraindications Sodium bicarbonate is contraindicated in patients with hypernatremia, severe pulmonary edema, hypocalcemia, and abdominal pain of unknown origin.

Cautions and Considerations Sodium bicarbonate is a vesicant at 8.4% and higher concentrations. Avoid extravasation and, in the event it occurs, discontinue the sodium bicarbonate solution. Extravasation may cause tissue necrosis (death) and skin sloughing. To prevent this condition, healthcare practitioners must administer sodium bicarbonate slowly. They should also observe for signs of extravasation and heed any patient complaint of pain during the infusion process. Extravasation requires prompt treatment.

In addition, controlled infusion rates and frequent laboratory tests are necessary to prevent dramatic swings in the pH and allow for the gradual and safe correction of acidosis or alkalosis.

Alkalosis

Alkalosis is typically caused by a loss in hydrogen ions from the GI tract (e.g., by vomiting) or in urine. This loss produces a relative increase in bicarbonate, which elevates the blood pH.

Metabolic alkalosis occurs when excess acid is excreted via the kidneys (such as in excess diuresis) or when acid is lost from the stomach (either from vomiting or gastric suction). **Respiratory alkalosis** is a condition in which patients have low levels of plasma carbon dioxide due to increased respiration.

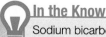
In the Know

Sodium bicarbonate, sometimes used to correct acid-base imbalances, can be found in the pharmacy and at the grocery store. Baking soda—used for cookies, cakes, and breads—is sodium bicarbonate. When combined with moisture and an acidic ingredient in baking, sodium bicarbonate undergoes a chemical reaction that produces bubbles of carbon dioxide. This reaction helps baked goods to rise.

Drug Regimens and Treatments

Acidic electrolyte products, most commonly ammonium chloride, may be used to treat alkalosis (see Table 26.5).

Ammonium Chloride

Ammonium chloride is an acidic substance used to treat metabolic alkalosis. It is typically administered in doses of 100–200 mEq mixed with 500–1,000 mL normal saline and then infused slowly over approximately 3 hours. This infusion prompts the kidneys to use ammonium in place of sodium in excretion processes. Less sodium is then available to combine to make sodium bicarbonate.

Side Effects Ammonium chloride can result in ammonium toxicity. Patients must be monitored for pallor, excess perspiration, irregular breathing, changes in heart rate, twitching, and seizures. If left untreated, coma and death could occur.

Contraindications Contraindications to ammonium chloride include liver or kidney dysfunction. Ammonium chloride should not be used in patients with metabolic alkalosis due to vomiting of hydrochloric acid that is accompanied by sodium loss.

Cautions and Considerations The concentrations and rates of infusion of ammonium chloride must be precise to avoid adverse effects. The maximum concentration of ammonium chloride when mixed with normal saline should be 1%–2%. The maximum infusion rate of ammonium chloride is 5 mL/minute to avoid venous irritation and ammonium toxicity.

Checkpoint 26.3

Take a moment to review what you have learned so far and answer these questions.

1. What is the difference between acidosis and alkalosis?

2. How would you describe the importance of the concentration and infusion rate of IV sodium bicarbonate and ammonium chloride?

Herbal and Alternative Therapies

Because electrolytes are essential trace minerals that are typically acquired from a nutritious diet, they are often categorized as dietary supplements rather than traditional OTC or prescription drug products. Oral dosage forms are indicated for situations in which immediate correction of an electrolyte imbalance is not necessary. Many electrolyte drinks are available on the market for rehydration after physical exercise, bouts of diarrhea, and vomiting associated with intestinal illness. Some of these products are listed in Table 26.3.

Chapter Review

Chapter Summary

Fluids and electrolytes are interdependent. Water is the primary body fluid and is compartmentalized into intracellular and extracellular spaces in the body. Extracellular fluid is located either in interstitial spaces or intravascular spaces. Electrolytes are molecular compounds that form ions when dissolved in water. Concentrations of electrolytes in the various fluid compartments are specific and help maintain equilibrium. When either fluid or molecules (such as electrolytes) are added or lost in one compartment, water shifts to compensate. Common electrolytes in the body include sodium, potassium, calcium, magnesium, chloride, bicarbonate, and phosphate. Excess or loss of any of these ions can produce significant illness if not addressed. Other ions, such as hydrogen ions (H^+) and bicarbonate, help maintain the acid-base balance in the body.

Dehydration is the excess loss of body fluids, primarily water. Edema is the accumulation of excess fluid in the interstitial space. Imbalances in electrolytes themselves may be related to fluid imbalances or other conditions. Each imbalance must be addressed individually for the patient and the electrolyte in question.

IV electrolyte products are used and prepared based on their tonicity (concentration compared with that of blood plasma). Hypertonic solutions have a higher concentration than blood plasma, and hypotonic solutions have a lower concentration. These solutions are used to hydrate patients and correct any other imbalances. Isotonic solutions have the same concentration as blood plasma and are used to maintain fluid status in the normal range.

Imbalances in electrolytes can cause changes in the blood pH. A decrease in pH produces acidosis, which is an excess of acidic molecules, such as carbon dioxide or a relative absence of basic molecules, such as bicarbonate. An increase in pH results in alkalosis, which involves depletion of acidic molecules or an increase in bicarbonate molecules. IV electrolyte solutions containing ammonium chloride and sodium bicarbonate are used to treat acid-base disorders.

IV fluids and electrolytes are products that allied health professionals may work with on a daily basis in the inpatient setting. Appreciation for the use, limitations, and special handling required for these products helps allied healthcare personnel deliver safe and effective care.

Chapter Checkup

The Navigator+ learning management system that accompanies this textbook offers many opportunities to help you master chapter content, including end-of-chapter exercises, a glossary of key terms, flash cards, and additional interactive activities.

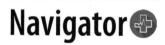

Career Exploration

If you enjoyed learning about fluids and electrolytes in this chapter, you may want to explore the following career options:

- athletic trainer
- certified clinical nutritionist
- clinical dietary specialist
- clinical laboratory scientist/technologist
- exercise physiologist
- intravenous (IV) pharmacy technician
- medical assistant
- medical laboratory technician
- medical laboratory technologist
- registered dietetic technician

27

Cancer and Chemotherapy

Andrea Iannucci and Tanja Monroe

Pharm Facts

- In the United States, one in two women and one in three men will develop cancer in their lifetime.

- The American Cancer Society's trademarked slogan, "The Official Sponsor of Birthdays," was registered in 2009 to support the belief that "a world with less cancer is a world with more birthdays."

- Seventy-eight percent of all cancer diagnoses are in individuals 55 years of age or older.

- The Global Burden of Disease Project, an independent research organization that tracks epidemiological levels and trends, reports that 34,000 cancer deaths per year worldwide are attributable to diets high in processed meats (ham, jerky, bacon, pepperoni, hot dogs, corned beef, sausages, canned meat).

- According to the American Cancer Society, cancer is the leading cause of death in the Hispanic population of the United States.

"I chose to become a chemotherapy technician because several of my family members and my best friend were diagnosed with cancer. I knew I wanted to make a difference in their lives and the lives of others who are battling this disease. As a chemotherapy technician, I prepare chemotherapy drugs using strict aseptic technique. Consequently, my work requires me to be meticulous, deliberate, and conscientious as I perform the sterile compounding procedures. Being part of a healthcare team that improves the lives of patients with cancer and, potentially, provides them with a cure is a rewarding experience."

—**Tanja Monroe**, CPhT
Hematology/Oncology Clinical
Pharmacy Technician

Learning Objectives

1 Explain the basic physiology of malignancy and tumor cell growth.

2 Identify and provide examples of traditional chemotherapy and cytotoxic drugs, hormonal drug therapies, and targeted drug therapies.

3 Identify the generic names, brand names, indications, dosage ranges, side effects, and cautions and considerations associated with the drugs commonly used to treat cancer.

4 Explain strategies that help prevent chemotherapy-related errors.

5 Identify current investigational therapies and alternative therapies used to treat cancer.

Each year, approximately 1.6 million individuals in the United States are diagnosed with cancer, and more than 500,000 patients will die from this disease. In fact, cancer is now the second-leading cause of death (behind heart disease) in the United States. These grim statistics are a reminder of the overwhelming impact cancer has on individuals, their families and caregivers, and the healthcare system. As part of this system, allied health professionals will most certainly be involved in caring for patients with cancer.

This chapter provides an overview of cancer and the arsenal of chemotherapy drugs used in the treatment of this disease. Chemotherapy drugs represent a complicated group of medications with a narrow window between safe therapeutic use and the potential for great toxicity. These medications are traditionally administered in a hospital or an out-patient chemotherapy infusion center by the intravenous (IV) route. Most IV chemotherapy drugs are prepared by pharmacists or pharmacy technicians in these settings. Over the past 10 years, however, the number of orally administered chemotherapy agents has increased; consequently, the care of patients with cancer is expanding into the community practice setting. This expansion has led to a greater number of healthcare personnel assisting patients with their chemotherapy regimens, including the management of the side effects from these toxic drugs.

In addition to having a good understanding of chemotherapy medications, allied health personnel must be cognizant of the safety measures that must be implemented during the preparation, handling, and administration of these medications. To that end, this chapter focuses on the potential hazards associated with chemotherapy so that healthcare personnel can protect their patients and themselves from harm.

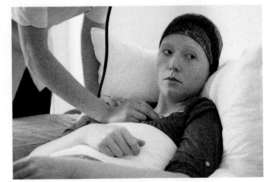

In the United States, breast cancer is the most common cancer among women.

Cancer and Its Development

Cancer is a term that describes a group of diseases characterized by the uncontrolled growth of dysfunctional cells. Normally, cells multiply only until there are enough of them to meet the needs of the body (for example, epidermal cells multiply to replace lost skin cells due to damage or aging). Cancer is thought to originate from a single cell (defined as **monoclonal**) that has lost its ability to control growth and proliferation.

This abnormal cell growth is caused by genetic changes that result from both external factors and internal factors. External factors include lifestyle choices, such as tobacco or alcohol use, sun exposure, poor nutrition, or physical inactivity; infectious disease processes; or exposure to environmental carcinogens, such as pesticides or asbestos. Internal factors include immune disorders, hormones, and genetic mutations. Although some cancers are hereditary, many more cancers result from some combination of lifestyle, environment, and genetic factors.

Pathophysiology of Cancer and Malignancy

In the past 20 years, scientists have discovered the role of genes in cancer development. Their research has established correlations between certain genetic mutations and the development of particular cancers. Identifying these correlations has been a catalyst for developing early cancer screening methods as well as targeting drug therapy for specific cancers. Both strategies continue to improve the early diagnosis and treatment of patients with cancer.

"Drivers" of Cancer

The two major classes of genes that play a role in cancer development are oncogenes and tumor-suppressor genes. Changes to these genes have been identified by scientists as the **"drivers" of cancer**, or genetic alterations that promote cancer progression.

Oncogenes

Oncogenes are genes that promote cancer formation. Oncogenes develop from **proto-oncogenes**, or genes that code for growth factors or their receptors (see Figure 27.1). All cells possess proto-oncogenes for normal function. Alterations of proto-oncogenes via exposure to chemicals, viruses, radiation, or hereditary factors can activate the oncogene that promotes abnormal cell growth. One example of an oncogene is the ERBB2 gene (also called the HER2/neu gene), which codes for a growth-factor receptor found in some forms of breast cancer.

FIGURE 27.1 Oncogenes and Cancer Formation

The activation of an oncogene converts a normal cell to a cancer cell.

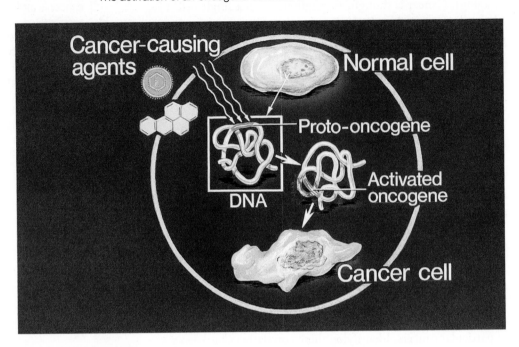

Tumor-Suppressor Genes

Tumor-suppressor genes turn off or down-regulate the proliferation of cancer cells. These genes are the brakes that inhibit inappropriate cell growth. Mutations or deletions of tumor-suppressor genes can also result in uncontrolled cell growth. One of the most common tumor-suppressor genes is *p53*. The normal gene product of *p53* halts cell division and induces **apoptosis**, or programmed cell death, in abnormal or aging cells. Mutations of *p53* are linked to resistance to many chemotherapy drugs.

Tumor Cell Proliferation

In general, tumor cells grow and divide with a high rate of proliferation. Growth of tumor cells is not, however, linear. Tumor cells exhibit an exponential rate of growth early on in tumor development, but the growth rate gradually slows over time. A model for **tumor cell proliferation** was developed by German mathematician Benjamin Gompertz. This model is now widely accepted as an approximation of tumor cell proliferation (see Figure 27.2). One cell divides into two cells; two cells divide into four cells; and so on. It typically takes about 30 divisions to make 1 g (about 1 cm^3) of tumor mass, which is the smallest clinically detectable tumor (1 g = 1 cm^3 = 10^9 = 1 billion cells).

During the exponential phase, a tumor is most sensitive to chemotherapy agents that attack and destroy rapidly dividing cells. After a tumor has reached a certain size, growth slows, possibly due to restrictions in space, decreased blood supply, and decreased nutritional supply. However, note that only 10 more divisions will make a 1-kg mass (about 10^{12} cells), which is considered a lethal tumor burden.

In the Know

Ancient Egyptian inhabitants believed that the appearance of a tumor, or swelling, on an individual's body was the result of an evil curse placed by the goddess Sekhmet. Therefore, they would perform elaborate rituals to rid the victim of this deadly disease.

FIGURE 27.2 Tumor Cell Growth

A tumor must reach a certain size before it can be detected. Unfortunately, chemotherapy drugs can kill only a percentage of cancer cells in the tumor after this point, instead of completely eradicating it.

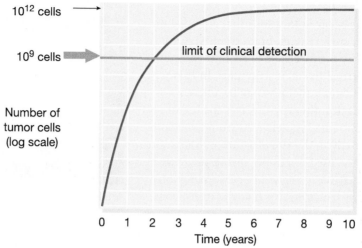

Adapted from Hoffman, Barbara, John Schorge, Joseph Schaffer, Lisa Halvorson, Karen Bradshaw, and F. Cunningham. 2012. *Williams Gynecology*, 2nd ed. New York: McGraw Hill Education.

Tumor Burden

Tumor burden is the number of cancer cells or the size of the tumor tissue. This measurement is a determining factor in the effectiveness of chemotherapy: The smaller the tumor burden, the more effective chemotherapy will be. A predominant hypothesis applied in cancer treatment is the **cell-kill hypothesis**. This hypothesis presumes that each cycle of chemotherapy kills a certain percentage of cancer cells. If a tumor has 10 billion cells and a chemotherapy cycle kills 95% of them, then 0.5 billion cells remain. The second cycle kills 95% more, leaving 25 million cells, and the third cycle would leave 1.25 million cells. Using this theory, tumor cell count will never reach zero from treatment alone, but once the number of cancer cells is low enough, normal host defense mechanisms take over to eradicate the remaining cells.

Treatments for Cancer

Treatments for cancer vary and are based on the type and location of the tumor as well as the extent of the disease. Tumors that are localized are generally easier to treat than tumors that have spread from the primary site to other parts of the body—a process known as **metastasis**.

There are four major modalities (methods) used to treat cancer. These methods include surgery, radiation therapy, immunotherapy, and chemotherapy. These treatments may be used alone or in combination to treat cancer.

Surgery

The most curable types of cancer are localized tumors that can be surgically removed or **resected**. Ideally, the tumor can be removed without leaving any cancer cells at the site of the resection. The surgeon typically removes a little bit of normal tissue around the site of the tumor—an area known as the **margin**. Once the tumor is completely resected, the surgeon assesses the site of removal for residual tumor cells. The absence of these tumor cells, a condition known as a **negative margin**, lowers the risk of tumor regrowth.

Radiation Therapy

Some tumors occur in locations that are difficult to reach with surgery (e.g., brain tumors). Other tumors may be too extensive to remove without damaging normal tissue or structures. In these situations, radiation therapy may be a better option. **Radiation therapy** involves the use of external beam radiation delivered from a machine outside the body to the site of a tumor. Radiation therapy may be used to rapidly shrink the mass of a tumor that is causing pain or impinging on vital organs or structures, such as the spinal cord. Sometimes, radiation therapy is used in conjunction with surgery to "clean up" areas of residual tumor that might have been left behind after surgery. This type of radiation therapy is called **adjuvant radiation therapy**.

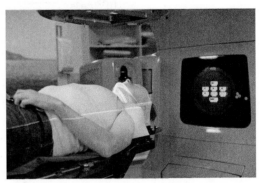

Almost half of all patients who have cancer undergo radiation therapy.

Immunotherapy

Immunotherapy is a type of cancer treatment that stimulates the immune system to stop or slow the growth of cancer cells. Two commonly used immunotherapy drugs are interferons and interleukins, which are used to treat **melanoma** (a frequently fatal type of skin cancer) and renal-cell carcinoma (an aggressive type of kidney cancer).

Immunotherapy in cancer treatment is being heavily researched. Newer immune-based therapies are being developed to prevent immune cells from being turned off by cancer cells. These novel therapies are called **immune checkpoint inhibitors** and represent a broad category of antineoplastic agents that are being studied on a number of tumor types.

Chemotherapy

Chemotherapy is the modality of administering drugs to treat cancer. This treatment method provides systemic exposure to anticancer therapy as a means of affecting the primary tumor as well as migrating tumor cells. Chemotherapy may be described as primary, adjuvant, or palliative, depending on the goals of therapy.

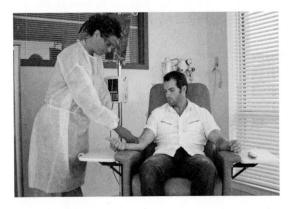

According to the American Cancer Society, prostate cancer is the most common cancer among men. Chemotherapy is sometimes used if the cancer has metastasized to other organs.

Primary Chemotherapy

Primary chemotherapy refers to the initial treatment of cancer with chemotherapy with **curative** intent. Examples of some of the cancers that can be cured with primary chemotherapy are Hodgkin's disease, lymphoma, leukemias, and testicular cancer.

Adjuvant Chemotherapy

Adjuvant chemotherapy refers to the treatment of residual cancer cells after removal or reduction of the tumor by surgery. Sometimes, if the tumor is too large to remove, a patient may be given **neoadjuvant chemotherapy** in an attempt to shrink the tumor so that it can be safely and completely removed with surgery. Both adjuvant and neoadjuvant chemotherapy can be curative if the tumor is effectively removed. One example of adjuvant therapy is administering chemotherapy and/or hormone therapy following a lumpectomy or mastectomy (types of surgical removal) in breast cancer. The patient is given adjuvant chemotherapy and radiation after surgery to ensure that any remaining cancer cells are eradicated.

Palliative Chemotherapy

Palliative chemotherapy is given for cancer that is not curable. The usual purpose of palliative chemotherapy is to prolong a patient's life and to improve his or her quality of life by decreasing the tumor size and reducing the symptoms caused by the tumor.

In the Know

In the late nineteenth century, German bacteriologist Paul Ehrlich used methylene blue stain to demonstrate cell pathology. His research in the use of chemical compounds to identify and treat diseases paved the way for genetic studies in cancer research and the development of drugs that interfere with the cell cycle. These drugs became known as *chemotherapy*, a term Ehrlich coined from the words *chemical* and *therapy*. For his pioneering work, Ehrlich won a Nobel Prize in 1908. Today, he is considered "The Father of Chemotherapy."

Checkpoint 27.1

Take a moment to review what you have learned so far and answer these questions.

1. How would you describe the cell-kill hypothesis?

2. What are the four major modalities of cancer treatment?

3. What are the treatment goals of primary chemotherapy, adjuvant chemotherapy, and palliative chemotherapy?

Chemotherapy Drugs

Multiple factors affect tumor response to chemotherapy drugs. Examples include the size of the tumor (tumor burden), cell resistance to the chemotherapy agent, the amount of chemotherapy administered, and the condition of the patient prior to chemotherapy. To reduce the potential for the cancer to become resistant to treatment, **combination chemotherapy** is usually administered. This type of regimen is designed to include drugs with the following characteristics:

- proven efficacy against the tumor being treated
- nonoverlapping toxicities
- different mechanisms of action

Sometimes combinations of drugs may have an enhanced response because the agents work together to amplify the individual effects of each drug. This is called a **synergistic effect**. The most important thing to know about combinations of anti-cancer drugs is that you cannot always predict the potential benefits or effects of the combination. Combination chemotherapy regimens must be selected based on proven safety and efficacy of the combination.

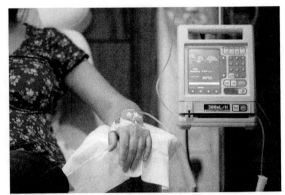

An infusion pump set delivers IV chemotherapy to a patient. The pump delivers medication at a controlled IV flow rate specified by the prescriber or pharmacist.

Cell Cycle and Mechanism of Action

Grasping how chemotherapy drugs work requires an understanding of the cell cycle. The **cell cycle** describes the process by which both normal cells and cancer cells divide. Because most cancer cells have lost their checks and balances on the rate of cellular replication, chemotherapy drugs are designed to interfere with the cell cycle at specific points.

Cell Cycle–Specific Drugs

Cell cycle–specific drugs exert their effects on rapidly dividing cancer cells, which are the most sensitive to the effects of chemotherapy. These drugs target cancer cells as they move into the susceptible phase of the cell cycle, while minimizing exposure to normal cells that may be in the resting phase of the cell cycle (see Figure 27.3). For this reason, these drugs are considered schedule dependent and are administered as continuous infusions (e.g., fluorouracil or cytarabine) or in repeated bolus doses (e.g., weekly bleomycin).

FIGURE 27.3 Cell Cycle

Often, multiple agents (shown in colored type) acting on different phases of cell growth and proliferation are used together to increase effectiveness and kill more cancer cells.

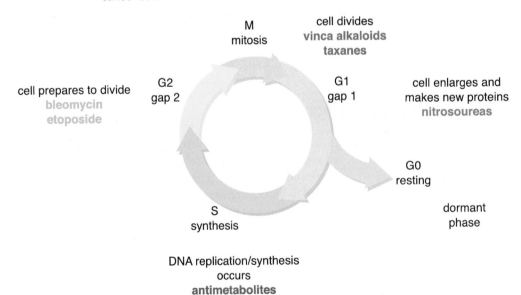

Cell Cycle–Nonspecific Drugs

Other chemotherapy agents can work at any point in the cell cycle and are called **cell cycle–nonspecific drugs**. The activity of these agents tends to be more dose dependent (higher dose provides higher cell kill) than schedule dependent. Cyclophosphamide, an alkylating agent, is an example of a cell cycle–nonspecific agent.

Kolb's Learning Styles

If you like collaborative learning, as Convergers do, get together with another student and describe the difference between cell cycle–specific and cell cycle–nonspecific chemotherapy. How do their mechanisms of action differ? How would changing the administration cycle of cell cycle–specific drugs enhance their cytotoxic effects on tumor cells? Think about how you would explain this process to a patient or family member who asks about how these drugs work.

Chemotherapy Drug Classifications

Chemotherapy drugs may be cytotoxic drugs (toxic to cells), hormonal therapies, immunotherapy, or one of the newer targeted anticancer therapies; however, many individuals consider cytotoxic drugs to be synonymous with the term *chemotherapy*.

Cytotoxic Drugs

Cytotoxic drugs work by interfering with some normal process of cell function or proliferation. Table 27.1 outlines the various categories of cytotoxic drugs and lists examples and major side effects of drugs within each category. Although cytotoxic drugs exert the majority of their effects on cancer cells, these agents do not target tumor cells specifically. As a result, chemotherapy drugs cause numerous side effects related to normal cell function. Side effects from traditional chemotherapy drugs might include **bone marrow suppression** (decreased production of blood cells, increased risks of infections and bleeding), **alopecia** (hair loss), nausea and vomiting, and **mucositis** (inflammation and ulceration of the mucous membranes lining the mouth and gastrointestinal [GI] tract). Table 27.2 describes some of the unique side effects of specific chemotherapy drugs as well as the preventive measures taken to avoid these toxicities. Although there are many risks associated with traditional chemotherapy agents, the use of these powerful drugs continues to either cure many patients of cancer or slow the progression of their disease, which prolongs their lives. Cytotoxic drugs remain a critical component of cancer treatment.

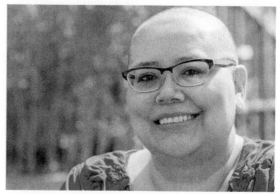

For patients with cancer, alopecia typically begins within the first two weeks of chemotherapy treatment and progressively worsens over the next two months.

TABLE 27.1 Traditional Chemotherapy and Cytotoxic Drug Categories

Category	Drugs	Major Side Effects
Alkylating agents	Bendamustine Busulfan Carboplatin Carmustine (BCNU) Chlorambucil Cisplatin Cyclophosphamide Dacarbazine Ifosfamide Lomustine Mechlorethamine Melphalan Oxaliplatin Procarbazine Temozolomide	Bone marrow suppression, alopecia, nausea and vomiting, infertility, secondary cancers
Antimetabolites	Capecitabine Cladribine Clofarabine Cytarabine Fludarabine Fluorouracil Gemcitabine Hydroxyurea Mercaptopurine Methotrexate Pemetrexed	Bone marrow suppression, immune system suppression, mucositis
Topoisomerase inhibitors	Daunorubicin Doxorubicin Epirubicin Etoposide Idarubicin Irinotecan Mitoxantrone Teniposide Topotecan	Bone marrow suppression, nausea and vomiting, mucositis, alopecia, diarrhea
Antimicrotubule agents	Docetaxel Eribulin Paclitaxel Vinblastine Vincristine Vinorelbine	Bone marrow suppression, mucositis, alopecia, nerve toxicity

TABLE 27.2 | Unique Toxicities of Chemotherapy Agents

Agent	Toxicity	Preventive Measures
Alkylating Agents		
Cisplatin	Kidney damage	• Administer aggressive IV fluids before and after each dose.
	Potassium and magnesium loss	• Provide potassium and magnesium supplements.
	Nerve pain and/or nerve damage	• Assess level of nerve damage with each treatment. Stop treatment at onset of symptoms. • Limit doses to $\leq$ 100 mg/m² for a cycle of treatment.
Ifosfamide	Hemorrhagic cystitis	• Administer IV fluids during and after treatment. • Give mesna (a bladder protectant) during and after treatment.
	Central nervous system (CNS) toxicity: confusion, delirium, paranoia, psychosis, coma	• Avoid ifosfamide in patients with severe kidney dysfunction to prevent CNS toxicity.
Oxaliplatin	Nerve pain and/or nerve damage (hands, feet, throat)	• Caution patients to avoid cold temperatures. • Advise patients to avoid cold beverages. • Limit doses or stop treatment if symptoms do not reverse.
Antimetabolites		
Capecitabine	Hand-foot syndrome	• Advise patients to use emollients on hands and feet.
	Diarrhea	• Limit doses or stop therapy if symptoms develop.
Cytarabine	Conjunctivitis	• Administer steroid eyedrops during treatment whenever patients receive doses > 1,000 mg/m².
Methotrexate	Kidney damage	• Administer aggressive IV fluids. • Provide urinary alkalinization using sodium bicarbonate.
	Severe bone marrow and mucosal toxicity	• Provide leucovorin rescue during the administration of methotrexate.
Pemetrexed	Severe bone marrow suppression	• Administer folic acid and vitamin B_{12} supplements, starting 5–7 days before treatment.
	Skin rash	• Give dexamethasone, starting 1 day before treatment.
Topoisomerase Inhibitors		
Anthracyclines: daunorubicin, doxorubicin, epirubicin, idarubicin	Cardiac toxicity: cardiomyopathy, congestive heart failure	• Track and limit cumulative doses. • Monitor heart function. • Stop treatment if symptoms develop.
Irinotecan	Severe diarrhea	• Administer atropine for diarrhea that occurs during drug administration. • Educate patients about how and when to take antidiarrheal agents (e.g., Imodium, Lomotil) after treatment.
Antimicrotubule Agents		
Paclitaxel	Allergic reaction	• Premedicate patients with diphenhydramine, famotidine, or another H2 blocker or with dexamethasone.
	Nerve pain and/or nerve damage	• Decrease dose or stop treatment if symptoms occur.
Vincristine	Nerve damage	• Cap individual doses at 2 mg. • Stop treatment if symptoms develop.
Miscellaneous Agent		
Bleomycin	Lung damage	• Track and limit cumulative doses to < 400 units. • Limit individual doses to $\leq$ 30 units. • Avoid giving to patients with kidney dysfunction.

Alkylating Agents

The oldest category of traditional cytotoxic drugs contains the **alkylating agents**. The first drug identified in this category as having anticancer activity was **mechlorethamine**, or nitrogen mustard, a derivative of mustard gas. The accidental release of mustard gas during World War II was only later discovered as playing a role in decreasing the activity of lymphocytes in soldiers who were exposed to the gas. The discovery of this reaction led to the development of this agent as a treatment for lymphoma, a cancer of the lymphatic system.

Alkylating agents work by binding to and damaging deoxyribonucleic acid (DNA) during the cell division process, ultimately preventing cell replication. Examples of alkylating agents are listed in Table 27.1. Alkylating agents have a broad spectrum of anticancer activity and are used to treat a variety of cancer types. **Cisplatin** is an alkylating agent that is used to treat many diseases, including lung, ovarian, and bone cancers. In addition, cisplatin is a critical component of the chemotherapy regimens for testicular cancer. **Cyclophosphamide** is an alkylating agent that plays an important role in treating lymphomas, leukemias, and breast cancer. **Carmustine**, also known as BCNU, and **lomustine** are in the category of alkylating agents known as **nitrosoureas**. These agents have the ability to penetrate the central nervous system (CNS) and are frequently used in the treatment of brain tumors. See Tables 27.3 and 27.4 for examples of other types of cancer that are treated with oral and injectable alkylating agents.

Side Effects The most common side effect of alkylating agents is bone marrow suppression. Alkylating agents also cause nausea, vomiting, and alopecia.

Many alkylating agents cause unique toxicities. Cisplatin is notorious for causing kidney damage and depleting potassium and magnesium levels. These side effects are minimized by providing patients with potassium and magnesium supplements as well as 1–2 L of IV fluid before and after administration of cisplatin. Cisplatin can also cause **peripheral neuropathy** (extremely painful damage to the nerves that affect the hands and feet) and **ototoxicity**, or damage to the nerves that affect hearing. Patients must be carefully assessed for these side effects between cycles of treatment, and doses should be decreased or stopped when symptoms develop. Maximum limits are placed on dosing cisplatin to avoid overdose

TABLE 27.3 Commonly Used Oral Chemotherapy Drugs

Generic (Brand)	Common Indication
Alkylating Agents	
Busulfan (Myleran)	Leukemia
Chlorambucil (Leukeran)	Chronic lymphocytic leukemia
Cyclophosphamide (Cytoxan)	Breast cancer, immune system diseases (e.g., arthritis, lupus)
Lomustine (Gleostine)	Brain tumor
Melphalan (Alkeran)	Multiple myeloma
Procarbazine (Matulane)	Brain tumor, Hodgkin's disease
Temozolomide (Temodar)	Brain tumor, melanoma
Antimetabolites	
Capecitabine (Xeloda)	Breast cancer, colon cancer
Hydroxyurea (Droxia, Hydrea)	Leukemia, sickle-cell anemia
Mercaptopurine (Purinethol)	Leukemia
Methotrexate (various brands)	Psoriasis, rheumatoid arthritis, systemic lupus erythematosus

TABLE 27.4 Commonly Used Injectable Chemotherapy Drugs

Generic (Brand)	Common Indication
Alkylating Agents	
Bendamustine (Treanda)	Chronic lymphocytic leukemia, lymphoma
Carboplatin (Paraplatin)	Breast cancer, lung cancer, ovarian cancer
Carmustine (BiCNU)	Brain tumor, lymphoma
Cisplatin (Platinol)	Bladder cancer, cervical cancer, ovarian cancer, sarcoma, testicular cancer
Cyclophosphamide (Cytoxan)	Breast cancer, immune system diseases, leukemia, lymphoma
Ifosfamide (Ifex)	Lymphoma, sarcoma, testicular cancer
Mechlorethamine (Mustargen)	Hodgkin's disease, lymphoma
Melphalan (Alkeran)	Multiple myeloma
Oxaliplatin (Eloxatin)	Colon cancer
Antimetabolites	
Cytarabine (Cytosar U)	Leukemia, lymphoma
Fludarabine (Fludara)	Leukemia, lymphoma
Fluorouracil (Adrucil)	Breast cancer, colon cancer, premalignant skin conditions (some), skin cancers (some)
Gemcitabine (Gemzar)	Bladder cancer, breast cancer, lung cancer, ovarian cancer, pancreatic cancer
Methotrexate (various brands)	Bone cancer, immune system diseases, leukemia, lymphoma
Pemetrexed (Alimta)	Lung cancer
Topoisomerase Inhibitors	
Daunorubicin (Cerubidine, Daunomycin)	Leukemia
Doxorubicin (Adriamycin)	Bone cancer, breast cancer, leukemia, lymphoma, multiple myeloma, sarcomas
Epirubicin (Ellence)	Breast cancer, esophageal/stomach cancers
Etoposide (VePesid)	Leukemia, lung cancer, lymphoma, testicular cancer
Idarubicin (Idamycin)	Acute leukemia
Irinotecan (Camptosar)	Brain tumor, colon cancer, lung cancer
Mitoxantrone (Novantrone)	Breast cancer, leukemia, lymphoma
Topotecan (Hycamtin)	Lung cancer, ovarian cancer
Antimicrotubule Agents	
Docetaxel (Taxotere)	Breast cancer, lung cancer, prostate cancer
Paclitaxel (Taxol)	Breast cancer, lung cancer, ovarian cancer
Vinblastine (Velban)	Lymphoma, testicular cancer
Vincristine (Oncovin)	Leukemia, lymphoma
Vinorelbine (Navelbine)	Breast cancer, lung cancer

and severe toxicities. **Ifosfamide** is known to cause **hemorrhagic cystitis**, or damage to and bleeding of the urinary bladder. This side effect can be prevented by coadministering the bladder-protective medication, **mesna**. Other unique toxicities of alkylating agents are outlined in Table 27.2.

Because alkylating agents cause damage to DNA, they are also **mutagenic**, meaning that they have the ability to cause changes in genetic material. As mutagens, these drugs have the potential to cause certain types of **secondary cancers** in patients who have received the drugs. The potential to cause secondary cancers is a rare but very serious side effect.

Alkylating agents are also known to cause damage to reproductive tissue, and patients who receive these medications may become infertile.

Drug Alert

Ifosfamide can cause severe hemorrhagic cystitis and must always be administered with the bladder-protective agent, mesna. Orders for administration of ifosfamide without mesna should *always* be questioned.

Contraindications Although alkylating agents are associated with several potential toxicities, there are very few absolute contraindications to the use of these agents in cancer treatment. Treatment decisions are always based on a risk/benefit assessment.

A history of allergic reaction would be one contraindication to the use of specific alkylating agents. Some alkylating agents such as cisplatin, **carboplatin**, and **oxaliplatin** are associated with a higher risk of allergic or hypersensitivity reaction. Patients who have exhibited an allergy to one of these agents may not be able to be treated with another agent in the *–platin* category. Skin tests to assess the risk of an allergic reaction and/or a protocol for administering sequentially escalating doses in a "desensitization" regimen may be considered as a means of managing patients who do not have other treatment options.

Other relative considerations to alkylating agents relate to avoiding some of the unique toxicities of these drugs. For example, patients with kidney dysfunction may not be good candidates for cisplatin therapy, which could worsen their kidney function, or ifosfamide therapy, which can cause serious CNS toxicity when given to patients with kidney dysfunction.

✚ *Note: Allied health professionals should be aware that an allergy to a particular drug contraindicates its use. This warning applies to all Contraindications sections in this chapter.*

Cautions and Considerations Alkylating agents are hazardous drugs and require special handling precautions for personnel who prepare and administer them. Some alkylating agents are absorbed through the skin, so extreme caution must be used when handling them. Healthcare personnel also need to be aware of the potential for exposure to these agents from patients' stool and contaminated body fluids such as urine.

Antimetabolites

Another class of cytotoxic drugs, known as **antimetabolites**, works in the synthesis phase of the cell cycle. These medications have differing mechanisms of action. Some antimetabolites inhibit enzyme production or activity that is needed for DNA or ribonucleic acid (RNA) synthesis. Methotrexate, cytarabine, and fluorouracil are antimetabolite drugs that interfere with the enzymes that are essential for tumor cell proliferation. Antimetabolites may also act as false **nucleotides** (the structural components of DNA and RNA) and, therefore, become falsely incorporated into DNA during synthesis because they resemble DNA nucleotides. **Mercaptopurine** is an antimetabolite drug that interferes with cell synthesis by replacing normal nucleotides in DNA/RNA production.

Antimetabolite drugs are used to treat a variety of cancers (see Tables 27.3 and 27.4). **Fluorouracil** and its oral counterpart, **capecitabine**, are commonly used to treat colon cancer. A topical form of fluorouracil also exists to treat some low-grade skin cancers and precancerous skin lesions. **Gemcitabine** is an antimetabolite drug that is used to treat lung and pancreatic cancers, and **pemetrexed** is an antimetabolite drug that is critical to the treatment of certain types of lung cancer. **Cytarabine** and **fludarabine** are drugs that are primarily used to treat different types of leukemia and lymphoma. One unique feature of cytarabine is that this agent is able to be safely administered directly into the CNS via a lumbar puncture (or "spinal tap") to patients who have leukemia cells in their cerebrospinal fluid. This procedure is referred to as **intrathecal (IT) administration. Hydroxyurea** is an orally administered antimetabolite drug that is commonly used to rapidly lower white blood cell counts in patients who have leukemia. Hydroxyurea is also used to help decrease painful crisis episodes for individuals with sickle-cell anemia.

Drug Alert

Even in very low doses, methotrexate can be extremely toxic, especially if it is administered incorrectly. Methotrexate is *never* administered daily for extended periods. Daily orders for even very low doses of methotrexate (e.g., 2.5 mg PO once a day) should *always* be questioned.

Methotrexate is commonly used to treat leukemia, bone cancer, breast cancer, and lymphomas, as well as a variety of nonmalignant immunologic conditions, such as psoriasis, rheumatoid arthritis, and systemic lupus erythematosus. (For more information about these nonmalignant immunologic conditions, see Chapters 9, 10, and 24, respectively.) Methotrexate suppresses immune system function and is one of the most complicated antimetabolites to administer. Methotrexate may be administered by different routes, including oral, IV, IT, intramuscular, and subcutaneous. It is given in a wide range of doses, from 5 mg once a week for rheumatoid arthritis to 20 g once or twice a month when used for bone cancer. If administered incorrectly, methotrexate can result in serious and sometimes fatal toxicities.

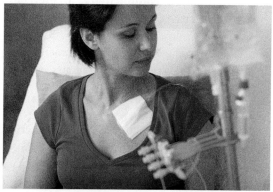
Methotrexate is frequently used to treat breast cancer in women. This drug is often administered through a central venous catheter into the subclavian vein.

Side Effects The major overlapping side effects of antimetabolite drugs include bone marrow suppression, immune system suppression, and mucositis.

Antimetabolite drugs also exhibit some unique toxicities (see Table 27.2). For example, one of the most serious side effects of methotrexate is kidney damage. When methotrexate is administered in doses above 1,000 mg, it can accumulate in the kidneys and form damaging renal crystals. To prevent such accumulation, patients are given IV fluids containing sodium bicarbonate or sodium acetate in order to alkalinize (increase the pH of) the urine. Increasing the urine pH makes methotrexate more soluble and prevents renal crystals from forming.

In high doses, methotrexate can also cause severe bone marrow suppression and mucosal injury in the GI tract. These side effects occur because methotrexate interferes with an enzyme that is important in normal bone marrow and mucosal cell development: dihydrofolate reductase. **Folinic acid** (also known as **leucovorin**) is a by-product of this enzyme. Therefore, the administration of folinic acid to patients who have received high-dose methotrexate rescues normal cells and allows the cells to resume their normal proliferation. This process, known as **leucovorin rescue**, is usually initiated 24 to 36 hours after the start of the methotrexate infusion, thus allowing methotrexate to exert its action on cancer cells. Timing is essential for leucovorin rescue because leucovorin cannot rescue cells that are exposed to high levels of methotrexate for more than 48 hours.

The oral antimetabolite capecitabine can cause a debilitating reaction called **palmar-plantar erythema**, better known as **hand-foot syndrome**. In hand-foot syndrome, patients experience painful sloughing and peeling of the skin on the palms of the hands and soles of the feet. The appearance of this condition in patients taking oral capecitabine necessitates a pause in treatment as well as a reduction in subsequent doses.

Cytarabine is an antimetabolite used in a wide range of doses. When it is administered at doses above 1,000 mg/m² of body surface area, cytarabine is excreted in tears and causes a chemical irritation of the eye. This irritation results in **conjunctivitis**. To prevent this side effect, patients receiving high-dose cytarabine must also receive steroid eyedrops (e.g., dexamethasone, prednisolone) during therapy and for 24 to 48 hours after completion of therapy.

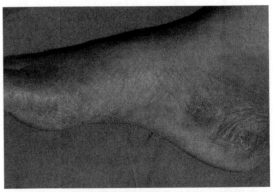

Hand-foot syndrome, a painful sloughing of the skin on the palms of the hands and soles of the feet, is a possible side effect of capecitabine.

Contraindications Similar to alkylating agents, antimetabolite drugs have very few absolute contraindications to their use.

For individuals who have a deficiency or a lack of an enzyme called *dihydropyrimidine dehydrogenase* (an enzyme that helps to break down and eliminate fluorouracil and capecitabine), a significant reduction in doses or a selection of alternative agents may be necessary. These individuals are extremely susceptible to the side effects of fluorouracil and capecitabine.

Methotrexate should not be administered as part of an anticancer treatment regimen to women who are pregnant. Because of its unique toxicity profile, methotrexate also should not be administered to patients with severe kidney dysfunction. Lastly, because methotrexate accumulates in interstitial spaces (a condition known as *third-space fluid shift*), this medication should be avoided or administered with extreme caution in patients who have ascites or pleural effusions.

Cautions and Considerations Antimetabolites are hazardous drugs and require special handling precautions for all personnel who prepare and administer them. As cell cycle–specific drugs, the cytotoxic effects of antimetabolite agents as well as their side effects may change, depending on how the agent is administered. Adjustments in the administration of these agents should only be made after considering the potential consequences.

Sometimes, the administration of these agents is manipulated to provide the best therapeutic effect. For example, in chemotherapy for patients with newly diagnosed acute leukemia, cytarabine is typically administered as a 24-hour continuous infusion for 7 days. By administering this cell cycle–specific agent continuously, the drug will be present in the synthesis phase of the cell cycle, where the cells are most susceptible to the toxic effects of this agent. In contrast, gemcitabine is a cell cycle–specific drug that is typically administered as a 30-minute infusion. Extending the duration of a gemcitabine infusion to 60 minutes might seriously increase the toxicity of this drug. Therefore, dosage schedules for antimetabolite drugs must be carefully followed to prevent excessive toxicity from these agents.

Topoisomerase Inhibitors

Some enzymes important in the process of DNA synthesis and cell replication are topoisomerases. DNA structure is tightly coiled and must be unwound during the replication process. Topoisomerases produce temporary breaks and repairs in DNA strands, which help unwind the DNA and allow the transcription process to occur.

There are two types of topoisomerase enzymes: **Topoisomerase I enzymes** produce single-strand DNA breaks, and **topoisomerase II enzymes** produce double-strand DNA breaks. Topoisomerase inhibitors interfere with the DNA repair function of topoisomerases and disrupt the cell replication process. These agents are very important components of cancer treatment and are used to treat many different types of cancer (see Table 27.4).

Topoisomerase I inhibitors include topotecan and irinotecan, both of which are derived from the *Camptotheca acuminata* tree. **Topotecan** is commonly used to treat ovarian cancer and lung cancer. **Irinotecan** is most frequently used to treat lung cancer and colon cancer. Both of these agents are also used to treat brain tumors or brain metastases because of their ability to penetrate the CNS.

Anthracyclines represent a large category of **topoisomerase II inhibitors** that are commonly used. Anthracyclines inhibit topoisomerase activity by inserting themselves (or intercalating) into strands of DNA. Anthracyclines are also referred to as DNA **intercalating agents**. These agents include daunorubicin, doxorubicin, epirubicin, and idarubicin. They are derived from a microorganism species, *Streptomyces*, which is found in soil and produces a red pigment. The *–rubicin* portion of their names comes from the French word *rubis*, which describes the red color of anthracycline agents. **Doxorubicin** is part of curative chemotherapy regimens for breast cancer and lymphoma. It is also used in treating bone cancer, leukemia, multiple myeloma, and sarcomas. **Daunorubicin** and **idarubicin** are primarily used to treat leukemia. **Epirubicin** is most frequently used to treat breast and esophageal/stomach cancers.

Etoposide and mitoxantrone are two other topoisomerase II inhibitors. **Etoposide** is derived from the American mayapple plant and is commonly used to treat leukemia, lung cancer, lymphoma, and testicular cancer. **Mitoxantrone** is similar in activity to the anthracyclines but has an inky blue color. This medication is frequently used to treat breast cancer, leukemia, and lymphoma.

Work Wise

Allied health professionals who work with chemotherapy patients may hear the acronym *CHOP* being used in the workplace. This acronym refers to a combination chemotherapy regimen:

Cyclophosphamide

Hydroxydaunorubicin (better known as doxorubicin)

Oncovin (brand name for vincristine)

Prednisone

Side Effects Topoisomerase inhibitors cause many of the same side effects common to other chemotherapy agents: bone marrow suppression, nausea and vomiting, mucositis, alopecia, and diarrhea.

Because these agents interfere with DNA, topoisomerase inhibitors also have the ability to cause secondary cancers such as acute leukemia. Although rare, the potential to cause secondary cancers is a serious side effect of topoisomerase inhibitors.

Another serious toxicity that can occur in patients who receive anthracyclines is **cardiac toxicity**. Cardiac toxicity from anthracyclines typically occurs many years after patients have received the drug. The risk of cardiac toxicity with anthracyclines is cumulative, increasing with each dose the patient receives. The best way to limit the risk of cardiac toxicity with these drugs is to track the patient's cumulative exposure and stop treatment after he or she has reached a **threshold dose**. The threshold dose is different for each anthracycline drug. For example, the lifetime cumulative dose limit for doxorubicin is approximately 450 mg/m^2, whereas the cumulative dose limit for idarubicin is approximately 225 mg/m^2.

Irinotecan causes the unique side effect of severe diarrhea (see Table 27.2). If not managed quickly, diarrhea from irinotecan can lead to serious complications. Patients who experience this type of diarrhea are treated with atropine, which is an injectable anticholinergic drug. The most serious form of diarrhea occurs in the days following administration of irinotecan. Patients must be adequately warned about the potential for this side effect and educated on how to appropriately administer antidiarrheal agents, such as loperamide, at the onset of symptoms.

Contraindications There are few absolute contraindications to the use of specific topoisomerase inhibitors. Patients who have a history of cardiac disease and/or evidence of congestive heart failure or cardiac dysfunction may not be good candidates for any of the anthracycline agents.

Many of the topoisomerase drugs are eliminated from the body through the liver and biliary systems. Therefore, patients who have significant liver dysfunction may not be able to tolerate drugs such as anthracyclines or irinotecan.

Topotecan is eliminated by the kidneys, so patients with significant kidney dysfunction are not good candidates for this agent.

Finally, patients who have a previous history of an allergic reaction to one of the topoisomerase inhibitors should not receive these medications.

Cautions and Considerations Patients who have a mutation in the liver enzyme UGT1a, the enzyme responsible for breaking down irinotecan, are susceptible to increased toxicity from irinotecan when this agent is administered in high doses. A commercial test is available to identify patients who have this genetic mutation. However, the clinical utility of this test is not widely established; therefore, it is not recommended for routine use.

Anthracyclines—such as daunorubicin, doxorubicin, epirubicin, and idarubicin— cause severe tissue damage if the infusion leaks under the skin during administration. This leaking and the related damage is called **extravasation**. Drugs that cause extravasation injury are referred to as **vesicants** (see Table 27.5). As such, anthracyclines require special precautions to prevent extravasation during administration. Veins must be chosen carefully for administration of vesicant drugs. In addition, patients must be carefully monitored during administration of chemotherapy vesicants so that the infusion can be stopped immediately if drug leakage is observed or if

TABLE 27.5 Chemotherapy Vesicant Drugs

Daunorubicin	Mitomycin
Doxorubicin	Vinblastine
Epirubicin	Vincristine
Idarubicin	Vinorelbine
Mechlorethamine	

patients complain of pain near the injection site. If vesicant drugs are to be administered in a prolonged infusion, patients must have central venous catheters or surgically placed implanted ports to decrease the risk of extravasation.

Some anthracycline drugs have been prepared in lipid formulations, known as **liposomal products**, to help decrease toxicity. Both daunorubicin and doxorubicin have liposomal formulations. Liposomal daunorubicin is known as DaunoXome, and liposomal doxorubicin is known as Doxil.

Antimicrotubule Agents

Microtubules are important to cell function. They play a role in maintaining cell shape and structure and are critical elements in the process of cell division or mitosis. **Antimicrotubule agents** interfere with the formation and function of microtubules, ultimately preventing cell growth and division.

Most antimicrotubule drugs are derived from plant sources. **Paclitaxel** and **docetaxel**—the **taxanes**—are derived from the bark and needles of yew trees. **Vincristine**, **vinblastine**, and **vinorelbine**—the **vinca alkaloids**—are derived from periwinkle plants. Antimicrotubule agents are important components in the treatment of lung, breast, ovarian, prostate, and testicular cancers, as well as for some types of leukemia and lymphoma.

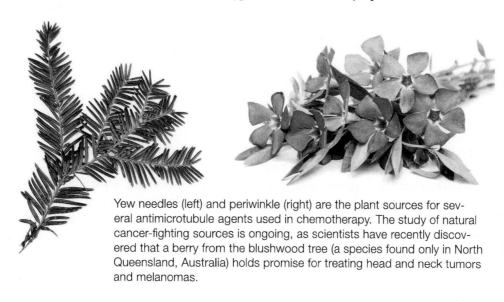

Yew needles (left) and periwinkle (right) are the plant sources for several antimicrotubule agents used in chemotherapy. The study of natural cancer-fighting sources is ongoing, as scientists have recently discovered that a berry from the blushwood tree (a species found only in North Queensland, Australia) holds promise for treating head and neck tumors and melanomas.

Side Effects Similar to other traditional cytotoxic drugs, antimicrotubule agents cause bone marrow suppression, mucositis, and alopecia. The degree of alopecia varies with these chemotherapy agents. For example, patients receiving paclitaxel may experience total body alopecia, including loss of eyelashes, eyebrows, and pubic hair. Nausea and vomiting with antimicrotubule agents may occur but is generally mild.

Because microtubules also play an important role in nerve function, many antimicrotubule agents cause peripheral neuropathy. Patients must be carefully assessed for this side effect while receiving paclitaxel or vincristine. Vincristine, in particular, can cause neurotoxicity to the GI tract. While on therapy with vincristine, patients must be closely monitored to make sure they do not develop an **ileus**, a condition in which GI motility is severely reduced.

Other unique side effects of taxanes include bone and muscle aches, which can occur for several days after an infusion. These side effects are typically managed with an over-the-counter (OTC) pain reliever such as acetaminophen or ibuprofen.

Contraindications The antimicrotubule agents paclitaxel and docetaxel are contraindicated in patients who have a history of a hypersensitivity reaction.

Vincristine should not be administered to patients who have a history of peripheral neuropathy. This medication may worsen the neuropathy.

Paclitaxel, docetaxel, vincristine, and vinblastine are contraindicated for patients with significant liver dysfunction because these agents are eliminated by the hepatic and biliary system.

 ## Drug Alert

Vincristine and vinblastine must *never* be administered by the intrathecal (IT) route. This warning is critical. Fatalities have been reported around the world when vincristine was inadvertently administered as an IT agent.

Cautions and Considerations Because they are plant derivatives, paclitaxel and docetaxel are commonly associated with allergic reactions during drug administration. Patients typically require premedication with antihistamines and corticosteroids to prevent severe allergic reactions to these drugs. Patients who have had allergic reactions to one or both of these agents may require additional premedication with corticosteroids or may not be able to tolerate reexposure to the agent, depending on the severity of the reaction.

Miscellaneous Cytotoxic Drugs

Two commonly used chemotherapy drugs that do not fit into the other cytotoxic drug categories are bleomycin and asparaginase.

Bleomycin works by causing cuts or breaks in DNA strands, preventing the process of cell proliferation. It is part of the curative chemotherapy regimens used to treat testicular cancer and Hodgkin's disease (a type of lymphoma).

Asparaginase is a drug with a very narrow spectrum of activity. Asparaginase is used to treat a common and often curable type of leukemia in children—acute lymphocytic leukemia. Leukemia cells require a large amount of the amino acid **asparagine** to proliferate. Unlike normal cells, leukemia cells are not able to make asparagine. Asparaginase is an enzyme that breaks down asparagine, depriving leukemia cells of this essential amino acid.

Side Effects Unlike many other cytotoxic drugs, one advantage to bleomycin is that it does not cause bone marrow suppression. However, this medication can cause a deadly type of lung toxicity known as **pulmonary fibrosis**. This condition occurs when the delicate tissue of the lung is damaged or scarred. It is important to track and limit cumulative doses of bleomycin to decrease the risk of pulmonary fibrosis.

Allergic reaction is one of the most common side effects of asparaginase therapy. Because asparaginase products are made from two different bacterial sources, patients who develop an allergic reaction to one product can often safely switch to the other product. Asparaginase can also interfere with normal protein synthesis in patients who are receiving it. Consequently, patients receiving asparaginase therapy have to be closely monitored for effects on clotting factors and might be at a higher risk for bleeding or clotting.

Contraindications Because of the risk for lung toxicity, patients older than age 60 may not be good candidates for treatment with bleomycin. Young patients who are athletes may also choose to limit their exposure to bleomycin in an effort to preserve their lung function.

Cautions and Considerations Patients who have received bleomycin may be at a higher risk for respiratory problems during surgery with general anesthesia. With that in mind, healthcare practitioners should educate patients about this risk and remind them to report prior exposure to bleomycin in all future preoperative assessments.

Hormonal Drug Therapies

Some types of cancer depend on naturally occurring hormones for growth (see Chapter 21 for human sex hormones). In tumors that are known to be dependent on specific hormones for proliferation, one treatment strategy is to block the activity of those hormones. Hormonal or endocrine drug therapies target the hormonal agent that is contributing to the growth of the specific type of tumor. For example, estrogen and progesterone are hormones that frequently stimulate breast tumors. Prostate cancer is often dependent on androgens, such as testosterone, for growth.

Antiestrogens

Antiestrogens—such as tamoxifen, anastrazole, letrozole, and exemestane—are commonly used to treat breast cancer. **Tamoxifen** works by blocking the estrogen receptor and can be used in the treatment of breast cancer for women of any age. **Anastrazole, letrozole,** and **exemestane** are **aromatase inhibitors**. These agents block the effects of estrogen by preventing synthesis of estrogen in the body. However, aromatase inhibitors only work in women who have experienced menopause. Younger women who have not undergone menopause will have too much ovarian production of estrogen that will counteract the effects of these agents.

Side Effects Side effects of antiestrogen therapy are very similar to menopausal symptoms, such as hot flashes, mood swings, and depression. In addition, the use of these agents can increase a woman's risk for blood clots and endometrial cancer.

Contraindications A history of blood clots may be a relative contraindication for therapy with an antiestrogen agent. However, physicians and patients may decide that the potential benefits of therapy outweigh the risks and choose to initiate therapy with enhanced monitoring for signs and symptoms of blood clots. Antiestrogen agents should also be avoided in patients who are pregnant or trying to become pregnant.

Cautions and Considerations Although associated with an increased risk of endometrial cancer, tamoxifen is approved for the *prevention* of breast cancer in women who have very high risk factors for developing the disease. Women using tamoxifen for breast-cancer prevention must be closely monitored for endometrial changes that are early indicators of cancer.

Antiandrogens

Antiandrogens work by blocking the activity of testosterone at the receptor level or interfering with the production of testosterone. These medications include **abiraterone, bicalutamide, enzalutamide,** and **flutamide,** and they are used to treat prostate cancer.

Side Effects Side effects of antiandrogen agents include hot flashes, breast tenderness, **gynecomastia** (enlargement of the breasts in men and boys), and decreased libido. Many antiandrogen agents also cause toxicity to the liver.

Contraindications There are no absolute contraindications to the use of antiandrogen agents.

Cautions and Considerations Patients taking antiandrogen agents must be educated about the potential for these agents to interact with other drugs. For example, both bicalutamide and flutamide can increase the anticoagulant effects of warfarin. For this reason, patients must be instructed not to add new drugs to their regimen without consulting a healthcare professional who is aware of all of their medications.

LHRH Agonists

Luteinizing hormone–releasing hormone (LHRH), also known as *gonadotropin-releasing hormone*, stimulates the production of both male and female reproductive hormones. LHRH initially stimulates the production of sex hormones, but, over time, continuous exposure to LHRH ultimately shuts down the production of sex hormones through a negative feedback loop (see Chapter 21). **Leuprolide** (Lupron) and **goserelin** (Zoladex) are analogs of naturally occurring LHRH. These drugs are called **LHRH agonists** and are frequently given to patients with hormone-sensitive tumors, such as breast and prostate cancers, to eliminate the source of endogenous estrogen, progesterone, and testosterone production.

Side Effects LHRH agonists cause many of the same side effects that are seen with antiandrogens. These side effects include hot flashes, gynecomastia, breast tenderness, decreased libido, and liver abnormalities. In addition, these agents can also cause local reactions or pain at the injection site.

Contraindications There are no absolute contraindications to the use of LHRH agonists in male patients. Women who are breast-feeding or pregnant should not be exposed to these drugs.

Cautions and Considerations Because LHRH analogs initially *stimulate* the production of testosterone, patients with prostate cancer can actually experience a flare of symptoms at the onset of therapy. This reaction can be significant if the tumor is in close proximity to vital structures (e.g., the spinal cord) or is associated with pain. To prevent this type of flare reaction, patients are commonly prescribed an antiandrogen such as bicalutamide to overlap with the first few weeks of LHRH agonist therapy.

LHRH agonists are available in a variety of dosage formulations that last for different durations. For example, these medications are available as injections that can provide an effect for days, weeks, or months. Healthcare practitioners who handle LHRH agonists must be cognizant of the different formulations of these agents.

Targeted Anticancer Therapies

As scientists have learned more about the biology of cancer, they have identified features of certain types of cancer that are critical for tumor cell growth. These critical components have become targets for more sophisticated cancer treatments. **Targeted anticancer therapies**, for example, are directed at specific molecular entities that are required for tumor cell development, proliferation, and growth. By targeting specific features of tumor cells, these therapies exert fewer effects on normal cells and are usually better tolerated than are traditional cytotoxic drugs.

Because targeted anticancer therapies are relatively new agents in the arsenal of cancer-fighting drugs, oncologists are still learning about them. Although these therapies have some serious and unusual side effects, they typically offer patients a much more direct treatment for their cancer, with fewer side effects than those that accompany traditional cytotoxic drugs. Targeted anticancer therapies are the future of anticancer treatment. For an overview of these therapies, see Table 27.6.

TABLE 27.6 Targeted Anticancer Therapies

Category	Anticancer Effect	Examples
Angiogenesis inhibitors	Prevent formation of blood vessels that allow for tumor growth and invasion of surrounding tissue	Bevacizumab (Avastin) Lenalidomide (Revlimid) Thalidomide (Thalomid)
Monoclonal antibodies	Target a specific marker or receptor on the surface of tumor cells, leading to destruction of those cells	Cetuximab (Erbitux) Panitumumab (Vectibix) Rituximab (Rituxan) Trastuzumab (Herceptin)
Signal transduction inhibitors	Prevent transmission of intracellular signals that stimulate cell proliferation	Axitinib (Inlyta) Bosutinib (Bosulif) Dasatinib (Sprycel) Erlotinib (Tarceva) Imatinib (Gleevec) Nilotinib (Tasigna) Sorafenib (Nexavar) Sunitinib (Sutent)

Angiogenesis Inhibitors

Although some targeted anticancer therapies have narrow therapeutic applications, many agents have been developed to target a wider variety of cancers. **Angiogenesis inhibitors** work by preventing tumor cells from building blood vessels that would supply the tumor with vital nutrients. By inhibiting new blood vessel formation at the site of the tumor, the tumor cells will eventually die.

Bevacizumab, for example, has significant anticancer activity in breast, lung, colon, and brain cancers. This medication also seems to enhance the effects of cytotoxic drugs when administered in combination with them.

Lenalidomide, another angiogenesis inhibitor, treats cancers of the blood. This medication targets mantle cell lymphoma and is used in combination with dexamethasone to treat multiple myeloma. Like lenalidomide, **thalidomide** is part of a combination drug therapy with dexamethasone for the treatment of multiple myeloma.

Side Effects Although most side effects associated with targeted anticancer therapies are less severe and more manageable than those seen with cytotoxic drugs, some of these drugs can cause very serious reactions.

Bevacizumab has the potential to interfere with wound healing and normal blood vessel formation. Bevacizumab may also cause bleeding, such as GI bleeding, nose bleeding, and CNS bleeding. Patients must be carefully monitored for bleeding, and treatment should be stopped if symptoms develop. Bevacizumab can also cause **hypertension** (high blood pressure) and kidney damage, so blood pressure measurements and urine samples must be evaluated prior to treatment.

Contraindications Bevacizumab is contraindicated in patients who have active bleeding (e.g., nosebleeds, blood in sputum) and in patients who have a significant risk of bleeding.

Cautions and Considerations Because bevacizumab interferes with normal wound healing, this medication must not be given to patients within four weeks of a surgical procedure.

Lenalidomide and thalidomide are reproductive toxins and should not be handled by healthcare personnel who are pregnant, possibly pregnant, or trying to conceive. Because of the high risk for reproductive toxicity, the prescribing and dispensing of these agents is strictly regulated. Prescribers, patients, and pharmacies must be registered with the manufacturers of these agents in order to access these drugs.

Monoclonal Antibodies

A **monoclonal antibody** is an antibody that has been developed from a single type of immune cell that was cloned from a parent cell. These antibodies are directed against a specific marker or antigen on target cells. Monoclonal antibodies are developed from a variety of sources, including mouse, bacterial, and human cell lines. Some of these medications designed to target specific markers on tumor cells have a limited range of activity.

Trastuzumab is a monoclonal antibody developed to target the HER2/neu receptor commonly found on breast cancer cells. However, this drug does not have as much activity in treating other types of tumors.

Rituximab was developed to treat non-Hodgkin's lymphoma and, therefore, targets a specific marker (CD20) on B lymphocytes. Because lymphocytes are active in various immunologic diseases, such as rheumatoid arthritis, rituximab has become a mainstay in treating many nonmalignant conditions by using the same mechanism of action—targeting CD20.

Cetuximab and **panitumumab** are monoclonal antibodies that target the epidermal growth factor receptor (EGFR), a growth factor receptor present on many types of cancer cells. Cetuximab has shown potential in treating head and neck, colon, lung, and pancreatic cancers. Panitumumab is used to treat colon and rectal cancers.

Side Effects Because monoclonal antibodies are frequently derived from animal sources, these medications can cause allergic reactions, such as a fever, chills, and flushing. Typically, these reactions occur during drug administration. Infusion reactions with rituximab and cetuximab can be prevented by premedicating patients with acetaminophen, diphenhydramine, or, possibly, corticosteroids. More serious allergic reactions, such as **anaphylaxis**, necessitate a change in therapy.

Drug Alert

Many monoclonal antibodies and some chemotherapy drugs pose a high risk of causing anaphylaxis in patients receiving these agents. Some institutions create policies or protocols that allow staff to initiate a rapid response to manage these allergic reactions. These protocols include procedures for additional monitoring as well as medication administration, including corticosteroids, antihistamines, bronchodilators, and epinephrine. Anaphylaxis kits containing these agents are created in portable cases that may be kept at the bedside while patients are receiving these high-risk medications. When using anaphylaxis kits, it is important that all members of the patient's healthcare team are aware of the content and location of the kits as well as the specific protocols for the use of these agents.

Contraindications Specific contraindications to monoclonal antibodies have not been determined.

Cautions and Considerations Many targeted anticancer therapies cause acnelike skin reactions. Sometimes, the rash that appears from the use of targeted therapies is a sign that the treatment is working. For example, patients who develop a rash while receiving cetuximab generally have a better response to treatment than those who do not develop a rash. These rashes can usually be managed with topical creams and antibiotic gels. On some occasions, the rash may be so severe that treatment must be stopped.

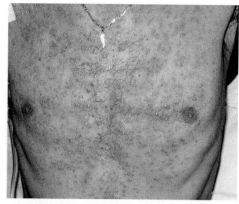

A skin rash is a known side effect of therapies that target epidermal growth factor receptors, such as cetuximab and erlotinib.

Signal Transduction Inhibitors

Certain targeted anticancer therapies were developed to affect the molecular abnormalities associated with specific tumor types. **Signal transduction inhibitors** are included in this category and were designed to target tumor-cell receptors. Typically, these medications are small-molecule oral agents that block or prevent communication and intracellular functions related to tumor growth and proliferation.

There are many types of signal transduction inhibitors being used and developed for cancer treatment. **Imatinib** and **dasatinib** were developed to target a specific chromosomal mutation associated with chronic myelogenous leukemia (CML). This type of cancer can be fatal if it is not managed in the early stage of the disease. These drugs have revolutionized the way CML is treated, and patients on oral therapy can maintain their disease state for many years without the risk of disease progression. However, because imatinib and dasatinib work against the specific abnormality associated with CML, these drugs have not been very useful in the treatment of other types of cancer. Newer agents in this same category of drugs include **nilotinib** and **bosutinib**.

Side Effects As previously mentioned, targeted anticancer therapies are generally better tolerated than traditional chemotherapy drugs. The side effects associated with signal transduction inhibitors vary greatly, depending on the specific target of the agent. **Edema**, or the swelling of tissues caused by excessive fluid retention, is one side effect of some of these agents. In addition, many signal transduction inhibitors can cause changes in normal cardiac conduction and hypertension. Medications used to treat CML can cause mild bone marrow suppression.

Contraindications There are no specific contraindications for signal transduction inhibitors. In general, there is limited experience in using these agents during pregnancy. Patients who become pregnant while taking a signal transduction inhibitor

In the Know

In the United States, 5,000 patients are diagnosed with CML every year. Prior to the approval of imatinib and the other tyrosine kinase inhibitors for CML treatment, the best chance for long-term survival with CML required bone marrow transplantation, an intensive procedure associated with a mortality rate as high as 25%. Now patients with CML are treated with oral signal transduction inhibitors and have long-term survival rates as high as 90%.

There are many other targeted anticancer therapies used in current cancer treatment. These therapies include drugs for treatment of lung cancer (erlotinib), breast cancer (lapatinib), and kidney cancer (pazopanib, sorafenib, and sunitinib). These agents have shown promising activity in the treatment of these diseases but have not yet accomplished the level of revolutionary therapy that signal transduction inhibitors have offered patients with CML.

must consult with their obstetrics/gynecology practitioner and medical oncologist to discuss the potential risks and benefits of continuing the agent during pregnancy.

Drug Alert

Many signal transduction inhibitors end with the suffix *-inib*. Consequently, a healthcare professional who sees a medication with this suffix should be alert for important drug interactions.

Cautions and Considerations Healthcare practitioners should have a heightened awareness of the potential for drug interactions during signal transduction inhibitor therapy. Prescription drugs as well as OTC and herbal or supplemental therapies have been shown to decrease the effectiveness of these agents. For example, histamine blockers or proton-pump inhibitors used for stomach acid suppression, such as famotidine or omeprazole, can decrease the absorption of dasatinib. Certain herbal therapies, such as St. John's wort, can decrease the efficacy of imatinib. Agents that interfere with the activity of these signal transduction inhibitors put patients at risk for disease progression. Other drug interactions can result in toxicity of these targeted anticancer therapies. Therefore, healthcare practitioners should discuss with their patients the importance of reporting any new drug or herbal therapy *before* taking it at the same time as a signal transduction inhibitor.

Patients who are taking oral signal transduction inhibitors to treat CML must continue their therapy without interruption to avoid progression to the accelerated phase of this disease.

Kolb's Learning Styles

No matter your preferred learning style, you may find it useful to approach learning chemotherapy drugs from the patient's point of view. Start with a list of common types of cancer (such as breast, prostate, colon, and lung). List the chemotherapy, hormonal therapies, and targeted drug therapies mentioned in this chapter that are used to treat each type of cancer. Then, for each drug, list the potential side effects the patient may experience when taking the medication. Organizing the information this way not only helps you recall these facts but also puts it into the patient's perspective. Imagine you are the patient and think about the choices you would make and the adverse effects you would face if given each therapy.

Investigational Therapies

Because knowledge of the causes of cancer is rapidly evolving, cancer therapy is a highly progressive field of research. Cancer researchers are constantly studying new approaches to improve cancer treatment outcomes. For many types of cancer, there are no curative therapies available. Even for cancers in which therapeutic options are plentiful, patients may not respond to currently available treatment options. As a result, many patients with cancer seek treatment with investigational drug therapies.

Investigational drugs are medications that are not yet approved by the US Food and Drug Administration (FDA) but are being studied as part of a clinical research program. There are thousands of clinical trials available to patients with all different stages and types of cancer. Healthcare personnel might suggest to their patients to discuss with their physicians what clinical trial options are available within their healthcare system. Patients who are interested in investigational therapies for cancer can also conduct their own research on the Internet. For example, the National Cancer Institute provides information on clinical trials online: http://PharmEssAH.emcp.net/CancerClinicalTrials.

Lastly, some investigational therapies for cancer may be approved for commercial use in another country or are currently under investigation for treatment of very rare or uncommon diseases. Frequently, these agents are made available to patients via expanded access or "compassionate use" approval. In this situation, the FDA allows the use of a particular investigational agent for a specific disease outside of a clinical trial. This type of approval is granted on a case-by-case basis and only in treatment of a serious medical illness or life-threatening condition. Institutional policies on how **expanded-access drugs** are handled may vary, so healthcare personnel who work with these medications should ensure that all local and institutional requirements are met before initiating therapy with these agents.

 ## Checkpoint 27.2

Take a moment to review what you have learned so far and answer these questions.

1. How are targeted anticancer therapies different from traditional, cytotoxic drugs?

2. Why is it important for patients on drug therapy for cancer treatment to consult with a healthcare professional before taking any new medications?

Handling and Administration of Chemotherapy Agents

Individuals involved in the handling and administration of chemotherapy risk possible accidental exposure to these hazardous agents and potential long-term effects as a result. Methods of possible accidental exposure include the following:

- inhalation, which can occur when (1) capsules or tablets are opened, broken, or crushed, or (2) hazardous drugs are prepared without adequate respiratory protection for the handler

- ingestion, which can occur when individuals are (1) eating or drinking in areas where hazardous drugs are stored or prepared, (2) placing food on contaminated surfaces, or (3) touching food or their mouths with contaminated hands

- injection, which can occur when healthcare personnel have a needle-stick injury during the preparation or administration of a chemotherapy agent

- topical absorption via the skin and/or eyes, which can occur when (1) handling oral or injectable chemotherapy agents without donning personal protective equipment (PPE), and (2) being exposed to accidental powder or liquid spillage from broken vials or leaky IV bags

Individuals who have been exposed to hazardous drugs should be evaluated by a physician. Contaminated clothing should be disposed of in chemotherapy waste containers, and exposed skin should be thoroughly washed with soap and water.

Personal Protective Equipment

Personal protective equipment (PPE) should be used at all times when handling both oral and injectable hazardous drugs. PPE protects the handler from being exposed to hazardous drugs or their residue (if left on the outside of vials, bottles, or IV bags). PPE also serves as product protection by keeping contaminants, such as lint or bacteria from the skin of the handler, away from the medication.

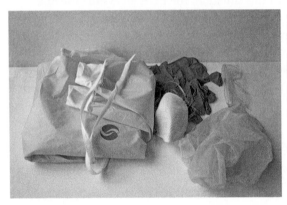

All healthcare personnel who prepare, handle, or administer chemotherapy drugs must don PPE including a single-use gown made of a thick, woven material that is impermeable to fluid; sterile, nitrile chemotherapy gloves; chemotherapy safety glasses; and a hair cover. A disposable respirator is also required.

PPE includes the following garments:

- shoe covers
- a disposable gown made of material that is impermeable to fluid
- sterile chemotherapy gloves
- chemotherapy safety glasses
- a hair cover
- a disposable respirator

Spill Kits

Individuals working with hazardous drugs should be trained to clean up small accidental spills to reduce exposure to hazardous drugs. To help with this task, healthcare personnel should have access to **spill kits** in all areas where hazardous drugs are prepared, administered, or transported. All cleanup supplies must be placed in sealed plastic bags and disposed of in appropriately labeled chemotherapy waste containers. Large spills may need to be cleaned up by the **hazardous materials (hazmat)** team.

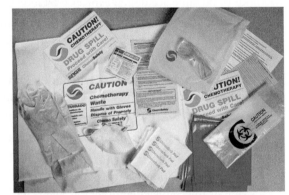

A chemotherapy spill kit is commercially available for purchase and should be used to clean up chemotherapy spills in both a healthcare setting and a home care setting.

In addition, every institution that prepares, dispenses, or administers hazardous medications is required to have a hazardous drugs communication program to identify drugs that require special handling and to outline the protocol for managing spills and other accidental exposure. Healthcare personnel should consult the Policy and Procedures (P&P) manual of their facility to learn these hazardous drug handling requirements.

If an accidental spill occurs, personnel should refer to **Safety Data Sheets (SDSs)**—formerly referred to as Material Safety Data Sheets—to guide the cleanup process (see Figure 27.4). SDSs are available from manufacturers for all potentially hazardous drugs

---

FIGURE 27.4 Safety Data Sheet

The Occupational Safety & Health Administration requires chemical manufacturers to provide SDSs for all hazardous chemical products.

spectrum®

SAFETY DATA SHEET

Preparation Date: 3/6//2013	Revision Date: 11/04/2015	Revision Number: G2

1. IDENTIFICATION

Product identifier

Product code: M1435
Product Name: METHOTREXATE, USP

Other means of identification

Synonyms: Amethopterin; (+)-Amethopterin; Amethopterine; 4-Amino-4-deoxy-N(sup 10)-methylpteroylglutamate; 4-Amino-4-deoxy-N(sup 10)-methylpteroylglutamic acid; 4-Amino-10-methylfolic acid; 4-Amino-N(sup 10)-methylpteroylglutamic acid; Antifolan; L-(+)-N-(p-(((2,4-Diamino-6-pteridinyl)methyl)methylamino)benzoyl)glutamic acid; N-(p-(((2,4-Diamino-6-pteridinyl)methyl)methylamino)benzoyl)-L-(+)-glutamic acid; N-(p-(((2,4-Diamino-6-pteridyl)methyl)methylamino)benzoyl)glutamic acid; N-Bismethylpteroylglutamic acid; Ledertrexate; Methylaminopterin; Methylaminopterinum; L-Glutamic acid, N-(4-(((2,4-diamino-6 pteridinyl)methyl)methylamino)benzoyl)- (9CI); Glutamic acid, N-(p-(((2,4-diamino-6-pteridinyl)methyl)methylamino)benzoyl)-, L-(+)-

CAS #:   59-05-2
RTECS #   MA1225000
CI#:   Not available

Recommended use of the chemical and restrictions on use

Recommended use: Medication.
Uses advised against   No information available

Supplier: Spectrum Chemical Mfg. Corp
     14422 South San Pedro St.
     Gardena, CA 90248
     (310) 516-8000
Order Online At: https://www.spectrumchemical.com

Emergency telephone number   Chemtrec 1-800-424-9300
Contact Person: Martin LaBenz (West Coast)
Contact Person: Ibad Tirmiz (East Coast)

2. HAZARDS IDENTIFICATION

Classification

This chemical is considered hazardous by the 2012 OSHA Hazard Communication Standard (29 CFR 1910.1200)

Acute toxicity - Oral	Category 3
Reproductive toxicity	Category 1B

Label elements

Product code: M1435   **Product name:** METHOTREXATE, USP   1 / 12

and chemical products. These sheets identify the drug or chemical and include its potential hazards, handling and storage requirements, first-aid measures for accidental exposure, and other critical information. There are a variety of Internet resources for obtaining SDSs for pharmaceutical products. Workplaces that handle hazardous drugs such as chemotherapy agents should keep copies of SDSs on file or have an established Internet link for each product they carry so that easy reference is possible when needed.

Preventing Chemotherapy-Related Medication Errors

Chemotherapy-related medication errors can occur at any step in processing an order. **Prescribing errors** occur when prescribers make an error in the order for a chemotherapy agent. **Transcription errors** occur when an order for a written chemotherapy order is incorrectly transcribed into the dispensing or computer system. (Transcription errors are virtually eliminated by the use of computerized provider order entry systems for chemotherapy drugs.) **Preparation errors** occur when a chemotherapy agent is prepared incorrectly. **Administration errors** occur when a chemotherapy agent is administered incorrectly.

Inventory and Storage Measures to Prevent Chemotherapy Errors

Several chemotherapy drugs have look-alike, sound-alike names or have similar packaging. To prevent inadvertent chemotherapy product mix-ups, healthcare personnel must implement storage and handling measures. Some of these measures include the following:

- not storing look-alike, sound-alike drugs next to each other

- affixing look-alike, sound-alike labels to certain medication containers to draw attention to the fact that there are other products with similar names or appearances (e.g., doxorubicin and liposomal doxorubicin [Doxil])

- using color-coded and/or labeled storage bins

- following manufacturers' warnings on hazardous drug products

- noticing tall-man lettering on medication labels (e.g., CISplatin vs. CARBOplatin, vinCRIStine vs. vinBLAStine). In tall-man lettering, the differing parts of two similar words are emphasized using capital letters (see Figure 27.5).

Work Wise

Everyone on the health-care team—including allied health professionals—plays a role in preventing medication errors with chemotherapy drugs. Whether involved in the preparation or administration of these highly toxic drugs, allied health personnel should be deliberate and methodical in their actions and should implement checks-and-balances procedures to ensure the safety of patients as well as themselves.

FIGURE 27.5 Carboplatin Medication Label

The medication label for carboplatin uses tall-man lettering to avoid confusion with another chemotherapy drug with a similar name: cisplatin.

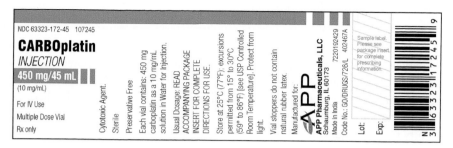

 Checkpoint 27.3

Take a moment to review what you have learned so far and answer these questions.

1. What are the four main types of errors that can occur when providing medication to a patient?

2. What are some inventory and storage measures healthcare professionals can take to prevent chemotherapy errors?

Herbal and Alternative Therapies

Many patients feel a loss of control when they are diagnosed with cancer or when their disease progresses. Consequently, some patients seek nontraditional or alternative approaches for treatment of their disease. Others simply prefer nontraditional therapies due to their holistic lifestyle or fundamental belief system. Although many herbal, supplemental, and complementary therapies are harmless, some are associated with significant toxicity and/or have the potential to negatively interact with traditional cancer treatments. In general, there is little scientific evidence to support many of the claims that are made for the curative potential of such supplemental and herbal therapies for cancer; however, some agents may provide effective symptom relief. Most of these agents are marketed as nutritional supplements, so they are not subject to the same regulatory standards as traditional, FDA-approved medications and can vary dramatically in quality and content. Most oncology practitioners discourage the indiscriminant use of herbal or supplemental therapies for cancer treatment. Healthcare personnel should encourage patients to discuss these agents with their oncology health professionals to determine if these medications are safe to use with their current cancer therapies.

 Patient Teaching

Discussions about the use of supplemental, complementary, or alternative therapies between patients and healthcare personnel may require a delicate approach. It is important not to make patients feel alienated over their beliefs or their desire to pursue the use of herbal or complementary agents.

Chapter Review

Chapter Summary

Chemotherapy agents have historically been administered to patients in a hospital or an outpatient chemotherapy infusion center by the IV route. With the introduction of orally administered chemotherapy drugs, cancer treatment is expanding into community settings. This expansion has led to a greater number of healthcare personnel assisting patients with their chemotherapy regimens. Because of the potential hazards associated with chemotherapy, it is important that healthcare personnel have a good understanding of chemotherapy drugs and the safety measures that must be implemented during the preparation, handling, and administration of these medications.

Cancer is a group of diseases characterized by the uncontrolled growth of dysfunctional cells. Two major classes of genes play a role in cancer development: oncogenes and tumor-suppressor genes. Oncogenes are genes that promote cancer formation; tumor-suppressor genes down-regulate the proliferation of cancer cells.

Tumor cells proliferate rapidly. During the exponential phase, the tumor is most sensitive to chemotherapy agents. A tumor burden is the number of cells or the size of the tumor tissue. The smaller the tumor burden, the more effective chemotherapy will be.

Treating cancer involves aggressive and rigorous therapy within multiple modalities, including surgery, radiation therapy, immunotherapy, and chemotherapy. These treatments may be used alone or together to treat cancer.

Chemotherapy may be described as primary, adjuvant, or palliative. Chemotherapy drugs are designed to interfere with the cell cycle at different points and have a narrow window between safe, therapeutic use and the potential for great toxicity.

Although cytotoxic drugs exert the majority of their effects on cancer cells, these agents do not target tumor cells specifically. As a result, chemotherapy drugs cause numerous side effects related to normal cell function, including bone marrow suppression, alopecia, nausea and vomiting, and mucositis.

Hormonal drug therapies target the hormonal agent that is contributing to the growth of the specific type of tumor. These therapies block the activity of that hormone.

Targeted anticancer therapies are relatively new agents in the arsenal of cancer-fighting drugs. Although these therapies have some serious and unusual side effects, they typically offer patients a much more direct treatment for their cancer.

Investigational therapies are also used for certain patients with cancer. Although not yet approved by the FDA, these therapies are used when no curative treatment regimens are available or when a patient is not responding to currently available treatment options.

All individuals who handle or administer chemotherapy medications must don PPE and have access to spill kits and SDSs. They must also implement safety measures for the storage and handling of these toxic agents, including separate storage areas for look-alike, sound-alike drugs; the application of labels to call attention to look-alike, sound-alike medications; and the use of color-coded storage bins. Healthcare personnel should also be alert to tall-man lettering and to the manufacturers' warnings on hazardous drug products.

Chapter Checkup

The Navigator+ learning management system that accompanies this textbook offers many opportunities to help you master chapter content, including end-of-chapter exercises, a glossary of key terms, flash cards, and additional interactive activities.

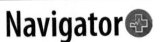

Career Exploration

If you enjoyed learning about chemotherapy and other cancer treatments in this chapter, you may want to explore the following career options:

- case manager
- certified clinical nutritionist
- chemotherapy technician
- computed tomography (CT) technician
- cytotechnologist
- diagnostic medical scientist
- genetic counselor
- histotechnologist
- magnetic resonance imaging (MRI) technician
- medical assistant
- medical dosimetrist
- occupational therapist
- positron emission tomography (PET) scan technician
- radiation therapist
- registered dietitian
- social worker

Pharmacotherapy for Special Patient Populations

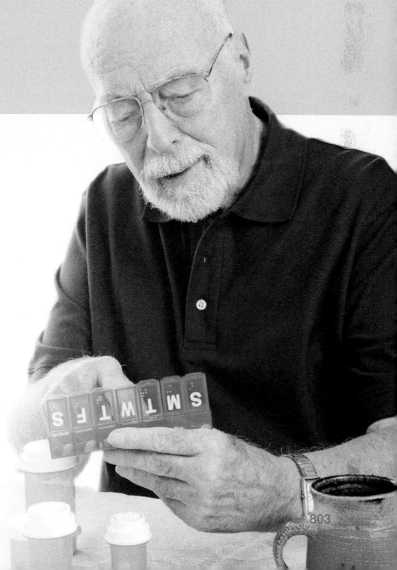

28 Pediatric Patients and Drug Therapy

Pharm Facts

- Less than 20% of medications are approved by the Food and Drug Administration for pediatric use; however, 89% of medications are used to treat children.

- Humans develop distinctive fingerprints by the age of three months. Fingerprints remain the same throughout life and are one of the last distinguishing characteristics to disappear after death.

- In 2015, the American Academy of Pediatrics recommended that children and young adults between 11 and 21 years of age be screened for high cholesterol levels due to rising obesity in this age-group.

- An average child triples his or her weight and grows one to one-and-a-half inches in height every month by one year of age. If human growth continued on that steep trajectory, a child who weighed 8 pounds and measured 20 inches in length at birth would weigh 315 pounds and be 25 feet tall by age 20.

"I began my career as an occupational therapist with the desire and passion to help others overcome both physical and mental obstacles that prevented them from accomplishing their dreams. One of my first clients was a young boy who lost both of his arms in an accident. I was struck by his resolve to not only accept his disability but to overcome it through grit and determination. Fitted with prosthetics, he was able to regain his independence and return to his normal school routine. His 'never-say-die' attitude continues to inspire me as I tackle personal obstacles in my life."

—**William C. Gielow**, MS, OTR /L
Program Chair/Occupational Therapist

Learning Objectives

1   Explain the unique healthcare challenges of neonatal and pediatric patients.

2   Understand the pharmacokinetics and pharmacodynamics of drugs in neonatal and pediatric patients.

3   Indicate specific drugs that are contraindicated or to be used with caution in neonatal and pediatric patients.

4   Know the common healthcare disorders that affect neonatal and pediatric patients and the drug therapies used to treat these conditions.

Pediatric medicine is a relatively new specialty in the medical community. Up until the nineteenth century, pediatric patients were primarily cared for by family members who had to rely on their own nurturing instincts as well as the advice of respected maternal figures in the community. With little understanding of pediatric anatomy and physiology, these untrained caregivers could sometimes do little to treat the healthcare needs of pediatric patients. Children were especially vulnerable to infectious diseases—such as smallpox, scarlet fever, and tuberculosis—due to their immature immune systems. To treat children who contracted these diseases, physicians would typically prescribe fresh air and cool fluids to rid the body of these germs. Other than these commonsense measures, no preventive therapies (such as vaccines) or cures existed. Consequently, infectious diseases claimed the lives of many thousands of children worldwide.

In response to the high mortality rates of children, pediatric hospitals in both London and Philadelphia were opened in the mid-1800s. These specialized hospitals catered to the illnesses and injuries of children. By the beginning of the twentieth century, the field of pediatric medicine had quickly become an established specialty. Early pediatric practitioners recognized that children have a unique physiology and, therefore, require medical treatment and medications to meet their specific healthcare needs.

Although the specialized diagnosis and treatment of children's health conditions underwent a significant transformation at the turn of the twentieth century, changes in drug therapy for children came slowly. Even well into the twentieth century, pediatric drug therapy was based on simply adjusting adult medication doses so that they were appropriate for a child's considerably smaller body size. Many different rules were developed by physicians to calculate the proper medication dose for a child. These rules contained calculations based on a child's weight, age, or a combination of both factors. The inconsistency of these rules led to inaccurate doses, and prescribers realized that a child's weight, not age, is a more reliable factor in determining a pediatric dosage. Today, some medications are formulated specifically for the physiology of pediatric patients.

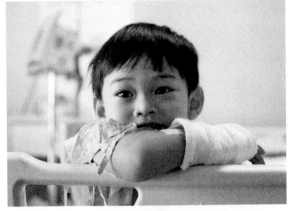

Pediatric patients have unique healthcare requirements. For this reason, children's hospitals offer state-of-the-art equipment sized for smaller patients and personnel who are educated and trained in treating children's physical, mental, and emotional needs.

This chapter addresses the unique challenges of pediatric patients and examines their specialized pharmacokinetics and pharmacodynamics processes. Understanding these distinct characteristics is essential to proper drug dosing. This chapter also focuses on disorders commonly seen in neonatal and pediatric patients and on their respective treatments, including safer alternative medications that should be used before other, more common drug therapies.

Unique Challenges of Pediatric Patients

Learning about the unique challenges of **pediatric patients** helps allied health professionals provide optimum care. Some of these challenges include the wide-ranging age-group of this patient population; communication issues among patients, their parents or caregivers, and healthcare practitioners; and an increased vulnerability of patients to medication errors.

Wide-Ranging Age-Group

The pediatric patient population spans a wide range of ages. Pediatric patients are categorized as follows:

- **fetus:** unborn offspring whose gestational age is determined by the number of weeks since conception (typically there are 40 gestational weeks in a pregnancy)
- **premature infant:** an infant born before the start of the 37th week of pregnancy
- **full-term infant:** an infant born during or after the 37th week of pregnancy
- **neonate:** an infant less than one month of age
- **infant:** a child whose age ranges from one month to one year of age
- **toddler:** a child whose age ranges from one to two years of age
- **preschooler:** a child whose age ranges from three to four years of age
- **grade-schooler:** a child whose age ranges from 5 to 12 years of age
- **adolescent:** a child whose age ranges from 13 to 18 years of age

Due to this wide range of ages, drug regimens and treatments must be catered to the physiology of the pediatric patient.

Communication Issues

The wide-ranging age-group of the pediatric population impacts healthcare communications. Unlike typical communications with adult patients, communications with pediatric patients are more complicated and involve a triad: the patient, his or her parents or caregivers, and the healthcare team. Collaborative decisions about medical care should involve the pediatric patient to the extent that is possible; consequently, all communications with a pediatric patient need to be developmentally based.

Vulnerability to Medication Errors

Children are far more vulnerable to medication errors than adults due to their unique pharmacokinetics, or the processing of medications in the body (see the section titled "Pharmacokinetics in Neonatal and Pediatric Patients" that follows). In fact, pediatric patients have a threefold risk of harm or death as a result of medication errors. Therefore, healthcare personnel must be vigilant in ensuring that the correct medication is administered in the correct dosage to the correct patient. All medications for pediatric patients should undergo multiple verification checks by healthcare staff members during the selection, preparation, and administration processes. (For more detailed information on medication errors, see Chapter 7.)

Pharmacokinetics in Neonatal and Pediatric Patients

The field of **pharmacokinetics** is devoted to observing and using mathematical models to predict how drugs enter, move around in, and leave the body. The pharmacokinetics process has four phases: absorption, distribution, metabolism, and excretion. This process impacts the effectiveness, dosing schedule, and use of medications. (For more detailed information on pharmacokinetics, see Chapter 3.)

Many factors need to be considered when determining drug therapy, including the specific characteristics of individual patients and how these characteristics might affect the pharmacokinetic properties of the drugs they take. Although some patient population generalizations can be made, no two patients are exactly alike. An awareness of these differences is important when choosing the best drug and an appropriate dose for each patient.

Age and liver and kidney functions are also significant factors when determining drug therapy. For this reason, prescribers and pharmacists are particularly challenged by the rapidly changing body systems of pediatric patients. These health professionals must be knowledgeable about pediatric physiology, dosing parameters, and drug properties to ensure the health and safety of children. Age-specific variation in the different stages of the pharmacokinetic processes can affect how rapidly and thoroughly certain types of drugs are processed (see Table 28.1).

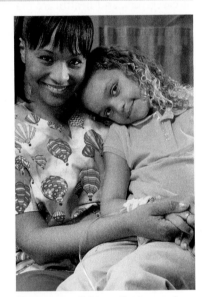

Because pediatric patients are at a high risk for medication errors, allied health professionals need to ensure that proper checks and balances are being followed during the preparation and administration of all drugs.

TABLE 28.1 Drugs Associated with Different Pharmacokinetic Processes

Pharmacokinetic Process	Affected Drugs
Absorption	pH-dependent drugs (e.g., penicillin), creams, ointments, IM injections
Distribution	Highly water-soluble drugs and highly protein-bound drugs
Metabolism	Acetaminophen (e.g., Tylenol), drugs processed by cytochrome P450 and UDP-glucuronosyltransferase enzymes
Excretion	Drugs eliminated by the kidneys

Safe and effective drug therapy requires that a drug is delivered to its target sites in concentrations that are sufficient to treat the disease state for which the agent is intended but not so high that drug levels can produce a state of toxicity. Patients experience toxic drug levels when they receive too much of a drug too fast, or when their bodies cannot get rid of a drug fast enough. In the pediatric patient population, premature infants, neonates, and infants are more vulnerable to drug toxicity than older children because of their size and immature physiology (liver and kidney functions). However, *all* children may be at risk for adverse drug reactions when their body weight has not been taken into account during drug dosing.

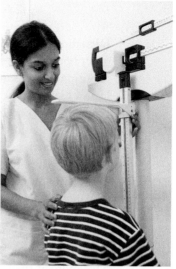

A child's body weight is an important measurement when determining drug dosing.

Absorption

Absorption is the process by which drugs enter the bloodstream. The absorption of drugs via different routes of administration is not the same in young children as it is in adults.

Oral Route of Administration

Because of slow gastric emptying, the rate at which oral medications are absorbed is slower in neonates and infants than in adults. Therefore, it takes longer for doses of drugs to achieve maximum plasma levels and reach full effect. Slow gastric emptying lasts until a child has reached approximately six to eight months of age.

The pH level in the gastrointestinal (GI) tract tends to be more alkaline in premature infants and neonates. (The pH level of the GI tract does not become more acidic until a child is between two and three years of age.) This higher gastric pH level affects the behavior of drugs that have pH-dependent absorption. Elevated pH levels can either increase absorption or decrease absorption, depending on the acid-base characteristics of a drug. For example, blood levels of penicillin, an acidic drug, in the alkaline GI tract of a neonate are five or six times higher than compared with blood levels of penicillin in older children.

Topical Route of Administration

Topical drugs such as creams and ointments may have a greater effect on children than adults because children may experience greater medication exposure. Children, especially the very young, have a higher ratio of body surface area to body mass than adults.

Rectal Route of Administration

In neonates and infants, liquid formulations are more likely to be effective than solid dosage forms (such as suppositories) because of the large number of bowel movements in this patient population. Frequent bowel evacuation increases the possibility of expulsion of the medication.

IM Route of Administration

Drugs delivered intramuscularly may be absorbed more effectively by infants than adults because of a higher density of skeletal-muscle capillaries in infants, but the rate of absorption is not very predictable because of differences in muscle mass, poor perfusion to various muscles, and other factors. Therefore, whenever possible, prescribers should avoid giving infants drugs via intramuscular (IM) injection.

Distribution

Distribution is the process by which drugs move around in the bloodstream and reach other body tissues. Factors such as body composition and protein binding affect distribution. Infants, for example, have a higher body water content than adults, so drugs that are highly water-soluble will distribute well, which could potentially lead to toxicity. In addition, neonates have lower levels of plasma proteins and an overall lower level of protein binding than adults have. Therefore, drugs that are highly protein bound will have more of their active form in circulation in neonates, and a dose that may seem appropriate for a neonate's weight might, in fact, be too high.

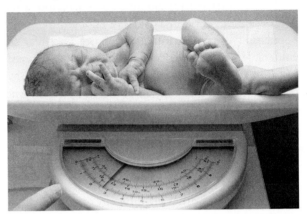

Because a neonate has a lower level of plasma proteins compared with an adult, a highly protein-bound drug will have more active drug in the bloodstream. Therefore, more drug will be distributed to body tissues.

Metabolism

Metabolism is a term that describes the way drugs are processed in the body, usually in the liver. In this process, the body breaks down and converts a medication into active chemical substances. In addition, metabolism serves to detoxify the blood. Many chemical gatekeepers in the body regulate metabolism, including cytochrome P450 enzymes (known as CYPs) and various transporter proteins. A given drug is generally processed by more than one of these gatekeepers.

In infants, drug metabolism is slower than the metabolism of older children and adults. This delayed metabolism occurs because certain CYP enzymes, such as CYP3A4, are present in very small numbers at birth. For this reason, a drug that is primarily processed via CYP3A4, such as simvastatin, would be more likely to build up to toxic levels in a very young patient whose enzyme levels are not at full strength, a process that is completed during the first year of life. Other enzymes, such as UDP-glucuronosyltransferases (UGTs), follow a similar pattern: small numbers at birth with a dramatic increase in the first year of life. UGTs affect the clearance of drugs such as acetaminophen. Consequently, infants are at risk for acetaminophen toxicity.

From 1 to 10 years of age, the rate at which drugs are cleared from the bloodstream by liver enzymes increases, and during that period the rates of clearance can be faster than adult rates.

Excretion

Excretion is the process by which drug molecules are removed from the bloodstream and leave the body, primarily in urine excreted from the kidneys. However, drug molecules can also be eliminated in bile, feces, perspiration, and exhalations. Although kidney function is low at birth, it increases rapidly and generally reaches adult levels by one year of age. When kidney function is low, the clearance of drugs from the body is slow. As a result, young infants may experience toxic levels of drugs that are primarily eliminated via the kidneys (e.g., aminoglycoside antibiotics, ibuprofen, and metformin). To avoid drug toxicity in infants, healthcare practitioners should prescribe lower doses of certain drugs and extend the intervals between doses.

As the pediatric patient's kidney function increases with age, the dosing of drugs that are primarily eliminated from the kidneys may need to be adjusted. For example, the kidney function of toddlers (children from one to two years of age) may reach a level of functioning that clears drugs via the kidneys more rapidly than in adults. Therefore, a larger dose or more frequent dosing may be required to treat a toddler.

Pharmacodynamics in Pediatric Patients

Whereas pharmacokinetics measures changes in drug levels in the body, **pharmacodynamics** studies the effects of drugs on the body. For example, pharmacokinetics measures the blood plasma level of an antihypertensive drug (a drug used to treat high blood pressure). Pharmacodynamics, on the other hand, measures the effect of the antihypertensive drug on a patient's blood pressure.

As you have already learned in this chapter, organ development and enzyme activity can lead to toxic drug levels in pediatric patients. To avoid these adverse effects, health practitioners need to be mindful of the following guidelines:

- Many drugs have not been tested on children, so the "safe" dose is not known.

- Some drugs should not be taken by children at any dose.

- Still other drugs should only be used to treat children after safer, alternative medications have been unsuccessful.

For drugs that have been extensively used to treat pediatric patients, health practitioners typically adjust the dose downward to avoid adverse events. To make this adjustment, prescribers sometimes use a chart called a *nomogram*, which assists them in calculating a child's dosage based on the child's height and weight (mass). (To view an example of a nomogram used in pediatric dosage calculations, see Chapter 6.)

Table 28.2 lists certain over-the-counter (OTC) and prescription drugs or drug classes that should be avoided or used with caution in children. Prescribers should turn to a pediatric dosing handbook (such as *The Harriet Lane Handbook of Pediatric Antimicrobial Therapy*) to assess the safety of each drug and to learn the appropriate dosing.

 Checkpoint 28.1

Take a moment to review what you have learned so far and answer these questions.

1. What are some of the unique challenges of providing health care to pediatric patients?

2. What happens to kidney function and the activity of metabolic enzymes in the liver during the first year of a child's life?

3. Why must health practitioners exercise caution when prescribing water-soluble drugs for infants?

TABLE 28.2 | Drugs to Avoid or Use with Caution in Pediatric Patients

Drug or Drug Class	Age Restriction	Risk(s) Posed by the Medication(s)
OTC Drugs		
Aspirin (Bayer, Bufferin, Ecotrin)	Do not use in children < 12 years of age who have flu symptoms or chicken pox.	Reye syndrome (potentially fatal)
OTC cough-and-cold medications	Do not use in children < 4 years of age.	Depends on individual product ingredients and may include oversedation and liver damage
Prescription Drugs		
Chloramphenicol (only available as a generic drug)	Use with caution in neonates; should only be used for serious infections that cannot be adequately treated with less toxic drugs.	Gray baby syndrome (potentially fatal)
Corticosteroids such as prednisone (Rayos) and steroid creams such as betamethasone (Luxiq)	Use with caution in all children; monitor growth rate during long-term use.	Slowed growth rate; more likely to cause adrenal crisis in children than in adults
Fluoroquinolone antibiotics such as cipro-floxacin (Cipro) and moxifloxacin (Avelox)	Use safer alternatives whenever possible.	Damage to joints and surrounding tissues
Promethazine (Phenergan)	Do not use in children < 2 years of age. In children ≥ 2 years of age, use cautiously at the lowest effective dose.	Potential for severe and possibly fatal respiratory depression
Sulfa antibiotics (e.g., sulfamethoxazole sold in a combination drug called trimethoprim/sulfamethoxazole [Bactrim])	Do not use in neonates; avoid use in infants < 2 months of age.	Hyperbilirubinemia, kernicterus
Tetracycline antibiotics such as minocycline (Minocin) and tetracycline (Sumycin)	Avoid use during tooth development (children < 8 years of age) unless alternatives are contraindicated.	Permanent tooth discoloration

Common Symptom Affecting Neonatal and Pediatric Patients

Fever, a symptom of the body's **febrile response**, is a common occurrence among pediatric patients. In fact, fever is one of the main reasons parents bring their children to pediatricians' offices, according to the American Academy of Pediatrics.

Fever

A **fever** is a higher-than-normal body temperature, defined as greater than 38° C (100.4° F). This symptom indicates that the body is fighting an illness. There is not always a correlation between a higher fever and a more serious illness: Some serious illnesses only cause a low fever, whereas milder infections may cause a high fever.

If an infant who is less than three months of age has a fever greater than

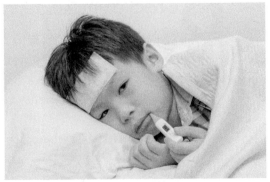

A fever from an infection typically does not rise above 103° F or 104° F.

38° C measured rectally, the parent or caregiver should call a physician. The temperature threshold for calling a physician is higher for children who are older than three months of age: greater than 39° C (102.2° F) measured rectally for children from ages 3 to 36 months, or greater than 39.5° C (103.1° F) measured orally for children older than 36 months.

Drug Regimens and Treatments

To treat a fever, a parent or caregiver should administer fluids to a child. If the child is uncomfortable, the parent or caregiver should administer an **antipyretic** (fever reducer) such as acetaminophen or ibuprofen, depending on the age of the child (see Table 28.3).

TABLE 28.3 Oral Liquid Antipyretics for Children

Generic (Brand)	Dosage Form	Age Restriction	Common Dosage	Maximum Dosage
Acetaminophen (Tylenol)	Capsule, oral suspension, oral syrup, tablet	For children < 3 months of age, consult a physician prior to administration	10–15 mg/kg* per dose every 4–6 hr	90 mg/kg a day; no more than 5 doses a day
Ibuprofen (Advil, Motrin)	Capsule, oral suspension, tablet	> 6 months of age	5–10 mg/kg* per dose every 6–8 hr	40 mg/kg a day

* For an obese child, it is possible that a weight-based dose could be a higher standard adult dose. In such cases, the standard adult dose is used.

Acetaminophen

Acetaminophen (Infants' Triaminic Fever Reducer, Tylenol) can be administered by a parent or caregiver to a child to reduce the fever. The parent or caregiver should follow the dosing guidelines that correspond to the child's age and weight. Children who are less than five years of age should only receive the liquid children's formulation of acetaminophen. Adult formulations of acetaminophen should *never* be administered to small children.

Ibuprofen

Another medication used to treat a fever in children who are older than six months of age is **ibuprofen** (Advil, Motrin). Ibuprofen should not be administered to children who are less than six months of age because of their reduced kidney function. Although both acetaminophen and ibuprofen are effective at reducing fever, acetaminophen is preferred in children because it has fewer side effects. Ibuprofen can cause gastritis (upset stomach) and should be taken with food, if possible.

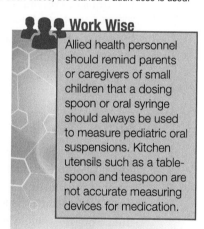

Work Wise

Allied health personnel should remind parents or caregivers of small children that a dosing spoon or oral syringe should always be used to measure pediatric oral suspensions. Kitchen utensils such as a tablespoon and teaspoon are not accurate measuring devices for medication.

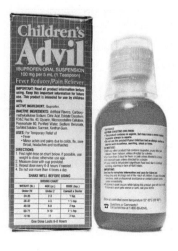

Children's Advil is a commonly used fever reducer and pain reliever. The medication label provides dosing guidelines for a child's weight and age.

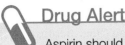
Common Conditions Affecting Neonatal and Pediatric Patients

A number of health conditions commonly occur in the pediatric patient population. These conditions affect several of the major body systems such as the sensory system (otitis media), cardiovascular system (iron-deficiency anemia), and respiratory system (asthma, croup, respiratory distress syndrome, respiratory syncytial syndrome, and pneumonia). Other common childhood disorders include infectious diseases that affect multisystems (diarrhea, streptococcal infections, acute bacterial meningitis, and bacteremia and sepsis).

Otic Disorder

According to the Centers for Disease Control and Prevention (CDC), the otic disorder **otitis media**—more widely known as a **middle ear infection**—is the most common pediatric outpatient diagnosis resulting in the dispensing of antibiotic prescriptions.

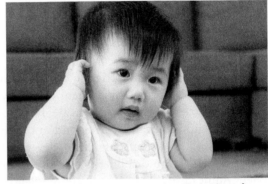

A baby pulling at his or her ear is a likely sign of a middle ear infection.

Otitis Media

The anatomic structure of children's ears plays a role in the frequent occurrence of otitis media. Because the **eustachian tube** in children is more horizontal than vertical as compared with adults, fluid from the middle ear does not drain well, allowing bacteria and viruses to flourish. Most middle ear infections are viral in nature and clear up on their own. Other infections develop after a child has contracted a viral respiratory tract infection in which mucus and fluid build up and provide a growing medium for pathogens. Symptoms of an ear infection include ear pain, jaw pain, sinus pain, itching, and fever. Pain is often severe enough to cause parents or caregivers to seek medical attention for their children.

Drug Regimens and Treatments

As mentioned earlier, otitis media is the most common reason antibiotics are prescribed for children. However, healthcare practitioners attempt to be judicious when prescribing antibiotics for ear infections so as to reduce **antibiotic resistance**. Antibiotics are given immediately for ear infections in infants who are less than 6 months of age and are suggested for ear infections in children who are 6 to 24 months of age. Children who are two years of age and older do not always receive antibiotics for middle ear infections. For this age-group, physicians consider the sever-ity of the infection and the child's medical history. (For more information on antibiotics, see Chapter 23.)

Oral drug therapy is the sole route of administration for the treatment of middle ear infections. Antibiotic eardrops will not effectively treat an infection of the middle ear because medica-tion applied to the external ear cannot reach the intended site of action. Table 28.4 shows a list of oral antibiotics used to treat otitis media. The drug of choice is the penicillin antibiotic amoxicillin, given at a high dose twice a day. However, children who have had more than one middle ear infection are given a different drug, amoxicillin/clavulanate, which covers additional types of bacteria. Because both drugs can cause diarrhea, it is helpful for patients to take these drugs with food.

Patients who have had an immediate allergy to penicillin drugs, such as amoxicillin, are given macrolide antibiotics, and patients who have experienced milder, delayed hypersensitivity to penicillins are prescribed cephalosporin antibiotics.

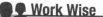

Work Wise

Healthcare personnel should recognize that many children have dif-ficulty swallowing tablets and capsules. To make a medication easier to swallow and better tast-ing for children, sprinkle the contents of a capsule into applesauce or use chocolate syrup to coat the oral medica-tion prior to swallowing. Some tablets may be ground into particles and disguised in flavorful liquids. Check with a pharmacist to determine if grinding a particular medication is safe.

Drug Alert

Semisynthetic penicillins such as amoxicillin are the preferred drugs used to treat infections such as otitis media. For this reason, allied health professionals should be sure to check a patient's medication history for any allergies to penicillin or its derivatives. Mild reactions to penicillin include hives, a rash, and itching; however, severe reactions such as anaphylaxis could be life threatening.

Patient Teaching

Most of the antibiotics prescribed for the treatment of otitis media are available as oral suspensions. Allied health personnel should remind parents or caregivers to shake the suspension container before measuring and administering a dose. If the bottle is not shaken, the patient will not receive a full dose of medication because the active ingredients in a suspension tend to settle at the bottom of the container.

Once a child is given antibiotics for the treatment of otitis media, the signs and symp-toms of infection usually clear up within one to three days. (However, allied health person-nel should remind parents or caregivers to administer the entire course of drug therapy.) The pain of ear infections is best treated with acetaminophen or ibuprofen at doses that are appropriate for the child's age and weight. In children who are two years of age or older, topical benzocaine (a numbing agent) may be used for pain; however, benzocaine should not be used if the patient has a ruptured tympanic membrane (eardrum). OTC deconges-tants and/or antihistamines should not be used to manage the symptoms of otitis media in children. In fact, the American Academy of Pediatrics recommends that no OTC cough-and-cold medications be administered to children who are less than four years of age.

Generic (Brand)	Dosage Form	Age Restriction	Common Dosage
Cephalosporins			
Cefdinir (Omnicef)	Capsule, oral suspension	6 months to 12 years of age	14 mg/kg a day, either in divided doses or dosed each day, max 600 mg a day
Cefpodoxime (Vantin)	Oral suspension, tablet	2 months to 12 years of age	10 mg/kg a day in divided doses, max 400 mg a day
Ceftriaxone (Rocephin)	Injection	2 months to 12 years of age	50 mg/kg a day dosed daily, max 1 g/dose
Cefuroxime (Zinacef)	Injection, oral suspension, tablet	≥ 3 months to 12 years of age	Injection: 50–100 mg/kg a day in divided doses, max 9 g a day Oral suspension: 30 mg/kg a day in divided doses, max 1 g a day Tablet: 250 mg twice a day
Macrolides			
Azithromycin (Zithromax)	Injection, oral suspension, tablet	≥ 6 months of age	10 mg/kg on day 1; 5 mg/kg on days 2–5
Clarithromycin (Biaxin)	Oral suspension, tablet	Not specified	15 mg/kg a day in divided doses
Penicillins			
Amoxicillin (Moxatag)	Capsule, chewable tablet, suspension, tablet	> 3 months of age and < 40 kg	90 mg/kg a day in divided doses
Amoxicillin/clavulanate (Augmentin)	Chewable tablet, suspension, tablet	≥ 3 months of age and < 40 kg	Amoxicillin: 90 mg/kg a day in divided doses, max 3 g a day Clavulanate: 6.4 mg/kg a day

Blood Disorder

One of the most common blood disorders among young children is iron-deficiency anemia. Iron is an essential nutrient for a child's growth and neurologic development. A deficiency of this nutrient results in decreased oxygen carried from the lungs to other parts of the body. (For more information on iron and nutrition, see Chapter 19.)

Iron-Deficiency Anemia

Iron-deficiency anemia is a lower-than-normal level of red blood cells (RBCs) in the body. Children with iron deficiency can experience impaired psychomotor and mental development that may have lifelong consequences. Whereas children who are born at full term have enough iron stored in their bodies to last the first five to six months of life, premature infants only have enough iron stores to last two to three months. Therefore, recommended guidelines to prevent iron-deficiency anemia are as follows:

- Infants who are born at full term (after the start of the 37th week of pregnancy) and are breast-fed should begin to receive iron supplementation at four months of age and continue this therapy until they are one year of age.

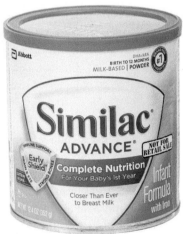

Premature infants and babies suffering from iron-deficiency anemia should receive iron supplementation such as an iron-fortified baby formula.

- Infants who are born prematurely (before the start of the 37th week of pregnancy) and are breast-fed should receive a higher dose of iron supplementation starting at one month of age.
- Infants who are fed formula should drink the iron-fortified variety.

Drug Regimens and Treatments

Children who are diagnosed with iron-deficiency anemia are given oral iron supplementation. There are several types of oral iron supplements that are effective, including ferrous sulfate, ferrous fumarate, and ferrous gluconate. Each form contains a different percentage of elemental iron content, which is important because dosing is based on the elemental iron content of the tablet, not the total milligrams in the tablet. (For more information on iron supplements, see Chapter 19.)

Patients will absorb more iron from each dose if the dose is taken with some source of vitamin C. In cases of severe iron deficiency, patients may be given iron dextran, an intravenous (IV) form of iron supplementation. Premature infants with severe iron deficiency may also be treated with a transfusion of RBCs or, in some cases, recombinant human erythropoietin (EPO).

Respiratory Disorders

Common childhood respiratory disorders include asthma, croup, respiratory distress syndrome, respiratory syncytial syndrome, and pneumonia. In fact, respiratory problems are one of the most common reasons for hospitalizations among children.

Asthma

Asthma is an inflammatory disorder of the airways and causes coughing, wheezing, breathlessness, and chest tightness. Inside the lungs, bronchioles constrict, mucus production increases, and tissue swells, making normal breathing difficult. Asthma affects more than 22 million individuals in the United States. Approximately six million of these asthma sufferers are children.

Each year, asthma accounts for thousands of emergency room (ER) visits, hospitalizations, and even deaths. The primary goal of treatment is to reduce acute and chronic troublesome symptoms, prevent exacerbations, and minimize hospitalizations or visits to the ER.

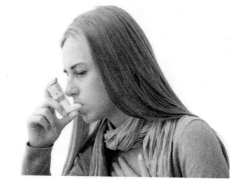

Asthma is a common chronic disorder among adolescents in the United States. For this reason, asthma is one of the leading causes of absenteeism in schools.

Drug Regimens and Treatments

Guidelines for the treatment of asthma divide pediatric patients into three age-groups:
- children who are younger than 5 years of age
- children who are 5 to 11 years of age
- children who are 12 to 18 years of age

Although there are fewer treatment options for the youngest group of patients, the treatment pattern is generally similar for the three age-groups (see Table 28.5). Children who are 12 to 18 years of age have the same treatment options as adults. The choice of treatment depends on how often a patient experiences symptoms and how severe those symptoms are.

TABLE 28.5 Preferred Treatment of Asthma in Pediatric Patients

	Increasing severity and frequency of symptoms					
	Step 1	Step 2	Step 3	Step 4	Step 5	Step 6
Age-Group	*Intermittent Asthma*	*Persistent Asthma: Continue using albuterol, plus add the following medications. . . .*				
< 5 years of age	Short-acting beta agonist as needed (e.g., albuterol)	Low-dose inhaled corticosteroid *or* montelukast, cromolyn	Medium-dose inhaled corticosteroid	Medium-dose inhaled corticosteroid *plus* long-acting beta agonist or montelukast	High-dose inhaled corticosteroid *plus* long-acting beta agonist or montelukast	Add oral corticosteroids
5–11 years of age	Same preferred treatment as age-group < 5 years of age	Same preferred treatment as age-group < 5 years of age	Low-dose inhaled corticosteroid *plus* long-acting beta agonist or montelukast or theophylline *or* medium-dose inhaled corticosteroid	Medium-dose inhaled corticosteroid *plus* long-acting beta agonist	High-dose inhaled corticosteroid *plus* long-acting beta agonist	Add oral corticosteroids
12–18 years of age	Same preferred treatment as age-group < 5 years of age	Same preferred treatment as age-group < 5 years of age	Low-dose inhaled corticosteroid *plus* long-acting beta agonist *or* medium-dose inhaled corticosteroid	Medium-dose inhaled corticosteroid *plus* long-acting beta agonist	High-dose inhaled corticosteroid *plus* long-acting beta agonist	Add oral corticosteroids

Patients with intermittent asthma use inhaled, short-acting beta agonist medications, such as albuterol, which relax the airway muscles and thus provide quick relief during asthma attacks.

Patients with more frequent and severe symptoms (**persistent asthma**) should continue to use the same short-acting medication for rescue from asthma attacks. However, they should also add a long-term control medication, such as an inhaled corticosteroid or an inhaled long-acting beta agonist, to their regimens. These long-term control medications reduce inflammation and prevent asthma attacks and are taken every day or twice a day rather than as needed. Generally, an inhaled corticosteroid such as fluticasone is added to a patient's regimen first, and then a long-acting beta agonist such as salmeterol is added later. Leukotriene receptor antagonists (LTRAs), such as montelukast, are also used as an alternative treatment starting at step 2 (see Table 28.5) of the treatment approach.

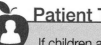
Patient Teaching

If children are prescribed both short-acting and long-acting asthma medications, allied health professionals should remind them—as well as their parents or caregivers—that they should administer the short-acting medication first, followed by the long-acting drug 5 to 10 minutes later. Allied health personnel should also warn patients that a long-term control medication should not be used for fast relief of asthmatic symptoms. Patients should rely on their short-acting beta agonist (such as albuterol) as a rescue inhalant.

Patients experiencing a severe **asthma exacerbation** are given a short course of oral corticosteroids such as prednisone, which helps decrease inflammation. A pediatric patient who is hospitalized for an asthma exacerbation may also receive inhaled ipratropium (an anticholinergic) and IV magnesium sulfate to help open up the airway passages.

These classes of medications used to treat asthma are discussed in greater detail in Chapter 17. However, specific medication classes and their appropriateness for children who are less than five years of age are highlighted in Table 28.6. In addition to the drugs listed in Table 28.6, cromolyn and theophylline are alternative medications that are sometimes used to treat children who are less than five years of age.

Quick Study

The names of most short-acting and long-acting beta agonist inhalers end in the suffix –terol, whereas the names of inhaled corticosteroids end in the suffixes –onide, –asone, or –olide.

TABLE 28.6 | **Medications Used to Treat Asthma in Children**

Drug Class	Generic (Brand)	Used to Treat Children < 5 Years of Age
Short-acting beta agonists	Albuterol (ProAir)	Yes
	Levalbuterol (Xopenex)	No
Inhaled corticosteroids	Beclomethasone (QVAR)	No
	Budesonide DPI (Pulmicort Flexhaler)	No
	Budesonide nebules (Pulmicort)	Yes
	Ciclesonide (Alvesco)	No
	Flunisolide (Aerospan)	No
	Fluticasone dry powder inhaler (Flovent Diskus)	No
	Fluticasone metered-dose inhaler (Flovent)	Yes
	Mometasone (Asmanex)	No
Combination products (long-acting beta agonists *plus* inhaled corticosteroids)	Budesonide/formoterol (Symbicort)	No
	Fluticasone/salmeterol (Advair)	No
Leukotriene receptor antagonists	Montelukast (Singulair)	Yes
	Zafirlukast (Accolate)	No
Oral systemic corticosteroids	Methylprednisolone (Medrol)	Yes
	Prednisolone (Orapred)	Yes
	Prednisone (Rayos)	Yes

Two types of devices are used to deliver inhaled asthma medications to pediatric patients: metered-dose inhalers and nebulizers. Children who have adequate coordination (typically children who are at least four years of age) can receive their medication via a **metered-dose inhaler** (MDI). This handheld device requires hand-eye coordination and timing of inhalation for optimum drug delivery. For this reason, a **spacer** is often recommended for use with pediatric patients. A spacer attaches to the MDI and suspends the medication mist in the air for a few seconds, allowing patients more time to coordinate the two required actions: breathing in and activating the inhaler. Use of a spacer allows patients to inhale a higher concentration of medication, thus providing better relief of symptoms. A **valved holding chamber** is a type of spacer that has a one-way valve at the end, which both traps the medication in the chamber and allows the user to inhale the medication slowly. Spacer devices may be packaged with the medication or dispensed separately and are available in small, medium, and large sizes for infants, children, and adults, respectively.

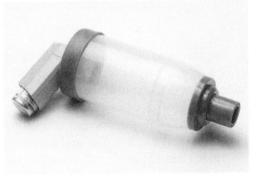

A spacer (the purple-and-transparent piece on the right) attaches to a metered-dose inhaler (on the left). The spacer suspends the medication aerosol for a few seconds, which provides a higher concentration of medication into the lungs of a child with asthma.

Very young patients who are unable to use MDIs (typically children younger than four years of age) use a **nebulizer** to deliver their asthma medication. A nebulizer sends a stream of air through the drug solution, creating a fine mist that patients inhale by breathing normally through a face mask.

After inhalation of a corticosteroid drug, a patient should rinse the mouth thoroughly to prevent an oral fungal infection known as **thrush**. Patients who use a face mask to inhale a corticosteroid should also wash the face after each treatment. The mouthpiece of the inhaler device itself should also be washed with soap and water at least once a week. (For tips on the proper use of an MDI, see Chapter 17.)

Croup

Croup is an inflammation of the larynx (voice box) and trachea, including the vocal cords. Croup symptoms include a barking cough and breathing problems such as **stridor** (a wheezing noise that occurs when breathing in). Older children with croup are more likely to have hoarseness than a barking cough. Symptoms are usually worse at night. In the most severe cases, croup can block the upper airway, hampering airflow, which can cause respiratory failure. Patients with severe croup may show signs of **retractions** (labored breathing) or even experience **cyanosis** (a bluish skin discoloration from lack of oxygenation of the blood) because of the decreased airflow.

Croup mainly affects children who are three months to five years of age, with the majority of cases occurring in patients between six months and three years of age. The condition is usually caused by parainfluenza or another virus such as respiratory syncytial virus. (See the section titled "Respiratory Syncytial Virus" later in this chapter.) Croup commonly occurs during the winter months.

Mild cases of croup can be managed at home. Parents or caregivers should humidify the air with a cool-air vaporizer, and administer oral antipyretics such as acetaminophen or ibuprofen at age-appropriate and weight-appropriate doses. In addition, they should encourage their child to ingest oral fluids. Parents or caregivers who seek out the care of a health professional to treat their child's croup will likely be given a single oral dose of the corticosteroid dexamethasone to reduce inflammation of the larynx and trachea.

A moderate case of croup, defined as croup accompanied by either stridor or retractions at rest, should be assessed by a health professional, either in a physician's office or—depending on symptoms—in an ER. Symptoms that indicate a patient with croup should go directly to the ER include cyanosis, lethargy, stridor or retractions with agitation, and marked sternal wall retractions.

Moderate-to-severe cases of croup require the administration of the corticosteroid dexamethasone orally or via injection. Oral dexamethasone is the preferred route of administration. However, because the oral liquid has a foul taste, healthcare personnel may need to administer an IM or IV injection.

Other treatments for moderate-to-severe croup include cool-mist humidified air, humidified oxygen, and inhaled epinephrine delivered via a nebulizer. These treatments would typically be given in an ER. Inhaled epinephrine usually decreases upper airway swelling within 30 minutes—a much shorter period than dexamethasone. Patients are observed for several hours after the initial treatment and may require additional doses of inhaled epinephrine during that time. If additional episodes of symptoms occur, the patient may need to be hospitalized.

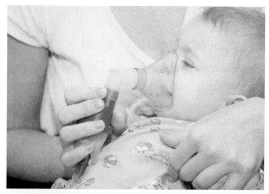

A child suffering from severe croup may require inhaled epinephrine delivered through a nebulizer.

Respiratory Distress Syndrome in Infants

Respiratory distress syndrome (RDS), also known as *hyaline membrane disease*, is a life-threatening condition that occurs shortly after birth in premature infants because the lungs of these neonates are not fully developed. In fully mature lungs, small air sacs called alveoli, which are located at the ends of the smallest airway passages, fill with air and allow for gas exchange with the blood. The surface area of the alveoli is extremely large, and respiratory tissue is well supplied with blood vessels, allowing gases such as oxygen and carbon dioxide to move easily into and out of the bloodstream.

Infants who are born prematurely do not have enough of a substance called **surfactant** in the lungs to keep the lung tissues as slippery as they need to be in order to remain inflated and functioning. (At approximately 36 weeks of gestational age, surfactant production reaches adequate levels in the lungs.) The result is RDS, which is signaled by collapsed alveoli and other areas of the lung, inflammation, and a deficiency of oxygen delivered to the body. Symptoms of RDS include rapid breathing, nasal flaring, audible grunting, retractions during inhalation (sucking in of the skin between the ribs, or just below the ribcage, or at the borders of the breastbone), and cyanosis.

Neonates with RDS are typically given replacement surfactant (either natural or synthetic). These patients are also connected to a machine that applies continuous positive airway pressure (CPAP) through the nasal passages, which helps keep the airways open. Some patients may also require mechanical ventilation, even though this treatment can damage the lungs of neonates.

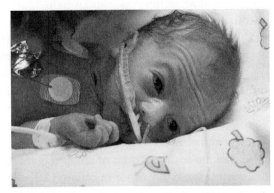

To prevent RDS, physicians administer prophylactic replacement surfactant and CPAP treatments. In addition, mothers who are 23 to 34 weeks pregnant and who seem likely to give birth within seven days may be given a corticosteroid, such as betamethasone, in order to speed the maturation of the fetal lungs and decrease the severity of the neonate's respiratory distress.

More than 90% of infants born before 28 weeks of gestation experience RDS. This disorder is treated using CPAP through the nasal passages of premature infants.

Respiratory Syncytial Virus

Respiratory syncytial virus (RSV) affects all age-groups, and most individuals who have mild respiratory symptoms recover within one to two weeks. However, the pediatric population—in particular, children who are immunocompromised, have underlying lung or congenital heart disease, or are premature (born before 37 weeks of gestation)—is much more vulnerable to severe respiratory symptoms if a virus is contracted. RSV is the most common cause of bronchiolitis and pneumonia among infants in the United States. RSV can also lead to croup and bronchitis. Symptoms of RSV include a runny nose and a decreased appetite, followed by a cough, sneezing, and a fever. Very young patients may present with only a few symptoms such as irritability, a decreased appetite, and difficulty breathing. In severe cases, children present with apnea and are hospitalized.

Drug Regimens and Treatments

Most patients recover from RSV without treatment. However, hospitalized children receive supplemental oxygen and other supportive care to treat severe cases of RSV. If the patient is wheezing, he or she will also receive a dose of an inhaled bronchodilator, such as albuterol or epinephrine. If the bronchodilator helps relieve symptoms, the patient will continue to use it throughout the bout of illness. Corticosteroids are not used to treat RSV in infants but may be used to treat RSV in older children. The antiviral medication ribavirin is used to treat severe RSV in immunosuppressed pediatric patients, but it is not routinely used for other infants and children.

For children who are less than two years of age and have a high risk for contracting severe RSV, health professionals may prescribe the monoclonal antibody palivizumab (Synagis) to prevent RSV. This medication is injected monthly during the annual RSV season, which runs from November to March.

Pneumonia

Pneumonia is a lower respiratory tract infection caused by bacterial, viral, or fungal pathogens. Pneumonia can be acquired from the general community or from exposure to pathogens during hospitalization. **Nosocomial pneumonia** is the term used to describe pneumonia that is acquired while a patient is hospitalized or living in a long-term care facility. This type of pneumonia is severe and difficult to treat because it is usually caused by more virulent pathogens. Patients in the inpatient setting encounter such pathogens because they are in close proximity to other sick patients who harbor these infections. Patients who get pneumonia from exposure outside of an inpatient facility have **community-acquired pneumonia (CAP)**. CAP is the most common serious childhood infection in the United States.

Drug Regimens and Treatments

Before selecting the appropriate therapy to treat pneumonia, health professionals must determine if a patient has CAP or nosocomial pneumonia. However, because determining the disease type takes time, a two-step treatment process is typically initiated.

First, the patient is treated according to **empirical therapy**, or a therapy based on common knowledge of the pathogens that typically cause certain types of pneumonia. This initial drug therapy is prescribed according to the patient's symptoms, general medical history, and the suspected location of exposure. These factors provide clues to the likely pathogen; therefore, drug therapy can be started immediately. An antibiotic that covers a broad range of pathogens will be chosen first to increase the chances that the appropriate pathogen is being targeted.

While the first therapy is in process, a second process, called **narrowing treatment**, begins. Laboratory tests and cultures are obtained to determine exactly what bacteria or fungus is present in the lungs. The patient and care providers must then wait a couple of days to receive the test results. Drug therapy is then changed, if necessary, to treat the found pathogen. Patients who have labored breathing may be administered bronchodilators and corticosteroids to assist breathing. For more detailed information on pneumonia and its related drug therapy, see Chapters 17 and 23.

In pediatric patients, the most likely pathogens that cause pneumonia vary by age-group; thus, empirical therapy depends on patient age (see Table 28.7). Newborns who have early-onset pneumonia (presenting in the first three to five days of life) are considered to have CAP, which is acquired from the mother, whereas neonates who present with pneumonia later in the first month of life are treated for nosocomial pneumonia. Infants between three and six months of age with CAP are typically hospitalized. For children with CAP who are not hospitalized, empirical therapy with oral antibiotics is often adequate. For these patients, laboratory tests and cultures are not usually necessary.

TABLE 28.7 Empirical Therapy for CAP in Children

Age-Group	Preferred Treatment	Alternative Treatments
0 to 1 month of age	IV ampicillin plus gentamicin	N/A
1 month to < 6 months of age	Oral erythromycin	N/A
6 months to < 5 years of age	Oral high-dose amoxicillin	• If the patient has an immediate penicillin allergy, azithromycin, clindamycin, linezolid, or levofloxacin may be used. • If the patient has a milder, delayed hypersensitivity to penicillins, cefdinir or another second-generation or third-generation cephalosporin antibiotic may be used.
≥ 5 years of age	Oral macrolide antibiotic such as azithromycin or clarithromycin	Fluoroquinolone antibiotic such as levofloxacin or moxifloxacin

Checkpoint 28.2

Take a moment to review what you have learned so far and answer these questions.

1. What medication is preferred for treatment of a fever in children?
2. What should a patient do after using an inhaled corticosteroid?
3. What are two drugs that can be used to treat asthma in children who are less than five years of age?

Common Infectious Diseases Affecting Neonatal and Pediatric Patients

Many infectious diseases affect neonatal and pediatric patients, including diarrhea, streptococcal infections, acute bacterial meningitis, and bacteremia and sepsis.

Diarrhea

Diarrhea is defined as excessive, soft, or watery stools. This condition can result from viruses, bacterial infections, or parasites. Common infectious causes of diarrhea include *Salmonella*, *Escherichia coli*, *Giardia*, and *Norovirus*. Drugs can be used to treat bacterial and parasitic infections, but not viral infections.

In addition to these infectious sources, drugs such as the antibiotic amoxicillin can cause diarrhea as a side effect. Diarrhea can also be a symptom of another illness outside the GI tract, such as an ear infection or pneumonia.

All children should be vaccinated for **rotavirus**, which causes vomiting and diarrhea in young children, particularly between six months and two years of age.

Drug Regimens and Treatments

In pediatric patients, diarrhea is mainly treated by using oral rehydration solutions such as Pedialyte to replace lost fluids and electrolytes. (For more information on oral rehydration solutions, see Chapter 26.) Patients who are extremely dehydrated may also be given IV fluids. Antibiotics are generally not used for mild diarrhea of bacterial origin. OTC antidiarrheal drugs such as loperamide (Imodium) and atropine/diphenoxylate (Lomotil) slow intestinal motility, but medications are contraindicated in children less than two years of age. These drugs are not recommended in young children because they do not treat the cause of the illness (infection) and are more likely to cause adverse effects in that patient population. For traveler's diarrhea, children may be treated with the macrolide antibiotic azithromycin.

A child who has blood in the stool should be seen by a physician so that serious and potentially life-threatening causes of diarrhea such as hemolytic uremic syndrome (HUS) can be ruled out. Caused by a strain of *E. coli*, HUS can be fatal in infants and small children. If a child has blood in the stool and has recently had a course of antibiotics, the child should be evaluated for pseudomembranous colitis, which can be caused by *Clostridium difficile (C. diff)* infection. Children who have had diarrhea for more than seven days should be further evaluated by a health professional.

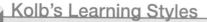
Streptococcal Infections

Pharyngitis (sore throat) is called *strep throat* when the condition is caused by a bacterial infection. Most cases of pharyngitis are caused by viruses and, therefore, should not be treated with antibiotics. However, group A streptococcal bacteria cause 15%–30% of pharyngitis cases in children, which is more than twice the rate found in adult patients. Streptococcal pharyngitis is most common among school-age children. Children less than three years of age may not present with a sore throat but may have only a low-grade fever and a runny nose, whereas infants may only present with a low-grade fever and fussiness.

Drug Regimens and Treatments

Strep throat is the only type of pharyngitis for which antibiotics are routinely prescribed. A swab of the patient's throat is quickly tested in a physician's office to confirm the presence of streptococcal bacteria before antibiotics are prescribed. Oral amoxicillin given at moderate doses (50 mg/kg a day) is the treatment of choice for pediatric patients, and oral cephalexin is an alternative treatment. Patients with a potentially severe allergy to penicillins and cephalosporins are given a macrolide antibiotic (azithromycin or clarithromycin) or clindamycin. To alleviate throat pain, patients may also take acetaminophen at age-appropriate and weight-appropriate doses.

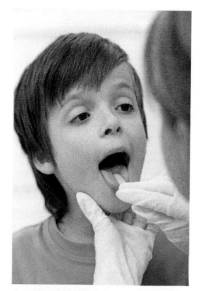

A patient who has been diagnosed with strep throat is generally asked to quarantine himself or herself for 24 hours after diagnosis to prevent contaminating others.

Acute Bacterial Meningitis

Meningitis is an inflammation of the meninges, which are the membranes that surround the brain and spinal cord. Meningitis can be caused by a bacterial, viral, or fungal infection, and its early symptoms include a sudden fever, a severe headache, and a stiff neck. **Bacterial meningitis** is a medical emergency and is deadly if it is not treated. Patients with this type of meningitis are hospitalized. Thanks to the *Haemophilus influenzae* type b (Hib) vaccine and the pneumococcal conjugate vaccine that was introduced in 1990, the number of bacterial meningitis infections has declined among all age-groups except infants who are less than two months of age. Both vaccines are given in multiple doses, starting in patients two months of age (see Figure 28.1).

The CDC publishes annual immunization schedules, based on medical and other indications, that are designed for use by healthcare professionals. To view these immunization schedules and the requisite, referenced footnotes, go to http://PharmEssAH.emcp.net/ChildImmunizationSched.

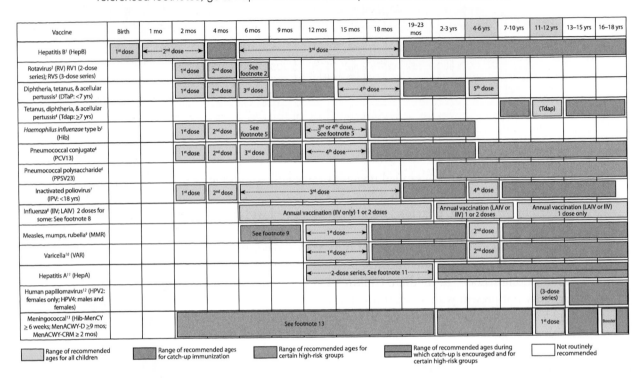

Drug Regimens and Treatments

Suspected bacterial meningitis is treated empirically with broad-spectrum IV antibiotics while laboratory tests are conducted to identify the bacterial cause of the infection. The preferred empirical therapy in children who are less than one month of age is a high dose of a third-generation cephalosporin, such as cefotaxime or ceftriaxone combined with vancomycin. Although the most likely pathogens vary with the patient's age, *Streptococcus pneumoniae* and *Neisseria meningitidis* are the most common causes of bacterial pneumonia in children. In addition to antibiotics, a pediatric patient may be given a single dose of the corticosteroid dexamethasone intravenously with the first dose of antibiotics in order to decrease brain swelling (cerebral edema).

As mentioned earlier, neonates are more likely to contract bacterial meningitis than members of any other age-group, and the children who survive the illness often suffer life-long complications such as seizures, developmental delays, and cerebral palsy. Neonates who present with suspected acute bacterial meningitis are treated empirically with ampicillin and the aminoglycoside antibiotic gentamicin. There are differences in treatment for neonates who present with meningitis early and those who present after the first week of life.

Bacteremia and Sepsis

The term **bacteremia** describes the presence of bacteria in the bloodstream, which is normally sterile. **Sepsis** is an inflammatory response to the invasion of bacteria into the bloodstream. This condition may result from a severe infection—in the respiratory tract, urinary tract, or other part of the body—that invades the blood. Infants and young children, the elderly, and individuals with compromised immune systems are more likely to get sepsis than other people. In up to 60% of pediatric cases, the pathogen causing sepsis is never identified. Children with sepsis typically have a fever; other common symptoms include a racing heart, rapid or labored breathing, cool extremities, and color changes.

Drug Regimens and Treatments

Sepsis can involve organ failure and lead to death (see Figure 28.2). Consequently, this condition is treated aggressively with IV antibiotics as well as drugs to correct low blood pressure, stabilize circulation, maintain blood glucose levels, and reduce inflammation. The choice of antibiotic depends on the age of the child, the suspected pathogens, and the child's medical history. Infants with sepsis may be treated with a combination of antibiotics, such as ampicillin and gentamicin, in order to combat a broad spectrum of bacteria types.

FIGURE 28.2 Sepsis

Sepsis is a life-threatening disorder that can trigger multiple organ dysfunction if not treated aggressively with IV antibiotics.

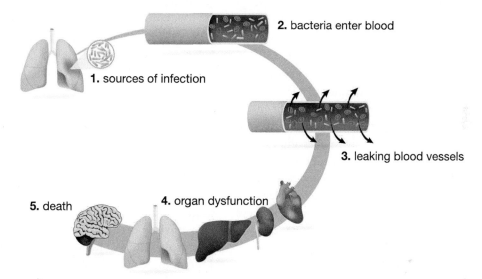

2. bacteria enter blood

1. sources of infection

3. leaking blood vessels

5. death

4. organ dysfunction

 Kolb's Learning Styles

If you enjoy collaboration, as Convergers do, work with classmates to learn more about pediatric treatment for a health condition that is not covered in this chapter (such as Type 1 diabetes, epilepsy, or another condition of your choice). First, use other chapters in this textbook to find out what drugs are used to treat the condition adults; then use a drug handbook to learn which of those drugs can be used to treat children. List the pediatric dosing for each drug, and compare your findings.

Checkpoint 28.3

Take a moment to review what you have learned so far and answer these questions.

1. What drug is used to treat streptococcal pharyngitis in children?

2. What are the three classic symptoms of meningitis?

Chapter Review

Chapter Summary

In the pediatric population, premature infants (born before 37 weeks of gestation), neonates (children who are less than one month of age), and infants (children whose ages range from one month to one year of age) are more vulnerable to drug toxicity than older children because of their size and immature physiology (liver and kidney functions). Because of slow gastric emptying, the rate at which medications are absorbed is slower in neonates and infants than in adults. Therefore, it takes longer for doses of drugs to achieve maximum plasma levels and reach full effect. Drug metabolism is also slower in infants than in older children and adults because some of the CYP enzymes and other gatekeepers of metabolism are only present in very small numbers at birth. These enzymes dramatically increase during the first year of life. Kidney function is low at birth but then increases rapidly and generally reaches adult levels by one year of age. When kidney function is low, the clearance of drugs from the body is slow. As a result, young infants may experience toxic levels of drugs that are primarily eliminated via the kidneys.

In some cases, drug dosing simply needs to be adjusted downward in order to avoid adverse events in pediatric patients. However, some drugs should not be taken by children at any dose. Other drugs should only be used to treat children after safer alternative medications have been tried and failed.

A fever is a common occurrence among pediatric patients and is a symptom that indicates the body is fighting an illness. A fever is a higher-than-normal body temperature, defined as greater than 38º C (100.4º F). If an infant who is less than three months of age has a fever greater than 38º C measured rectally, the parent or caregiver should call a physician. The temperature threshold for calling a physician is higher for children who are older than three months of age: greater than 39º C (102.2º F) measured rectally for children from 3 to 36 months of age or greater than 39.5º C (103.1º F) measured orally for children older than 36 months of age.

Several other health conditions commonly occur in the pediatric patient population. These conditions affect many of the major body systems such as the sensory system (otitis media), cardiovascular system (iron-deficiency anemia), and respiratory system (asthma, croup, RDS, RSV, and pneumonia).

Otitis media is the most common pediatric outpatient diagnosis resulting in the dispensing of antibiotic prescriptions. Antibiotics are given immediately for ear infections in infants who are less than 6 months of age and are suggested for ear infections in children who are 6 to 24 months of age. Children who are two years of age and older do not always receive antibiotics for middle ear infections. The drug of choice is the penicillin antibiotic amoxicillin, given at a high dose twice a day.

Iron-deficiency anemia is a lower-than-normal level of RBCs in the body. Children with iron deficiency can experience impaired psychomotor and mental development that may have lifelong consequences. Therefore, premature infants and full-term infants who are breast-fed should be given iron supplementation. Infants who are fed formula should drink the iron-fortified variety. Children who are diagnosed with iron-deficiency anemia should also receive oral iron supplementation.

Asthma is an inflammatory disorder of the airways and causes coughing, wheezing, breathlessness, and chest tightness. Inside the lungs, bronchioles constrict, mucus production increases, and tissue swells, making normal breathing difficult. Guidelines for the treatment of asthma divide pediatric patients into three age-groups: children who are younger than 5 years of age, children who are 5 to 11 years of age, and children who are 12 to 18 years of age. Short-acting beta agonists, such as albuterol and inhaled corticosteroids, are the mainstays of asthma treatment in young children.

Croup, RDS, and RSV are three respiratory conditions that affect small children more often than adults. Croup is an inflammation of the larynx (voice box) and trachea, including the vocal cords. Croup symptoms include a barking cough and breathing problems such as stridor. Patients with severe croup may show signs of retractions or even experience cyanosis. The condition is usually caused by parainfluenza or another virus such as RSV. Mild cases of croup can be managed at home. Moderate-to-severe cases of croup require the administration of the corticosteroid dexamethasone orally or via injection. Other treatments for moderate-to-severe croup include humidified air or humidified oxygen and inhaled epinephrine delivered via a nebulizer.

RDS is a life-threatening condition that occurs shortly after birth in premature infants because the lungs of these neonates are not fully developed. Infants who are born prematurely do not have enough surfactant in the lungs to keep the lung tissues as slippery as they need to be in order to remain inflated and functioning. Symptoms of RDS include rapid breathing, nasal flaring, audible grunting, retractions during inhalation, and cyanosis. Neonates with RDS are typically given replacement surfactant and are connected to a machine that applies CPAP through the nasal passages.

In the pediatric population, RSV is the most common cause of bronchiolitis and pneumonia among infants in the United States. RSV can also lead to croup and bronchitis. Symptoms of RSV include a runny nose and a decreased appetite, followed by a cough, sneezing, and a fever. Most patients recover from RSV without treatment. However, hospitalized children receive supplemental oxygen and a dose of an inhaled bronchodilator such as albuterol or epinephrine. Corticosteroids are not used to treat RSV in infants but may be used to treat older children. The antiviral medication ribavirin is used to treat severe RSV in immunosuppressed pediatric patients.

Pneumonia is a lower respiratory tract infection caused by bacterial, viral, or fungal pathogens. Pneumonia can be acquired from the general community or from exposure to pathogens during hospitalization. Before selecting the appropriate therapy to treat pneumonia, health professionals must determine if a patient has CAP or nosocomial pneumonia. In pediatric patients, the most likely pathogens that cause pneumonia vary by age-group. Neonates who have early-onset pneumonia (presenting in the first three to five days of life) are considered to have CAP, which is acquired from the mother, whereas newborns who present with pneumonia later in the first month of life are treated for nosocomial pneumonia. Infants

between three to six months of age with CAP are typically hospitalized. For children with CAP who are not hospitalized, empirical therapy with oral antibiotics is often adequate.

Other common childhood disorders include infectious diseases that affect multisystems (diarrhea, streptococcal infections, acute bacterial meningitis, sepsis, and bacteremia).

Diarrhea is defined as excessive, soft, or watery stools. This condition can result from viruses, bacterial infections, or parasites. In pediatric patients, diarrhea is mainly treated by using oral rehydration solutions such as Pedialyte to replace lost fluids and electrolytes. Patients who are extremely dehydrated may also be given IV fluids. OTC antidiarrheal drugs such as loperamide (Imodium) and atropine/diphenoxylate (Lomotil) slow intestinal motility, but medications are contraindicated in children who are less than two years of age. For traveler's diarrhea, children may be treated with the macrolide antibiotic azithromycin. Children who have had diarrhea for more than seven days should be further evaluated by a health professional.

Most cases of pharyngitis (sore throat) are caused by viruses and, therefore, should not be treated with antibiotics. However, group A streptococcal bacteria causes 15%–30% of pharyngitis cases in children and must be treated with antibiotics. Oral amoxicillin given at moderate doses (50 mg/kg a day) is the treatment of choice for pediatric patients, and oral cephalexin is an alternative treatment. Patients with a potentially severe allergy to penicillins or cephalosporins are given a macrolide antibiotic (azithromycin or clarithromycin) or clindamycin.

Meningitis is an inflammation of the meninges, which are the membranes that surround the brain and spinal cord. Meningitis can be caused by a bacterial, viral, or fungal infection, and its early symptoms include a sudden fever, a severe headache, and a stiff neck. Bacterial meningitis is contracted by neonates more than any other age-group. Suspected bacterial meningitis is treated empirically with broad-spectrum IV antibiotics while laboratory tests are conducted to identify the bacterial cause of the infection. The preferred empirical therapy in children who are less than one month of age is a high dose of a third-generation cephalosporin such as cefotaxime or ceftriaxone combined with vancomycin. In addition to antibiotics, a pediatric patient may be given a single dose of the corticosteroid dexamethasone intravenously with the first dose of antibiotics in order to decrease brain swelling (cerebral edema).

Bacteremia describes the presence of bacteria in the bloodstream, which is normally sterile. Sepsis is an inflammatory response to the invasion of bacteria into the bloodstream. This condition may result from a severe infection—in the respiratory tract, urinary tract, or other part of the body—that invades the blood. In up to 60% of pediatric cases, the pathogen that causes sepsis is never identified. This condition is treated aggressively with IV antibiotics as well as drugs to correct low blood pressure, stabilize circulation, maintain blood glucose levels, and reduce inflammation. The choice of antibiotic depends on the age of the child, the suspected pathogens, and the child's medical history. Infants with sepsis may be treated with a combination of antibiotics: ampicillin and gentamicin.

Chapter Checkup

The Navigator+ learning management system that accompanies this textbook offers many opportunities to help you master chapter content, including end-of-chapter exercises, a glossary of key terms, flash cards, and additional interactive activities.

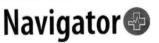

 ## Career Exploration

If you enjoyed learning about pediatric care in this chapter, you may want to explore the following career options:

- behavioral specialist
- certified clinical nutritionist
- genetic counselor
- medical assistant
- pediatric occupational therapist
- pharmacy technician
- registered dietitian

29 Geriatric Patients and Drug Therapy

Pharm Facts

- The world's population is getting older. In 2000, there were 605 million individuals over 60 years old. By 2050, the World Health Organization estimates that there will be more than 2 billion individuals who have reached this milestone.

- According to the US Department of Health & Human Services, the ratio of women to men over 65 years old is 100:76. That ratio changes dramatically by age 85 to 100:49.

- Among older adults, 80% have been diagnosed with a chronic health condition, such as a cardiovascular disorder, arthritis, or osteoporosis. At least 50% of that patient population has a minimum of two chronic conditions.

- Japan has the highest elderly population in the world, with 25% of its citizens over age 65. By 2030, 33% of its population will be older adults.

- One in five geriatric patients is readmitted to a hospital within 30 days of leaving the facility.

"As a medical social worker in the geriatrics field, the daily interaction with patients and families is the most fulfilling aspect of my career. I am part of an interdisciplinary team, working with healthcare professionals and family caregivers to meet the patient's goals. On any given day, I may arrange for post-hospital services, visit a hospice patient, provide counseling, or facilitate a care conference. I also work with the medical team and community services to help patients access programs that can reduce out-of-pocket costs. I take pride in helping older adults and their families reach their goals for care and better understand available resources."

—**Karen Arnold Truax**, MSW, LCSW
Medical Social Worker

Learning Objectives

1 Explain the unique healthcare challenges of geriatric patients.

2 Describe the physiologic and pathophysiologic changes in the human body that occur with the aging process.

3 Identify the factors that can contribute to polypharmacy and the possible consequences of this practice.

4 Identify measures through which the allied health professional can help prevent polypharmacy.

5 Understand the effects that the aging process has on each phase of pharmacokinetics.

6 Understand the effects that the aging process has on pharmacodynamics.

7 Know the common healthcare disorders that affect the geriatric patient population and the drug therapies used to treat these conditions.

8 Become familiar with the Beers Criteria and its importance to drug therapy in geriatric patients.

The march of time takes a toll on the human body. With advancing age, individuals experience declines in cardiovascular function and strength as well as in brain function, bone density, and muscle mass. Kidney and liver function decrease; tissues lose elasticity; and visual and hearing acuity diminish. Generally, the ability to respond to stressors is reduced in old age. Interestingly, many of the problems that are common among older patients start with the letter *i:* immobility, isolation, incontinence, infection, impaired senses, instability, intellectual impairment, impotence, immunodeficiency, insomnia, and iatrogenesis (medical problems caused by medical treatment).

This chapter provides a brief overview of the physiologic changes in aging and how they affect specific body systems. In particular, the chapter focuses on the distinct drug therapies used to treat disorders of these systems, including medications that should be used with caution or not at all in geriatric patients.

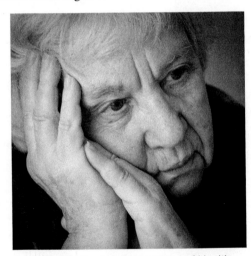

According to the US Department of Health & Human Services, there will be 72.1 million individuals age 65 or older by 2030—more than double the figure from 2000. As the population ages, allied health professionals will need to have a greater understanding of the needs of this patient population.

Unique Challenges of Geriatric Patients

Learning about the unique challenges of **geriatric patients** helps allied health professionals provide optimal care. Some of these challenges include the wide-ranging age-group of this patient population, the variability in lifestyle and living accommodations, the atypical clinical presentations of geriatric patients, and the widespread issue of drug-therapy nonadherence.

Wide-Ranging Age-Group

Generally speaking, the characteristics and healthcare needs of geriatric patients at the younger end of the spectrum (in their 60s and 70s) are not the same as the healthcare needs of those individuals age 80 or older, or of those who are age 85 or older (a demographic group known as "the oldest old"). Medical needs of geriatric patients grow exponentially with age.

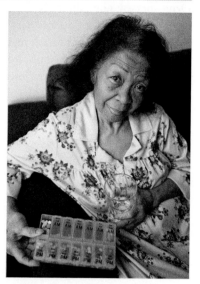

Using a pill organizer can help a geriatric patient organize and track medications.

Variable Lifestyle and Living Accommodations

Lifestyle and living accommodations also play a role in geriatric-patient care. For example, older people living in institutions are often more frail than those living in the community and are at risk for different types of bacterial infections. In addition, institutionalized older adults are more likely to take multiple drugs (often more than six medications a day), a practice known as **polypharmacy**. This practice puts patients at increased risk for adverse drug reactions and drug interactions. If a patient has an especially long list of prescribed drugs, some of the drugs may be unnecessary or may be causing undesirable symptoms such as confusion. With that in mind, healthcare professionals should be alert to the widespread problem of polypharmacy and should monitor for side effects whenever a patient starts a new medication, stops an old medication, or changes doses.

Work Wise

Because of the widespread practice of polypharmacy among the elderly, healthcare professionals should be vigilant in monitoring all medications and supplements that a geriatric patient is taking.

Atypical Clinical Presentations

Health problems in older adults (65 years of age and older) may have atypical presentations, which can make diagnosis challenging. For example, a urinary tract infection may present initially as confusion rather than as a patient complaint of the most common symptom—painful urination. An acute myocardial infarction (heart attack) may not be heralded by chest pain. In fact, only about 50% of older patients complain of chest pain during a heart attack. Being cognizant of the potential for these discrepancies is important. An older patient's complaints may not match the standard complaints for a given diagnosis.

Drug-Therapy Nonadherence

Drug-therapy nonadherence in the geriatric patient population has a number of contributing factors. Older patients may have multiple diseases requiring multiple medications, may be forgetful or confused, may have trouble reading the fine print on medication labels, and may experience unpleasant medication side effects that encourage nonadherence. The allied health professional can help geriatric patients adhere to their drug therapy by projecting a caring, patient attitude when instructing older individuals about their medications.

Physiologic and Pathophysiologic Aging

To begin to understand the healthcare needs of the geriatric patient population, allied health professionals need to know the **physiologic** and **pathophysiologic** aging processes of the body systems.

Integumentary, Muscular, and Skeletal Systems

The integumentary system undergoes some evident changes during the aging process. The skin wrinkles, thins, and becomes dry. In addition, other physiologic changes take place that are not visible to the naked eye: a decrease in the number of blood vessels, a loss of subcutaneous fat, and **atrophy** (shrinking or wasting away) of the sweat glands. These changes affect the regulation of body temperature and cause delays in wound healing.

The muscular and skeletal systems undergo physiologic changes as well. An individual's strength declines as muscle mass decreases, and his or her mobility is hampered by the deterioration of joint cartilage and its resulting pain. Bone mass decreases, so older adults are at an increased risk for fractures.

Nervous and Sensory Systems

The aging process causes various physiologic changes in the nervous system. In the brain, the number of neurons decreases; nerves and nerve fibers decline; and atrophy results in **cranial dead space** (the area in the skull that is left empty or inactive as the brain shrinks). These changes can lead to an increased risk of neurologic problems, a decline in short-term memory, Parkinsonism (a set of movement abnormalities characteristic of Parkinson's disease but not always caused by that disease), and a slower transmission of signals in the nervous system.

The sensory system is also affected by aging in a number of ways. An individual's sense of taste changes as the salivary glands and taste buds atrophy. The tongue's sensory taste receptors for bitterness and sourness are unaltered in old age, but the receptors for sweetness and saltiness are changed, leading to a decrease in appetite. The senses of smell and touch are also affected by the aging process. A reduced number of nerve fibers in the nose can hamper

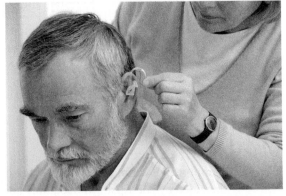

According to the US National Institutes of Health, approximately one-third of older adults between the ages of 65 and 74 have hearing loss; after age 75, that statistic climbs to one-half.

the ability to smell noxious odors. Overall, a decreased sense of touch puts older adults at a higher risk for falls and other accidents.

The eyes have several associated problems including loss of visual acuity, distorted depth perception, and an elevated risk of glaucoma. A decrease in rod and cone function impairs night vision and affects color perception. The discrimination of colors, particularly blue and green, is also affected by atrophy of the ciliary muscles. Lastly, decreased tear secretion and changes in the lens result in an increase in eye dryness and irritation.

Hearing acuity decreases with age because of the loss of auditory neurons. Older adults may experience a loss of hearing from high to low frequency sounds and may have more difficulty hearing when there is background noise. Cerumen (earwax) production increases, and its buildup can result in hearing loss.

Cardiovascular and Respiratory Systems

As the cardiovascular system ages, muscle fibers in the tissues of the heart's chambers atrophy or degenerate; the arteries harden; and systolic blood pressure increases. The left ventricle of the heart loses some flexibility (compliance); the number of pacemaker cells in the heart's sinoatrial node decreases; and the sensitivity of the **baroreceptors**, or sensors in the arteries that regulate the cardiovascular system, is reduced. These physiologic changes can lead to increased blood pressure, arrhythmias, a decreased tolerance for exercise, and an increased risk for **orthostatic hypotension**, or a sudden drop in blood pressure that causes dizziness and fainting when rising from a standing or sitting position.

In the respiratory system, the elasticity of lung tissue decreases with age, and the muscles contributing to respiration lose strength. The tiny fibers called *cilia*, which that line the airways and are responsible for removing irritants, atrophy. In addition, the flexibility of the chest wall decreases. Because of these and other changes, the respiratory systems of older adults are less efficient and more vulnerable to infection. Older adults also have a greater risk of **aspiration**, which is the inhalation of foreign objects such as food or vomit into the airways. Aspiration can lead to pneumonia, which is so common among geriatric patients that the Centers for Disease Control and Prevention (CDC) recommends that all individuals age 65 or older receive the pneumococcal polysaccharide vaccine to provide protective immunity against bacterial forms of pneumonia.

Gastrointestinal and Endocrine Systems

The gastrointestinal (GI) system undergoes many changes as people age. In addition to the atrophy of the salivary glands and the taste buds, the liver becomes smaller, and muscle tone in the bowel decreases. Esophageal emptying slows, and the secretion of hydrochloric acid and gastric acid decreases. The mucosal lining of the GI tract shrinks. Decreased appetite is common in older patients, as is discomfort after eating related to slowed passage of food through the GI tract. These patients also have an increased risk for constipation, esophageal spasm, and diverticular disease. Changes in the GI tract such as shifts in the acid-base balance can alter the **efficacy** of drugs, a topic that will be discussed in more detail in the section titled "Pharmacokinetics in Geriatric Patients."

In the endocrine system of an older adult, the levels of several hormones that regulate the body's processes decrease. These hormones include testosterone, estrogen, growth hormone, insulin, adrenal androgens, aldosterone, and thyroid hormone. The decline in thyroid hormone levels contributes to the decrease in basal metabolic rate that occurs in old age, a change that can be a factor in weight gain. Changes in the endocrine system, such as the decreased insulin response, leave older patients less well equipped to tolerate major stressful events such as surgery. Finally, for complex reasons that are not fully understood, the ability to regulate body temperature decreases in old age. Consequently, older adults are less likely to respond to infection with fever.

Reproductive and Renal Systems

The reproductive system also undergoes changes in old age. For women, the elasticity and lubrication of the vaginal tissue decline. Men experience enlargement of the prostate as well as decreased seminal fluid volume and force of ejaculation.

In the renal system, the kidneys lose mass and the number of functioning nephrons declines with age. These physiologic changes hinder the kidneys' ability to clear or eliminate drugs from the body. The bladder's capacity and muscle tone diminish as well, resulting in an increased urgency to void. In addition, older patients are not as effective at completely emptying the bladder.

Immune System

Age-related changes affect several cell types in the immune system. Changes also occur in the thymus, lymphocytes, lymphatic system organs, and elements of the innate immune system (such as epithelial barriers [the skin and the blood-brain barrier] and blood cells that attack foreign bodies). As a result, older adults are more susceptible to infectious diseases and tend to experience more severe symptoms for longer periods. They have a higher risk of secondary complications following infections. In light of these risks, vaccination is very important for these vulnerable patients, even though vaccines tend to be less effective in this population.

Work Wise

Because of a decline in function of the immune system, older adults are more susceptible to infectious diseases and have a higher risk of secondary complications following infections. Consequently, allied health professionals must take precautions to prevent the spread of infectious diseases, including proper handwashing technique and the use of personal protective equipment.

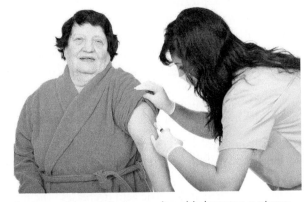

Because older adults have vulnerable immune systems, routine vaccinations must be administered and health records must be kept up to date.

Checkpoint 29.1

Take a moment to review what you have learned so far and answer these questions.

1. What are three physiologic changes that occur in the cardiovascular system of older adults?

2. What are some sensory changes that occur in old age?

Kolb's Learning Styles

If you like to learn from others, as Accommodators do, one activity that may help you learn about the age-related changes older adults encounter is to interview someone 80 years old or older. Perhaps find a grandparent who would be willing to talk about some of these physiologic changes and the challenges they present. Design your interview guide from the information in this chapter to make sure you ask about the changes as outlined in this text.

Drug Alert

Shingles is the common term for herpes zoster, an infection that occurs following reactivation of the varicella-zoster virus. The infection causes a rash and painful burning sensation that follows the line of a set of nerves as it travels around the trunk, a phenomenon known as "the ring of fire." This nerve pain can persist long after the rash has healed.

Shingles affects older patients more frequently because immunodeficiency is common in this patient population. For this reason, the Centers for Disease Control and Prevention (CDC) recommends that all individuals 60 years of age or older receive a single dose of the herpes zoster vaccine (Zostavax). The vaccine decreases the risk of herpes zoster infection for the remainder of the patient's life.

Pharmacokinetics in Geriatric Patients

The field of **pharmacokinetics** is devoted to observing and using mathematical models to predict how drugs enter, move around in, and leave the body. (For detailed information on this topic, see Chapter 3.) Pharmacokinetic processes impact the effectiveness, dosing schedule, and use of medications. Safe and effective drug therapy requires that a drug is delivered to its target sites in concentrations that are sufficient to treat the disease state for which the agent is intended but not so high that drug levels can produce a state of toxicity.

Adverse drug reactions tend to occur when drug levels are too high. Patients also experience effects of toxic drug levels when they get too much of a drug too fast, or when they cannot get rid of a drug fast enough. These causative factors for drug toxicity result from the following: (1) too much of the dose was taken into the body, or the dose was taken in too quickly, or the drug was converted from its inactive form to its active form too quickly; or (2) levels in the body became too high because the patient was not able to metabolize or eliminate the drug from the body as quickly as expected.

The pharmacokinetics process has four phases: absorption, distribution, metabolism, and excretion. An understanding of these processes provides an important framework for researchers who are developing drugs and for healthcare personnel who are prescribing and administering them. Patients react differently to drugs and therefore must be monitored closely. Although data on pharmacokinetics in older adults are limited, healthcare personnel must be aware of the effects of the aging process on pharmacokinetics and be vigilant in monitoring the responses of geriatric patients to medications.

Absorption

Absorption is the process by which drugs enter the bloodstream. The absorption of most drugs is not changed in older adults because most drugs taken orally are absorbed via passive diffusion, which does not decline as the body ages. However, the absorption of certain drugs *is* altered in older patients because of the decreased acidity of the GI tract in that patient population.

Because substances that are absorbed from the GI tract into the bloodstream are first carried via the hepatic portal vein to the liver before entering the rest of the body's circulation, many drugs undergo the **first-pass effect**. This effect refers to the liver metabolizing drugs as they "pass" or travel through it. As a result, the full dose of a drug does not reach its targets in the body, and its systemic effect is lessened or effectively eliminated. In old age, the liver does not block as much drug from entering systemic circulation during that first pass. Consequently, some drugs in geriatric patients have a higher **bioavailability**, or the percentage of drug that reaches the bloodstream. Two such drugs are morphine and propranolol (see Table 29.1).

TABLE 29.1	Drugs Commonly Affected By Age-Related Changes in Absorption, Distribution, and Metabolism
Pharmacokinetic Process	**Drugs Affected by Age-Related Changes**
Absorption	Morphine (Kadian) Propranolol (Inderal LA)
Distribution	Naproxen (Aleve) Phenytoin (Dilantin) Warfarin (Coumadin)
Metabolism	Imipramine (Tofranil) Lidocaine (Xylocaine) Morphine (Kadian) Propranolol (Inderal LA)

Distribution

Distribution is the process by which drugs move around in the bloodstream and reach other body tissues. Typically, the **blood-brain barrier** protects the brain from drugs, but, as patients age, that barrier becomes more porous when the activity of a group of gatekeepers called P-glycoproteins decreases. As a result, older people may experience higher than normal amounts of drug reaching the brain.

In addition, geriatric patients may need to have different loading doses of drugs because volume of distribution changes with age. Some older adults may have lower levels of plasma proteins, such as albumin, which can lead to more of the active form of a drug in circulation. This heightened drug activity can occur in patients who are taking drugs such as naproxen, phenytoin, and warfarin. However, other health conditions, such as the presence of inflammatory disease or cancer, can have the opposite effect: decreasing the amount of the active form of a drug in circulation.

Metabolism

Metabolism is a term that describes the way drugs are processed in the body, usually in the liver. In this sequence of steps, the body breaks down and converts a medication into active chemical substances. In addition, metabolism serves to detoxify the blood. The metabolic process is affected by aging in a couple of ways. First, the volume of the liver decreases with age, which may account for slowed clearance in the liver. Second, blood-flow in the liver decreases as an individual ages, which can slow the metabolism of drugs that are mainly extracted via the liver. These drugs include imipramine, lidocaine, morphine, and propranolol. The activity of the group of chemical gatekeepers located in the liver, known as cytochrome P450 enzymes, does not seem to decline with age.

Excretion

Excretion is the process by which drug molecules are removed from the bloodstream and leave the body, primarily in urine excreted from the kidneys. However, drug molecules can also be eliminated in bile, feces, perspiration, and exhalations. Kidney function declines with age, so drugs that are cleared primarily through the kidneys may need to be given in lower doses or less frequently in older patients. However, the decline is not predictable. Up to one-third of older adults have kidney function in the normal range as measured by the **creatinine clearance (CrCl) rate**. Because the decline in kidney function is variable from patient to patient, the kidney function of geriatric patients should be tested so that dosing can be lowered for patients with impaired kidney function. Aminoglycosides, atenolol, digoxin, lithium, and vancomycin are just a few of the drugs that are cleared mainly by the kidneys and that may require dosing adjustments in patients with very low kidney function. (For a listing of these drugs, see Table 29.2.)

TABLE 29.2 Drugs Commonly Affected by Impaired Kidney Function

Allopurinol
Amantadine
Antibiotics: aminoglycosides, cephalexin, sulfamethoxazole/trimethoprim
Atenolol
Cetirizine
Digoxin
Fluconazole
Gabapentin
Lithium
Methotrexate
Metoclopramide
Nitrofurantoin
Nonsteroidal anti-inflammatory drugs (NSAIDs)
Ranitidine

Pharmacodynamics in Geriatric Patients

Whereas pharmacokinetics measures changes in drug levels in the body, **pharmacodynamics** studies the effects of drugs on the body. The aging process can affect pharmacodynamics in a variety of ways. For example, older adults are more sensitive to the sedating effects of benzodiazepines than younger patients are and may experience a greater analgesic response to opioids. In addition, the effects of warfarin and anticoagulants on blood thinning are greater in older adults, so they may need lower doses of these medications. Finally, the reduction of baroreceptor function that occurs in old age can lead to an increased response to some blood pressure medications (calcium-channel blockers) but a decreased response to other blood pressure medications (beta blockers). Allied health professionals should be aware of these pharmacodynamic changes in older patients and be vigilant for any changes related to their drug regimens. For example, personnel should closely monitor blood pressure for any older patients who are taking beta blockers or calcium-channel blockers.

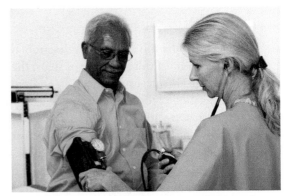

An allied health professional must monitor blood pressure readings of an older patient who is taking an antihypertensive medication.

 Checkpoint 29.2

Take a moment to review what you have learned so far and answer these questions.

1. How do changes in the first-pass effect impact the absorption process of medications in older adults?

2. What physiologic change affects the distribution of drugs in geriatric patients, thereby making them more vulnerable to the effects of drugs?

Common Disorders Affecting Geriatric Patients

A number of health conditions commonly occur in the geriatric patient population. These ailments affect several of the major body systems such as the skeletal system, the sensory system, the cardiovascular system, and the nervous system.

Arthritis

Arthritis is an inflammation of the joints. Two types of arthritis—osteoarthritis and rheumatoid arthritis—are commonly seen in older patients. Drug therapy used to treat these two disorders is provided in Table 29.3.

Osteoarthritis

Osteoarthritis is a degenerative disease in which cartilage in joints becomes thinner and less elastic. The gradual wearing of cartilage can lead to changes in the underlying bone surfaces. This condition is related to both age and trauma and typically affects synovial joints. The most commonly affected joints are the acromioclavicular joint (shoulder), hips, knees, fingers, and big toes. The joints of the knees and fingers have a higher likelihood of being impaired by this disorder because of weight bearing (knees) and repetition of movements (fingers).

The disease is characterized by progressive pain, stiffness, limited range of motion, and deformed joints. Stiffness in the morning is the most prevalent complaint; stiffness is also common after inactivity such as sitting. Osteoporosis leads to limitations in mobility in older adults, and osteoarthritis of weight-bearing joints increases the risk of falls and

TABLE 29.3 Drug Therapy for Treatment of Arthritis in Geriatric Patients

Generic (Brand)	Indication
Analgesic	
Acetaminophen (Tylenol)	Osteoarthritis
Biologic Disease-Modifying Antirheumatic Drugs (DMARDs)	
Adalimumab (Humira)	Rheumatoid arthritis
Etanercept (Enbrel)	Rheumatoid arthritis
Nonbiologic DMARDs	
Methotrexate (Rheumatrex)	Rheumatoid arthritis
Sulfasalazine (Azulfidine)	Rheumatoid arthritis
NSAIDs	
Ibuprofen (Advil, Motrin)	Osteoarthritis
Naproxen (Aleve, Naprosyn)	Osteoarthritis
Topical Agent	
Capsaicin cream (Trixaicin)	Osteoarthritis

fractures. Osteoarthritis generally appears after age 40, and advanced age is the greatest risk factor for this condition.

Drug Regimens and Treatments

Drug treatment options for osteoarthritis include topical agents such as capsaicin creams, analgesics such as acetaminophen, and nonsteroidal anti-inflammatory drugs (NSAIDs) such as ibuprofen (see Chapter 10). NSAIDs should be used with additional caution in older adults because of the risks of GI bleeding and the development of peptic ulcers. In addition, NSAIDs should be used with caution in patients with hypertension or renal impairment, which are common among older adults. When simple analgesics are not adequate or NSAIDs are contraindicated, other treatment options include opioid pain relievers and the injection of steroids or other medications into the joint. There are several surgical options, including joint replacement.

Rheumatoid Arthritis

Whereas osteoarthritis is a caused by the degeneration of the joint, **rheumatoid arthritis** involves an abnormal process in which the immune system destroys the synovial membrane and produces inflammation within the joint itself (see Figure 29.1). Rheumatoid arthritis tends to affect small joints first, such as those in the fingers, wrists, and elbows. It is not known why the incidence of this autoimmune condition increases with age. In younger patients, rheumatoid arthritis is much more common in women than in men; however, there is no gender difference in incidence among patients who have the elderly-onset form of the disease (60 years of age or older).

In the Know

Capsaicin creams contain the ingredient that makes chili peppers hot. These products work by desensitizing the nerve endings in the area of application. Capsaicin creams cause a burning sensation the first few times they are applied to the affected area; however, this reaction diminishes after several days. If the cream is not applied regularly (three to four times per day), the burning sensation recurs. Patients should be advised to wear gloves when applying capsaicin cream, to avoid contact with their eyes, and to wash their hands thoroughly after each application.

Osteoarthritis results from the wear and tear of aging joints. Rheumatoid arthritis, on the other hand, is a chronic autoimmune disorder that affects not only the joints but also other body tissues. Osteoarthritis is more common in the geriatric patient population.

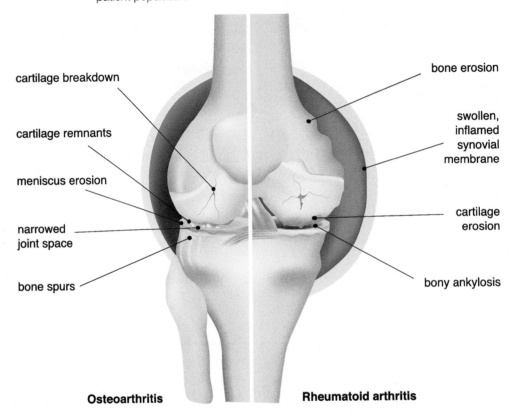

cartilage breakdown

cartilage remnants

meniscus erosion

narrowed joint space

bone spurs

bone erosion

swollen, inflamed synovial membrane

cartilage erosion

bony ankylosis

Osteoarthritis

Rheumatoid arthritis

In geriatric patients, rheumatoid arthritis is more likely to affect the larger joints and to have a faster onset of symptoms. In addition to pain and inflammation, older patients are more likely to have systemic symptoms including weight loss, fever, and night sweats. Diagnosis is challenging because the symptoms can be nonspecific in the older population and easily confused with other, more common conditions. For example, in a geriatric patient, weight loss, fever, and night sweats could also be caused by influenza or a bacterial infection.

Drug Regimens and Treatments

Treatment of the disease is similar in older and younger adults. NSAIDs relieve pain but pose higher risks to older patients than to younger adults. Disease-modifying antirheumatic drugs (DMARDs) work by suppressing the immune system, which treats the condition but also leaves patients more vulnerable to infection (see Chapter 10). For example, the commonly used DMARD methotrexate (Rheumatrex) is eliminated via the kidneys; therefore, older patients are more likely to experience side effects such as infections, anemia, liver damage, and hair loss. In addition, older patients are more likely to experience toxic effects from biologic DMARDs used to treat rheumatoid arthritis. These toxic effects include fungal infections, tuberculosis, and atypical mycobacterial infections.

Osteoporosis

Osteoporosis is a condition whose hallmarks are reduced bone mineral density, disrupted microarchitecture of bone structure, and increased likelihood of fracture (see Figures 29.2 and 29.3). As adults age, resorption of bone tissue exceeds the deposit of new bone. Furthermore, newly formed bone is less dense and more fragile than original bone. This reduction or weakening of bone mass increases the risk for bone fracture in geriatric patients. For adults older than age 50, these bone-aging processes occur at a faster rate for women than for men.

Osteoporosis occurs as a result of the physiologic processes described earlier as well as deficiencies in estrogen, calcium, and vitamin D. The reduction in bone mass is accelerated and more severe in women who have had an early, total hysterectomy in which the ovaries have been removed along with the uterus, because without ovaries a woman's body produces less estrogen. With less estrogen, lower amounts of calcium are taken up into bony tissue. Daily calcium with vitamin D is essential to the prevention of bone loss. Gender, ethnicity, heredity, and age are the risk factors for osteoporosis that cannot be modified.

FIGURE 29.2 Osteoporosis Close-Up	**FIGURE 29.3** Normal and Osteoporotic Vertebrae
The interior of a bone resembles a honeycomb. In osteoporosis, the areas inside these compartments enlarge, reducing bone density and strength.	Age-related kyphosis, or curving of the spine, often accompanies severe osteoporosis. Kyphosis results from compressed, weakened vertebrae.

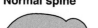

Normal bone   **Bone with osteoporosis**

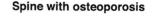

Normal spine   **Spine with osteoporosis**

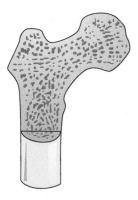
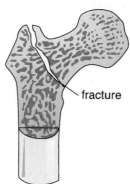
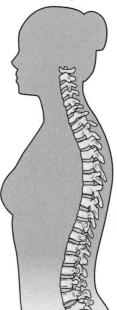
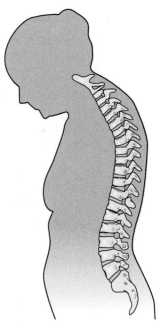

fracture

close-up view   close-up view

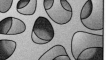
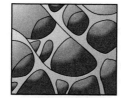

Drug Alert

Chronic use of corticosteroids can deplete bone mass. Older adults who have taken corticosteroids for significant durations may be at increased risk for developing osteoporosis. It is recommended that older adults undergo bone density screening, especially those who have taken corticosteroids on a long-term basis.

Patients with osteoporosis are prescribed bisphosphonate drugs such as alendronate (Fosamax), which increase bone mineral density by decreasing the rate of bone resorption (see Chapter 10). To avoid throat irritation, esophagitis, and esophageal ulceration, patients should take each dose of a bisphosphonate with a full glass of water and then remain upright for 30 minutes.

Patient Teaching

Allied health professionals should encourage patients to make lifestyle changes to reduce the risk of osteoporosis. These changes may include smoking cessation, increased calcium intake, and avoidance of alcohol. In addition, healthcare personnel should teach patients strategies for preventing falls and should recommend that patients perform weight-bearing exercises (if their overall health allows) and take supplemental calcium and vitamin D.

Ophthalmic Disorders

Physiologic changes in old age commonly lead to presbyopia and dry eye syndrome and can cause more serious problems such as glaucoma and cataracts.

Presbyopia

Presbyopia is the most common cause of visual impairment in the United States. As part of the normal aging process, the lenses of the eyes lose elasticity over time. This loss of flexibility makes it more difficult to focus on objects that are nearby, or less than an arm's length away. Presbyopia typically affects patients age 40 or older and is often diagnosed with a chief complaint of difficulty discerning printed material. By age 65, the lenses have lost all flexibility. There is no medical treatment for presbyopia, but glasses or contact lenses can be used to correct vision.

Dry Eye Syndrome

Old age and female gender are the top risk factors for keratoconjunctivitis sicca, commonly known as **dry eye syndrome (DES)**. This condition results when the eyes are unable to produce sufficient tears to lubricate and nourish the eye. DES affects between 5%–30% of individuals who are age 50 or older, and its prevalence increases with age.

Drug Regimens and Treatments

Topical cyclosporine (Restasis) for ophthalmic use is commonly prescribed to treat DES and is approved for patients with chronic dry eye (see Chapter 14). This local medication increases tears by means of anti-inflammatory and immune-modulating effects. Restasis is provided by the manufacturer in single-use vials and is instilled in the eyes every 12 hours. In addition to topical cyclosporine, patients with dry eye syndrome can also use artificial tears (over-the-counter [OTC] eyedrops) as needed.

Glaucoma

Glaucoma is the second-leading cause of blindness in the United States. This chronic disorder is characterized by abnormally high internal eye pressure that destroys the optic nerve and causes partial-to-complete loss of vision. The increased intraocular pressure is due to an imbalance between production and drainage of aqueous humor in the front portion of the eye. This imbalance is typically caused by an obstruction that impedes normal drainage. Initially, a patient with glaucoma loses parts of the peripheral vision; if untreated, the vision loss can spread slowly to the entire field of vision.

Open-angle glaucoma is the most common type of glaucoma, and its incidence increases with age. In open-angle glaucoma, the angle of the anterior chamber remains open, but filtration is gradually diminished in the tissues for reasons that are not well understood. In chronic open-angle glaucoma, the goals of treatment are gradual reduction and long-term normalization of intraocular pressure, prevention of optic nerve damage, and preservation of vision.

Drug Regimens and Treatments

Several types of eyedrops are used to treat glaucoma, including prostaglandins, beta blockers, alpha-adrenergic (primarily alpha-2) agonists, and carbonic anhydrase inhibitors (see Chapter 14). Although eyedrops deliver only very small doses of medication, it is possible for them to have systemic effects. For example, it is possible that the beta blocker eyedrop medication timolol could lower systemic blood pressure or lead to bradycardia in a patient already taking heart medications such as diltiazem or digoxin. Although these systemic effects are unlikely, older patients using eyedrops should be monitored for adverse effects. Allied health professionals should also be aware that patients who have been diagnosed with glaucoma should avoid taking certain drugs that increase intraocular pressure or could potentially cause closure of the angle through which fluids drain. These drugs include the following:

- OTC cold remedies
- appetite suppressants
- motion sickness medications
- sleep aids

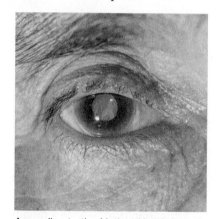

According to the National Institutes of Health, one-half of individuals age 80 or older have a cataract or have undergone cataract surgery. In addition to age, other risk factors for cataracts include smoking, diabetes, and prolonged sun exposure.

Cataracts

A **cataract** is an area of opacity in the lens of the eye that can cause cloudy or fuzzy vision. This condition is the leading cause of blindness, and its prevalence increases with age. The relationship between the increased incidence of cataracts and the aging process is not clear. The treatment for cataracts is surgical removal of the cloudy cataract and lens replacement with a clear, artificial lens.

Cardiovascular Disease

Cardiovascular disease or heart disease is widespread among older adults, affecting 70%–79% of individuals who are ages 60 to 79 and 79%–86% of individuals who are 80 years of age and older. In the United States, more than 80% of adults who are 65 years of age or older die of cardiovascular disease. Drug regimens used to treat various cardiovascular conditions in geriatric patients are listed in Table 29.4.

TABLE 29.4	Drug Therapy for Common Cardiovascular Conditions in Geriatric Patients

Patients with cardiovascular conditions often must take drugs from several different classes. For example, a patient with hypertension will typically start drug therapy with a thiazide diuretic and then, if the blood pressure remains too high, the healthcare practitioner will add an angiotensin-converting enzyme (ACE) inhibitor or angiotensin receptor blocker (ARB).

Condition	Prescribed Drug Therapy
Hypertension	Thiazide diuretics ACE inhibitors ARBs Calcium-channel blockers Beta blockers
Angina	Nitrates Beta blockers Calcium-channel blockers Antiplatelet therapy (e.g., clopidogrel) Statins
Congestive Heart Failure	Diuretics ACE inhibitors ARBs Beta blockers Digoxin Vasodilators
Stroke	Drugs to treat underlying disorder (e.g., hypertension, heart failure) Antiplatelet therapy Anticoagulants

Hypertension

Approximately two-thirds of adults ages 65 to 74 have **hypertension** or high blood pressure (defined as systolic pressure over 140 mm Hg and/or diastolic pressure over 90 mm Hg). Hypertension is considered a modifiable risk factor for serious cardiovascular conditions such as stroke, heart failure, and coronary artery disease. Elevated systolic pressure poses a greater risk than elevated diastolic pressure for adverse cardiovascular events. This is noteworthy because isolated systolic hypertension is very common in older patients, occurring in 90% of patients older than 80 years of age.

Drug Regimens and Treatments

Treatment of hypertension in older adults reduces the risks of disability and death from stroke and other cardiovascular causes. It is treated with thiazide diuretics, followed by the addition of beta blockers, angiotensin-converting enzyme (ACE) inhibitors, angiotensin receptor blockers (ARBs), and calcium-channel blockers. These drugs are discussed in detail in Chapter 15.

The choice of antihypertensive medications depends on the older patient's kidney function; **comorbidity**, or the simultaneous presence of two conditions; and tolerability. For example, thiazide diuretics are not effective for patients with very low kidney function and may exacerbate gout. Although beta blockers may not be as effective as other classes of antihypertensive drugs at reducing mortality, they are used as first-line therapy in many older patients who have other conditions that require the use of a beta blocker, such as heart failure, angina, or a history of myocardial infarction. Beta blockers pose a particular risk of **bradycardia**, or a slowed heart rate below 60 beats per minute, in patients 65 years of age and older. The effects of antihypertensive drugs on the central nervous system (CNS) may be greater in older adults. Beta blockers can cause somnolence and depression in older adults, and the alpha-2 adrenergic agonist clonidine (Catapres) is not recommended as a first-line treatment for hypertension in older patients because of the high risk of CNS adverse effects.

Angina and Coronary Heart Disease

Angina pectoris—or, simply, angina—is a symptom of coronary heart disease. Angina is chest pain caused by **myocardial ischemia**, or inadequate bloodflow and insufficient oxygen supply to a portion of the heart. Ischemia usually occurs because of a blockage in the coronary arteries that supply the heart with blood. Tissue damage from this blockage is not sufficiently extensive to be considered a heart attack but does cause recurring chest pain episodes. The hallmarks of angina are the same for both younger and older adults: tightness, burning, or squeezing sensation in the chest. In older patients, these symptoms may present as weakness, confusion, or dizziness.

Drug Regimens and Treatments

The treatment for angina is the use of sublingual nitroglycerin. Individuals should be in a sitting position when they place the drug under their tongue in order to avoid the risk of orthostatic hypotension. Patients with stable angina should take a regular regimen of beta blockers and aspirin and receive drugs for any of their risk factors for coronary heart disease such as hypertension and high cholesterol. If beta blockers do not adequately control angina, long-acting nitrates and calcium-channel blockers may be added, but older patients taking those medications are at an increased risk for orthostatic hypotension. (For more information on drugs used to treat angina, see Chapter 15.) Revascularization surgery is also an option for older adults with symptomatic coronary artery disease, but the risks associated with such surgery increase with age and comorbidities.

Acute Myocardial Infarction

An **acute myocardial infarction (MI)**, or *heart attack*, occurs when one or more of the coronary arteries become significantly blocked (usually by 70% or more), resulting in extensive tissue damage. Older adults experiencing an acute MI are more likely to present with weakness, confusion, syncope (fainting), and abdominal pain than with the classic symptom of chest pain.

Drug Regimens and Treatments

The treatment for an acute MI in geriatric patients is the same as for younger adults: beta blockers, aspirin, ACE inhibitors, and statins to lower cholesterol (see Chapter 15).

Congestive Heart Failure

Congestive heart failure (CHF) is a complex cardiovascular disorder in which the heart does not pump blood as well as it should to meet the body's needs. Heart failure is caused by damage to the heart (for example, MI) and results in fluid buildup, shortness of breath, and fatigue. The symptoms of CHF may present differently in the geriatric patient population. Instead of complaining of shortness of breath, an older patient may have symptoms of hypoxia (such as light-headedness), tiredness/sleepiness, restlessness, and confusion.

Drug Regimens and Treatments

Diastolic dysfunction is the main cause of CHF in older adults. Diastolic dysfunction is treated with beta blockers to control heart rate and diuretics to treat pulmonary congestion and peripheral edema. Treatment of older adults with systolic dysfunction is the same as for younger adults with the condition: diuretics, ACE inhibitors or ARBs, beta blockers, and aldosterone blockers (see Chapter 15). Although digoxin may reduce mortality in older patients with CHF, these patients must be monitored for signs of digoxin toxicity such as vision changes (blurred or yellowish vision), dizziness, vomiting, and confusion.

Cerebrovascular Disease

A **cerebrovascular accident**, more commonly known as a **stroke**, occurs when an event interrupts or severely reduces the oxygen supply to an area of the brain, leading to the death of brain tissue. A stroke causes a sudden neurologic deficit and can present with symptoms such as loss of coordination, difficulty speaking, headache, changes in vision, or paralysis of the face, arm, or leg.

Advanced age is an important risk factor for stroke. The risk doubles every 10 years after age 55, with 75% of all strokes occurring in patients 65 years of age and older. Stroke is a major cause of disability: Among stroke survivors, 40% report mild dysfunction, 40% report significant dysfunction, 10% report no dysfunction, and 10% require institutional care.

A stroke may be caused by one of two primary events: (1) an ischemic stroke or cerebral infarction, or (2) a cerebral hemorrhage. An ischemic stroke and a cerebral hemorrhage differ significantly. An i**schemic stroke** is the result of obstruction of bloodflow, whereas a **cerebral hemorrhage** involves primary rupture of a blood vessel. Ischemic strokes are by far the most common type of strokes. Stroke can be considered as a finite event, an ongoing event, or a series of protracted occurrences. A stroke may evolve over several hours, days, or months. In a **transient ischemic attack (TIA)**, the patient experiences temporary neurologic changes during a brief period. TIAs may be important warning signs and predictors of imminent stroke. A **reversible ischemic neurologic deficit (RIND)** is an event that reverses spontaneously but less rapidly than a TIA does. RINDs

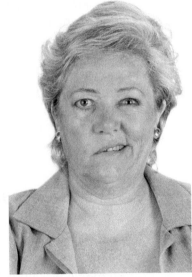

A stroke can damage the area of the brain that is responsible for sending nerve signals to the facial muscles. The resulting paralysis may be permanent.

last more than 24 hours and resolve in less than 21 days. In most cases, however, RINDs resolve within a matter of days, rather than weeks.

Risk factors for ischemic stroke include several conditions that are common in the older population such as high cholesterol level, cardiac arrhythmia, coronary artery disease, prosthetic heart valve, diabetes, hypercoagulable states, obesity, and physical inactivity. These conditions increase the likelihood of blood clots forming and traveling to the brain.

Drug Regimens and Treatments

Because brain-cell death is irreversible, most drug therapy for stroke is aimed at prevention rather than treatment. Anticoagulation and antiplatelet therapies are used to prevent stroke, and thrombolytic therapy is sometimes used to break up an ischemic clot that has caused a massive stroke (see Chapter 16).

Cancer

The incidence of **cancer** and mortality rates from cancer increase with age. The median age range for diagnosis of major tumors is 68 to 74 years, and the median age range for death from cancer is 70 to 79 years. Many theories exist as to why the incidence of cancer increases with age. In addition to having experienced longer exposure to carcinogens, the geriatric patient may have an increased cellular susceptibility to carcinogens, decreased immune function, and a decreased ability to repair deoxyribonucleic acid (DNA).

The symptoms of cancer can easily be confused with normal age-related changes, so clinicians must be vigilant for the warning signs of cancer and follow cancer screening recommendations. For example, rectal bleeding, a symptom of colon or rectal cancer, could be mistaken for blood caused by hemorrhoids, and skin cancer could be mistaken for age spots.

Drug Regimens and Treatments

Chemotherapy drugs represent a complicated group of medications with a narrow window between safe therapeutic use and the potential for high toxicity. Prescribers must carefully weigh the benefits of treatment against the risks, and consider quality of life when devising treatment plans. This analysis should take into account the geriatric patient's functional status (degree of frailty) and comorbidities (other disease states), as those factors play a large role in a patient's ability to survive chemotherapy. Older adults also may need lower doses of chemotherapy drugs because of decreased kidney and liver functions. These physiologic changes can make geriatric patients more likely to experience adverse reactions. In addition, older patients are more susceptible to bone marrow suppression, an adverse effect of several classes of chemotherapy agents. Finally, because many chemotherapy agents cause nausea and vomiting, patients should be adequately hydrated and given antiemetic medications to prevent nausea and vomiting prior to each round of chemotherapy. (To learn more about chemotherapy drugs and their treatment regimens, refer to Chapter 27.)

Quick Study

Allied health professionals should be aware that serotonin (5-HT3) receptor antagonists, a class of drugs used to prevent and treat chemotherapy-induced nausea and vomiting, have a similar ending: –*setron*. Examples of these medications include palonosetron (Aloxi) and ondansetron (Zofran).

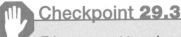

Checkpoint 29.3

Take a moment to review what you have learned so far and answer these questions.

1. What is the major risk posed by osteoporosis?

2. What is the difference between glaucoma and a cataract? Which one is treated surgically?

3. What symptoms of CHF may be more common among geriatric patients than the classic complaint of shortness of breath?

Drug Considerations for Geriatric Patients

The **Beers Criteria**, published by the American Geriatrics Society (AGS), is a list of drugs that many prescribers consider potentially dangerous for patients who are 65 years of age or older because of an increased risk of adverse effects or a potential to exacerbate disease states that are common in older adults. The updated version (2012) of the Beers Criteria can be viewed at the following website: http://PharmEssAH.emcp.net/BeersCriteria. Table 2 of the Beers Criteria summarizes why each drug or class of drugs on the list is potentially inappropriate for older adults. Many of the drugs are on the list because they cause anticholinergic effects, which can be much worse in older patients. When a drug blocks cholinergic activity in the parasympathetic system, dry mouth, dry eyes, constipation, and urinary retention may occur. Blood pressure also increases. Some other drugs are on the list because they can cause orthostatic hypotension, exacerbate heart failure, or cause CNS adverse effects such as confusion.

The Beers Criteria is intended only as a guide for prescribers. For each geriatric patient, the prescriber must carefully consider whether the clinical benefits of the drug outweigh the potential risks. Although there is some debate concerning which drugs belong on the Beers Criteria, this list is a valuable tool for all allied health professionals who care for older adults.

CNS Medications

Several CNS drugs, such as sedative-hypnotics, antidepressants, and antipsychotics, must be used cautiously in older adults. The effects of these medications can be heightened because of a decreased clearance from the body and the normal aging processes of the brain. As mentioned earlier in this chapter, the blood-brain barrier, which protects the brain from drugs, becomes more porous in the geriatric population, allowing more medications to reach the brain.

Sedative-Hypnotics

Sedative-hypnotics such as alprazolam (Xanax) should not be used to induce sleep or treat delirium in geriatric patients because these drugs increase the risk of cognitive impairment and delirium in that patient population. It may seem strange that a drug that is used for its calming effects can cause delirium, but it is true. Short-acting benzodiazepines such as lorazepam are sometimes used to treat delirium in younger patients. Zolpidem (Ambien) and other nonbenzodiazepines should

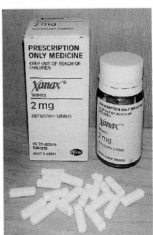

The American Geriatrics Society recommends that Xanax be used cautiously in geriatric patients because of its adverse effects: cognitive impairment, risk for falls, and delirium.

not be used long term for sleep (more than 90 days) in older adults because they have an increased tendency to cause delirium, falls, and fractures in those patients. (For more specific information on benzodiazepines and sleep aids, see Chapter 13.)

Antidepressants

Tricyclic antidepressants (TCAs)—especially amitriptyline and doxepin—should be avoided in older patients because they are highly anticholinergic (sedating and constipating) and because they can cause orthostatic hypotension. In addition, TCAs can also cause or exacerbate the **syndrome of inappropriate secretion of antidiuretic hormone (SIADH)** and hyponatremia. **Hyponatremia** is a lower-than-normal concentration of sodium in the blood that produces symptoms such as nausea, vomiting, and malaise.

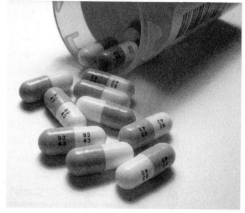

Prescribers may start geriatric patients on a lower dose of a selective serotonin reuptake inhibitor (SSRI) antidepressant such as fluoxetine (Prozac) or citalopram (Celexa). In fact, the maximum recommended dose of citalopram in patients who are age 60 or older is 20 mg a day because of the risk of cardiac arrhythmia (QT prolongation).

In addition to SSRIs, other classes of antidepressants such as serotonin-norepinephrine reuptake inhibitors should be used with caution in older patients because of their potential to exacerbate or cause SIADH and hyponatremia. (For more information on antidepressants, see Chapter 13.)

Healthcare practitioners need to carefully assess the risks versus the benefits of prescribing fluoxetine (Prozac) for their geriatric patients diagnosed with depression.

Antipsychotics

Antipsychotics cause an increased risk for stroke and cerebrovascular death in patients with dementia. Consequently, the use of these medications should be avoided in that patient population. In addition, antipsychotics can worsen constipation, a common complaint of older patients. Furthermore, antipsychotics should be used with caution in geriatric patients because of their potential to cause or exacerbate SIADH and hyponatremia as well as to incite changes in mental status.

Drug Alert

Federal guidelines from Medicare govern the use of antipsychotic medications for geriatric patients in a nursing care facility. These drugs should not be administered to an agitated patient who is calling out or displaying another form of attention-seeking behavior unless he or she shows signs of self-harm or the intent to harm others. Using antipsychotic medications to sedate a patient who is being a nuisance is not considered ethical.

Drugs for Alzheimer's Disease

Drug therapy for Alzheimer's disease does not alter the disease's progression. The goal of drug therapy is to maintain cognitive function and alertness for as long as possible.

Several drugs are used for this disease including anticholinesterase inhibitors such as donepezil (Aricept) and the N-methyl-D-aspartate (NMDA) receptor antagonist memantine (Namenda). The **anticholinesterase inhibitors**, which are used to treat mild-to-moderate Alzheimer's disease, work by inhibiting enzymes that break down acetylcholine, a neurotransmitter thought to be deficient in early Alzheimer's disease. **Memantine** is reserved for treatment of moderate-to-severe Alzheimer's disease. Later in the disease, antidepressants can be used for depression. Benzodiazepines

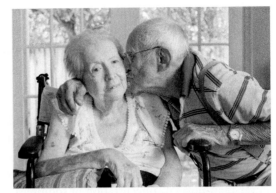

According to the Alzheimer's Association, Alzheimer's disease is the sixth leading cause of death in the United States. Two-thirds of its victims are women.

have been used for anxiety and sleep problems in this patient population, but their long-term use is no longer recommended. Although antipsychotic medications such as haloperidol (Haldol) have been used to treat hallucinations in patients with Alzheimer's disease, those drugs increase the risk of cardiovascular disease and death in patients with dementia. (For more information on Alzheimer's disease and its treatment, refer to Chapter 12.)

Cardiovascular System Medications

Heart disease is the leading cause of death among patients age 65 years or older in the United States, and cardiovascular system drugs such as diuretics and beta blockers are among the most commonly prescribed medications in this age-group. Consequently, allied health professionals will encounter drugs used for hypertension, arrhythmias, and stroke prevention in practice every day.

Antihypertensives

Several **antihypertensives** should be used with caution in geriatric patients. Spironolactone dosages should be restricted to less than 25 mg a day for patients with heart failure or low kidney function. Higher dosages of this medication can cause elevated potassium levels. Thiazide diuretics are not effective for patients with very low kidney function and may exacerbate gout. Although beta blockers may not be as effective as other classes of antihypertensive drugs at reducing mortality, they are used as first-line therapy in many older patients who have other conditions that call for the use of a beta blocker, such as heart failure, angina, or a history of MIs. Beta blockers pose a particular risk of bradycardia (slowed heart rate) in patients 65 years of age or older.

The CNS effects of antihypertensive drugs may be greater in geriatrics than in other patient populations. Beta blockers can cause somnolence and depression in older adults, and the alpha-2 adrenergic clonidine (Catapres) is not recommended as a first-line treatment for hypertension in older patients because of the high risk of CNS adverse effects. (For more information on antihypertensives, see Chapter 15.)

Cardiac Glycosides

Cardiac glycosides such as digoxin are used to treat certain cardiovascular disorders, and older patients must be monitored carefully for any adverse effects. Digoxin (Lanoxin) is used to restore the force of myocardial contraction without increasing oxygen demands and to slow the heart. Digoxin should be used with caution because of the risk of drug accumulation in the blood. This condition is commonly known as **digoxin toxicity**, or **digitalis toxicity**, and geriatric patients are particularly vulnerable. The three primary signs and symptoms of digitalis toxicity are nausea, vomiting, and arrhythmias. However, the patient may also experience vertigo, general weakness, and visions of yellow-green halos around objects. If any of these signs and symptoms occur, the drug should be discontinued immediately. As a general guideline, the AGS recommends avoiding digoxin doses greater than 0.125 mg a day because there is not enough additional benefit to outweigh the increased risk of toxicity. (For more information on digoxin, see Chapter 15.)

Anticoagulants

Older patients often require lower doses of warfarin (Coumadin), the most commonly used **anticoagulant**, than the general patient population. Dosing is based on the results of a laboratory test value known as the **international normalized ratio (INR)**. Because warfarin interacts with many drugs and supplements, and because increased or decreased efficacy can have serious consequences for older patients, patients taking warfarin should ensure that their prescribers know about any changes in their medication regimens, including changes in intake of herbal supplements.

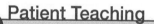 Patient Teaching

Allied health professionals should inform patients who are taking warfarin therapy that significant changes in their dietary intake of green, leafy vegetables can affect the efficacy of the drug. These types of vegetables contain large amounts of vitamin K, a substance involved in the clotting cascade. Consequently, a large change in the quantity of green, leafy vegetables in the diet may require a warfarin dosage change. To maintain a consistent level of medication, patients should monitor their daily intake of these vegetables. In addition, patients will undergo periodic laboratory tests to check their warfarin levels.

No dose adjustment is required for dabigatran (Pradaxa) in geriatric patients unless they have very poor kidney function. Dabigatran is used only with extreme caution in patients 75 years old or older because of the known risk of hemorrhage in that patient population. (For more information about anticoagulants, see Chapter 16.)

GI System Medications

GI system medications such as phenothiazines pose risks for older patients because these drugs tend to cause sedation and confusion. Commonly prescribed GI system medications for geriatric patients include treatments for constipation.

Phenothiazines

Promethazine (Phenergan) belongs to the drug class known as **phenothiazines**. This medication is highly anticholinergic and is used as an antiemetic. Whenever possible, its use should be avoided in patients 65 years of age or older because of an increased risk for confusion, dry mouth, and constipation in that patient population. (For more information on promethazine, see Chapter 18.)

Laxatives

Geriatric patients are at a higher risk of constipation because of their physical inactivity, low-fiber diets, and low fluid intake. In addition, muscle tone in the bowel decreases with age. Furthermore, many of the medications that are commonly prescribed for this age-group can cause constipation. To combat constipation, patients should be encouraged to eat a high-fiber diet and to drink plenty of water. If constipation persists, **laxatives** such as bulk-forming laxatives, stool softeners, and stimulant laxatives are ordered. (A more detailed discussion of laxatives can be found in Chapter 18.)

Anticholinergics

Because older adults are at an increased risk for adverse effects such as confusion, constipation, and dry mouth from anticholinergic medications, and because clearance of those drugs is reduced with age, it is best to avoid their use whenever possible. Anticholinergics include first-generation antihistamines such as the antinausea medication meclizine, the antiemetic drug hydroxyzine, and allergy medications such as diphenhydramine (see Table 29.5).

TABLE 29.5 Anticholinergic Drugs

Generic (Brand Name)	Dispensing Status
Antihistamines (First-Generation)	
Chlorpheniramine (Aller-Chlor)	OTC
Diphenhydramine (Benadryl)	OTC
Doxylamine (Doxytex)	OTC
Hydroxyzine (Vistaril)	Rx
Meclizine (Antivert)	OTC
Antiparkinson Agents	
Benztropine (Cogentin)	Rx
Procyclidine	Rx
Trihexyphenidyl	Rx
Drugs for Overactive Bladder	
Fesoterodine (Toviaz)	Rx
Tolterodine (Detrol)	Rx
Trospium (Sanctura)	Rx

Drugs for Infection

Nitrofurantoin is not recommended for the treatment or prevention of urinary tract infections in older patients because it is not effective in patients with low kidney function and has a potential for pulmonary toxicity. Older patients with poor kidney function may need to take lower doses or less frequent doses of other antibiotics such as sulfamethoxazole/trimethoprim, ciprofloxacin, and gentamicin. (For more information on drugs used for urinary tract infections, see Chapter 22.)

Drugs for Pain

Many pain relievers such as ibuprofen are used by older adults, even though these NSAIDs pose an increased risk of GI bleeding and peptic ulcer disease in this vulnerable patient population. Patients with heart failure should avoid taking NSAIDs because of their potential to promote fluid retention and exacerbate the condition. Aspirin at doses greater than 325 mg a day should be avoided for the same reasons. Among the NSAIDs, indomethacin has the most adverse effects. Opioids (such as oxycodone) are sedating and constipating, and older patients may be more sensitive to these adverse effects. (For more information on pain medications, see Chapter 25.)

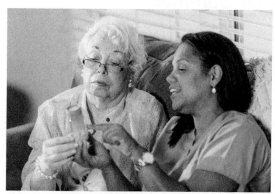

An allied health professional should discuss all drug therapy (both over-the-counter and prescription medications) with a patient and should inquire about any adverse effects the patient is experiencing.

Kolb's Learning Styles

Assimilators like to work with details and lists. Convergers prefer hands-on manipulation of information. These kinds of learners may find creating their own flash cards useful for studying the common conditions and drug therapy regimens associated with geriatric patients. Before creating the flash cards, students should gather different colors of cards or ink and assign certain colors to particular disease states or drug classes. They should then write the name of a drug class on one side of the card and the condition that drug class is used to treat on the other side of the card. Once the cards are completed, students should quiz themselves or work with partners to test their drug knowledge.

Checkpoint 29.4

Take a moment to review what you have learned so far and answer these questions.

1. What CNS drugs must be used cautiously in older adults?

2. What cardiovascular system drugs are among the most commonly prescribed medications for the geriatric patient population?

3. What are some examples of anticholinergic drugs, and why is it best to avoid their use in older adults whenever possible?

Chapter Review

Chapter Summary

With advancing age, people experience declines in cardiovascular function and strength as well as in brain function, bone density, and muscle mass. Kidney and liver functions decline; tissues lose elasticity; and visual and hearing acuity decrease. Because of these physiologic changes, drugs that are metabolized in the liver or eliminated through the kidneys often need dosage adjustments to avoid adverse effects in this patient population. Normally, the blood-brain barrier protects the brain from drugs, but that barrier becomes more porous in old age when the activity of a group of gatekeepers called p-glycoproteins decreases.

Polypharmacy is the use of multiple drugs at the same time, and it is a common problem among older patients. This practice puts patients at increased risk for adverse drug reactions and drug interactions. Through different mechanisms, older adults are more sensitive to the sedating effects of benzodiazepine drugs and may experience a greater analgesic response to opioids than that in younger patients. The effects of warfarin and other anticoagulants are greater in older adults, so they may need lower doses of these blood thinners.

The Beers Criteria is a list of drugs that many prescribers consider inappropriate for patients who are age 65 or older because of an increased risk of adverse effects or a potential to exacerbate disease states that are common among older adults. Many of the drugs are on the list because they cause anticholinergic effects, which can be much worse in geriatric patients.

Chapter Checkup

The Navigator+ learning management system that accompanies this textbook offers many opportunities to help you master chapter content, including end-of-chapter exercises, a glossary of key terms, flash cards, and additional interactive activities.

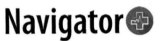

Career Exploration

If you enjoyed learning about geriatric care in this chapter, you may want to explore the following career options:

- audiologist
- case manager
- certified bone densitometry technologist (CBDT)
- certified clinical nutritionist
- certified nursing assistant
- clinical dietitian specialist
- dementia care specialist
- home care assistant/aide
- medical assistant
- medical social worker
- occupational therapist
- pharmacy technician
- physical therapist
- recreational therapist
- registered dietitian

A | Checkpoint Answer Keys

Chapter 1

Checkpoint 1.1

1. Hippocrates proposed that disease was caused by natural rather than supernatural causes and published numerous texts that categorized diseases, signs, and symptoms. He also established a lexicon of medical terminology.

2. Oswald Schmiedeberg (1838-1921)

3. Paracelsus advocated the use of individual drugs (rather than mixtures or potions) based on his theory that treating a disease with individual drugs would make it easier to determine which agents were effective and which agents harmed patients.

Checkpoint 1.2

1. Insulin, chloroquine, and arsphenamine (used to treat syphilis) were all developed in the first half of the twentieth century.

2. Vaccines, antidepressants, oral contraceptives, human immunodeficiency virus (HIV) medications

3. The US Pharmacopeia (USP) was the first official listing of drugs in the United States. Today, a revision of this early formulary exists and is written by the US Pharmacopeial Convention.

Checkpoint 1.3

1. Generic name and brand name

2. All the drugs within a specific class typically have generic names that look similar to one another. For example, the generic names of beta blockers end in *-olol* (such as atenolol).

Checkpoint 1.4

1. Kolb's Learning Styles include Accommodators, Divergers, Assimilators, and Convergers. The categories in Kolb's Learning Styles are based on the idea that students tend to be better at two of the four learning stages: learning by being involved in the world (concrete experience), thinking about those experiences (reflective observation), making generalizations and developing theories based on those experiences (abstract conceptualization), and testing those theories while solving problems (active experimentation).

2. The websites for the American Cancer Society, American Diabetes Association, American Heart Association, and American Lung Association are reliable sources.

Chapter 2

Checkpoint 2.1

1. Streptomycin, digitalis, morphine, codeine, acetylsalicylic acid (aspirin), thyroid, and others

2. A synthetic drug is a drug that has been created from a series of chemical reactions to produce a specific pharmacologic effect. A semisynthetic drug is a natural drug that has been modified chemically in the laboratory to do one or more of the following actions: (1) improve the efficacy of the natural product; (2) reduce its side effects; (3) overcome developing bacterial resistance; or (4) broaden the spectrum of bacteria against which a product can be effective. Both classifications of drug are produced in the laboratory but by different processes.

3. Pharmacogenomics is a field of study that examines the relationship between an individual's genes and his or her body's response to drugs.

Checkpoint 2.2

1. Prescription drugs are dispensed from the pharmacy upon receipt of a prescription from a prescriber. In the United States, prescription or legend drugs are considered to be too dangerous to be used without medical supervision, so they are available to patients only upon prescription from a prescriber. Medications that can be bought without a prescription are called over-the-counter (OTC) medications.

2. Medications that have potential for abuse and dependence are categorized by the US Drug Enforcement Administration (DEA) as controlled substances. These drugs are placed in one of five schedules, based on their degree of potential for abuse. Some examples of controlled substances in each of the schedules include:

   - Schedule I: heroin, crack, LSD
   - Schedule II: morphine, methadone, oxycodone, fentanyl, Ritalin
   - Schedule III: steroids, codeine
   - Schedule IV: benzodiazepines, sleep aids (such as zolpidem), appetite suppressants
   - Schedule V: codeine combination products, cough syrup

3. Items that are considered behind-the-counter products include medications containing pseudoephedrine, codeine cough syrups, insulin syringes, and certain asthma medications.

Chapter 3

Checkpoint 3.1

1. Drugs used for the treatment of a disease cure or eliminate effects of the disease. Examples of a curative drug would be antibiotics. Examples of drugs used to eliminate the effects of a disease would include blood pressure medications. These medications would be considered disease management medications in that they may not completely cure the condition but their mechanisms of action can eliminate the effects of the condition. Drugs used for palliative care are used for terminally ill patients. In these situations, the disease cannot be cured or treated, but the unwanted effects or symptoms can be managed so that the patient is more comfortable and has a higher quality of life. Pain medications used for end-stage cancer are examples of palliative drug therapy.

2. Drug molecules connect with receptors already within the body to produce physiologic effects. Drug molecules are similarly shaped to substances within the body that already connect with receptors. So, agonists can be considered to mimic normal physiologic effects in that they connect with receptors to stimulate action. Antagonists are considered "blockers" because they connect with receptors that block a normal physiologic response.

3. The therapeutic range is the concentration range in the bloodstream that is high enough to produce an effect but low enough to avoid toxic effects. Doses and schedules are designed to bring drug concentrations into this range to achieve the optimal results for a particular drug therapy. The time-response curve depicts this range graphically to show the increase in blood concentration when a dose is taken and the decrease in blood concentration as the medication is eliminated from the body.

Checkpoint 3.2

1. Absorption is the process of bringing a drug into the body. It is affected by dosage form and method of administration among other things. Distribution is the process of moving a drug around the body, usually in the bloodstream. Bloodflow and protein content within the blood can affect the distribution of a drug. Metabolism is the process of breaking down or changing drug molecules to deactivate them. This process happens primarily in the liver. Excretion is the process of eliminating drug molecules from the bloodstream and body. This process happens primarily in the kidneys.

2. The first-pass effect refers to what happens as drugs "pass" or travel through the liver and encounter metabolizing enzymes. As a result, the full drug dose does not reach the body, and its systemic effect is lessened or effectively eliminated. For those drugs that are quickly and easily metabolized by liver enzymes, this first-pass effect is especially problematic, and alternative routes of administration that bypass the liver must be used.

3. Many liver enzymes are involved in metabolism; the cytochrome P450 enzyme system most frequently deactivates drugs. Cytochrome P450 enzymes that metabolize drugs are numbered. Common ones include 1A2, 2A6, 2C9, 2D6, and 3A4. Two drugs that use the same enzyme system, when given together, can compete for elimination and increase potential for drug toxicity.

4. Some common allergic reactions to drugs include nasal secretions, swelling, wheezing, an excessively rapid heart rate, urticaria (hives), pruritus (itching), angioedema (an abnormal accumulation of fluid in tissue), wheals (red, elevated areas on the body), and—in rare cases—even death.

Checkpoint 3.3

1. A systemic effect occurs when a drug is absorbed and then circulated throughout the bloodstream. Effects throughout the body can be achieved using systemic routes of administration (buccal, implant, oral, parenteral, rectal, and transdermal). A local effect occurs when a drug remains at the site of administration rather than being absorbed into the bloodstream. Thus, the drug action is confined or localized in that area only. Local routes of administration include dermal, inhalation, intranasal, ophthalmic, otic, and vaginal.

2. *Intramuscular:* An injection that administers a drug into the muscle tissue. A 1-inch needle is typically used and inserted at a 90-degree angle.

   Intravenous: An injection of a drug directly into a vein. The size of the needle may vary, and the insertion angle is usually 15 to 20 degrees from the surface of the skin.

   Subcutaneous: An injection of a drug into the layer of fat just below the skin. If a 1-inch needle is used, a 45-degree angle is implemented. Smaller insulin needles can be inserted at a 90-degree angle.

   Intrathecal: An injection of a drug directly into the cerebrospinal fluid. This type of injection is used to deliver regional anesthesia.

   Intradermal: An injection of a drug just under the top layer of skin. This type of injection is used for tuberculosis screening.

3. Nitroglycerin

Checkpoint 3.4

1. Tablet, capsule, caplet, gelcap, powder, troche, lozenge, implant

2. Suppository, ointment, cream, gel, lotion, paste, patch

3. Syrup, solution, elixir, tincture, emulsion, suspension, aerosol

Chapter 4

Checkpoint 4.1

1. A health professional is an individual who has been educated, trained, and state-licensed to diagnose and/or treat the medical problems of patients whom they see on a routine basis. Health professionals include physicians, doctors of osteopathy, podiatrists, dentists, pharmacists, chiropractors, physician assistants, and nurse practitioners. An allied health professional is an individual who has been educated, trained, and licensed and/or certified to provide a range of diagnostic, technical, therapeutic, and direct and indirect patient care services. He or she also provides support services that are critical to other health professionals.

2. Allied health professionals work in a variety of settings, including hospitals, ambulatory clinics, laboratories, schools, creative arts studios, counseling centers, pharmaceutical and medical equipment companies, and health technology firms.

3. Allied health professionals fall into two distinct categories: (1) technicians and assistants; and (2) technologists and therapists.

Checkpoint 4.2

1. Allied health professionals should have good critical thinking skills; a high degree of professionalism; effective communication skills; an aptitude for technology; and an awareness of and sensitivity to cultural and linguistic diversity.

2. To present a professional appearance, allied health professionals should follow commonsense guidelines including clean, neat clothing; close-toed shoes with nonskid soles; simple jewelry that does not impede work tasks; clean, modestly manicured nails; light and natural makeup; and no fragrance.

3. Ethics is the study of standards of conduct and moral judgment that outline the rights and wrongs of human conduct and behavior.

Checkpoint 4.3

1. Licensure is the process by which the state board grants permission to an individual to engage in a given occupation upon finding that the applicant has attained the minimum degree of competency necessary to safeguard the public. Certification is a recognition by a private board or professional organization that an individual has taken an assessment that demonstrates understanding of the qualifications of a particular profession.

2. A preceptorship is an opportunity for allied health students to apply what they have learned in the classroom to a clinical setting. It allows students to interact with patients and healthcare staff, use critical

thinking skills, and complete real-world documentation. Preceptorships also help build confidence and reinforce the importance of good communication and professionalism skills in a career position.

Checkpoint 4.4

1. Some of the clinical duties of allied health professionals include interprofessional communication, direct patient care, clinical documentation, patient safety, protection of personal and private health information, and patient education. Some nonclinical duties performed by allied health professionals include the updating and filing of patient medical records, completion of insurance forms, patient billing and bookkeeping tasks, and inventory of supplies and equipment.

2. To obtain a thorough medication history, an allied health professional must document all prescription drugs, over-the-counter (OTC) drugs, and herbal and alternative therapies that a patient takes. In addition to this information, an allied health professional must also record the patient's use of alcohol and/or recreational drugs.

3. Health literacy is "the degree to which an individual has the capacity to obtain, communicate, process, and understand basic health information and services to make appropriate health decisions."

Chapter 5

Checkpoint 5.1

1. A prescription is an order of medication issued by a prescriber for a valid medical condition. This form is taken by the patient to his or her pharmacy to be filled. A medication order is a set of instructions given by a prescriber that specifies patient medications within an institutional or a hospital setting.

2. Signa

3. Standing order

4. Inscription

Checkpoint 5.2

1. Responses may vary. Some possible responses include *ad* (right ear), *as* (left ear), *au* (both ears), *od* (right eye), *os* (left eye), *ou* (each eye), *po* (by mouth), *pr* (by rectum), *sl* (sublingually), *top* (topically), or *vag* (vaginally).

2. q6h

3. Take 10 milligrams by mouth twice daily.

4. Advantages of adopting a CPOE system include elimination of poor handwriting, a decrease in spelling errors, the avoidance of nonstandard abbreviations, immediate access to patients' medical records,

streamlined workflow processes, improved documentation, and enhanced coordination of patient care.

Checkpoint 5.3

1. Information on a medication container label includes patient identification information; the name, address, and phone number of the pharmacy; dosage directions; the Rx number; the number of refills; the prescriber's name; the drug name; and the drug's manufacturer. If the medication is a scheduled drug, the label must also contain a transfer warning.

2. An auxiliary label is a small, colorful label that is added to a dispensed medication to supplement the directions on the medication container label. This label addresses how to take the medication, how to store the medication, or how to handle the medication. Auxiliary labels also warn patients about possible side effects and drug interactions. For a patient, knowing and following this information will improve the efficacy and safety of drug administration, thus improving patient outcome.

Chapter 6

Checkpoint 6.1

1. The denominator is the number on the bottom of the fraction.

2. It is equal to 9 because numbers of lower value that are to the left of numbers of higher value should be subtracted from the number of higher value.

3. Multiply the fraction $^5/_6$ by the reciprocal of the fraction $^2/_3$, which is $^3/_2$.

Checkpoint 6.2

1. 28.35 g

2. 1 mL

3. mg/mL

Checkpoint 6.3

1. Every country in the world uses 24-hour time with the exception of the United States and Canada.

2. Celsius temperature scale

3. 24-hour time

Checkpoint 6.4

1. A nomogram is a chart that is used to compare the height and weight of a patient in order to determine the patient's body surface area (BSA).

2. Pediatric patients

3. The first rule is that 3 of the 4 amounts must be known. The second rule is that the numerators must have the same units. The third rule is that the denominators must have the same units.

Chapter 7

Checkpoint 7.1

1. Omission error, wrong-dose error, extra-dose error, wrong-dosage-form error, wrong-time error

2. Patients should know the following information about each of their medications: purpose of medication, generic and brand names of the medication, appearance of the medication, correct dose and dosage (frequency) of the medication, actions to take when a dose is missed, duration of treatment, medications or foods that interact with the medication, common side effects, special precautions necessary for drug therapy, and proper storage of the medication.

3. A work environment that is disorganized, poorly lit, unsanitary, noisy, or full of distractions could increase the likelihood of medication errors.

Checkpoint 7.2

1. The Poison Prevention Packaging Act of 1970 required that prescription drugs be packaged in child-resistant containers.

2. Tall-man lettering is used by manufacturers to help prevent medication selection errors.

3. Automation such as bar-coding technology decreases medication selection errors. E-prescribing eliminates illegible prescriptions. Integrated, automated systems decrease the likelihood of several types of medication errors.

Checkpoint 7.3

1. A sentinel event is an unexpected occurrence involving death, serious physical or psychological injury, or the potential for such occurrences to happen in a medical setting. For example, a medication error that results in death would be a sentinel event.

2. Some examples of high-alert medications include warfarin, amiodarone, and digoxin.

3. The mission of the Institute for Safe Medication Practices (ISMP) is to understand the causes of medication errors and to provide and communicate time-critical error-reduction strategies to the healthcare community, policymakers, and the public.

Chapter 8

Checkpoint 8.1

1. The Drug Enforcement Administration (DEA) regulates controlled substances, whereas the Food and Drug Administration (FDA) enforces the packaging, labeling, advertising, and marketing guidelines for medications. The Occupational Safety and Health Administration (OSHA) establishes and enforces safety and health regulations and standards in the workplace.

2. Schedule II: morphine; Schedule III: barbiturates; Schedule IV: zolpidem

3. Pseudoephedrine does not require a prescription, but the medication is kept behind the counter in a pharmacy because the drug has been used to make methamphetamine, which is an illegal type of stimulant.

Checkpoint 8.2

1. US Pharmacopeial Convention (USP)

2. An accreditation agency provides guidance on an educational institution's curriculum and instruction and awards a "seal of approval" to programs that meet its standards.

Checkpoint 8.3

1. Because laws governing the practice of medicine do not always dictate the proper behavior in every situation, the allied health professional must have a set of professional ethics that guide his or her behavior.

2. Allied health professionals should not divulge patient-protected health information outside the workplace. Inside the workplace, allied health personnel should limit disclosures to the minimum amount of information that is required for the intended purpose. They should also ensure that computer screens are not in view of the public. Finally, allied health professionals should not leave phone messages containing detailed medical information for patients.

3. DEA Form 222

Chapter 9

Checkpoint 9.1

1. The Sun Protection Factor (SPF) estimates the amount of resistance to burning that a product provides. So, if an individual selects a sunscreen with an SPF of 15, it generally means that he or she can spend 15 times longer in the sun than the typical time it would take to burn. This rating system is based on skin type in unprotected exposure to sun for 45 to 60 minutes.

2. Benzoyl peroxide and salicylic acid

3. Retinoid medications such as acitretin, adapalene, tretinoin, isotretinoin, alitretinoin, and tazarotene

Checkpoint 9.2

1. Bacitracin, bacitracin/neomycin/polymyxin B, clindamycin, erythromycin, mupirocin, neomycin, retapamulin

2. *Lindane:* This lotion is used for scabies, and the shampoo is used for lice. Lindane has significant central nervous system (CNS) toxicities and can cause seizures, so it is limited to prescription use only. It

should be used only with great caution to treat infants or children. Patients must follow instructions closely and avoid getting the lotion in the eyes or on mucous membranes. Lindane should be washed off in 8 to 12 hours. Repeat applications can cause dermatitis, so reapplication is not recommended. Patients or caregivers applying lindane should wear gloves or wash their hands thoroughly after application.

Malathion: This medication is a prescription product used to treat head lice. Malathion kills both the adult lice and the nits. To use malathion, apply the lotion to dry hair until fully wetted and then leave it on the hair to dry naturally for 8 to 12 hours. Afterward, the hair can be shampooed and all nits removed with a fine-tooth comb. If lice are present in seven days, repeat this procedure.

Pyrethrin and permethrin: These medications are considered first-line therapies because they are available over the counter. Pyrethrin is used, however, only for head lice. Permethrin, depending on the formulation, can be used for either lice or scabies and has residual activity for up to 14 days. Neither of these products kills both the lice and the nits, so repeat application is often needed in seven days.

3. Minoxidil and finasteride

Checkpoint 9.3

1. Dermatitis is an itchy rash usually caused by local irritation and an allergic reaction. It is a short-term problem that is treated by using topical anti-inflammatory products and by removing the source of irritation. Eczema is a severe drug skin condition that may be related to an allergy, but not always. It is a chronic condition that comes and goes and is worse when the skin naturally dries out. Psoriasis is an autoimmune condition in which the scaly, itchy patches appear on the skin.

2. Corticosteroids are used to treat both dermatitis and eczema. These drugs are listed in Table 9.6.

3. Once an ulcer has developed, treatment involves wound cleaning and removal of necrotic or dead tissue (a process known as *debridement*) while the wound heals on its own. These wounds, especially deep ones, can take significant time to heal. Some drugs promote regranulation, which is the process of building new skin layers over a wound area.

Checkpoint 9.4

1. Urticaria (hives), pruritus, or a diffuse redness on the trunk of the body; anaphylaxis; Stevens-Johnson syndrome; heparin-induced thrombocytopenia (HIT)

2. Any of the drugs listed in Table 9.9 can cause photosensitivity.

3. Aloe vera

Chapter 10

Checkpoint 10.1

1. Bones provide structure and support for the body, help muscles effectively move parts of the body, protect delicate organs, and help produce blood cells.

2. Bone density declines.

Checkpoint 10.2

1. Medications that treat osteoarthritis (OA) include acetaminophen; nonsteroidal anti-inflammatory drugs (NSAIDs) such as diclofenac, etodolac, ibuprofen, indomethacin, ketoprofen, ketorolac, meloxicam, nabumetone, naproxen, oxaprozin, piroxicam, and sulindac; and COX-2 inhibitors (celecoxib).

2. Severe liver impairment or severe active liver disease are the contraindications to acetaminophen use.

3. Rheumatoid arthritis (RA) treatment options include auranofin, azathioprine, cyclophosphamide, cyclosporine, hydroxychloroquine, leflunomide, methotrexate, sulfasalazine, adalimumab, anakinra, certolizumab, etanercept, golimumab, and infliximab.

4. Gouty arthritis treatment options include NSAIDs (naproxen, indomethacin), colchicine, triamcinolone, prednisone, allopurinol, febuxostat, and probenecid.

Checkpoint 10.3

1. Nausea, vomiting, and constipation

2. Bisphosphonates work by inhibiting osteoclasts from removing calcium from bone tissue. They prevent bone breakdown.

Chapter 11

Checkpoint 11.1

1. Skeletal muscles are muscles used for voluntary movement such as walking, clapping, and chewing. They are connected to bones and joints by tendons. Cardiac muscle is found only in the heart. These muscle cells are specifically designed for the pumping and squeezing action required for each heartbeat. Smooth muscle can be found in the stomach, intestines, bladder, uterus, blood vessel walls, and other hollow organs. These muscles are designed for involuntary movement such as peristalsis, a process in which food progresses through the intestines or blood flows through the vasculature.

2. Acetylcholine (ACh), a neurotransmitter, is released from the nerve cell, travels across the neuromuscular junction (the tiny space between the nerve cell and the muscle cell), and stimulates muscle cell receptors to cause cell membrane depolarization. Depolarization changes the balance of positive and negative electrical charges along the membrane surface and opens ion channels, allowing sodium (Na^+) to enter the cells.

Sodium influx causes the release of the intracellular calcium stores that stimulate muscle fiber contraction. Muscle fibers contract and shorten the muscle, which in turn pulls on attached bones and joints, thereby creating movement. Muscle contraction stops when ACh is deactivated in the neuromuscular junction by the enzyme acetylcholinesterase.

3. Deltoid (in the arms), gluteus medius (in the buttocks), and vastus lateralis (a muscle in the quadriceps group of the legs)

Checkpoint 11.2

1. The drugs listed in Table 11.1 (baclofen, carisoprodol, chlorzoxazone, cyclobenzaprine, metaxalone, methocarbamol, orphenadrine citrate, and tizanidine) are all drugs used for muscle spasms caused by injury or lower back pain.

2. Dantrolene is used to treat spasticity from spinal cord injury. This medication is also used to treat malignant hyperthermia due to anesthesia.

3. Neuromuscular blocking agents cause temporary paralysis. These agents are used with anesthesia for short-term muscle relaxation during endotracheal intubation, mechanical respiration, and surgical procedures.

Checkpoint 11.3

1. For patients who have myasthenia gravis, neostigmine and pyridostigmine enhance muscle strength. The immunosuppressants azathioprine and cyclophosphamide are used to slow the progression of the disorder.

2. The polio vaccine is a required vaccination for all children entering kindergarten in the United States. The vaccine is given to children in four doses at the following ages: 2 months, 4 months, 6 to 18 months, and 4 to 6 years. For US adults, the Centers for Disease Control and Prevention (CDC) recommends the polio vaccine for only those individuals who are traveling to a country where polio is present or for those individuals who are caring for a patient with polio.

3. Rhabdomyolysis is a syndrome in which muscle breakdown occurs and releases toxic cell contents into the bloodstream. This syndrome is a rare but serious side effect of the cholesterol-lowering class of drugs called *statins*. Symptoms can include muscle aches and pain, red- to brown-colored urine, and muscle weakness.

Chapter 12

Checkpoint 12.1

1. *Cerebral cortex:* higher cognitive functions such as memory and thinking
   Cerebellum: movement and coordination

Thalamus and hypothalamus: body temperature and hormonal regulation
Pons and medulla: autonomic and reflex functions of the body

2. Nerve signal conduction occurs when a nerve cell is stimulated and produces chemical neurotransmitters. These neurotransmitters are released into the synaptic cleft (space between nerve cells) and travel to the neighboring cell. The neurotransmitters connect to receptors on the neighboring cell, and this process repeats itself, thus carrying along the signal.

3. *Acetylcholine:* acts within the autonomic nervous system to control blood pressure, digestion, heart function, and various glands
   Dopamine: controls mood and coordinated movement
   Epinephrine: acts within the sympathetic nervous system to control cardiac function and bronchodilation (breathing)
   GABA: acts within the brain to control nerve signal delivery
   Norepinephrine: acts within the central nervous system (CNS) and sympathetic nervous system to control mood, emotions, blood pressure, cardiac function, and digestion
   Serotonin: acts in the CNS and peripheral nervous systems to control mood, emotions, blood pressure, and digestion

Checkpoint 12.2

1. Sodium-channel blockers, calcium-channel blockers, GABA enhancers, glutamate inhibitors

2. *Dopamine agonists:* apomorphine, bromocriptine, levodopa/carbidopa, pramipexole, ropinirole amantadine
   Anticholinergics: benztropine, trihexyphenidyl
   COMT inhibitors: entacapone, tolcapone
   MAOIs: rasagiline, selegiline

3. Typically, therapy starts with a dopamine agonist or an anticholinergic. Then amantadine, entacapone, tolcapone, or selegiline is added as needed to control symptoms.

Checkpoint 12.3

1. Donepezil, galantamine, and rivastigmine

2. Attention-deficit/hyperactivity disorder (ADHD) is characterized by inattention, impulsivity, and hyperactivity. To be diagnosed with ADHD, an individual must exhibit six or more symptoms of inattention and six or more hyperactivity/impulsivity symptoms that impair daily life in at least two settings for at least six months.

3. To treat ADHD, health practitioners prescribe stimulants such as amphetamine, dexmethylphenidate, dextroamphetamine, and methylphenidate, and the nonstimulant atomoxetine.

Checkpoint 12.4

1. Alpha blockers inhibit alpha receptors in the autonomic system to control blood pressure and bladder emptying. Beta blockers inhibit beta receptors in the autonomic nervous system to control blood pressure, heart rate, and heart rhythm. They can reduce stress on the heart.

2. Alpha blockers are especially useful for treating men with both high blood pressure and benign prostatic hyperplasia. Beta blockers are used for high blood pressure and cardiac arrhythmias. They are especially useful for patients who have had a heart attack because they can reduce stress on the heart.

3. Common side effects of beta blockers include headache, dizziness, light-headedness, nausea, fatigue/weakness, increased incidence of depression, and slowed heart rate.

Chapter 13

Checkpoint 13.1

1. SSRIs, SNRIs, TCAs, and MAOI inhibitors are all drug classes that are used to manage depression.

2. Selective serotonin reuptake inhibitors (SSRIs) and serotonin-norepinephrine reuptake inhibitors (SNRIs) both block reuptake of serotonin in the neuronal synapse.

3. TCAs can cause drowsiness, especially at higher doses. Other side effects include anticholinergic effects (e.g., dry mouth, blurred vision, constipation, and urinary retention). Some of these agents can also cause priapism.

Checkpoint 13.2

1. Benzodiazepines and buspirone are used to treat anxiety. Also, some SSRIs such as sertraline can be used for treatment of anxiety associated with posttraumatic stress disorder (PTSD) and obsessive-compulsive disorder (OCD).

2. Insomnia is treated with over-the-counter (OTC) antihistamines and sleep aids.

3. Aripiprazole, clozapine, olanzapine, paliperidone, quetiapine, risperidone, ziprasidone

4. Eszopiclone, ramelteon, zaleplon, zolpidem

Checkpoint 13.3

1. Lithium is the drug of choice for the treatment of bipolar disorder, but antidepressants and antipsychotics may also be used.

2. Aripiprazole, clozapine, olanzapine, paliperidone, risperidone, ziprasidone

3. Common side effects of atypical antipsychotics include drowsiness, headache, constipation, dry mouth, urinary incontinence or retention, rash, excitation, and, occasionally, frequent hiccups. Decreases in blood pressure, especially when standing or sitting up, can also occur. Significant weight gain occurs for many patients on these medications. Some atypical antipsychotics can cause arrhythmias and QT-wave prolongation.

Chapter 14

Checkpoint 14.1

1. Cone cells sense color and are responsible for day vision. Rod cells are responsible for night vision, as well as for black-and-white vision.

2. The eardrum separates the middle ear from the external ear. The bones inside the middle ear are the malleus, incus, and stapes. The stapes in effect taps on the oval window, the entrance to the inner ear. The eustachian tube connects the middle ear to the throat.

3. Presbycusis is caused by damage to the sensory hairs in the inner ear. This damage occurs naturally with age and exposure to loud noise.

Checkpoint 14.2

1. Prostaglandin agonists, beta blockers, alpha receptor agonists, miotics

2. Aminoglycosides, macrolides, sulfonamides, quinolones, and antivirals

3. Ophthalmic corticosteroids are useful for calming inflammation related to eye infections. These agents can reduce pain, redness, and irritation.

Checkpoint 14.3

1. Ophthalmic antivirals

2. Topical antihistamines, decongestants, mast cell stabilizers, nonsteroidal anti-inflammatory drugs (NSAIDs)

3. Hormonal changes (especially menopause), autoimmune disorders that affect tear production (Sjögren's syndrome, collagen vascular disease, rheumatoid arthritis, lupus), any condition that impedes proper closing of the eyes or impairs the blink reflex (stroke), and environmental causes (dry air from air conditioning or heat)

Checkpoint 14.4

1. To treat otitis media, healthcare practitioners prescribe antibiotics to eradicate the infection and topical analgesics to relieve the pain. Drugs for otitis externa include drying agents and earwax removers.

2. Otitis externa

3. Ototoxicity is damage to the ear caused by chemical or drug exposure.

Chapter 15

Checkpoint 15.1

1. These blood vessels circulate blood throughout the body, bringing needed oxygen and nutrients to tissues and carrying away carbon dioxide and toxic by-products. Arteries carry blood away from the heart, and veins carry blood back to the heart. Capillaries are the tiny blood vessels in which critical fluids, gases, and nutrients are exchanged between the blood and body tissues.

2. Sinoatrial (SA) node

3. Blood pressure is measured with an instrument called a sphygmomanometer and a cuff that is wrapped around a patient's arm and inflated to apply pressure. When blood starts flowing again, the first or upper number reported in a blood pressure result is obtained. This number is called the systolic reading or the systolic blood pressure (SBP). The diastolic reading or the diastolic blood pressure (DBP), the lower number in a blood pressure reading, is obtained at the point at which the cuff is loose enough that blood flows freely through the artery without turbulence.

Checkpoint 15.2

1. Recommendations include treating high blood pressure when it exceeds 150/90 for individuals 60 years of age and older and 140/90 for individuals less than 60 years of age. Patients with diabetes or kidney disease should begin treatment for high blood pressure when it exceeds 140/90, no matter what age they are. Healthy lifestyle modifications, such as weight loss and regular exercise, are used to treat hypertension at all stages.

2. Angiotensin-converting enzyme (ACE) inhibitors, angiotensin receptor blockers (ARBs), calcium-channel blockers, thiazide diuretics, alpha blockers, and beta blockers

3. *ACE inhibitors:* cough, headache, dizziness, fatigue, mild diarrhea, angioedema

ARBs: headache, dizziness, fatigue, mild diarrhea, respiratory tract infections

Calcium-channel blockers: headache, dizziness, fatigue, constipation, nausea, heartburn, flushing

Thiazide diuretics: hypotension, dizziness, rash, hair loss (alopecia), upset stomach, diarrhea, constipation

Alpha blockers: headache, dizziness, nausea, fatigue

Beta blockers: headache, dizziness, nausea, fatigue, weakness

Checkpoint 15.3

1. *Class I:* membrane-stabilizing agents

Class II: beta blockers

Class III: potassium-channel blockers

Class IV: calcium-channel blockers

2. Responses will vary. Medications that interact with antiarrhythmic agents can be found in Table 15.5.

3. Digoxin is used to treat atrial fibrillation and flutter.

Checkpoint 15.4

1. Vasodilators: long-acting and short-acting nitrates, angiotensin-converting enzyme (ACE) inhibitors, calcium-channel blockers, beta blockers

2. Loop diuretics, ACE inhibitors, beta blockers

3. HMG-CoA reductase inhibitors (statins), fibrates, ezetimibe, niacin

Chapter 16

Checkpoint 16.1

1. The blood is made up of cells suspended in liquid plasma. Blood plasma contains water, protein (albumin and immunoglobulins), and various dissolved substances. Drug molecules are carried by the blood either as dissolved substances in the plasma or as substances bound to proteins such as albumin. Three types of cells are found in the blood: erythrocytes, leukocytes, and platelets or thrombocytes.

2. The Rh factor is a protein that may be present on red blood cells (RBCs). Those individuals who have the protein marker are considered Rh-positive; those individuals who are missing the marker are considered Rh-negative. If a mother is Rh-negative and her fetus is Rh-positive, the mother's blood will form antibodies against the baby's RBCs and jeopardize its survival. Therefore, mothers who are Rh-negative must receive an immunoglobulin injection (RhoGAM) that inhibits the production of these antibodies.

3. Thrombin, fibrinogen, and fibrin are necessary to form a functional blood clot.

Checkpoint 16.2

1. *Iron-deficiency anemia:* This disorder can happen relatively quickly, but replenishing these iron stores in the body can take several months.

Folate-deficiency anemia: This condition is commonly seen in patients who are alcoholics because they tend not to get proper nutrition.

Pernicious anemia: This disorder, caused by a deficiency in vitamin B_{12}, may take weeks or months to develop, but replenishing vitamin B_{12} takes only days or weeks.

Anemia of chronic disease: This condition is most often caused by chronic kidney disease.

Hemolytic anemia: This type of anemia is caused by the rapid destruction of red blood cells (RBCs) and can be triggered by infection, malignancy, or drug therapy.

Rapid-onset anemia: This condition results from rapid blood loss.

Chronic anemia: This disorder results from chronic blood loss—for example, from stomach ulcers.

Sickle-cell anemia: This type of anemia is a genetic disorder that causes malformation of RBCs.

2. Symptoms of anemia may include an accelerated heart rate, light-headedness, and breathlessness. Chronic anemia produces fatigue, weakness, headache, vertigo, light-headedness, sensitivity to cold, pallor, and loss of skin tone.

3. Iron, folic acid (folate), and vitamin B_{12} are used to treat anemia. The hematopoietic agents erythropoietin and darbepoetin can also be used to treat anemia.

Checkpoint 16.3

1. An ischemic stroke results from an obstruction of bloodflow, and a hemorrhagic stroke results from a rupture in a blood vessel that supplies an area of the brain.

2. Anticoagulation and antiplatelet therapies are used more often to prevent stroke rather than to break up a clot once it has already caused a stroke.

3. Anticoagulants can cause bruising, bleeding due to excessive anticoagulation, thrombocytopenia (low platelet count), fever, pain at the injection site, nausea, anemia, headache, back pain, hair loss, skin lesions, and purple/blue toe syndrome.

4. Factors VIIa, VIII, and IX as well as von Willebrand factor are used to treat hemophilia.

Chapter 17

Checkpoint 17.1

1. The upper respiratory tract includes the nasal passages; sinuses; pharynx, which is comprised of the nasopharynx, oropharynx, and laryngopharynx; and the larynx, where the epiglottis is located.

2. The lower respiratory tract includes the trachea (windpipe) and lungs, which are comprised of the bronchi, bronchioles, and alveoli.

3. The gas-exchange process occurs in the alveoli of the lungs.

Checkpoint 17.2

1. *First-generation antihistamines:* chlorpheniramine, clemastine, diphenhydramine

Second-generation antihistamines: cetirizine, desloratadine, fexofenadine, loratadine

2. *Sinus congestion:* phenylephrine and pseudoephedrine

Runny nose: antihistamines, decongestants, and cough remedies. Antihistamines and nasal corticosteroids are used to treat symptoms including runny nose, watery/itchy eyes, and sneezing, whether the symptoms are caused by allergies or infection (see Table 17.1 for commonly used antihistamines).

Cough: codeine phosphate, dextromethorphan, hydrocodone, guaifenesin

Checkpoint 17.3

1. Short-acting beta agonists, corticosteroids, leukotriene inhibitors, mast cell stabilizers, xanthine agents, and omalizumab

2. Common side effects of short-acting beta agonists include dizziness, nervousness, heartburn, nausea, and tremors. They can also have cardiac effects including increased blood pressure and tachycardia.

3. Asthma medications can be administered via a metered-dose inhaler (with a spacer attachment), nebulizer, or dry powder inhaler.

Checkpoint 17.4

1. Anticholinergics, long-acting beta agonists, and inhaled corticosteroids (in combination with other therapies) are used to treat chronic obstructive pulmonary disease (COPD).

2. *Anticholinergics:* aclidinium, ipratropium, ipratropium/albuterol, tiotropium, umeclidinium/vilanterol

Long-acting beta agonists: arformoterol, formoterol, indacaterol, salmeterol

Checkpoint 17.5

1. Empirical therapy is using treatment based on common knowledge of pathogens typically causing pneumonia. Empirical treatment helps guide initial drug therapy.

2. Bupropion, nicotine, and varenicline

Chapter 18

Checkpoint 18.1

1. Food starts in the mouth and is propelled into the stomach via the esophagus. Acid and enzyme secretions in the stomach digest large particles and proteins in ingested food. Food then travels to the small intestine where further digestion takes place. Food then moves to the large intestine or colon. Waste material exits the body via the rectum and anus via defecation.

2. The liver is a major site of drug metabolism in the body. After orally administered drugs are absorbed,

they pass through the liver. The liver metabolizes them before they reach their target in the body. This process is called the *first-pass effect*.

Checkpoint 18.2

1. Acute diarrhea can be caused by infections such as traveler's diarrhea and food poisoning, as well as certain drugs (see Table 18.1). Infectious causes of diarrhea include *Salmonella, Escherichia coli (E. coli), Giardia,* and *Norovirus.* Constipation is often caused by a diet low in fiber or fluid intake. Constipation can also be caused by certain foods or drugs (see Table 18.3).

2. Opiate derivatives are used to treat diarrhea. They work by inhibiting peristalsis and slowing the progression of food through the gastrointestinal (GI) tract. Bismuth subsalicylate is also used to treat diarrhea. This medication works via antibacterial, antisecretory, and anti-inflammatory mechanisms.

3. Bulk-forming laxatives are used to treat constipation. They work by drawing water and other electrolytes into the GI system. Increased volume in the GI tract triggers peristalsis and facilitates bowel movements. Stool softeners are used to treat constipation as well. These medications work by increasing water and electrolyte secretions in the GI tract, which makes stools softer and easier to pass. Another drug class used to treat constipation is stimulant laxatives. These drugs work by stimulating parasympathetic neurons that control bowel muscles, thereby enhancing peristalsis and GI motility. Finally, bowel preparation (osmotic) laxatives treat constipation by drawing water and electrolytes into the GI tract. They prepare the bowel for examination by completely cleaning it out.

Checkpoint 18.3

1. Peptic ulcers are most often caused by a bacterial parasite, *H. pylori.* Stress ulcers occur in critically ill patients who are bedridden. The exact mechanism by which they form is not well understood, but it is thought that serious illness, stress, and trauma lead to a decrease in the protective mucous layer of the stomach and an increase in acid secretion in the stomach.

2. Antacids, proton pump inhibitors, H2 blockers, sucralfate, misoprostol

Checkpoint 18.4

1. Anticholinergic antiemetics, general antiemetics, serotonin type 3 (5-HT3) receptor antagonists, dronabinol, neurokinin-1 receptor antagonists

2. Linaclotide, lubiprostone, polyethylene glycol 3350, alosetron, bile acid sequestrants, dicyclomine, hyoscyamine

3. Crohn disease is similar to ulcerative colitis in that it involves inflammation of the gastrointestinal (GI) tract and causes chronic diarrhea. It differs in that it is an autoimmune disease in which the immune system malfunctions and attacks tissue lining of the entire GI tract.

Chapter 19

Checkpoint 19.1

1.

Vitamin	DRIs for Men	DRIs for Women
A (as retinol activity equivalents)	900 mcg	700 mcg
D (as cholecalciferol)	15 mcg	15 mcg
E (as alpha-tocopherol)	15 mg	15 mg
K (as phytonadione)	120 mcg*	90 mcg*

Red type indicates that the value is an RDA; an asterisk indicates that the value is an AI.

2.

Vitamin	DRIs for Men	DRIs for Women
B₁ (thiamine)	1.2 mg	1.1 mg
B₂ (riboflavin)	1.3 mg	1.1 mg
B₃ (niacin)	16 mg	14 mg
B₅ (pantothenic acid)	5 mg*	5 mg*
B₆ (pyridoxine)	1.3 mg	1.3 mg
B₇ (biotin)	30 mcg*	30 mcg*
B₉ (folate or folic acid)	400 mcg	400 mcg
B₁₂ (cyanocobalamin)	2.4 mcg	2.4 mcg
C (ascorbic acid)	90 mg	75 mg

Red type indicates that the value is an RDA; an asterisk indicates that the value is an AI.

3. Vitamin K sources include green vegetables such as spinach, broccoli, and Brussels sprouts, and fats such as plant oils and margarine.

Checkpoint 19.2

1. Diarrhea, vomiting, metallic taste in the mouth, and cirrhosis

2. Iodine deficiency can lead to goiter, hypothyroidism, neuromuscular problems, deafness, decreased mental function, and bone softening/slowed growth.

Checkpoint 19.3

1. A BMI range from 19–25

2. IBW (kg) = 50 + (2.3 × height in inches over 5 feet)

3. IBW (kg) = 45.5 + (2.3 × height in inches over 5 feet)

Checkpoint 19.4

1. Lipase inhibitors, serotonin agonists, and sympathomimetics
2. Orlistat

Checkpoint 19.5

1. Anorexia, food allergies/intolerance, chronic infection or inflammatory conditions, cancer, endocrine disorders, pulmonary disease, cirrhosis of the liver, renal failure, nausea/vomiting/diarrhea, trauma, burns, sepsis, inflammatory bowel disease, Crohn disease, short-bowel syndrome, inadequate parenteral or enteral nutrition, psychiatric or psychological conditions

2. Enteral nutrition uses the gastrointestinal (GI) tract, whereas parenteral nutrition avoids the GI tract. Enteral nutrition should never be administered through an intravenous (IV) line, whereas parenteral nutrition is always administered through an IV line. Finally, parenteral nutrition carries a risk of precipitation, whereas enteral nutrition does not.

Chapter 20

Checkpoint 20.1

1. The glands and structures of the endocrine system include the pancreas, pituitary, hypothalamus, thyroid, parathyroid, and adrenal glands.

2. *Pancreas:* insulin and glucagon

   Pituitary: antidiuretic hormone (ADH), adrenocorticotropic hormone (ACTH), growth hormone (GH), gonadotropic hormones, thyroid-stimulating hormone (TSH), oxytocin (OT), prolactin (PRL), melanocyte-stimulating hormone (MSH)

   Thyroid: tri-iodothyronine (T3) and thyroxine (T4)

   Parathyroid: parathyroid hormone

   Adrenal glands: corticosteroids

   Hypothalamus: corticotropin-releasing factor

Checkpoint 20.2

1. Metformin, insulin secretagogues (sulfonylureas, meglitinides), TZDs, incretins (GLP-1 agonists, DPP-4 inhibitors), sodium glucose transporter-2 inhibitors
2. Metformin, glimepiride, glipizide, glyburide, nateglinide, repaglinide, pioglitazone, rosiglitazone, exenatide, liraglutide, pramlintide, saxagliptin, sitagliptin, canagliflozin, dapagliflozin
3. Insulin secretagogues (sulfonylureas, meglitinides)

Checkpoint 20.3

1. Insulin is released into the bloodstream from the pancreas or it is injected. Insulin triggers receptors on the surface of cells in the body to open channels that allow glucose to enter the cell where it can be used for energy. Glucose in the blood decreases.

2. *Aspart:* 1 to 2 hours

   Glulisine: 1 hour

   Lispro: 1 to 2 hours

   Regular: 4 hours

   NPH: 6 to 8 hours

   Detemir: 24 to 36 hours

   Glargine: 24 to 36 hours

3. Symptoms of hypoglycemia include shakiness, dizziness, sweating, headache, irritability, confusion, vision changes, and hunger. Patients with hypoglycemia should ingest 15–30 g of carbohydrate in the form of simple sugar. Fruit juice, nondiet soda, hard candy, and glucose tablets are good sources of such carbohydrates.

Checkpoint 20.4

1. Symptoms of hypothyroidism include constipation; bradycardia; depression; fatigue; dry skin, nails, and scalp; tremors; reduced mental acuity; memory loss; intolerance to cold; lower voice pitch; and weight gain.
2. Synthroid, Tirosint, Cytomel, Triostat, Thyrolar, Armour Thyroid
3. Addison's disease is a deficiency of glucocorticosteroid production from the adrenal glands. Cushing's syndrome is the overproduction of glucocorticoid hormones often caused by an adrenal gland tumor.

Chapter 21

Checkpoint 21.1

1. Testis, epididymis, ductus deferens (also called vas deferens), seminal vesicle, prostate gland, urethra, penis
2. Ovary, fallopian tube, uterus, cervix, vagina
3. *Estrogen:* Primary effects include breast enlargement, endometrial growth, production of cervical mucus, vaginal mucosa maintenance, bone health, and cessation of growth in height for women. Other effects include sodium retention, function of the skin's blood vessels, cholesterol levels, blood coagulation, calcium utilization, and carbohydrate metabolism.

   Progesterone: Progesterone suppresses luteinizing hormone (LH) production, thickens cervical mucus, and alters the endometrial lining to support implantation. It has effects on insulin levels, glucose tolerance, fat deposition, body temperature, and maintenance of pregnancy.

Follicle-stimulating hormone (FSH): Stimulates follicle development in the ovaries to produce mature ovum and stimulates ovaries to produce estrogen.

Luteinizing hormone (LH): Causes the most mature follicle (in the ovary) to burst and release an ovum.

Checkpoint 21.2

1. Hypogonadism, sometimes called low testosterone, is the underproduction of testosterone in men. Insufficient testosterone production can contribute to infertility in men. Symptoms include fatigue, low sexual desire, weakness, erectile dysfunction, poor sleep, depression, irritability, and memory loss. Many men attribute these symptoms to getting older. Men with hypogonadism are given exogenous testosterone to supplement the hormone that is missing. Dosing is adjusted individually and guided by laboratory tests and relief of symptoms.

2. Avanafil (Stendra), sildenafil (Viagra), tadalafil (Cialis), vardenafil (Levitra), yohimbine (Aphrodyne, Yocon)

3. Smoking cessation, reduced alcohol consumption, and avoidance of street drugs can help enhance male fertility. Men with low sperm counts should wear loose-fitting underclothes (i.e., boxer shorts) to decrease the internal temperature in the testes. Hot tubs, saunas, and other activities that can raise body temperature should be avoided when trying to conceive if male fertility is a concern.

Checkpoint 21.3

1. In addition to clomiphene, these gonadotropin therapy agents are often used to treat infertility in women: FSH, hCG and r-hCG, and progestins.

2. Menopause is the cessation of sex hormone production in women. It is a permanent cessation of menstruation, defined by the absence of menses for at least 12 months. This life change occurs during the fifth or sixth decade of a woman's life. The lack of estrogen causes vasomotor spasms (hot flashes), irregular menstrual bleeding, vaginal dryness and atrophy (tissue shrinkage), weight gain, insomnia, fatigue, loss of libido, depression, mood swings, and memory impairment. To mitigate the impact of these effects, many women take estrogen supplements, or hormone replacement therapy.

3. A home pregnancy test is used when a woman suspects she might be pregnant, such as when she misses a menstrual cycle. A home ovulation test is used when a woman wants to become pregnant. A home ovulation kit measures hormonal fluctuation, which predicts when ovulation is about to occur. This test signals the time of highest possibility for fertilization and can help couples attempting to conceive to know when intercourse is most likely to result in pregnancy.

Checkpoint 21.4

1. Male condom, female condom, diaphragm, cervical cap

2. The vaginal ring is a combination birth control that contains synthetic estrogen and progesterone. The ring is inserted into the vagina where the hormones are absorbed through the vaginal mucosa. This device is left in place for three weeks and then removed for a week while menstruation occurs.

3. Oral contraceptives manipulate hormones to prevent ovulation and change the texture of cervical mucus. Oral contraceptives that contain synthetic estrogens work by suppressing production of luteinizing hormone (LH), the hormone that triggers ovulation. Oral contraceptives that contain progesterones suppress LH production and thicken cervical mucus, making travel difficult for sperm. Oral contraceptives are taken daily at the same time to maintain a steady and elevated hormone level.

Checkpoint 21.5

1. Gender reassignment begins with counseling to ensure proper diagnosis and to discuss the risks and benefits of gender reassignment therapy. Hormonal therapy, which suppresses characteristics of the native sex and enhances characteristics of the desired gender, is often the next step. This therapy allows the patient to transition in appearance to the new gender and provides time for the patient to experience life as a member of the opposite sex. The last step is to undergo surgical intervention to remove sexual organs of the natal sex and to create anatomic features of the new gender.

2. *Bacterial sexually transmitted infections (STIs):* chlamydia, gonorrhea, syphilis, vaginosis

   Viral STIs: genital herpes, human papillomavirus (HPV), human immunodeficiency virus (HIV)/acquired immunodeficiency syndrome (AIDS)

3. *Genital herpes:* acyclovir, famciclovir, valacyclovir

   Chlamydia: doxycycline, azithromycin, erythromycin

   Vaginosis (bacterial): metronidazole, clindamycin

   Vaginosis (yeast): Over-the-counter (OTC) or prescription vaginal candidiasis products

Chapter 22

Checkpoint 22.1

1. The kidneys clear the blood of metabolic by-products and waste substances; balance fluids and electrolytes, such as sodium, potassium, and calcium, in the body; regulate the blood pH and blood pressure; and produce hormones that regulate systemic and kidney hemodynamics (renin, angiotensin II, and prostaglandins), red blood cell production (erythropoietin), and mineral metabolism.

2. Aldosterone and antidiuretic hormone

Checkpoint 22.2

1. Examples of nephrotoxic or potentially nephrotoxic drugs include nonsteroidal anti-inflammatory drugs (NSAIDs), amphotericin B, contrast media (dye for imaging procedures), aminoglycosides, and cisplatin and carboplatin.
2. Dry mouth, constipation, blurred vision, and urine retention are all potential side effects of antimuscarinic drugs.

Checkpoint 22.3

1. Medications commonly used to treat chronic kidney disease (CKD) are angiotensin-converting enzyme (ACE) inhibitors, angiotensin receptor blockers (ARBs), and diuretics.
2. Thiazide diuretics, potassium-sparing diuretics, loop diuretics, and carbonic anhydrase inhibitors
3. Hemodialysis is accomplished by diverting bloodflow through a machine that mechanically filters the blood and returns the blood to the body. Peritoneal dialysis is accomplished by putting dialysate into the abdominal cavity and leaving it there for a certain period—typically, a few days.

Chapter 23

Checkpoint 23.1

1. Bone marrow is an important lymphoid tissue. It is the primary source of erythrocytes, leukocytes, and thrombocytes.
2. Proper hand washing and hand hygiene minimize touch contamination and reduce the transmission of infectious agents. These processes are important for infection control and prevention.

Checkpoint 23.2

1. The main classes of antibiotics include penicillins, cephalosporins, carbapenems and monobactams, vancomycin, aminoglycosides, tetracyclines, macrolides, fluoroquinolones, sulfonamides, nitrofurantoin, and metronidazole.
2. Patients taking cephalosporins or metronidazole should avoid alcohol products or beverages.

Checkpoint 23.3

1. NRTIs, NtRTIs, NNRTIs, PIs, fusion inhibitors, CCR5 inhibitors, and integrase inhibitors are the drug classes used to treat human immunodeficiency virus (HIV).
2. PIs that are used to treat HIV have the side effect of fat redistribution.

Checkpoint 23.4

1. The antifungals clotrimazole, nystatin, and posaconazole are used to treat oral thrush.
2. Azoles and echinocandins are associated with the suffixes *–azole* and *–fungin*, respectively.

Chapter 24

Checkpoint 24.1

1. Female patients should receive three doses of the human papillomavirus (HPV) vaccine.
2. Common side effects of vaccines include fever, headache, upset stomach, local injection-site irritation, mild skin rash, and irritability.

Checkpoint 24.2

1. The interferons available for treating multiple sclerosis (MS) include interferon beta-1a and interferon beta-1b.
2. The common side effects of corticosteroids include headache, dizziness, insomnia, and hunger.

Chapter 25

Checkpoint 25.1

1. Acetaminophen, aspirin, nonsteroidal anti-inflammatory drugs (NSAIDs), and COX-2 inhibitors
2. When taken in doses over 4 g a day or used chronically at daily maximum dose levels, acetaminophen can cause liver toxicity.

Checkpoint 25.2

1. *Natural opiates:* morphine, codeine
   Semisynthetic opiates: hydrocodone, hydromorphone, oxycodone
   Synthetic opiates: fentanyl, methadone, tramadol
2. Common side effects of opioids include sedation, dizziness, upset stomach, fatigue, headache, and constipation.

Checkpoint 25.3

1. Preventing migraines requires that the patient avoid known triggers including certain foods, stress, sleep deprivation, medications, and environmental irritants.
2. For best results, triptans should be used at the first sign that a headache is starting.

Checkpoint 25.4

1. A general anesthetic affects the entire body and causes a loss of consciousness. Skeletal muscle relaxes, breathing slows, respiratory mucous production increases, and urination stops. Indications for general anesthesia include surgery and certain diagnostic procedures. A local anesthetic depresses the nerve activity

in a defined area of the body. This action results in loss of sensation in that area. Indications for local anesthesia include dental work and sutures.

2. Naloxone (Evzio)

Chapter 26

Checkpoint 26.1

1. Approximately two-thirds of total body water is housed in the intracellular fluid, and the other one-third of water is found in extracellular fluid. Three-quarters of the extracellular fluid resides in the interstitial spaces between the cells in tissues, and the remaining quarter is part of the intravascular space.

2. Potassium is the most abundant cation found in the intracellular fluid. Sodium is the most abundant cation in the extracellular fluid.

Checkpoint 26.2

1. Isotonic solution

2. Hyperphosphatemia

Checkpoint 26.3

1. Acidosis occurs when plasma contains excess hydrogen ions, which causes the pH to drop below the normal range. Alkalosis occurs when there is a loss of hydrogen ions, which causes the pH to increase above the normal range.

2. When infused intravenously, sodium bicarbonate may cause extravasation. Ammonium chloride may cause venous irritation and ammonium toxicity. Making sure concentrations and infusion rates are low helps prevent these unwanted side effects.

Chapter 27

Checkpoint 27.1

1. The "cell-kill hypothesis" presumes that each cycle of chemotherapy kills a certain percentage of cancer cells. If a tumor has 10 billion cells and a chemotherapy cycle kills 95% of them, then 0.5 billion cells remain. The second cycle kills 95% more, leaving 25 million cells, and the third cycle would leave 1.25 million cells. Using this theory, tumor cell count will never reach zero from treatment alone, but once the number of cancer cells is low enough, normal host defense mechanisms take over to eradicate the remaining cells.

2. Surgery, radiation therapy, immunotherapy, and chemotherapy

3. Primary chemotherapy is typically administered with curative intent, whereas palliative chemotherapy is administered to provide symptom relief. Adjuvant

chemotherapy refers to the treatment of residual cancer cells after removal or reduction of the tumor by surgery.

Checkpoint 27.2

1. Targeted anticancer therapies focus on a specific abnormality or entity that is associated with a certain type of cancer. Traditional chemotherapy targets cells that exhibit characteristics of cancer cells, or cells with a high rate of proliferation. Targeted anticancer therapies tend to have less of an effect on normal cells than traditional chemotherapy agents do, thus they are frequently associated with fewer side effects.

2. It is important that patients who are receiving drug therapy for cancer treatment do not take medications that might (1) interact with their treatment, (2) interfere with the treatment's effects, or (3) increase the treatment's side effects.

Checkpoint 27.3

1. Prescribing errors, transcription errors, preparation errors, and administration errors

2. Healthcare personnel should store look-alike, sound-alike drugs apart from each other; affix look-alike, sound-alike labels to certain medication containers; use color-coded and/or labeled storage bins; follow manufacturers' warnings on hazardous drug products; and observe tall-man lettering on medication labels.

Chapter 28

Checkpoint 28.1

1. The unique challenges of providing health care to pediatric patients include the wide-ranging age-group; the implementation of developmentally-based communication among the patient, his or her parent or caregiver, and the healthcare practitioner; and the increased vulnerability of the pediatric patient to medication errors.

2. Kidney function is low at birth, but it increases rapidly and generally reaches adult levels by one year of age. When kidney function is low, the clearance of drugs from the body is slow. As a result, young infants may experience toxic levels of drugs that are primarily eliminated via the kidneys.

3. Infants have a higher body water content than adults. Consequently, drugs that are highly water-soluble distribute well, which may result in a higher risk of drug toxicity for infants.

Checkpoint 28.2

1. Acetaminophen is preferred to treat a fever in children because it has fewer side effects.

2. After inhalation of a corticosteroid drug, a patient should rinse his or her mouth thoroughly to prevent thrush.

3. Albuterol, budesonide nebules, fluticasone metered-dose inhaler, montelukast, methylprednisolone, prednisolone, prednisone

Checkpoint 28.3

1. Amoxicillin

2. A sudden fever, a severe headache, and a stiff neck

Chapter 29

Checkpoint 29.1

1. Muscle fibers in the tissues of the heart's chambers atrophy or degenerate; the arteries harden; and systolic blood pressure increases. The left ventricle of the heart loses some flexibility; the number of pacemaker cells in the heart's sinoatrial (SA) node decreases; and the sensitivity of the baroreceptors is reduced.

2. Taste buds atrophy; the ability to smell noxious odors is hampered; the sense of touch decreases; visual acuity is reduced (e.g., impaired night vision and affected color perception); and hearing acuity decreases.

Checkpoint 29.2

1. In older adults, the first-pass effect is altered because the liver does not block as much drug from entering the circulation. Consequently, certain drugs have a higher bioavailability, or the percentage of drug that reaches the bloodstream.

2. The blood-brain barrier becomes more porous.

Checkpoint 29.3

1. The reduction or weakening of bone mass increases the risk for bone fracture.

2. Both glaucoma and cataracts are common vision problems in old age that can lead to blindness. Glaucoma is a type of vision loss caused by optic nerve damage due to increased intraocular pressure. This condition is treated with eyedrops. A cataract is an area of opacity in the lens of the eye that can cause cloudy or fuzzy vision. This condition is treated with surgery.

3. An older patient with congestive heart failure (CHF) may complain of symptoms of hypoxia (such as light-headedness), tiredness/sleepiness, restlessness, and confusion.

Checkpoint 29.4

1. Sedative-hypnotics, antidepressants, and antipsychotics

2. Diuretics and beta blockers

3. Any drug listed in Table 29.5 is an example of an anticholinergic drug. Anticholinergic adverse effects include confusion, constipation, and dry mouth, and clearance of these drugs is reduced with age.

Kolb's Learning Styles Inventory

HayGroup®

Excerpts from the
Kolb Learning Style Inventory Workbook
Version 3.1

How do we learn?

We all learn in different ways. The Kolb Learning Style Inventory (LSI) is designed to help you understand how you learn best in educational settings and everyday life.

Learning can be described as a cycle made up of four basic phases. The LSI takes you through those four phases to give you a better understanding of how you learn. Knowing more about your learning style can help you understand:

- how to maximize your learning from educational programs
- how you solve problems
- how you work in teams
- how to manage disagreement and conflict
- how you make career choices
- how to improve personal and professional relationships

What does the LSI Workbook cover?

Your current situation

The LSI will be more helpful to you if you think first about a real situation. Take a few moments to reflect on a recent time when you learned something new.

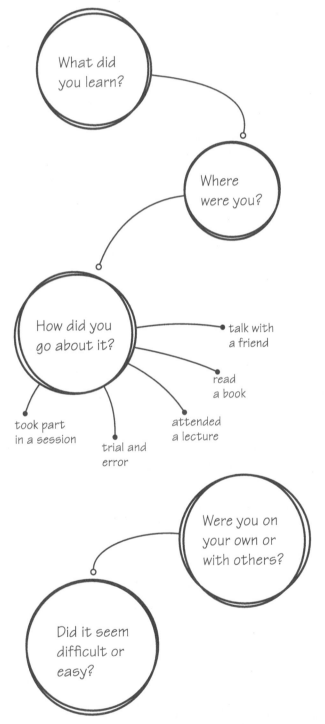

Completing the LSI

- Now find the two-part questionnaire in this workbook. It asks you to complete 12 sentences that describe learning. Each sentence has four endings. To respond to these sentences, consider the recent learning situation you've just reflected on.

- Rank the endings for each sentence according to how well you think each ending describes the way you learned. Write 4 next to the sentence ending that describes how you learned best, and so on down to 1 for the sentence ending that seems least like the way you learned. Be sure to rank all the endings for each sentence. Do not give two endings the same number.

Some people find it easiest to decide first which phrase best describes them (4 – careful) and then to decide which phrase is least like them (1 – fast). Then they give a 3 to that word in the remaining pair that is more like them (3 – logical) and a 2 to the word that is left over (2 – happy).

> **Step 1:** Complete Sheet 1 of the questionnaire
>
> **Step 2:** Go to Sheet 2 to calculate your scores
>
> **Step 3:** Add up your scores for each shape
>
> **Step 4:** Enter your scores for each shape at the top right of Sheet 2

Each shape should have a score in the range of 12 to 48. Your four shape scores should add up to a total of 120.

Sheet 1

LEARNING-STYLE INVENTORY

The Learning-Style Inventory describes the way you learn and how you deal with ideas and day-to-day situations in your life. Below are 12 sentences with a choice of endings. Rank the endings for each sentence according to how well you think each one fits with how you would go about learning something. Try to recall some recent situations where you had to learn something new, perhaps in your job or at school. Then, using the spaces provided, rank a "4" for the sentence ending that describes how you learn *best*, down to a "1" for the sentence ending that seems least like the way you learn. Be sure to rank all the endings for each sentence unit. Please do not make ties.

Example of completed sentence set:

1. When I learn:　　2 I am happy.　　1 I am fast.　　3 I am logical.　　4 I am careful.

Remember:　　**4** = *most* like you　　**3** = *second most* like you　　**2** = *third most* like you　　**1** = *least* like you

	A	B	C	D
1. When I learn:	___ I like to deal with my feelings.	___ I like to think about ideas.	___ I like to be doing things.	___ I like to watch and listen.
2. I learn best when:	___ I listen and watch carefully.	___ I rely on logical thinking.	___ I trust my hunches and feelings.	___ I work hard to get things done.
3. When I am learning:	___ I tend to reason things out.	___ I am responsible about things.	___ I am quiet and reserved.	___ I have strong feelings and reactions.
4. I learn by:	___ feeling.	___ doing.	___ watching.	___ thinking.
5. When I learn:	___ I am open to new experiences.	___ I look at all sides of issues.	___ I like to analyze things, break them down into their parts.	___ I like to try things out.
6. When I am learning:	___ I am an observing person.	___ I am an active person.	___ I am an intuitive person.	___ I am a logical person.
7. I learn best from:	___ observation.	___ personal relationships.	___ rational theories.	___ a chance to try out and practice.
8. When I learn:	___ I like to see results from my work.	___ I like ideas and theories.	___ I take my time before acting.	___ I feel personally involved in things.
9. I learn best when:	___ I rely on my observations.	___ I rely on my feelings.	___ I can try things out for myself.	___ I rely on my ideas.
10. When I am learning:	___ I am a reserved person.	___ I am an accepting person.	___ I am a responsible person.	___ I am a rational person.
11. When I learn:	___ I get involved.	___ I like to observe.	___ I evaluate things.	___ I like to be active.
12. I learn best when:	___ I analyze ideas.	___ I am receptive and open-minded.	___ I am careful.	___ I am practical.

Sheet 2

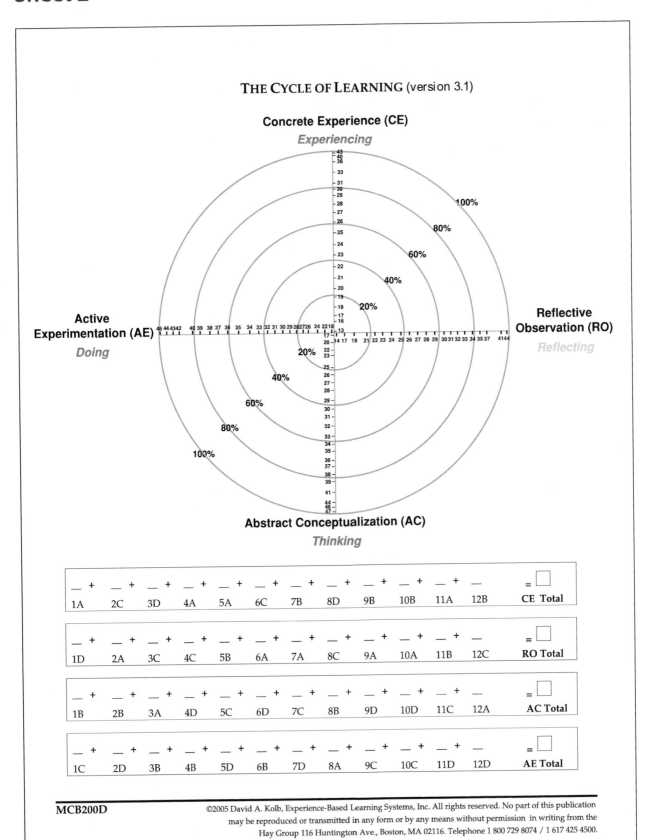

THE CYCLE OF LEARNING (version 3.1)

Concrete Experience (CE)

Experiencing

Active Experimentation (AE)

Doing

Reflective Observation (RO)

Reflecting

Abstract Conceptualization (AC)

Thinking

__ +	__ +	__ +	__ +	__ +	__ +	__ +	__ +	__ +	__ +	__ +	__	= ☐
1A	2C	3D	4A	5A	6C	7B	8D	9B	10B	11A	12B	CE Total

__ +	__ +	__ +	__ +	__ +	__ +	__ +	__ +	__ +	__ +	__ +	__	= ☐
1D	2A	3C	4C	5B	6A	7A	8C	9A	10A	11B	12C	RO Total

__ +	__ +	__ +	__ +	__ +	__ +	__ +	__ +	__ +	__ +	__ +	__	= ☐
1B	2B	3A	4D	5C	6D	7C	8B	9D	10D	11C	12A	AC Total

__ +	__ +	__ +	__ +	__ +	__ +	__ +	__ +	__ +	__ +	__ +	__	= ☐
1C	2D	3B	4B	5D	6B	7D	8A	9C	10C	11D	12D	AE Total

Recording your scores on the Learning Cycle

On the diagram below, mark a dot on the corresponding line to indicate your CE, RO, AC, and AE scores. Then connect the dots to form a kite-shaped pattern on the diagram.

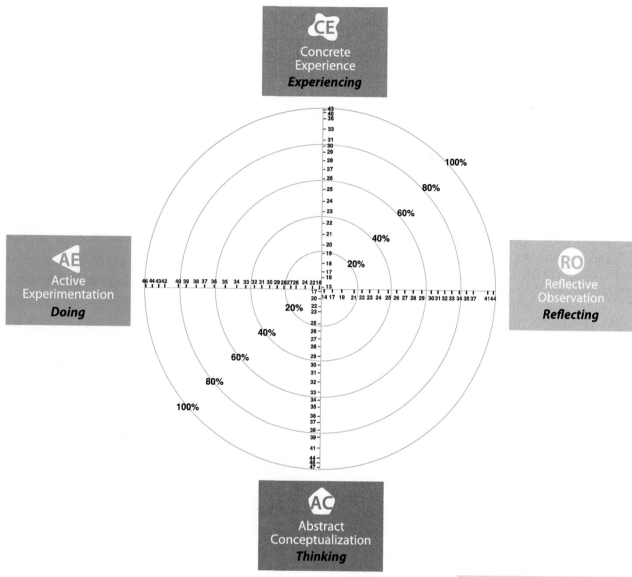

Example:

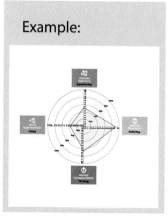

What do my scores mean?

Your scores indicate how much you rely on each of the four different learning modes: Concrete Experience, Reflective Observation, Abstract Conceptualization, and Active Experimentation. These learning modes make up a four-phase learning cycle. Different learners start at different places in this cycle. Effective learning eventually involves all four phases. You can see by the placement of your dots which of the four learning phases you tend to prefer in a learning situation. The closer your dots are to the 100% ring on the circle, the more you tend to use that way of learning.

What do the percentages mean?

Another way to understand the placement of your dots is to compare them with the scores of others. The percentile labels on the concentric circles represent the norms on the four basic scales (CE, RO, AC, AE) for 6,977 men and women ranging in age from 17–75.

For example, on the vertical line in the diagram (CE): if you were to score 26, then you would have scored higher on CE than 60% of the people in the normative sample. You can compare your scores for each of the other learning modes with the sample group.

Who is included in this sample group?

This sample group includes college students and working adults in a wide variety of fields. It is made up of users living in 64 countries, with the largest representations from US, Canada, UK, India, Germany, Brazil, Singapore, France, and Japan. A wide range of occupations and educational backgrounds is represented. For complete information about the normative comparison group and other validity research, consult the LSI Technical Specifications available at www.learningfromexperience.com or www.haygroup.com/TL

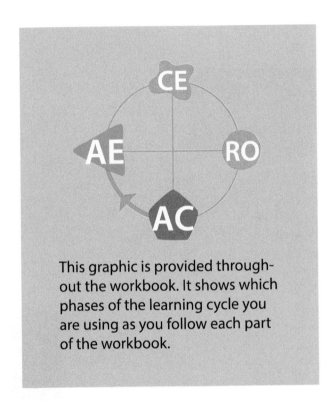

This graphic is provided throughout the workbook. It shows which phases of the learning cycle you are using as you follow each part of the workbook.

Understanding the Learning Cycle

The model below describes the four phases of the learning cycle.

There are two ways you can take in experience – by Concrete Experience or Abstract Conceptualization. There are also two ways you deal with experience – by Reflective Observation or Active Experimentation. When you use both the concrete and abstract modes to take in your experience, and when you both reflect and act on that experience, you expand your potential to learn.

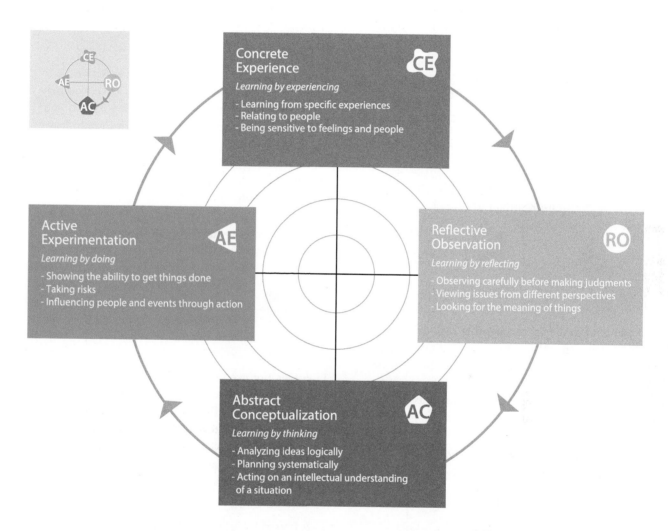

Concrete Experience
Learning by experiencing
- Learning from specific experiences
- Relating to people
- Being sensitive to feelings and people

Active Experimentation
Learning by doing
- Showing the ability to get things done
- Taking risks
- Influencing people and events through action

Reflective Observation
Learning by reflecting
- Observing carefully before making judgments
- Viewing issues from different perspectives
- Looking for the meaning of things

Abstract Conceptualization
Learning by thinking
- Analyzing ideas logically
- Planning systematically
- Acting on an intellectual understanding of a situation

You may begin a learning process in any of the four phases of the learning cycle. Ideally, using a well-rounded learning process, you would cycle through all four phases. However, you may find that you sometimes skip a phase in the cycle or focus primarily on just one. Think about the phases you tend to skip and those you tend to concentrate on.

Identifying your preferred learning style

Now that you've plotted your scores on the graph (page 3), you can see that the connected dots form the general shape of a kite. Because each person's learning style is unique, everyone's kite shape will be a little different. The learning preferences indicated by the shape of your kite tell you about your own particular learning style and how much you rely on that style.

For example, if you have both Concrete Experience and Reflective Observation learning preferences, you will tend to have a Diverging style. Your preference may be to consider a situation from differing perspectives. You tend to diverge from conventional solutions, coming up with alternative possibilities.

If you have the **Diverging** style, your kite shape might look similar to one of these:

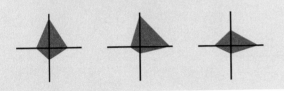

If you tend to use approaches that include Reflective Observation and Abstract Conceptualization, you probably prefer the Assimilating style. You may be interested in absorbing the learning experience into a larger framework of ideas. You tend to assimilate information into theories or models.

If you have the **Assimilating** style, your kite shape might look similar to one of these:

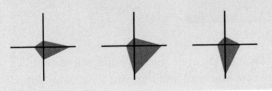

If you tend to approach the learning process by focusing on Abstract Conceptualization and Active Experimentation, you probably prefer the Converging style. You may enjoy gathering information to solve problems. You tend to converge on the correct solution.

If you have the **Converging** style, your kite shape might look similar to one of these:

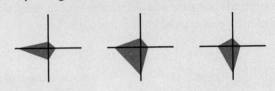

If your primary learning modes involve Active Experimentation and Concrete Experience, you may find yourself using the Accommodating style. If you prefer Accommodating, you may want to put ideas that you have practiced into action, finding still more uses for whatever has been learned. You tend to accommodate, or adapt to, changing circumstances and information.

If you have the **Accommodating** style, your kite shape might look similar to one of these:

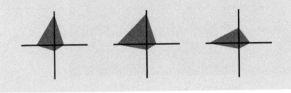

However, not everyone falls into one of the four dominant styles. You may have a profile that balances along two or more dimensions of the learning cycle. Current research suggests that some people learn through one or more of the 'balancing' styles. A balancing style may indicate a person who is comfortable with a variety of learning modes.

A few samples of a balancing style kite are shown below:

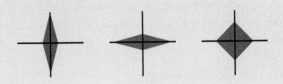

Scoring your preferred learning style

Understanding your preferred learning style, and the strengths and weaknesses inherent in that style, is a major step toward increasing your learning power and getting the most from your learning experiences.

To determine your learning style, take your scores for the four learning phases, AC, CE, AE, and RO (listed on the second sheet of the questionnaire) and subtract as follows to get your two combination scores:

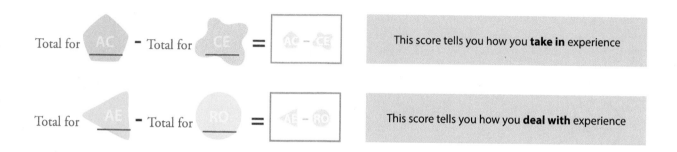

Total for AC — Total for CE = AC – CE | This score tells you how you **take in** experience

Total for AE — Total for RO = AE – RO | This score tells you how you **deal with** experience

Now mark your AC-CE score on the vertical dimension of the Learning Style Type Grid on page 8. Mark your AE-RO score on the horizontal dimension. Then place a dot marking the intersection of the two scores on the grid.

Example: If your AC - CE score is -2 and your AE - RO score is +15, your style falls into the Accommodating quadrant.

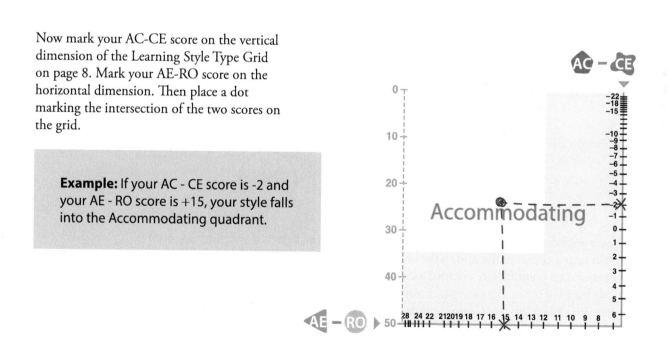

Your Learning Style grid

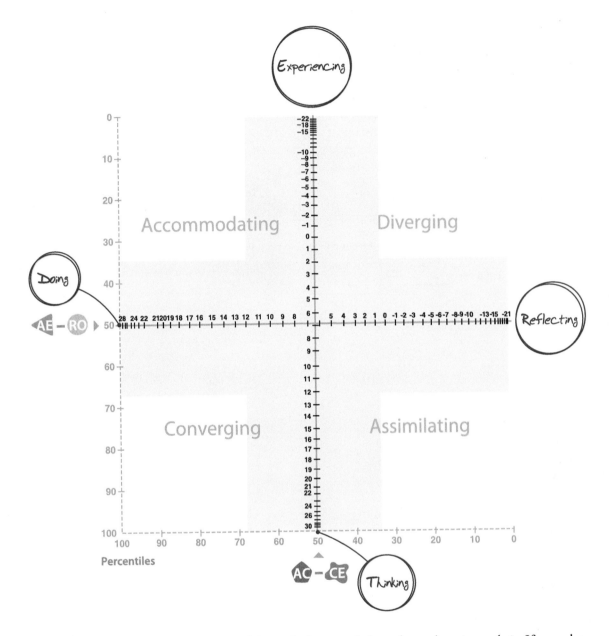

The closer your data point is to the center of the grid, the more balanced your learning style is. If your data point falls near a corner of the grid in the unshaded area, you tend to rely heavily on that particular learning style. If your data point falls in a shaded area then your style is characterized by a combination of the two adjoining learning styles. For example, if your data point falls in the shaded area between the Accommodating and Diverging quadrants your learning style is characterized by a strong orientation to Concrete Experience (CE) with an equal emphasis on Active Experimentation (AE) and Reflective Observation (RO), and with little emphasis on Abstract Conceptualization (AC). If your data point falls in the middle of the shaded area then you balance experiencing, thinking, reflection and action.

What each learning style means

The Diverging style

Combines the Concrete Experience and Reflective Observation phases

People with this learning style are best at viewing concrete situations from many different points of view. Their approach to situations is to observe rather than take action. If this is your style, you may enjoy situations that call for generating a wide range of ideas, such as brainstorming sessions. You probably have broad cultural interests and like to gather information. In formal learning situations you may prefer working in groups to gather information, listening with an open mind and receiving personalized feedback.

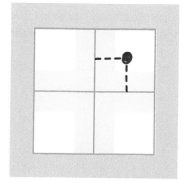

The Assimilating style

Combines the Reflective Observation and Abstract Conceptualization phases

People with this learning style are best at understanding a wide range of information and putting it into concise, logical form. If this is your learning style, you probably are less focused on people and more interested in abstract ideas and concepts. Generally, people with this learning style find it more important that a theory have logical soundness than practical value. In formal learning situations you may prefer lectures, readings, exploring analytical models and having time to think things through on your own.

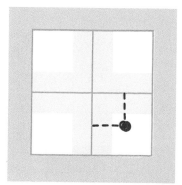

The Converging style

Combines the Abstract Conceptualization and Active Experimentation phases

People with this learning style are best at finding practical uses for ideas and theories. If this is your preferred learning style, you have the ability to solve problems and make decisions based on finding solutions to questions or problems. You would rather deal with technical tasks and problems than with social and interpersonal issues. In formal learning situations you may prefer experimenting with new ideas, simulations, laboratory assignments and practical applications.

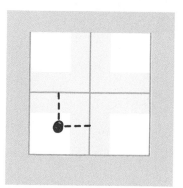

The Accommodating style

Combines the Active Experimentation and Concrete Experience phases

People with this learning style have the ability to learn primarily from 'hands-on' experience. If this is your style, you probably enjoy carrying out plans and involving yourself in new and challenging experiences. Your tendency may be to act on intuition rather than on logical analysis. In solving problems, you may rely more heavily on people for information than on your own technical analysis. In formal learning situations you may prefer to work with others to get assignments done, to set goals, to do field work and to test out different approaches to completing a project.

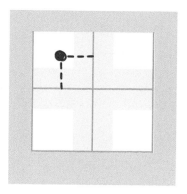

Note: The names of the learning style types are adopted from several established theories of thinking and creativity. Assimilating and Accommodating originate in Jean Piaget's definition of intelligence as the balance between the process of adapting concepts to fit the external world (Accommodating) and the process of fitting observations of the world into existing concepts (Assimilating). Converging and Diverging are the two essential creative processes identified in J. P. Guilford's structure-of-intellect model and other theories of creativity.

The basic strengths of each learning style

The chart below identifies the strengths of each learning style.

Draw your own kite shape on this chart to help you see where your relative learning strengths are. You can also see those learning strengths that fall outside of your kite shape.

Are there areas not emphasized by your kite shape that you would like to develop?

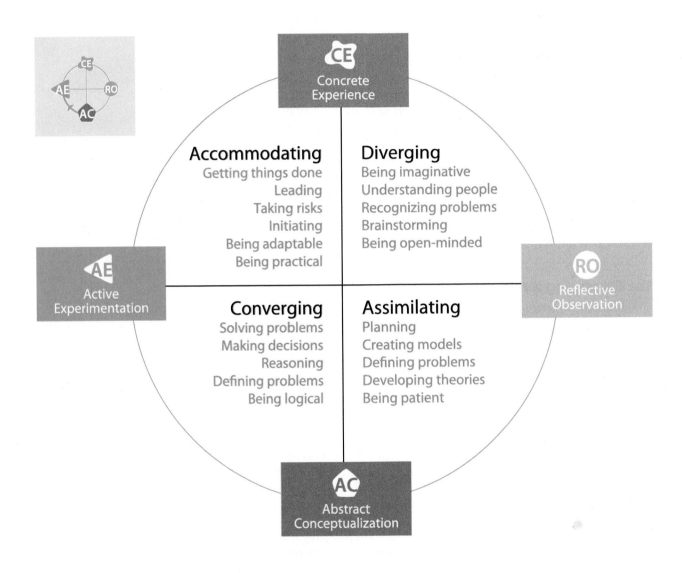

Strengthening and developing each learning style

When you completed the questionnaire you thought about a real situation in which you learned something new. But remember, you are learning lots of different things in different situations; at home, at work, in your hobbies, in school, college or university, on training courses or with friends and colleagues. Different situations place different demands on us.

If you rely too heavily on one learning style, you run the risk of missing out on important ideas and experiences. So it's also helpful to consider how you use other learning styles.

For example, at work you may be a wonderful decision maker, but perhaps you see a need to strengthen your 'people skills'. At home you might be the one who always gets things done, but sometimes your actions need more planning, or perhaps you need more imagination in your day-to-day work.

Tips for strengthening your use of the Diverging style:

- tune in to people's feelings
- be sensitive to values
- listen with an open mind
- gather information
- imagine the implications of ambiguous situations

Tips for strengthening your use of the Assimilating style:

- organize information
- test theories and ideas with others
- build conceptual models
- design experiments
- analyze data

Tips for strengthening your use of the Converging style:

- create new ways of thinking and doing
- experiment with new ideas
- choose the best solution
- set goals
- make decisions

Tips for strengthening your use of the Accommodating style:

- commit yourself to objectives
- seek new opportunities
- influence and lead others
- become personally involved
- deal with people

General tips for developing your learning style

Whatever learning style you choose to develop, the following tips will help you:

Develop relationships with people whose learning styles are different from your own.

You may feel drawn to people who have a similar approach to learning. But you will experience the learning cycle more completely with those whose learning style is different from your own. It is essential to value different learning styles – problems are solved more effectively by working with others.

This is the easiest way to develop your learning styles.

Try to learn in ways that are the opposite of your current preferences.

Try to become a more flexible learner by consciously choosing to use the learning style opposite to your own preference. For example, if you have an Assimilating style, focus on using skills associated with the Accommodating style (taking risks, getting things done, being adaptable).

This approach may seem awkward to you at first – it is the most challenging approach to take, but it can also be the most rewarding. In the long run your increased flexibility will allow you to cope with challenges of all kinds.

Improve the fit between your learning style and the demands you face.

Concentrate on tasks that fit your learning strengths, and rely on other people where you have weaknesses. For example, if your preferred learning style is Diverging, spend your time gathering information and thinking of all the options. Get someone with the Converging style to choose the best solution.

This strategy can help you perform at your best and achieve greatest satisfaction.

Remember:

- develop a long term plan – look for improvements over months, not right away
- look for safe ways to practice new skills
- reward yourself – becoming a flexible learner is hard work!

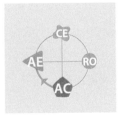

Image Credits

613 © Pfizer Inc. Used with permission; 614 © JPC-PROD/ Shutterstock.com; 617 © www.royaltystockphoto.com/Shutterstock.com; 623 © Paradigm Publishing, Inc.; 624 © Paradigm Publishing, Inc.; 625 © Paradigm Publishing, Inc.; 626 © Paradigm Publishing, Inc.; 630 *both* © Paradigm Publishing, Inc.; 632 © Tibanna79/Shutterstock.com; 633 © Paradigm Publishing, Inc.; 638 © Paradigm Publishing, Inc.; 640 *both* Reprinted with permission of Mylan Pharmaceuticals Inc. All rights reserved.; 643 *top* © Paradigm Education Solutions; *bottom* © Paradigm Publishing, Inc.; 644 © iStock.com/sturti; 645 © iStock.com/Boogich; 648 *top* © iStock.com/humonia; *bottom* © iStock.com/urfinguss; 649 © iStock.com/Eraxion; 653 *icons* © MiAdS/Shutterstock.com and © extender_01/Shutterstock.com; 654 © Paradigm Publishing, Inc.; 655 © Paradigm Publishing, Inc.; 656 © Paradigm Publishing, Inc.; 658 © iStock.com/ Wicki58; 659 *top* © Paradigm Publishing, Inc.; *bottom* © toeytoey/shutterstock.com; 661 Centers for Disease Control and Prevention (public domain); 662 *top* © Eric Braem/Paradigm Publishing, Inc.; *bottom* © iStock.com/Triton21; 664 Gregory Moran, MD/Centers for Disease Control and Prevention (public domain); 669 © iStock.com/HeikeKampe; 670 © Eric Braem/ Paradigm Publishing, Inc.; 671 © Paradigm Publishing, Inc.; 672 *top* Macrobid container label used with permission. Macrobid is a registered trademark of Almatica Pharma, Inc.; *bottom* © iStock.com/Oktay Ortakcioglu; 674 © Paradigm Publishing, Inc.; 676 © Francis James Grogan/Dreamstime.com; 677 Courtesy of Gilead Sciences, Inc.; 683 © Adam J/Shutterstock.com; 685 © Paradigm Publishing, Inc.; 686 © Juan Gaertner/Shutterstock.com; 688 © Samuel Cohen/Shutterstock.com; 693 © Paradigm Publishing, Inc.; 694 © iStock.com/gokhan ilgaz; 695 © Paradigm Publishing, Inc.; 696 © iStock.com/Christopher Futcher; 697 © Yuganov Konstantin/Shutterstock.com; 698 *top* Centers for Disease Control and Prevention (public domain), modified; *bottom* © Constantine Pankin/Shutterstock.com; 700 © Sherry Yates Young/Shutterstock.com; 701 © iStock.com/ dra_schwartz ; 702 © iStock.com/KarenMower; 705 © 2015 Novartis Pharmaceuticals Corporation; 707 Niklas D (CC BY-SA 3.0); 709 © Jeffrey B. Banke/Shutterstock.com; 710 © iStock.com/Pamela Moore; 712 © iStock.com/MJJATE; 713 © iStock.com/PetePattavina; 716 *top* © iStock.com/Eraxion; *bottom* © Paradigm Publishing, Inc.; 717 © iStock.com/Ingram_Publishing; 720 © Odua Images/Shutterstock.com; 721 © Blamb/ Shutterstock.com; 722 *left* © SARAPON/Shutterstock.com; *right* © Mike Focus/Shutterstock.com; 723 © iStock.com/Jan-Otto; 724 *top* © Paradigm Publishing, Inc.; *middle* © Paradigm Publishing, Inc.; *bottom* © Sunshine_Art/Shutterstock.com; 725

© Eric Braem/Paradigm Publishing, Inc.; 727 © Eric Braem/ Paradigm Publishing, Inc.; 728 © Sherry Yates Young/Shutterstock.com; 730 © iStock.com/Marc Dufresne; 732 © iStock.com/JannHuizenga; 735 Vincent van Gogh (public domain); 737 © LunaseeStudios/Shutterstock.com; 739 © iStock.com/STEEX; 740 JohnOyston/Wikimedia Commons (CC BY-SA 3.0); 741 © iStock.com/NoDerog; 743 © iStock.com/jiangjunyan; 747 © Paradigm Publishing, Inc.; 748 © Paradigm Publishing, Inc.; 749 © Paradigm Publishing, Inc.; 751 A.D.A.M., a business unit of Ebix, Inc.; 752 © Paradigm Publishing, Inc.; 753 © iStock.com/dtimiraos; 755 James Heilman, (CC BY-SA 3.0); 756 © LunaseeStudios/Shutterstock.com; 759 Image used with permission from Fresenius Kabi USA, LLC; 760 © Evan Lorne/ Shutterstock.com; 763 © riggsby/Shutterstock.com; 770 © iStock.com/KatarzynaBialasiewicz; 772 National Cancer Institute (public domain); 773 © The McGraw-Hill Companies, Inc.; 774 *top* © iStock.com/Lighthousebay; *bottom* © iStock.com/Trish233; 776 *top* © Brian A. Jackson/Shutterstock.com; *bottom* © Paradigm Publishing, Inc.; 777 © Emerald Raindrops/Shutterstock.com; 783 © Image Point Fr/Shutterstock.com; 784 © DermNetNZ.org; 787 *left* © Africa Studio/Shutterstock.com; *right* © almaje/Shutterstock.com; 793 © AlphaMed Press 2011; 796 *both* © Paradigm Publishing, Inc.; 797 Courtesy of Spectrum Laboratory Products Inc., 2015; 799 Image used with permission from Fresenius Kabi USA, LLC; 802 *top* © iStock.com/areeya_ann; *bottom* © iStock.com/simonmasters; 803 © Lisa F. Young/Shutterstock.com; 806 © Yongcharoen_kittiyaporn/Shutterstock.com; 808 © iStock.com/XiXinXing; 809 © bikeriderlondon/Shutterstock.com; 810 © Luke Schmidt/ Shutterstock.com; 812 © parinyabinsuk/Shutterstock.com; 813 © iStock.com/evemilla; 814 © iStock.com/leungchopan; 816 © Rob Hainer/Shutterstock.com; 817 © Alexander Raths/ Shutterstock.com; 820 © xshot/Shutterstock.com; 821 © Dmitriy Sudzerovskiy/Shutterstock.com; 822 © Gert Vrey/ Shutterstock.com; 825 © Ilike/Shutterstock.com; 826 Centers for Disease Control and Prevention (public domain); 827 © Designua/Shutterstock.com; 832 © Oleg Golovnev/Shutterstock.com; 833 © iStock.com/michellegibson; 834 © Alexander Raths/ Shutterstock.com; 836 © Blaj Gabriel/Shutterstock.com; 840 © iStock.com/gchutka; 842 © Designua/Shutterstock.com; 843 *both* © Paradigm Publishing, Inc.; 845 © ARZTSAMUI/ Shutterstock.com; 848 © Jo Ann Snover/Shutterstock.com; 850 Editor182/Wikipedia (public domain); 851 Tom Varco (CC BY-SA 3.0); 852 © Fotoluminate LLC/Shutterstock.com; 855 © iStock.com/kali9

Generic and Brand-Name Drugs Index

Note: Page numbers followed by an *f* indicate that the reference appears in a figure; page numbers followed by a *p* indicate that the reference appears in a photo; and page numbers followed by a *t* indicate that the reference is found in a table.

Information about scheduled drugs can be found in Chapters 2 and 8 as well as in the Subject Index.

Navigator Paradigm Education Solutions' *Pocket Drug Guide* provides the generic names and brand names of the drugs listed below.

A

abacavir, 677*t*, 678, 678*t*
Abelcet, 684*t*
Abilify, 356*t*
abiraterone, 789
Abstral, 729*t*
Accolate, 463*t*, 819*t*
Accupril, 396*t*, 397, 637*t*
acebutolol, 330, 330*t*, 401*t*, 402, 404*t*
Aceon, 396*t*, 637*t*
acetaminophen, 266–267, 266*p*, 270, 279, 451, 513, 628, 711, 725–726, 725*p*, 725*t*, 726, 728, 729*t*, 731, 737, 737*t*, 738, 787, 808*t*, 810, 813, 813*t*, 821, 841*t*
acetazolamide, 639*t*, 640
acetic acid, 379*t*
acetylcysteine, 471
AcipHex, 397, 498*t*, 502*t*
acitretin, 242*t*, 242*t*.
aclidinium, 466*t*, 467
Aclovate, 253*t*
ActHIB, 699*t*
Acticin, 246*t*
Acticort, 253*t*
Activase, 443*t*
Activella, 601*t*
Actonel, 280*t*
ACTOplus Met, 561*t*
Actos, 564*t*
Acular, 375*t*
acyclovir, 374, 616*t*, 675*t*, 676, 676*p*
Adalat, 398*t*
adalimumab, 251, 272, 273*t*, 274, 841*t*
adapalene, 242*t*
Adderall, 324*t*, 325
Adderall XR, 324*t*, 325
Addyi, 602–603, 603*t*
Adipex-P, 540*t*
Adrenaline, 332*t*, 553
Adriamycin, 781*t*
Adrucil, 781*t*
Advair, 462*t*, 463, 819*t*
Advil, 267, 268*t*, 269, 813, 813*p*, 813*t*, 841*t*
AeroBid, 462*t*

Aerospan, 819*t*
Afluria, 699*t*
A-Hydrocort, 512*t*, 709*t*
AK-Con, 375*t*
AK-Dilate, 375*t*
Akne-Mycin, 241*t*.
Akten, 366*t*
Ala-Cort, 253*t*
Alaway, 375*t*
albuterol, 460*t*, 461, 466*t*, 467, 819*t*, 822
Alcaine, 366*t*
alclometasone, 253*t*
alcohol, 379*t*, 590*t*
Aldactazide, 639*t*
Aldactone, 639*t*
aldosterone, 641
alendronate, 279, 280, 280*t*, 495*t*, 844
Alesse, 608*t*
Aleve, 267, 268*t*, 838*t*, 841*t*
alfuzosin, 634, 634*t*, 680, 681
Alimta, 781*t*
aliskiren, 397, 398, 413
Alitretinoin, 242*t*
Alkeran, 780*t*, 781*t*
Allegra, 452*t*
Aller-Chlor, 854*t*
Alli, 539*p*, 539*t*
allicin, 420
allopurinol, 275, 276, 276*t*, 277, 839*t*
almotriptan, 736*t*
Alocril, 375*t*
aloe vera, 259
Alomide, 375*t*
alosetron, 319, 342, 510, 510*t*, 511
Aloxi, 506*t*, 849
Alphagan P, 368*t*
alpha-tocopherol, 420, 520*t*, 522
alprazolam, 293, 348*t*, 679, 686, 850
alprostadil, 590, 591
Alrex, 372*t*
Altabax, 245*t*
Altacaine, 366*t*
Altace, 396*t*, 637*t*
Altafrin, 375*t*
Altazine, 375*t*
alteplase, 443, 443*t*
ALternaGEL, 497*t*

aluminum chloride, 765
aluminum hydroxide, 497*t*
Alupent, 460*t*
Alvesco, 819*t*
amantadine, 318, 319*t*, 320, 675*t*, 676, 839*t*
Amaryl, 563*t*
Ambien, 351*t*, 850
AmBisome, 684*t*
amcinonide, 253*t*
Amerge, 736*t*
A-MethaPred, 512*t*, 709*t*
Amethia, 608*t*
Amidate, 740*t*
amides, 742
amifostine, 629
amikacin, 471, 668*t*
amiloride, 639*t*, 641
aminoglycoside, 370, 371, 381, 381*t*, 470, 628, 664, 668, 669, 811, 826, 839*t*
aminophylline, 464
aminoquinoline, 274
aminosalicylates, 512, 513
amiodarone, 320, 356, 404*t*, 406, 406*f*, 407, 438*t*, 680, 681
Amitiza, 510*t*
amitriptyline, 343*t*, 734, 734*t*, 851
amlodipine, 398*t*, 399
ammonium chloride, 764*t*
Amnesteem, 242*t*
amoxapine, 317
amoxicillin, 502*t*, 661, 662, 662*p*, 663*t*, 816*t*, 823*t*, 825
Amphotec, 684*t*
amphotericin B, 628, 684*t*, 685, 685*f*, 686
ampicillin, 663*t*, 823*t*, 826, 827
amprenavir, 405, 406
Anacaine, 741*t*
Anafranil, 343*t*
anakinra, 272, 273*t*, 274
Anaspaz, 510*t*
anastrazole, 789
Anbesol, 741*t*
Ancef, 665*t*
Ancobon, 684*t*
AneCream, 741*t*
Anectine, 295*t*
Angiomax, 436*t*
Anoro Ellipta, 463, 466*t*

antacids, 489, 497, 633*t*
Antara, 417*t*
anthracyclines, 779*t*, 786
antiandrogens, 789–790
antibiotics, 258*t*, 471*p*, 486, 486*t*, 503*t*, 523, 659–661, 702, 812*t*
anticholinergics, 320, 354, 466, 495*t*, 504–505, 631, 633*t*
anticoagulants, 434, 435, 437, 439, 442, 496, 514, 688, 846*t*
anticonvulsants, 312, 488, 723, 733, 739, 740
antidepressants, 258*t*, 323, 340, 346, 352, 474, 590*t*, 592, 723, 734
antiemetics, 489*t*, 740
antiepileptics, 312, 733
antiestrogens, 789
antifungals, 488, 501, 618, 683
antihistamines, 251, 258, 258*t*, 344, 350, 374, 451, 452, 453, 455, 489*t*, 504
antimalarials, 708
antimuscarinics, 622, 631–632
antioxidants, 527*p*
antiplatelet drugs, 434, 441, 442
antipsychotics, 258*t*, 317, 352, 354, 354*p*, 355, 356, 357
antipyrine, 379*t*, 380
antispasmodics, 511
antistaphylococcal penicillins, 664
antitoxins, 712–713
antivenoms, 712–713, 713*p*
Antivert, 854*t*
antivirals, 618, 674*f*, 676
Anu-Med, 332*t*
Anusol, 509*t*
Anzemet, 506*t*
Aphrodyne, 591*t*
Apidra, 568*t*
Aplenzin, 345
Apokyn, 318*t*
apomorphine, 318, 318*t*, 319
aprepitant, 507, 508, 508*p*
Apri, 608*t*
Apriso, 512*t*
Aptiom, 313*t*
Aptivus, 680*t*
Aralen, 707*t*
Aranesp, 432*t*
Arava, 273*t*

Arcapta Neohaler, 463, 467*t*
Aredia, 280*t*
arformoterol, 467*t*, 468
argatroban, 436*t*, 438
Aricept, 323*t*, 852
aripiprazole, 356, 356*t*
Aristospan, 276*t*
Arixtra, 436*t*
Armour Thyroid, 573, 573*t*
aromatase inhibitors, 789
arsenic trioxide, 356
ascorbic acid, 523*t*, 527, 628, 688
Asmanex, 462*t*, 463, 819*t*
asparaginase, 788
asparagine, 788
aspart, 568*t*
aspirin, 269, 270, 271, 276, 316,
  334, 381*t*, 418–419, 434, 438,
  441*p*, 441*t*, 442, 445, 489,
  495, 495*t*, 496*p*, 514, 525,
  721, 725*t*, 726–727, 727*p*,
  729*t*, 731, 737, 737*t*, 738,
  812*t*, 814, 847, 855
Astelin, 456*t*
astemizole, 668, 679
Astepro, 456*t*
Astroglide, 605
Atacand, 398*t*, 637*t*
Atarax, 504*t*
atazanavir, 680, 680*t*
atenolol, 329, 330, 330*t*, 401,
  401*t*, 402, 839*t*
Ativan, 348*t*, 738
atomoxetine, 324*t*, 325, 326
atorvastatin, 325, 417*t*, 686
atovaquone, 687
atracurium, 295*t*
Atralin, 242*t*
Atripla, 677, 677*t*, 678*t*
atropine, 366*t*, 412*t*, 467, 487,
  487*t*, 488, 824
Atropine Care, 366*t*
Atrovent, 466*t*
Aubagio, 705*t*
Augmentin, 663*t*, 816*t*
auranofin, 272*t*, 274
Aurodex, 379*t*
Auro-Dri, 379*t*
Avage, 242*t*
avanafil, 591*t*
Avandamet, 561*t*
Avandia, 564*t*
Avapro, 398*t*, 637*t*
Avastin, 791*t*
Avelox, 670*t*, 812*t*
Aventyl, 343*t*, 734*t*
Aviane, 608*t*
Avita, 242*t*, 521
Avodart, 635*t*
Avonex, 705*t*
Axert, 736*t*
Axid, 500*t*, 502*t*
axitinib, 791*t*
azathioprine, 251, 272, 272*t*, 296*t*,
  297, 512, 512*t*, 514, 524, 707,
  707*t*, 708
azelaic acid, 241, 241*t*

azelastine, 375*t*, 456*t*
Azelex, 241*t*
Azilect, 321
azilsartan, 398*t*, 637*t*
azithromycin, 616*t*, 617*p*, 667,
  667*t*, 668, 816*t*, 823*t*, 825
Azmacort, 462*t*
azole antifungals, 686
aztreonam, 471, 666
Azulfidine, 273*t*, 512*t*, 841*t*
Azurette, 608*t*

B

bacitracin, 245*t*, 371*t*
baclofen, 291, 291*t*
Bactrim, 672*t*, 812*t*
Bactroban, 245*t*
balsam of Peru, 250
barbiturates, 495*t*, 609, 738, 740
Baycadron, 709*t*
Bayer, 725*t*, 812*t*
beclomethasone, 456*t*, 462*t*, 819*t*
Beconase AQ, 456*t*
belladonna alkaloids, 504
Belviq, 541*p*
Benadryl, 412*t*, 452*t*, 854*t*
benazepril, 396*t*, 637*t*
bendamustine, 778*t*, 781*t*
Benefiber, 491*t*
Benicar, 398*t*, 637*t*
Bentyl, 510*t*
Benzac, 241*t*.
benzocaine, 379*t*, 380, 741*p*, 741*t*,
  742, 815
benzodiazepines, 312, 323, 346,
  347, 348, 349, 350, 351, 354,
  357, 381*t*, 686, 728, 738, 739,
  742, 852
benzoyl peroxide, 240, 241, 241*t*.
benzphetamine, 540*t*
benztropine, 319*t*, 320, 354, 854*t*
benzyl alcohol, 432, 504
bepridil, 679, 680, 681
beta blockers, 329, 400–402, 400*p*,
  413, 414, 845, 846, 846*t*,
  847, 848
beta-carotene, 381
Betagan, 368*t*
betamethasone, 253*t*, 684*t*, 709,
  709*t*, 812*t*
betamethasone dipropionate, 253*t*
betamethasone valerate, 253*t*
Betapace, 330*t*, 401*t*, 404*t*
Betaseron, 705*t*
beta-sitosterol, 419, 420
Beta-Val, 253*t*
betaxolol, 329, 330, 330*t*, 368*t*,
  401*t*, 402
Betoptic, 368*t*
bevacizumab, 791, 791*t*
Biaxin, 667*t*, 816*t*
bicalutamide, 789
BICNU, 781*t*
bifidobacteria, 515
bile acid sequestrants, 510, 510*t*
bimatoprost, 368, 368*t*

biotin, 523*t*, 526
bisacodyl, 491*t*, 492
bismuth subsalicylate, 487*t*,
  488–489, 488*p*, 502*t*
bisoprolol, 329, 330, 330*t*, 401*t*,
  402
bisphosphates, 279, 280
bivalirudin, 436*t*, 438
black cohosh, 358, 619
bleomycin, 779*t*, 788, 789
Bleph-10, 371*t*
Blephamide, 371*t*
Blocadren, 330*t*, 401*t*
Bonine, 504*t*
Boniva, 280*t*
Bontril, 540*t*
bosentan, 563
Bosulif, 791*t*
bosutinib, 791*t*, 793
Botox, 286, 293, 293*p*, 294
botulinum toxin, 286, 293, 294
bretylium, 412*t*
Brevibloc, 330*t*, 401*t*, 404*t*
Brevicon, 608*t*
Brevital, 740*t*
Brevoxyl, 241*t*.
brimonidine, 368*t*, 369
Bromday, 375*t*
bromfenac, 375*t*
bromocriptine, 318*t*, 319
bronchodilators, 465, 469, 471,
  633*t*, 822
Brovana, 467*t*
budesonide, 456*t*, 462*t*, 512, 512*t*,
  513, 709, 709*t*, 819*t*
Bufferin, 812*t*
bumetanide, 414, 639*t*, 640, 641
Bumex, 641
bupivacaine, 741*t*, 742
bupropion, 326, 340, 344–345,
  473*t*, 474
buspirone, 344, 349
busulfan, 778*t*, 780*t*
butalbital, 737, 737*t*, 738
butenafine, 684*t*, 686
butoconazole, 684*t*
butorphanol, 737, 737*t*, 738
Bydureon, 565*t*
Byetta, 565*t*
Bystolic, 330*t*, 401*t*

C

caffeine, 344, 737, 737*t*, 738, 743
calamine, 254
Calan, 398*t*, 405*t*
calciferol, 521
calcipotriene, 254
calcitonin, 280*t*, 281
Cal-Citrate, 757*t*
calcium, 278*p*
calcium acetate, 278*t*
calcium carbonate, 278*t*, 497,
  497*t*, 757*t*
calcium chloride, 412*t*, 757*t*
calcium citrate, 278*t*, 757*t*
calcium glubionate, 278*t*

calcium gluconate, 278*t*, 757*t*
calcium lactate, 278*t*, 757*t*
calcium phosphate, 278*t*
Cal-Lac, 757*t*
Caltrate, 757*t*
Camila, 608*t*
camphor, 250
Camptosar, 781*t*
Camrese Lo, 608*t*
canagliflozin, 571, 571*t*
Canasa, 512*t*
Cancidas, 684*t*
candesartan, 398*t*, 637*t*
cannabinoid, 507
Cannabis sativa, 743
capecitabine, 483, 778*t*, 779*t*,
  780*t*, 784
Capex, 253*t*
Capoten, 396*t*, 637*t*
capsaicin, 743*p*, 841, 841*t*
captopril, 396*t*, 637*t*
carbachol, 368*t*, 369
carbamate, 315
carbamazepine, 313*t*, 315, 316,
  321, 344, 346, 438*t*, 503*t*,
  603, 609
carbamide peroxide, 379*t*, 380
carbapenems, 661, 666
carbidopa, 318, 318*t*, 319
Carbocaine, 741*t*
carbonic anhydrase inhibitors, 638,
  640, 845
carboplatin, 628, 629, 778*t*, 781*t*,
  782, 799*f*
Cardene, 398*t*
Cardizem, 398*t*, 405*t*
Cardura, 329*t*, 401*t*, 634*t*
carisoprodol, 291*t*, 292, 292*p*, 293
Carmustine, 778*t*, 781*t*, 790
Carteolol, 330, 330*t*, 368*t*, 369
Cartrol, 330*t*
carvedilol, 330, 330*t*
caspofungin, 684*t*
Catapres, 847, 852
catechol-O-methyltransferase, 318
Caziant, 608*t*
Ceclor, 665*t*
Cedax, 665*t*
cefaclor, 665*t*
cefazolin, 471, 665*t*
cefdinir, 665, 665*t*, 816*t*
cefditoren, 664, 665*t*
cefepime, 471, 664, 665*t*
cefixime, 665, 665*t*
cefotaxime, 665*t*, 826
cefotetan, 665*t*
cefoxitin, 665*t*
cefpodoxime, 816*t*
ceftaroline, 664, 665*t*
ceftazidime, 471, 665*t*
ceftibuten, 665*t*
ceftriaxone, 616*t*, 617*p*, 664, 665*t*,
  816*t*, 826
cefuroxime, 665*t*, 816*t*
Celebrex, 270, 271*p*
celecoxib, 270, 271
Celestone, 709*t*

ketoconazole, 243, 346, 348, 407, 499, 500, 589, 590*t*, 634, 684*t*, 685, 736
ketoprofen, 268*t*
ketorolac, 268*t*, 269, 269*f*, 375*t*
Ketorolac tromethamine, 269*f*
ketotifen, 375*t*
Kineret, 272, 273*t*
Klonopin, 348*t*
K-Lor, 642, 757*t*
Klor-Con, 642, 757*t*
K-Lyte, 642, 757*t*
Konsyl Fiber, 491*t*
Korlym, 595
K-Phos, 757*t*
K-Tab, 642
K-Y Jelly, 605
Kytril, 506*t*

L

labetalol, 594
lacosamide, 313*t*, 315
LactiCare, 253*t*
lactulose, 494
Lamictal, 314*t*, 488
Lamisil, 488
Lamisil AT, 684*t*
lamivudine, 677*t*, 678, 678*t*
lamotrigine, 314*t*, 315, 352, 609
Lanacane, 741*p*, 741*t*
Lanacort, 253*t*
lanolin, 259
Lanoxin, 408*t*, 852–853
lansoprazole, 498, 498*t*, 499, 502*t*
Lantus, 568*t*
Lasix, 412*t*, 639*t*, 640
latanoprost, 368*t*
laxatives, 489–490
Lazanda, 729*t*
leflunomide, 273*t*, 274
lenalidomide, 791, 791*t*, 792
Lescol, 417*t*
Lessina, 608*t*
letrozole, 789
leucovorin, 784
Leukeran, 780*t*
leuprolide, 790
levalbuterol, 460*t*, 461, 819*t*
Levaquin, 670*t*
Levatol, 330*t*
Levbid, 510*t*
Levemir, 568*t*
levetiracetam, 314*t*, 315, 503*t*
Levitra, 413, 591*t*
Levlite, 608*t*
levobunolol, 368*t*, 369
levodopa, 318, 318*t*, 319, 320, 321, 429
levofloxacin, 371*t*, 429, 670, 670*t*, 671, 823*t*
levomethadyl, 356
levomilnacipran, 341*t*
levonorgestrel, 601*t*, 608*t*, 609, 610, 614
Levophed, 332*t*
levothyroxine, 438*t*, 501, 572*p*, 573, 573*t*

Levsin, 510*t*
Lexapro, 341*t*
Lexiva, 680*t*
Lialda, 512*t*
Lidex, 253*t*
lidocaine, 366*t*, 403*t*, 405, 412*t*, 680, 741*t*, 742, 838*t*
linaclotide, 509, 510*t*, 511
lincosamides, 667
lindane, 246*t*, 247–248
linezolid, 342, 343, 345, 471, 474, 734, 823*t*
Linzess, 510*t*
Lioresal, 291*t*
liothyronine, 573, 573*t*
liotrix, 573*t*
Lipitor, 417*t*
liposome, 685
liraglutide, 541, 541*t*, 542, 565*t*, 566
lisinopril, 396*p*, 396*t*, 637*t*
lispro, 568*t*, 570
lithium, 317, 352, 400, 839*t*
Lithobid, 352
Livalo, 417*t*
Lo, 608*t*
Locoid, 253*t*
Lodine, 268*t*
lodoxamide, 375*t*
Loestrin, 608*t*
Lofibra, 417*t*
LoKara, 253*t*
Lo Minastrin Fe, 608*t*
Lomotil, 487, 487*t*, 488, 823
lomustine, 778*t*, 780*t*, 790
Lonox, 487*t*
loperamide, 487, 487*t*, 488, 510, 679, 823
lopinavir, 680, 680*t*
Lopressor, 330*t*, 401*t*
Loprox, 684*t*
loratadine, 452, 452*t*
lorazepam, 312, 348, 348*t*, 738
lorcaserin, 540, 541
Lortab, 729*t*
losartan, 398*t*, 637*t*
Lotemax, 372*t*
Lotensin, 396*t*, 637*t*
loteprednol, 372, 372*t*
Lotrimin AF, 684*t*
Lotrimin Ultra, 684*t*
Lotrisone, 253*t*, 684*t*
Lotronex, 510*t*, 511
lovastatin, 417*t*, 438*t*, 668, 680, 681, 686
Lovaza, 419
Lovenox, 436*t*
lubiprostone, 509, 510, 510*t*
Lucentis, 366, 377
Lumigan, 368, 368*t*
Luminal, 314*t*
Lunesta, 351*t*
Lupron, 790
Lutera, 608*t*
Luvox, 341*t*
Luxiq, 253*t*, 812*t*
Lyrica, 314*t*, 734*t*
Lyza, 608*t*

M

Maalox, 497, 497*t*
Macrobid, 672*f*, 672*t*
Macrodantin, 672*t*
macrolides, 346, 381*t*, 667, 668, 825
Mag-200, 757*t*
Mag-Cap, 757*t*
Mag-G, 757*t*
magnesium chloride, 757*t*, 761
magnesium citrate, 493
magnesium gluconate, 757*t*, 761
magnesium hydroxide, 497*t*
magnesium lactate, 757*t*, 761
magnesium oxide, 757*t*, 761
magnesium sulfate, 412*t*, 594, 757*t*, 761
Magonate, 757*t*
Mag-Ox, 757*t*
Mag-Tab, 757*t*
Magtrate, 757*t*
ma huang, 334, 546
malathion, 246*t*, 247, 248
Maltsupex, 491*t*
manganese, 528*t*, 530–531
mannitol, 706
Maox, 757*t*
maprotiline, 258*t*
maraviroc, 681, 682*t*
Marcaine, 741*t*
marijuana, 743
Marplan, 344*t*
Matulane, 780*t*
Mavik, 396*t*, 637*t*
Maxair, 460*t*
Maxalt, 736*t*
Maxidex, 372*t*
Maxipime, 665*t*
Maxitrol, 371*t*
Maxivate, 253*t*
Maxzide, 638, 639*t*
mechlorethamine, 778*t*, 780, 781*t*, 786*t*
meclizine, 504, 504*t*, 594, 610, 854*t*
Medrol, 512*t*, 709*t*, 819*t*
medroxyprogesterone, 601*t*, 613, 615
mefloquine, 356, 687
Mefoxin, 665*t*
megestrol, 407
meglitinides, 562, 563
melatonin, 350, 357, 358
meloxicam, 268*t*
melphalan, 778*t*, 780*t*, 781*t*
memantine, 323, 323*t*, 852
Menactra, 699*t*
Menest, 601*t*
Menomune, 699*t*
Menopur, 593, 597
Mentax, 684*t*
menthol, 250
meperidine, 321, 344
Mephyton, 440*t*
mepivacaine, 741*t*, 742
meprobamate, 292
mercaptopurine, 276, 483, 524,

778*t*, 780*t*
meropenem, 471, 666
mesalamine, 512, 512*t*
Mestinon, 296, 296*t*
Metaglip, 561*t*
Metamucil, 491*p*, 491*t*
metaproterenol, 460*t*, 461
metaxalone, 291*t*
metformin, 315, 561, 561*t*, 562, 564, 571, 598, 811
methadone, 321, 728, 729*t*, 731–732
methamphetamine, 325, 454
methicillin, 664
methimazole, 574, 575
methocarbamol, 291*t*, 292
methohexital, 740, 740*t*
methotrexate, 251, 270, 273*t*, 274, 483, 483*p*, 707, 707*t*, 711, 711*t*, 712, 778*t*, 779*t*, 780*t*, 781*t*, 782, 784, 797*f*, 839*t*, 841*t*
methyclothiazide, 639*t*
methylcellulose, 491*t*
methyldopa, 429, 590*t*
methylene blue, 342, 343, 345, 474, 734
Methylin, 324*t*
methylphenidate, 324*t*, 325
methylprednisolone, 512, 512*t*, 513, 704, 707, 709, 709*t*, 710, 819*t*
metipranolol, 368*t*
metoclopramide, 317, 505, 505*t*, 594, 610, 839*t*
metolazone, 639*t*, 642
metoprolol, 329, 330, 330*t*, 331, 401*t*, 402
metoprolol succinate salt, 402
metoprolol tartrate, 402
MetroCream, 241*t*., 245*t*
MetroGel, 241*t*, 245*t*, 673
MetroLotion, 241*t*., 245*t*
metronidazole, 241, 241*t*., 245, 245*t*, 438*t*, 502*t*, 616*t*, 673, 687
Mevacor, 417*t*
Mexican yam, 619
mexiletine, 404*t*, 405
Miacalcin, 280*t*
micafungin, 684*t*
Micardis, 398*t*, 637*t*
Micatin, 684*t*
miconazole, 684*t*, 686
Micro-K, 642, 757*t*
Micronase, 563*t*
Microzide, 639*t*
midazolam, 412*t*, 679, 680, 681, 738
midodrine, 332*t*, 333
Midrin, 737*t*
Mifeprex, 595
mifepristone, 595
Milk of magnesia, 494
milnacipran, 342
Minipress, 329*t*, 401*t*
Minocin, 669*t*, 812*t*
minocycline, 241, 669*t*, 812*t*

minoxidil, 248–249
Miostat, 368*t*
mirabegron, 631, 631*t*, 632
MiraLAX, 493, 493*p*, 510*t*
Mirapex, 318*t*
Mircette, 608*t*
mirtazapine, 343*t*
misoprostol, 501, 595
mitomycin, 786*t*
mitoxantrone, 705*t*, 706, 778*t*, 781*t*, 785
Mobic, 268*t*
moexipril, 396*t*, 637*t*
mometasone, 253*t*, 456*t*, 462*t*, 463, 819*t*
monacolins, 420
Monistat, 684*t*
monobactams, 661, 666
MonoNessa, 608*t*
Monopril, 396*t*
montelukast, 463, 463*t*, 464, 818, 819*t*
morphine, 503*t*, 728, 728*p*, 729*t*, 730, 838*t*
Motrin, 267, 268*t*, 269, 813, 813*t*, 841*t*
Moxatag, 663*t*, 816*t*
moxifloxacin, 356, 670*t*, 671, 812*t*, 823*t*
MS Contin, 729*t*
Mucinex, 454*t*
mucolytics, 471
Multaq, 405*t*
mupirocin, 245, 245*t*
Murine, 375*t*
muscle relaxants, 290
mustargen, 781*t*
Myambutol, 470*t*
Mycamine, 684*t*
Mycelex, 684*t*
Mycogen, 253*t*
Mycolog, 253*t*
Myconel, 253*t*
mycophenolate, 711*t*, 712
Mycostatin, 684*t*
Myco-Triacet, 253*t*
Mydral, 366*t*
Mydriacyl, 366*t*
mydriatics, 366*t*
Myfortic, 711*t*, 712
Mylan, 640*f*
Mylanta, 497*t*
Myleran, 780*t*
Myrbetriq, 631*t*
Mysoline, 314*t*

N

nabumetone, 268*t*
nadolol, 330*t*, 401*t*
Nafarelin, 593, 597
nafcillin, 471, 663*t*
Nallpen, 663*t*
naloxone, 412*t*, 742
Namenda, 323*t*, 852
naphazoline, 374, 375*t*
Naphcon, 375*t*

Naprosyn, 268*t*, 841*t*
naproxen, 275, 838, 838*t*, 841*t*
naproxen sodium, 267, 268*t*
naratriptan, 736, 736*t*
Narcan, 412*t*
Nardil, 344*t*
Nasacort AQ, 456*t*
Nascobal, 430*t*
Nasonex, 456*t*
natalizumab, 704, 705*t*, 706
nateglinide, 563, 563*t*
Naturalyte, 756*t*
Navelbine, 781*t*
nebivolol, 330, 330*t*, 401, 401*t*, 402
Necon, 608*t*
nedocromil, 375*t*
nefazodone, 315, 348, 736
nelfinavir, 680, 680*t*, 736
NeoBenz, 241*t.*
Neofrin, 332*t*, 375*t*
neomycin, 245*t*, 298, 371*t*, 378, 378*t*, 381*t*, 701
Neoral, 272, 272*t*, 296*t*, 297, 512*t*, 711*t*
Neosporin, 245*t*
Neosporin AF, 684*t*
neostigmine, 296, 296*t*, 297
Neo-Synephrine, 332*t*, 453*t*
nepafenac, 375*t*
Nesacaine, 741*t*
Neurontin, 313*t*, 734*t*
Neutrogena, 241*t.*
Nevanac, 375*t*
nevirapine, 679, 679*t*, 680
Nexavar, 791*t*
Nexium, 498*t*, 502*t*
Next Choice, 609, 609*p*, 610
niacin, 418, 419*t*, 523*t*, 524, 525
Niacor, 419*t*
Niaspan, 419, 419*t*
nicardipine, 398*t*, 399
NicoDerm, 473*t*
Nicorette, 473*t*
nicotine, 323, 472, 473–475, 473*t*, 495*t*, 590*t*
Nicotrol, 473*t*
nifedipine, 398*t*, 399, 500
nilotinib, 791*t*, 793
Nimbex, 295*t*
nisoldipine, 398*t*, 399
nitrates, 411, 412, 413, 495*t*, 591, 846*t*
Nitro-Bid, 411*t*
Nitro-Dur, 411*t*
nitrofurantoin, 429, 629, 671, 672, 672*t*, 839*t*, 854
Nitrogard, 411*t*
nitrogen mustard, 790
nitroglycerin, 411*t*, 412, 412*t*, 413
Nitrolingual, 411*t*
nitrosoureas, 790
Nitrostat, 411*t*
nitrous oxide, 739, 740*t*
Nix, 246*t*
nizatidine, 500*t*, 502*t*
Nizoral, 243, 684*t*

nonnucleoside, 315
nonoxynol 9, 611*t*
nonsteroidal anti-inflammatory drugs (NSAIDS), 258*t*, 267–270, 271, 275, 323, 352, 374, 381*t*, 429, 438, 442, 495–496, 495*t*, 496*p*, 501, 628, 721, 731, 735, 738
norelgestromin, 611*t*
norepinephrine, 309*t*, 332*t*, 333
norepinephrine reuptake inhibitors (SNRIs), 340, 341*t*, 342, 344, 345
norethindrone, 601*t*, 608*t*
Norflex, 291*t*
norgestimate, 608*t*
norgestrel, 608*t*
Norinyl, 608*t*
Noritate, 245*t*
Norpace, 403*t*
Norpramin, 343*t*
Nor-QD, 608*t*
Nortrel, 608*t*
nortriptyline, 326, 343*t*, 734*t*
Norvasc, 398*t*
Norvir, 680*t*
Novantrone, 781*t*
Novarel, 592, 597
Novolin N, 568*t*
Novolin R, 568*t*
NovoLog, 568*t*
NovoSeven RT, 444*p*
NPH insulin, 568*t*
NuvaRing, 611*t*
Nyamyc, 684*t*
nystatin, 253*t*, 684*t*, 685, 686
Nystop, 684*t*

O

Ocella, 608*t*
Ocuflox, 371*t*
Ocuvite, 381
Ofirmev, 725*t*
ofloxacin, 371*t*, 378*t*
Ogestrel, 608*t*
olanzapine, 356, 356*t*
Oleptro, 345
olmesartan, 398*t*, 637*t*
olopatadine, 375*t*
Olux, 253*t*
omalizumab, 464
omeprazole, 498, 498*t*, 499, 502*t*
Omnaris, 456*t*
Omnicef, 665, 816*t*
Oncovin, 781*t*
ondansetron, 319, 506, 506*t*, 507*f*, 849
Onglyza, 565*t*
Onsolis, 729*t*
opiate derivatives, 487, 488
opiates, 489, 503*t*
opioids, 855
Opti-Clear, 375*t*
OptiPranolol, 368*t*
Optivar, 375*t*, 456*t*

oral contraceptives, 606–607, 607*p*
Oralyte, 487
Orapred, 709*t*, 819*t*
orlistat, 538, 539*p*, 539*t*
orphenadrine, 292
orphenadrine citrate, 291*t*
Ortho-Cyclen, 608*t*
Ortho Evra, 611*t*
Ortho Micronor, 608*t*
Ortho-Novum, 608*t*
Ortho Tri-Cyclen, 608*t*
Ortho Tri-Cyclen Lo, 608*t*
Os Cal, 757*t*
Oscimin, 510*t*
oseltamivir, 675*t*, 676
Otrexup, 707*t*
Ovcon, 608*t*
Ovide, 246*t*
Ovidrel, 592, 597
Ovral, 608*t*
oxacillin, 663*t*
oxaliplatin, 778*t*, 779*t*, 781*t*, 782
oxaprozin, 268*t*
oxazepam, 348, 348*t*
oxcarbazepine, 313*t*, 315, 321
Oxy, 241*t.*
oxybutynin, 631*t*
oxycodone, 503*t*, 728, 729*t*, 730–731, 855
OxyContin, 729*t*
oxymetazoline, 375*t*
Ozurdex, 372*t*

P

paclitaxel, 778*t*, 779*t*, 781*t*, 787, 788
paliperidone, 356, 356*t*, 357
palivizumab, 822
palonosetron, 506, 506*t*, 849
Pamelor, 343*t*, 734*t*
pamidronate, 280*t*
pancuronium, 295*t*
Pandel, 253*t*
panitumumab, 791*t*, 792
PanOxyl, 241*t.*
Panretin, 242*t*
pantoprazole, 498*t*, 502*t*
pantothenic acid, 523*t*, 525*p*
para-aminobenzoic acid (PABA), 239, 240
Parafon Forte, 291*t*
Paraplatin, 781*t*
Parcaine, 366*t*
Parlodel, 318*t*
Parnate, 344*t*
paroxetine, 341*t*, 600
Pataday, 375*t*
Patanol, 375*t*
Paxil, 341*t*, 600
PediaCare, 453*t*, 454*t*, 487
Pedialyte, 487, 756*t*, 823
Pediapred, 709*t*
Pediazole, 667*t*
pediculicide, 247, 248
PedvaxHIB, 699*t*
PEG, 510*t*

rocuronium, 295t
Rogaine, 248–249
Rolaids, 497t
Romazicon, 412t, 742
ropinirole, 318t, 319
Rosadan, 245t
rosiglitazone, 561t, 564t
rosuvastatin, 417t, 438t
Rotarix, 699t
RotaTeq, 699t
Rozerem, 351t
RU-486, 595
Ryanodex, 294p
Rythmol, 404t

S

Sabril, 313t
St. John's wort, 299, 321, 342, 603, 609, 619, 679, 680, 681
Sal-Clens, 241t.
salicylate, 274, 381t, 523
salicylic acid, 241, 241t.
salmeterol, 462t, 463, 467t, 819t
SAMe, 358
Sanctura, 631t, 854t
Sancuso, 506t
Sandimmune, 272, 272t, 296t, 297, 512t, 711t
saquinavir, 420, 680, 680t
Sarafem, 341t
saw palmetto, 645p
saxagliptin, 565t
Saxenda, 541t
scabicides, 247
Scalpicin, 253t
Scopace, 504t
scopolamine, 366t, 504, 504p, 504t
Seasonale, 607, 608t
Seasonique, 607, 608t
Sectral, 330t, 401t, 404t
sedatives, 347, 350, 474
seed oil, 259
selective estrogen receptor
    modulators (SERMs), 281
selective serotonin reuptake
    inhibitors (SSRIs), 317, 340,
    341t, 342, 344, 345, 633t
selegiline, 318, 321, 321t, 732
selenium, 528t, 531
selenium sulfide, 243
Selzentry, 681, 682t
senna, 491t, 492
Septra, 672t
Serevent Discus, 467t
Seromycin, 470t
Seroquel, 356t
serotonin, 309t, 319
serotonin receptor antagonists,
    506, 849
sertraline, 258t, 341t, 342
sildenafil, 412, 680, 681
Silenor, 343t
silver nitrate, 616
silver sulfadiazine, 257
Simply Stuffy, 453t

Simponi, 273t
simvastatin, 417t, 418, 438t, 668, 680, 681, 686, 810
Sinemet, 318t
Singulair, 463t, 819t
sirolimus, 712
sitagliptin, 561t, 565t
sitosterol, 420
Skelaxin, 291t
Slo-Niacin, 419t
Slo-Salt, 757t
Slow Fe, 530
Slow iron, 430t
sodium bicarbonate, 412t, 764t, 765
sodium chloride, 757t
sodium phosphate, 493
sodium polystyrene sulfonate, 642
solifenacin, 631t
Solu-Cortef, 512t, 709t
Solu-Medrol, 512t, 709t
Soma, 291t, 292
Sonata, 351t
sorafenib, 791t
Soriatane, 242t
sotalol, 330, 330t, 331, 356, 401, 401t, 404t, 406
soy, 619
Spectracef, 665t
spermicides, 604, 606p
Spiriva, 463, 466t
spironolactone, 397, 590t, 615, 638, 639t, 640f, 641, 852
Sporanox, 684t
Sprintec, 608t
Sprycel, 791t
Stadol, 737t
Starlix, 563t
statins, 299, 322, 416–417, 846t, 847
stavudine, 678, 678t
Stendra, 591t
Sterapred, 512t
steroid, 371
Strattera, 324t, 326
streptomycin, 470, 470t
Stribild, 677, 677t
Stridex, 241t.
Subsys, 729t
succinimides, 315
succinylcholine, 295
sucralfate, 500, 501, 633t
Sucrets, 531p, 741t
Sudafed, 453t
SudoGest, 453t
Sudogest PE, 332t
Sufenta, 740t
sufentanil, 740, 740t
Sular, 398t
sulbactam, 663t
sulfacetamide, 370, 371t
sulfamethoxazole, 438t, 629, 672, 672t, 812t, 839t, 854
sulfas, 258t, 671, 672
sulfasalazine, 273t, 274, 512, 512t, 513, 841t
Sulfazine, 512t

sulfonamides, 257, 259, 271, 315, 523, 640, 641–642, 671
sulfonylureas, 497, 562, 563, 564, 565
sulindac, 268t, 628
sumatriptan, 736, 736t
Sumycin, 812t
sunitinib, 791t
Suprane, 740t
Suprax, 665, 665t
Suprenza, 540t
Sustain, 757t
Sustiva, 679t
Sutent, 791t
Symbicort, 462t, 819t
Symlin, 565t
Symmetrel, 319t, 675t
sympathomimetics, 344, 539–540
Synacort, 253t
Synagis, 822
Synalar, 253t
Synthroid, 572p, 573t

T

Taclonex, 254
tacrolimus, 252, 356, 711t, 712
tadalafil, 412, 591t
tafluprost, 368t
Tagamet, 500t, 502t
Take Action, 609, 610
talc, 250
Tambocor, 403t
Tamiflu, 675t
tamoxifen, 438t, 789
tamsulosin, 634, 634t
Tarceva, 791t
Tasigna, 791t
Tasmar, 320t
Tavist, 452t
Taxol, 781t
Taxotere, 781t
tazarotene, 242t
Tazicef, 665t
tazobactam, 471, 663t
Tazorac, 242t
Tecfidera, 705t
Teflaro, 665t
Tegretol, 313t
telmisartan, 398t, 637t
temazepam, 348, 348t
Temodar, 780t
Temovate, 253t
temozolomide, 778t, 780t
tenecteplase, 443t, 444
teniposide, 778t
tenofovir, 677p, 677t, 678, 678t
Tenormin, 330t, 401t
terazosin, 329t, 401t, 634, 634t
terbinafine, 684t, 685, 686
terfenadine, 668, 679
teriflunomide, 704, 705t, 706
teriparatide, 280t, 281, 282
testosterone, 615
Tetcaine, 366t
tetracaine, 366t, 741t, 742
tetracycline, 241, 242, 258t, 259,

431, 489, 495t, 497, 502t, 609, 616t, 669p, 669t, 670, 687, 812t
tetrahydrozoline, 375t
TetraVisc, 366t
Teveten, 398t, 637t
Texacort, 253t
thalidomide, 791, 791t, 792
Thalomid, 791t
theophylline, 323, 464, 471, 500, 503t, 628
thiamine, 523t, 524
thiazide, 399–400, 400p, 590t, 638, 638f, 641–642, 846t
thiazolidinediones, 564, 565
thioridazine, 342, 354t, 355, 356
Thorazine, 354t, 505t
thrombolytics, 434
thyroid extract, 573t
Thyrolar, 573t
tiagabine, 291, 314t, 315
ticarcillin, 663t
ticlopidine, 441t, 442, 445
Tikosyn, 405t
Timentin, 663t
timolol, 330, 330t, 368t, 401, 401t
Timoptic, 368t
tinzaparin, 436t, 438
tioconazole, 684t
tiotropium, 466t, 467, 467p
tipranavir, 680t, 681
Tirosint, 573t
Tisit, 246t
Tivicay, 682t
tizanidine, 291, 291t, 292, 342, 671
TNKase, 443t
TOBI, 668t
TobraDex, 371t
tobramycin, 370, 371t, 471, 668, 668t
Tobrex, 371t, 668t
tocopherol, 522
Today, 611t, 612p
Tofranil, 838t
tolcapone, 320, 320t, 321
tolterodine, 631t, 854t
Topamax, 314t
Topicaine, 741t
Topicort, 253t
topiramate, 312, 314t, 315, 540t
topotecan, 778t, 781t, 785, 786
Toprol, 330t, 401t
Toradol, 268t
torsemide, 414, 639t
Toviaz, 631t, 854t
tramadol, 321, 729t, 731–732
trandolapril, 396t, 637t
Transderm Scop, 504t
Tranxene, 348t
tranylcypromine, 344t
trastuzumab, 791t, 792
Travatan, 368t
travoprost, 368t
trazodone, 340, 345, 680
Treanda, 781t
Trental, 441t

tretinoin, 242*t*, 521
Tretin-X, 521
triamcinolone, 253*t*, 275, 276, 276*t*, 372, 372*t*, 456*t*, 462*t*
Triaminic, 453*t*
triamterene, 638, 639*t*, 641
Triaz, 241*t*.
triazolam, 348, 348*t*, 679, 680, 681
tribasic, 278*t*
TriCor, 417*t*
tricyclic antidepressants, 258*t*, 321, 340, 342–343, 344, 345, 381*t*, 633*t*, 733, 734
Triesence, 372*t*
trifluoperazine, 354*t*, 355
trifluridine, 373*t*, 374
Triglide, 417*t*
Trihexy, 319*t*
trihexyphenidyl, 319*t*, 320, 854*t*
Trilafon, 354*t*
Trileptal, 313*t*
Tri-Levlen, 608*t*
trimethoprim, 370, 371*t*, 407, 629, 672, 672*t*, 812*t*, 839*t*, 854
TriNessa, 608*t*
Tri-Norinyl, 608*t*
Triostat, 573*t*
Triphasil, 608*t*
triptans, 735, 736
Tri-Statin, 253*t*
Trixaicin, 841*t*
Trizivir, 678*t*
troleandomycin, 736
tropicamide, 366*t*
trospium, 631*t*, 854*t*
Truvada, 677*p*, 677*t*, 678*t*
Tucks, 253*t*, 509*t*
Tudorza Pressair, 463, 466*t*
Tums, 497, 497*t*, 757*t*
Tylenol, 266*p*, 725*t*, 729*t*, 808*t*, 813, 813*t*, 841*t*
Typhim Vi, 699*t*
tyramine, 344
Tysabri, 705*t*

U

ulipristal, 609, 610
Uloric, 276*t*
Ultiva, 740*t*
Ultracet, 729*t*
Ultram, 729*t*
Ultravate, 253*t*
umeclidinium, 466*t*, 467
Unasyn, 663*t*
unfractionated heparin, 436*t*

Unifiber, 491*t*
Univasc, 396*t*, 637*t*
unoprostone, 368*t*
Uro-KP, 757*t*
Uro-Mag, 757*t*
Uroxatral, 634*t*

V

vaginal ring, 611
vaginal sponge, 612
Vagistat-1, 684*t*
valacyclovir, 616*t*, 675*t*, 676
Valcyte, 373*t*
valerian, 299
valganciclovir, 373*t*, 374
Valium, 348*t*, 412*t*, 738
valproate, 315, 316
valproate sodium, 313*t*
valproic acid, 312, 313*t*, 315, 316, 352, 381*t*
valsartan, 398*t*, 637*t*
Valtrex, 675*t*
vancomycin, 471, 666, 668
Vandazole, 673
Vanos, 253*t*
Vantin, 816*t*
Vaqta, 699*t*
vardenafil, 412, 591*t*
varenicline, 473*t*, 474–475
Varivax, 699*t*
Vasotec, 396*t*, 637*t*
Vectibix, 791*t*
vecuronium, 295*t*
Velban, 781*t*
Velivet, 608*t*
venlafaxine, 326, 341*t*, 342
Venofer, 430*t*, 530
Ventolin, 460*t*
VePesid, 781*t*
Veramyst, 456*t*
verapamil, 279, 329*t*, 398*t*, 399, 401, 405*t*, 407, 412*t*, 414
Verdeso, 253*t*
Verelan, 398*t*, 405*t*
Versed, 412*t*, 738
VESIcare, 631*t*
Vexol, 372*t*
Vfend, 684*t*
Viagra, 413, 591*p*
Vibramycin, 669*t*
Vicks 44, 454*t*
Vicodin, 728, 729*t*
Vicoprofen, 729*t*
Victoza, 565*t*
Videx, 678*t*
vigabatrin, 313*t*, 315
Vigamox, 670*t*

vilanterol, 466*t*
Vimpat, 313*t*
vinblastine, 778*t*, 781*t*, 786*t*, 787, 788
vincristine, 778*t*, 779*t*, 781*t*, 786*t*, 788
vinorelbine, 778*t*, 781*t*, 786*t*, 787
Viorele, 608*t*
Viracept, 680*t*
Viramune, 679*t*
Virazole, 675*t*
Viread, 678*t*
Viroptic, 373*t*, 374
Visine, 375*t*
Visken, 330*t*
Vistaril, 504*t*, 854*t*
Vistide, 373*t*, 374
Vitekta, 682*t*
Vivotif Berna, 699*t*
Voltaren, 268*t*, 375*t*
voriconazole, 438*t*, 684*t*, 685
VoSpire ER, 460*t*
Vytorin, 417*t*

W

warfarin, 270, 334, 346, 420, 434, 436*t*, 437, 438, 439, 440, 445, 489, 500, 508, 514, 523, 688, 838, 838*t*, 853
Welchol, 510*t*
Wellbutrin, 345, 473*t*
Westcort, 253*t*
wheat dextrin, 491*t*
wild yam, 619
witch hazel, 508, 509, 509*t*

X

Xalatan, 368*t*
Xanax, 348*t*, 850, 850*p*
xanthine, 442, 464
Xeloda, 780*t*
Xenical, 539*t*
Xgeva, 280*t*
Xopenex, 460*t*, 819*t*
xylocaine, 403*t*, 412*t*, 741*t*, 838*t*

Y

Yasmin, 608*t*
Yaz, 608*t*
YF-Vax, 699*t*
Yocon, 591*t*
yohimbine, 591*t*, 592

Z

Zaditor, 375*t*
zafirlukast, 463, 463*t*, 464, 819*t*

zaleplon, 350, 351*t*
Zanaflex, 291*t*
zanamivir, 675*t*, 676
Zantac, 500*t*, 502*t*
Zarontin, 313*t*
Zaroxolyn, 639*t*
Zebeta, 330*t*, 401*t*
Zelapar, 321*t*
Zemuron, 295*t*
Zenzedi, 324*t*
Zephrex, 453*t*
Zerit, 678*t*
Zestril, 396*t*, 637*t*
Zetia, 417*t*, 420
zidovudine, 677*t*, 678, 678*t*
zileuton, 463, 463*t*, 464
Zinacef, 665*t*, 816*t*
zinc, 475, 528*t*, 531, 688
zinc oxide, 250, 254
Zioptan, 368*t*
ziprasidone, 356*t*
Zirgan, 373*t*
Zithromax, 667*t*, 816*t*
Zocor, 417*t*
ZoDerm, 241*t*.
Zofran, 506*t*, 849
Zoladex, 790
zoledronic acid, 280, 280*t*
zolmitriptan, 736, 736*t*
Zoloft, 341*t*
zolpidem, 350, 351*t*, 850
Zomig, 736*t*
Zonegran, 313*t*
zonisamide, 313*t*, 315
Zostavax, 244, 699*t*
Zosyn, 663*t*
Zovia, 608*t*
Zovirax, 675*t*
Zyban, 345, 473*t*
Zydis, 356*t*
Zyflo, 463*t*
Zyprexa, 356, 356*t*
Zyrtec, 452*t*

Subject Index

Note: Page numbers followed by an *f* indicate that the reference appears in a figure; page numbers followed by a *p* indicate that the reference appears in a photo; and page numbers followed by a *t* indicate that the reference is found in a table.

Drugs are covered in the "Generic and Brand-Name Drugs Index."

A

abbreviated new drug application (ANDA), 42, 839–840
abbreviations
    common medical, 134–135
    common prescription, 135, 136t
    error-prone abbreviation list, 135
ABCDEs, 238
ablation, 574
absence (petit mal) seizure, 311t
absorption, in GI system, 482
absorption, of drug, 64–67, 65f
    bloodflow and surface area of absorption site, 67, 67f
    chemical properties and absorption sites, 65–66
    dosage form, 65
    drug transport mechanisms and, 66–67, 66f
    geriatric patients, 838
    pediatric and neonatal patients and, 809
    route of administration, 64
abstinence, 603
Accommodator learning style, 19–20, 19t, 20f
accreditation
    accreditation organizations, 118, 118t–120t, 225–226
    defined, 118, 225
Accrediting Bureau of Health Education Schools (ABHES), 118, 225–226
ACE inhibitors, 396–397, 396t
    for angina and heart attack, 413–414
    common drug name stems for, 48t
acetaminophen
    for mild pain and fever, 725–726, 725t
    for osteoarthritis treatment, 266–267, 266p
    Stevens-Johnson syndrome, 267
    for treating fever in children, 813, 813t
acetylcholine (ACh)
    action of, 309t
    Alzheimer's disease and, 323

muscle contraction and, 287–288, 287f
acetylcholinesterase, 288
acid-base balance, 763
acid-base imbalance, 763–765
acid-base pair buffer, 763
acidic drugs
    absorption in stomach and, 66
    elderly patients and, 89
acidity, 763
acidosis, 764–765
acid reflux disease, proton pump inhibitor for, 83
acne
    characteristics of, 240
    drug treatments for, 240–243, 669
acne vulgaris, 240
acquired immune response, 693, 694t
acquired immunity
    defined, 655
    immunoglobulins, 693, 694t
    physiology of, 693, 694t
    T cells and B cells, 693, 693f
actinic keratosis, 238
active immunity, 696–697
active transport mechanisms, 66, 66f
actual body weight (ABW), 532–533, 532t
acupuncture therapy, 299
acute gout attack, 275
acute kidney injury, 636
acute myocardial infarction (MI), geriatric patients, 847
acute pain, 722
adaptive immunity, 655
addiction, 72
    centrally acting muscle relaxants and, 292
    characteristics of, 728
    defined, 51
    methadone for withdrawal, 728, 731
    opioid analgesics and, 728
Addison's disease, 574–575
addition
    decimals, 155
    fractions, 150–151
adenosine triphosphate (ATP), 524
adequate intakes (AIs), 519
adipose tissue, 237, 237f

adjuvant chemotherapy, 775
adjuvant radiation therapy, 774
administration errors, 798
admission order, 129, 130f
adrenal cortex, 553, 554f
adrenal glands, 551f, 554f
    Addison's disease, 574–575
    Cushing's syndrome, 575
    role of, 553
adrenaline (epinephrine), 34
    "fight-or-flight" response, 553
    production of, 553
adrenal medulla, 553, 554f
adrenergic agonists
    defined, 328
    sympathomimetics, 331–332
adrenergic inhibitors
    alpha blockers, 328–329, 329t
    beta blockers, 329–331, 330t
    defined, 328
adrenergic receptors, 327–328
adrenocorticotropic hormone (ACTH), 553
adulterated product, 43–44
adverse drug reaction (ADR), 46
    reporting, 219–220
    skin and, 257–259
    Vaccine Adverse Event Reporting System (VAERS), 298
Adverse Event Reporting System (FAERS), 207
advertising of drugs, 46
aerobic bacteria, 658
aerosol, 87
afferent arteriole, 624
affinity, drug action and, 62
age, as drug response factor, 88–89
aging. *See also* geriatric patients
    physiologic and pathophysiologic process, 834–836
    skin and, 238
agonist, 62
agranulocytes, 652–653, 653f
Aguilar, Abelardo, 15
albumin, 425, 425f, 750, 753
alchemy, 8
aldosterone, 625
aldosterone antagonists, 641
alimentary tract, 482
AliveCor Mobile ECG, 106
alkalinity, 763

alkalosis, 765
alkylating agents, 778t–779t, 780–782
allergen, 71
allergic reaction, 113
    drug-allergy rashes, 258–259
    heparin-induced thrombocytopenia (HIT), 259
    severe, and EpiPen, 34
    types of hypersensitivity reactions, 694, 694p
allergic response, 71
allergies
    chronic rhinitis, 455–457, 456t
    eye allergies, 374, 375t
    histamine release and, 455
    penicillin, 662
allicin, 420
allied health professional
    accreditation, 118, 118t–120t
    appearance of, 101
    attitude, 102
    career outlook for, 120
    certification, 109
    clinical duties, 111–116
    communication skills, 103–104
    critical thinking skills of, 100
    cultural and linguistic competence, 107
    defined, 97
    educational requirements, 108
    ethics and, 230
    legal responsibilities of, 226–230
    licensure, 108
    medication errors, 196–201
    nonclinical duties, 116–117
    number of, 97
    personal code of conduct and ethics, 102–103
    personal medication error prevention strategies, 200–201
    personal qualities of, 100–107
    pharmacology study for, 16–18
    preceptorship, 110
    professionalism and, 100–103
    registration, 109
    scope of practice, 110–117, 226–227
    self-direction, 100
    specialties and positions, 99t

decimal point, 154
decimals
    adding and subtracting, 155
    decimal units and values, 154, 154f
    defined, 154
    as fractions, 154
    fractions as, 150
    leading zero, 154
    multiplying and dividing, 155–156
    percent as, 159, 160
    rounding, 156–157
decongestants
    cautions for, 454
    for common cold, 453–454, 453t
    for eye allergies, 374, 375t
    as pharmacodynamic agent, 59, 59p
    side effects, 453
decubitus ulcers, 254–255
deep-vein thrombosis (DVT), 434
defecation, 484
De Humani Corporis Fabrica (On the Fabric of the Human Body) (Vesalius), 9
dehydration, 751–755, 752f, 752t
    hypertonic solutions, 754–755
    hypotonic solutions, 755
    isotonic solutions, 753–754
    symptoms of, 751, 751f
deltoid muscle, 288
delusional disorder, 353
De Materia Medica (On Medical Matters) (Dioscorides), 7
dementia
    drug therapy for, 322–323, 323t
    incidence of, 322
dendrites, 308, 309f
denominator, 148
    common, 150, 150t
deoxyribonucleic acid (DNA), 15, 15p, 34–35, 35f
dependence
    centrally acting muscle relaxants and, 292
    psychological and physical, 51
dependence, drug, 72
depolarization, 288
depression, 308, 340–346
    bupropion, 344–345
    drug treatment for, 340–346
    monoamine oxidase inhibitors (MAOIs), 344, 344t
    SSRIs and SNRIs, 340–342
    symptoms and signs of, 340
    trazodone, 345–346
    tricyclic antidepressants (TCAs), 342–344, 343t
dermal route of administration, 80
dermatitis
    drug treatments for, 251–254, 253t
    types and symptoms, 249–251, 249p, 250p

dermatophytes, 244, 683
dermis, 237, 237f
descending colon, 483f, 484
De Sedibus et Causis Morborum per Anatomen Indagatis (The Seats and Causes of Disease) (Morgagni), 9
designer drugs, 34
destructive agent, 60
detrusor muscles, 626
dexamethasone, 574, 821
dextrans, 753
dextrose, 752, 752t
DHA, 419
diabetes, 555–571
    ACE inhibitors for, 396
    blood glucose measurement, 560
    drug discoveries for, 15
    drug treatment for, 561–571
    gestational diabetes, 558
    herbal therapies, 576
    hypoglycemia symptoms/treatment, 559–560
    incretin therapies, 564–566, 565t
    insulin secretagogues, 562–563, 563t
    insulin treatment, 567–570, 568t
    lifestyle modifications, 561
    medical costs of, 556
    metabolic syndrome, 557
    metformin, 561–562, 561t
    microvascular/macrovascular complications of untreated, 559, 559t
    retinopathy, 376
    risk factors for, 558
    sodium-glucose linked transporter-2 (SGLT-2) inhibitors, 571, 571t
    symptoms of, 558–559
    thiazolidinediones (TZDs), 564, 564t
    Type 1 diabetes, 556–557, 557f
    Type 2 diabetes, 557, 558f
diabetes mellitus, 556
diabetic neuropathy, 723p
diagnostic agent, 59
dialysate, 643
dialysis, 643–644, 643f
diaper rash, 250
diaphragm, 606, 606p
diarrhea
    acute, 486
    antidiarrheal medications, 486–489, 487t
    bismuth subsalicylate, 487t, 488–489
    drugs that cause, 486t
    infections that cause, 486
    opiate derivatives, 487–488, 487t
    pediatric and neonatal patients, 824
diastole, 389

diastolic blood pressure (DBP), 393
dietary reference intakes (DRIs)
    defined, 519
    for fat-soluble vitamins, 520t
    for water-soluble vitamins, 523t
dietary supplement, 53, 53p
    defined, 220
    false claims, 220
    FDA monitoring of, 220
    USP standards for, 220, 225
    USP Verified Mark, 220
Dietary Supplement Health and Education Act (DSHEA), 53
diffusion, 67
digestion. *See also* gastrointestinal (GI) system
    defined, 482
    lower GI system and, 484
    sphincters and, 484
    upper GI system and, 482–483
digitalis toxicity, 853
digoxin, 407–408, 407p, 408t
digoxin toxicity, 853
dihydropyrimidine dehydrogenase, 784
dilation, of blood vessels, 392
dimensional analysis method, 179
Dioscorides, Pedanius, 7
dipeptidyl peptidase-4 (DPP-4) inhibitors, 565, 565t
diphtheria, pertussis and tetanus vaccine, 698f, 699t, 700, 826t
direct-acting muscle relaxants, 294, 294p
direct patient care, 112–113
direct thrombin inhibitors, 435, 436t
discharge order, 132
disease-modifying antirheumatic drugs (DMARDs)
    arthritis treatment, 841t, 842
    cautions and considerations, 274
    commonly used, 272t–273t
    contraindications, 274
    overview of, 272
    side effects, 274
disease-modifying therapies, 704, 705t, 706
distribution, drug, 67–68, 68f
    affinity for protein molecules, 68
    blood-brain barrier, 68, 68f
    drug solubility, 68
    geriatric patients, 838
    pediatric and neonatal patients, 810
diuresis, 758
diuretics
    carbonic anhydrase inhibitor, 638, 638f, 639t, 640
    commonly used, 639t
    discovery of, 15
    for edema, 755–756, 755p
    loop, 414, 415f, 638, 638f,

    639t, 640–641
    photosensitivity, 258t
    potassium-sparing, 638, 638f, 639t, 641
    sites of action, 638f
    thiazide, 399–400, 638, 638f, 639t, 641–642
Diverger learning style, 19–20, 19t, 20f
dividend, 156
division
    decimals, 155–156
    fractions, 152–153
divisor, 156
documentation, legal requirements for, 228–230
Domagk, Gerhard, 15
dopamine (DA)
    action of, 309t
    as neurotransmitter, 338
    Parkinson's disease and, 316–317, 317f
dopamine agonists, for Parkinson's disease treatment, 318–319, 318t
dosage calculations. *See* medication calculation methods
dosage formulation (dosage form), 82–87
    absorption and, 65
    liposome dosage form, 685, 685f
    liquid, 86–87
    prescription abbreviations for, 136t
    semisolid, 84–86
    solid, 82–84
dose
    dose-response relationship, 62–64
    drug concentrations and steady state, 62–64, 63f
    loading dose, 62
    peak and trough, 63
    therapeutic range, 62, 63f
    toxic concentration, 62, 63f
dose-response relationship
    drug concentrations and steady state, 62–64, 63f
    time-response curve, 62, 63f
    toxic concentration, 62, 63f
doshas, 5, 5f
dram, 162, 163t
Dr. Bernard Lo's Clinical Model, 103
drivers of cancer, 771–772
dronabinol, 507
drug(s)
    action of, 61–70
    allergic response, 71
    approval process for, 38–42
    beneficial effects of, 70
    biotechnologically engineered drugs, 16
    brand or trade name, 17, 37
    chemical name, 36–37
    classifications for, 47–53
    clearance, 69

defined, 4
designer drugs, 34
as destructive agent, 60
as diagnostic agent, 59
disposal of, by patients,
    193–194
expiration date, 193–194
FDA's role in development,
    42–47
generic name, 17, 37
half-life, 69
handling and storage of, 114
indication and
    contraindication, 70
interactions, 71–72
marketing and advertising of
    drugs, 46
natural sources of, 32–33
orphan drugs, 41, 219
packaging and labeling of,
    43–45
as pharmacodynamic agent, 59
as prophylactic agent, 59–60
safety and efficacy of, 42–43
scheduled drugs, 221–222
semisynthetic, 33
side effects of, 70
sources of, 32–34
synthesized, 34
synthetic, 32
therapeutic agent, 58–59
therapeutic effect, 70
uses of, 58–60
drug abuse, 72
drug action
    absorption, 64–67, 65f
    affinity and, 26
    agonists and antagonists, 62
    distribution, 67–68, 68f
    dose-response relationship,
        62–64
    drug concentrations and steady
        state, 62–64, 63f
    elimination, 69–70
    excretion, 69–70
    loading dose, 62
    mechanisms of, 61–64
    metabolism, 59
    onset of action, 62
    receptors, 61, 61f
    time-response curve, 62, 63f
drug administration
    medication errors during, 197
    six "rights" of correct drug
        administration, 197
drug-allergy rashes, 258–259, 258p
drug approval process, 38–42
    abbreviated new drug
        application (ANDA), 42
    clinical trials, 39
    FDA's role in, 38, 219
    new drug application (NDA),
        39–40
    overview of, 41f
    postmarketing surveillance, 46
    preclinical testing, 38

risk and cost of drug
    development, 41–42
timeline for, 41
drug classes
    controlled substances, 48–51
    defined, 47
    dietary supplement, 53, 53p
    homeopathic medications,
        52–53, 52p
    mechanism of action, 47
    naming rules for generic
        names, 18
    over-the-counter (OTC) drug,
        51–52
    prescription drug, 48
    therapeutic classes, 47
drug dependence, 72
drug-drug interaction, 71–72
Drug Enforcement Administration
    (DEA), 48, 217
    controlled substance
        restrictions by, 221–223
    defined, 221
    Electronic Prescriptions for
        Controlled Substances
        (EPCS) program, 126
    inspection of pharmacies by,
        223
    prescribers of controlled
        substances registration,
        223–224
    Prescription Drug Take-Back
        Day, 194
    role and responsibilities of, 221
Drug Enforcement Administration
    (DEA) number, 127–128
Drug Facts box, 52, 52p
drug-food interaction, 72
drug handbook, 24, 25t
drug interactions, 71–72
drug literacy, 199
drug nomenclature, 36–37
drug-package insert, 44, 44f
drug recall, 46, 47t
drug-resistant TB, 470
drug response factor, 88–90
    age, 88–89
    gender, 89
    GI system function, 90
    kidney function, 90
    liver function, 90
    nutritional status, 90
    weight, 89
drug-seekers, 50
drug sponsor, 38
drug therapy
    defined, 4
    patient's understanding of,
        192, 193t
drug tolerance, 50
drug transport mechanisms,
    66–67, 66f
dry eye, chronic, 366, 375–376,
    375t
dry eye syndrome (DES), 844
drying agents, 379t, 380–381

dry macular degeneration,
    376–377
dry powder inhaler (DPI), 462,
    462p
ductus deferens, 584
duodenal ulcers, 495
dyskinesias, 319
dyslipidemia, 524

E

eardrops, 379–380, 380f
ears, 377–381
    common disorders of, 377–381
    drying agents, 379t, 380–381
    earwax removers, 379t,
        380–381
    external ear infection (otitis
        externa), 379–380
    herbal and alternative
        medicines for, 381
    middle ear infection (otitis
        media), 377–379, 378t–379t
    otic analgesics, 378, 379t
    otic antibiotics, 378–379, 378t
    ototoxicity, 381, 381t
    patient education for ear drop
        administration, 380, 380f
    structures and functions of,
        354f, 364–365, 365f
    swimmer's ear, 379
earwax removers, 379t, 380–381
Eastern medicine. See traditional
    Eastern medicine
Ebers Papyrus, 5, 5p
echinacea
    to boost immune function, 687
    for respiratory tract infections,
        475, 475p
echinocandin, 685
eclampsia, 593
ectopic pregnancy, 595
eczema
    drug treatments for, 251–254,
        253t
    symptoms of, 250–251, 250p
edema, 755–756, 755p
educational requirements, 108
efferent arteriole, 624
Ehrlich, Paul, 14
elastin, 238
elderly patients. See geriatric
    patients
electrocardiogram (ECG or EKG)
    machine, 390, 391f
electrocardiogram (ECG)
    technicians, 112, 112p
electrolytes/electrolyte balance
    acid-base imbalance, 763–765
    defined, 748
    disorders of imbalance,
        756–762
    herbal and alternative therapies,
        766
    hypocalcemia/hypercalcemia,
        759–760
    hypochloremia/

hyperchloremia, 762
hypokalemia/hyperkalemia,
    758–759
hypomagnesemia/
    hypermagnesemia, 760–761
hyponatremia/hypernatremia,
    757–758
hypophosphatemia/
    hyperphosphatemia,
    761–762
list of, and normal
    concentrations, 749–750,
    749t
physiology of, 748–750
replacement products, 756,
    757t
electronic health records (EHRs)
    benefits of, 104, 105f
    confidentiality and, 227f
    e-prescription, 126f
    linked to patient health record,
        113
    medication safety and, 205
electronic medication
    administration records (eMARs),
    206
electronic prescription
    (e-prescription), 125, 126f
    for controlled substances, 126
    minimizing medication errors
        and, 204, 205f
Electronic Prescriptions for
    Controlled Substances (EPCS)
    program, 126
Eli Lilly and Company, 15
elimination, 622
elimination, of drug, 69–70
elixir, 87
embolus, 434
embryo, 582
emergency contraceptives,
    609–610, 609p
emergency room drug kit, 411,
    412t
emesis, 503
emollient laxative, 491t, 492
emphysema, 465, 465f
empirical therapy, 468–469, 823
emulsion, 87
encounter form, 117
endocrine system
    Addison's disease, 574–575
    aging process and, 835–836
    anatomy and physiology of,
        550–555, 551f–555f
    circadian rhythm and, 553,
        554f
    Cushing's syndrome, 575
    diabetes, 555–571
    herbal and alternative therapies,
        576
    hyperthyroidism, 573–574
    hypothyroidism, 571–573,
        572f, 573t
endogenous chemical messengers,
    61, 61f

Institute of Medicine (IOM), 188, 189
institutional review board (IRB), 38
insulin
  basal and bolus, 567, 567f
  cautions for, 570
  commonly used, 567, 568t
  first extraction of, 14
  glucose metabolism and, 554, 555f
  injections sites for, 568–569, 569f
  medication errors and, 570
  onset and duration of action for, 567, 568f
  route of administration, 77
  side effects of, 569–570
  Type 2 diabetes and, 557
insulin pumps, 569
insulin resistance, 557
insulin secretagogues, 562–563, 563t
insurance forms, 117
integrase inhibitors, 681, 682t
integumentary system, 235–259
  adverse drug reactions affecting, 257–259
  aging process and, 834
  anatomy and physiology of, 236–237, 237f
  common skin disorders and drug treatments, 237–257
  herbal and alternative therapies, 259
  overview, 236
interferon betas, 704, 705t
interferons, for melanoma treatment, 774
interleukin-1 (IL-1), 272
interleukins, for melanoma treatment, 774
intermediate acting insulin, 567, 568f, 568t
internal urinary sphincter, 626
international normalized ratio (INR), 434, 853
international units (IUs), 519
interprofessional communication, 111–112
interstitial spaces, 747, 747f
intracellular calcium stores, 288
intracellular fluid, 746, 747f
intradermal (ID) route of administration, 78, 79f
intramuscular (IM) injections, 288
intramuscular (IM) route of administration, 78, 78f
intranasal route of administration, 81
intraocular pressure, 366, 367f
intrathecal (IT) route of administration, 79, 783
intrauterine device (IUD), 614–615, 614p
intravascular space, 747, 747f
intravenous route of

administration, 76, 77f
  absorption, 64
  central IV line, 76
  peripheral IV line, 76
intravitreal implant, 79
intrinsic aging, 238
intrinsic pathway, 426, 427f
inventory, of supplies and equipment, 117
investigational drugs, for cancer treatment, 794–795
investigational new drug (IND) application, 38
in virtro fertilization (IVF), 597, 597f
iodine, 528t, 529–530, 529p
iPLEDGE, 242–243, 242p
iris, 362, 363f
iron
  in blood, 425
  DRI values for, 528t
  overview of, 530
  supplementation for anemia treatment, 430–431, 430t, 816–817
iron-deficiency anemia, 428, 530
  children and, 816–817
irritable bowel syndrome (IBS), 509–511, 510t
ischemic stroke, 433, 848
isotonicity, 749
isotonic solutions, 753–754
IV fluid products, 751–752

J

Japanese encephalitis vaccine, 699t, 701
jaundice, 672, 672p
jejunostomy (J) tube, 543, 544f
Jenner, Edward, 10, 10f
jock itch, 244
Joint Commission, 118
  accreditation and medication safety standards, 210–211
  error-prone abbreviation list, 135
  Sentinel Event Policy, 207–208
  SPEAK UP program, 211
  standards set by, 225
joints
  anatomy and function of, 264, 265f
  gouty arthritis, 274–277
  osteoarthritis, 265–271, 266f, 842f
  rheumatoid arthritis, 271–274, 842f

K

kava, 358
Keats, John, 12
keratin, 236
keratolytic agent, 241
keratomalacia, 521
ketoacidosis, 557
ketoconazole, 243

ketones, 555
kidney disease
  ACE inhibitors and ARBs, 636–638, 637t
  anemia of chronic disease, 428–429
  dialysis, 643–644, 643f
  diuretics, 638–642, 638f, 639t
  end-stage, 644
  kidney transplantation, 644
  potassium supplements, 642
  stages of chronic, 636t
kidneys
  acute kidney injury, 636
  anatomy and physiology of, 622–625, 623f–625f
  children and drug therapy, 810–811
  chronic kidney disease, 636–644
  drugs commonly affected by impaired, 839t
  elderly patients and drug therapy, 89, 839
  excretion of drugs, 69–70
  function of, as drug response factor, 90
  kidney function assessment, 627
  kidney stones and calcium, 279
  kidney transplantation, 644
  nephrons and urine formation, 624–625, 625f
  nephrotoxicity and renal dosing, 627–629
  NSAIDS use and, 270, 628
  renin-angiotensin system, 392, 392f
  role of, 622–623
  susceptibility to medication errors and function of, 198
kidney stones, 760, 760p
killer T cells, 656, 656f, 693, 693f
Kolb, David, 19
Kolb's Learning Styles Inventory, 19–20, 19t, 20f
kwashiorkor, 542

L

labeler code, 45
labels, drug
  black box warning, 44, 44f, 204
  for controlled substance, 49f
  design for safety, 203
  Drug Facts box, 52, 52p
  drug-package insert, 44, 44f
  FSA requirements, 43–45
  National Drug Code (NDC) number, 45, 45f
  over-the-counter (OTC) drug, 52
  pregnancy labeling system, 43
labels, medication, 139–141
  auxiliary labels, 141, 141f
  information on, 140, 140f

national drug code (NDC) number, 203
  tall-man lettering, 203, 203p
laboratory information management system (LIMS), 106
laboratory information system (LIS), 106
lactic acidosis, 562
lactobacilli, 515
lactulose, 494
lanolin, 259
laparoscopic banding, 538, 538f
large intestine, 483f, 484
laryngopharynx, 448, 449f
larynx, 448, 449f
laws/legal issues, 216–230
  accreditation standards and organizations, 225–226
  confidentiality, 227–228
  defined, 217
  documentation and handling of medication, 228–230
  healthcare standards, 224–225
  legal responsibilities of allied health professionals, 226–230
  professional ethics, 230
  regulatory agencies, 217–224
  scope of practice, 226–227
  significant healthcare legislation, 217, 218t
laxatives
  bowel preparation ("prep") laxatives, 492–493, 493p
  bulk-forming laxatives, 490–491, 491p, 491t
  emollient laxative, 491t, 492
  geriatric patients and, 854
  miscellaneous, 494
  overview of, 489–490
  stimulant laxatives, 491t, 492
  stool softeners, 491t, 492
leading zero, 154, 210
learning styles
  Kolb's Learning Styles Inventory, 19–20, 19t, 20f
  preferred learning styles, 21
  types of, 19
legend drug, 48
lens, 362, 363f
lesions, 238
leucovorin, 784
leucovorin rescue, 784
leukocytes, 425f, 426, 652–653, 653f
leukotriene inhibitors, 463–464, 463t
leukotriene receptor antagonists, 818, 819t
leukotrienes, 463
Levin tube, 544f
lexicon, 6
Leydig cells, 584
LHRH agonists, 790
lice, 245–248, 246t

determining understandability, 23
onset of action, 62
oocytes, 586
open-angle glaucoma, 366, 367f
ophthalmic alpha receptor agonists, 366–369, 367t
ophthalmic anti-infective agents, 370–371, 371t
ophthalmic beta blockers, 366–369, 367t
ophthalmic corticosteroids, 372, 372t
ophthalmic drops, patient education for administration, 366, 367
ophthalmic glaucoma agents, 366–369, 367t
ophthalmic local anesthetics, 366t
ophthalmic ointments, 370
ophthalmic route of administration, 81, 81p
opiate derivatives, for diarrhea, 487–488, 487t
opioid analgesics, 728–732, 729t
    natural opioids, 728–730, 729t
    semisynthetic opioids, 729t, 730–731
    synthetic opioids, 729t, 731–732
opioid receptor antagonist, 742
opioids, 728
opioid tolerant, 731
opthalmic antivirals, 373–374, 373t
optic nerve, 363f, 366
oral contraceptives, 15
    acne amelioration and, 607
    cautions and considerations, 608–609
    common products, 607–608, 608t
    overview of, 606–607
oral corticosteroids, 462
oral disintegrating tablet, 83
oral route of administration
    absorption, 64, 74
    advantages of, 74
    buccal route, 75
    GI track and, 74
    pediatric and neonatal patients and, 809
    sublingual route, 74–75
oral thrush, 463, 683, 683p, 684t
oral thyroid supplementation, 574
organizational policies and procedures, to prevent organizational failure, 191
organization failure, 190–191
organ of Corti, 364f, 365, 365f
organ rejection, 710
organ transplantation, immune suppression and, 710–712
oropharynx, 448, 449f
orphan drugs, 41, 219
orthostatic hypotension, 398, 634, 835

osmolarity, 753
osmosis, 748
osteoarthritis (OA)
    acetaminophen, 266–267, 266p
    chondroitin, 282
    COX-2 Inhibitors, 270–271
    drug treatments for, 266–271
    geriatric patients and, 840–841, 841t
    glucosamine, 282
    incidence of, 265
    of knee joint, 266, 266f
    nonsteroidal anti-inflammatory drugs (NSAIDs), 267–270, 268f, 268t, 269f
    other osteoporosis agents, 280f, 281–282
    selective estrogen receptor modulators (SERMs), 280t, 281
    symptoms of, 265–266
osteoblasts, 264, 264f
osteoclasts, 262, 263, 264f
osteomalacia, 522
osteopenia, 278
osteoporosis, 277–282, 600
    bisphosphonates, 279–280, 280t
    calcium and vitamin D, 277–278, 278t
    drug treatment for, 278–282
    geriatric patients, 843–844, 843f
    hormone replacement therapy (HRT), 278
    incidence of, 262
    risk factors for, 277–278
    symptoms of, 277, 277p
otic analgesics, 378, 379t
otic route of administration, 81
otitis externa, 379–380
otitis media, 377–379, 378t–379t
    treating pediatric patients, 814–815, 816t
ototoxicity, 381, 381t, 666
    alkylating agents and, 780
ova, 582
oval window, 364, 364f, 365f
ovaries, 551f, 582, 583f
overactive bladder, 631
overflow incontinence, 631
overnutrition, 532
over-the-counter (OTC) drugs
    for acne, 240–241, 241t
    advertising of, 46
    to avoid for pediatric patients, 812t
    behind the-counter products, 51, 51p
    Drug Facts box, 52, 52p
    FDA and, 219
    overview of, 51
    product labeling, 52
    sale of precursor's to methamphetamine, 222–223
ovulation, 586, 587f

ovulation induction, 597
ovulation stimulants, 598–599, 599t
ovum, 585, 586f
oxygen
    bloodflow in circulatory system, 388, 389f
    gas-exchange process, 450, 450f

P

package code, 45
packages, drug
    black box warning, 44, 44f
    drug-package insert, 44, 44f
    FDA requirements, 43–45
    safety and design of, 203
Paget's disease, 279
pain, 720–743
    acute, 722
    analgesic and anesthetic antagonist, 742
    anatomy and physiology of, 721, 721f
    anesthesia, 738–742, 740t
    assessment scales for, 723–724f
    chronic, 722
    fear of addiction and control of, 728
    as fifth vital sign, 720
    geriatric patients and drugs for, 855
    herbal and alternative therapies, 743
    mild-to-moderate pain disorders, 725–727, 725t
    moderate-to-severe pain disorders, 727–738, 729t, 734t, 736t, 737t
    neuropathic, 723
    neuropathic pain agents, 733–734, 734t
    nonopioid analgesics for, 725–727, 725t
    NSAID blocking pathway, 267, 268f
    opioid analgesics for, 728–732, 729t
    perception of, 721, 721f
    selective serotonin receptor agonists for, 735–736, 736t
    somatic, 722
    triptans for, 735–736, 736t
    types of, 722–723
    visceral, 723
pain receptors, 721
palmar-plantar erythema, 784, 784p
palliative chemotherapy, 775
pancreas, 551f
    function in GI tract, 483f, 484, 485f
    glucose metabolism, 554–555, 555f
    role of, 554
pancreatic enzyme supplements, 471
panic disorder, 345–346

pantothenic acid, 523t, 525
para-aminobenzoic acid (PABA), 239
Paracelsus, 8
parasites, 686, 686p
parasitic infections, 686–687, 687t
parasympathetic nervous system, 307, 327f, 328
parathyroid glands, 551f, 552, 553f
parathyroid hormone, 281, 552
parenteral nutrition, 545–546
parenteral route of administration, 76–79
    benefits of, 76
    epidural route, 79
    intradermal route, 78, 79f
    intramuscular route, 78, 78f
    intrathecal route, 79
    intravenous route, 76, 77f
    subcutaneous route, 76–77, 77f
parietal cells, 483
Parkinson's disease (PD)
    anticholinergics and amantadine, 319–320, 319t
    COMT inhibitors, 320–321, 321t
    dopamine agonists, 318–319, 318t
    drugs that cause symptoms that mimic, 317
    incidence of, 316
    mechanism of, 316–317, 317f
    monoamine oxidase inhibitors (MAOIs), 321, 321t
    symptoms of, 316–317
partial seizure, 310, 311f, 311t
partial thromboplastin time (PTT), 434
passive immunity, 695
passive transport mechanisms, 66f, 67
paste, 86
patent, 37, 219
pathogenic bacteria, 658
patient adherence, 115
patient-centered approach, 113
patient education
    anticoagulation therapy, 437
    asthma medication for children, 819
    ear drop administration, 380, 380f
    eye drop/ointment administration, 366, 367, 370
    glucose meters, 560
    health literacy, 115
    home ovulation test, 596
    home pregnancy testing, 594
    hyperphosphatemia, 761
    injection-site reaction prevention, 706
    insulin injections, 569
    medication error prevention and, 199
    medication measurement, 165
    metered-dose inhaler use, 461

reproductive systems, 581–619. *See also* female reproductive system; male reproductive system
  aging process and, 836
  anatomy and physiology of, 583–588, 584*f*, 585*f*
  conditions and disorders of, 588–603
  contraception, 603–615
  gender reassignment, 615
  herbal and alternative therapies, 619
  sex hormone production and reproduction, 582–583, 583*f*
  sexually transmitted infections, 616–619
rescue therapies, 458
resected, 773
respiratory acidosis, 764
respiratory alkalosis, 765
respiratory depression, 730
respiratory distress syndrome (RDS), 821–822, 822*p*
respiratory syncytial virus (RSV), 822
respiratory system, 447–475
  aging process and, 835
  anatomy and physiology of, 448, 449*f*, 450
  asthma, 457–464, 458*f*, 460*t*, 462*t*, 463*t*, 817–820
  chronic obstructive pulmonary disease (COPD), 465–468, 465*f*, 466*t*, 467*t*
  common cold, 451–455, 452*t*, 453*t*, 454*t*
  croup, 820–821
  cystic fibrosis (CF), 471–472
  herbal and alternative therapies, 475
  lower respiratory tract, 449*f*, 450, 450*f*
  pediatric patients and disorders of, 817–823
  pneumonia, 468–469, 822–823, 823*t*
  respiratory distress syndrome (RDS), 821–822, 822*p*
  respiratory syncytial virus (RSV), 822
  rhinitis and nasal congestion, 455–457, 456*t*
  smoking and, 472–475
  tuberculosis, 469–470, 470*t*
  upper respiratory tract, 448, 449*f*
reticulocyte count, 432, 432*t*
retina, 362, 363*f*
retinoic acids, 520
retinoids, 242–243, 242*p*, 242*t*
  iPLEDGE, 242–243, 242*p*
retinopathy, 366, 376, 559*t*
retractions, 820
retrovirus, drug treatment for, 676–677
reuptake, 338
reverse peristalsis, 502

reverse transcriptase, 676
reversible ischemic neurologic deficit (RIND), 848–849
rhabdomyolysis, 299
rhabdomyolysis., 739
rheumatoid arthritis (RA)
  biologic response modifiers, 272, 273*t*
  disease-modifying antirheumatic drugs (DMARDs), 272, 272*t*–273*t*, 274
  geriatric patients, 841–842, 842*f*
  lab test for, 271
  symptoms of, 271, 271*p*
rheumatologist, 707
Rh factor, 427–428, 713
rhinitis, 455–457, 456*t*
riboflavin, 523*t*, 524
ribonucleic acid (RNA), 34
rickets, 522, 522*p*
rights, six "rights" of correct drug administration, 197
ringworm, 244
rod cells, 362–363, 363*f*
rod-shaped bacteria, 659*f*
Roman numeral system, 146–148, 147*t*
root-cause analysis, 196
root word, 111
Rosacea, 240, 240*p*
rotavirus, 824
  vaccine for, 699*t*, 701, 826*t*
routes of administration, 73–81
  absorption and, 64
  local routes, 79–81, 80*t*
  pediatric and neonatal patients and, 809
  systemic routes, 73–79, 74*t*

S

Saccharomyces boulardii (S. boulardii), 515
safety. *See also* medication safety
  child-resistant container, 202, 202*p*
  drug disposal by patients, 193–195
  drug handling and storage, 114, 199
  medication safety measures, 201–206
  package, label and medication design for, 203–204
  patient safety, 114
  preprinted prescription forms, 202
Safety Data Sheets (SDSs), 797–798, 797*f*
St. John's wort, 358, 619
salicylates, ototoxicity, 381*t*
salicylic acid, 241, 241*t*
saliva, 484
salivary glands, 483*f*, 484
Salk, Jonas, 15

Salmonella, as cause of diarrhea, 486
SAMe, 358
satiety, 536, 564
saturated fats, 535
saw palmetto, 645
scabicides, 247–248
scabies, 246–248, 246*t*
scheduled drugs, 48–49, 49*t*, 221–222, 222*t*
  disposing, 229
  ordering, 228–229
  storing, 229
  tracking, 229
Schedule I drugs, 49*t*, 221, 222*t*
Schedule II drugs, 49*t*, 221, 222*t*, 223–224
  disposing of, 229
  documentation requirements, 228
  prescription for, 126–127
  tracking, 229
Schedule III drugs, 49*t*, 221, 222*t*, 223
Schedule IV drugs, 49*t*, 221, 222*t*, 223
Schedule V drugs, 49*t*, 221, 222*t*, 223
schedule, of controlled substances, 48, 49*t*, 218*t*
schizophrenia, 308, 338
  drug treatment for, 353–357, 354*t*, 356*t*
  symptoms of, 353
schizophreniform disorder, 353
Schmiedeberg, Oswald, 11
Schwann cells, 308
sciatic nerve, 723
sclera, 362, 363*f*
scope of practice, 110–117, 226–227
  clinical documentation, 113–114
  clinical duties, 111–116
  defined, 110
  direct patient care, 112–113
  interprofessional communication, 111–112
  nonclinical duties, 116–117
  patient education, 115–116
  patient safety, 114
  protected health information, 115
scrotum, 584, 584*f*
scrubs, 101
scruple, 162, 163*t*
scurvy, 527
sebaceous glands, 237
seborrheic dermatitis, 249–250
sebum, 240
secondary cancer, 782
secretion, 624
sedative, 347
sedative-hypnotics, geriatric patients and, 850–851
seizure disorders, 310–316
  antiepileptic drugs (AEDs),

312–316, 313*t*–314*t*
  drug treatment for, 312–316
  epilepsy, 310
  symptoms and causes, 310
  types of seizures, 310, 311*t*
seizures (convulsions)
  causes of, 310
  defined, 310
  generalized, 310, 311*f*, 311*t*
  partial, 310, 311*f*, 311*t*
seizure threshold, 732
selection error, 196
selective estrogen receptor modulators (SERMs), 280*t*, 281
selective serotonin receptor agonists
  common drug name stems for, 48*t*
  for migraine headaches, 735–736, 736*t*
  triptans, 735–736, 736*t*
selective serotonin reuptake inhibitors (SSRIs), 340–342, 341*f*, 341*t*
selenium, 528*t*, 531
selenium sulfide, 243
self-direction, 100
self-injector pens, 567*p*, 569
semen, 584
semicircular canals, 364*f*, 365, 365*f*
seminal vesicles, 584, 584*f*
semisolid formulation, 84–86
  cream, 85
  gel, 85
  lotion, 86
  ointment, 85
  paste, 86
  suppository, 85
  transdermal patch, 86
semisynthetic drug, 33
semisynthetic opioids, 729*t*, 730–731
Semmelweis, Ignaz, 11
sensation, 721, 721*f*
sensory system. *See also* pain
  aging process and, 834–835
  defined, 362
  ears, 377–381
  eyes, 362–377
sentinel event, 207–208
Sentinel Event Policy, 207–208
sepsis, 826–827, 827*f*
serotonin, 540
  as neurotransmitter, 338
  selective serotonin reuptake inhibitors (SSRIs), 340–342, 341*f*, 341*t*
  serotonin-norepinephrine reuptake inhibitors (SNRIs), 340–342, 341*f*, 341*t*
serotonin (5-HT), 309*r*
serotonin agonists, 540–541, 541*t*
serotonin-norepinephrine reuptake inhibitors (SNRIs), 340–342, 341*f*, 341*t*
serotonin syndrome, 342, 539–540
serotonin type 3 (5-HT3) receptor antagonists, 506, 506*t*, 507*f*

Serturner, Friedrich Wilhelm, 728p
serum creatinine (SCr), 627
Seven-Step Decision Model, 103
severe pain, 727
sexually transmitted infections
    (STIs)
        bacterial, 616–618
        chlamydia, 616
        common drug therapy for,
            616, 616t
        genital herpes, 618
        gonorrhea, 617
        human immunodeficiency
            virus (HIV), 618–619
        human papillomavirus (HPV),
            618
        syphilis, 617
        vaginosis, 617–618
        viral, 618–619
sharps disposal, 195, 195p
shingles, 244
short-acting beta agonists,
    460–461, 460t, 818, 818t, 819t
short-acting insulin, 567, 568f,
    568t
sickle-cell anemia, 429, 429f
side effect
    defined, 70
    most common, 70
sigmoid colon, 483f, 484
signa, 127f, 128
signal conduction, 338, 339f
signal transduction inhibitors,
    793–794
silver sulfadiazine, 257
single order, 129
sinoatrial (SA) node, 390, 391f
sinuses, 448, 449f
sinus rhythm, 402
site of administration, prescription
    abbreviations for, 136t
six "rights" of correct drug
    administration, 197
skeletal muscles, 286, 287f
skeletal system
    aging process and, 834
    anatomy and physiology of,
        262–264, 263f–265f
    arthritis, 262
    bone structure and function,
        262–264, 263f, 264f
    gouty arthritis, 274–277
    herbal and alternative therapies,
        282
    osteoarthritis, 265–271
    osteoporosis, 262, 277–282
    overview, 262
    rheumatoid arthritis, 271–274
skin
    acne and dandruff, 240–243
    adverse drug reactions
        affecting, 257–259
    aging, sun exposure and skin
        cancer, 238–240
    anatomy and physiology of,
        236–237, 237f
    burns, 255–257

cancer, 238, 238f
common disorders and drug
    treatments, 237–257
decubitus ulcers, 254–255
dermatitis, eczema and
    psoriasis, 249–254
drug-allergy rashes, 258–259,
    258p
hair loss, 248–249
herbal and alternative therapies,
    259
infections of, 244–245, 683,
    684t
lice and scabies infestation,
    245–248
photosensitivity, 258, 258t
rash, as drug side effect, 70
sleep aids, 350–351, 351t
sleep hygiene, 349
small intestines
    in digestive process, 482, 483f,
        484
    drug absorption in, 67, 67f, 72,
        74, 484
smallpox, 9–10
smartphone applications (apps),
    106
smoking
    nicotine dependence, 472
    respiratory system and, 472
smoking cessation
    benefits of, 472
    drug treatments for, 473–475,
        473t
    nicotine withdrawal, 472–473
smooth muscles, 287, 287f
sodium
    electrolyte role, 749
    hypertonic solutions and,
        754–755
    hyponatremia/hypernatremia,
        757–758
    normal concentration of, 749t
    replacement products, 757t
sodium bicarbonate, 763,
    764–765, 764t
sodium-channel blockers
    as antiepileptic agents, 313t
    contraindications, 315
sodium-glucose linked
    transporter-2 (SGLT-2)
    inhibitors, 571, 571t
sodium influx, 288
sodium phosphate, 493
sodium/potassium exchange pump,
    66
solid formulation
    absorption and, 65
    caplet, 84
    capsule, 83
    gelcap, 84
    implant, 84
    lozenge or troche, 84
    powder, 84
    tablet, 82–83, 83f
solubility, 68
solute, 87, 746

solution, 86–87
solvent, 87, 746
somatic nervous system, 306–307
somatic pain, 722
sound waves, 364
soy, 619
spacer, for inhaler, 460, 820, 820p
SPEAK UP program, 211
spectrum of activity, 659
sperm, 582
spermicide, 604
spherical-shaped bacteria, 659f
sphincters, digestive process and,
    484
sphygmomanometer, 393
spill kits, 796, 796p
spinal realignment, 299
spiral-shaped bacteria, 659f
spirochetes, 659f
spleen, 654, 654f
squamous cell carcinoma, 238
stable angina, 409
standard
    defined, 224
    organizations providing,
        224–225
standard time, 172, 173t
standing order, 132, 133f
stapes, 364–365, 364f, 365f
Staphylococcus aureus, 244
State Boards of Pharmacy,
    medication error reporting, 207
statins, 416–417, 417t
stat order, 132
status epilepticus, 311t, 312
steady state, 62–64, 63f
steatorrhea, 471
stents, coronary artery, 410, 410f
Stevens-Johnson syndrome,
    258–259, 258p, 267, 672
stimulant laxatives, 491t, 492
stomach, 482, 483f. See also
    gastrointestinal (GI) system
        acid environment and drug
            absorption, 65–66, 483
        drug absorption in, 74
        elderly patients and drug
            therapy, 89
        NSAIDS and, 269
stool, 484
stool softeners, 491t, 492
strep throat, 825
streptococcal infections, 825
Streptomyces erythreus, 15
stress ulcers, 495
striated muscles, 286, 287f
stridor, 820
stroke, 848–849
    anticoagulant agents, 435–440,
        436t
    anticoagulation antagonists,
        440–441, 440t
    antiplatelet agents, 441–442,
        441t
    prevention and treatment
        overview, 434
    thrombolytic agents, 442–444,

443t
    types of, 433
subcutaneous route (sub-Q) route
    of administration, 76–77, 77f
subcutaneous tissue, 237, 237f
sublingual route of administration,
    74–75
    absorption and, 65
subscription, 127f, 128
substance P, 507
substantia nigra, 316–317, 317f
subtherapeutic dose, 192
subtraction
    decimals, 155
    fractions, 150–151
sucralfate, 500–501
suffix, 111–112
sulfa drugs, 671–672, 672t
    cautions for pediatric use, 812t
sulfonamides
    for eye infection, 371t
    jaundice, 672, 672p
    overview of, 671–672, 672t
    Stevens-Johnson syndrome,
        259, 672
sulfonylureas, 562–563, 563t
sun exposure
    skin and, 238
    sunscreen and, 238–240
sun protection factor (SPF), 239
sunscreens, 238–240, 239t
super bill, 117
suppositories
    for constipation, 490
    as dosage form, 85, 85p
    glycerin suppositories, 494
    insertion, 490, 490f
surfactant, 821
surgical advances, 11
Sushruta, 5
Sushruta Samhita, 5
suspension, 87
sustained-release (SR) medications,
    83
sweat glands, 237, 237f
swimmer's ear, 379
sympathetic-mediated pain, 723
sympathetic nerves, 327
sympathetic nervous system, 307,
    327–328, 327f
    "fight-or-flight" response, 327
sympathomimetic drugs, 539–540,
    540p, 540t
synaptic cleft, 338, 339f
synaptic space, 308
syndrome of inappropriate
    secretion of antidiuretic hormone
    (SIADH), 851
synergistic drug therapy, 668, 725
synergistic effect, 776
synovial fluid, 264, 265f
synovial membrane, 264, 265f
synthesized drug, 34
synthetic drugs, 33
synthetic opioids, 729t, 731–732
syphilis, 617
syrup, 86

Système International (SI), 165–166, 166t
systemic corticosteroids, 708–710, 709t
systemic effect, 73
systemic lupus erythematosus (SLE), 707–708, 707t
systemic routes of administration, 73–79, 74t
  implantation route, 79
  oral route, 74–75
  overview of, 73–74, 74t
  parenteral route, 76–79, 77f–79f
  rectal route, 76
  transdermal route, 75, 75f
systems of measurement
  apothecary system, 162–163, 163t
  avoirdupois system, 163
  conversions between, 169, 169t–170t
  historical overview of, 162
  household system, 164, 164t
  metric system, 165–168
  temperature, 171–172
systole, 389
systolic blood pressure (SBP), 393

T

tablet coating, 82
tablets
  characteristics of, 82
  chewable tablet, 83
  compression tablet, 82–83, 83f
  multiple-compression tablet, 83, 83f
  oral disintegrating tablet, 83
tachycardia, 402, 403f
Takeaway Environmental Return System, 194
tall-man lettering, 203, 203p, 798, 799f
tardive dyskinesia, 355
Target, 203
targeted anticancer therapies, 790–794
  angiogenesis inhibitors, 791–792, 791t
  monoclonal antibodies, 791t, 792–793
  signal transduction inhibitors, 793–794
T cells, 653, 653f, 655–656, 656f, 693, 693f
TeamSTEPPS, 212
technical failure, 201
technology, up-to-date, to prevent organizational failure, 191
technology skills, 104–106, 105f
telemedicine, 106
telephone prescription, 125
temperature
  equivalencies, 171–172, 171t
  Fahrenheit and Celsius, 171
temporary abstinence, 603

testes, 551f, 582, 583f, 584f
testosterone, 583, 583f
  exogenous testosterone, 589–590
  as primary male hormone, 584–585
tetanus vaccine, 699t
tetany, 759
tetracyclines
  cautions for pediatric use, 812t
  common drug name stems for, 48t
  overview of, 669–670, 669t
  Stevens-Johnson syndrome, 259
thalamus, 307, 308f
therapeutic agent, 58–59
therapeutic classes, 47
therapeutic effect, 70
therapeutic range, 62, 63f
therapeutic window', 408
thiamine, 523t, 524
thiazide diuretics, 399–400, 638, 638f, 639t, 641–642
thiazolidinediones (TZDs), 48t, 564, 564t
third-hand smoke, 101
third-space fluid shift, 784
three-in-one TPN mixtures, 545
threshold dose, 786
thrombin, 426, 426f
thrombocytes, 425f, 426, 653
thrombolytic agents, 442–444, 443t
thrombolytic therapy, 434
thrush, 820
thymus gland, 551f, 653, 654f
thyroid gland, 551f, 553f
  feedback loop with pituitary gland, 571–572, 572f
  hyperthyroidism, 573–574
  hypothyroidism, 571–573, 573t
  role of, 552
  thyroid pill color-coding, 574f
thyroid hormone products, 572–573, 573t
thyroid-stimulating hormone (TSH), 552
thyroxine (T₄), 552
time
  military time, 172–173, 173t
  standard time, 172, 173t
  24-hour time system, 172–173, 173t
time of administration, prescription abbreviations for, 136t
time-response curve, 62, 63f
tincture, 87
tinea, 244
Tinea, 683t
tinnitus, 640
tocopherol, 522
tolerable upper intake levels, 519
tolerance, 72

centrally acting muscle relaxants and, 292
tonic-clonic (grand mal) seizure, 311t
tonicity, 752–753, 752f
tonsils, 654, 654f
topical acne agents, 241, 241t
topical antibiotic agents, 245, 245t
topical antihistamines, 374, 375t
topical anti-infectives, 370–371, 371t
topical corticosteroids, 251–252, 253t
topical hemorrhoid agents, 508–509, 509t
topical nasal antihistamines, 456–457, 456t
topical nasal corticosteroids, 456–457, 456t
topical route
  absorption, 64
  pediatric and neonatal patients and, 809
topoisomerase I/II enzymes, 785
topoisomerase inhibitors, 778t–779t, 785–787
total parenteral nutrition (TPN), 545–546, 545p, 751
toxic concentration, 62, 63f
trace minerals, 527–531, 528t
trachea, 449f, 450
trade name, 37
traditional Eastern medicine
  Ayurvedic medicine, 5, 5f
  Li Shizhen, 6
  roots of, 5–6
traditional Western medicine
  Dioscorides, 7
  Galen, 7, 7f
  Hippocrates, 6, 6f
  roots of, 6–7
transcription errors, 798
transdermal contraceptives, 610–611, 611t
transdermal patch, 86
  disposal of, 195
transdermal route of administration, 75, 75f, 75p
trans fat, 535
transient ischemic attack (TIA), 433, 848
transplantation, kidney, 644
transsexualism, 615
transverse colon, 483f, 484
traveler's diarrhea, 486
travel vaccines, 698, 700
trazodone, 345–346
Treatise on Scurvy, A (Lind), 9
Treponema pallidum, 617
Trichomonas vaginalis, 617
tricyclic antidepressants (TCAs)
  common, for insomnia, 350
  common drug name stems for, 48t
  for depression, 342–344, 343t
  geriatric patients and, 851

ototoxicity, 381t
trigeminal nerve, 723
triglycerides, 415
tri-iodothyronine (T₃), 552
triptans, 735–736, 736t
troche, 84
trough, drug dose, 63
T-score, 277
tuberculosis (TB)
  cause and drug treatment for, 469–470, 470t
  drug-resistant, 470
  incidence of, 469, 470
tuberculosis (TB) skin tests, 78
tumor burden, 773
tumor cell proliferation, 772, 773f
tumor lysis syndrome, 761
tumor necrosis factor (TNFs), biologic response modifiers, 272
tumor necrosis factor alpha (TNF-alpha) inhibitors, 251
tumor-suppressor genes, 772
turgor, 751, 751f
24-hour time system, 172–173, 173t
two-in-one TPN mixtures, 545
tympanic membrane, 364, 364f, 365f
Type 1 diabetes, 556–557, 557f
Type 2 diabetes, 557, 558f
Type I hypersensitivity, 694
Type II hypersensitivity, 694
Type III hypersensitivity, 694
Type IV hypersensitivity, 694
typhoid vaccine, 699t, 701
typical antipsychotic agents, 353–355, 354t
tyramine, 344

U

UDP-glucuronosyltransferases (UGTs), 808t, 810
ulcerative colitis
  aminosalicylates for, 512–513, 512t
  corticosteroids for, 512t, 513
  immunosuppressants for, 512t, 513–514
  symptoms of, 511
ulcers
  antacids, 497, 497t
  decubitus, 254–255
  decubitus ulcers, 254–255
  duodenal ulcers, 495
  H2 blockers, 499–500, 499p, 500p, 500t
  H. pylori and, 495, 501, 502t
  misoprostol and NSAID-induced ulcer, 501
  NSAIDs and prostaglandins, 495–496
  peptic ulcer disease (PUD), 495, 496f
  proton pump inhibitors (PPIs), 498–499, 498t
  stress ulcers, 495

wheals, 71, 78
white blood cells (WBCs), 425*f,*
  426, 652–653, 653*f*
whiteheads, 240
wild yam, 619
Wilkins, Maurice, 15
Witch hazel, 508
withdrawal symptoms, 51
Withering, William, 9
work ethic, 102
written communication, 104

written prescription, 125
  challenges of reading,
    137–138, 138*f*
wrong-dosage-form error, 190
wrong-dose error, 190
wrong-time error, 190

X

xanthine agents, 464

Y

yeast, 683
yellow fever vaccine, 699*t,* 701

Z

zinc
  to boost immune system, 688
  DRI values for, 528*t*
  eye health and, 381
  overview of, 531

  for respiratory tract infections,
    475
zinc oxide, 254
zoonotic diseases, 656
zoster, vaccine for, 698*f,* 699*t,*
  701, 837
zygote, 582, 585, 586*f*